Hoffbrand's Essential Haematology

Ninth Edition

A. Victor Hoffbrand
MA DM FRCP FRCPath FRCP(Edin) DSc FMedSci
Emeritus Professor of Haematology
University College London

Contributing Authors

Pratima Chowdary
MBBS MD MRCP FRCPath
Professor of Haemophilia and
Haemostasis, University College London
And
Consultant Haematologist
KD Haemophilia and Thrombosis Centre
Royal Free Hospital, London, UK

Graham P. Collins
MA MBBS FRCP FRCPath DPhil
Associate Professor of Haematology and Haematology Consultant
Oxford Cancer and Haematology Centre
Churchill Hospital, Oxford, UK

Justin Loke
BM BCh PhD MRCP FRCPath
AACR-CRUK Transatlantic Fellow
Dana-Farber Cancer Institute, Boston, USA and
University of Birmingham, UK

WILEY Blackwell

This ninth edition first published 2024
© 2024 John Wiley & Sons Ltd

Edition History
1e 1980, Blackwell Publishing; 2e 1984 - Blackwell Publishing; 3e 1993, Blackwell Publishing; 4e 2001, Blackwell Publishing; 5e 2006, Blackwell Publishing; 6e 2011, Wiley-Blackwell; 7e 2015, Wiley-Blackwell; 8e 2020, John Wiley & Sons Ltd

All rights reserved. No part of this publication may be reproduced, stored in a retrieval system, or transmitted, in any form or by any means, electronic, mechanical, photocopying, recording or otherwise, except as permitted by law. Advice on how to obtain permission to reuse material from this title is available at http://www.wiley.com/go/permissions.

The right of A. Victor Hoffbrand, Pratima Chowdary, Graham P. Collins and Justin Loke to be identified as the authors of this work has been asserted in accordance with law.

Registered Offices
John Wiley & Sons, Inc., 111 River Street, Hoboken, NJ 07030, USA
John Wiley & Sons Ltd, The Atrium, Southern Gate, Chichester, West Sussex, PO19 8SQ, UK

For details of our global editorial offices, customer services, and more information about Wiley products visit us at www.wiley.com.

Wiley also publishes its books in a variety of electronic formats and by print-on-demand. Some content that appears in standard print versions of this book may not be available in other formats.

Trademarks: Wiley and the Wiley logo are trademarks or registered trademarks of John Wiley & Sons, Inc. and/or its affiliates in the United States and other countries and may not be used without written permission. All other trademarks are the property of their respective owners. John Wiley & Sons, Inc. is not associated with any product or vendor mentioned in this book.

Limit of Liability/Disclaimer of Warranty
The contents of this work are intended to further general scientific research, understanding, and discussion only and are not intended and should not be relied upon as recommending or promoting scientific method, diagnosis, or treatment by physicians for any particular patient. In view of ongoing research, equipment modifications, changes in governmental regulations, and the constant flow of information relating to the use of medicines, equipment, and devices, the reader is urged to review and evaluate the information provided in the package insert or instructions for each medicine, equipment, or device for, among other things, any changes in the instructions or indication of usage and for added warnings and precautions. While the publisher and authors have used their best efforts in preparing this work, they make no representations or warranties with respect to the accuracy or completeness of the contents of this work and specifically disclaim all warranties, including without limitation any implied warranties of merchantability or fitness for a particular purpose. No warranty may be created or extended by sales representatives, written sales materials or promotional statements for this work. This work is sold with the understanding that the publisher is not engaged in rendering professional services. The advice and strategies contained herein may not be suitable for your situation. You should consult with a specialist where appropriate. The fact that an organization, website, or product is referred to in this work as a citation and/or potential source of further information does not mean that the publisher and authors endorse the information or services the organization, website, or product may provide or recommendations it may make. Further, readers should be aware that websites listed in this work may have changed or disappeared between when this work was written and when it is read. Neither the publisher nor authors shall be liable for any loss of profit or any other commercial damages, including but not limited to special, incidental, consequential, or other damages.

Library of Congress Cataloging-in-Publication Data
Names: Hoffbrand, A. V., author. | Chowdary, Pratima, author. | Collins, P. Graham (Hematologist) author. | Loke, Justin, 1984– author.
Title: Hoffbrand's essential haematology / A. Victor Hoffbrand ; contributing authors, Pratima Chowdary, Graham P. Collins, Justin Loke.
Other titles: Essential haematology
Description: Ninth edition. | Hoboken, NJ : Wiley-Blackwell 2024. | Includes bibliographical references and index.
Identifiers: LCCN 2024005129 (print) | LCCN 2024005130 (ebook) | ISBN 9781394168156 (paperback) | ISBN 9781394168163 (adobe pdf) | ISBN 9781394168170 (epub)
Subjects: MESH: Hematologic Diseases
Classification: LCC RC633 (print) | LCC RC633 (ebook) | NLM WH 120 | DDC 616.1/5–dc23/eng/20240311
LC record available at https://lccn.loc.gov/2024005129
LC ebook record available at https://lccn.loc.gov/2024005130

Cover Design: Wiley
Cover Image: © Science Photo Library/Alamy Stock Photo

Set in 10/12pt Adobe Garamond Pro by Straive, Pondicherry, India

SKY10075182_051624

Contents

Preface to the Ninth Edition

Advances in the understanding the pathogenesis of blood diseases and improvements in their treatment have continued apace in the 5 years since the eighth edition of *Hoffbrand's Essential Haematology* was published. Gene mutations are increasingly used to define and classify inherited and acquired haematological diseases, as a guide to therapy and to predict prognosis. Mutations underlying many rarer blood diseases have been identified, allowing appropriate panels of DNA probes to be established, facilitating the diagnosis of future cases. Many more drugs directed against specific sites in the cell signalling pathways have been approved.

The past five years have also seen substantial advances in immunological treatment for malignant haematological diseases. Mono- and bi-specific antibodies are increasingly incorporated into frontline therapy as well into treatment of relapsed disease. Chimeric antigen receptor (CAR)-T cells are challenging stem cell transplantation for potential cure for relapsed B-cell lymphoid neoplasms.

New drugs have also been introduced for treatment of benign (now termed in the United States 'classical') haematological diseases. These include mitapivat for pyruvate kinase deficiency, sutimlimab for cold agglutinin disease, luspatercept for anaemia in thalassaemia and myelodysplasia and pegcetacoplan for paroxysmal nocturnal haemoglobinuria. Drugs inhibiting prolyl hydroxylase in the hypoxia-inducible factor pathway are being developed to treat anaemia. They are already in illegal use for 'doping' of athletes to enhance their performance.

The fifth edition of the World Health Organisation (2022) Classification of the Haemato-lymphoid Tumours has been incorporated throughout this new edition and is given as an Appendix. The International Consensus Classification (ICC) of Myeloid Neoplasms, Acute Leukaemias and Mature Lymphoid Neoplasms was also published in 2022. It is beyond the scope of this book to compare and contrast the WHO and ICC classifications. Reference to the ICC classification are given in the Appendix.

David Steensma, the remarkable co-author of HEH8 stepped down for this new edition when he was appointed Global Head of Haematology at Novartis Institute for Biological Research. For the first time for *Essential Haematology*, there will be co-authorship by a specialist in the coagulation field. Professor Pratima Chowdary, Director of the Katherine Dormandy Haemophilia and Thrombosis Centre at the Royal Free Hospital, London, has ensured that the major section of the book dealing with bleeding and thrombotic disorders is authoritative and up to date. Graham Collins, Associate Professor of Haematology, Oxford Haematology and Cancer Centre has had the monumental task of updating the sections of HEH dealing with the lymphoid malignancies. Dr Justin Loke, AACR-CRUK Transatlantic Fellow, University of Birmingham, UK, now at the Dana-Farber Cancer Institute, Boston, USA, has undertaken the parallel task of updating the chapters dealing with the myeloid malignancies.

We are grateful to Dr Connor Sweeney, Professor Ashutosh Wechelaker and Professor Irene Roberts for their expert contributions to chapters 17 (acute lymphoblastic leukaemia), 23 (amyloid) and 34 (pregnancy and neonatal haematology), respectively. We are also grateful to Professor Barbara Bain who kindly checked the validity of our accompanying MCQs and to Dr Kirollos Kamel for his valuable contributions to chapters 30 and 31 (thrombosis and its management). We thank our publishers Wiley-Blackwell and especially Sophie Bradwell, Mandy Collison, Neelukiran Sekar and Kimberly Monroe-Hill for their unstinting help and support at all stages of production of this new edition. We also thank Jane Fallows for producing again such beautiful, clear diagrams.

Essential Haematology began life in 1980 as a textbook for medical students. We hope medical and other undergraduate students will continue to use it and share our excitement about one of the most advanced fields in medicine. With the vast expansion of knowledge of blood and its diseases over the past 44 years, the book has inevitably expanded. It is now also suitable for those beginning a career in haematology, for clinical and non-clinical scientists and nurses with an interest in blood and its diseases and for those working in closely related fields.

A. Victor Hoffbrand
London, 2024

About the Companion Website

Don't forget to visit the companion website for this book:

www.wiley.com/go/haematology9e 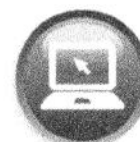

There you will find invaluable material designed to enhance your learning, including:

Multiple Choice Questions
Figures (PPT)
Tables (PDF)

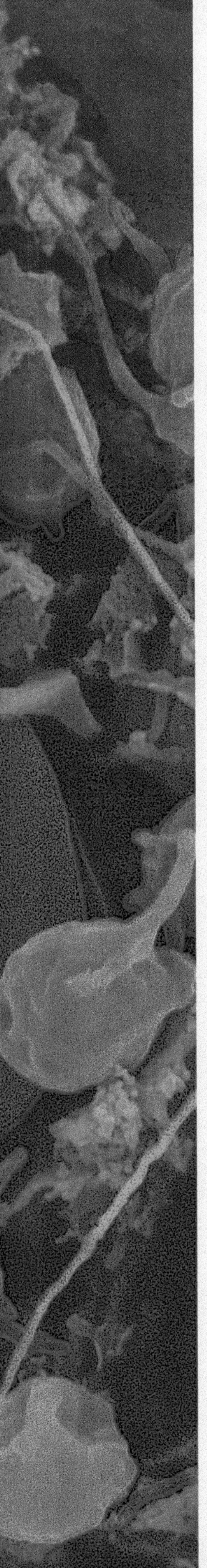

CHAPTER 1

Haemopoiesis

Key topics

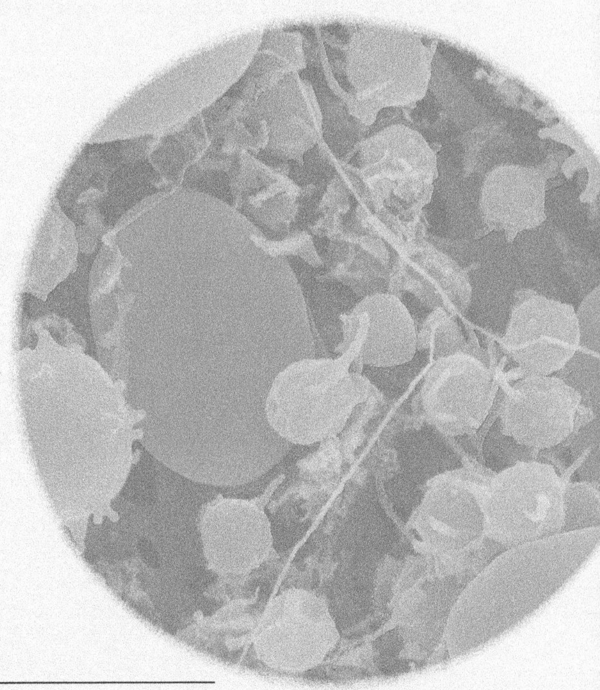

Hoffbrand's Essential Haematology, Ninth Edition. A. Victor Hoffbrand, Pratima Chowdary, Graham P. Collins, and Justin Loke.

© 2024 John Wiley & Sons Ltd. Published 2024 by John Wiley & Sons Ltd.

Companion website: www.wiley.com/go/haematology9e

This chapter deals with the general aspects of blood cell formation (haemopoiesis). The processes that regulate haemopoiesis and the early stages of formation of red cells (erythropoiesis), granulocytes and monocytes (myelopoiesis) and platelets (thrombopoiesis) are also discussed.

Site of haemopoiesis

In the first few weeks of gestation, the embryonic yolk sac is a transient site of primitive haemopoiesis. Definitive haemopoiesis derives from a population of stem cells first observed in the aorta–gonads–mesonephros (AGM) region of the developing embryo. These common precursors of endothelial and haemopoietic cells are called haemangioblasts and seed the liver, spleen and bone marrow.

From 6 weeks until 6–7 months of foetal life, the liver and spleen are the major haemopoietic organs and continue to produce blood cells until about 2 weeks after birth (Table 1.1; see Fig. 7.1b). The placenta also contributes to foetal haemopoiesis. The bone marrow takes over as the most important site from 6 to 7 months of foetal life. During normal childhood and adult life, the marrow is the only source of new red cells, granulocytes, monocytes and platelets. The developing cells are situated outside the bone marrow sinuses; mature cells are released into the sinus spaces, the marrow microcirculation and so into the general circulation.

In infancy all the bone marrow is haemopoietic, but during childhood and beyond there is progressive replacement of marrow throughout the long bones with fat cells, so that in adult life haemopoietic marrow is confined to the central skeleton and proximal ends of the femurs and humeri (Table 1.1). Even in these active haemopoietic areas, approximately 50% of the marrow consists of fat in the middle-aged adult (Fig. 1.1). The remaining fatty marrow is capable of reversion to haemopoiesis, and in many diseases there is also expansion of haemopoiesis down the long bones. Moreover, in certain disease states, the liver and spleen can resume their foetal haemopoietic role ('extramedullary haemopoiesis').

Table 1.1 Dominant sites of haemopoiesis at different stages of development.

Foetus	0–2 months (yolk sac)
	2–7 months (liver, spleen)
	5–9 months (bone marrow)
Infants	Bone marrow (practically all bones); dwindling contribution from liver/spleen that ceases in the first few months of life
Adults	Vertebrae, ribs, sternum, skull, sacrum and pelvis, proximal ends of femur

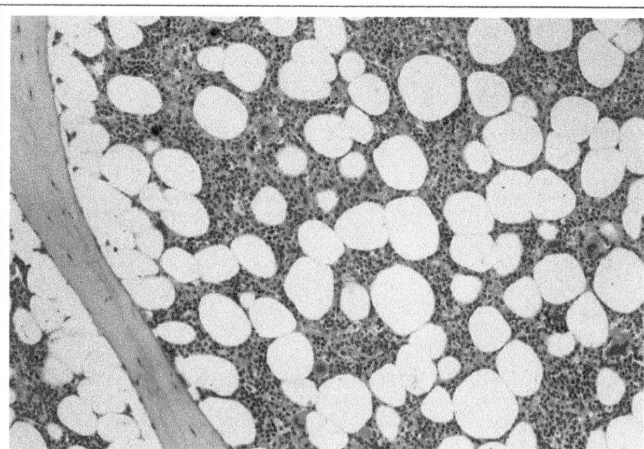

Figure 1.1 Normal bone marrow trephine biopsy (posterior iliac crest). Haematoxylin and eosin stain; approximately 50% of the intertrabecular tissue is haemopoietic tissue and 50% fat.

Haemopoietic stem and progenitor cells

Haemopoiesis starts with a pluripotent stem cell that can self-renew by asymmetrical cell division but also gives rise to the precursor of the separate cell lineages. The stem cells are able to repopulate a bone marrow from which all stem cells have been eliminated by lethal irradiation or chemotherapy. Self-renewal and repopulating ability define the **haemopoietic stem cell** (HSC). HSCs are rare perhaps 1 in every 20 million nucleated cells in bone marrow. Newer DNA sequencing techniques suggest that a typical adult has approximately 50 000 HSCs.

HSCs are heterogeneous, with some able to repopulate a bone marrow for more than 16 weeks, called **long-term HSCs**, while others, although able to produce all haemopoietic cell types, engraft only transiently for a few weeks and are called **short-term HSCs**. Although the exact cell surface marker phenotype of the HSC is still unknown, on immunological testing these cells are positive for the markers cluster of differentiation 34 (CD34), CD49f and CD90 and negative for CD38 and CD45RA and for cell lineage-defining markers (Lin). Morphologically, HSCs have the appearance of small- or medium-sized lymphocytes.

Cell differentiation occurs from the stem cells via committed **haemopoietic progenitors**, which are restricted in their developmental potential (Fig. 1.2). The existence of the separate progenitor cells can be demonstrated by *in vitro* culture techniques. Stem cells and very early progenitors are assayed by culture on bone marrow stroma as long-term culture-initiating cells, whereas later progenitors are generally assayed in semi-solid media. As examples, in the erythroid series progenitors can be identified in special cultures as burst-forming units (BFU-E, describing the 'burst' with which they form in culture) and

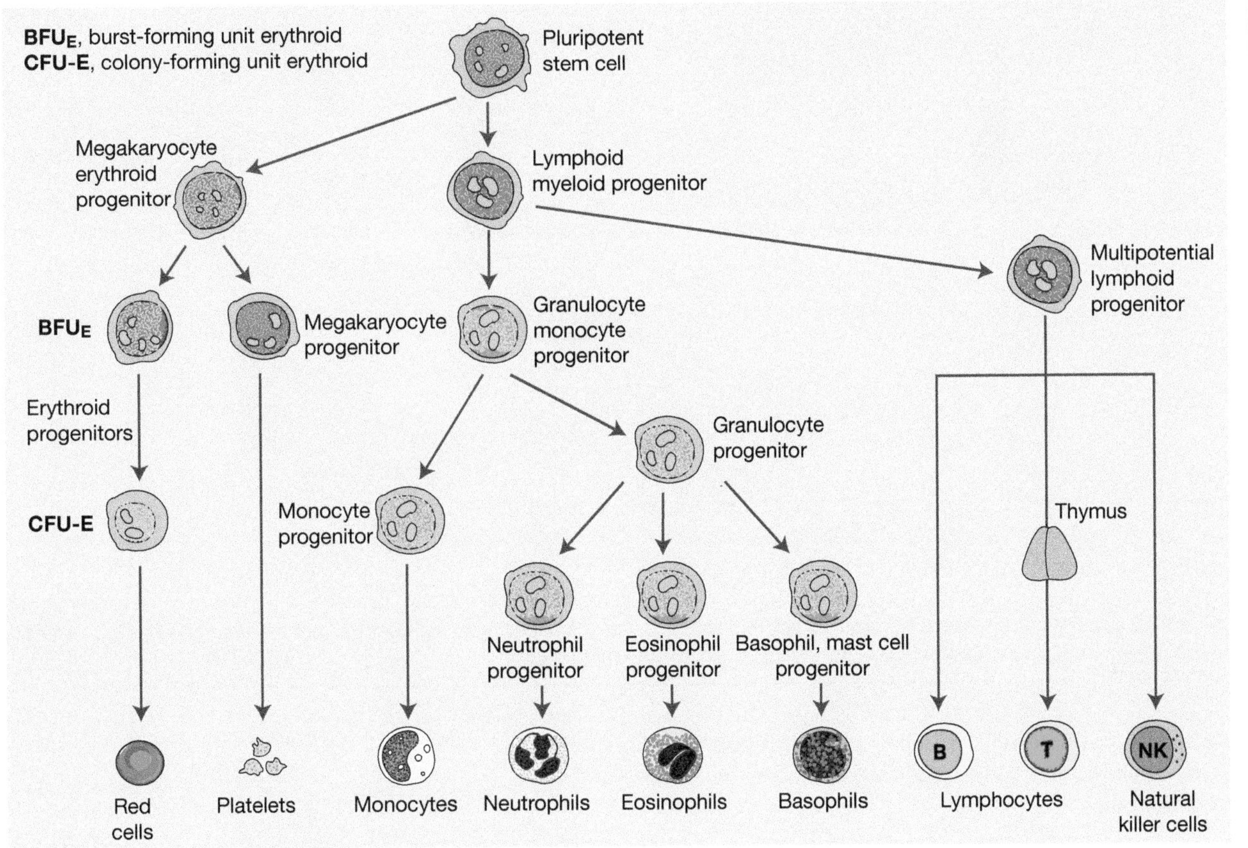

Figure 1.2 Diagrammatic representation of the bone marrow pluripotent stem cells (haemopoietic stem cells, HSC) and the cell lines that arise from them. A megakaryocytic/erythroid progenitor (MkEP) and a mixed lymphoid/myeloid progenitor are formed from the pluripotent stem cells. Each gives rise to more differentiated progenitors. BFU-E, burst-forming unit erythroid; CFU-E, colony-forming unit erythroid.

colony-forming units (CFU-E; Fig 1.2); the mixed granulocyte/monocyte progenitor is identified as a colony-forming unit-granulocyte/monocyte (CFU-GM) in culture. Megakaryocytes derive from a megakaryocyte progenitor, itself derived from an earlier mixed erythroid–megakaryocyte progenitor.

In the haemopoietic hierarchy, the pluripotent stem cell gives rise to a **mixed erythroid and megakaryocyte progenitor**, which then divides into separate erythroid and megakaryocyte progenitors. The pluripotent stem cell also gives rise to a **mixed lymphoid, granulocyte and monocyte progenitor**, which divides into a progenitor of granulocytes and monocytes and a mixed lymphoid progenitor, from which B- and T-cell lymphocytes and natural killer (NK) cells develop (Fig. 1.2). The spleen, lymph nodes and thymus are secondary sites of lymphocyte production (Chapter 9).

As the stem cell has the capability for **self-renewal** (Fig. 1.3), the marrow cellularity remains constant in a normal, healthy steady state. There is considerable amplification in the system: one stem cell is capable of producing about 10^6 mature blood cells after 20 cell divisions (Fig. 1.3). In humans, HSCs are capable of about 50 cell divisions (the 'Hayflick limit'), with progressive telomere shortening with each division affecting viability.

Under normal conditions most HSCs are dormant, with at most only a few percent active in cell cycle on any given day. Any given HSC enters the cell cycle approximately once every 3 months to 3 years in humans. By contrast, progenitor cells are much more numerous and highly proliferative. With ageing, the number of stem cells falls and the relative proportion giving rise to lymphoid rather than myeloid progenitors also falls. Stem cells also accumulate genetic mutations with age, an average of 8 exonic coding mutations by age 60 years (1.3 per decade). These, either passengers without oncogenic potential or drivers that cause clonal expansion, may be present in neoplasms arising from these stem cells (Chapters 11, 16).

The progenitor and precursor cells are capable of responding to haemopoietic growth factors with increased production of one or other cell line when the need arises. The development

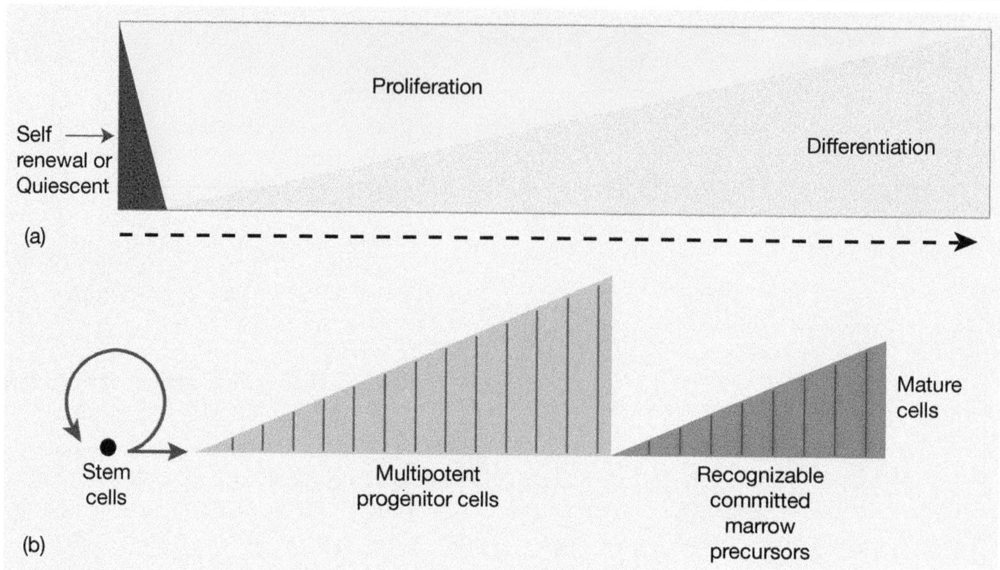

Figure 1.3 (a) Bone marrow cells are increasingly differentiated and lose the capacity for self-renewal as they mature. **(b)** A single stem cell gives rise, after multiple cell divisions (shown by vertical lines), to $>10^6$ mature cells.

of the mature cells (red cells, granulocytes, monocytes, megakaryocytes and lymphocytes) is considered further in other sections of this book.

Bone marrow stroma and niches

The bone marrow forms a suitable environment for stem cell survival, self-renewal and formation of differentiated progenitor cells. It is composed of various types of stromal cells and a microvascular network (Fig. 1.4). **The stromal cells include adipocytes, fibroblasts, macrophages, megakaryocytes, osteoblasts, osteoclasts, endothelial cells and mesenchymal stem cells (which have the capacity to self-renew and differentiate into osteocytes, adipocytes and chondrocytes).** The stromal cells secrete extracellular molecules such as collagen, glycoproteins (fibronectin and thrombospondin) and glycosaminoglycans (hyaluronic acid and chondroitin derivatives) to form an extracellular matrix.

The HSCs reside in two types of niche. These provide some of the growth factors, adhesion molecules and cytokines which support stem cells, maintaining their viability and reproduction, e.g. stem cell factor (SCF) expressed by stromal and endothelial cells binds to its receptor, KIT (CD117), on stem cells. The niches are either vascular, including arterioles and sinusoids that converge on a central vein, or endosteal with osteoblasts and osteoclasts closely associated with bone. Sympathetic nerves and non-myelinated Schwann cells are important regulators of stem cell quiescence or release.

Haemopoietic stem cells (as well as mesenchymal stem cells) traffic around the body. They are found in peripheral blood in low numbers. In order to exit the bone marrow, cells must cross the blood vessel endothelium, and this process of mobilization is enhanced for HSCs by the administration of growth factors such as granulocyte colony-stimulating factor (G-CSF). The reverse process, stem cell homing, depends on a chemokine gradient in which stromal-derived factor 1 (SDF-1), which binds to its receptor CXCR4 on HSC, is critical.

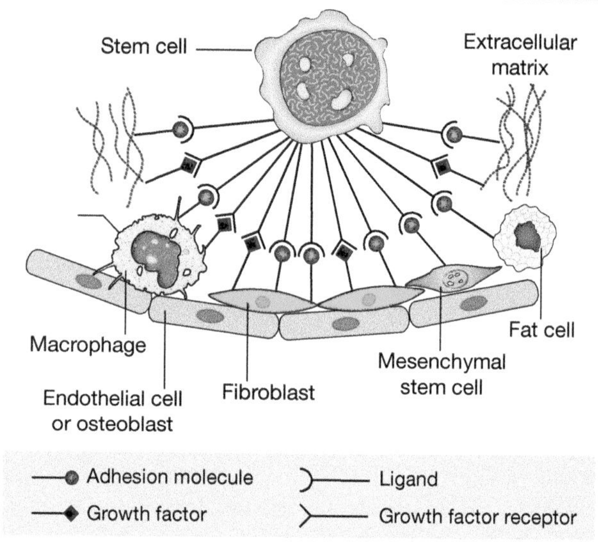

Figure 1.4 Haemopoiesis occurs in a suitable microenvironment ('niche') provided by a stromal matrix on which stem cells grow and divide. The niche may be vascular (lined by endothelium) or endosteal (lined by osteoblasts). There are specific recognition and adhesion sites; extracellular glycoproteins, e.g. fibronectin, collagen and other compounds, form a matrix and are involved in stem cell binding (see text).

The regulation of haemopoiesis

Transcription factors

Haemopoiesis starts with stem cell division in which one cell replaces the stem cell (*self-renewal*) and the other is committed to differentiation. These early committed progenitors express low levels of transcription factors that commit them to discrete cell lineages.

Transcription factors regulate gene expression by controlling the transcription of specific genes or gene families (Fig. 1.5). Typically, they contain at least two domains: a DNA-binding domain, such as a leucine zipper or helix–loop–helix motif which binds to a specific DNA sequence, and an activation domain, which contributes to the assembly of the transcription complex at a gene promoter. The transcription factors interact, so that reinforcement of one transcription programme may suppress that of another lineage

Which cell lineage is selected for differentiation depends on both chance and the external signals received by progenitor cells. Examples of transcription factors involved in haemopoiesis include RUNX1, GATA2 and MT2A in the earliest stages; GATA1, GATA2 and FOG1 in erythropoiesis and megakaryocytic differentiation; PU.1 and the CEBP family in granulopoiesis; PAX5 in B lymphocyte and NOTCH1 in T lymphocyte development. The transcription factors induce synthesis of proteins specific to a cell lineage. For example, GATA1 binds to specific motifs on the erythroid genes for globin and haem synthesis and so activates these genes. Mutation, deletion or translocation of transcription factor genes underlies many cases of haematological neoplasms (Chapter 11).

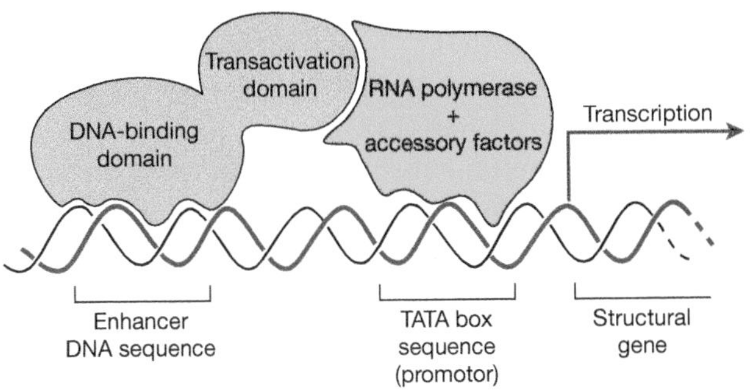

Figure 1.5 Model for control of gene expression by a transcription factor. The DNA-binding domain of a transcription factor binds a specific enhancer sequence adjacent to a structural gene. The transactivation domain then binds a molecule of RNA polymerase, thus augmenting its binding to the TATA box. The RNA polymerase now initiates transcription of the structural gene to form mRNA. Translation of the mRNA by the ribosomes generates the protein encoded by the gene. Transcription factors work in combination to both activate and repress the expression of a large number of genes.

Haemopoietic growth factors

The haemopoietic growth factors are a group of glycoproteins that regulate the proliferation and differentiation of haemopoietic progenitor cells and the function of mature blood cells. **They may act locally at the site where they are produced by cell–cell contact, e.g. SCF, or circulate in plasma, e.g. G-CSF or erythropoietin (EPO)**. They also bind to the extracellular matrix to form niches to which stem and progenitor cells adhere. The growth factors may cause cell proliferation, but can also stimulate differentiation and maturation, prevent apoptosis and affect the function of mature cells (Fig. 1.6).

The growth factors share a number of common properties (Table 1.2) and act at different stages of haemopoiesis (Table 1.3; Fig. 1.6). **Stromal cells are the major source of growth factors except for EPO, 90% of which is synthesized in the kidney, and thrombopoietin (TPO), made largely in**

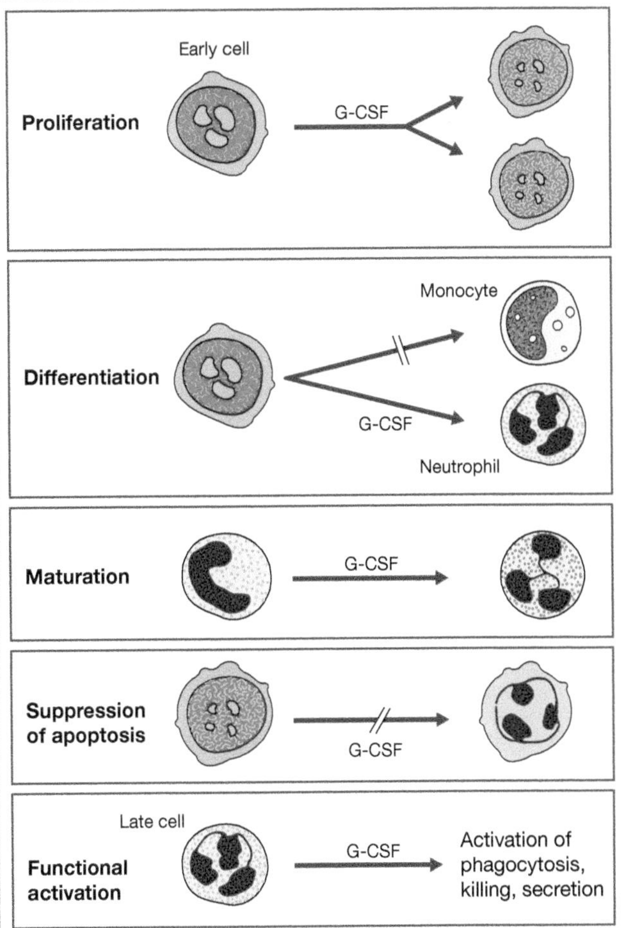

Figure 1.6 Growth factors may stimulate the proliferation of early bone marrow cells, direct differentiation to one or other cell type, stimulate cell maturation, suppress apoptosis or affect the function of mature non-dividing cells, as illustrated here for granulocyte colony-stimulating factor (G-CSF) for an early myeloid progenitor and a mature neutrophil.

Table 1.2 General characteristics of myeloid and lymphoid growth factors.
Glycoproteins that act at very low concentrations
Act hierarchically
Usually produced by many cell types
Usually affect more than one lineage
Usually active on stem/progenitor cells and on differentiated cells
Usually show synergistic or additive interactions with other growth factors
Often act on the neoplastic equivalent of a normal cell
Multiple actions: proliferation, differentiation, maturation, prevention of apoptosis, functional activation

Table 1.3 Haemopoietic growth factors (see also Fig. 1.7).
Act on stromal cells IL-1, TNF
Act on pluripotential stem cells SCF, TPO, FLT3-, NOTCH1
Act on multipotent lymphoid/myeloid progenitor cells IL-3, IL-7, SCF, FLT3-L, TPO, GM-CSF
Act on lineage-committed progenitor cells Granulocyte/monocyte production: IL-3, GM-CSF, G-CSF, M-CSF, IL-5 (eosinophil CSF) Mast cell production: KIT-ligand Red cell production: IL-3, EPO Platelet production: IL-3, TPO Lymphocyte/NK cell production: IL-1, IL-2, IL-4, IL-7, IL-10, other ILs

CSF, colony-stimulating factor; EPO, erythropoietin; FLT3-L, FLT3 ligand; G-CSF, granulocyte colony-stimulating factor; GM-CSF, granulocyte–macrophage colony-stimulating factor; IL, interleukin; M-CSF, macrophage/monocyte colony-stimulating factor; NK, natural killer; SCF, stem cell factor (also known as TAL1); TNF, tumour necrosis factor; TPO, thrombopoietin.

the liver. An important feature of growth factor action is that two or more factors may synergize in stimulating a particular cell to proliferate or differentiate. Moreover, the action of one growth factor on a cell may stimulate production of another growth factor or growth factor receptor.

SCF, TPO.NOTCH1 and FLT3 ligand act locally on the pluripotential stem cells and on myeloid/lymphoid progenitors (Fig. 1.7). Interleukin-3 (IL-3) has widespread activity on lymphoid/myeloid and megakaryocyte/erythroid progenitors. Granulocyte–macrophage colony-stimulating factor (GM-CSF), G-CSF and macrophage colony-stimulating factor (M-CSF) enhance neutrophil and macrophage/monocyte production, IL-5 eosinophil, KIT mast cell, TPO platelet and EPO red cell production. These lineage-specific growth factors also enhance the effects of SCF, FLT3-L and IL-3 on the survival and differentiation of early haemopoietic cells. Interleukin-7 is involved at all stages of lymphocyte production, and various other interleukins and toll-like receptor ligands (not shown) direct B and T lymphocyte and NK cell production (Fig. 1.7).

These factors maintain a pool of haemopoietic stem and progenitor cells on which later-acting factors, EPO, G-CSF, M-CSF, IL-5 and TPO, act to increase production of one or other cell lineage in response to the body's need. Granulocyte and monocyte formation, for example, can be stimulated by infection or inflammation through release of IL-1 and tumour necrosis factor (TNF), which then stimulate stromal cells to produce growth factors in an interacting network (Fig. 8.4). In contrast, cytokines, such as transforming growth factor-β (TGF-β) and γ-interferon (IFN-γ), can exert a negative effect on haemopoiesis and may have a role in the development of aplastic anaemia (p. 313).

Growth factor receptors and signal transduction

The biological effects of growth factors are mediated through specific receptors on target cells. Many receptors, such as the EPO receptor (EPO-R) and GM-CSF-R, are from the **haemopoietin receptor superfamily** which dimerize after binding their ligand.

Dimerization of the receptor leads to activation of a complex series of intracellular signal transduction pathways, of which the three major ones are the JAK/STAT (signal transducer and activator of transcription) pathway, the mitogen-activated protein (MAP) kinase and the phosphatidylinositol 3-kinase (PI3K) pathways (Fig. 1.8; see also Fig 9.4, Fig 15.2). The Janus-associated kinase (JAK) proteins are a family of four tyrosine-specific protein kinases that associate with the intracellular domains of the growth factor receptors (Fig. 1.8). A growth factor molecule binds simultaneously to the extracellular domains of two or three receptor molecules, resulting in their aggregation. Receptor aggregation induces activation of the JAKs, which then phosphorylate members of the STAT family of transcription factors. This results in their dimerization and translocation from the cell cytoplasm across the nuclear membrane to the cell nucleus. Within the nucleus STAT dimers activate the transcription of specific genes. A model for the control of gene expression by a transcription factor is shown in Fig. 1.5. The clinical importance of this pathway is revealed for example by the finding of an activating mutation of the *JAK2* gene as a cause of polycythaemia vera and related myeloproliferative neoplasms (p. 195).

JAK can also activate the MAPK pathway, which is regulated by RAS and controls proliferation. PI3 kinases phosphorylate

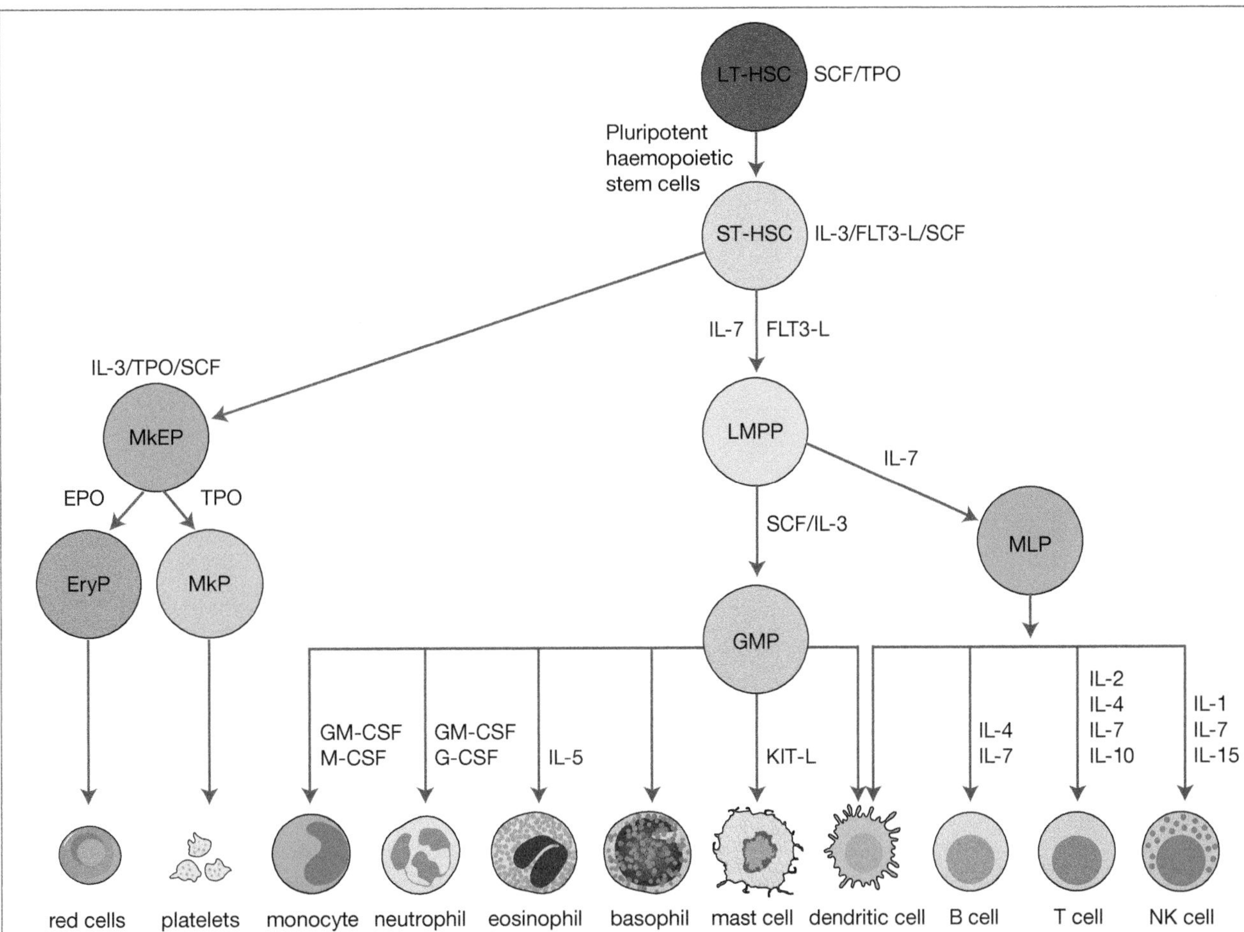

Figure 1.7 The role of growth factors in normal haemopoiesis. Multiple growth factors act on the earlier marrow stem and progenitor cells. EPO, erythropoietin; EryP, erythroid progenitor; FLT3-L, FLT3 ligand; G-CSF, granulocyte colony-stimulating factor; GM-CSF, granulocyte–macrophage colony-stimulating factor; GMP, granulocyte–macrophage progenitor; HSC, haemopoietic stem cells; IL, interleukin; LMPP, lymphoid-primed multipotential progenitor; LT, long-term; M-CSF, macrophage/monocyte colony-stimulating factor; MkEP, megakaryocyte–erythroid progenitor; MkP, megakaryocyte progenitor; MLP, multipotential lymphoid progenitor; NK, natural killer; PSC, pluripotential stem cell; SCF, stem cell factor; ST, short-term; TLR, toll-like receptor; TPO, thrombopoietin. Source: Adapted from A.V. Hoffbrand *et al.* (2019) *Color Atlas of Clinical Hematology: Molecular and Cellular Basis of Disease,* 5th edn. Reproduced with permission of John Wiley & Sons.

inositol lipids, which have a wide range of downstream effects, including activation of AKT. This results in a block of apoptosis and other actions (Figs. 1.8, 15.2). Different domains of the intracellular receptor protein may signal for the different processes e.g. proliferation or suppression of apoptosis, mediated by growth factors.

A second, smaller group of growth factors, including SCF, FLT3L and M-CSF (Table 1.3), bind to receptors that have an extracellular immunoglobulin-like domain linked via a transmembrane bridge to a cytoplasmic tyrosine kinase domain. Growth factor binding results in dimerization of these receptors and consequent activation of the tyrosine kinase domain. Phosphorylation of tyrosine residues in the receptor itself generates binding sites for signalling proteins which initiate complex cascades of biochemical events, resulting in changes in gene expression, cell proliferation and prevention of apoptosis.

Adhesion molecules

Cell adhesion molecules (CAMs) are glycoprotein molecules which mediate the attachment of cells to each other, to the extracellular matrix and play roles in cell-cell synapse formation. They typically are composed of three domains: intracellular, transmembrane and extracellular. They are divided into four large families: integrins, immunoglobulin super family, selectins and cadherins. They function as 'molecular glue' maintaining tissue structure and function. The integrins are particularly

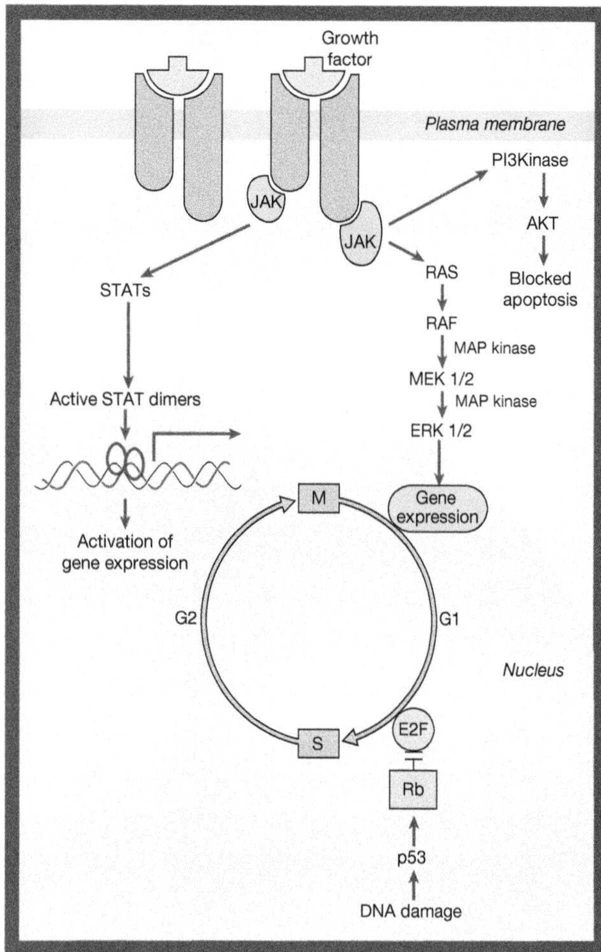

Figure 1.8 Control of haemopoiesis by growth factors. The factors act on cells expressing the corresponding receptors. Binding of a growth factor to its receptor activates the JAK/STAT, MAPK and phosphatidyl-inositol 3-kinase (PI3K) pathways (see also Fig. 15.2), which leads to transcriptional activation of specific genes. E2F is a transcription factor needed for cell transition from G1 to S phase. E2F is inhibited by the tumour suppressor gene Rb (retinoblastoma), which can be indirectly activated by p53. The synthesis and degradation of different cyclins stimulate the cell to pass through the different phases of the cell cycle. The growth factors may also suppress apoptosis by activating AKT (protein kinase B).

important in linking the extracellular environment including collagen, fibronectin and fibrinogen to intracellular signalling pathways. The selectins which include E (endothelial)-selectin, L (leucocyte)-selectin and P (platelet)-selectin are particularly important in the immune system in helping white cells in trafficking and homing.

In the bone marrow CAMs attach haemopoietic precursors, leucocytes and platelets to various components of the extracellular matrix, to endothelium, to other surfaces and to each other. The CAMs on the surface of leucocytes and platelets are termed receptors and these interact with proteins termed ligands on the surface of target cells, e.g. endothelium. The molecules are important in the development and maintenance of inflammatory as well as immune responses, and in platelet–vessel wall and leucocyte–vessel wall interactions. Glycoprotein IIb/IIIa, for example, is a CAM, also called integrin IIβ/IIIα and involved in platelet adhesion to vessel walls and to each other (Chapter 26).

The pattern of expression of adhesion molecules on tumour cells may determine their mode of spread and tissue localization e.g. the pattern of metastasis of carcinoma cells to specific visceral organs or bone or of non-Hodgkin lymphoma cells into a follicular or diffuse pattern. The adhesion molecules may also determine whether or not cells circulate in the bloodstream or remain fixed in tissues. They may also partly determine whether or not tumour cells are susceptible to the body's immune defences. Attempts to treat cancer and other diseases with drugs which inhibit specific adhesion molecules have so far been unsuccessful.

The cell cycle

The cell division cycle, generally known simply as the **cell cycle**, is a complex process that lies at the heart of haemopoiesis. Dysregulation of cell proliferation is also the key to the development of malignant disease. The duration of the cell cycle is variable between different tissues, but the basic principles remain constant. The cycle is divided into the mitotic phase (**M phase**), during which the cell physically divides, and **interphase**, during which the chromosomes are duplicated and cell growth occurs prior to division (Fig. 1.8). The M phase is further partitioned into classical **mitosis**, in which nuclear division is accomplished, and **cytokinesis**, in which cell fission occurs.

The interphase is divided into three main stages: a **G_1 phase**, in which the cell begins to commit to replication, an **S phase**, during which DNA content doubles and the chromosomes replicate, and the **G_2 phase**, in which the cell organelles are copied and cytoplasmic volume is increased. If cells rest prior to division, they enter a G_0 state where they can remain for long periods of time. The number of cells at each stage of the cell cycle can be assessed by exposing cells to a chemical or radiolabel that gets incorporated into newly generated DNA.

The cell cycle is controlled by two **checkpoints,** which act as brakes to coordinate the division process, at the end of the G_1 and G_2 phases. Two major classes of molecules control these checkpoints, **cyclin-dependent protein kinases** (Cdk), which phosphorylate downstream protein targets, and **cyclins**, which bind to Cdk and regulate their activity. An example of the importance of these systems is demonstrated by mantle cell lymphoma, which results from the constitutive activation of cyclin D1 as a result of a chromosomal translocation (p. 279).

Epigenetics

Epigenetics refers to changes in DNA and chromatin that affect gene expression other than those that affect DNA sequence (Fig. 16.1).

Cellular DNA is packaged by wrapping it around histones, a group of specialized nuclear proteins. The complex is tightly compacted as chromatin. In order for the DNA code to be read, transcription factors and other proteins need to physically attach to DNA. Histones act as custodians for this access and so for gene expression. Histones may be modified by methylation, acetylation and phosphorylation, which can result in increased or decreased gene expression and so changes in cell phenotype.

Epigenetics also includes changes to DNA itself, such as methylation of DNA bases. The methylation of cytosine residues to methylcytosine results in inhibition of gene transcription. The DNA methyltransferase genes *DNMT3A* and *B* are involved in this methylation. *TET1, 2, 3* and *IDH1* and *IDH2* are involved in the hydroxylation and breakdown of methylcytosine and restoration of gene expression (Fig. 16.1). These genes are frequently mutated in the myeloid malignancies, especially myelodysplastic syndromes and acute myeloid leukaemia (Chapters 13, 15 and 16).

Apoptosis

Apoptosis (programmed cell death) is a regulated process of physiological cell death in which individual cells are triggered to activate intracellular proteins that lead to the death of the cell. Morphologically it is characterized by cell shrinkage, condensation of the nuclear chromatin, fragmentation of the nucleus and cleavage of DNA at inter-nucleosomal sites. It is an important process for maintaining tissue homeostasis in haemopoiesis and lymphocyte development.

Apoptosis results from the action of intracellular cysteine proteases called **caspases**, which are activated following cleavage and lead to endonuclease digestion of DNA and disintegration of the cell skeleton (Fig. 1.9). There are two major pathways by which caspases can be activated. The first is by activation through membrane proteins such as Fas or TNF receptor via their intracellular death domain. An example of this mechanism is shown by activated cytotoxic T cells expressing Fas ligand, which induces apoptosis in target cells. The second pathway is via the release of cytochrome c from mitochondria. Cytochrome c binds to APAF-1, which then activates caspases. DNA damage induced by irradiation or chemotherapy may act through this pathway.

The protein p53 encoded by the *TP53* gene on chromosome 17 has an important role in sensing DNA damage. It activates apoptosis by raising the cell level of BAX, which then increases cytochrome c release (Fig. 1.9). p53 also shuts down the cell cycle to stop the damaged cell from dividing (Fig. 1.8). The cellular level of p53 is controlled by a second protein, MDM2. Following death, apoptotic cells display molecules that lead to their ingestion by macrophages. Loss of TP53 is a major mechanism by which malignant cells evade controls that would induce cell death.

As well as molecules that mediate apoptosis, there are several intracellular proteins that protect cells from apoptosis.

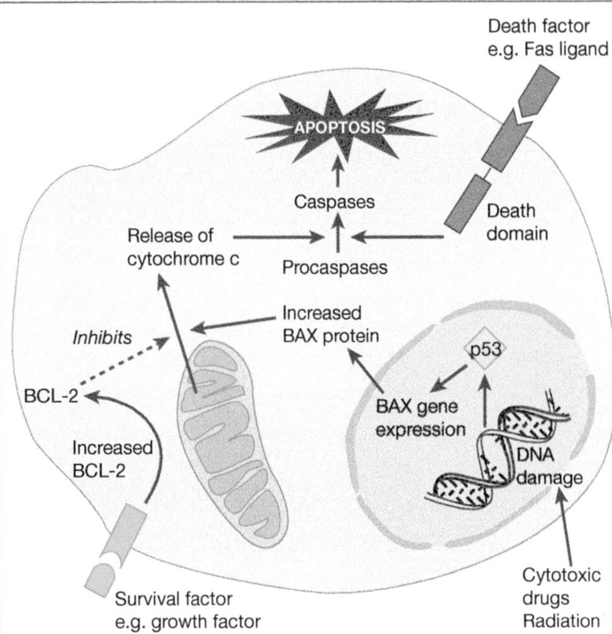

Figure 1.9 Representation of apoptosis. Apoptosis is initiated via two main stimuli: (i) signalling through cell membrane receptors such as FAS or tumour necrosis factor (TNF) receptor; or (ii) release of cytochrome c from mitochondria. Membrane receptors signal apoptosis through an intracellular death domain leading to activation of caspases which digest DNA. Cytochrome c binds to the cytoplasmic protein Apaf-1 leading to activation of caspases. The intracellular ratio of pro-apoptotic, e.g. BAX, or anti-apoptotic, e.g. BCL-2, members of the BCL-2 family may influence mitochondrial cytochrome c release. Growth factors raise the level of BCL-2, inhibiting cytochrome c release, whereas DNA damage, by activating p53, raises the level of BAX, which enhances cytochrome c release.

The best-characterized example is BCL-2. BCL-2 is the prototype of a family of related proteins, some of which are anti-apoptotic and some, like BAX, pro-apoptotic. The intracellular ratio of BAX and BCL-2 determines the relative susceptibility of cells to apoptosis, e.g. determines the lifespan of platelets, and may act through regulation of cytochrome c release from mitochondria.

Many of the genetic changes associated with malignant disease lead to a reduced rate of apoptosis and hence prolonged cell survival. The clearest example is the translocation of the *BCL2* gene to the immunoglobulin heavy chain locus in the t(14;18) translocation in follicular lymphoma (p. xxx). Overexpression of the BCL-2 protein makes the malignant B cells less susceptible to apoptosis. The drug venetoclax which inhibits BCL-2 is now widely used to treat both myeloid and lymphoid malignant diseases. Apoptosis is the normal fate for most B cells undergoing selection in the lymphoid germinal centres.

Several translocations leading to the generation of fusion proteins, such as t(9;22), t(11;14) and t(15;17), also result in inhibition of apoptosis (Chapter 11). In addition, genes encoding proteins that are involved in mediating apoptosis following DNA damage, such as p53 and ATM, are also frequently mutated and therefore inactivated in haemopoietic malignancies.

Necrosis is death of cells and adjacent cells due to ischemia, chemical trauma or hyperthermia. The cells swell and the plasma membrane loses integrity. There is usually an inflammatory infiltrate in response to spillage of cell contents. Autophagy is the digestion of cell organelles by lysosomes. It may be involved in cell death, but in some situations also in maintaining cell survival by recycling nutrients.

SUMMARY

- Haemopoiesis (blood cell formation) arises from pluripotent stem cells in the bone marrow. Haemopoietic stem cells give rise to mixed and then single lineage progenitor and precursor cells which, after multiple cell divisions and differentiation, form red cells, granulocytes (neutrophils, eosinophils and basophils), monocytes, platelets, B and T lymphocytes and natural killer (NK) cells.
- Haemopoietic tissue occupies about 50% of the marrow space in normal adult marrow. Haemopoiesis in adults is confined to the central skeleton, but in infants and young children haemopoietic tissue extends down the long bones of the arms and legs.
- Stem cells reside in the bone marrow in osteoblastic or endothelial niches formed by stromal cells. They also circulate in the blood.
- Growth factors attach to specific cell surface receptors and produce a cascade of phosphorylation events in the cell nucleus.
- Transcription factors are molecules that bind to DNA and control the transcription of specific genes or gene families. They carry the message to those genes that are to be 'switched on or off', to stimulate cell division, differentiation or functional activity or to suppress apoptosis.
- Adhesion molecules are a large family of glycoproteins that mediate the attachment of marrow precursors and mature leucocytes and platelets to extracellular matrix, to endothelium and to each other.
- Epigenetics refers to changes in DNA and chromatin that affect gene expression other than those that affect DNA sequence. Histone modification and DNA (cytosine) methylation are two important examples relevant to haemopoiesis and haematological malignancies.
- Apoptosis is a physiological process of cell death resulting from activation of caspases. The intracellular ratio of pro-apoptotic proteins, e.g. BAX, to anti-apoptotic proteins, e.g. BCL-2, determines the cell susceptibility to apoptosis.

Now visit **www.wiley.com/go/haematology9e** to test yourself on this chapter.

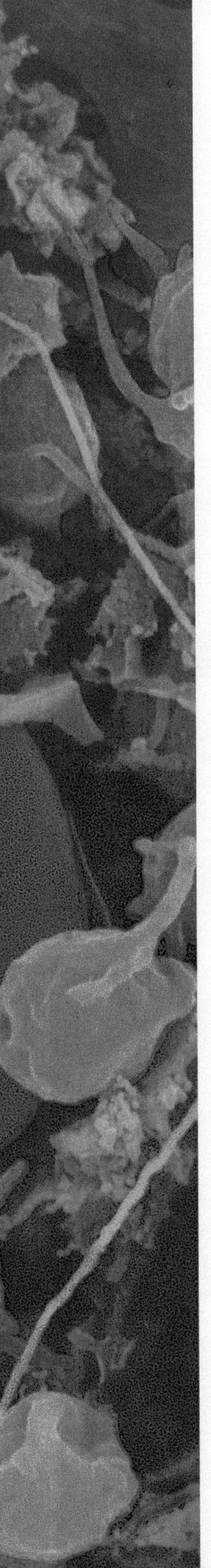

CHAPTER 2

Erythropoiesis and general aspects of anaemia

Key topics

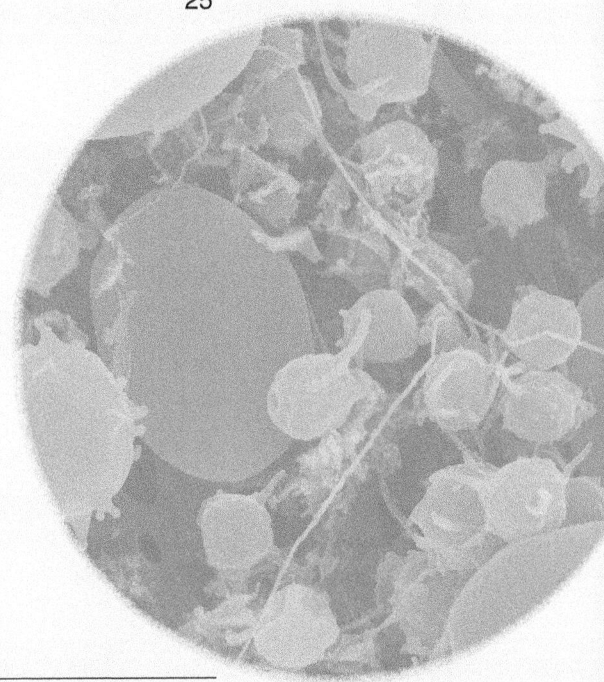

Hoffbrand's Essential Haematology, Ninth Edition. A. Victor Hoffbrand, Pratima Chowdary, Graham P. Collins, and Justin Loke.

© 2024 John Wiley & Sons Ltd. Published 2024 by John Wiley & Sons Ltd.

Companion website: www.wiley.com/go/haematology9e

Blood cells

All the circulating blood cells derive from pluripotential stem cells in the marrow. They divide into three main types. The most numerous are **red cells (erythrocytes)**, specialized for the carriage of oxygen from the lungs to the tissues and of carbon dioxide in the reverse direction (Table 2.1). They have a 4-month life span, whereas the smallest cells, **platelets** involved in haemostasis, circulate for only 10 days. **The white cells are made up of four main types of phagocyte: neutrophils, eosinophils, basophils and monocytes**, which protect against bacterial and fungal infections (Chapter 8); and of **lymphocytes**, which include **B cells**, involved in antibody production, **T cells** (CD4 helper and CD8 suppressor), concerned with the immune response and in protection against viruses and foreign cells, and **natural killer (NK) cells**, a subset of CD8 T cells (Chapter 9). White cells have a wide range of life span (Table 2.1).

The red cells and platelets are counted and their diameter and other parameters measured by an automated cell counter (Fig. 2.1). The counter also enumerates the different types of white cell by flow cytometry and detects abnormal cells.

Erythropoiesis

We each make approximately 10^{12} new erythrocytes each day by the complex and finely regulated process of erythropoiesis. This progresses from the stem cell through progenitor cells, the erythroid and megakaryocyte colony-forming unit (CFU_{MkE}), burst-forming unit erythroid (BFU_E) and erythroid CFU (CFU-E; Fig. 1.2) to the first recognizable erythrocyte precursor in the bone marrow, the pronormoblast (Fig. 2.2). This process occurs in an erythroid niche in which about 30 erythroid cells at various stages of development surround a central macrophage.

The pronormoblast is a large cell with dark blue cytoplasm, a central nucleus with nucleoli and slightly clumped chromatin (Fig. 2.2). It gives rise to a series of progressively smaller normoblasts by a number of cell divisions. These also contain

Table 2.1 The blood cells.

Cell	Diameter (μm)	Life span in blood	Number	Function
Red cells	6–8	120 d	Male: 4.5–6.5 × 10^{12}/L Female: 3.9–5.6 × 10^{12}/L	Oxygen and carbon dioxide transport
Platelets	0.5–3.0	10 d	140–400 × 10^9/L	Haemostasis
Phagocytes				
Neutrophils	12–15	6–10 h	1.8–7.5 × 10^9/L	Protection from bacteria, fungi
Monocytes	12–20	20-40 h	0.2–0.8 × 10^9/L	Protection from bacteria, fungi
Eosinophils	12–15	Days	0.04–0.44 × 10^9/L	Protection against parasites
Basophils	12–15	Days	0.01–0.1 × 10^9/L	
Lymphocytes B T	7–9 (resting) 12–20 (active)	Weeks or years	1.5–3.5 × 10^9/L	B cells: immunoglobulin synthesis T cells: protection against viruses; immune functions
Natural killer cells NK	10 (resting) 10–20 (active)	Hours or days	0.1–0.4	Protection against virus-infected and neoplastic cells

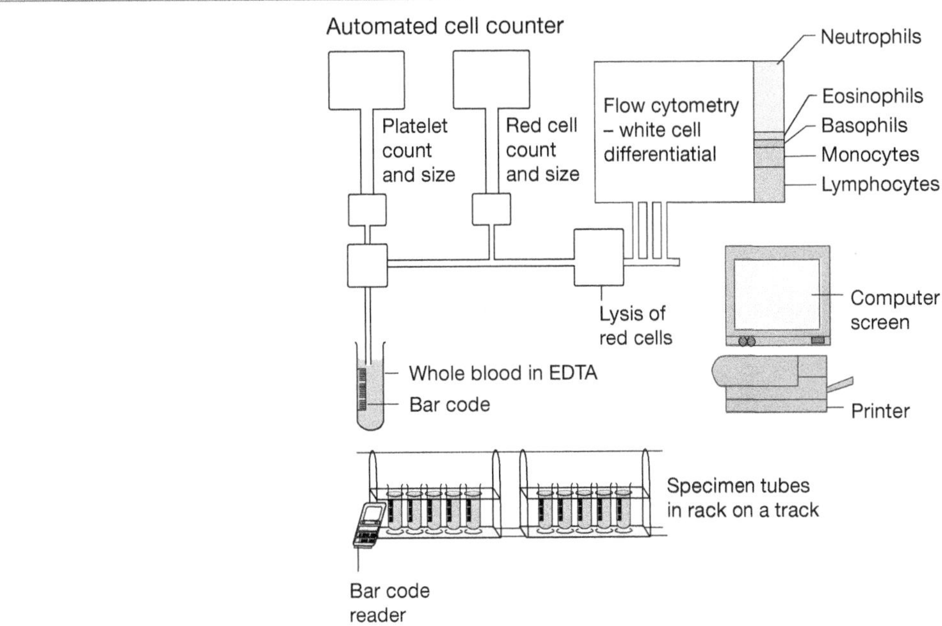

Figure 2.1 Automated blood cell counter. Source: A.B. Mehta, A.V. Hoffbrand (2014) *Haematology at a Glance*, 4th edn. Reproduced with permission of John Wiley & Sons.

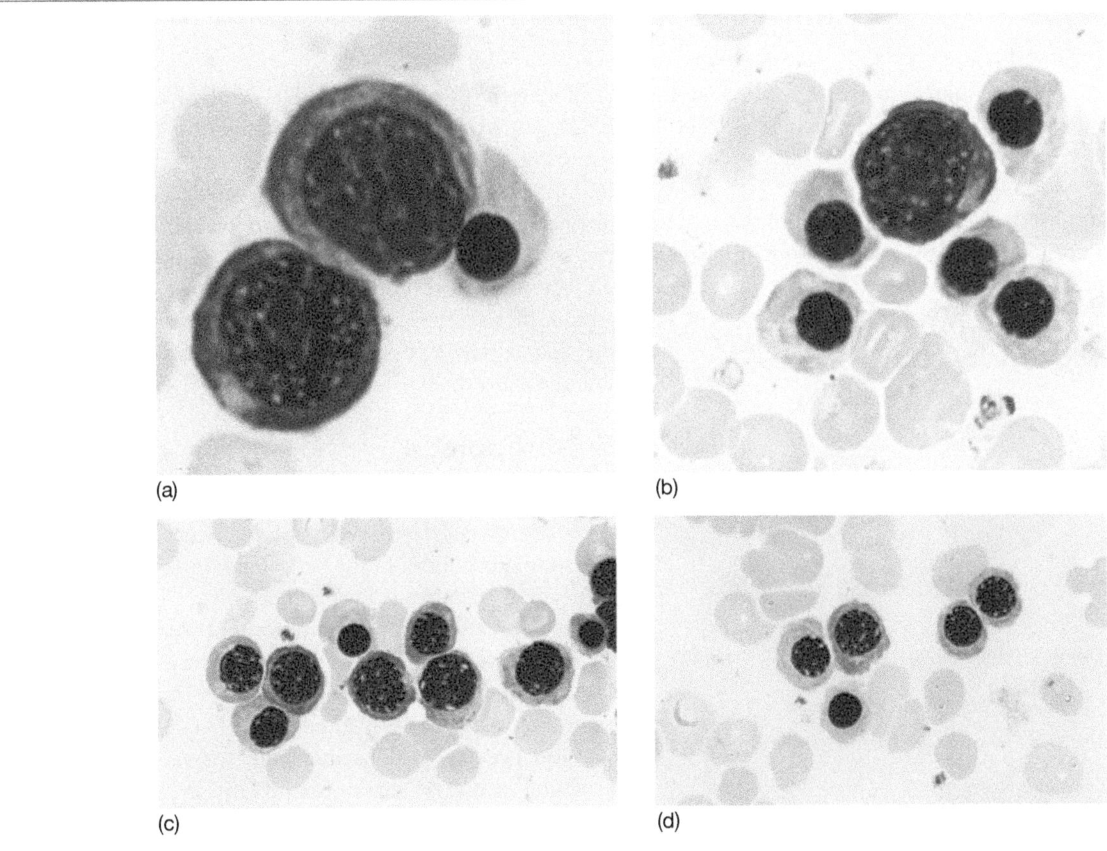

Figure 2.2 Erythroblasts (normoblasts) at varying stages of development. The earlier cells are larger, with more basophilic cytoplasm and a more open nuclear chromatin pattern **(a, b)**. The cytoplasm of the later cells is paler blue and more eosinophilic as a result of haemoglobin formation **(c, d)**.

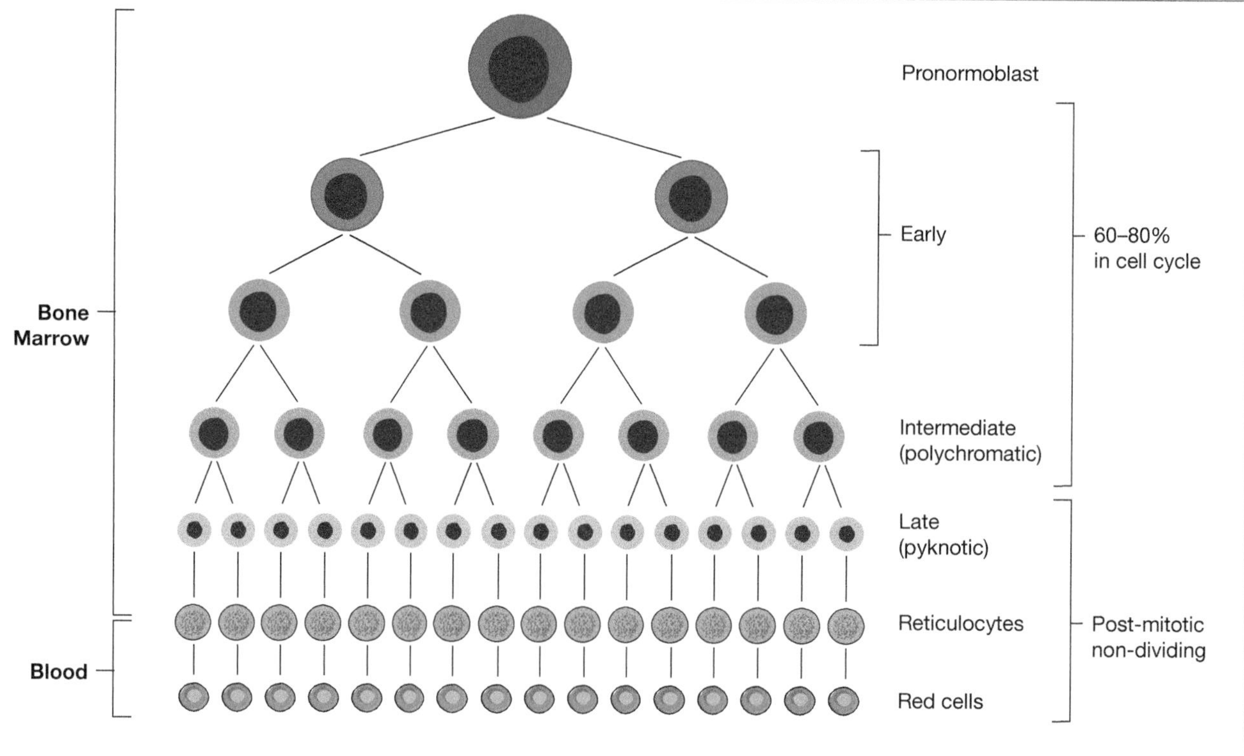

Figure 2.3 The amplification and maturation sequence in the development of mature red cells from the pronormoblast.

progressively more haemoglobin (which stains pink) in the cytoplasm; the cytoplasm also stains paler blue as it loses its RNA and protein synthetic apparatus, while nuclear chromatin becomes more condensed (Figs. 2.2 and 2.3). The nucleus is finally extruded from the late normoblast within the marrow and a reticulocyte results. This still contains some ribosomal RNA and so is still able to synthesize haemoglobin (Fig. 2.4).

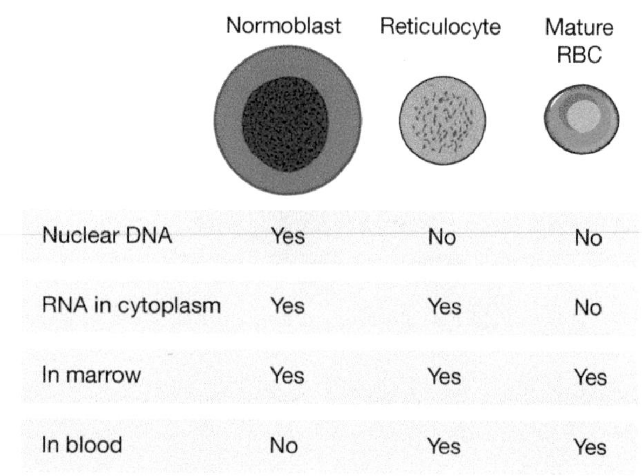

	Normoblast	Reticulocyte	Mature RBC
Nuclear DNA	Yes	No	No
RNA in cytoplasm	Yes	Yes	No
In marrow	Yes	Yes	Yes
In blood	No	Yes	Yes

Figure 2.4 Comparison of the DNA and RNA content, and marrow and peripheral blood distribution, of the erythroblast (normoblast), reticulocyte and mature red blood cell (RBC).

The **reticulocyte** is slightly larger than a mature red cell. It circulates in the peripheral blood for 1–2 days before maturing, when RNA is completely lost. A completely pink-staining mature erythrocyte results, which is a non-nucleated biconcave disc (Fig. 2.4). One pronormoblast usually gives rise to 16 mature red cells (Fig. 2.3). Normoblasts are not present in normal human peripheral blood (Fig. 2.4). They appear in the blood if erythropoiesis is occurring outside the marrow (extramedullary erythropoiesis) and also with some marrow diseases.

Erythropoietin

Erythropoiesis is regulated by the hormone erythropoietin, a heavily glycosylated polypeptide. Ninety percent of the hormone is produced in the peritubular interstitial cells of the kidney and 10% in the liver and elsewhere. There are no preformed stores. The stimulus to erythropoietin production is the oxygen (O_2) tension in the tissues of the kidney (Fig. 2.5a). Erythropoietin production increases with decreased O_2 delivery to the kidney. This is caused most frequently by anaemia, but also occurs when haemoglobin for some metabolic or structural reason is unable to give up O_2 normally, when atmospheric O_2 is low or with defective cardiac or pulmonary function or damage to the renal circulation.

Hypoxia induces stabilization of the hypoxia-inducible factor (HIF-1α) which then forms a dimer with HIFβ, the dimer stimulating erythropoietin production. The dimer also

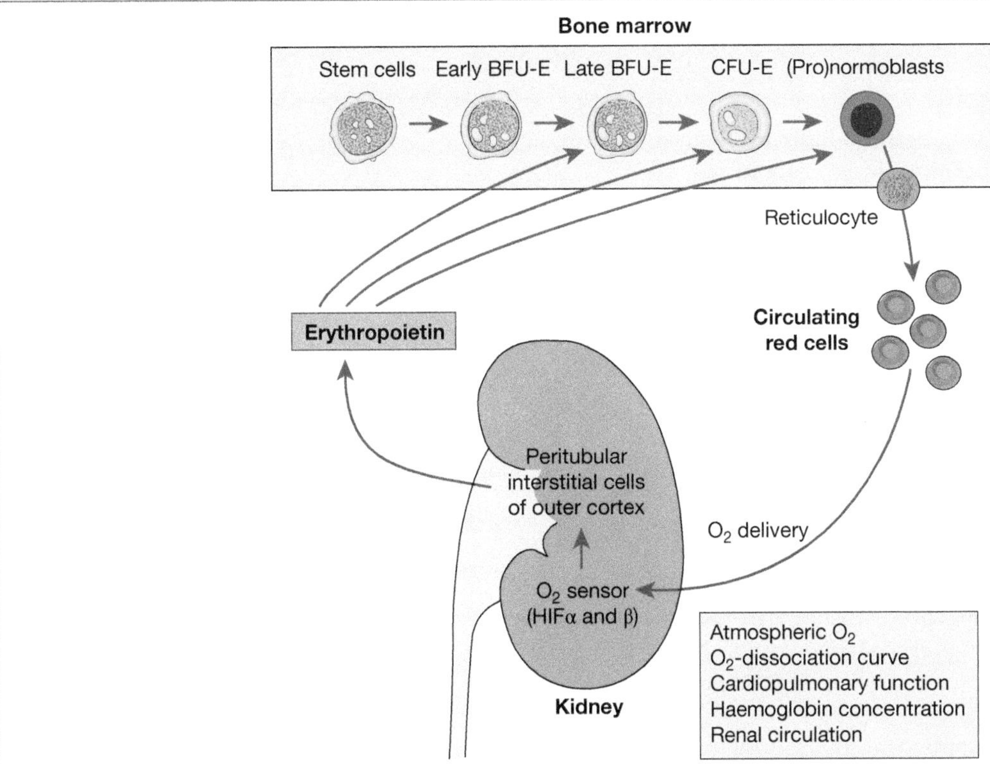

Figure 2.5a The production of erythropoietin by the kidney in response to its oxygen (O_2) supply. Erythropoietin stimulates erythropoiesis and so increases O_2 delivery. BFU_E, erythroid burst-forming unit; CFU-E, erythroid colony-forming unit.

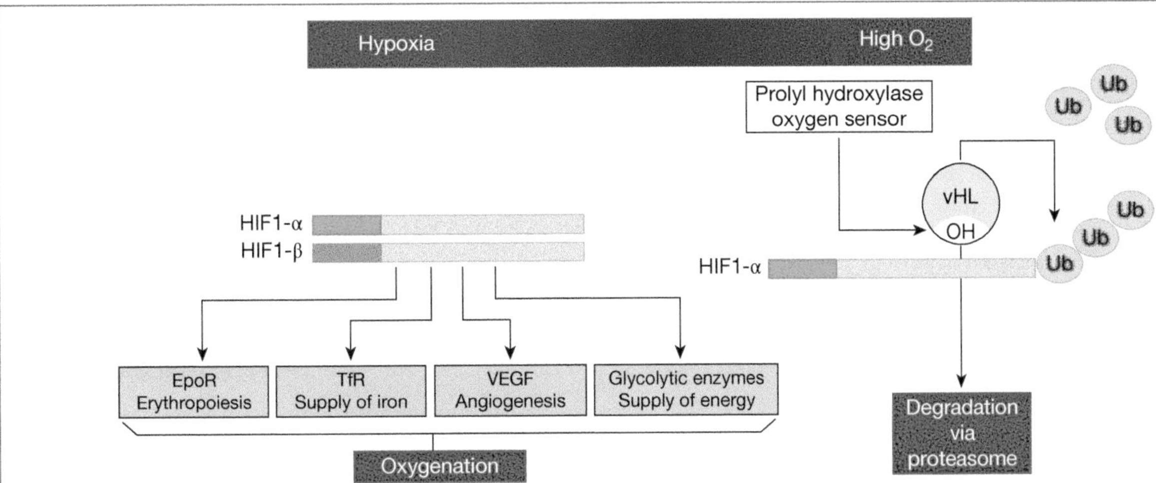

Figure 2.5b The oxygen sensor: hypoxia stabilises hypoxia inducible factor (HIF)α which then forms a dimer with HIFβ, which stimulates erythropoietin production. PHD2 (prolyl hydroxylase), the oxygen sensor, uses molecular oxygen to hydroxylate HIF-1α. This hydroxylation allows von Hippel-Lindau (vHL) binding to HIFα and stimulates its breakdown by ubiquitination. Source: D.R. Higgs *et al*. In A.V. Hoffbrand *et al*. (eds) (2016) *Postgraduate Haematology*, 7th edn. Reproduced with permission of John Wiley & Sons.

stimulates new vessel formation, glycolytic enzyme and transferrin receptor synthesis and increased iron absorption by reducing hepcidin synthesis. Prolyl hydroxylase (PHD2) is a key oxygen sensor. It uses molecular oxygen to hydroxylate HIFα. Hydroxylation allows the von Hippel-Lindau (vHL) protein to break down HIFα by ubiquitination (Fig. 2.5b). Mutations in the genes *vHL, PHD2* and *HIF2α* are rare causes of congenital polycythaemia (Chapter 15). Daprodustat, roxadustat and vadadustat which inhibit PDH2 and raise endogenous erythropoietin production are in clinical trials for treating the anaemia of chronic renal failure and as a result of chemotherapy for cancer.

Erythropoietin stimulates erythropoiesis by increasing the number of progenitor cells committed to erythropoiesis.

The transcription factor GATA2 is involved in initiating erythroid differentiation from pluripotential stem cells. Subsequently the transcription factors GATA1 and FOG1 are activated by erythropoietin receptor stimulation and are important in enhancing expression of erythroid-specific genes, e.g. of globin, haem biosynthetic and red cell membrane proteins, and also enhancing expression of anti-apoptotic genes and of the transferrin receptor1 (CD71). Late BFU_E and CFU-E, which have erythropoietin receptors, are stimulated to proliferate, differentiate and produce haemoglobin. The proportion of erythroid cells in the marrow increases and, in the chronic state, there is anatomical expansion of erythropoiesis into fatty marrow and sometimes into extramedullary sites. In infants, the marrow cavity may expand into cortical bone, resulting in bone deformities with frontal bossing and protrusion of the maxilla (Chapter 7).

Conversely, increased O_2 supply to the tissues (because of an increased red cell mass or because haemoglobin is able to release its O_2 more readily than normal) reduces the erythropoietin drive. Plasma erythropoietin levels can be valuable in clinical diagnosis. They are high in anaemia, unless this is due to renal failure or if a tumour-secreting erythropoietin is present, but low in severe renal disease or polycythaemia vera (Fig. 2.6).

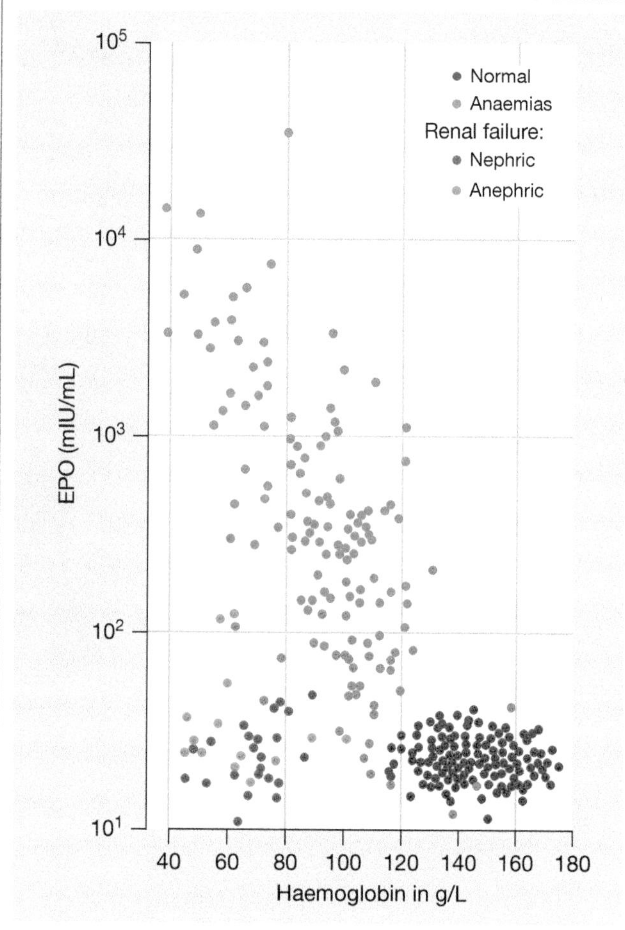

Figure 2.6 The relation between the concentration of erythropoietin (EPO) in plasma and haemoglobin concentration. Anaemias in this figure exclude conditions shown to be associated with impaired production of EPO. Source: Modified from M. Pippard *et al.* (1992) *Br. J. Haematol.* 82: 445. Reproduced with permission of John Wiley & Sons.

Indications for erythropoietin therapy

Recombinant erythropoietin is needed for treating anaemia resulting from renal disease or from various other causes. It is given subcutaneously either three times weekly, once every 1–2 weeks or every 4 weeks, depending on the indication and on the preparation used (erythropoietin alpha or beta; darbepoetin alpha, a heavily glycosylated longer-acting form; or Micera, the longest-acting preparation). The main indication is end-stage renal disease (with or without dialysis). The patients often also need oral or intravenous iron. Other indications are listed in Table 2.2. The haemoglobin level and quality of life may be improved. A low serum erythropoietin level prior to treatment is valuable in predicting an effective response. Side effects include a rise in blood pressure, thrombosis and local injection site reactions. Erythropoietin has been associated with progression of some tumours which express EPO receptors and so with reduced survival. It is only indicated as an alternative to blood transfusion in cancer patients with symptomatic anaemia where the benefits outweigh the risks of tumour progression and of venous thrombosis. Prolyl hydroxylase inhibitors (see above) are undergoing trials for treating anaemia in cancer patients.

Table 2.2 Clinical indications (in selected subjects) for erythropoietin.

Anaemia of chronic renal disease
Myelodysplastic syndrome
Anaemia associated with malignancy and chemotherapy
Anaemia of chronic diseases, e.g. rheumatoid arthritis
Anaemia of prematurity
Perioperative uses

The marrow requires many other substances for effective erythropoiesis. These include metals iron and cobalt, vitamins (vitamin B_{12}, folate, vitamin C, vitamin E, vitamin B_6, thiamine and riboflavin) and hormones androgens and thyroxine. Deficiency in any of these may be associated with anaemia.

Haemoglobin

Haemoglobin synthesis

Each molecule of normal adult **haemoglobin** A (Hb A, the dominant haemoglobin in blood after the age of 3–6 months) consists of four polypeptide chains, $\alpha_2\beta_2$, each with its own haem group. Normal adult blood also contains small quantities of two other haemoglobins: Hb F and Hb A_2. These also contain α chains, but with γ and δ chains, respectively, instead of β (Table 2.3). The synthesis of the various globin chains in the foetus and adult is discussed in Chapter 7.

Haem synthesis occurs largely in mitochondria by a series of biochemical reactions, commencing with the condensation of glycine and succinyl coenzyme A under the action of the key rate-limiting enzyme δ-aminolaevulinic acid synthase (ALAS) (Fig. 2.7). Pyridoxal phosphate (vitamin B_6) is a coenzyme for this reaction. The main sources of succinyl CoA are glutamine and glucose, which are converted to alpha-ketoglutarate, a succinate precursor inside the erythroid cells. Ultimately, protoporphyrin combines with iron in the ferrous (Fe^{2+}) state to form haem (Fig. 2.8). A tetramer of four globin chains, each with its own haem group in a 'pocket', is then formed to make up a haemoglobin molecule (Fig. 2.9). An enzyme eIF2alpha kinase, also known as haem-regulated inhibitor (HRI), senses intracellular haem concentration. If this is low as in iron deficiency, HRI phosphorylates its substrate eIF2alpha which then reduces globin synthesis by inhibiting its mRNA translation.

An adjacent gene *Nprl3* shares some enhancers with the α-globin gene and so the control of expression of the two genes is coupled. *Nprl3* provides negative regulation of mTORC1, a critical controller of cellular metabolism. Nprl3 is essential for optimal erythropoiesis and for responding to fluctuating nutrient (including iron) and growth factor concentrations.

Table 2.3 Normal haemoglobins in adult blood.

	Hb A	Hb F	Hb A_2
Structure	$\alpha_2\beta_2$	$\alpha_2\gamma_2$	$\alpha_2\delta_2$
Normal (%)	96–98	0.5–0.8	1.5–3.2

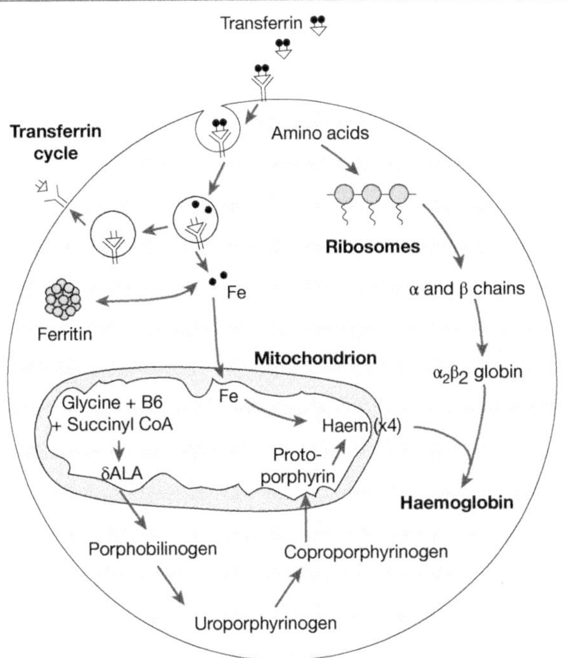

Figure 2.7 Haemoglobin synthesis in the developing red cell. The mitochondria are the main sites of protoporphyrin synthesis, iron (Fe) is supplied from circulating transferrin and globin chains are synthesized on ribosomes. δ-ALA, δ-aminolaevulinic acid; CoA, coenzyme A.

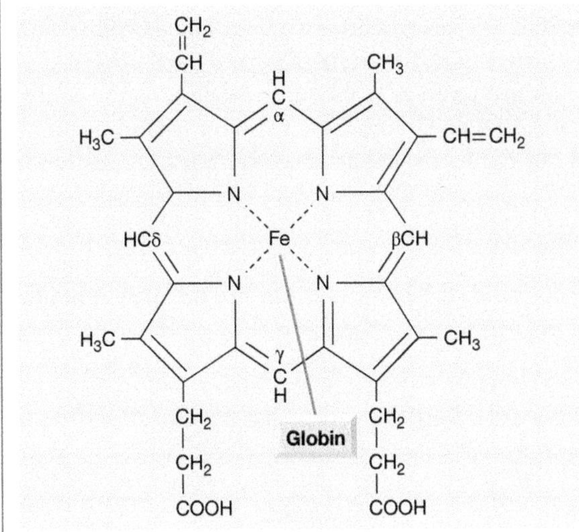

Figure 2.8 The structure of haem.

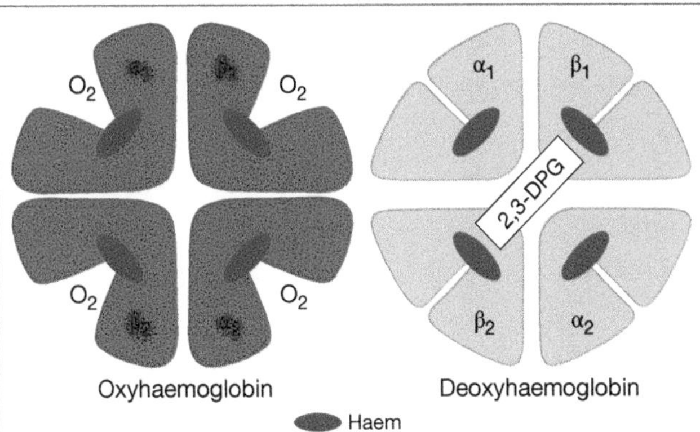

Figure 2.9 The oxygenated and deoxygenated haemoglobin molecule. α, β, globin chains of normal adult haemoglobin (Hb A); 2,3-DPG, 2,3-diphosphoglycerate.

Haemoglobin function

The red cells in systemic arterial blood carry O_2 from the lungs to the tissues and return in venous blood with CO_2 to the lungs. As the haemoglobin molecule loads and unloads O_2, the individual globin chains move on each other (Fig. 2.9). The $\alpha_1\beta_1$ and $\alpha_2\beta_2$ contacts stabilize the molecule. When O_2 is unloaded the β chains are pulled apart, permitting entry of the metabolite 2,3-diphosphoglycerate (2,3-DPG), resulting in a lower affinity of the molecule for O_2. This movement is responsible for the sigmoid form of the haemoglobin O_2 dissociation curve (Fig. 2.10). The P_{50} (the partial pressure of O_2 at which haemoglobin is half saturated with O_2) of normal blood is 26.6 mmHg. With increased affinity for O_2, the curve shifts to the left (the P_{50} falls), while with decreased affinity for O_2, the curve shifts to the right (the P_{50} rises).

Normally, *in vivo*, O_2 exchange operates between 95% saturation (arterial blood) with a mean arterial O_2 tension of 95 mmHg and 70% saturation (venous blood) with a mean venous O_2 tension of 40 mmHg (Fig. 2.10).

The normal position of the curve depends on the concentration of 2,3-DPG, H^+ ions and CO_2 in the red cell and on the structure of the haemoglobin molecule. High concentrations of 2,3-DPG, H^+ or of CO_2, and the presence of sickle haemoglobin (Hb S), shift the curve to the right (oxygen is given up more easily), whereas foetal haemoglobin (Hb F) – which is unable to bind 2,3-DPG – and certain rare abnormal haemoglobins associated with polycythaemia shift the curve to the left because they give up O_2 less readily than normal.

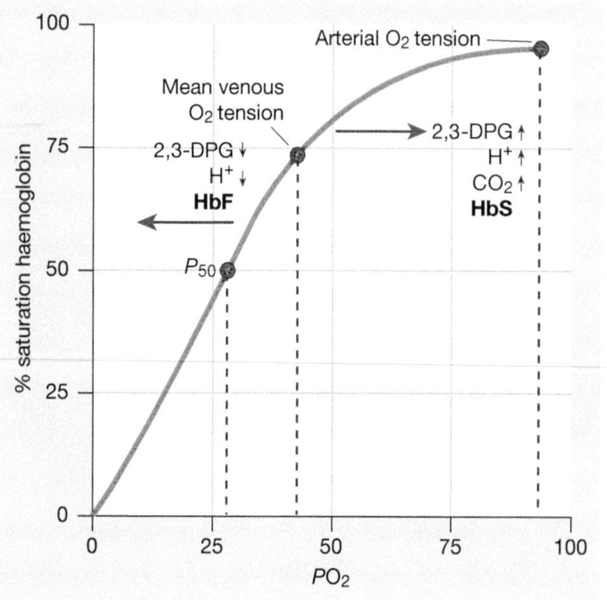

Figure 2.10 The haemoglobin oxygen (O2) dissociation curve. 2,3-DPG, 2,3-diphosphoglycerate.

Methaemoglobinaemia

This is a clinical state in which circulating haemoglobin is present with iron in the oxidized Fe^{3+} instead of the usual Fe^{2+} state. It may arise because of a hereditary deficiency of the enzyme methaemoglobin reductase or inheritance of a structurally abnormal haemoglobin (Hb M). Hb Ms contain an amino acid substitution affecting the haem pocket of the globin chain. Toxic methaemoglobinaemia and/or sulphaemoglobinaemia occurs when a drug or other toxic substance oxidizes haemoglobin. In all these states, the patient is likely to show cyanosis.

The red cell

In order to carry haemoglobin into close contact with the tissues and for successful gaseous exchange, the red cell, 8 μm in diameter, must pass repeatedly through the microcirculation, whose minimum diameter is 3.5 μm. It must maintain haemoglobin in a reduced (ferrous) state and maintain osmotic equilibrium despite the high concentration of protein (haemoglobin) in the cell. A single journey round the body takes 20 seconds and its total journey throughout its 120-day life span has been estimated to be 480 km (300 miles). To fulfil these functions, the cell is a flexible biconcave disc with an ability to generate energy as adenosine triphosphate (ATP) by the anaerobic glycolytic (Embden–Meyerhof) pathway (Fig. 2.11) and to generate reducing power both as nicotinamide adenine dinucleotide (NADH) by this pathway and as reduced nicotinamide adenine dinucleotide phosphate (NADPH) by the hexose monophosphate shunt (Fig. 2.11, Fig. 6.6).

Red cell metabolism

Embden–Meyerhof pathway

In this series of biochemical reactions, glucose that enters the red cell from plasma by facilitated transfer is metabolized to lactate (Fig. 2.11). For each molecule of glucose used, two molecules of ATP and thus two high-energy phosphate bonds are generated. This ATP provides energy for maintenance of red cell volume, shape and flexibility.

The Embden–Meyerhof pathway generates NADH, which is needed by the enzyme methaemoglobin reductase to reduce functionally dead methaemoglobin containing ferric iron, produced by oxidation of approximately 3% of haemoglobin each day, to functionally active haemoglobin containing ferrous ions. The Rapoport–Luebering shunt, or side-arm, of this pathway (Fig. 2.11) generates 2,3-DPG, important in the regulation of haemoglobin's oxygen affinity (Fig. 2.10).

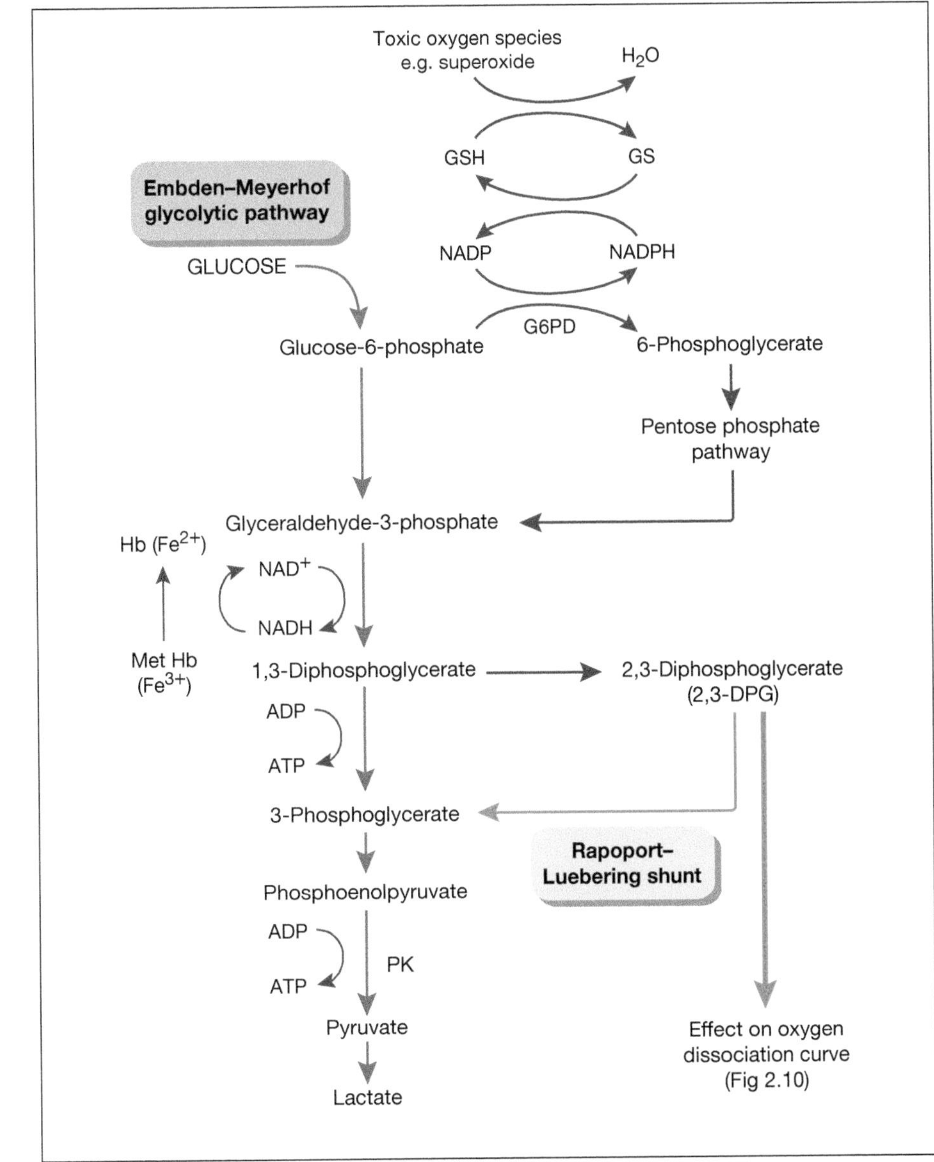

Figure 2.11 The anaerobic Embden–Meyerhof pathway generates energy as ATP and reducing power as NADH. The pentose-phosphate shunt pathway generates additional reducing power as NADPH. Further down the main pathway the Rapoport–Luebering shunt generates 2,3 DPG which effects oxygen binding and release by haemoglobin (Fig 2.10). GS, glutathione; GSH, reduced glutathione; G6PD, glucose-phosphate dehydrogenase; PK, pyruvate kinase; NAD, NADP, ADP, ATP see text.

Hexose monophosphate (pentose phosphate) shunt

Approximately 10% of glycolysis occurs by this oxidative pathway in which glucose-6-phosphate is converted to 6-phosphogluconate and so to a pentose-5-phosphate (Fig. 2.11, Fig. 6.6). NADPH is generated and is linked with glutathione, which maintains sulphydril (SH) groups intact in the cell, including those in haemoglobin and in the red cell membrane. In one of the most common inherited abnormalities of red cells, glucose-6-phosphate dehydrogenase (G6PD) deficiency, the red cells are extremely susceptible to oxidant stress (Chapter 6).

Red cell membrane

The red cell membrane comprises a lipid bilayer, membrane integral proteins and a membrane skeleton (Fig. 2.12). Approximately 50% of the membrane is protein, 20% phospholipids, 20% cholesterol molecules and up to 10% is carbohydrate. Carbohydrates occur only on the external surface, while proteins are either integral, penetrating the lipid bilayer, or form a skeleton on the inner surface of the membrane. Several red cell proteins have been numbered according to their mobility on polyacrylamide gel electrophoresis (PAGE), e.g. band 3, proteins 4.1, 4.2 (Fig. 2.12).

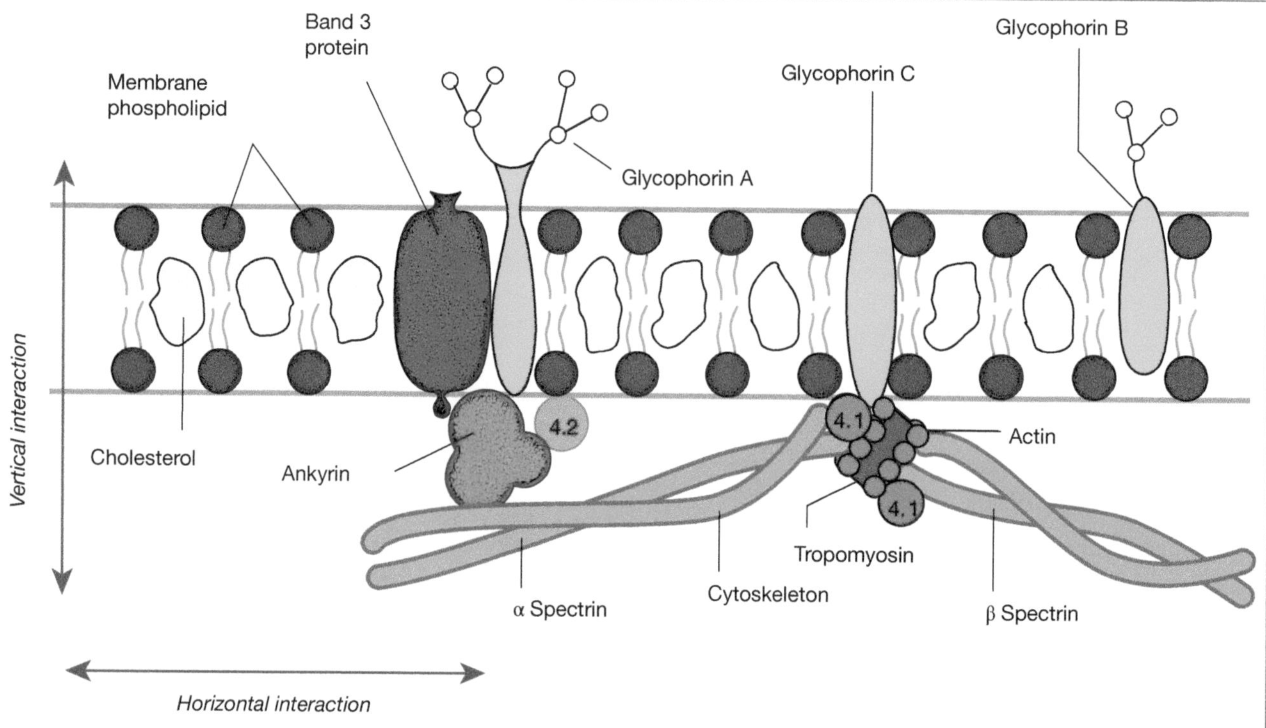

Figure 2.12 The structure of the red cell membrane. Some of the penetrating and integral proteins carry carbohydrate antigens; other antigens are attached directly to the lipid layer.

The membrane skeleton is formed by structural proteins that include α and β spectrin, ankyrin, protein 4.1 and actin. These proteins form a horizontal lattice important in maintaining the biconcave shape. Spectrin is the most abundant and consists of two chains, α and β, wound around each other to form heterodimers, which then self-associate head to head to form tetramers. These tetramers are linked at the tail end to actin and attached there to protein band 4.1. At the head end, the β spectrin chains attach to ankyrin, which connects them to band 3, the transmembrane protein that acts as an anion channel ('vertical connection'; Fig. 2.12). Protein 4.2 enhances this interaction.

Defects of the membrane proteins explain some of the abnormalities of shape of the red cell membrane, e.g. hereditary spherocytosis and elliptocytosis (Chapter 6), while alterations in lipid composition because of congenital or acquired abnormalities in plasma cholesterol or phospholipid may be associated with other membrane abnormalities (Fig. 2.16).

Anaemia

Anaemia is defined as a reduction in the haemoglobin concentration of the blood below normal for age and sex (Table 2.4). Although normal values can vary between laboratories, typical values would be less than 135 g/L in adult males and less than 115 g/L in adult females (Fig. 2.13). The World Health Organisation (WHO) defines anaemia as a haemoglobin level < 130 g/L for adult males, < 120 g/L for adult non-pregnant females and <110 g/L from the age of 6–59 months. Newborn infants have a high haemoglobin level; 140 g/L is taken as the lower limit at birth (Fig. 2.13). Anaemia in pregnancy and neonates is discussed in Chapter 34.

Alterations in total circulating plasma volume as well as in total circulating haemoglobin mass determine the haemoglobin concentration. Reduction in plasma volume as in dehydration may mask anaemia or even cause apparent (pseudo) polycythaemia (Chapter 15). Conversely, an increase in plasma volume as with splenomegaly or pregnancy may cause anaemia even with a normal total circulating red cell and haemoglobin mass.

After acute major blood loss, anaemia is not immediately apparent because the total blood volume is reduced. It takes up to a day for the plasma volume to be replaced and so for the degree of anaemia to become apparent. Regeneration of red cells and haemoglobin mass takes substantially longer. The initial clinical features of major blood loss are therefore a result of reduction in blood volume rather than of anaemia.

Global incidence

On the basis of the WHO definitions, anaemia was estimated in 2010 to occur in about 33% of the global population. Prevalence was greater in females than males at all ages and most frequent in children less than 5 years old. Anaemia was most frequent in

Table 2.4 Normal values for blood cells and haematinics.

	Males	Females
Haemoglobin (g/L)	135.0–175.0	115.0–155.0
Red cells (erythrocytes) ($\times10^{12}$/L)	4.5–6.5	3.9–5.6
PCV (haematocrit) (%)	40–52	36–48
Mean cell volume (MCV) (fL)	80–95	
Mean cell haemoglobin (MCH) (pg)	27–34	
Reticulocyte count ($\times10^9$/L)	50–150	
White cells (leucocytes)		
Total ($\times10^9$/L)	4.0–11.0	
Neutrophils ($\times10^9$/L)	1.8–7.5 (Caucasians 1.5–7.5 (Africa and Middle-East)	
Lymphocytes ($\times10^9$/L)	1.5–3.5	
Monocytes ($\times10^9$/L)	0.2–0.8	
Eosinophils ($\times10^9$/L)	0.04–0.44	
Basophils ($\times10^9$/L)	0.01–0.1	
Platelets ($\times10^9$/L)	150–400	
Serum iron (μmol/L)	10–30	
Total iron-binding capacity (μmol/L)	40–75 (2.0–4.0 g/L as transferrin)	
Serum ferritin* (μg/L)	40–340	14–150
Serum vitamin B_{12}* (ng/L)	160–925 (20–680 pmol/L)	
Serum folate* (μg/L)	3.0–15.0 (4–30 nmol/L)	
Red cell folate** (μg/L)	160–640 (360–1460 nmol/L)	

PCV, packed cell volume.
* Normal ranges differ between laboratories.
** Normal ranges differ between different laboratories.

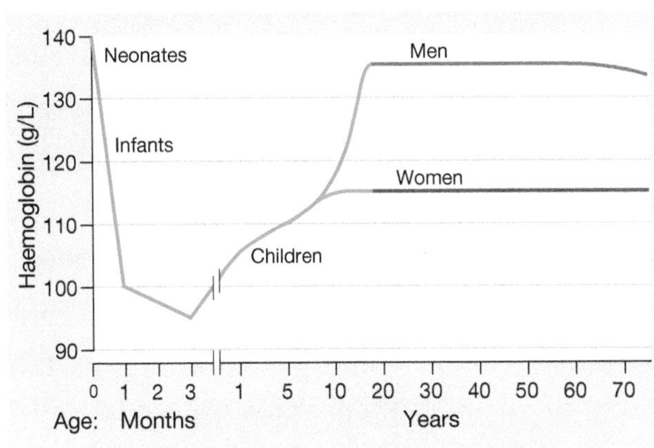

Figure 2.13 The lower limit of blood haemoglobin concentration in healthy men, women and children of various ages.

South Asia, and in Central, West and East Sub-Saharan Africa. The main causes are iron deficiency (caused by life-long poor diet combined with menstruation and/or repeated pregnancies, hookworm, schistosomiasis), the anaemia of inflammation (Chapter 3), sickle cell diseases, thalassaemia (Chapter 7), malaria (Chapter 32).

Clinical features of anaemia

The major adaptations to anaemia are in the cardiovascular system with increased cardiac stroke volume and tachycardia and in the haemoglobin O_2 dissociation curve. In some patients with quite severe anaemia, there may be no symptoms or signs, whereas others with mild anaemia may be severely incapacitated. The presence or absence of clinical features depends on:

1 ***Speed of onset*** Rapidly progressive anaemia causes more symptoms than anaemia of slow onset. This is because there is less time for adaptation in the cardiovascular system and in the O_2 dissociation curve of haemoglobin.
2 ***Severity*** Mild anaemia often produces no symptoms or signs, but these are usually present when the haemoglobin is less than 90 g/L. Even severe anaemia (haemoglobin concentration as low as 60 g/L) may produce remarkably few symptoms, when there is very gradual onset in young subjects who are otherwise healthy.
3 ***Age*** The elderly tolerate anaemia less well than the young because normal cardiovascular compensation is impaired.
4 ***Haemoglobin O_2 dissociation curve*** Anaemia, in general, is associated with a rise in 2,3-DPG in the red cells and a shift in the O_2 dissociation curve to the right, so that oxygen is given up more readily to tissues. This adaptation, which takes days to occur, is particularly marked in some anaemias that either raise 2,3-DPG directly, e.g. pyruvate kinase deficiency (Chapter 6), or that are associated with a low-affinity haemoglobin, e.g. Hb S (Fig. 2.10).

Symptoms

If the patient does have symptoms, these are usually shortness of breath, particularly on exertion, weakness, lethargy, palpitation and headaches. In older subjects, symptoms of cardiac failure, angina pectoris, intermittent claudication or confusion may be present. Visual disturbances because of retinal haemorrhages may complicate very severe anaemia, particularly of rapid onset (Fig. 2.14).

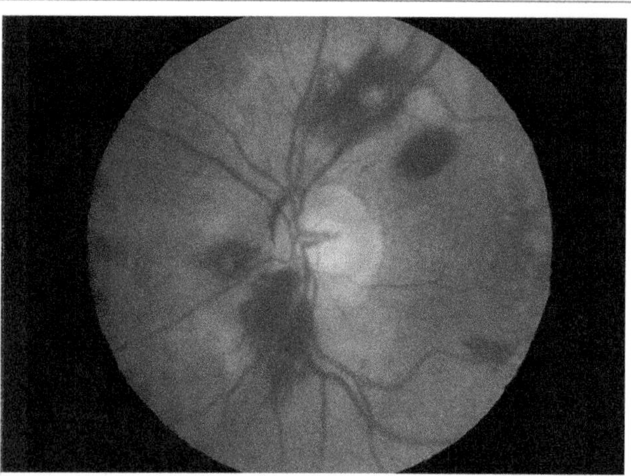

Figure 2.14 Retinal haemorrhages in a patient with severe anaemia (haemoglobin 25 g/L) caused by severe haemorrhage.

Signs

These may be divided into general and specific. General signs include pallor of mucous membranes or nail beds, which occurs if the haemoglobin level is less than 90 g/L (Fig. 2.15). Conversely, skin colour is not a reliable sign. A hyperdynamic circulation may be present with tachycardia, a bounding pulse, cardiomegaly and a systolic flow murmur. Particularly in the elderly, features of congestive heart failure may be present.

Specific signs are associated with particular types of anaemia, e.g. koilonychia (spoon nails) with iron deficiency, jaundice with haemolytic or megaloblastic anaemias, leg ulcers with sickle cell and other haemolytic anaemias, or bone deformities with thalassaemia major.

The association of features of anaemia with excess infections or spontaneous bruising suggests that neutropenia or thrombocytopenia may be present, possibly as a result of bone marrow failure.

Classification of anaemia

Red cell indices

The most useful classification is based on the red cell indices, especially MCV. This divides the anaemia into microcytic, normocytic and macrocytic (Table 2.5). As well as suggesting the nature of the primary defect, this classification may also indicate an underlying abnormality before overt anaemia has developed.

In two common physiological situations, the mean corpuscular volume (MCV) may be outside the normal adult range. In the newborn for a few weeks, the MCV is high, but in infancy it is low, e.g. 70 fL at 1 year of age and rises slowly throughout childhood to the normal adult range. In normal pregnancy there is a slight rise in MCV, even in the absence of other causes of macrocytosis, e.g. folate deficiency.

Other laboratory findings

Although the red cell indices will indicate the type of anaemia, further useful information can be obtained from the initial blood sample.

Leucocyte and platelet counts

Measurement of these helps to distinguish 'pure' anaemia from 'pancytopenia' (subnormal levels of red cells, neutrophils and platelets), which suggests a more general marrow defect or destruction of cells, e.g. hypersplenism. In anaemias caused by haemolysis or haemorrhage, the neutrophil and platelet counts are often raised; in infections and leukaemias, the leucocyte count is also often raised, and there may be abnormal leucocytes or neutrophil precursors present.

Reticulocyte count

The normal percentage is 0.5–2.5%, and the absolute count 50–150 × 10^9/L (Table 2.4). This should rise in anaemia because of erythropoietin increase and be higher the more

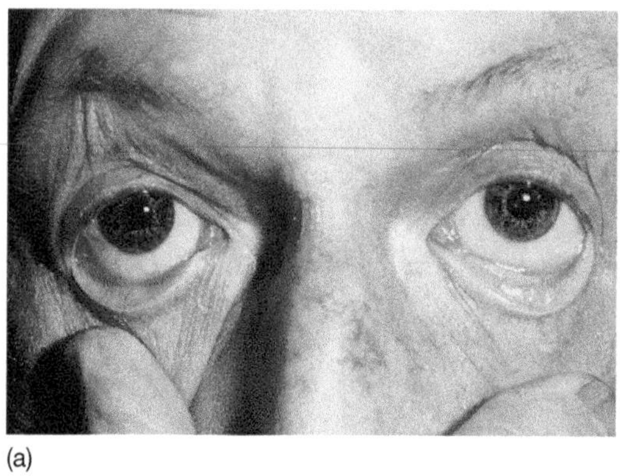

(a)

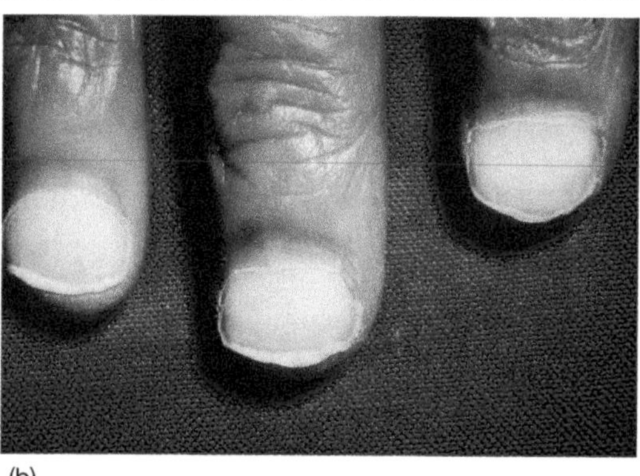

(b)

Figure 2.15 Pallor of the conjunctival mucosa **(a)** and of the nail bed **(b)** in two patients with severe anaemia (haemoglobin 60 g/L).

Table 2.5 Classification of anaemia.

Microcytic, hypochromic	Normocytic, normochromic	Macrocytic
MCV <80 fL	MCV 80–95 fL	MCV >95 fL
MCH <27 pg	MCH ≥27 pg	Megaloblastic: vitamin B_{12} or folate deficiency. Non-megaloblastic: alcohol, liver disease, myelodysplasia, aplastic anaemia, etc. (Table 5.10)
Iron deficiency	Many haemolytic anaemias	
Thalassaemia Anaemia of chronic disease (some cases) Lead poisoning Sideroblastic anaemia (some cases)	Anaemia of chronic disease (some cases)	
	After acute blood loss	
	Renal disease	
	Mixed deficiencies	
	Bone marrow failure e.g. post-chemotherapy, infiltration by carcinoma, etc.	

MCH, mean corpuscular haemoglobin; MCV, mean corpuscular volume.

severe the anaemia. This is particularly so when there has been time for erythroid hyperplasia to develop in the marrow as in chronic haemolysis. After an acute major haemorrhage, there is an erythropoietin response in 6 hours, and the reticulocyte count rises within 2–3 days, reaches a maximum in 6–10 days and remains raised until the haemoglobin returns to the normal level. If the reticulocyte count is not raised in an anaemic patient, this suggests impaired marrow function, lack of erythropoietin (renal disease) or lack of erythropoietin stimulus (Table 2.6).

Table 2.6 Factors impairing the normal reticulocyte response to anaemia.

Marrow diseases, e.g. hypoplasia, infiltration by carcinoma, lymphoma, myeloma, acute leukaemia, tuberculosis
Deficiency of iron, vitamin B_{12} or folate
Lack of erythropoietin, e.g. renal disease
Reduced tissue O_2 consumption, e.g. myxoedema, protein deficiency
Ineffective erythropoiesis, e.g. thalassaemia major, megaloblastic anaemia, myelodysplasia, myelofibrosis
Chronic inflammatory or malignant disease

Blood film

It is important to examine the blood film in all cases of anaemia. Abnormal red cell morphology (Fig. 2.16) or red cell inclusions (Fig. 2.17) may suggest a particular diagnosis. During the blood film examination, white cell abnormalities are sought, platelet number and morphology assessed and the presence of abnormal cells, e.g. normoblasts, granulocyte precursors or blast cells, is noted.

Bone marrow examination

This is needed when the cause of anaemia or other abnormality of the blood cells cannot be diagnosed from the blood count, film and other blood tests alone. It may be performed by aspiration or trephine biopsy (Fig. 2.18). For bone marrow aspiration, a needle is inserted into the marrow cavity and a liquid sample of marrow is sucked into a syringe. This sample is then spread on a slide for microscopy and stained by the usual Romanowsky technique. The detail of the developing cells can be examined, e.g. normoblastic or megaloblastic and the proportion of the different cell lines assessed (myeloid: erythroid ratio), the proportion of granulocyte precursors to red cell precursors in the bone marrow, normally 2.5 : 1 to 12 : 1. The presence of cells foreign to the marrow, e.g. secondary carcinoma, can also be observed. The cellularity of the marrow can be viewed provided fragments are obtained. An iron stain is performed routinely so that the amount of iron in reticuloendothelial stores (macrophages) and as fine

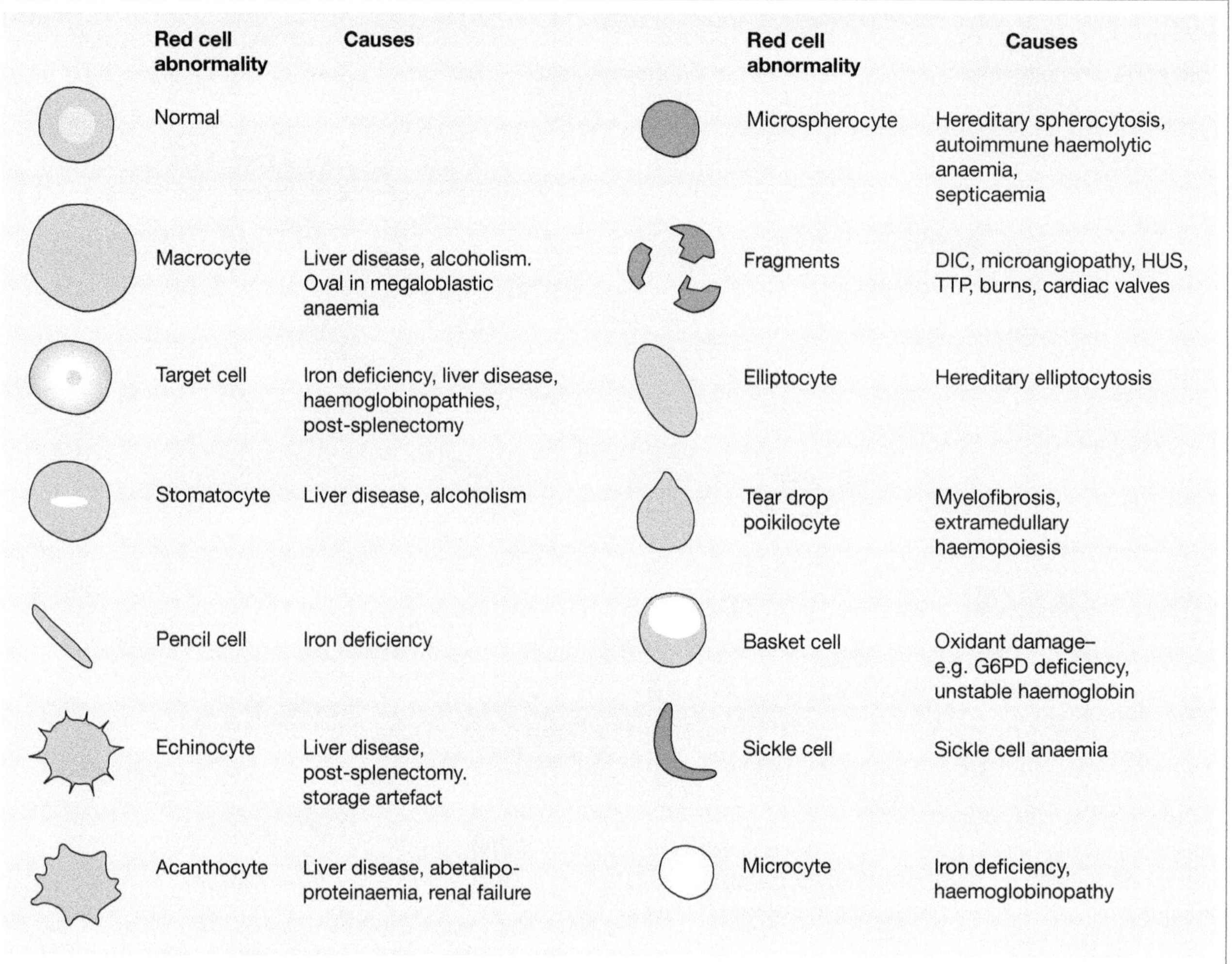

Red cell abnormality	Causes	Red cell abnormality	Causes
Normal		Microspherocyte	Hereditary spherocytosis, autoimmune haemolytic anaemia, septicaemia
Macrocyte	Liver disease, alcoholism. Oval in megaloblastic anaemia	Fragments	DIC, microangiopathy, HUS, TTP, burns, cardiac valves
Target cell	Iron deficiency, liver disease, haemoglobinopathies, post-splenectomy	Elliptocyte	Hereditary elliptocytosis
Stomatocyte	Liver disease, alcoholism	Tear drop poikilocyte	Myelofibrosis, extramedullary haemopoiesis
Pencil cell	Iron deficiency	Basket cell	Oxidant damage– e.g. G6PD deficiency, unstable haemoglobin
Echinocyte	Liver disease, post-splenectomy. storage artefact	Sickle cell	Sickle cell anaemia
Acanthocyte	Liver disease, abetalipoproteinaemia, renal failure	Microcyte	Iron deficiency, haemoglobinopathy

Figure 2.16 Some of the more frequent variations in size (anisocytosis) and shape (poikilocytosis) that may be found in different anaemias. DIC, disseminated intravascular coagulopathy; G6PD, glucose-6-phosphate dehydrogenase; HUS, haemolytic-uraemic syndrome; TTP, thrombotic thrombocytopenic purpura.

granules ('siderotic' granules) in the developing erythroblasts can be assessed (Fig. 3.10).

An aspirate sample may also be used for a number of other specialized investigations (Table 2.7).

A trephine biopsy provides a solid core of bone including marrow and is examined as a histological specimen after fixation in formalin, decalcification and sectioning. Usually immunohistology is performed, depending on the diagnosis suspected (Chapter 11). A trephine biopsy specimen is less valuable than aspirate when individual cell detail is to be examined, but provides a panoramic view of the marrow, from which overall marrow architecture, cellularity and presence of fibrosis or abnormal infiltrates can, with immunohistology if needed, be reliably determined.

Ineffective erythropoiesis

Erythropoiesis is not entirely efficient since approximately 10–15% of developing erythroblasts die within the marrow without producing mature cells. This is termed ineffective erythropoiesis and it is substantially increased in a number of chronic anaemias (Fig. 2.19). The serum unconjugated bilirubin (derived from breaking down haemoglobin) and lactate dehydrogenase (LDH, derived from breaking down cells) are usually raised when ineffective erythropoiesis is marked. The reticulocyte count is low in relation to the degree of anaemia and to the proportion of erythroblasts in the marrow.

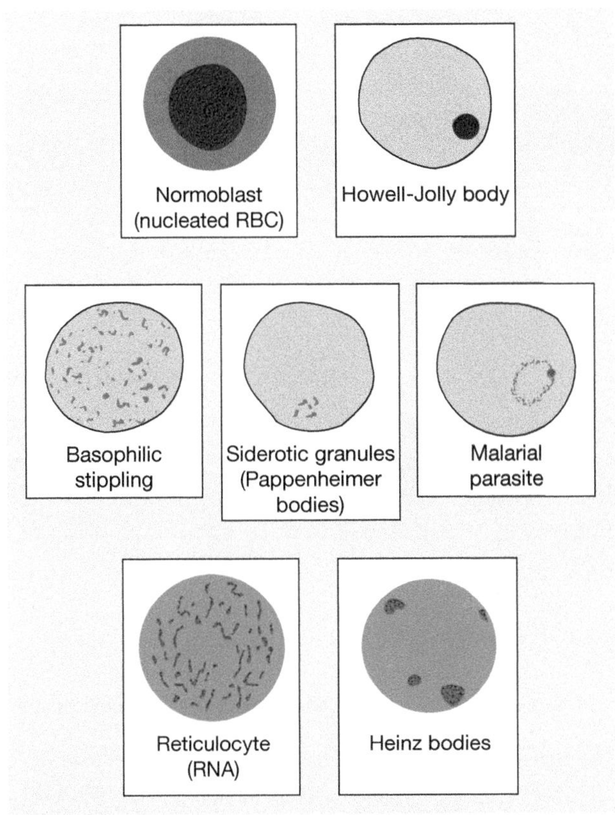

Figure 2.17 Red blood cell (RBC) inclusions which may be seen in the peripheral blood film in various conditions. The reticulocyte RNA and Heinz bodies are only demonstrated by supravital staining, e.g., with new methylene blue. Heinz bodies are oxidized denatured haemoglobin. Siderotic granules (Pappenheimer bodies) contain iron. They are purple on conventional staining, but blue with Perls' stain. The Howell–Jolly body is a DNA remnant. Basophilic stippling is denatured RNA.

Assessment of erythropoiesis

Total erythropoiesis and the amount of erythropoiesis that is effective in producing circulating red cells can be assessed by examining the bone marrow, haemoglobin level and reticulocyte count.

Total erythropoiesis is assessed from the marrow cellularity and the myeloid: erythroid ratio. This ratio falls and may be reversed when total erythropoiesis is selectively increased.

Effective erythropoiesis is assessed by the reticulocyte count. This is raised in proportion to the degree of anaemia when erythropoiesis is effective, but is low when there is ineffective erythropoiesis or an abnormality preventing normal marrow response (Table 2.6).

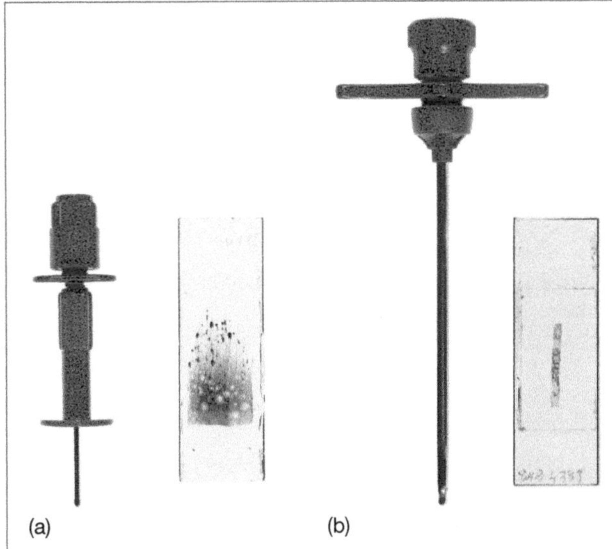

Figure 2.18 **(a)** The bone marrow aspiration needle and a smear made from a bone marrow aspirate. **(b)** The bone marrow trephine biopsy needle and a normal trephine biopsy section.

Table 2.7 Indications for bone marrow aspiration and trephine biopsy.

	Aspiration	**Trephine biopsy**
Site	Posterior iliac crest (sternum if obese; tibia in infants)	Posterior iliac crest
Stains	Romanowsky; Perls' reaction (for iron)	Haematoxylin and eosin; reticulin (silver stain)
Result available	1–2 h	1–7 d (according to decalcification method)
Indications	Investigation of unexplained anaemia, neutropenia, thrombocytopenia, suspicion of leukaemia, myeloproliferative disorders, myelodysplasia, aplastic anaemia, lymphoma, myeloma, amyloid, secondary carcinoma, cases of splenomegaly or pyrexia of undetermined cause	
Special tests	Flow cytometry, cytogenetics, FISH and molecular tests including DNA or RNA analysis for gene abnormalities. Consider microbiological culture, cytochemical markers and progenitor cell culture	Immunohistology

FISH, fluorescence *in situ* hybridization.

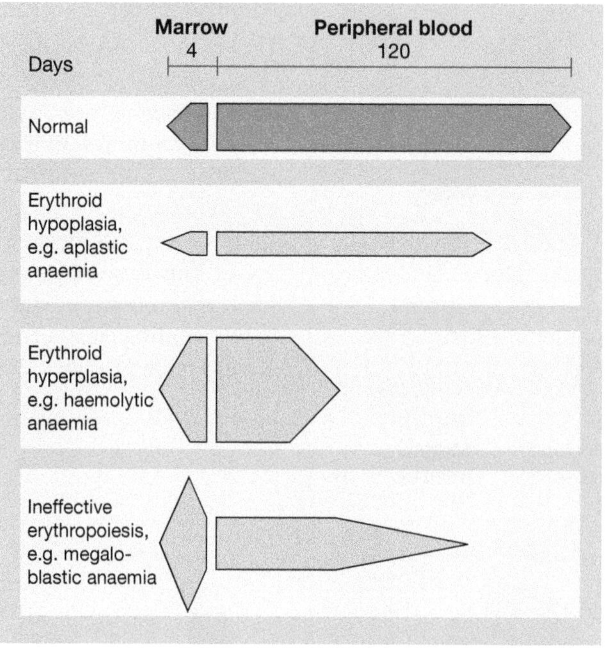

Figure 2.19 The relative proportions of marrow erythroblastic activity, circulating red cell mass and red cell lifespan in normal subjects and in three types of anaemia.

SUMMARY

- Erythropoiesis (red cell production) is regulated by erythropoietin, which is secreted by the kidney in response to hypoxia. Erythropoiesis occurs from mixed progenitor cells through a series of nucleated red cell precursors (normoblasts) to a reticulocyte stage, containing RNA but not DNA.
- Various short- or long-acting preparations of erythropoietin are used clinically to treat anaemia in renal failure and other diseases.
- Haemoglobin is the main protein in red cells. It consists of four polypeptide (globin) chains, in adults dominantly 2α and 2β, each containing an iron atom bound to protoporphyrin to form haem.
- The red cell has two biochemical pathways for metabolizing glucose, the Embden–Meyerhof pathway, which generates ATP, needed for maintenance of red cell shape and flexibility, and NADH, which prevents oxidation of haemoglobin; and the hexose monophosphate pathway, which generates NADPH, important for maintaining glutathione, which protects haemoglobin and proteins in the red cell membrane from oxidation.
- The Luebering–Rapoport shunt, or side arm, of the Embden–Meyerhof pathway generates 2,3-DPG, important in the regulation of haemoglobin's oxygen affinity
- The red cell membrane consists of a lipid bilayer, proteins which form a membrane skeleton and are integral to the membrane, and carbohydrate surface antigens.
- Anaemia is defined as a haemoglobin level in blood below the normal level for age and sex. It is classified according to the size of the red cells (MCV) into macrocytic, normocytic and microcytic. The reticulocyte count, morphology of the red cells and changes in the white cell and/or platelet count also help in the diagnosis of the cause of anaemia.
- The general clinical features of anaemia include fatigue, headaches, shortness of breath on exertion, pallor of mucous membranes and tachycardia.
- Other features relate to particular types of anaemia, e.g. jaundice, glossitis, leg ulcers, bone changes.
- Bone marrow examination by aspiration or trephine biopsy may be important in the investigation of anaemia as well as of many other haematological diseases. Special tests, e.g. immunology by flow cytometry or immunohistology, cytogenetics or molecular genetics, can be performed on the cells or core of bone obtained.

Now visit **www.wiley.com/go/haematology9e** to test yourself on this chapter.

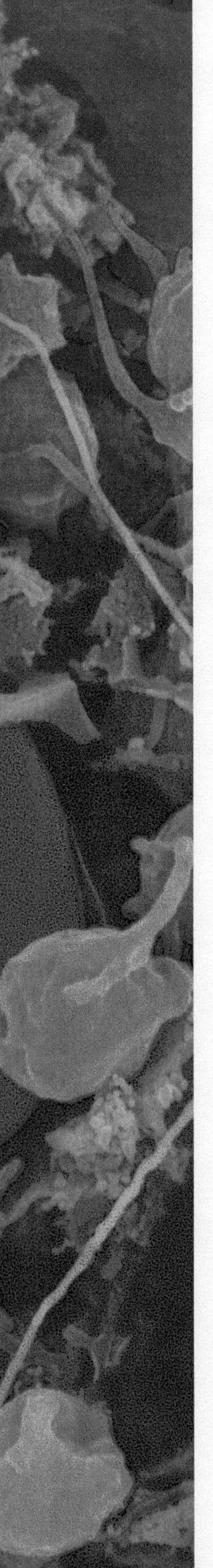

CHAPTER 3

Hypochromic anaemias

Key topics

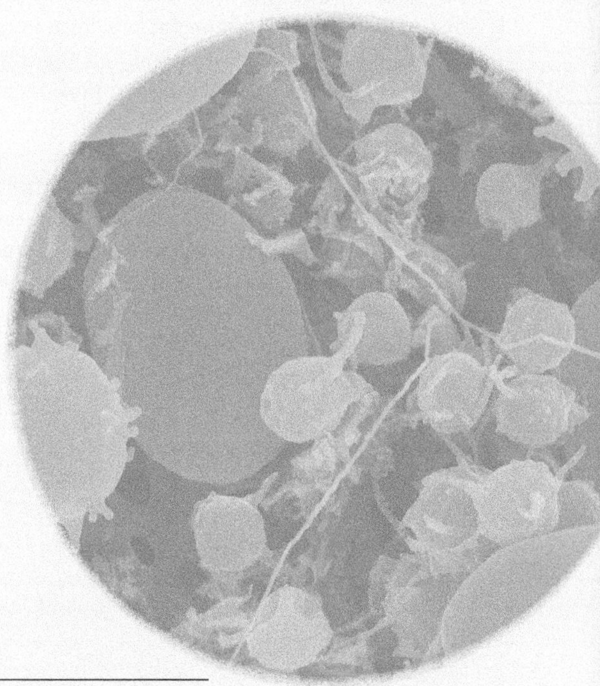

Hoffbrand's Essential Haematology, Ninth Edition. A. Victor Hoffbrand, Pratima Chowdary, Graham P. Collins, and Justin Loke.

© 2024 John Wiley & Sons Ltd. Published 2024 by John Wiley & Sons Ltd.

Companion website: www.wiley.com/go/haematology9e

Iron is one of the most common elements in the Earth's crust, yet iron deficiency is the most common cause of anaemia, affecting about 500 million people worldwide. It is particularly frequent in low-income populations, such as in sub-Saharan Africa or South Asia, where the diet is frequently of poor quality and parasites, e.g. hookworm or schistosomiasis, which cause iron loss due to haemorrhage, may be present. Moreover, the body has limited ability to absorb iron. **Iron deficiency is the major cause of a microcytic, hypochromic anaemia, in which the mean corpuscular volume (MCV) and mean corpuscular haemoglobin (MCH) are both reduced and the blood film shows small (microcytic) and pale (hypochromic) red cells.** This appearance is caused by a defect in haemoglobin synthesis. The major differential diagnosis of a microcytic, hypochromic anaemia is between iron deficiency, the anaemia of chronic disease, which are both dealt with in this chapter, and thalassaemia, which is considered in Chapter 7 (Fig. 3.1).

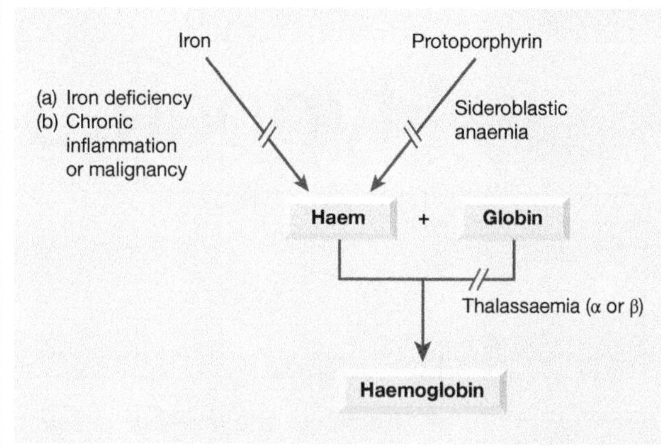

Figure 3.1 The causes of a hypochromic microcytic anaemia. These include lack of iron (iron deficiency) or of iron release from macrophages to serum (anaemia of chronic disease), failure of protoporphyrin synthesis (sideroblastic anaemia) or of globin synthesis (α- or β-thalassaemia). Lead also inhibits haem and globin synthesis.

Nutritional and metabolic aspects of iron

Body iron distribution and transport

The transport and storage of iron are largely mediated by three proteins: transferrin, transferrin receptor 1 (TFR1) and ferritin.

Each transferrin molecule can contain up to two atoms of iron in the ferric form. Transferrin delivers iron to tissues that have transferrin receptors (TFR1s), especially erythroblasts in the bone marrow, which incorporate the iron into haemoglobin (Figs. 2.7 and 3.2). The transferrin is then reutilized. At the end of their life, red cells are broken down in the macrophages of the reticuloendothelial system and the iron released from haemoglobin enters the plasma and provides most of the iron attached to transferrin. Only a small proportion of plasma transferrin iron comes from dietary iron, absorbed each day through the duodenum. Iron in excess of that needed for haemoglobin synthesis is also released from erythroblasts and erythrocytes to plasma transferrin. There is a diurnal variation in serum iron, highest in the mornings or noon and then falling to lowest levels in the evening.

Some iron is stored in the macrophages as **ferritin and haemosiderin**, the amount varying widely according to overall body iron status. **Ferritin** is a water-soluble protein–iron complex. It is made up of an outer protein shell, apoferritin, consisting of 22 subunits and an iron–phosphate–hydroxide core. It contains up to 20% of its weight as iron and is not visible by light microscopy. Specialized intracellular carrier proteins transfer iron to ferritin and from ferritin to phagolysosomes for its degradation and release of its iron.

Haemosiderin is an insoluble protein–iron complex of varying composition containing approximately 37% iron by weight. It is derived from partial lysosomal digestion of ferritin molecules and is visible in macrophages and other cells by light microscopy after staining by Perls' (Prussian blue) reaction (Fig. 3.10). Iron in ferritin and haemosiderin is in the ferric form. It is mobilized after reduction to the ferrous form. A copper-containing enzyme caeruloplasmin catalyses oxidation of the iron to the ferric form for binding to plasma transferrin.

Most body iron is in haemoglobin. Iron is also present in muscles as myoglobin and in most body cells in iron-containing enzymes, e.g. cytochromes or catalase (Table 3.1). This tissue iron

Table 3.1 The distribution of body iron.

Amount of iron in average adult	Male (g)	Female (g)	Percentage of total
Haemoglobin	2.4	1.7	65
Ferritin and haemosiderin	1.0 (0.3–1.5)	0.3 (0–1.0)	30
Myoglobin	0.15	0.12	3.5
Haem enzymes, e.g., cytochromes, catalase, peroxidases, flavoproteins	0.02	0.015	0.5
Transferrin-bound iron	0.004	0.003	0.1

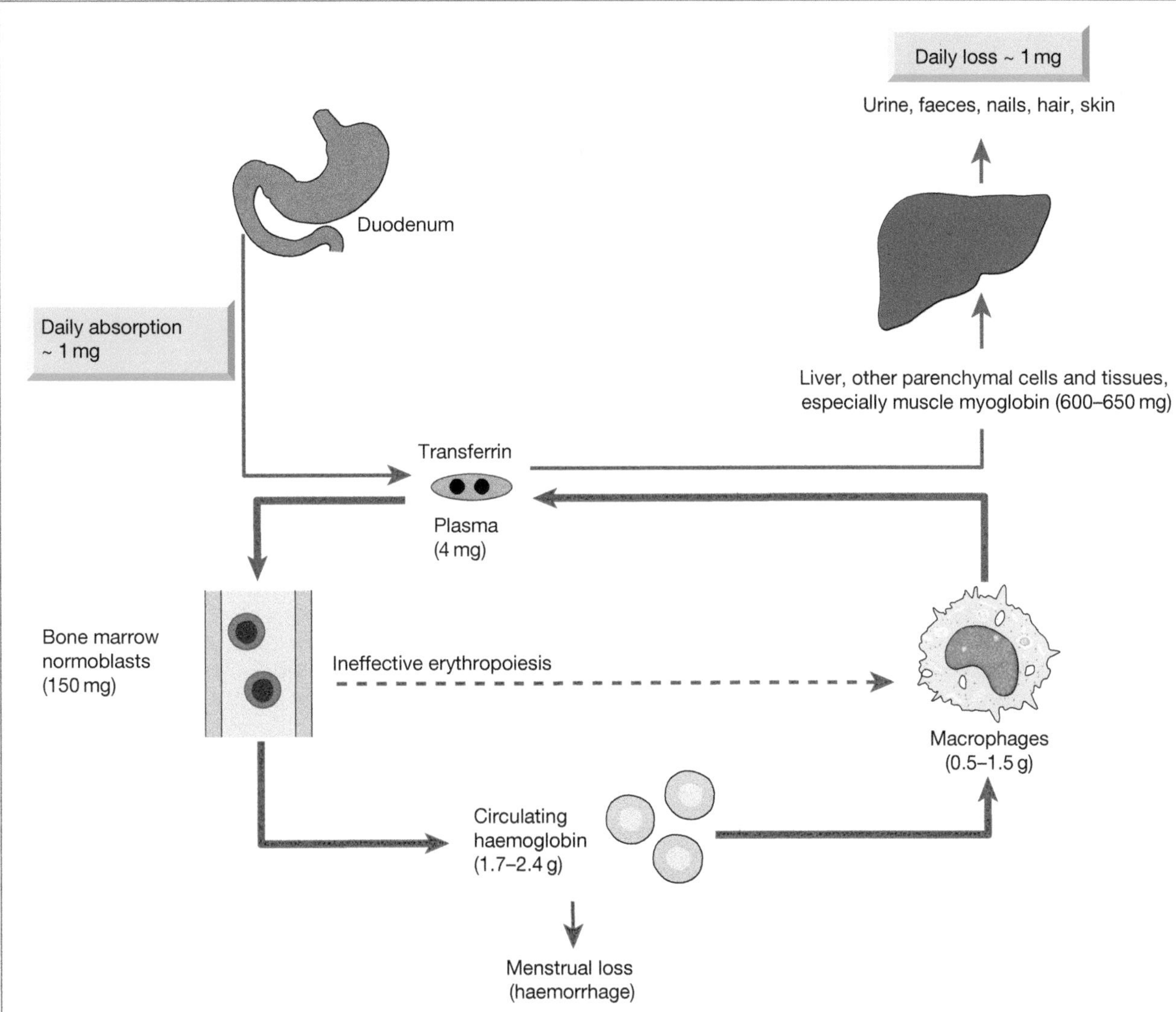

Figure 3.2 Daily iron cycle. Most of the iron in the body is contained in circulating haemoglobin and is reutilized for haemoglobin synthesis after the red cells die. Iron is transferred from macrophages to plasma transferrin and so to bone marrow erythroblasts. Iron absorption is normally just sufficient to make up for iron loss. The dashed line indicates ineffective erythropoiesis.

is less likely to become depleted than haemosiderin, ferritin and haemoglobin in states of iron deficiency, but some reduction of tissue haem-containing enzymes may also occur.

Regulation of ferritin and transferrin receptor 1 synthesis

The levels of ferritin, TFR1, δ-aminolaevulinic acid synthase (ALAS) and also of the divalent metal transporter 1 (DMT1), important in iron absorption, are linked to iron status, so that iron overload causes a rise in tissue ferritin and a fall in TFR1 and DMT1, whereas in iron deficiency ferritin and ALAS are low and TFR1 and DMT1 increased. This linkage arises through the binding of an iron regulatory protein (IRP) to iron response elements (IREs) on the ferritin, TFR1, ALAS and DMT1 mRNA molecules. Iron deficiency increases the ability of IRP to bind to the IREs, whereas iron overload reduces the binding. The site of IRP binding to the IREs determines whether the amount of the individual mRNAs and so protein produced is increased or decreased (Fig. 3.3). Upstream binding reduces translation, whereas downstream binding stabilizes the mRNA, increasing translation and so protein synthesis.

When plasma iron is raised and transferrin is saturated, the amount of iron transferred to parenchymal cells e.g. those of the liver, endocrine organs and heart is increased and this is the basis of the pathological changes associated with iron loading conditions. There may also be free iron in plasma (non-transferrin bound iron) which is toxic to different organs (Chapter 4).

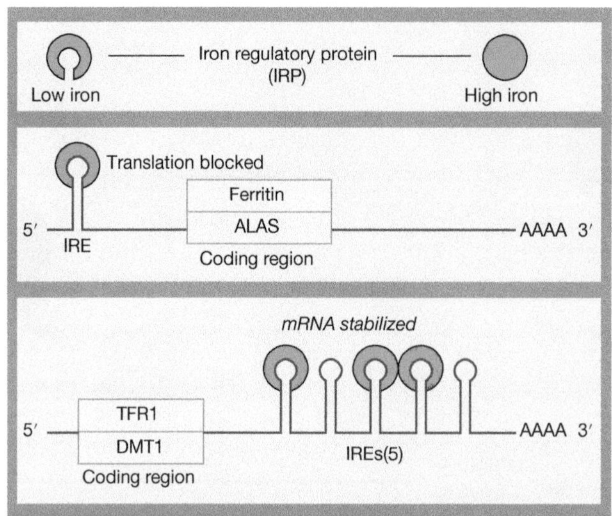

Figure 3.3 Regulation of transferrin receptor 1 (TFR1), δ-aminolaevulinic acid synthase (ALA-S), divalent metal transporter 1 (DMT1) and ferritin expression by iron regulatory protein (IRP) sensing of intracellular iron levels. IRPs are able to bind to stem-loop structures called iron response elements (IREs). IRP binding to the IRE within the 3′ untranslated region of TFR1 and DMT1 leads to stabilization of the mRNA and increased protein synthesis, whereas IRP binding to the IRE within the 5′ untranslated region of ferritin and ALA-S mRNA reduces translation. IRPs can exist in two states: at times of high iron levels the IRP binds iron and exhibits a reduced affinity for the IREs, whereas when iron levels are low the binding of IRPs to IREs is increased. In this way, synthesis of TfR, ALAS, DMT1 and ferritin is coordinated to physiological requirements.

Hepcidin

Hepcidin is a 25 amino acid polypeptide produced by liver cells. It is the major hormonal regulator of iron homeostasis (Fig. 3.4a). It inhibits iron release from macrophages, from intestinal epithelial cells and from other cells by its interaction with the transmembrane iron exporter, ferroportin. It accelerates degradation of ferroportin protein by lysosomes and so directly inhibits iron export from ferroportin. Raised hepcidin levels therefore profoundly affect iron metabolism by reducing its absorption and its release from macrophages and hepatocytes.

Control of hepcidin expression

The synthesis of hepcidin in the liver is stimulated or inhibited by several factors. These include iron status, plasma cytokines, erythropoiesis and hypoxia (Fig. 3.4a). Control of hepcidin synthesis and so of iron status is best considered by comparing the control in iron overload when, except in genetic haemochromatosis, plasma hepcidin levels are high with that in iron deficiency when plasma hepcidin levels are low (Fig. 3.4c).

In **iron overload**, diferric transferrin stimulates liver sinusoidal cells to secrete bone morphogenetic proteins (BMPs) (Fig. 3.4b). Among them BMP2 controls basal hepcidin levels while BMP6 is especially increased in iron overload. The BMPs bind to their receptors (BMPRs) on the hepatic cell membrane. Diferric transferrin also binds to and stabilizes the transferrin receptor 2 (TFR2) on the cell membrane. Binding of BMPs to BMPRs results in the formation of a signalling complex consisting of BMPRs and three proteins TFR2, hemojuvelin (HJV) and HFE. This complex stimulates hepcidin synthesis via the signalling proteins SMADs, which transfer the message to the cell nucleus. Diferric transferrin also binds to TFR1 to provide the cell with iron.

In **iron deficiency** there is little if any circulating diferric transferrin. This results in reduced synthesis of BMPs by the liver sinusoidal cells (Fig. 3.4c). Also in the absence of binding to diferric transferrin, TFR2 is degraded or shed from the cell membrane and HFE is deviated to bind to the unoccupied TFR1. Iron deficiency also stimulates the protease matriptase 2 (TMPRSS6) to cleave HJV from the cell surface. The result of all these reactions is failure to form the necessary complex to signal for hepcidin synthesis. Finally, iron deficiency stimulates a histone deacetylase which acts on the hepcidin locus to suppress the transcription of hepcidin.

Erythroblasts secrete **erythroferrone** and probably other proteins, which suppress BMP-mediated signalling for hepcidin secretion (Fig. 3.4a). This results in low plasma hepcidin levels in conditions with increased numbers of early erythroblasts in the marrow, e.g. conditions of ineffective erythropoiesis, such as thalassaemia major, so iron absorption is inappropriately increased despite the presence of iron overload due to transfusions. Hypoxia also suppresses hepcidin synthesis, whereas in inflammation interleukin 6 (IL-6) and other cytokines increase hepcidin synthesis (Fig. 3.4a). This results in lowering of plasma iron and helps to protect against infection by depriving bacteria of non-transferrin-bound iron in plasma.

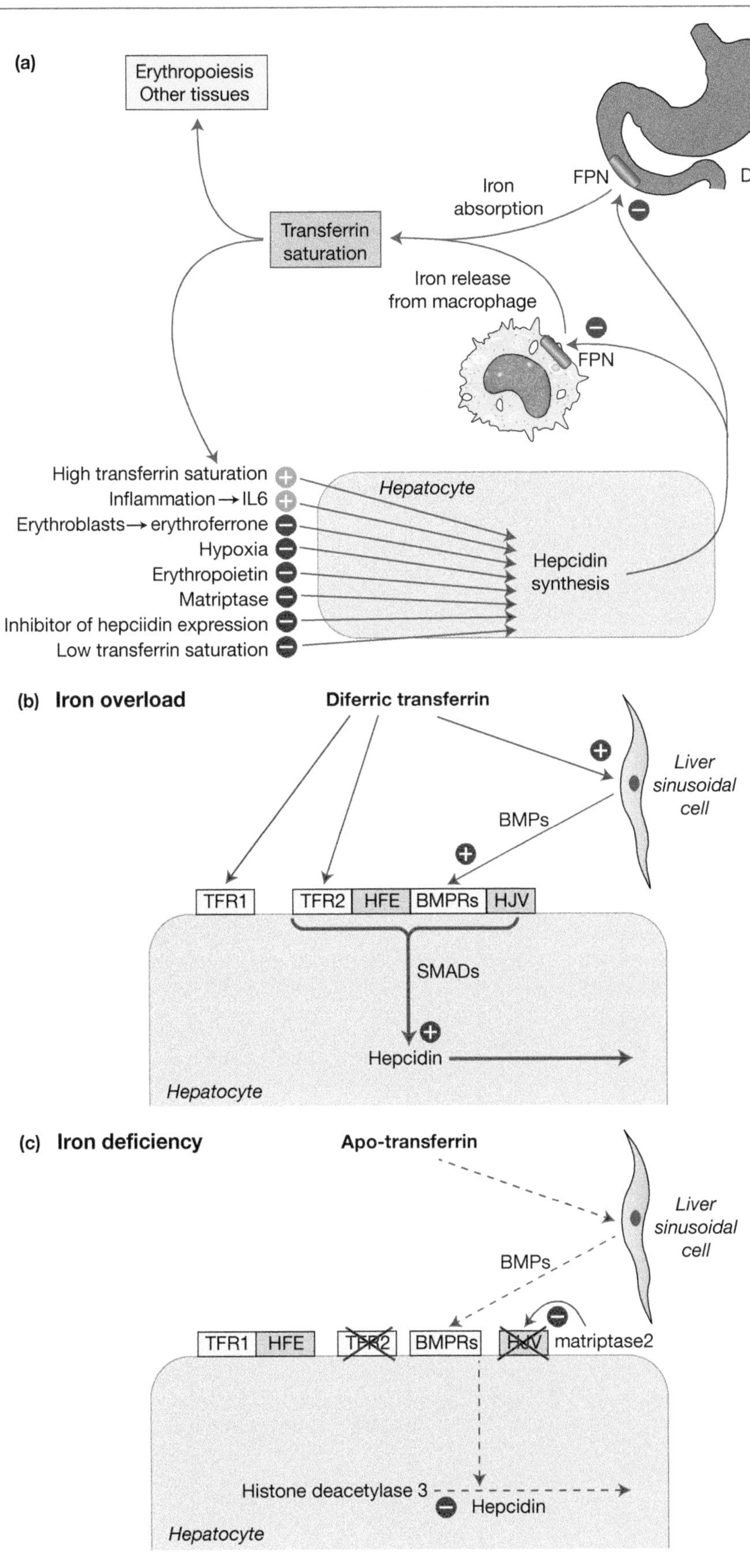

Figure 3.4 **(a)** Hepcidin reduces iron absorption and release from macrophages by stimulating degradation of ferroportin. Its synthesis is increased by diferric transferrin and by inflammation, but reduced by increased erythropoiesis and hypoxia. **(b)** The proposed mechanism by which the degree of transferrin saturation by iron in iron overload stimulates hepcidin synthesis (see also text). BMP synthesis by liver sinusoidal cells is stimulated by diferric transferrin, which also stabilizes TFR2 and by binding to TFR1 prevents HFE being deviated by attaching to TFR1. Binding of BMPs to BMPRs stimulates, in a complex with HFE, TFR2 and HJV on the hepatic cell membrane, hepcidin synthesis by signalling through SMAD proteins. **(c)** In iron deficiency low concentrations of diferric transferrin result in reduced BMP synthesis. Also lack of diferric iron to bind to TFR2 results in degradation or shedding of TFR2 from the cell membrane. Additionally, failure of diferric transferrin to bind to TFR1 results in HFE binding to TFR1. Iron deficiency also activates matriptase2, which cleaves HJV. The result of all these actions is failure to form the necessary complex to stimulate hepcidin synthesis. In addition in iron deficiency, a histone deacetylase 3 is activated and this suppresses transcription of hepcidin. BMP, bone morphogenetic protein; BMPR, bone morphogenetic protein receptor; HJV, hemojuvelin; TFR1 and 2, transferrin receptor 1 and 2. Source: (b and c) Courtesy of Professor Clara Camaschella.

Table 3.2 Iron absorption.

Factors favouring absorption	Factors reducing absorption
Inorganic iron	Haem iron
Ferrous form (Fe^{2+})	Ferric form (Fe^{3+})
Acids (hydrochloric acid, vitamin C)	Alkalis – antacids, pancreatic secretions
Solubilizing agents, e.g. sugars, amino acids	Precipitating agents, e.g. phytates, phosphates, tea
Reduced serum hepcidin e.g. iron deficiency	Increased serum hepcidin e.g. inflammation
Ineffective erythropoiesis (increased plasma erythroferrone)	Decreased erythropoiesis (decreased plasma erythroferrone)
Pregnancy	Iron overload (acquired)
Hereditary haemochromatosis	

Dietary iron

Iron is present in food as ferric hydroxides and as ferric–protein and haem–protein complexes. Both the iron content and the proportion of iron absorbed differ from food to food; in general meat, in particular liver, is a better source than vegetables, eggs or dairy foods. The average Western diet contains 10–15 mg iron daily, from which only 5–10% is normally absorbed. The proportion can be increased to 20–30% in iron deficiency or pregnancy (Table 3.2), but even in these situations most dietary iron remains unabsorbed.

Iron absorption

Organic dietary iron is partly absorbed as haem and partly broken down in the stomach and duodenum to inorganic iron. Absorption occurs through the duodenum. Haem is absorbed through a receptor on the apical membrane of the duodenal enterocyte. It is then broken down to release its iron. Inorganic iron absorption is favoured by factors such as acid and reducing agents that keep iron in the gut lumen in the Fe^{2+} rather than the Fe^{3+} state (Table 3.2). The protein DMT1 is involved in transfer of inorganic iron from the lumen of the gut across the enterocyte microvilli (Fig. 3.5). Ferroportin at the basolateral surface controls the exit of iron from the cell into portal plasma. The amount of iron absorbed is regulated according to the body's needs by changing the levels of DMT1 and ferroportin. For DMT1 this occurs by the IRP/IRE binding mechanism (Fig. 3.3) and for ferroportin by hepcidin (Fig. 3.4a). Ferroportin is also present in liver, heart, kidney, brain and placenta, where it is important in exporting iron.

Ferrireductase present at the enterocyte's apical surface converts iron from the Fe^{3+} to Fe^{2+} state and another enzyme, hephaestin (ferrioxidase), converts Fe^{2+} to Fe^{3+} at the basal surface prior to its binding to transferrin.

Iron requirements

The amount of iron required each day to compensate for losses from the body and for growth varies with age and sex; it is highest in pregnancy, adolescent and menstruating females (Table 3.3). Therefore these groups are particularly likely to develop iron deficiency if there is any additional iron loss or prolonged reduced dietary intake.

Table 3.3 Estimated daily iron requirements. Units are mg/day.

	Urine, sweat, faeces	Menses	Pregnancy	Growth	Total
Adult male	0.5–1				0.5–1
Postmenopausal female	0.5–1				0.5–1
Menstruating female*	0.5–1	0.5–1			1–2
Pregnant female*	0.5–1		1–2		1.5–3
Children (average)	0.5			0.6	1.1
Female (age 12–15)*	0.5–1	0.5–1		0.6	1.6–2.6

*These groups are more likely to develop iron deficiency.

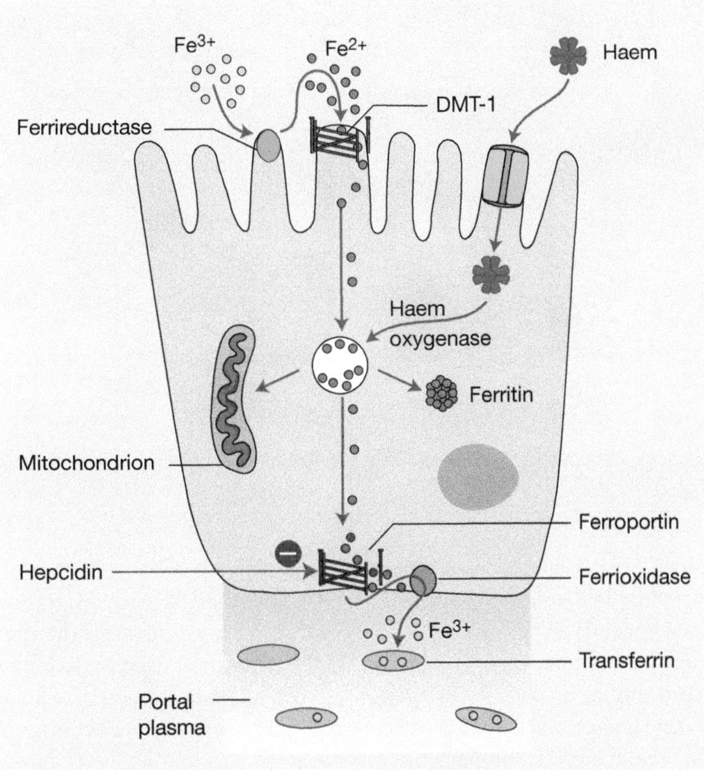

Figure 3.5 The regulation of iron absorption. Dietary ferric (Fe^{3+}) iron is reduced to Fe^{2+} by ferrireductase and its entry to the enterocyte is through the divalent cation binder DMT-1. Its export into portal plasma is controlled by ferroportin. It is oxidized by hephaestin (ferrioxidase) before binding to transferrin in plasma. Haem is absorbed after binding to its receptor protein.

Iron deficiency

Clinical features

When iron deficiency is developing, the reticuloendothelial stores (haemosiderin and ferritin) become completely depleted before anaemia occurs (Fig. 3.6). As the deficiency progresses, the individual may show the general symptoms and signs of anaemia (Chapter 2); and also painless glossitis, angular stomatitis, brittle, ridged or spoon nails (koilonychia; Fig. 3.7), hair loss and unusual dietary cravings (pica). Fatigue and depression are frequent and may occur even before anaemia is present. Oral or parenteral iron has been shown to reduce fatigue in iron-deficient (low serum ferritin) non-anaemic women. The cause of the epithelial cell changes may be related to reduction of tissue iron-containing enzymes. Neonatal iron deficiency is associated with cognitive and behavioural abnormalities, while in children it can cause irritability, poor cognitive function and a decline in psychomotor development.

Causes of iron deficiency

In developed countries, chronic blood loss, especially uterine or from the gastrointestinal tract, is the dominant cause of iron deficiency (Table 3.4) and dietary deficiency is rarely the sole cause. Five hundred millilitres of blood contain approximately 250 mg iron and, despite the increased absorption of iron at an early stage of iron deficiency, negative iron balance is usual in chronic blood loss.

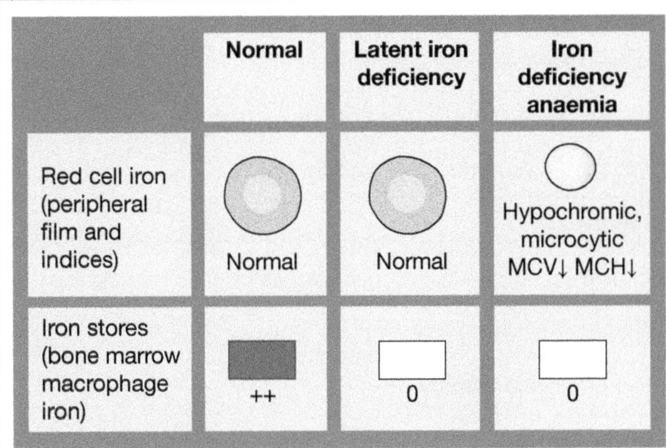

	Normal	Latent iron deficiency	Iron deficiency anaemia
Red cell iron (peripheral film and indices)	Normal	Normal	Hypochromic, microcytic MCV↓ MCH↓
Iron stores (bone marrow macrophage iron)	++	0	0

Figure 3.6 The development of iron deficiency anaemia. Reticuloendothelial (macrophage) stores are lost completely before anaemia develops. MCH, mean corpuscular haemoglobin; MCV, mean corpuscular volume.

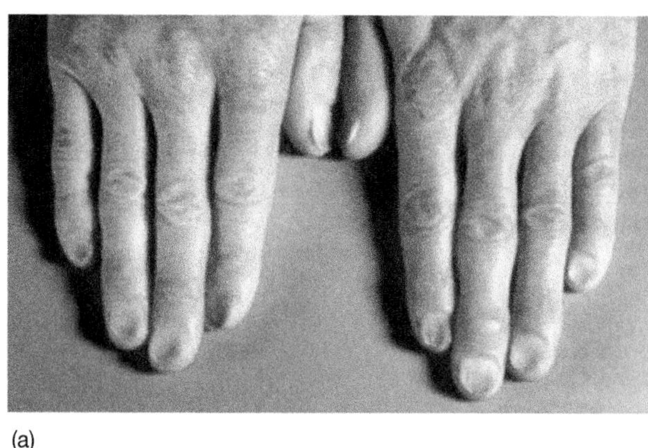

(a)

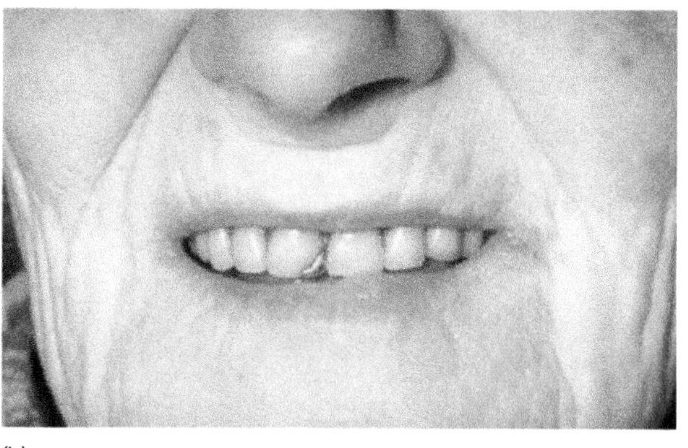

(b)

Figure 3.7 Iron deficiency anaemia. **(a)** Koilonychia: typical 'spoon' nails. **(b)** Angular cheilosis: fissuring and ulceration of the corner of the mouth.

Increased demands for iron during infancy, adolescence, pregnancy, lactation and in menstruating women account for the high risk of iron deficiency anaemia in these particular clinical groups. Newborn infants have a store of iron derived from delayed clamping of the cord and the breakdown of excess red cells. From 3 to 6 months, there is a tendency for a negative iron balance because of growth. From 6 months, supplemented formula milk and mixed feeding, particularly with iron-fortified foods, prevent iron deficiency.

In pregnancy increased iron is needed for an increased maternal red cell mass requiring approximately 600 mg iron, transfer of 300 mg of iron to the foetus and because of blood loss at delivery (Chapter 34). Menorrhagia (a loss of 80 mL or more of blood at each cycle) is difficult to assess clinically, although the loss of clots, the use of large numbers of pads or tampons or prolonged periods all suggest excessive loss.

It takes about 8 years for an adult male starting with normal iron stores to develop iron deficiency anaemia solely as a result of a poor diet or malabsorption resulting in no iron intake. In developed countries inadequate intake or malabsorption is only rarely the sole cause of iron deficiency anaemia. Gluten-induced enteropathy, partial or total gastrectomy and atrophic gastritis (often auto-immune and with *Helicobacter pylori* infection) may, however, predispose to iron deficiency.

Table 3.4 Causes of iron deficiency.
Chronic blood loss
Uterine
Gastrointestinal, e.g. peptic ulcer; oesophageal varices; aspirin (or other non-steroidal anti-inflammatory drugs) ingestion; gastrectomy; carcinoma of the stomach, caecum, colon or rectum; hookworm; schistosomiasis; angiodysplasia; inflammatory bowel disease; piles; diverticulosis
Rarely, haematuria, haemoglobinuria, pulmonary haemosiderosis, self-inflicted blood loss
Increased demands (see also Table 3.3)
Prematurity
Growth
Pregnancy
Erythropoietin therapy
Malabsorption
Gluten-induced enteropathy, gastrectomy, autoimmune gastritis, bariatric surgery, Helicobacter infection
Poor diet
A major factor in many developing countries, but rarely the sole cause in developed countries

In developing countries, iron deficiency may occur as a result of a life-long poor diet, consisting mainly of cereals and vegetables. Hookworm or schistosomiasis may aggravate iron deficiency, as may repeated pregnancies, growth in children and menorrhagia in young females.

Laboratory findings

These are summarized and contrasted with those in other hypochromic anaemias in Table 3.7.

Red cell indices and blood film

Even before anaemia occurs, the red cell indices fall, and they fall progressively as the anaemia becomes more severe. The blood film usually shows hypochromic, microcytic red cells with occasional target cells and pencil-shaped poikilocytes (Fig. 3.8). Rarely the red cell indices may be normal. The reticulocyte count is low in relation to the degree of anaemia. When iron deficiency is associated with severe folate or vitamin B_{12} deficiency, a 'dimorphic' film occurs with a dual population of red cells of which one is macrocytic and the other microcytic and hypochromic; the indices may be normal. A dimorphic blood film is also seen in patients with iron deficiency anaemia who have received recent iron therapy and produced a population of new haemoglobinized normal-sized red cells (Fig. 3.9) and when the patient has been transfused. The platelet count is often moderately raised in iron deficiency, particularly when haemorrhage is continuing. Low iron promotes megakaryocyte commitment of megakaryocytic-erythroid bone marrow progenitors.

Bone marrow iron

Bone marrow examination is not needed to assess iron stores except in complicated cases. In iron deficiency anaemia, there is a *complete* absence of iron from stores (macrophages) and from developing erythroblasts (Fig. 3.10). The erythroblasts are small and have a ragged cytoplasm.

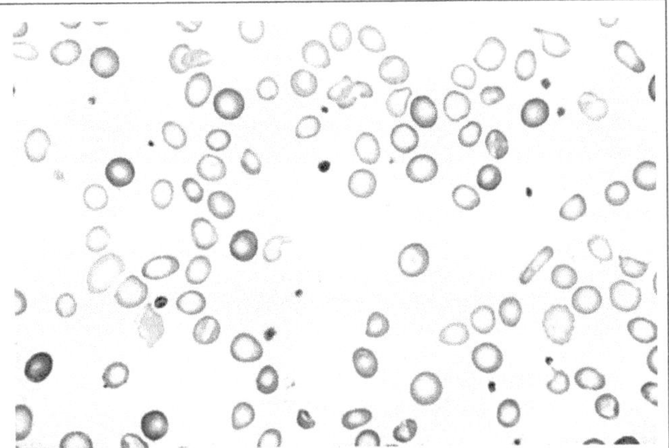

Figure 3.8 The peripheral blood film in severe iron deficiency anaemia. The cells are microcytic and hypochromic with occasional target cells.

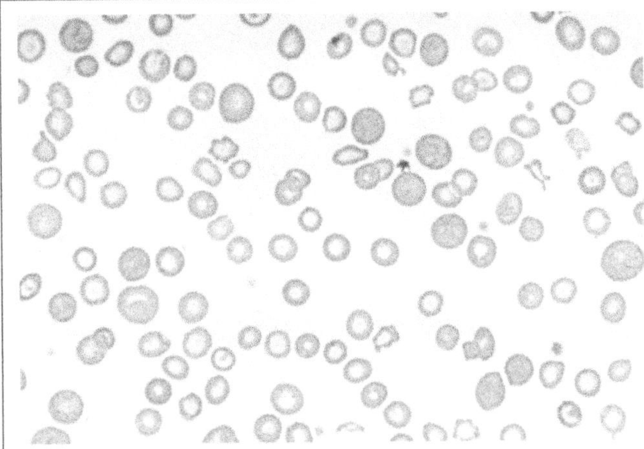

Figure 3.9 Dimorphic blood film in iron deficiency anaemia responding to iron therapy. Two populations of red cells are present: one microcytic and hypochromic, the other normocytic and well haemoglobinized.

Serum iron, total iron-binding capacity (TIBC) and transferrin saturation (TSAT)

The serum iron falls but this assessment alone is not useful. The total iron-binding capacity (TIBC) (or transferrin level) rises so that the TSAT (the ratio between serum iron and TIBC or transferrin expressed as a percentage) is <16% though some take <20% as abnormal (Fig. 3.11). This contrasts both with the anaemia of chronic disease (see below), when the serum iron and the TIBC are both reduced, and with other hypochromic anaemias where the serum iron is normal or even raised. Because of the diurnal fluctuations in serum iron, the TSAT may also fluctuate.

Serum ferritin

A small fraction of body ferritin circulates in the serum, the concentration being related to tissue, particularly reticuloendothelial, iron stores. The normal range in men is higher than in women (Fig. 3.11). In iron deficiency anaemia, the serum ferritin is very low <15 μg/L. A raised serum ferritin indicates iron overload, excess release of ferritin from damaged tissues or an acute phase response, e.g. in inflammation. The serum ferritin is normal or raised in the anaemia of chronic disorders so it cannot exclude iron deficiency in this setting. If an active inflammatory state is present, a serum ferritin <150 ug/L suggests iron deficiency may also be present.

i

Other tests

Plasma soluble transferrin receptors and red cell zinc protoporphyrin levels are raised in iron deficiency but neither are sufficiently specific or sensitive to be recommended for routine use. Assays of serum hepcidin have been developed and are likely to become available in the routine clinical laboratory.

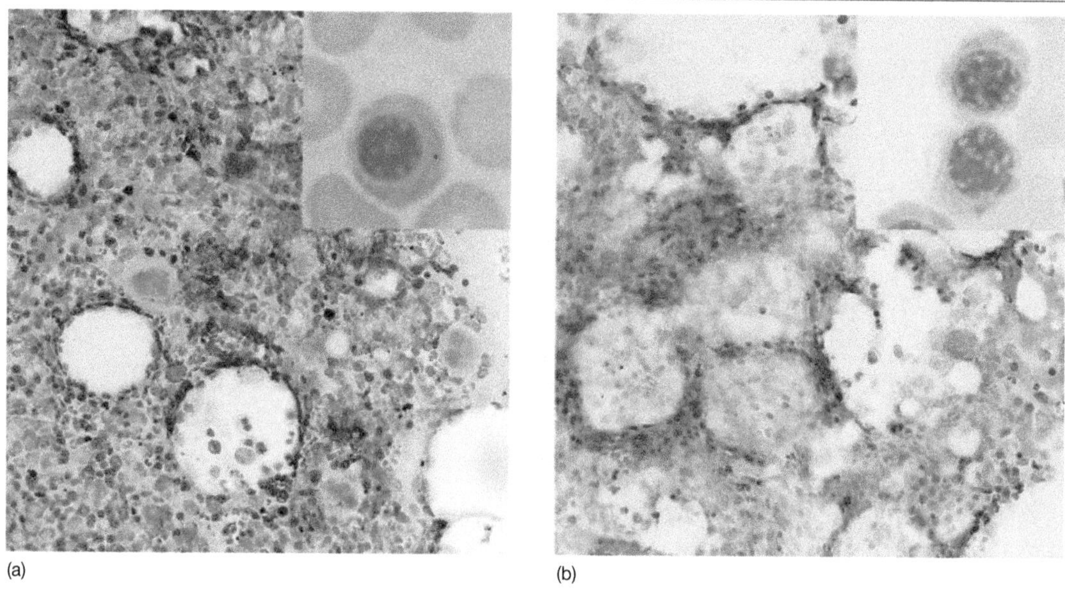

Figure 3.10 Bone marrow iron assessed by Perls' stain. **(a)** Normal iron stores indicated by blue staining in the macrophages. Inset: normal siderotic granule in erythroblast. **(b)** Absence of blue staining (absence of haemosiderin) in iron deficiency. Inset: absence of siderotic granules in erythroblasts.

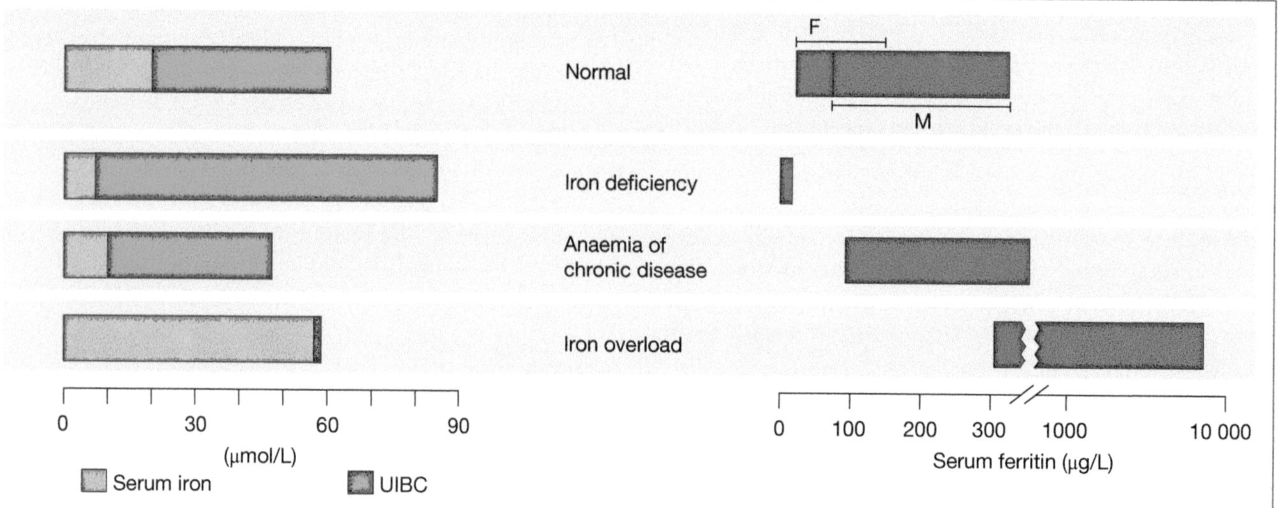

Figure 3.11 The serum iron, unsaturated serum iron-binding capacity (UIBC) and serum ferritin in normal subjects and in those with iron deficiency, anaemia of chronic disease and iron overload. The total iron-binding capacity (TIBC) is made up of the serum iron and the UIBC. In some laboratories, the transferrin content of serum is measured directly by immunodiffusion, rather than by its ability to bind iron, and is expressed in g/L. Normal serum contains 2–4 g/L transferrin (1 g/L transferrin = 20 μmol/L binding capacity). Normal ranges for serum iron are 10–30 μmol/L; for TIBC, 40–75 μmol/L; for serum ferritin, male, 40–340 μg/L; female, 14–150 μg/L.

Investigation of the cause of iron deficiency (Fig. 3.12)

In premenopausal women, menorrhagia and/or repeated pregnancies are the usual causes. If these are not present, other causes must be sought. In some patients with menorrhagia, a clotting or platelet abnormality, e.g. von Willebrand disease is present. In poor countries, the combination of prolonged inadequate intake of iron with expansion of blood volume with growth, and the onset of menstruation and repeated pregnancies in young women, is the major cause of iron deficiency in childhood, adolescence and fertile adult females. In men and postmenopausal women, gastrointestinal blood loss is the main cause of iron deficiency and the exact site is sought from the clinical history, physical and rectal examination, by occult blood tests, and by appropriate use of upper and lower gastrointestinal endoscopy and/or radiology, e.g. computed tomography (CT) of the pneumocolon, or virtual colonoscopy using the 3D colon system (Figs. 3.12 and 3.13). In difficult cases, a camera in a capsule can be swallowed, which relays pictures of the gastrointestinal tract electronically. Tests for parietal cell antibodies, *Helicobacter* infection and serum gastrin level may help to diagnose autoimmune gastritis. Tests for transglutaminase antibodies and duodenal biopsy to look for gluten-induced enteropathy may be needed. Hookworm and schistosomiasis ova are sought in stools of subjects from areas where these infestations are endemic. Serological tests for schistosomiasis can also be performed. Rarely, a coeliac axis angiogram is needed to demonstrate angiodysplasia.

If gastrointestinal blood loss is excluded, loss of iron in the urine as haematuria or haemosiderinuria (resulting from chronic intravascular haemolysis) is considered. A normal chest X-ray excludes the rare condition of pulmonary haemosiderosis. Rarely, patients bleed themselves, producing iron deficiency.

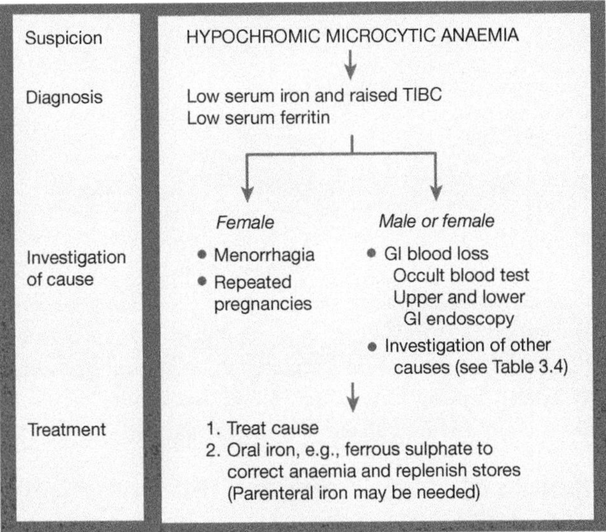

Figure 3.12 Investigation and management of iron deficiency anaemia. GI, gastrointestinal; TIBC, total iron-binding capacity.

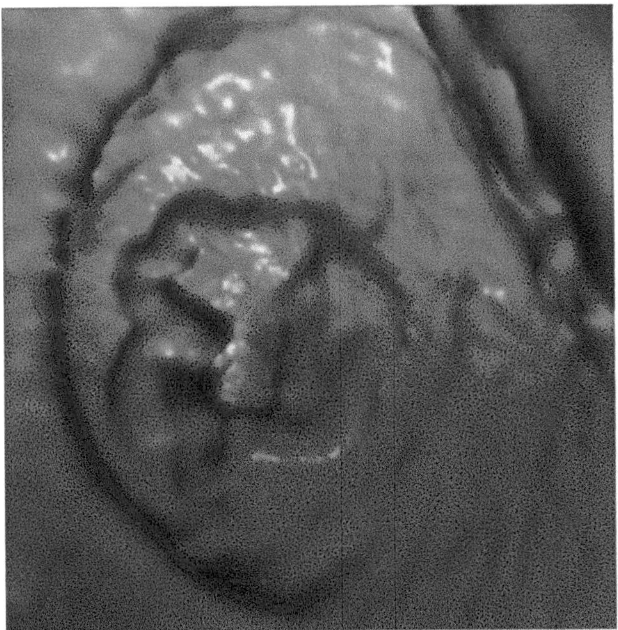

Figure 3.13 Virtual colonoscopy showing carcinoma of colon causing colonic obstruction and iron deficiency.

Treatment

The underlying cause is treated as far as possible. In addition, iron is given to correct the anaemia and replenish iron stores.

Oral iron

The best preparations are ferrous sulphate (200 mg) and ferrous fumarate (210 mg), which are cheap and contain 67 mg iron in each tablet. Iron is best absorbed if they are taken on an empty stomach. In the past doses two or three times daily were used to overcome limited absorption. Once daily doses are now advocated based on the rise in plasma hepcidin level (which blocks further iron absorption) within hours of a single oral dose of iron. For those without anaemia or only mildly anaemic, alternate day dosing may be used. For those with more severe anaemia, daily doses or even intravenous iron are needed to correct the anaemia more quickly. If side effects occur, e.g. nausea, abdominal pain, constipation or diarrhoea, these can be reduced by giving iron with food or by using a preparation with a lower iron content, e.g. ferrous gluconate, which contains only 37 mg per 300 mg tablet. An elixir of iron is available for children. Slow-release preparations should not be used.

Oral iron therapy should be given for long enough both to correct the anaemia and to replenish body iron stores, which usually means for at least up to 6 months. The haemoglobin should rise at the rate of approximately 20 g/L every 3 weeks. Failure of response to oral iron has several possible causes (Table 3.5). These should all be considered before parenteral

Table 3.5 Failure of response to oral iron.
Continuing haemorrhage
Failure to take tablets
Wrong diagnosis – especially thalassaemia trait, sideroblastic anaemia, IRIDA
Mixed deficiency – associated folate or vitamin B_{12} deficiency
Another cause for anaemia e.g. malignancy, inflammation
Malabsorption – see Table 3.4
Use of slow-release preparation
IRIDA, iron-refractory iron deficiency anaemia.

Table 3.6 Intravenous iron preparations.

Trade name	Cosmofer (Europe) INFeD (USA)	Ferinject (Europe) Injectafer (USA)	Feraheme	Monofer, Diafer (Europe) Monoferric (USA)	Ferrlecit	Venofer (Europe only)
Carbohydrate	Low molecular weight dextran	Carboxymaltose	Ferumoxytol	Derisomaltoside	Gluconate in sucrose solution	Sucrose
Vial	50 mg/μL	50 mg/ml	30 mg/mL	100 mg/mL or 50 mg/mL	5 mL (12.5 mg/mL)	20 mg/mL
Total dose	Yes	Yes	Yes	Yes	No	No
Test dose required	Yes	No	No	No	No	No
Infusion time	1 h	15 min	15 min	20 min	60 min	15 min
Slow intravenous injection	Yes	Yes	No	Yes	Yes	Yes

iron is used. Iron fortification of the diet in infants in Africa reduces the incidence of anaemia, but increases susceptibility to malaria.

Parenteral iron

Many different preparations are available with varying licensing arrangements in different countries (Table 3.6). The dose may be calculated according to body weight and degree of anaemia, but it is more usual in order not to waste costly drugs to give 1000 mg as a single dose to moderately anaemic patients and 1500 mg divided into two doses, given at least 48 hours apart, to those more severely anaemic or of large body mass. All the preparations contain ferric (usually ferric hydroxide) iron. Iron dextran can be given in small doses by slow intravenous injection or by infusion as a total dose in one day. Ferric carboxymaltose and ferric isomaltoside may be given as a total dose in one day by intravenous infusion or by slow intravenous injections. Ferumoxytol is given only by intravenous infusion. Ferric hydroxide–sucrose, which releases iron from its sugar more rapidly than the other preparations, is administered by slow intravenous injection or infusion, to a maximum of 200 mg iron in each dose.

Rarely there may be hypersensitivity or anaphylactoid reactions to parenteral iron, especially in those with a previous reaction, multiple drug allergies and severe atopy. If the reaction is severe, it is treated with intravenous hydrocortisone and possibly adrenaline.

Parenteral iron is given when there are high iron requirements, as in gastrointestinal bleeding, severe menorrhagia, middle or late pregnancy (avoided in the first trimester), chronic haemodialysis and chronic renal failure with erythropoietin therapy, post-operative after major surgery. It is also given when oral iron is ineffective, e.g. iron malabsorption (Table 3.4), if IRIDA (see below) is present, or when oral iron causes intolerable side effects or is impractical, e.g. active inflammatory bowel disease. The haematological response to parenteral iron is no faster than to adequate dosage of oral iron, but the iron stores are replenished faster. Intravenous iron may increase functional capacity and quality of life in some patients with congestive heart failure, even in the absence of anaemia (see p. xxx). It may also be effective in restless leg syndrome. Early trials show it can reduce blood transfusion needs in chemotherapy-induced anaemia in cancer patients.

Anaemia of chronic disease (inflammation)

One of the most common anaemias occurs in patients with a variety of chronic inflammatory and malignant diseases (Table 3.7). With iron deficiency it accounts for about two-thirds of the world's anaemias. The characteristic features are:

1. Normochromic, normocytic or mildly hypochromic (MCV rarely <75 fL) indices and red cell morphology.
2. Mild and non-progressive anaemia (haemoglobin rarely <90 g/L) – the severity being related to the severity of the underlying disease.

Table 3.7 Causes of the anaemia of chronic disease.

Chronic inflammatory diseases
Infections, e.g. pulmonary abscess, tuberculosis, osteomyelitis, pneumonia, bacterial endocarditis
Non-infectious, e.g. rheumatoid arthritis, systemic lupus erythematosus and other connective tissue diseases, sarcoidosis, inflammatory bowel disease
Other chronic disorders
Congestive heart failure Chronic pulmonary disease Chronic renal disease Obesity Anaemia in the elderly Anaemia in critical illness (accelerated course)
Malignant diseases
Carcinoma, lymphoma, sarcoma

Table 3.8 Laboratory diagnosis of a hypochromic anaemia.

	Iron deficiency	Chronic disease	Thalassaemia trait (α or β)	Sideroblastic anaemia	IRIDA
MCV/ MCH	Reduced in relation to severity of anaemia	Normal or mild reduction	Reduced; low for degree of anaemia	Usually low in congenital type but MCV usually raised in acquired type	Reduced in relation to severity of anaemia
Serum iron	Reduced	Reduced	Normal	Raised	Reduced
TIBC	Raised	Reduced	Normal	Normal	Reduced
Serum ferritin	Reduced	Normal or raised	Normal	Raised	Raised
Bone marrow iron stores	Absent	Present	Present	Present	Present
Erythroblast iron	Absent	Absent	Present	Ring forms	Absent
Haemoglobin electrophoresis	Normal	Normal	Hb A_2 raised in β form	Normal	Normal

Hb, haemoglobin; IRIDA, non-refractory iron deficiency anaemia; MCH, mean corpuscular haemoglobin; MCV, mean corpuscular volume; TIBC, total iron-binding capacity.

3 Both the serum iron and TIBC are reduced.
4 The serum ferritin and hepcidin levels are normal or raised.
5 Bone marrow storage (reticuloendothelial) iron is normal, but erythroblast iron is reduced (Table 3.8).
6 Raised plasma levels of hepcidin and inflammation-induced cytokines block intestinal iron absorption and cause iron retention in the reticuloendothelial cells.
7 Shortened reduced red cell life span, suppressed erythropoietin response to anaemia and inhibited erythroid cell differentiation.

The pathogenesis of this anaemia is related to decreased release of iron from macrophages to plasma, because of raised serum hepcidin levels stimulated by IL-6 and IL-1β and lipopolysaccharide, a mechanism to protect the host against bacteria which need iron to multiply. There is also an inadequate erythropoietin response to anaemia caused by the effects of cytokines such as IL-1, IL-6, IL-10 interferon-gamma and tumour necrosis factor. These cytokines directly damage red cells whose life span is also reduced both by activation of macrophages and by deposition of antibody and complement on their surface. Interferon-γ further impairs haemopoiesis by binding to thrombopoietin, inhibiting thrombopoietin binding to its receptor on marrow cells.

The anaemia is corrected by successful treatment of the underlying disease. It does not respond to iron therapy but diagnosis of the anaemia when there is coexisting iron deficiency may be difficult. If the serum ferritin is <100 ug/L or saturation of the TIBC <20%, co-existing iron deficiency is suspected. The combination of iron therapy and erythropoietin injections improve the anaemia in some cases. In many conditions, this anaemia is complicated by anaemia resulting from other causes, e.g. vitamin B_{12} or folate deficiency, renal failure, bone marrow failure, hypersplenism, endocrine abnormality or leucoerythroblastic anaemia. These are discussed in Chapter 32.

Measurement of serum hepcidin and drugs to inhibit hepcidin, both being developed, would be major advances in the diagnosis and treatment of the anaemia of chronic disease.

Iron refractory iron deficiency anaemia (IRIDA)

This rare autosomal recessive syndrome presents with an hypochromic microcytic anaemia. The serum iron is low with <5% saturation of the iron binding capacity (Table 3.8). It is caused by inherited mutations of matriptase 2, which allow uninhibited hepcidin secretion, or even more rarely mutations of *DMT1* genes (Figs. 3.4 and 3.5). There may be a haematological response to intravenous but usually not to oral iron.

Sideroblastic anaemia

This is an uncommon refractory anaemia defined by the presence of many pathological ring sideroblasts in the bone marrow (Fig. 3.14). These are erythroblasts containing numerous iron granules arranged in a ring or collar around the nucleus, instead of the one or two randomly distributed iron granules in normal erythroblasts (Fig. 3.10). There is also usually erythroid hyperplasia with ineffective erythropoiesis. Primary sideroblastic anaemia is diagnosed when 15% or more of marrow erythroblasts are ring sideroblasts but in the presence of the *SF3B1*mutation as few as 5% ring sideroblasts in

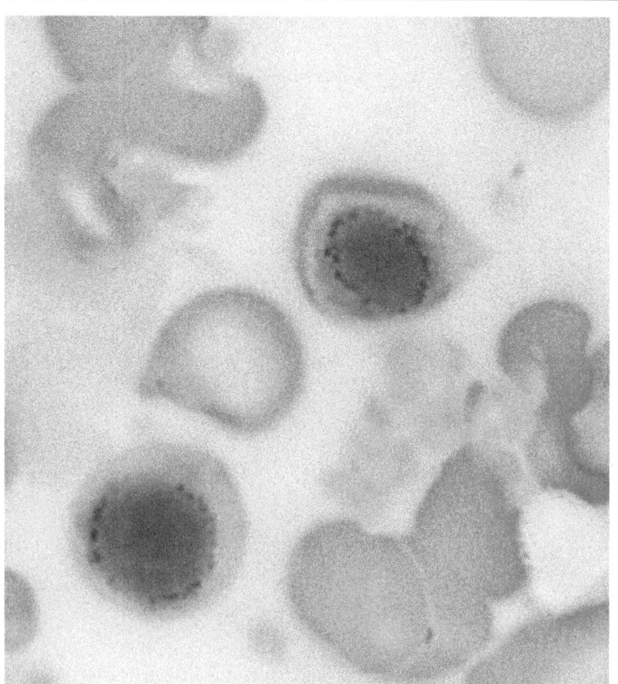

Figure 3.14 Ring sideroblasts with a perinuclear ring of iron granules in sideroblastic anaemia.

patients with myelodysplasia is still classified as a 'primary' sideroblastic anaemia (see below). Ring sideroblasts can also be found at lower numbers in a variety of other anaemias.

Sideroblastic anaemia is classified into different types (Table 3.9), the common link is a defect in haem synthesis. In the **hereditary forms,** the anaemia is usually markedly hypochromic and microcytic but some types show normocytic or macrocytic red cells. The most common mutations are in the *ALAS* gene, which is on the X chromosome. Pyridoxal-6-phosphate is a coenzyme for ALAS. Other rare types include an X-linked mitochondrial disease with spino-cerebellar degeneration and ataxia, mutations in other mitochondrial genes with the triad of anaemia, deafness and diabetes or Pearson syndrome (when there is also pancreatic insufficiency). Thiamine-responsive anaemia with both megaloblastic and sideroblastic erythropoiesis, accompanied by deafness and diabetes is due to mutations of the gene which codes for a thiamine transporter. Various congenital malformations of the limbs, face, nervous system, heart and other organs may be present in these rare syndromes.

The most frequent of the acquired sideroblastic anaemias is **refractory anaemia with ring sideroblasts** with the *SF3B1* mutation, a subtype of myelodysplasia (Chapter 16). Acquired reversible forms may be due to alcohol, lead and drugs, e.g. isoniazid.

In some patients, particularly with the hereditary *ALAS* mutated type, there is a response to pyridoxine therapy. High doses of thiamine (vitamin B1) improve those with the thiamine transporter gene mutation. Luspatercept (Chapters 7, 16) can be tried. Folate deficiency may occur and folic acid therapy may also be tried. Other treatments, e.g. erythropoietin and luspatercept, are effective in some patients with the myelodysplasia form (Chapter 16). In many severe cases, however, repeated blood transfusions are the only method of maintaining a satisfactory haemoglobin concentration, and transfusional iron overload requiring iron chelation therapy becomes a major problem.

Lead poisoning

Lead inhibits both haem and globin synthesis at a number of points. In addition, it interferes with the breakdown of RNA by inhibiting the enzyme pyrimidine 5′ nucleotidase, causing accumulation of denatured RNA in red cells, the RNA giving

Table 3.9 Classification of sideroblastic anaemia.
Hereditary
X chromosome-linked *ALAS* mutation
usually occurs in males, transmitted by females; also occurs rarely in females
X-linked mitochondrial gene mutation with spino-cerebellar ataxia.
Other rare autosomal types usually involving mitochondrial proteins or thiamine phosphorylation; deafness and diabetes often present
Acquired
Primary
Myelodysplasia (refractory anaemia with ring sideroblasts, as low as 5% with *SF3B1* mutation; see Chapter 16). N.B. Ring sideroblast formation (<15% of erythroblasts) may also occur in the bone marrow inother malignant diseases of the marrow, e.g. other types of myelodysplasia, myelofibrosis, myeloid leukaemia, myeloma, drugs, e.g. anti-tuberculosis (isoniazid, cycloserine), alcohol, lead other benign conditions, e.g. haemolytic anaemia, megaloblastic anaemia, rheumatoid arthritis
ALAS, δ-aminolaevulinic acid synthase.

an appearance called basophilic stippling on the ordinary (Romanowsky) stain (Fig. 2.17). The anaemia may be hypochromic or predominantly haemolytic, and the bone marrow may show ring sideroblasts. Free erythrocyte protoporphyrin is raised.

Differential diagnosis of hypochromic anaemia

Table 3.8 lists the laboratory investigations that may be necessary. The clinical history is particularly important, as the source of the haemorrhage leading to iron deficiency or the presence of an inflammatory or other chronic disease may be revealed. The ethnic group and the family history may suggest a possible diagnosis of thalassaemia or other genetic defect of haemoglobin. Physical examination may also be helpful in determining a site of haemorrhage, features of a chronic inflammatory or malignant disease, koilonychia or, in some haemoglobinopathies, an enlarged spleen or bony deformities.

In thalassaemia trait the red cells tend to be very small, often with an MCV of 70 fL or less, even when anaemia is mild or absent; the red cell count is usually over 5.5×10^{12}/L. Conversely, in iron deficiency anaemia the indices fall progressively with the degree of anaemia and when anaemia is mild the indices may be normal or only just reduced, e.g. MCV 75–80 fL. In the anaemia of chronic disorders, the indices are also not markedly low, an MCV in the range 75–82 fL being usual.

It is usual to measure serum iron and TIBC, and/or serum ferritin to confirm iron deficiency. Haemoglobin high-performance liquid chromatography (HPLC) or electrophoresis with an estimation of Hb A_2 and Hb F is carried out in all patients suspected of thalassaemia or other genetic defect of haemoglobin, because of the family history, ethnic group, red cell indices and blood film. Iron deficiency or the anaemia of chronic disorders may also occur in these subjects. β-Thalassaemia trait is characterized by a raised Hb A_2 above 3.5%, but in α-thalassaemia trait there is no abnormality on simple haemoglobin studies, so the diagnosis is usually made by exclusion of all other causes of hypochromic red cells and by the presence of a red cell count $>5.5 \times 10^{12}$/L. DNA studies confirm the diagnosis.

Bone marrow examination is essential if a diagnosis of sideroblastic anaemia is suspected, but is not usually needed in diagnosis of the other hypochromic anaemias.

SUMMARY

- Iron is present in the body in haemoglobin, myoglobin, haemosiderin and ferritin, and in iron-containing enzymes. Transferrin is the main transport protein in blood.
- Hepcidin is the main regulator of iron absorption and iron release from macrophages and other cells.
- Iron metabolism is regulated according to iron status by intracellular iron regulatory proteins and by control of hepcidin synthesis. Hepcidin synthesis is also affected by erythroferrone secreted by erythroblasts and by inflammation.
- Iron deficiency is the most common cause of anaemia throughout the world. The red cells are hypochromic and microcytic. The serum ferritin, serum iron and saturation of the iron-binding capacity are reduced.
- In Western countries, it is usually caused by haemorrhage from the gastrointestinal or the female genital tract.
- Prolonged reduced dietary intake may cause the anaemia, particularly in developing countries, where hookworm and schistosomiasis may also be important causes of blood loss.
- It is treated by oral or less frequently parenteral iron to correct the anaemia and to restore body stores of iron, and by treating, as far as possible, the underlying cause.
- Other frequent causes of a hypochromic, microcytic anaemia are the anaemia of chronic disease, which occurs in patients with chronic inflammatory or malignant diseases, and α- or β-thalassaemia. Less common causes include sideroblastic anaemia (some cases), iron refractory iron deficiency anaemia and lead poisoning.
- Sideroblastic anaemias characterized by ring sideroblasts in the marrow are rare. They may be inherited or acquired; the most common subtype is myelodysplasia with the *SF3B1* mutation.

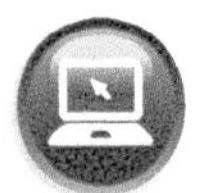

Now visit **www.wiley.com/go/haematology9e** to test yourself on this chapter.

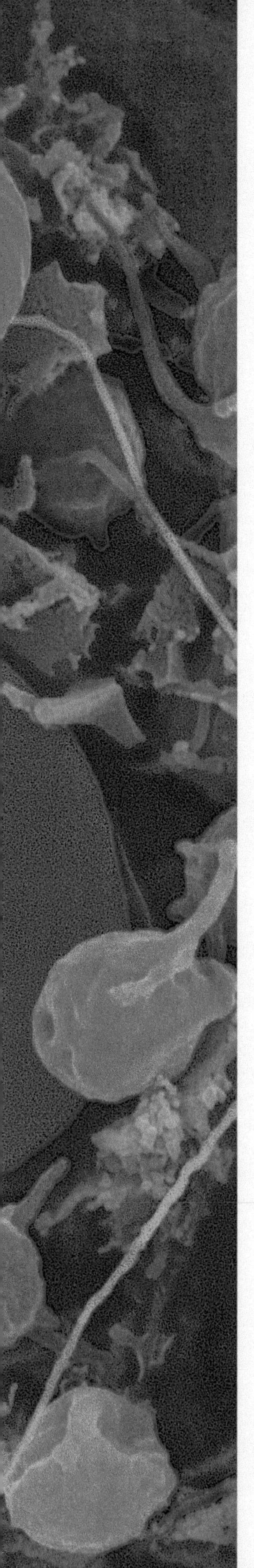

CHAPTER 4

Iron overload

Key topics

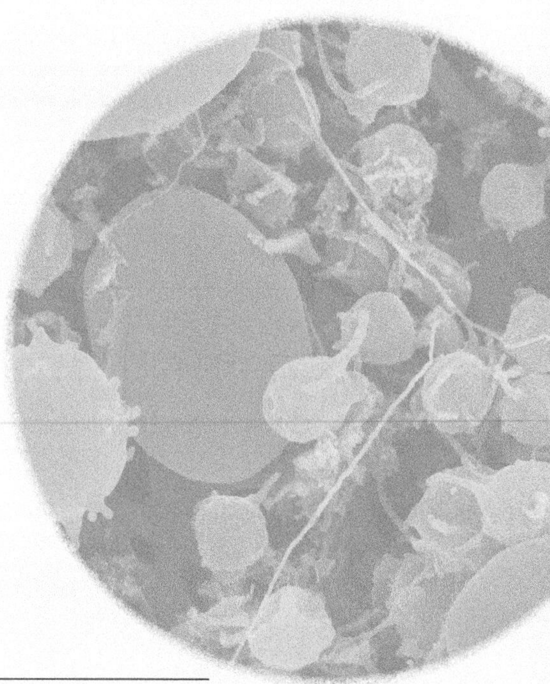

Hoffbrand's Essential Haematology, Ninth Edition. A. Victor Hoffbrand, Pratima Chowdary, Graham P. Collins, and Justin Loke.

© 2024 John Wiley & Sons Ltd. Published 2024 by John Wiley & Sons Ltd.

Companion website: www.wiley.com/go/haematology9e

There is no physiological mechanism for eliminating excess iron from the body. Iron absorption is carefully regulated to avoid accumulation of excess iron. Iron overload (haemosiderosis) occurs in genetic disorders associated with inappropriately increased iron absorption (haemochromatosis), or in patients with severe chronic anaemias, especially those who receive regular blood transfusions. Excessive iron deposition in tissues may result in serious damage particularly to the heart, liver and endocrine organs. The causes of iron overload are listed in Table 4.1 and causes of hereditary haemochromatosis in Table 4.2.

Table 4.1 The causes of iron overload.

Increased iron absorption	Hereditary (genetic) haemochromatosis Ineffective erythropoiesis, e.g. non-transfusion-dependent thalassaemia or myelodysplastic syndromes Chronic liver disease
Increased iron intake	African siderosis (dietary and genetic components)
Repeated red cell transfusions	Transfusion siderosis

Table 4.2 Genetic causes of haemochromatosis and of hyperferritinaemia.

Type	Inheritance	Clinical condition	Gene defect
1	AR	Classical hereditary haemochromatosis	*HFE*
2	AR	Juvenile haemochromatosis	Hemojuvelin (*HJV*) Hepcidin (*HAMP*)
3	AR	Hereditary haemochromatosis	Transferrin receptor 2 (*TFR2*)
4a	AD	RE iron loading	Ferroportin (*SLC11A3*)
4b	AD	Parenchymal iron loading	Ferroportin (*SCL11A3*) (mutation at the hepcidin binding site)
5	AD	Hereditary hyperferritinaemia – cataract syndrome (no iron deposition)	Ferritin light chain (*FTL*)

AD, autosomal dominant; AR, autosomal recessive; RE, reticuloendothelial.

Assessment of iron status and organ function

The tests to assess iron overload and the degree of damage caused by iron are listed in Table 4.3. The serum ferritin is the most widely used test to assess iron overload and to monitor its treatment, although inflammatory and other diseases may increase serum ferritin levels even in the absence of iron overload. The percentage saturation of the iron-binding capacity (transferrin) is also valuable. Serum non-transferrin-bound (NTBI) iron, also known as labile plasma iron, is a toxic form of iron that occurs in severe transfusional iron overload but tests for NTBI are not widely available.

Aceruloplasminaemia is another rare genetic cause of iron loading.

Table 4.3 Assessment of iron overload.

Assessment of iron stores	
Serum ferritin	
Serum iron and percentage saturation of iron-binding capacity (transferrin)	
Serum non-transferrin-bound iron (NTBI)	
Bone marrow biopsy (Perls' stain) for iron within reticuloendothelial(RE) stores	
Liver biopsy (parenchymal and RE stores)	
Liver CT scan or MRI (T_2* or Ferriscan technique)	
Cardiac MRI (gated T_2* technique)	
Pancreas and pituitary MRI (not widely available) Annual transfusional calculated iron loading	
Assessment of tissue damage caused by iron overload	
Cardiac	Clinical; chest X-ray; ECG (24-h monitor); echocardiography (ECHO) to assess left and right ventricular ejection fraction at rest and with stress
Liver	Liver function tests, alpha-fetoprotein; liver ultrasound; MRI, fibroscan
Endocrine and bone	Clinical examination (including for growth and sexual development); oral glucose tolerance test; thyroid, parathyroid, gonadal, adrenal function and growth hormone assays; radiology for bone age; isotopic bone density study, vitamin D
Musculoskeletal	Hand X-rays with assessment of metacarpophalangeal joints

CT, computed tomography; ECG, electrocardiography; MRI, magnetic resonance imaging.

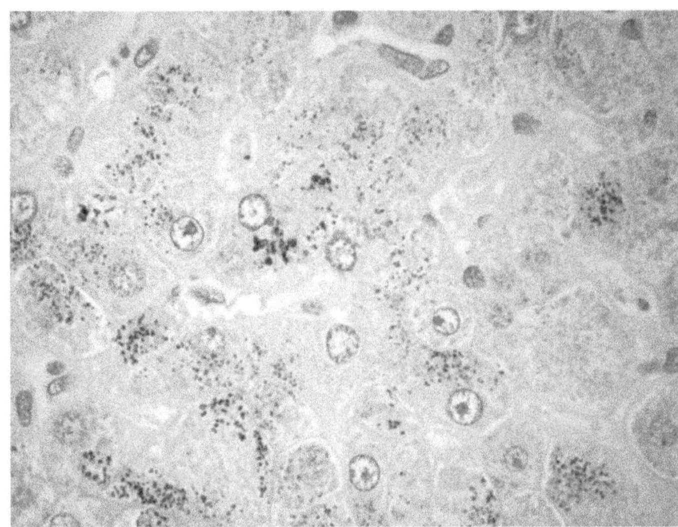

Figure 4.1 Liver biopsy in genetic haemochromatosis. Iron loading of hepatic parenchymal cells (Perls' stain). Source: Courtesy of Professor A.P. Dhillon.

Liver biopsy with staining for iron (Fig. 4.1) and chemical analysis of iron content is useful for assessment of both parenchymal iron (within hepatic cells) and reticuloendothelial iron (within Kupffer cells). Magnetic resonance imaging (MRI) using the T_2* technique is the best non-invasive guide to liver and cardiac iron. A commercial Ferriscan MRI technique is widely used for measuring liver iron. Liver biopsy also allows estimation of the degree of fibrosis. Fibroscan (transient elastography) is a non-invasive ultrasound method of assessing liver fibrosis from any cause, including iron overload. Serum alpha-fetoprotein and liver ultrasound are used for serial screening for hepatocellular carcinoma in patients with known iron overload, previous hepatitis C or liver fibrosis typically on an annual basis. Monitoring for cardiac iron overload and of cardiac function are discussed on page xx under the heading of transfusional iron overload where cardiac disease is a major complication. Other complications of transfusional iron overload including liver, endocrine and bone disease are also discussed further under the heading thalassaemia major in Chapter 7.

Hereditary (genetic, primary) haemochromatosis

Hereditary haemochromatosis is a group of diseases in which there is from birth excessive absorption of iron from the gastrointestinal tract leading to iron overload of the parenchymal cells, dominantly of the liver (Fig. 4.1). At later stages endocrine and heart complications occur. In contrast to transfusional iron overload, the macrophages are not iron overloaded.

Most patients are homozygous for a missense mutation (C282Y) in the *HFE* gene, which leads to insertion of a tyrosine residue rather than cysteine in the mature protein. This allele has the highest prevalence (approximately 1 in 10) within populations of Northern European origin. However, gene penetrance is low; only a small proportion of this ethnic group who are homozygous for the mutation (about 1 in 300) present with clinical features of the disease. Affected individuals usually show a serum ferritin greater than 1000 μg/L. A second mutation H63D resulting in a histidine to aspartic acid substitution is found with the C282Y mutation in approximately 5% of patients with genetic haemochromatosis. Homozygotes for the H63D mutation usually do not have the disease. The H63D mutation has a broader global distribution than C282Y.

HFE is involved in regulation of hepcidin synthesis (Fig. 3.4). The C282Y mutation causes low plasma levels of hepcidin and so high levels of ferroportin in enterocytes, macrophages and other cells. Iron absorption and iron release from macrophages is therefore increased. Iron overload develops over decades and damages parenchymal cells, so that patients may present in adult life with hepatic disease (fibrosis, cirrhosis, hepatocellular carcinoma), endocrine disturbances (diabetes mellitus, hypothyroidism or impotence) or melanin skin pigmentation (Fig. 4.2). In some severe cases, there is cardiac failure or arrhythmia but these are more dominant features of transfusional iron overload. Homozygosity for the *HFE* mutation also underlies an arthropathy due to calcium pyrophosphate deposition and not related to the degree of iron overload. Most commonly affected are the second and third metacarpophalangeal joints.

Other non-*HFE* genetic factors as well as dietary iron intake, alcohol consumption, pregnancies, menstrual blood loss, other blood loss, e.g. gastrointestinal bleeding or blood donation affect the phenotype and time of presentation of the

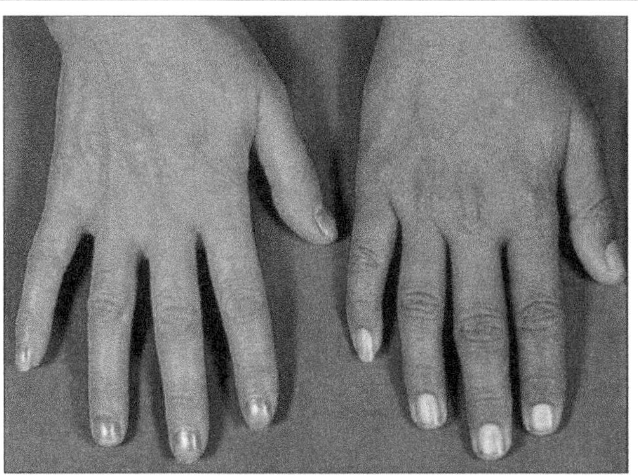

Figure 4.2 Melanin skin pigmentation. The right hand is of a teenager with iron overload caused by thalassaemia major. The left hand is of her mother, who has normal iron status.

disease. Regular blood donors on average present several years later than individuals who never donate blood.

The initial clinical presentation is often with non-specific symptoms such as fatigue, loss of libido or arthralgias. Diagnosis is suspected by the presence of increased levels of serum iron, serum transferrin saturation and ferritin. The diagnosis is confirmed by testing for the *HFE* mutation, but a negative result does not exclude the diagnosis, since mutations of other genes may cause a similar disease phenotype (Table 4.2 and below). Liver biopsy is useful to quantify the degree of iron overload and assess liver damage, but is associated with risks, including bleeding. MRI can be used instead to measure liver and cardiac iron.

Treatment is with regular venesection, initially at 1–2-week intervals, each unit of blood removing 200–250 mg of iron. Organ function may improve and liver fibrosis resolve, but the arthropathy does not respond to iron removal and response of the endocrine damage is variable. There are differences of opinion as to whether patients without evidence of organ dysfunction due to iron overload should be treated. Venesections are generally started when the serum ferritin is raised to over 1000 μg/L but some recommend starting if the serum ferritin is >300 μg/L in males or >200 μg/L in females. Venesection is monitored by serum ferritin and the aim is to restore this to normal, <100 μg/L, and then keep it there with further less frequent venesections, e.g. a few times per year. Some patients elect to become blood donors, but some blood banks and regulatory agencies do not allow blood donation from patients with haemochromatosis. Those with abnormal liver tests are excluded from donating due to the inability to exclude viral causes of hepatic enzyme elevation.

Rarer forms of genetic haemochromatosis are caused by mutations in genes for other iron regulatory proteins, including hemojuvelin, hepcidin and transferrin receptor 2. All (types II and III; Table 4.2) are associated, like homozygous *HFE* disease, with low plasma levels of hepcidin. They often present below the age of 30 years as severe (especially for Type II) iron overload with cardiomyopathy in children, adolescents or young adults. Hypogonadism is another particular feature, whereas arthropathy is absent. Genetic iron overload in Asian populations is usually due to these mutations rather than mutation of *HFE*.

On the other hand, ferroportin gene mutations (type IV disease) usually cause reticuloendothelial but not parenchymal cell iron overload. They do rarely cause parenchymal overload if the mutations in the ferroportin gene are at the hepcidin binding site. Aceruloplasminaemia is another rare genetic cause of iron loading. Mutations of the ferritin light chain gene (type V disease) cause a raised monoclonal serum ferritin with cataracts resulting from ferritin deposition in the eye, but no other tissue iron overload.

African iron overload

This occurs in sub-Saharan Africa through a combination of increased iron absorption due to a genetic defect, possibly in the ferroportin gene, and consumption of beverages, especially beer, with a high iron content due to the use of iron brewing or cooking pots.

Non-transfusion-dependent thalassaemia (thalassaemia intermedia)

Moderately severe forms of thalassaemia may lead to increased iron levels even in patients who do not need regular blood transfusions (Chapter 7). This is due to increased iron absorption due to raised plasma erythroferrone. This leads to increased levels of iron in the liver. The heart is spared. Blood transfusions at times of increased anaemia, e.g. with intercurrent infections, may increase the iron burden. Iron chelation is indicated if the liver iron concentration is above 5 mg/g dry weight or when the serum ferritin reaches 800 μg/L or when the iron leads to organ damage (see also Chapter 7). Other haemolytic anaemias including pyruvate kinase deficiency may also lead to iron loading due to low serum hepcidin levels caused by raised plasma erythroferrone due to ineffective erythropoiesis.

Transfusional iron overload

This develops in patients with chronic severe anaemia not due to haemorrhage who need regular blood transfusions. Each 500 mL of transfused blood contains 200–250 mg iron so iron overload is inevitable unless iron chelation therapy is given (Table 4.4). To make matters worse, iron absorption from food is increased in β-thalassaemia major and other anaemias secondary to ineffective erythropoiesis despite tissue iron overload. This is due to release from early erythroblasts of erythroferrone and of other proteins that inhibit hepcidin synthesis (Fig. 3.4). Non-transferrin-bound iron may appear in plasma when transferrin is >70% saturated. It causes widespread iron deposition in parenchymal tissues.

Table 4.4 Causes of anaemia that may lead to transfusional iron overload.

Congenital	Acquired
β-Thalassaemia major	Myelodysplastic neoplasias
β-Thalassaemia/Hb E disease	Red cell aplasia
Congenital dyserythropoietic anaemias	Acute leukaemias
Sickle cell anaemia (some cases)	Aplastic anaemia
Red cell aplasia (Diamond–Blackfan)	Primary myelofibrosis
Congenital sideroblastic anaemia	
Dyserythropoietic anaemia	

Hb, haemoglobin.

Cardiac damage due to iron is a dominant problem in transfusional iron overload. As for hereditary haemochromatosis, iron also damages the liver (Fig. 4.3) and the endocrine organs, including the hypothalamus and pituitary, with failure of growth, delayed or absent puberty, diabetes mellitus, hypothyroidism and hypoparathyroidism. Skin pigmentation as a result of excess melanin and haemosiderin gives a slate grey appearance even at an early stage of iron overload.

In the absence of intensive iron chelation, death occurs in the second or third decade of life in thalassaemia major, usually from congestive heart failure or cardiac arrhythmias. **T_2* MRI is a valuable measure of cardiac and liver iron loading (Fig. 4.4).**

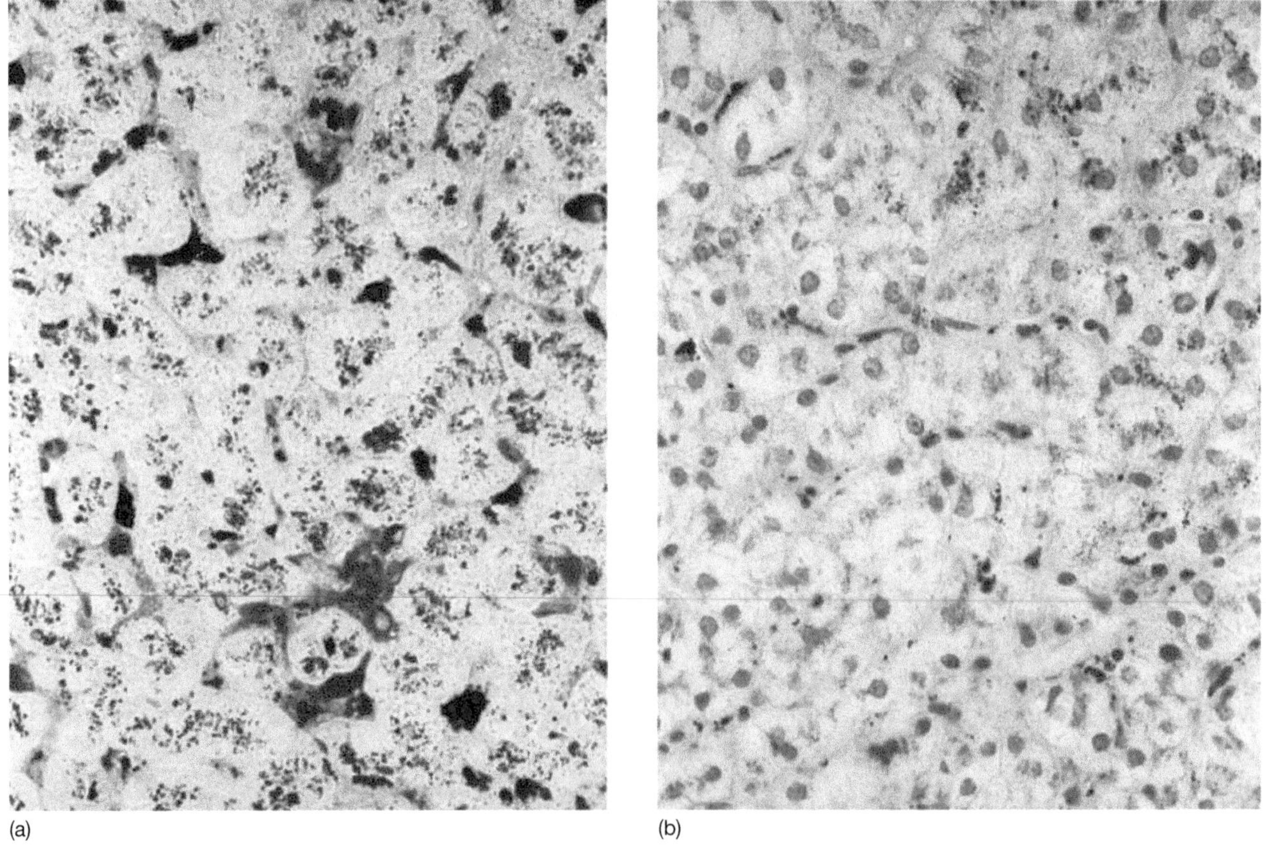

Figure 4.3 β-Thalassaemia major: needle biopsy of liver. **(a)** Grade IV siderosis with iron deposition in the hepatic parenchymal cells, bile duct epithelium, macrophages and fibroblasts (Perls' stain). **(b)** Reduction of iron excess in liver after intensive chelation therapy.

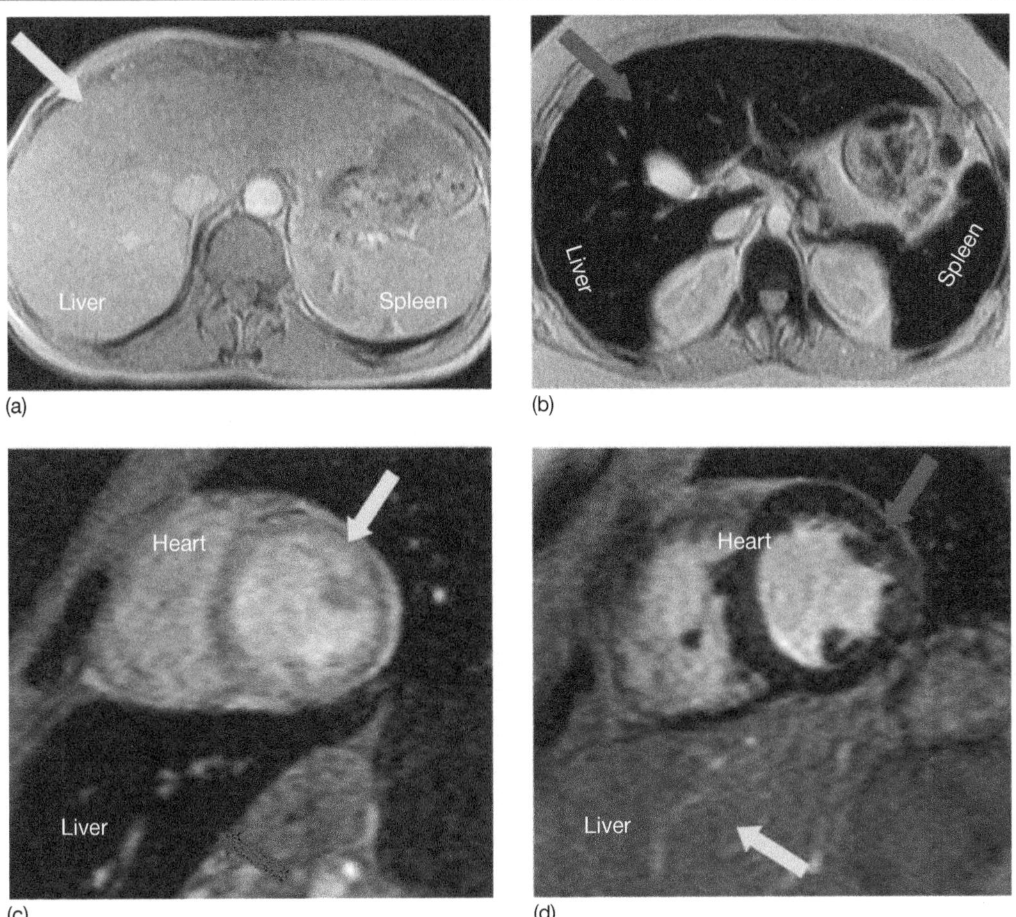

Figure 4.4 T_2* magnetic resonance images (MRIs) showing tissue appearance in iron overload: **(a)** normal volunteer, **(b)** severe iron overload. Green arrow, normal appearance; red arrow, iron overload. Lack of correlation: liver and cardiac iron in two cases of thalassaemia major, **(c)** and **(d)**.

It can detect increased cardiac iron and predict for cardiac failure or arrhythmia before sensitive tests detect impaired cardiac function. The shorter the relaxation time, the greater the cardiac iron burden and the greater risk of subsequent cardiac failure or arrhythmia (Fig. 4.5). Serum ferritin and liver iron correlate poorly with cardiac iron (Figs. 4.4 and 4.5). Moreover, serum ferritin is raised in viral hepatitis and other inflammatory disorders and should therefore be interpreted in conjunction with more accurate tests of iron status, such as T_2* MRI, Ferriscan R2 or liver biopsy. It is, however, useful for monitoring changes in iron burden when this is being treated by chelation therapy. It is important to monitor LVEF annually by echocardiography or MRI from the age of 8 in thalassaemia major. Monitoring for liver, endocrine and bone disease is also needed.

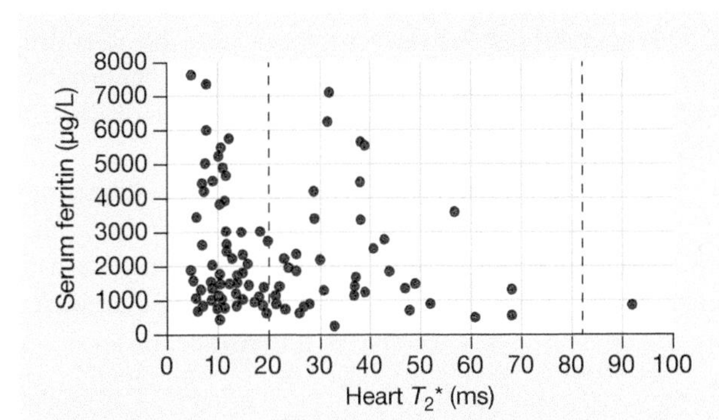

Figure 4.5 Comparison of T_2* magnetic resonance imaging (MRI) measurement of cardiac iron and serum ferritin in thalassaemia major patients. There are substantial numbers of patients with very high serum ferritin (>3000 µg/L) but normal heart iron (T_2* >20 msecs) and, conversely, many patients with serum ferritin levels <1000 µg/L with severe cardiac iron loading (T_2* <10 msecs). Source: L.J. Anderson *et al.* (2001) *Eur. Heart J.* 22: 2171–79.

Iron chelation therapy

Iron chelation therapy is used to treat transfusional iron overload. Three effective drugs are available: orally administered deferasirox and deferiprone, and parenterally administered

Table 4.5 Characteristics of desferrioxamine, deferiprone and deferasirox.

	Desferrioxamine (DFO)	Deferiprone (DFP)	Deferasirox (DFX)
Structure	Hexadentate	Bidentate	Tridentate
Molecular weight (Da)	560	139	373
Iron–chelator complex	1 : 1	1 : 3	1 : 2
Plasma clearance ($t_{1/2}$)	20 min	1–3 h	1–16 h
Absorption	Negligible	Peak 45 min	Peak 1–2.9 h
Iron excretion	Urine + faecal	Urine	Faecal
Therapeutic daily dose	40 mg/kg	75–100 mg/kg	20–40 mg/kg (dispersible tablet) 7–21 mg/kg (coated tablet)
Route	Parenteral	Oral	Oral
Clinical experience	>45 y	>35 y	>20 y
Side effects	Ototoxicity, retinal toxicity, growth defects, cartilage and bone abnormalities	Agranulocytosis, arthropathy, gastrointestinal disturbance, transient transaminitis, zinc deficiency	Skin rashes, gastrointestinal disturbance, rising serum creatinine

deferoxamine (Table 4.5). Thalassaemia major is the most frequent indication worldwide, but chelation is also used for iron overloaded, usually heavily transfused patients with the other anaemias (Table 4.4) and with other iron loading anaemias such as non-transfusion-dependent thalassaemia (Chapter 7) and pyruvate kinase deficiency (Chapter 6).

Deferasirox is given orally once daily and leads to iron loss in the faeces. Skin rashes and transient changes in liver enzymes and rise in serum creatinine are the main side effects. Licensing for young children and lack of major side effects have resulted in its widespread use, but high cost means that the other drugs may be preferred in some countries. Deferasirox removes iron primarily from the liver and is the least effective of the three drugs for eliminating cardiac iron.

Deferiprone is also an oral chelator and causes predominantly urinary iron excretion. It was usually given in three doses daily but a twice daily delayed release formulation has now been approved. It is licensed for first line treatment at varying starting ages in children in different countries. It may be used alone or, if this is inadequate, in combination with deferoxamine infused on one or more days a week, since the drugs have an additive or even synergetic effect on iron excretion. Alone it is the most effective of the three drugs at removing cardiac iron and improving left and right heart function. Side effects include an arthropathy, agranulocytosis (in about 1%), neutropenia, gastrointestinal disturbance and, rarely in patients with diabetes, zinc deficiency. Monitoring of the blood count weekly for the first 6 months, fortnightly for the next 6 months and then every 2–4 weeks or at time of blood transfusion is recommended for all patients receiving deferiprone. Combination therapy with the two orally active chelators, if either alone is not sufficiently effective, has been effective without unexpected toxicity in several trials, but is not yet licensed in any country.

The third drug, **deferoxamine**, was the first of the three drugs to be used in clinical practice. It is not active orally and is usually given by subcutaneous infusion over 8–12 hours for 5–7 days each week; vitamin C is given to increase iron excretion. Most iron is lost in the urine, but up to one-third is also excreted in the stools. Because of the difficult administration, lack of patient adherence is a major problem. It may be given on one or more each days each week in combination with daily deferiprone or deferasirox and can be used intravenously in combination with oral deferiprone in patients with severe iron overload at risk of dying from cardiac failure. Side effects are particularly frequent if high doses are used in children and in adults without heavy iron overload. These include high tone deafness, retinal damage, bone abnormalities and growth retardation. Patients receiving deferoxamine should have auditory and fundoscopic examinations annually.

All three chelators can be given in children. Deferasirox is most frequently used and a liquid formulation of deferiprone and a sprinkle form of deferasirox are available.

Chelation is typically started in thalassaemia major after 10–12 units have been transfused or the serum ferritin is >1000 μg/L. In other conditions such as myelodysplastic neoplasias, there is controversy about when to initiate chelation and hepatic and cardiac T_2* MRI may help guide this decision.

Chelation is given to keep the cardiac T_2^* at >20 msecs, liver at <7 mg/g dry weight and serum ferritin level at <1000–1500 µg/L, when the body iron stores are approximately 5–10 times normal. MRI assesses cardiac and liver iron accurately and should be repeated annually or more frequently if there is definite cardiac or liver damage (Fig. 4.5). Serum ferritin is useful in monitoring changes in iron stores, but as it is an acute phase reactant it may be elevated in the presence of recent infection trauma or surgery and this may falsely suggest inadequate chelation.

Serial tests of heart, liver and endocrine function are also needed to monitor therapy.

Life expectancy has improved dramatically for thalassaemia major patients since the introduction of iron chelation. Chelation may even reverse liver, endocrine and cardiac damage in cases where this has developed before effective chelation has been started.

SUMMARY

- Iron overload may be caused by excessive absorption of iron from food because of low plasma hepdidin levels due to hereditary (genetic) haemochromatosis or because of raised plasma erythroferrone levels due to ineffective erythropoiesis.
- Iron overload may also result from repeated blood transfusions in patients with refractory anaemias. Each unit of transfused blood contains 200–250 mg of iron.
- Excess iron absorbed from the gastrointestinal tract in hereditary haemochromatosis accumulates in the parenchymal cells of the liver, the endocrine organs and, in severe cases, the heart.
- Hereditary haemochromatosis is usually caused by homozygous mutation C282Y of the *HFE* gene resulting in the HFE protein change and a low serum hepcidin level. Rarer forms are caused by mutations of other genes coding for proteins hemojuvelin, hepcidin, transferrin receptor 2 and ferroportin involved in iron regulation.
- Repeated venesections are used to reduce the body iron burden in hereditary haemochromatosis.
- Transfusional iron overload most frequently occurs in thalassaemia major, but also in other transfusion-dependent refractory anaemias, e.g. some cases of myelodysplastic neoplasias, sickle cell anaemia, primary myelofibrosis, red cell aplasia and aplastic anaemia.
- Transfusional iron overload causes damage to the liver, endocrine organs and heart, with iron accumulation also in macrophages of the reticuloendothelial system.
- Cardiac failure or arrhythmia caused by cardiac siderosis, best detected by T_2^* MRI, is the most frequent cause of death from transfusional iron overload.
- Treatment is with iron chelating drugs: deferasirox and deferiprone which are active orally, or with deferoxamine, given subcutaneously or intravenously.
- Life expectancy has improved dramatically in thalassaemia major as a result of iron chelation therapy and the use of T_2^* MRI to accurately measure cardiac and liver iron.

Now visit **www.wiley.com/go/haematology9e** to test yourself on this chapter.

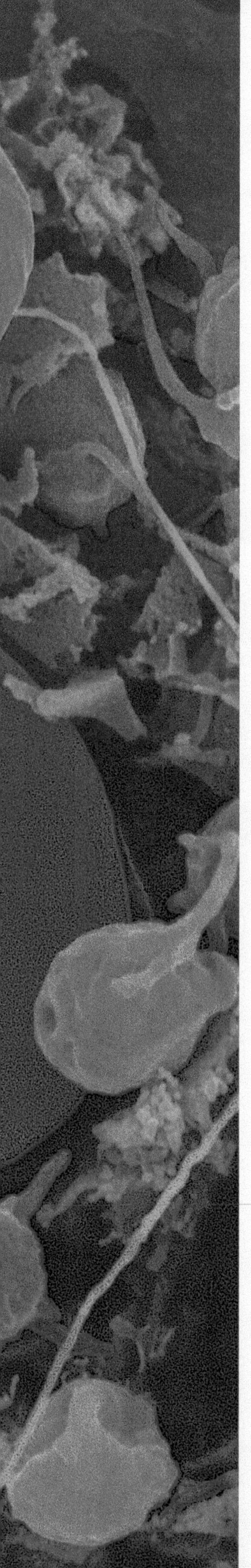

CHAPTER 5

Megaloblastic anaemias and other macrocytic anaemias

Key topics

Hoffbrand's Essential Haematology, Ninth Edition. A. Victor Hoffbrand, Pratima Chowdary, Graham P. Collins, and Justin Loke.

© 2024 John Wiley & Sons Ltd. Published 2024 by John Wiley & Sons Ltd.

Companion website: www.wiley.com/go/haematology9e

Introduction to macrocytic anaemia

In macrocytic anaemia, the red cells are abnormally large (mean corpuscular volume, MCV >98 fL). There are several causes (Table 2.5) broadly subdivided into megaloblastic and non-megaloblastic (Table 5.10), based on the appearance of developing erythroblasts in the bone marrow. An elevated MCV may also be an artefact reported by an automated cell counter if red cell agglutination or a paraprotein is present.

Megaloblastic anaemias

This is a group of anaemias in which the erythroblasts in the bone marrow show a characteristic abnormality: maturation of the nucleus is delayed relative to that of the cytoplasm. The underlying defect is defective DNA synthesis. This is usually caused by deficiency of vitamin B_{12} or folate. Less commonly, inherited or acquired, e.g. by drugs, abnormalities of the metabolism of these vitamins or inherited or acquired lesions in DNA synthesis may cause an identical haematological appearance (Table 5.1). Morphologically, this developmental asynchrony is manifest by a persistently open, loosely organized chromatin in the erythropoietic cell nucleus, while the cytoplasm exhibits staining changes of haemoglobinization typical of later stages of maturation (Fig 5.14).

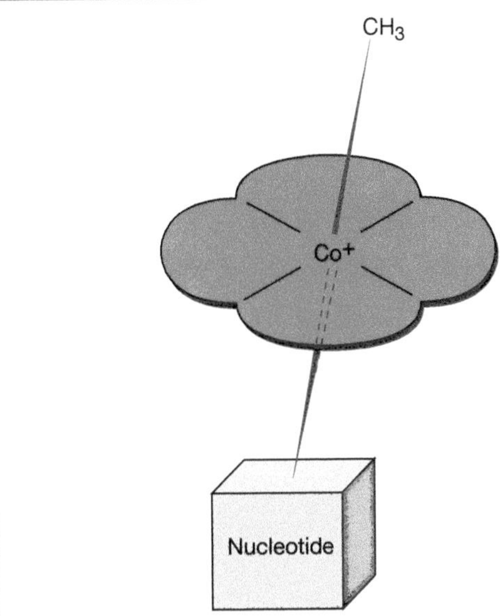

Figure 5.1 The structure of methylcobalamin, the main form of vitamin B_{12} in human plasma. Other forms include deoxyadenosylcobalamin, the main form in human tissues; hydroxocobalamin and cyanocobalamin, the main forms used in treatment of vitamin B_{12} deficiency and in multivitamin supplements.

Vitamin B_{12} (B_{12}, cobalamin)

Vitamin B_{12} is synthesized in nature by microorganisms. Animals acquire it by eating food of animal origin, by internal production from intestinal bacteria (not in humans) or by eating bacterially contaminated foods. Vitamin B_{12} consists of a small group of compounds, the cobalamins, which have the same basic structure, a cobalt atom at the centre of a corrin ring (Fig. 5.1). The reactive centre of the molecule is attached to either a cyano group (-CN, cyanocobalamin), a hydroxyl group (-OH, hydroxocobalamin), a methyl group (-CH_3, methylcobalamin) or 5-deoxyadenosyl (adenosylcobalamin). The vitamin is found in foods of animal origin such as liver, meat, fish and dairy produce, but does not occur in fruit, cereals or vegetables, except in small amounts due to contamination by insect parts in harvesting or by micro-organisms in a natural environment (Table 5.2).

Table 5.1 Causes of megaloblastic anaemia.
Vitamin B_{12} deficiency (causes are listed in Table 5.3)
Folate deficiency (causes are listed in Table 5.5)
Combined folate and B_{12} deficiency
Abnormalities of vitamin B_{12} or folate metabolism, e.g. transcobalamin deficiency, nitrous oxide, anti-folate drugs such as methotrexate, phenytoin or trimethoprim
Inherited defects of DNA synthesis
Congenital enzyme deficiencies, e.g. orotic aciduria, which impairs pyrimidine synthesis
Acquired enzyme deficiencies, e.g. due to hydroxyurea, purine synthesis antagonists such as 6-mercaptopurine, pyrimidine antagonists such as cytarabine

Absorption

A normal diet contains a large excess of B_{12} compared with daily needs (Table 5.2). B_{12} is released from protein binding in food by pepsin in the stomach. It is then mainly combined with the protein, **intrinsic factor (IF)**. IF is synthesized by the gastric parietal cells. The IF–B_{12} complex subsequently binds in the ileum to a specific surface receptor for IF, **cubam**, a complex of proteins cubilin and amnionless. Amnionless directs endocytosis of the cubilin IF–B_{12} complex into the ileal cell so that B_{12} is absorbed and IF destroyed (Fig. 5.2). The maximum amount of B_{12} that can be absorbed from a single oral dose (either in the form of food or a supplement) via the IF–cubam mechanism is about 1–2 µg.

Some dietary B_{12}, after release from food, binds to the glycoprotein haptocorrin (also known as R-factor, R-protein, or transcobalamin I) (Fig 5.2). This glycoprotein is present in plasma, milk, saliva and gastric juice. Release of dietary B_{12} from haptocorrin, making it available for binding to IF, depends largely on proteases from the pancreas.

Table 5.2 Vitamin B_{12} and folate: nutritional aspects.

	Vitamin B_{12}	Folate
Typical daily dietary intake	7–30 μg	200–400 μg
Food sources	Animal products only	Many foods, especially liver, greens and yeast
Effect of cooking	Little effect	Easily destroyed
Minimal adult daily requirement	2 μg	100–200 μg
Body stores when replete	2–3 mg (sufficient for 2–4 years)	10–12 mg (sufficient for 4 months)
Absorption		
Site	Ileum	Duodenum and jejunum
Mechanism	Bound to intrinsic factor, absorbed by cubam	Conversion to methyltetrahydrofolate
Limit	2–3 μg/day	50–80% of dietary content
Enterohepatic circulation	5–10 μg/day	90 μg/day
Transport in plasma	Most bound to haptocorrin; TC essential for cell uptake	Weakly bound to albumin
Major intracellular physiological forms	Methyl- and deoxyadenosyl-cobalamin	Reduced polyglutamate derivatives
Usual therapeutic form	Hydroxocobalamin or cyanocobalamin	Folic (pteroylglutamic) acid

TC, transcobalamin (transcobalamin II); haptocorrin = transcobalamin 1.

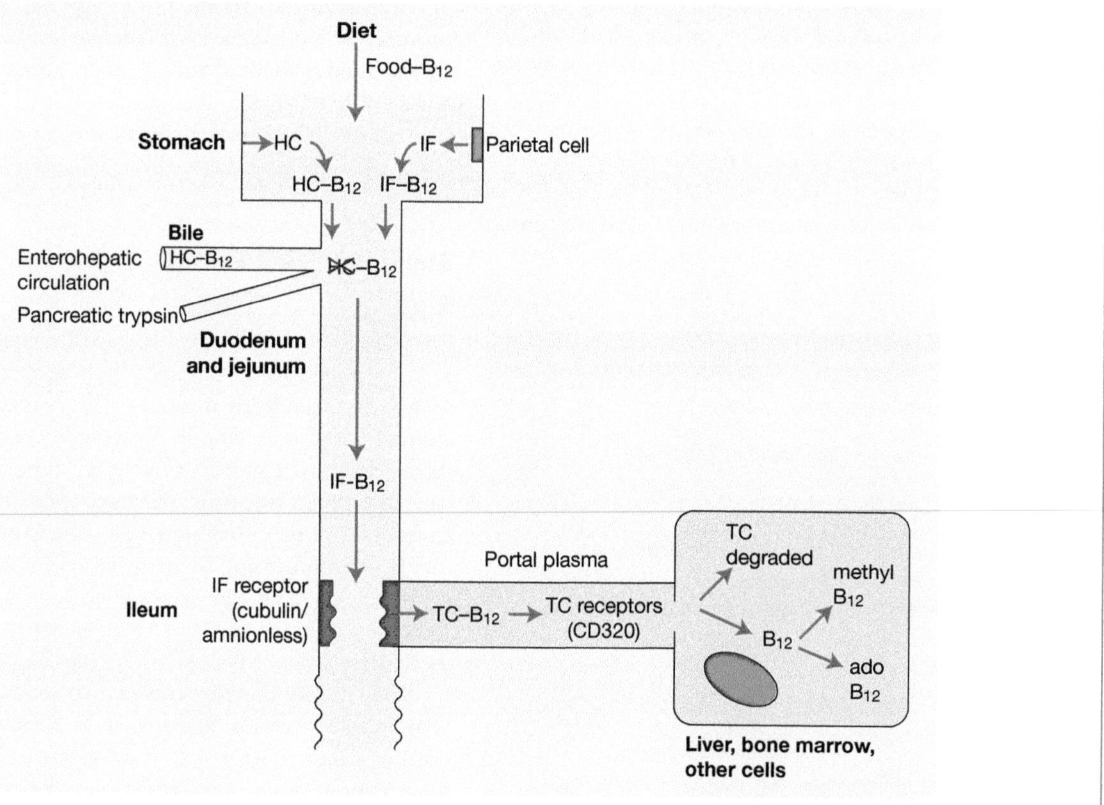

Figure 5.2 The absorption of dietary vitamin B_{12} after combination with intrinsic factor (IF), through the ileum. TC, transcobalamin; IF, intrinsic factor; HC, haptocorrin; ado B_{12}, see text.

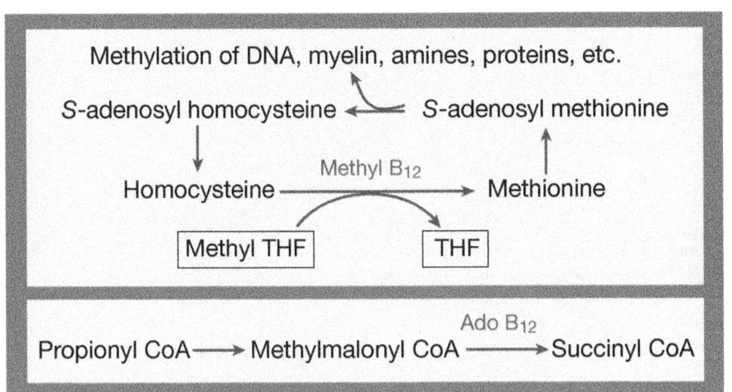

Figure 5.3 The biochemical reactions of vitamin B_{12} in humans. Ado B_{12}, deoxyadenosylcobalamin; CoA, coenzyme A; THF, tetrahydrofolate.

Transport of vitamin B_{12}: the transcobalamins

Vitamin B_{12} is absorbed from the ileal cell into portal blood, where it attaches to the plasma-binding protein transcobalamin (TC, also called transcobalamin II), which delivers B_{12} to the bone marrow and all other tissues. Although TC is the essential plasma protein for transferring B_{12} into the cells of the body, the amount of B_{12} on TC is normally very low (<50 ng/L).

Congenital TC deficiency due to germline mutations in the *TCN2* gene causes megaloblastic anaemia because of failure of B_{12} to enter marrow (and other cells) from plasma, but the serum B_{12} level in TC deficiency is normal. This is because most B_{12} in plasma is bound to haptocorrin. This glycoprotein is synthesized by granulocytes and macrophages. In myeloproliferative neoplasms where granulocyte production may be greatly increased, the haptocorrin and B_{12} levels in plasma both rise considerably. This also occurs in some liver diseases. B_{12} bound to haptocorrin in the blood does not transfer to marrow; the B12 is functionally 'dead'.

Biochemical functions

Vitamin B_{12} is a coenzyme for two biochemical reactions. First, as methyl B_{12} it is a cofactor for methionine synthase, the enzyme responsible for methylation of homocysteine to methionine which uses methyltetrahydrofolate (methylTHF) as methyl donor (Fig. 5.3). Second, as deoxyadenosyl B_{12} (ado B_{12}) it is coenzyme in the conversion of methylmalonyl coenzyme A (CoA) to succinyl CoA, a key intermediate in the citric acid cycle (Fig. 5.3).

Folate

Folic (pteroylglutamic) acid is the parent compound of a large group of compounds, the folates (Fig. 5.4). This family of compounds is also known as vitamin B9, a name which often appears on the packets of cereals that have been fortified with the vitamin.

Absorption, transport and function

Dietary folates are a complex mixture of variously reduced and polyglutamated folates. They are all converted to one compound, methylTHF, a reduced monoglutamate form which circulates in plasma (Fig. 5.5a). After entering cells, methylTHF is de-methylated to THF, and then converted to folate polyglutamate forms by addition of usually four, five or six glutamate moieties (Fig. 5.6). Folic (pteroylglutamic) acid itself is a poor substrate for reduction by dihydrofolate reductase. It is mainly converted during absorption to methylTHF at doses of 200–400 μg, larger oral doses of folic acid enter portal plasma unchanged and are then converted to physiological forms in the liver or excreted in the urine (Fig 5.5b).

Folates are needed in a variety of biochemical reactions in the body involving single carbon unit transfer, in amino acid interconversions, e.g. homocysteine conversion to methionine (Figs. 5.3 and 5.6) and serine to glycine, or in synthesis of pyrimidine and purine precursors of DNA.

Biochemical basis for megaloblastic anaemia

DNA is formed by polymerization of the four deoxyribonucleoside monophosphates derived from their triphosphates (Fig 5.6). Folate deficiency is thought to cause megaloblastic anaemia by limiting synthesis of thymidine monophosphate (dTMP) from deoxyuridine monophosphate, a rate-limiting step in DNA synthesis. This reaction needs 5,10-methylene THF polyglutamate as coenzyme. Consequent starvation of the precursor dTTP leads to prolongation of the S phase during mitosis, failure to form new double-stranded DNA and apoptotic cell death.

The role of B_{12} in DNA synthesis is indirect. B_{12} is needed in the conversion of methylTHF, which enters marrow and other cells from plasma, to THF and other active folates. In this reaction, homocysteine is converted to methionine. THF (but not methylTHF) is a substrate for folate polyglutamate synthesis. The folate polyglutamates are the intracellular folate coenzymes. B_{12} deficiency therefore reduces the supply of the critical folate coenzyme 5,10-methylene THF polyglutamate, needed for synthesis of thymidine monophosphate (dTMP) (Fig. 5.6). The block caused by B_{12} deficiency in the conversion of methylTHF either mono- or poly-glutamate, to other forms of folate has been termed the 'methylfolate trap'. Other congenital or acquired causes of megaloblastic anaemia, e.g. antimetabolite drug therapy, mainly inhibit purine or pyrimidine synthesis at one or another step. The result is a reduced supply of one or other of the four precursors needed for DNA synthesis.

Folate reduction

During the synthesis of dTMP, the folate polyglutamate coenzyme becomes oxidized from the THF to the dihydrofolate (DHF) state (Fig. 5.6). The enzyme dihydrofolate reductase regenerates active THF from DHF. Inhibitors of this enzyme,

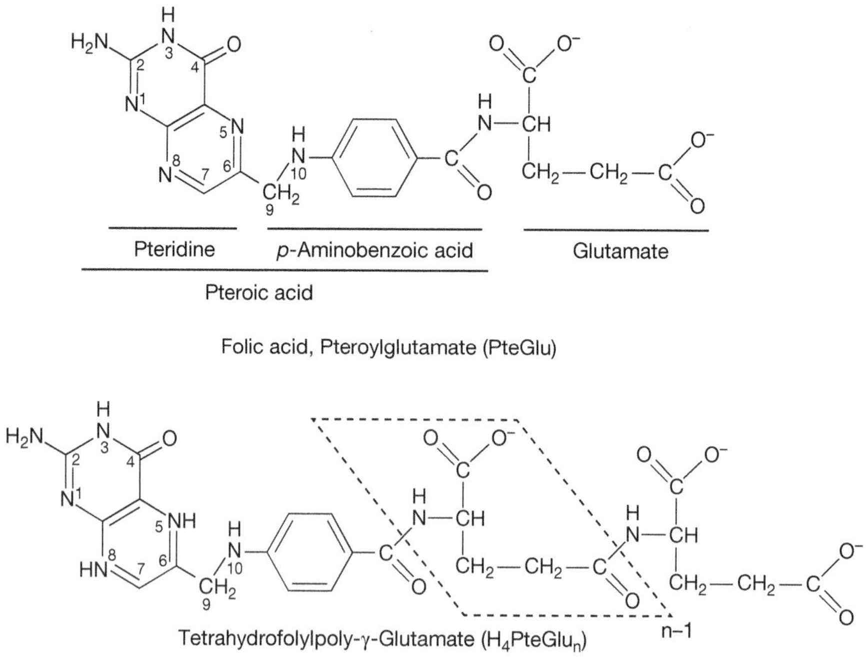

Pteridine p-Aminobenzoic acid Glutamate

Pteroic acid

Folic acid, Pteroylglutamate (PteGlu)

Tetrahydrofolylpoly-γ-Glutamate ($H_4PteGlu_n$)

One carbon substituent		Position	Oxidation state
Methyl	$—CH_3$	N-5	Methanol
Methylene	$—CH_2—$	N-5, N-10	Formaldehyde
Methenyl	—CH=	N-5, N-10	Formate
Formyl	—CHO	N-5 or N-10	Formate
Formimino	HN=CH—	N-5	Formate

Figure 5.4 The upper panel shows the chemical structure of folic acid (pteroylglutamic acid). The middle panel shows the structure of folic acid reduced to the tetrahydrofolate form and with one additional glutamic acid. The lower panel shows the five single carbon units that may be added to the folate molecule. Source: Courtesy of Professor Barry Shane.

e.g. methotrexate, inhibit folate-mediated biochemical reactions including in DNA synthesis (Fig. 5.6). Methotrexate is a useful drug, mainly in the treatment of malignant, e.g. acute lymphoblastic leukaemia (Chapter 17) or inflammatory disease, e.g. rheumatoid arthritis, psoriasis with excessive cell turnover. The weaker antagonist, pyrimethamine, is used primarily against toxoplasmosis. Trimethoprim, active against bacterial DHF reductase but only very weakly against the human enzyme, is used alone or in combination with a sulphonamide, as cotrimoxazole, especially to treat urinary tract infections. Toxicity caused by methotrexate or pyrimethamine may be reversed by the reduced folate, folinic acid (5-formyl THF). In the protocols used, this reversal does not eliminate the effectiveness of methotrexate when used in anti-cancer chemotherapy.

Causes of severe vitamin B_{12} deficiency

In developed countries, severe deficiency is usually caused by the auto-immune disease, pernicious anaemia (Table 5.3). Less commonly, severe deficiency may be caused by extreme lack of B_{12} in the diet (as in strict veganism without dietary supplements), total gastrectomy or small intestinal lesions. In vegetarians and people subsisting on a poor-quality diet low in B_{12}-rich foods, an intact entero-hepatic circulation usually but not invariably helps to protect them from severe B_{12} deficiency. The deficiency takes at least 2 years to develop, i.e. the time needed for body stores to deplete at the rate of 1–2 μg/day when there is severe malabsorption of B_{12}. There is no syndrome of B_{12} deficiency as a result of increased utilization or loss of the vitamin. Nitrous oxide, however, may rapidly inactivate body B_{12} (p. 63).

Pernicious anaemia

Pernicious anaemia (PA) is caused by autoimmune attack on the gastric mucosa, leading to atrophy of the stomach. The wall of the stomach becomes thin, with a plasma cell and lymphoid infiltrate of the lamina propria. Intestinal metaplasia may occur. Destruction of parietal cells results in achlorhydria and lack of secretion of IF. Serum gastrin levels are raised. *Helicobacter pylori* infection may initiate an autoimmune

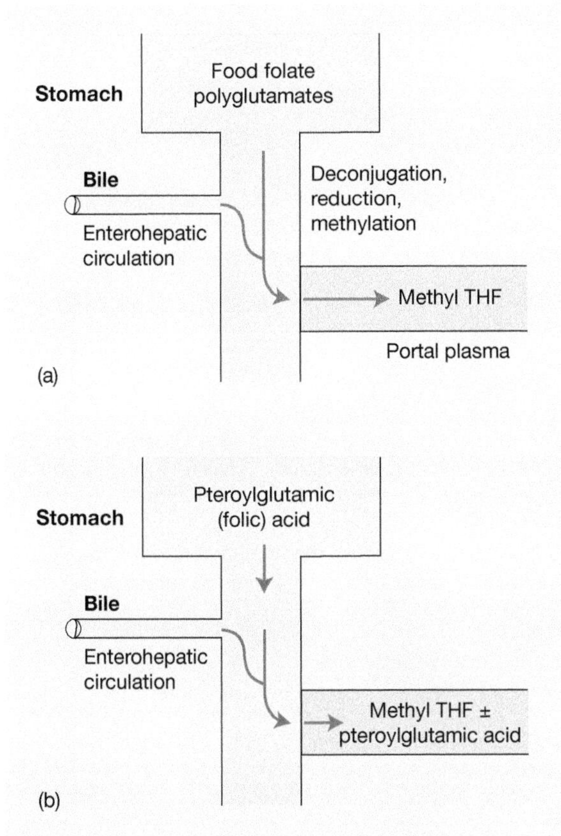

Figure 5.5 **(a)** The absorption of dietary folates; **(b)** The absorption of pteroylglutamic (folic) acid. At doses up to 400 μg, most pteroylglutamic (folic) acid is converted to methyltetrahydrofolate (methylTHF). At higher doses, unchanged pteroylglutamic acid enters portal plasma.

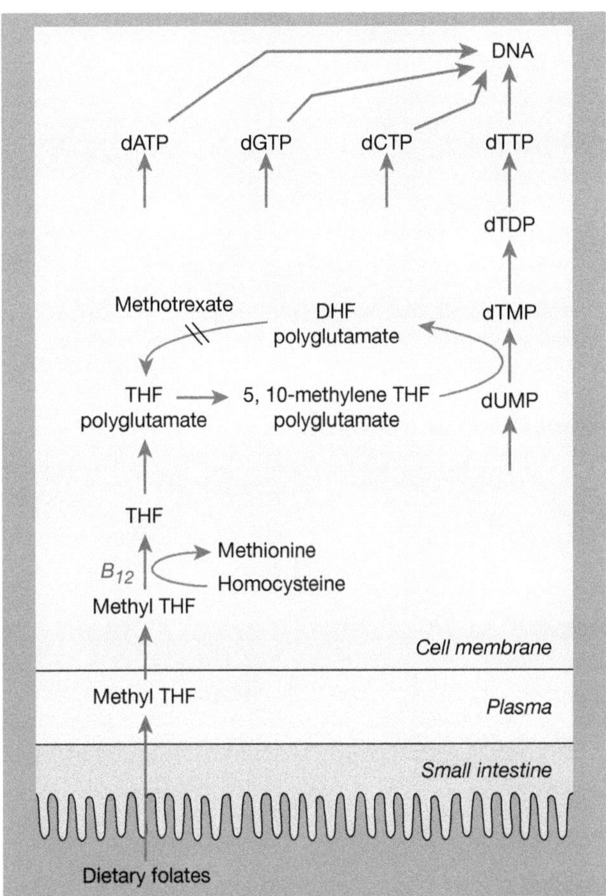

Figure 5.6 The biochemical basis of megaloblastic anaemia caused by vitamin B_{12} or folate deficiency. Folate is required in one of its coenzyme forms, 5,10-methylenetetrahydrofolate polyglutamate, in the synthesis of thymidine monophosphate from its precursor deoxyuridine monophosphate. Vitamin B_{12} is needed to convert methyltetrahydrofolate (methylTHF), which enters the cells from plasma, to THF, from which polyglutamate and other forms of folate are synthesized. Dietary folates are all converted to methylTHF (a monoglutamate) by the small intestine. The block in conversion of methylTHF to THF at the monoglutamate and polyglutamate levels and so to other forms of folate has been called the 'methylfolate trap'. A, adenine; C, cytosine; d, deoxyribose; DHF, dihydrofolate; DP, diphosphate; G, guanine; MP, monophosphate; T, thymine; TP, triphosphate; U, uracil.

gastritis, which presents in younger subjects as iron deficiency and in the elderly as PA.

More females than males are affected (1.6: 1), with a peak occurrence at 60 years, and there may be associated autoimmune disease, particularly thyroid diseases (Table 5.4). The disease is found in all races, but is most common in Northern Europeans. It tends to occur in families. There is also an increased incidence of carcinoma of the stomach (approximately 2–3% of all cases of pernicious anaemia).

Antibodies

Ninety per cent of patients with PA show in the serum parietal cell antibody directed against the gastric proton pump H^+/K^+-AT Pase. The antibody, however, is not specific for PA. PA is distinguished from simple atrophic (non-PA) autoimmune gastritis by the presence of antibodies to IF. **Fifty to seventy percent of PA patients show in serum an antibody to IF which inhibits IF binding to B_{12}.** An antibody blocking IF attachment to its ileal binding site is less frequent. IF antibodies also occur in PA in gastric juice, where they block any remaining IF binding B_{12}. IF antibodies are specific for PA, but as they occur in the serum of only half of patients, their absence from serum does not exclude the diagnosis. The more common parietal cell antibody is less specific, as it occurs quite commonly in older subjects, e.g. 16% of normal women over 60 years even without PA.

Other causes of severe vitamin B_{12} deficiency

Congenital lack or abnormality of IF due to mutations of its gene usually presents at approximately 2 years of age, when

Table 5.3 Causes of severe vitamin B_{12} deficiency.

Nutritional Especially strict vegans
Malabsorption *Gastric causes* Pernicious anaemia Congenital lack or abnormality of intrinsic factor Total or partial gastrectomy
Intestinal causes Intestinal stagnant loop syndrome – jejunal diverticulosis, blind-loop, stricture, etc. Chronic tropical sprue Ileal resection and Crohn's disease Congenital selective malabsorption with proteinuria (autosomal recessive megaloblastic anaemia) Fish tapeworm

Table 5.4 Pernicious anaemia: associations.

Female	Vitiligo
Blue eyes	Myxoedema
Early greying	Hashimoto's disease
Northern European	Thyrotoxicosis
Familial	Addison's disease
Blood group A	Hypoparathyroidism Type I diabetes Hypogammaglobulinaemia Carcinoma of the stomach

stores of B_{12} derived from the mother *in utero* have been exhausted. Specific malabsorption of B_{12} is due to genetic mutation of the IF–B_{12} receptor proteins, cubilin or amnionless. It usually presents in infancy or childhood and is associated with proteinuria in 90% of cases. Infants born to and breast fed by B_{12}-deficient mothers may also develop symptomatic B_{12} deficiency.

Causes of mild vitamin B_{12} deficiency

The two most frequent causes worldwide of mild B_{12} deficiency, almost always insufficient to cause anaemia or a neuropathy, are an inadequate diet and malabsorption of food B_{12} due to atrophic gastritis (particularly in the elderly and with *Helicobacter* pylori infection). Less frequent causes are bariatric surgery, chronic pancreatitis, gluten-induced enteropathy, HIV infection, and prolonged treatment with proton pump inhibitors, metformin or cholestyramine. In the Zollinger–Ellison syndrome, the pH in the duodenum falls so low that pancreatic enzymes that normally release B_{12} from haptocorrin are inactivated. These malabsorption conditions do not usually lead to B_{12} deficiency sufficient to cause anaemia or neuropathy. In pregnancy, serum B_{12} levels may fall to below the normal range, but spontaneously return to normal after delivery (Chapter 34).

Table 5.5 Causes of folate deficiency.

Nutritional Especially old age, institutions, poverty, famine, special diets, goat's milk anaemia etc.
Malabsorption Tropical sprue, gluten-induced enteropathy (adult or child). Possible contributory factor to folate deficiency in some patients with partial gastrectomy, extensive jejunal resection or Crohn's disease
Excess utilization
Physiological Pregnancy and lactation, prematurity
Pathological Haematological diseases: haemolytic anaemias, myelofibrosis Malignant disease: carcinoma, lymphoma, myeloma Inflammatory diseases: Crohn's disease, tuberculosis, rheumatoid arthritis, psoriasis, exfoliative dermatitis, malaria
Excess urinary folate loss Active liver disease, congestive heart failure
Drugs Anticonvulsants, sulfasalazine
Mixed Liver disease, alcoholism, intensive care

Folate deficiency

This is most often a result of a poor dietary intake of folate alone or in combination with a condition of increased folate utilization or malabsorption (Table 5.5). Excess cell turnover of any sort, including pregnancy, is a cause of an increased need for folate. Some of the folate coenzyme involved in synthesis of thymidine monophosphate is degraded at the C_9—N_{10} bond during the reaction. Consequently when DNA synthesis and so thymidine synthesis is increased, destruction of folate in increased. The mechanism by which anticonvulsants and barbiturates cause the deficiency is controversial.

Clinical features of megaloblastic anaemia

The onset is usually insidious, with gradually progressive symptoms and signs of anaemia (Chapter 2). The patient may be mildly jaundiced (lemon yellow; Fig. 5.7) because of the

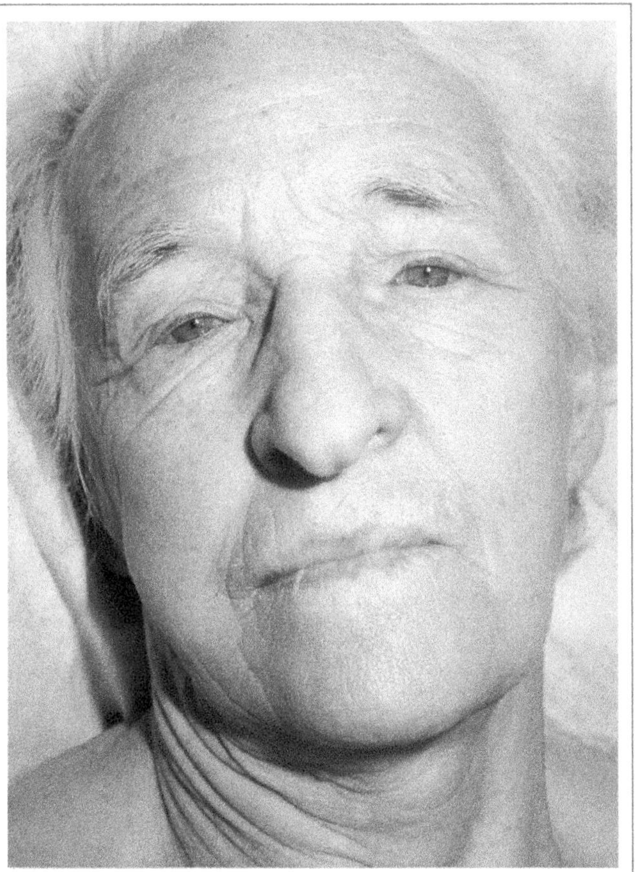

Figure 5.7 Megaloblastic anaemia: pallor and mild icterus in a patient with a haemoglobin count of 70.0 g/L and a mean corpuscular volume of 132 fL.

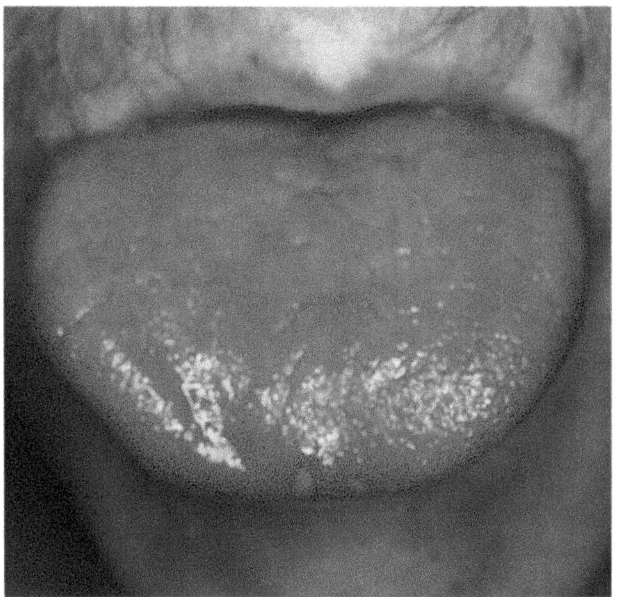

Figure 5.8 Megaloblastic anaemia: glossitis – the tongue is beefy red and painful.

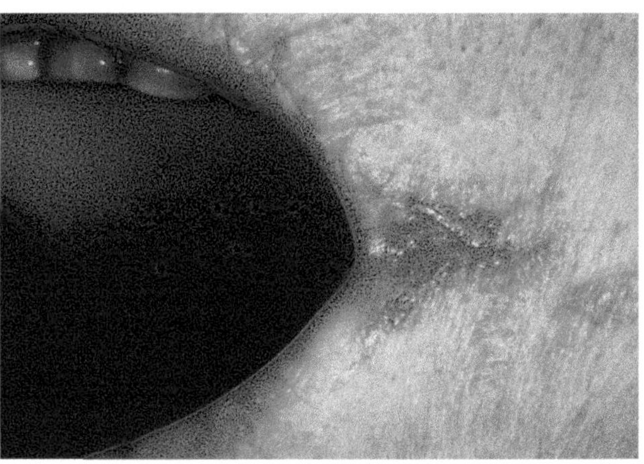

Figure 5.9 Megaloblastic anaemia: angular cheilosis (stomatitis).

excess breakdown of haemoglobin resulting from increased ineffective erythropoiesis in the bone marrow. Glossitis (a beefy-red sore tongue; Fig. 5.8), angular cheilosis (Fig. 5.9) and mild symptoms of malabsorption with loss of weight because of the epithelial abnormality may be present. Purpura as a result of thrombocytopenia and widespread melanin pigmentation (the cause of which is unclear) are less frequent presenting features (Table 5.6). Many asymptomatic patients are diagnosed when a blood count performed for another reason reveals macrocytosis.

Vitamin B_{12} neuropathy (subacute combined degeneration of the cord)

Severe B_{12} deficiency can cause a progressive neuropathy affecting the peripheral sensory nerves and posterior and lateral spinal columns (Fig. 5.10). The neuropathy is symmetrical and affects the lower more than the upper limbs. The patient notices tingling in the feet, difficulty in walking, and may fall over in the dark due to loss of positional sense. Rarely, optic atrophy or severe psychiatric symptoms are present. Anaemia may be severe, mild or even absent. The

Table 5.6 Effects of vitamin B_{12} or folate deficiency.
Megaloblastic anaemia
Macrocytosis of epithelial cell surfaces
Neuropathy (for B_{12} deficiency only)
Sterility
Rarely, reversible melanin skin pigmentation
Decreased osteoblast activity
Neural tube defects in the foetus

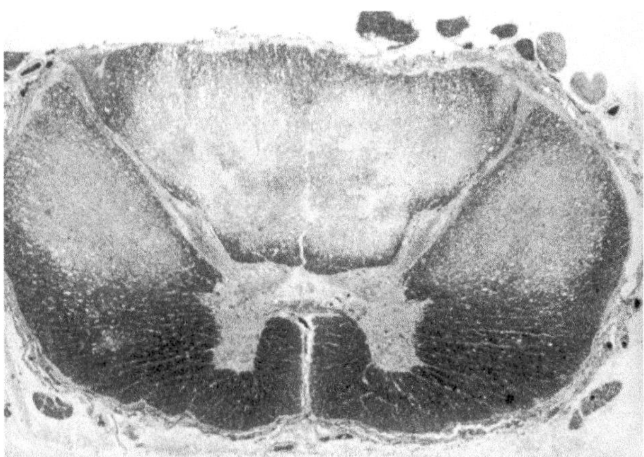

Figure 5.10 Cross-section of the spinal cord in a patient who died with subacute combined degeneration of the cord (Weigert–Pal stain). There is demyelination of the dorsal and dorsolateral columns.

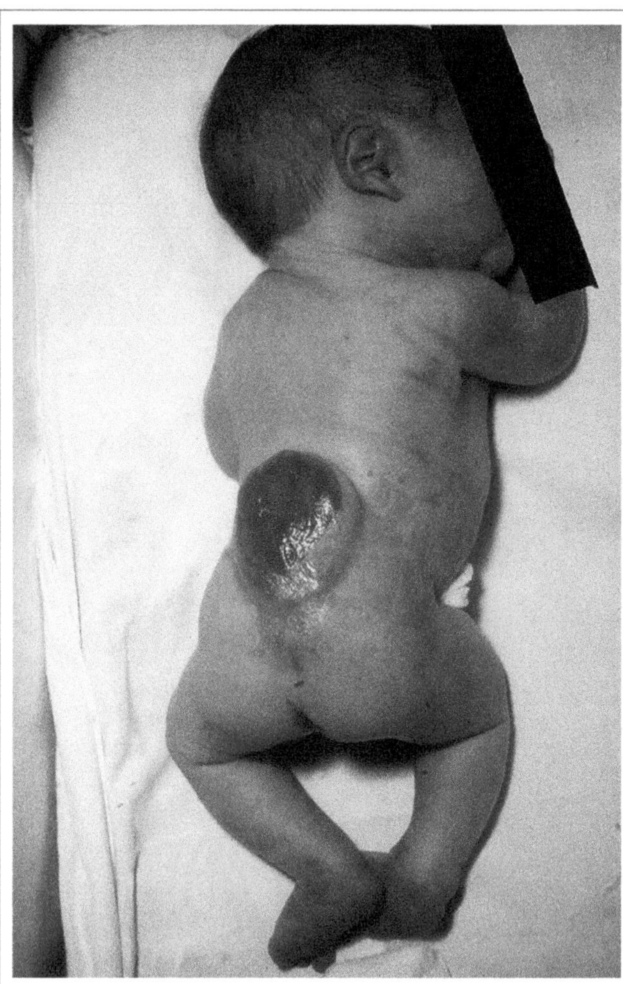

Figure 5.11 A baby with neural tube defect (spina bifida). Source: Courtesy of Professor C.J. Schorah.

duration and severity of the neurological defects predict the outcome. The peripheral neuropathy is usually reversible with B_{12} therapy, but spinal cord recovery is usually incomplete, especially if the neuropathy has been present for more than a few months. Prolonged deficiency in infants impairs motor function, which also may be irreversible.

The cause of the neuropathy is likely to be related to the accumulation of *S*-adenosyl homocysteine and reduced levels of *S*-adenosyl methionine in nervous tissue, resulting in defective methylation of myelin and other substrates.

Neural tube defect

Folate deficiency in the mother predisposes to the neural tube defects (NTDs) anencephaly, spina bifida or encephalocoele in the foetus. The neural tube is formed in the foetus from a plate of cells in the early embryo. It gives rise to the brain and spinal cord and their covering skull and spinal bones. The defect can affect the head when part or all the brain and skull are missing. More frequently it is the spine which is defective with failure of closure, often with protrusion of the spinal cord and its covering meninges in the lower back region (Fig. 5.11). The abnormality may be detected by ultrasound during the pregnancy when a therapeutic abortion can be performed. The foetus may also die *in utero* or soon after birth. An infant born with spina bifida often has paralysis of the lower limbs and may have urinary and faecal incontinence. Hydrocephalus due to obstruction of flow of cerebrospinal fluid is another serious complication.

The lower the maternal serum or red cell folate (or serum B_{12}) levels, the higher the incidence of NTDs (Fig. 5.12). Moreover, supplementation of the diet with folic acid at the time of conception and in early pregnancy reduces the incidence of NTD by up to 83%. The exact mechanism is uncertain, but is thought to be related either to a fault in DNA synthesis or to the build-up of homocysteine and *S*-adenosyl homocysteine in the foetus, which may impair methylation of various proteins and lipids. A common polymorphism (677C→T) in the enzyme 5,10-methylene tetrahydrofolate reductase (5,10-MTHFR), which reduces conversion of 5,10-MTHF to methylTHF, results in higher serum homocysteine and lower serum and red cell folate levels compared with controls. The incidence of the mutation is higher in foetuses with NTD than in controls.

Other tissue abnormalities

Sterility is frequent in either sex with severe B_{12} or folate deficiency. Macrocytosis, excess apoptosis and other morphological abnormalities of cervical, buccal, bladder and other epithelia occur. Widespread reversible melanin pigmentation may also occur. B_{12} deficiency is associated with reduced osteoblastic activity.

Raised serum homocysteine levels and low serum or red cell folate and the polymorphism in the MTHFR enzyme (see

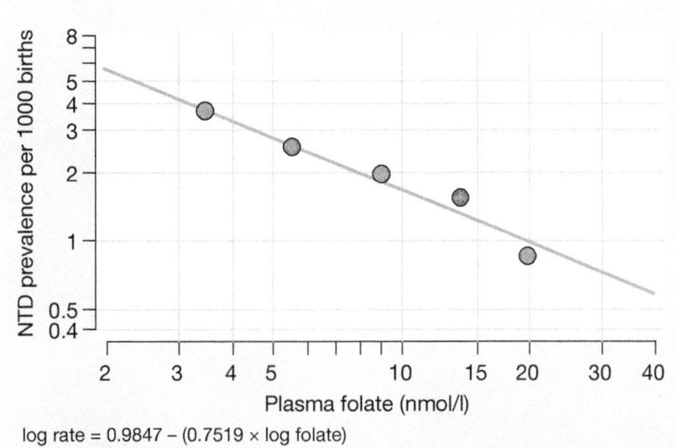

Figure 5.12 Linear relation between maternal plasma folate level and prevalence of a neural tube defect (NTD) birth. The lower the plasma folate, the higher the prevalence of an NTD pregnancy with no threshold. A similar linear relation is found between maternal red cell folate and prevalence of NTD births. 10 nmol/L = 3.8 μg/L. Source: N.J. Wald *et al.* (1998) Folic acid food fortification to prevent neural tube defects. *Lancet* 351: 834. N.J. Wald, J. Noble. In C.H. Rodeck, M.J. Whittle (eds) (1999) *Primary Prevention of Neural Tube Defects in Fetal Medicine: Basic Science and Clinical Practice*. London: Churchill Livingstone, pp. 283–90. L.E. Dale *et al.* (1995) Folate levels and neural tube defects: implications for prevention. *Journal of the American Medical Association* 274: 215–9.

above) have been associated with an increased incidence of cardiovascular diseases, including myocardial infarct, peripheral vascular diseases, stroke and venous thrombosis (Chapter 30). Folic acid prophylaxis, however, has not reduced the incidence of the arterial diseases or cardiovascular events, except for stroke in hypertensive subjects, where a reduction of 15% has been shown in large-scale controlled studies in China.

Various associations have been found between folate status and malignant diseases, but meta-analysis of subjects randomized to take folic acid or placebo in trials lasting two years or more does not show any difference in cancer incidence between those taking folic acid and the controls.

Laboratory findings

The anaemia is macrocytic (MCV >98 fL by definition and often as high as 120–140 fL in severe cases). The macrocytes are typically oval (Fig. 5.13a,b). In severe cases, megaloblasts

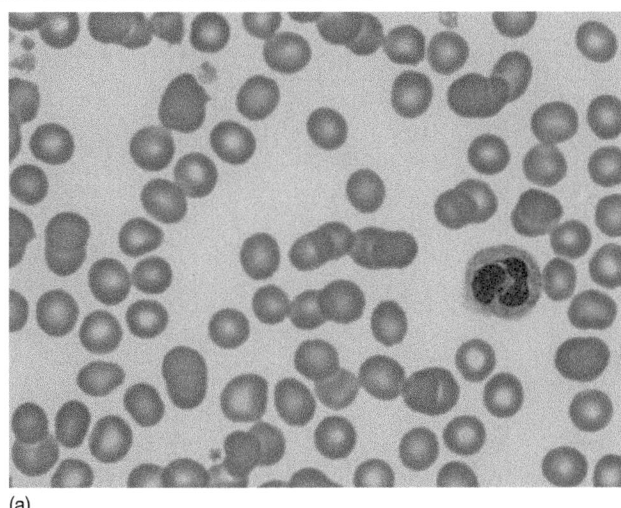
(a)

Figure 5.13(a) Normal blood film. The red cells are similar in shape (circular) and size. The white cell (neutrophil) to the right of the film has a nucleus with two major lobes.

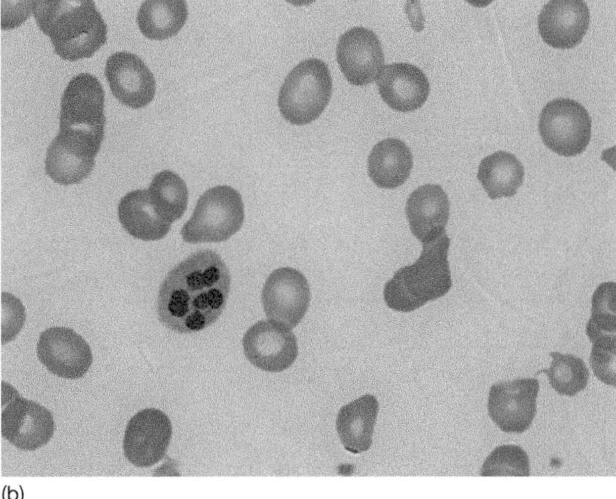
(b)

Figure 5.13(b) Blood film from a patient with severe megaloblastic anaemia. Compared to a normal blood film at the same magnification, the red cells are larger and fewer in number. Many of the red cells are oval and misshapen. The neutrophil to the left of the centre has a nucleus with six lobes. Source: Courtesy (a) and (b) *Professor Barbara Bain*.

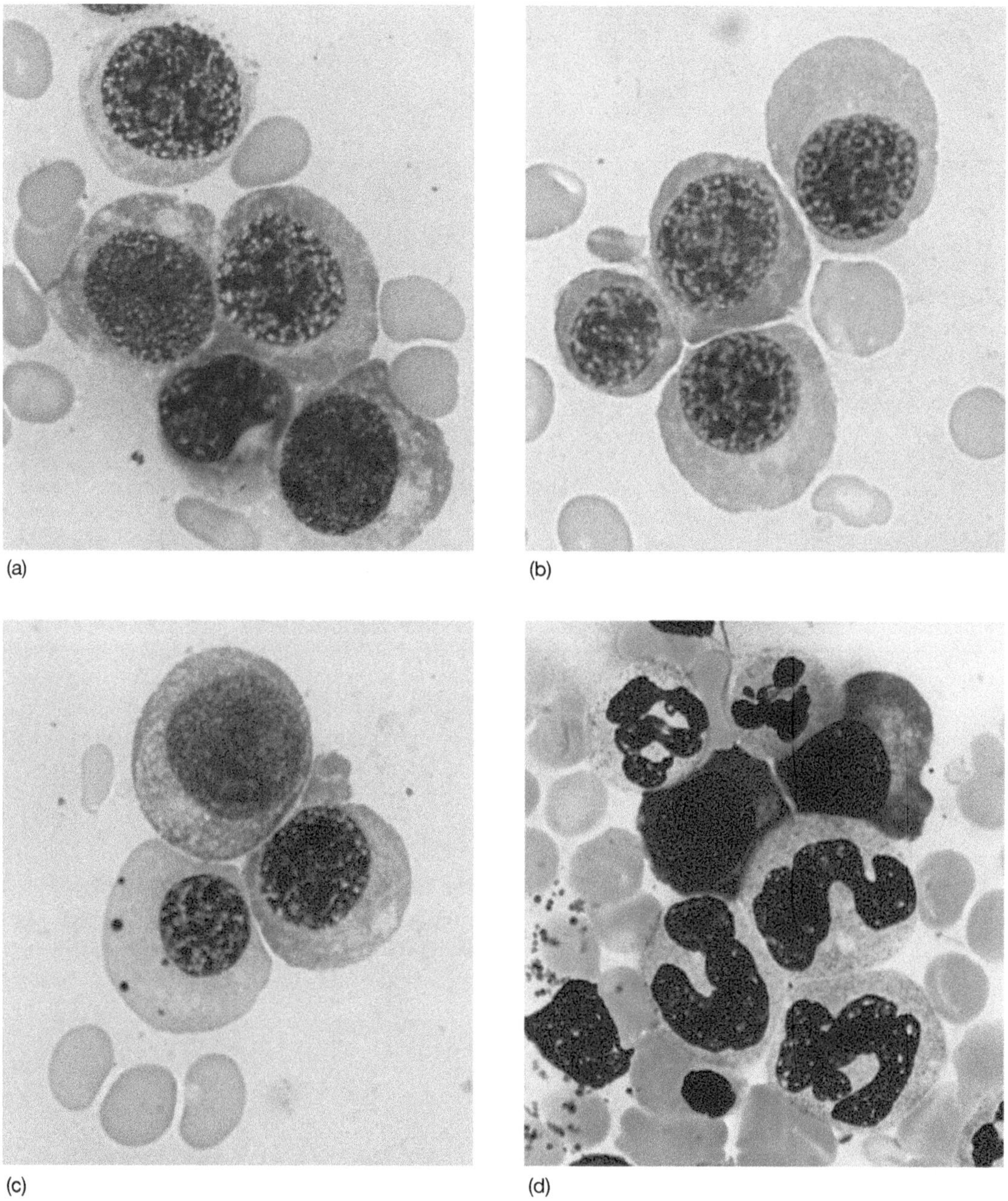

(a) (b)

(c) (d)

Figure 5.14 Megaloblastic changes in the bone marrow in a patient with severe megaloblastic anaemia. **(a–c)** Erythroblasts showing fine, open stippled (primitive) appearance of the nuclear chromatin even in late cells (pale cytoplasm with some haemoglobin formation). **(d)** Abnormal giant metamyelocytes and band forms.

may appear in the peripheral blood due to extramedullary haemopoiesis. If iron deficiency is also present the MCV may be normal, but the red cell distribution width (RDW) in such cases will be very wide and the blood film dimorphic, with distinct populations of large and small cells. The reticulocyte count is low and the total white cell and platelet counts may be reduced, especially in severely anaemic patients. **A proportion of the neutrophils show hypersegmented nuclei (six or more nuclear lobes)**. The bone marrow is usually hypercellular and the erythroblasts are large and show an open, fine, lacy primitive chromatin pattern despite normal cytoplasmic haemoglobinization (Fig. 5.14). Giant and abnormally shaped metamyelocytes are characteristic.

The serum unconjugated bilirubin and lactate dehydrogenase are raised as a result of marrow cell breakdown (ineffective haemopoiesis).

Table 5.7 Laboratory tests for vitamin B_{12} and folate deficiency.

			Result in	
Test	**Normal values***		**Vitamin B_{12} deficiency**	**Folate deficiency**
Serum vitamin B_{12}	160–925 ng/L	120–680 pmol/L	Low	Normal or borderline low
Serum folate	3.0–15.0 μg/L	4–30 nmol/L	Normal or raised	Low
Red cell folate	160–640 μg/L	360–1460 nmol/L	Normal or low	Low

*Normal values differ with different commercial kits.

Diagnosis of vitamin B_{12} or folate deficiency

It is usual to assay serum B_{12} and folate and in many laboratories also red blood cell folate (Table 5.7). The serum B_{12} is low in megaloblastic anaemia or neuropathy caused by B_{12} deficiency. In B_{12} deficiency, the serum folate tends to rise but the red cell folate falls. In the absence of B_{12} deficiency, however, the red cell folate is a more accurate guide to tissue folate status than the serum folate. Serum and red cell folate are both low in megaloblastic anaemia caused by folate deficiency. Serum folate in contrast to red cell folate is more labile, and even one or two nutritious meals in a hospitalized patient admitted with severe deficiency may normalize serum folate. However, red cell folate will remain low for some time.

Measurement of serum or urine methylmalonic acid is a test for B_{12} deficiency and measurement of homocysteine is a test for either folate or B_{12} deficiency. These are not specific, however, and it is difficult to establish normal levels in different age groups. These biochemical tests are also not widely available.

Tests for cause of vitamin B_{12} or folate deficiency

Useful tests are listed in Table 5.8. For B12 deficiency these are mainly concerned with assessing gastric function and testing for antibodies to gastric antigens. In all cases of pernicious anaemia, endoscopy studies should be performed at diagnosis to confirm the presence of gastric atrophy and exclude carcinoma of the stomach. For folate deficiency, the dietary history is most important, although it is difficult to estimate folate intake accurately. Unsuspected gluten-induced enteropathy or other underlying conditions should also be considered (Table 5.5).

Table 5.8 Tests for cause of vitamin B_{12} or folate deficiency.

Vitamin B_{12}	**Folate**
Diet history	Diet history
Serum gastrin	Tests for intestinal malabsorption
IF, parietal cell antibodies	Anti-transglutaminase and endomysial antibodies
Endoscopy	Duodenal biopsy Underlying disease

IF, intrinsic factor.

Treatment

Most cases only need therapy with the appropriate vitamin (Table 5.9). Patients with megaloblastic anaemia or neuropathy due to B_{12} deficiency should be treated initially with injections of B_{12}. If large doses of folic acid, e.g., 5 mg/day are given in B_{12} deficiency they cause a haematological response, but will allow a neuropathy to appear or progress as the B12 deficiency progresses. Folic acid in 5mg doses should therefore not be given alone for any prolonged period unless B_{12} deficiency has been excluded. In severely anaemic patients who need treatment urgently, it may be safer to initiate treatment with both vitamins after blood has been taken for B_{12} and folate assays. In the elderly, the presence of heart failure should be corrected with diuretics. Blood transfusion should be avoided if possible, as it may cause circulatory overload.

Parenteral B_{12} therapy is usually used for subsequent lifelong maintenance (Table 5.9). Large oral doses are needed daily to achieve sufficient B_{12} absorption for maintenance in PA and compliance with long-term therapy may be a problem. Oral therapy is more appropriate for those with mild degrees of B_{12} deficiency, e.g. dietary deficiency or with malabsorption of food B_{12}.Also for those with such disorders as haemophilia which make injections unsafe.

For folate deficiency, an oral dose of 5 mg daily is indicated initially, with parenteral therapy reserved for those receiving parenteral nutrition. It is usual to continue for 4 months and then to decide whether or not to continue this long term (Table 5.9).

Response to therapy

The patient usually begins to feel better after 24–48 hours of correct vitamin therapy, with increased appetite and well-being. The haemoglobin should rise by 20–30 g/L each fortnight. The white cell and platelet counts become normal in 7–10 days (Fig. 5.15) and the marrow is normoblastic in about 48 hours, although giant metamyelocytes persist for up to 12 days.

Table 5.9 Treatment of megaloblastic anaemia.

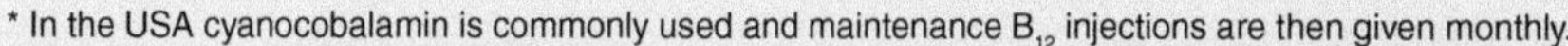

	Vitamin B_{12} deficiency	Folate deficiency
Compound	Hydroxocobalamin*	Folic acid
Route	Intramuscular**	Oral
Dose	1000 μg	5 mg
Initial dose	6 × 1000 μg over 2–3 weeks	Daily for 4 months
Maintenance	1000 μg every 3 months*; usually life-long or daily large (500–1000 μg) oral doses of B_{12}	Depends on underlying disease; life-long therapy e.g. 5 mg once weekly may be needed in chronic inherited haemolytic anaemias, myelofibrosis, renal dialysis
Prophylactic	Following total gastrectomy or ileal resection Daily oral B_{12} for vegans and in developing countries during pregnancy and lactation	Pregnancy, severe haemolytic anaemias, dialysis, prematurity In over 80 countries the diet (grain, flour or rice) is fortified with folic acid to reduce the incidence of neural tube defect affected pregnancies and births

* In the USA cyanocobalamin is commonly used and maintenance B_{12} injections are then given monthly.
** Some clinicians recommend daily oral or sublingual therapy of vitamin B_{12} deficiency (see text).

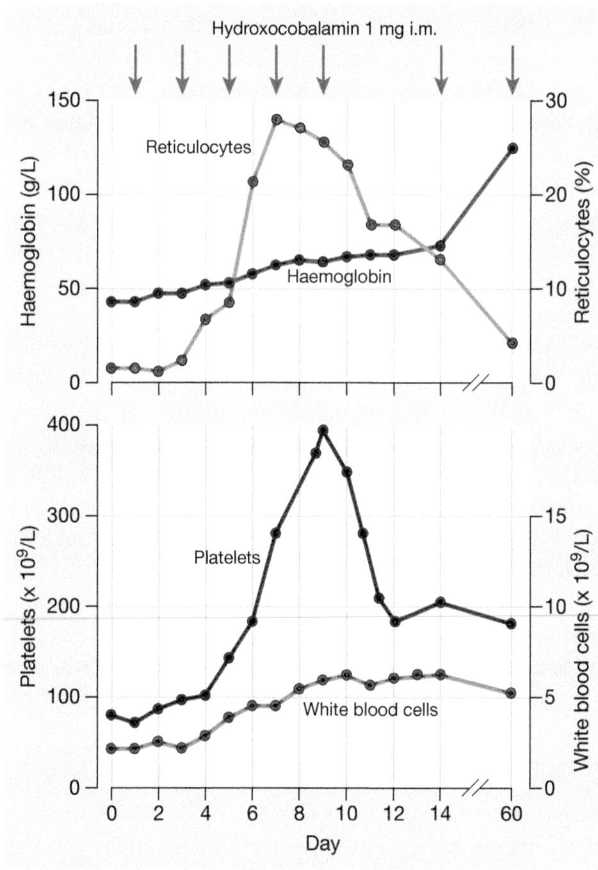

Figure 5.15 Typical haematological response to vitamin B_{12} (hydroxocobalamin) therapy in pernicious anaemia.

Prophylactic therapy

Vitamin B_{12} is given 3-monthly to those who have had a total gastrectomy or ileal resection. Oral supplements and consumption of dairy products or of foods fortified with B_{12} are recommended for vegetarians and those living because of poverty on a diet low in B_{12}-rich foods. In developing countries oral B_{12} supplements are recommended for all pregnant and lactating women.

Folic acid is given before and in pregnancy for the first 3 months at a typical dosage of 400 μg/day to reduce the risk of an NTD. The neural tube is formed within the first 4–6 weeks of gestation. In the UK a larger dose 5 mg daily is recommended throughout pregnancy for those considered at high risk e.g. having had a previous NTD pregnancy, with diabetes or sickle cell disease. This two dose recommendation seems unnecessary; all women should take the larger dose if they may become pregnant and in the first 3 months of pregnancy to get the greater benefit. All women of child-bearing age are also recommended to have an intake of at least 400 μg/day (by increased intake of folate-rich or folate-supplemented foods or as folic acid) to prevent a first occurrence of an NTD foetus. There have been no trials aimed at showing whether vitamin B12 fortification of the diet would also be beneficial in reducing the incidence of NTD pregnancies

Food fortification with folic acid, e.g., 150–220 ug/100 g of flour or grain is mandated in about 80 countries (including North America since 1998) and has reduced the prevalence of NTDs with no untoward effects reported. Folic acid supplementation of foods has not been approved in Europe though in 2021, the UK announced that it intended to introduce this. Many breakfast cereals are voluntarily fortified with folic acid by the manufacturers.

Folic acid is also given to patients undergoing chronic dialysis, with severe chronic haemolytic anaemias, e.g. sickle cell anaemia, and to premature babies.

Other megaloblastic anaemias

The most frequent (Table 5.1) causes are drugs inhibiting DNA synthesis, e.g. hyroxycarbamide (hydroxyurea), cytarabine, or drugs inhibiting dihydrofolate reductase, e.g. methotrexate or pyrimethamine. Myelodysplastic neoplasias are also a relatively frequent cause in the elderly. Congenital deficiencies of enzymes involved in DNA synthesis, e.g. orotic aciduria, are extremely rare.

Abnormalities of vitamin B_{12} or folate metabolism

These include rare congenital deficiencies of enzymes concerned in B_{12} or folate intracellular trafficking or metabolism, or of the serum transport protein for B_{12}, TC. Nitrous oxide (N_2O) anaesthesia causes rapid inactivation of body B_{12} by oxidizing the reduced cobalt atom of methyl B_{12}. Megaloblastic marrow changes occur with several days of N_2O administration and can cause pancytopenia. Chronic exposure (as in dentists and anaesthetists) has been associated with neurological damage resembling B_{12} deficiency neuropathy. Antifolate drugs, particularly those which inhibit DHF reductase, e.g. methotrexate and pyrimethamine, may also cause megaloblastic change.

Other macrocytic anaemias

There are many non-megaloblastic causes of macrocytic anaemia (Table 5.10). The exact mechanism creating large red cells in each of these conditions is not clear, although increased lipid deposition on the red cell membrane or alterations of erythroblast maturation time in the marrow may be implicated. Alcohol is the most frequent cause of a raised MCV in the absence of anaemia. Reticulocytes are bigger than mature red cells, so haemolytic anaemia is a cause of macrocytic anaemia. Antimetabolite drugs such as hydroxycarbamide (Table 12.1) cause macrocytosis and the marrow may show megaloblastic changes. The other underlying conditions listed in Table 5.10 are usually easily diagnosed provided that they are considered and the appropriate investigations to exclude B_{12} or folate deficiency are carried out.

Table 5.10 Causes of macrocytosis other than megaloblastic anaemia.
Alcohol
Liver disease
Myxoedema
Myelodysplastic neoplasias; VEXAS (see page xxx)
Antimetabolite drugs, e.g. hydroxycarbamide
Aplastic anaemia
Pregnancy
Smoking
Reticulocytosis
Myeloma and paraproteinaemia
RBC agglutination (artefactual)

Differential diagnosis of macrocytic anaemias

The clinical history and physical examination may suggest B_{12} or folate deficiency as the cause. Diet, drugs, alcohol intake, family history, history suggestive of malabsorption, presence of autoimmune diseases or other associations with pernicious anaemia (Table 5.4), previous gastrointestinal disease or operations are all important. The presence of jaundice, glossitis or symmetrical neuropathy are also important indications of megaloblastic anaemia.

The laboratory features of particular importance are the shape of macrocytes (oval in megaloblastic anaemia), the presence of hypersegmented neutrophils, leucopenia and thrombocytopenia in megaloblastic anaemia, and the bone marrow appearance. Assays of serum B_{12} and folate are essential. Exclusion of alcoholism (particularly if the patient is not anaemic), liver and thyroid function tests, and bone marrow examination for myelodysplasia, aplasia or myeloma are important in the investigation of macrocytosis not caused by B_{12} or folate deficiency.

SUMMARY

- Macrocytic anaemias show an increased size of circulating red cells (MCV >98 fL). The bone marrow erythropoiesis may be megaloblastic or normoblastic.
- Vitamin B_{12} or folate deficiency causes megaloblastic anaemia, in which the bone marrow erythroblasts have a typical abnormal appearance with delayed maturation of the nucleus compared to the degree of cytoplasmic haemoglobinization.
- Folates take part in biochemical reactions in DNA synthesis. B_{12} has an indirect role in DNA synthesis by its involvement in folate metabolism.
- B_{12} deficiency may also cause a neuropathy due to damage to the spinal cord and peripheral nerves.
- Severe B_{12} deficiency is usually caused by B_{12} malabsorption due to pernicious anaemia in which there is autoimmune gastritis, resulting in failure of synthesis of intrinsic factor, a protein made in the stomach which facilitates B_{12} absorption by the ileum.
- Other gastrointestinal diseases as well as a vegan diet may cause B_{12} deficiency.
- Folate deficiency may be caused by a poor diet, malabsorption, e.g. gluten-induced enteropathy, or

by excess cell turnover, e.g. pregnancy, haemolytic anaemias, malignancy.

- Treatment of B_{12} deficiency is usually with injections of hydroxocobalamin and of folate deficiency with oral folic (pteroylglutamic) acid.
- Folate deficiency predisposes to neural tube defect (NTD) affected pregnancies. Supplements of folic acid before and during the early weeks of pregnancy and fortification of the diet with folic acid in about 80 countries that have mandated for this have successfully reduced the incidence of NTD affected pregnancies and births.
- Rare causes of megaloblastic anaemia include inborn errors of B_{12} or folate transport or metabolism, and defects of DNA synthesis not related to B_{12} or folate.
- Causes of macrocytic red cells with or without anaemia and usually with normoblastic erythropoiesis include alcohol, liver disease, hypothyroidism, myelodysplasia, paraproteinaemia, cytotoxic drugs, aplastic anaemia, pregnancy and the neonatal period. In the non-anaemic patient, alcohol is the most frequent cause.

Now visit **www.wiley.com/go/haematology9e** to test yourself on this chapter.

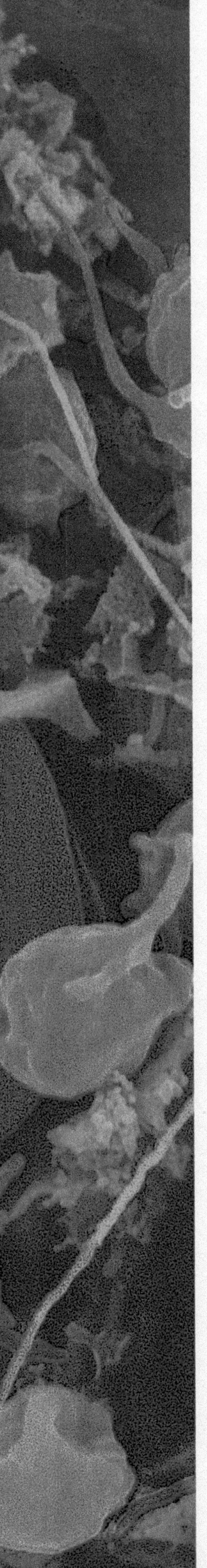

CHAPTER 6

Haemolytic anaemias

Key topics

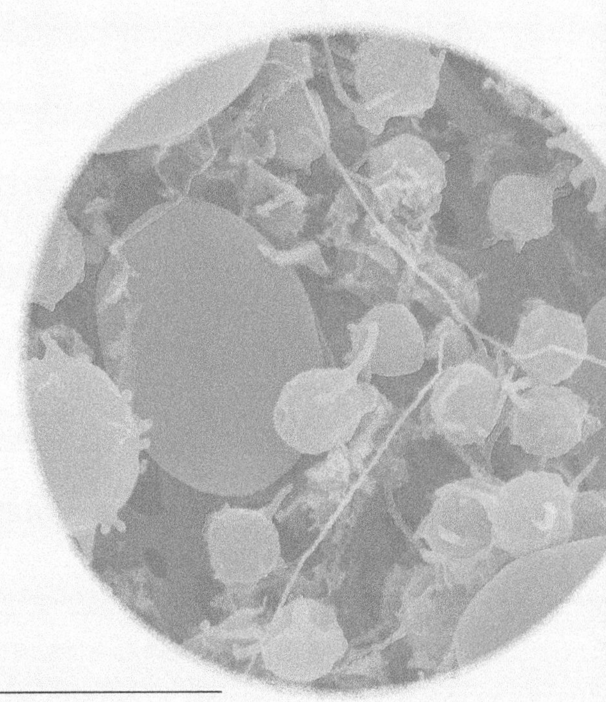

Hoffbrand's Essential Haematology, Ninth Edition. A. Victor Hoffbrand, Pratima Chowdary, Graham P. Collins, and Justin Loke.

© 2024 John Wiley & Sons Ltd. Published 2024 by John Wiley & Sons Ltd.

Companion website: www.wiley.com/go/haematology9e

Normal red cell destruction

Normal (physiological) red cell destruction occurs after a mean life span of 120 days. Aged cells are removed extravascularly by the macrophages of the reticuloendothelial (RE) system, especially in the marrow but also in the liver and spleen. As red cells have no nucleus and therefore cannot synthesize new RNA and proteins, cell metabolism gradually deteriorates as enzymes are degraded, and the cells also become stiffer and less deformable in the microcirculation when structural proteins are degraded. Eventually senescent red cells become non-viable.

Breakdown of haem from haemoglobin liberates iron which macrophages export via ferroportin bound to plasma transferrin into plasma for recirculation. Protoporphyrin, the organic ring into which ferrous iron is embedded to form haem, is broken down in the macrophages to biliverdin and then to bilirubin. Bilirubin, which is lipid soluble, circulates bound to albumin to the liver where it is conjugated to glucuronides to make it water soluble and facilitate its excretion. Bilirubin glucuronides are excreted via bile into the gut where they are converted to stercobilinogen and stercobilin, which are brown in colour and excreted in faeces (Fig. 6.1). Stercobilinogen and stercobilin are partly reabsorbed after reduction by bacterial action in the intestines to urobilinogen and urobilin (also known as urochrome) which are excreted in the urine, urobilin being responsible for urine's yellow colour. Globin chains of haemoglobin are broken down to individual amino acids, which are reutilized for general protein synthesis in the body.

Haptoglobins are proteins in normal plasma which bind haemoglobin if either intravascular or significant extravascular haemolysis is present. The haemoglobin–haptoglobin complex is removed from plasma by the RE system. Intravascular haemolysis, i.e. the breakdown of red cells within blood vessels, plays little or no part in normal red cell destruction, but is important in some pathological states, discussed later.

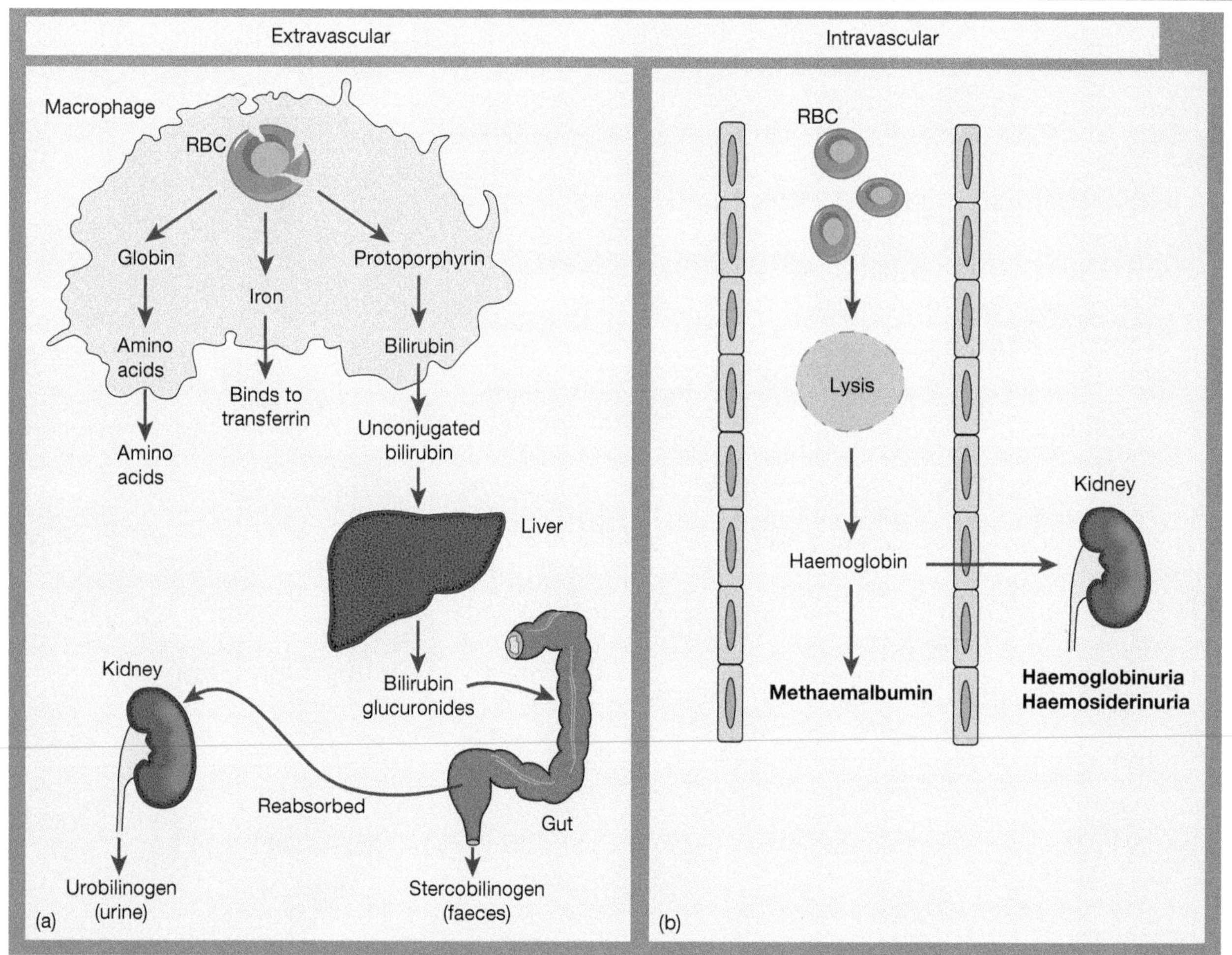

Figure 6.1 **(a)** Normal red blood cell (RBC) breakdown. This takes place extravascularly in the macrophages of the reticuloendothelial system. **(b)** Intravascular haemolysis within the blood vessel occurs in some pathological disorders, and is associated with haemoglobinaemia, haemoglobinuria and haemosiderinuria.

Introduction to haemolytic anaemias

Haemolytic anaemias are defined as anaemias that result from an increase in the rate of red cell destruction. Because of erythropoietic hyperplasia and anatomical extension of bone marrow, red cell destruction may increase several-fold before anaemia develops – this is called compensated haemolytic disease. The normal adult marrow, after full expansion, is able to produce red cells at 6–8 times the normal rate. Therefore, anaemia due to haemolysis may not be seen until the red cell life span drops to less than 30 days. The expanded red cell production leads to a marked reticulocytosis.

Classification

Table 6.1 is a simplified classification of the haemolytic anaemias. **Hereditary haemolytic anaemias are typically the result of 'intrinsic' red cell defects, whereas acquired haemolytic anaemias are usually the result of an 'extracorpuscular' or 'environmental' change**. Paroxysmal nocturnal haemoglobinuria (PNH) is an exception because, although it is an acquired disorder, the PNH red cells have an intrinsic defect. PNH is associated with marrow hypoplasia and is discussed with aplastic anaemia in Chapter 24.

Clinical features

The patient may show pallor of the mucous membranes, mild fluctuating jaundice and splenomegaly. There is no bilirubin in urine, but the urine may turn dark on standing because of excess urobilinogen, which is colourless but oxidizes in light to highly coloured urobilin. Pigment (bilirubin) gallstones may complicate the condition (Fig. 6.2).

Some patients with haemolysis develop disease-specific complications. For instance, patients with sickle cell disease, hereditary spherocytosis, or rarely other haemolytic anaemias may develop ulcers around the ankle (Fig. 7.20), while those with thalassaemia major who do not receive regular transfusions develop bone deformities (Figs. 7.9 and 7.10). Patients with cold-reactive autoantibodies may exhibit discoloration in peripheral (acral) regions of the body such as the earlobes or fingertips, and patients with PNH may develop thrombosis.

Aplastic crises may occur, usually precipitated by infection with parvovirus, which 'switches off' erythropoiesis. These crises are characterized by a sudden fall in haemoglobin level and in reticulocyte count (Fig. 24.7). Rarely, folate deficiency may cause an aplastic crisis in which the bone marrow becomes megaloblastic.

Laboratory findings

The laboratory findings are conveniently divided into three groups.

1 **Features of increased red cell breakdown:**
   (**a**) serum bilirubin raised, unconjugated and bound to albumin;
   (**b**) urine urobilinogen increased;
   (**c**) serum haptoglobins absent because the haptoglobins become saturated with haemoglobin and the complex is removed by RE cells.

Table 6.1 Classification of haemolytic anaemias.

Hereditary	Acquired
Membrane defects Hereditary spherocytosis, hereditary elliptocytosis, others *Metabolic disorders* G6PD deficiency, pyruvate kinase deficiency	*Autoimmune* Warm antibody type (see Table 6.5) Cold antibody type
Haemoglobinopathies and thalassaemias Hb SS, Hb SC, Hb CC, unstable haemoglobins, thalassaemia major and others; Chapter 7	*Alloimmune* Haemolytic transfusion reactions (acute or delayed) Haemolytic disease of the newborn Allografts, especially in stem cell transplantation Drug-associated *Red cell fragmentation syndromes* (Table 6.6) Microangiopathy, e.g. disseminated intravascular coagulation March haemoglobinuria *Infections:* malaria, clostridia, tick-borne illnesses such as babesiosis *Chemicals:* especially drugs, industrial/domestic substances, e.g. naphthalene in moth balls Severe burns *Secondary:* severe liver and renal disease *Paroxysmal nocturnal haemoglobinuria* (Chapter 24)

G6PD, glucose-6-phosphate dehydrogenase; Hb, haemoglobin.

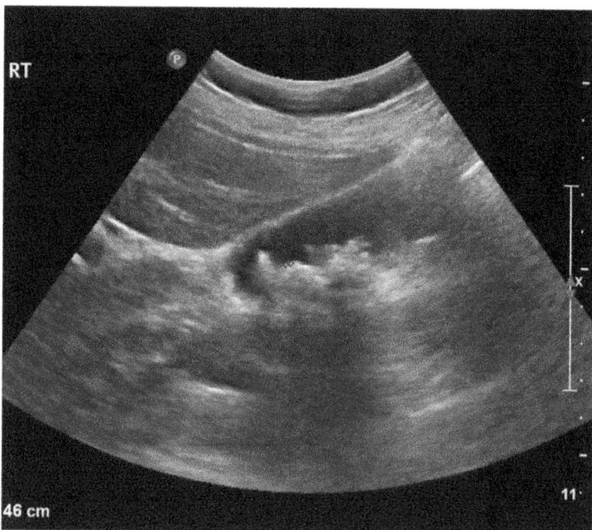

Figure 6.2 Ultrasound of multiple small pigment gallstones typical of those associated with hereditary spherocytosis. Source: Courtesy of Dr P. Wylie.

(d) Serum lactate dehydrogenase (LDH) may be raised in both severe extravascular and in intravascular haemolysis

2 Features of increased red cell production:

(a) reticulocytosis;

(b) bone marrow erythroid hyperplasia – the normal marrow myeloid: erythroid ratio of 2 : 1 to 12 : 1 is reduced to 1 : 1 or reversed.

3 Damaged red cells, visualized by:

(a) routine blood film morphology e.g. microspherocytes, elliptocytes, fragments;

(b) flow cytometry after eosin-5-maleimide (EMA) staining, see Fig 6.5;

(c) specific enzyme, protein or DNA tests.

Table 6.2 Causes of intravascular haemolysis.
Mismatched blood transfusion (usually ABO)
G6PD deficiency with oxidant stress
Red cell fragmentation syndromes
Some severe autoimmune haemolytic anaemias
Some drug- and infection-induced haemolytic anaemias
Paroxysmal nocturnal haemoglobinuria
March haemoglobinuria
Unstable haemoglobin
G6PD, glucose-6-phosphate dehydrogenase.

Intravascular and extravascular haemolysis

There are two mechanisms whereby red cells are destroyed in haemolytic anaemias. There may be excessive removal of red cells by cells of the RE system (**extravascular haemolysis**) or red cells may be broken down directly in the circulation (**intravascular haemolysis**) (Fig. 6.1; Table 6.2). Whichever mechanism dominates will depend on the pathology involved.

In intravascular haemolysis, free haemoglobin is released, which rapidly saturates plasma haptoglobins. The excess free haemoglobin is filtered by the glomerulus. If the rate of haemolysis saturates the renal tubular reabsorptive capacity, free haemoglobin enters urine (Fig. 6.3). Iron released from haemoglobin in the renal tubules is seen as haemosiderin in a urinary deposit. Oxidized haem bound to albumin (methaemalbumin) is also formed from the process of intravascular haemolysis.

The main laboratory features of intravascular haemolysis therefore are (Fig. 6.3):

1 Haemoglobinaemia and haemoglobinuria.

2 Haemosiderinuria.

3 Methaemalbuminaemia (detected spectrophotometrically).

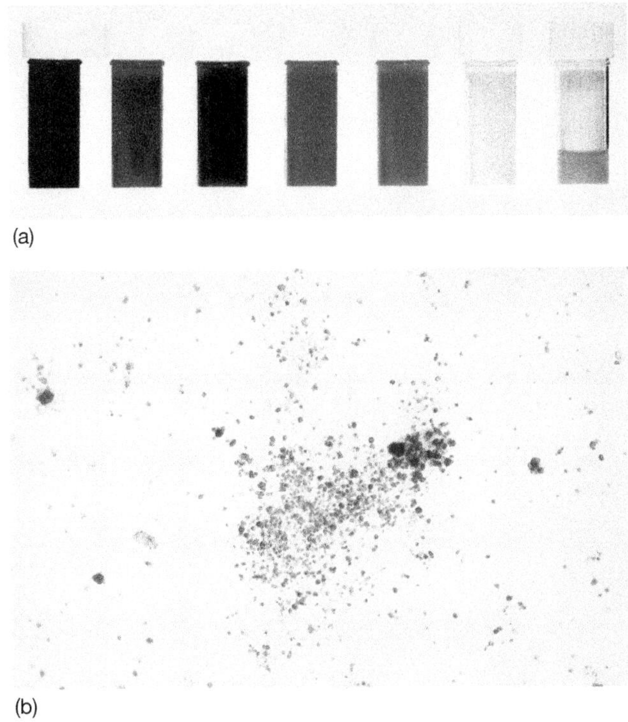

Figure 6.3 **(a)** Progressive urine samples in an acute episode of intravascular haemolysis showing haemoglobinuria of decreasing severity. **(b)** Prussian blue-positive deposits of haemosiderin in a urine spun deposit (Perls' stain).

Hereditary haemolytic anaemias

Membrane defects

Hereditary spherocytosis

Hereditary spherocytosis (HS) is the most common hereditary haemolytic anaemia in Northern Europeans.

Pathogenesis

HS is usually caused by defects in the proteins involved in the vertical interactions between the membrane skeleton and the lipid bilayer of the red cell (Table 6.3; Fig. 2.12). The marrow produces red cells of normal biconcave shape, but these lose membrane and become increasingly spherical (loss of surface area relative to volume) as they circulate through the spleen and the rest of the RE system. The loss of membrane may be caused by the release of parts of the lipid bilayer that are not supported by the skeleton. Ultimately, the spherocytes are unable to pass through the microcirculation, especially in the spleen, and die prematurely.

Clinical features

The inheritance is usually autosomal dominant with variable expression; rarely, it may be autosomal recessive. In about 25% of cases the mutation is new (spontaneous) with no family history of the disease. The anaemia may present at any age from infancy to old age. Jaundice is typically fluctuating and is particularly marked if the haemolytic anaemia is associated with Gilbert's disease (a defect of hepatic conjugation of bilirubin). Splenomegaly occurs in most patients. Pigment gallstones are

Table 6.3 Molecular basis of hereditary spherocytosis and elliptocytosis.

Hereditary spherocytosis

- Ankyrin deficiency or abnormalities (most common cause – about 50% of patients)
- α- or β-spectrin deficiency or abnormalities
- Band 3 abnormalities
- Pallidin (protein 4.2) abnormalities

Hereditary elliptocytosis

- α- or β-spectrin mutants leading to defective spectrin dimer formation
- α- or β-spectrin mutants leading to defective spectrin–ankyrin associations
- Protein 4.1 deficiency or abnormality
- Southeast Asian ovalocytosis due to a band 3 deletion

frequent (Fig. 6.2); aplastic crises, usually precipitated by parvovirus infection, may cause a sudden increase in the severity of anaemia (Fig. 24.8).

Haematological findings

Anaemia is usual but not invariable; its severity tends to be similar in members of the same family. Reticulocytes are usually 5–20%. The blood film shows microspherocytes (Fig. 6.4a), which are densely staining with smaller diameters than normal red cells.

Investigation and treatment

A rapid flow cytometric analysis of eosin-5-maleimide (EMA) bound to erythrocytes is used as a test for HS and membrane protein deficiency (Fig. 6.5). EMA is a dye that binds specifically to band 3 of the red blood cell cytoskeleton and measures the content of erythrocyte structural proteins, which is altered in HS. The EMA test has replaced the osmotic fragility test, which showed the red cells to be excessively fragile compared to normal red cells in dilute saline solutions. Identification of the exact molecular defect is not needed for management, but electrophoresis of membrane proteins is carried out in difficult cases. The direct antiglobulin (Coombs') test is normal in HS, excluding an autoimmune cause of spherocytosis and haemolysis.

The principal form of treatment is splenectomy, preferably laparoscopic, although this should not be performed unless clinically indicated by symptomatic anaemia or gallstones, leg

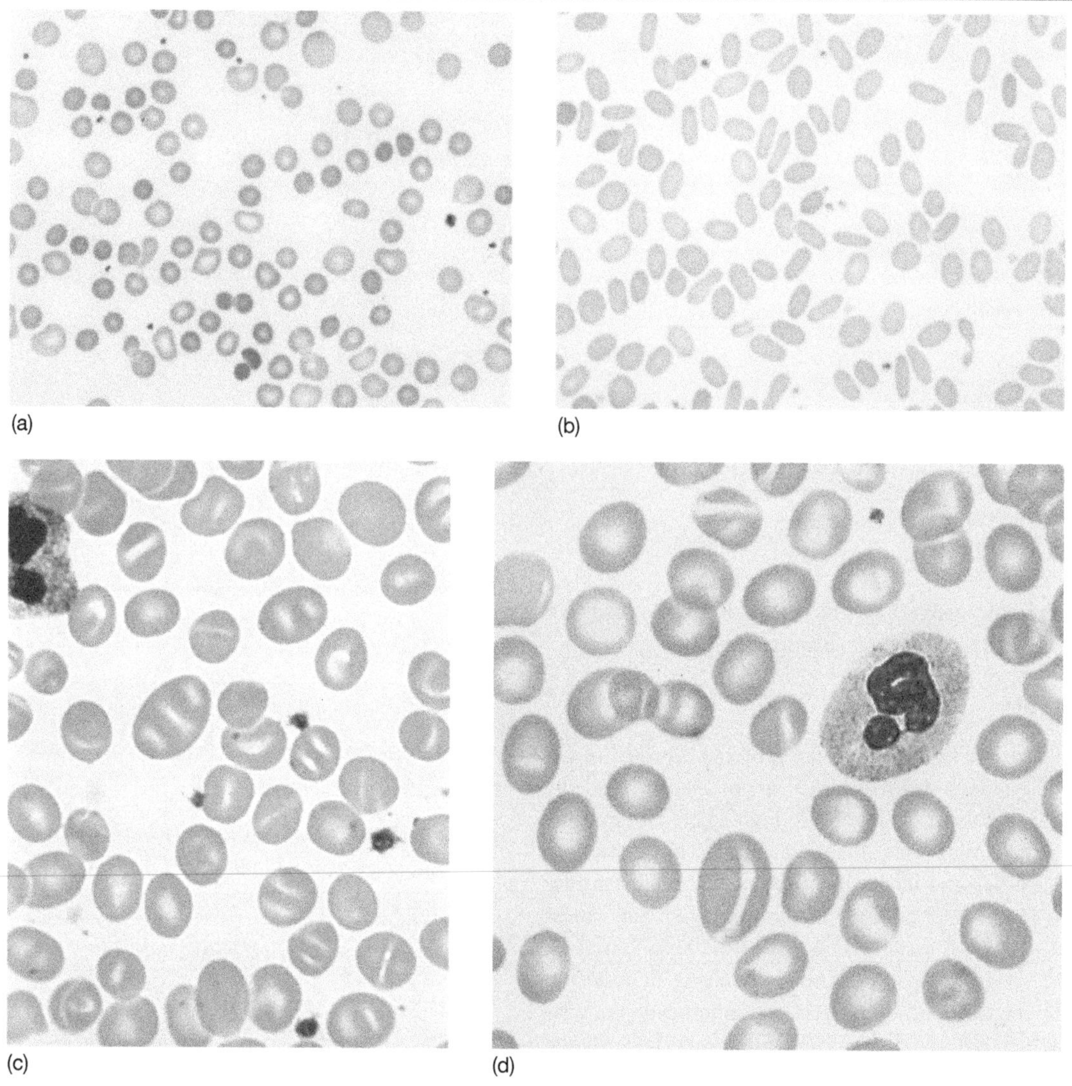

Figure 6.4 **(a)** Blood film in hereditary spherocytosis. The spherocytes are deeply staining and of small diameter. Larger polychromatic cells are reticulocytes (confirmed by supravital staining). **(b)** Blood film in hereditary elliptocytosis. **(c)** Hereditary stomatocytosis: peripheral blood film showing many cells with the characteristic loosely folded appearance of the membrane. **(d)** Southeast Asian ovalocytosis. Source: A.V. Hoffbrand *et al.* (2019) *Color Atlas of Hematology*, 5th edn. Reproduced with permission of John Wiley & Sons.

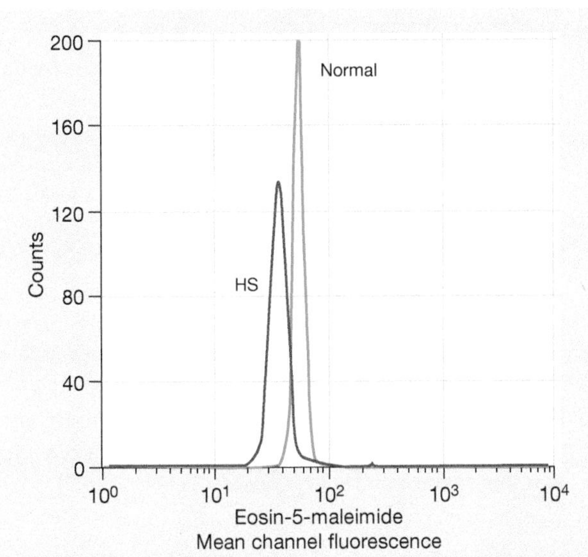

Figure 6.5 Eosin-5-maleimide (EMA) staining in hereditary spherocytosis (HS) showing reduced mean channel fluorescence due to membrane band 3 protein deficiency. Source: Courtesy of Mr G. Ellis.

ulcers or growth retardation. Because of the risk of post-splenectomy sepsis, particularly in early childhood (Chapter 10), the frequency of splenectomy has fallen over recent decades and the age at splenectomy has risen. Cholecystectomy should be performed with splenectomy if symptomatic gallstones are present. Unless there is additional pathology, splenectomy in HS should always produce a rise in the haemoglobin level to normal, even though microspherocytes formed in the rest of the RE system will remain. Folic acid, e.g. 5 mg weekly, is given in severe cases to prevent folate deficiency.

Hereditary elliptocytosis

Hereditary elliptocytosis (HE) has similar clinical and laboratory features to HS, except for the appearance of the blood film (Fig. 6.4b). HE is usually a clinically mild disorder and is predominantly discovered by chance on a blood film. There may be no evidence of haemolysis. Occasional patients require splenectomy. The basic defect is a failure to form normal spectrin heterodimers. Genetic mutations affecting horizontal interactions of red cell skeletal proteins have been detected (Table 6.3).

Patients with homozygous or doubly heterozygous elliptocytosis present with a severe haemolytic anaemia termed hereditary pyropoikilocytosis; this is most common in patients of African descent. In severe cases, splenectomy can be performed which results in clinical improvement. Folic acid supplementation is also appropriate.

Hereditary stomatocytosis

This is a group of rare red cell membrane defects including xerocytosis and overhydrated stomatocytosis, in which the red cells have mouth-like slits in a stained blood film (Fig 6.4c). The cells leak cations and anaemia is variable. Stomatocytosis may also occur as an artefact if blood films are badly prepared.

Southeast Asian ovalocytosis

This is common in Melanesia, Malaysia, Indonesia and the Philippines and is caused by a 9-amino acid deletion at the junction of the cytoplasmic and transmembrane domains of the band 3 protein. The cells are rigid and resist invasion by malarial parasites. The blood film shows ovalocytes and stomatocytes (Fig 6.4d). Most cases are not anaemic and asymptomatic. Treatment is rarely required.

Defective red cell metabolism

Glucose-6-phosphate dehydrogenase deficiency

Glucose-6-phosphate dehydrogenase (G6PD) functions to reduce nicotinamide adenine dinucleotide phosphate (NADP) to NADPH. This reaction is the only source of NADPH needed for the production of reduced glutathione. The gene coding G6PD is on the X chromosome. G6PD deficiency renders the red cell susceptible to oxidant stress (Fig. 6.6).

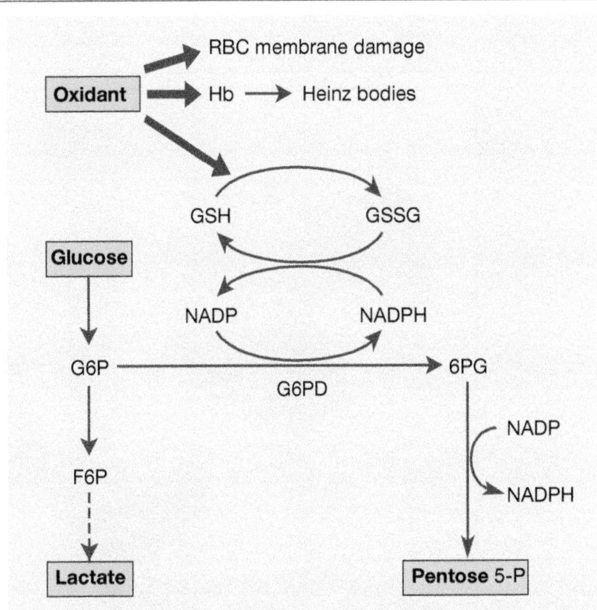

Figure 6.6 Haemoglobin and red blood cell (RBC) membranes are usually protected from oxidant stress by reduced glutathione (GSH). In G6PD deficiency, NADPH and GSH synthesis is impaired. F6P, fructose-6-phosphate;G6P, glucose-6-phosphate; G6PD, glucose-6-phosphate dehydrogenase; 6-PG, 6-phosphogluconate; GSSG, glutathione (oxidized form); NADP, NADPH, nicotinamide adenine dinucleotide phosphate.

Epidemiology

There is a wide variety of normal genetic variants of the enzyme G6PD. The most common isoforms are type B and type A, which is predominant in Africans. They have the same enzyme activity. In addition, more than 400 variants caused by point mutations or deletions that alter the activity of the G6PD enzyme have been characterized, and worldwide over 400 million people are G6PD deficient (Fig. 6.7).

The inheritance is sex-linked, dominantly affecting males, and carried by females who show approximately half the normal red cell G6PD values. Because of lyonization, heterozygote females may have a substantial proportion of G6PD deficient red cells and be susceptible to haemolysis. The female heterozygotes have an advantage of resistance to potentially lethal *Falciparum* malaria. The degree of deficiency varies with ethnic group and G6PD genotype, often being mild (10–60% of normal activity) in black Africans, more severe in Middle Eastern and South-East Asians, and most severe in Mediterranean populations, e.g. <10% of normal activity with G6PD Mediterranean. The degree of enzyme activity and the clinical severity of the syndrome do not always correlate. Severe deficiency occurs occasionally in Northern European people.

Clinical features

G6PD deficiency is usually asymptomatic, with a normal blood count between attacks of haemolysis. The main clinical syndromes that occur with red cell G6PD levels between 2% and 60% of normal are:

1 **Acute haemolytic anaemia in response to oxidant stress**, e.g. drugs, fava beans or infections (Table 6.4). Fava beans (*Vica fava*) contain an oxidant chemical, divicine. The degree of anaemia it causes is dose related. The acute haemolytic anaemia is caused by rapidly developing intravascular haemolysis with haemoglobinuria (Fig. 6.3a). Depending on the G6PD genotype, the anaemia may be self-limiting, as new young red cells are made with near normal enzyme levels, or may be life-threatening.
2 **Neonatal jaundice**, usually without haemolysis.
3 **Rarely, a congenital non-spherocytic haemolytic anaemia.** This chronic anaemia may result from different types of severe enzyme deficiency (levels <2% of normal).

Diagnosis

During a crisis the blood film may show contracted and fragmented cells, 'bite' cells and 'blister' cells (Fig. 6.8), which have had Heinz bodies removed by the spleen. Heinz bodies (oxidized, denatured and insoluble haemoglobin that precipitates in the red cell) may be seen in the reticulocyte preparation, particularly if the spleen is absent (Fig. 2.17). There are also features of intravascular haemolysis.

Between acute crises (except in the rare cases of congenital non-spherocytic haemolytic anaemia) the blood count is

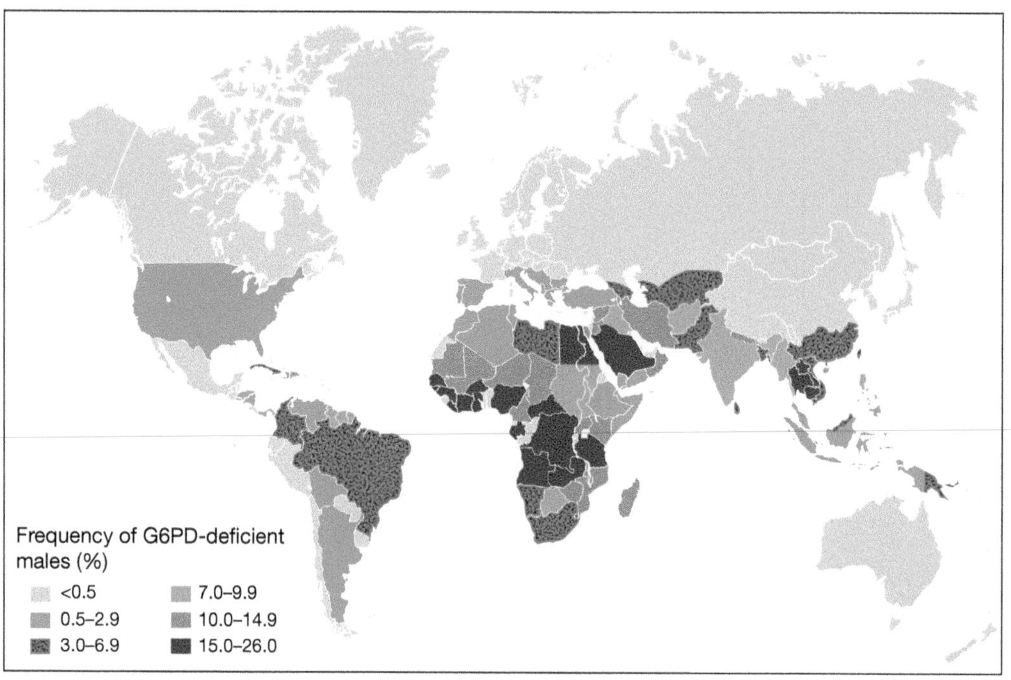

Figure 6.7 Global distribution of *G6PD* gene variants causing glucose-6-phosphate dehydrogenase (G6PD) deficiency. Shaded areas indicate the prevalence of G6PD deficiency. The distribution is similar to that of malaria; in countries where endogenous G6PD deficiency is not found, the distribution reflects immigration patterns. Source: Adapted from L. Luzzatto, R. Notaro (2001) *Science* 293: 442.

Table 6.4 Agents that may cause haemolytic anaemia in glucose-6-phosphate dehydrogenase (G6PD) deficiency.

Infections and other acute illnesses, e.g. diabetic ketoacidosis
Drugs ■ Antimalarials, e.g. primaquine, pamaquine, chloroquine, Fansidar, Maloprim, quinine ■ Sulphonamides and sulphones, e.g. co-trimoxazole, sulfanilamide, dapsone, sufasalazine ■ Other antibacterial agents, e.g. quinolones, nitrofurans, nalidixic acid, chloramphenicol, ciprofoxcin, ■ Analgesics, e.g. aspirin (moderate doses are safe) ■ Anti-helminths, e.g. β-naphthol, stibophen ■ Miscellaneous, e.g. vitamin K analogues, rasburicase, glibenclamide, isoniazid, naphthalene (mothballs), probenecid
Fava beans
Chemical oxidants

N.B. Many common drugs have been reported to precipitate haemolysis in G6PD deficiency in some patients, e.g. aspirin, quinine and penicillin, but not at conventional dosage.

normal. The enzyme deficiency is detected by one of a number of screening tests or by direct enzyme assay of red cells. Because of the higher enzyme level in young red cells in some G6PD genotypes, red cell enzyme assay may give a 'false' normal level in the phase of acute haemolysis with a reticulocyte response. Subsequent assay after the acute phase reveals the low G6PD level when the red cell population is of normal age distribution.

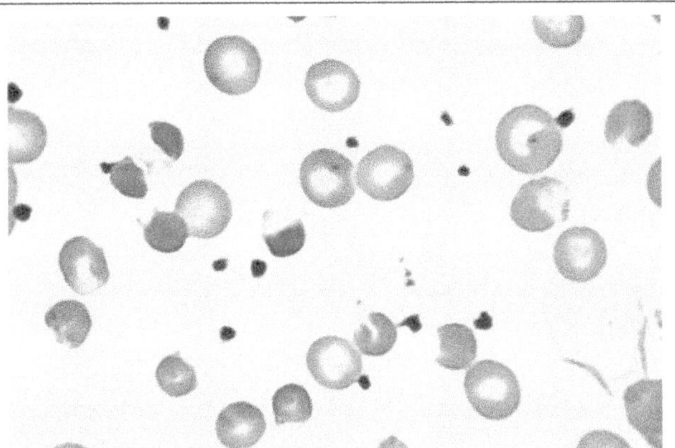

Figure 6.8 Blood film in glucose-6-phosphate dehydrogenase (G6PD) deficiency with acute haemolysis after an oxidant stress. Some of the cells show loss of cytoplasm with separation of remaining haemoglobin from the cell membrane ('blister' cells). There are also numerous contracted and deeply staining cells. Supravital staining (as for reticulocytes) showed the presence of Heinz bodies (Fig. 2.17).

Treatment

The offending drug is stopped, any underlying infection is treated, a high urine output is maintained with fluid supplementation. Blood transfusion is undertaken where necessary for severe anaemia. G6PD-deficient babies are prone to neonatal jaundice and in severe cases phototherapy and exchange transfusion is needed to avoid kernicterus (Chapter 34). The jaundice is usually not caused by excess haemolysis, but by deficiency of G6PD affecting neonatal liver function. Gilbert's syndrome (the genetic defect reducing the liver's ability to metabolise bilirubin) may also be present.

Glutathione deficiency and other syndromes

Other defects in the pentose phosphate pathway leading to similar syndromes to those of G6PD deficiency have been described – particularly defects causing glutathione deficiency.

Glycolytic (Embden–Meyerhof) pathway defects

These are all uncommon and lead to a congenital non-spherocytic haemolytic anaemia. In some there are defects of other systems e.g. a myopathy.

Pyruvate kinase deficiency

The most frequently encountered is the autosomal recessive condition pyruvate kinase deficiency (Fig. 2.11). The affected patients are homozygous or more frequently doubly heterozygous for mutations in the gene *PKLR*. Over 350 different mutations have been described. The red cells become rigid as a result of reduced adenosine triphosphate (ATP) formation. The severity of the anaemia varies widely (haemoglobin 40–100 g/L). It results in relatively mild symptoms because of a shift to the right in the oxygen-dissociation curve caused by a rise in intracellular 2,3-diphosphoglycerate (2,3-DPG). Clinically, jaundice is usual and gallstones are frequent. Frontal bossing and leg ulcers (Chapter 7) may be present. Iron loading occurs not only from transfusions but also due to raised plasma erythroferrone levels, consequent on the increased and ineffective erythropoiesis, which inhibit hepcidin synthesis. Perinatal complications including hydrops, prematurity, neonatal jaundice and anaemia are common.

The blood film shows poikilocytosis and distorted 'prickle' cells, particularly post-splenectomy. Direct enzyme assay and genomic sequencing are needed to make the diagnosis.

Treatment is with the drug Mitapivat, a small-molecule oral activator of wild and most mutant pyruvate kinases. It is associated with a rapid increase in haemoglobin in 40–50% of adults with PK deficiency. Features of haemolysis are reduced. It has only low grade and transient side effects. Responses have been durable for up to a year and longer follow up studies in adults and studies in children are ongoing. It is unclear whether the genotype predicts for response. Splenectomy may alleviate the anaemia but does not cure it. It increases the risk of infections and of venous thrombosis so is indicated only in those patients who need frequent transfusions. Iron chelation may be needed. Trials of lentivital mediated gene therapy are in progress for severe PKD deficiency.

Genetic disorders of haemoglobin synthesis

Many of these cause clinical haemolysis. They are discussed in Chapter 7.

Acquired haemolytic anaemias

Immune haemolytic anaemias

Autoimmune haemolytic anaemias

Autoimmune haemolytic anaemias (AIHAs) are caused by antibody production by the body against its own red cells. They are characterized by a positive direct antiglobulin test (DAT), also known as the Coombs' test (Fig 33.5), and divided into 'warm' and 'cold' types (Table 6.5) according to whether the antibody reacts more strongly with red cells at 37°C or 4°C.

Warm autoimmune haemolytic anaemias

In warm AIHA, red cells are coated with immunoglobulin (Ig), usually IgG alone or IgG together with complement (C3d, the degraded fragment of C3). They are taken up by RE macrophages which have receptors for the Ig Fc fragment. Part of the coated membrane is lost, so the cells becomes progressively more spherical to maintain the same volume and are ultimately prematurely destroyed, predominantly in the spleen. When the cells are coated both with IgG and complement or with complement alone, red cell destruction occurs more generally in the RE system.

Clinical features

The disease may occur at any age, with a preponderance of female patients. It presents as a haemolytic anaemia of varying severity. The spleen is often enlarged. The disease tends to remit and relapse. It may occur alone or in 50–70% of cases in association with other diseases, particularly lymphoid malignancies, infection and auto-immune disorders (Table 6.5). When associated with immune thrombocytopenic purpura (ITP), a similar condition affecting platelets (p. XXX), it is called Evans' syndrome. When secondary to systemic lupus erythematosus, the cells typically are coated with IgG and complement. A subtype typically associated with SLE or lymphoma occurs with both warm and cold type antibodies which may be lytic and cause intravascular haemolysis. In all 'idiopathic' cases, an underlying lymphoproliferative disease should be considered, and computed tomography (CT) scan of the chest, abdomen and pelvis performed.

Table 6.5 Immune haemolytic anaemias: classification.

Warm type	Cold type
Autoimmune	*Primary* ■ Cold agglutinin disease
Primary *Secondary* ■ SLE, other immune dysregulation diseases – ulcerative colitis, primary biliary cirrhosis, post-allogeneic stem cell transplantation ■ Infections, e.g. hepatitis C, HIV, Covid, pneumococcal ■ Malignancy – CLL, lymphomas, thymoma, solid organ ■ Drugs, e.g. fludarabine, cephalosporins, penicillin, methyldopa, Rh(D) immune globulin, alpha interferon ■ Pregnancy	*Secondary* ■ Infections – *Mycoplasma* pneumonia, infectious mononucleosis ■ Malignancy – lymphoma, CLL, solid organ ■ Post-allogeneic stem cell transplantation *Paroxysmal cold haemoglobinuria* (rare, sometimes associated with infections, e.g. adenovirus, influenza, Covid, syphilis)
Alloimmune	
Induced by red cell antigens	
■ Haemolytic transfusion reactions ■ Haemolytic disease of the newborn ■ Post-allogeneic stem cell grafts	
Drug induced	
■ Drug–red cell membrane complex ■ Immune complex	

CLL, chronic lymphocytic leukaemia; HIV, human immunodeficiency virus; SLE, systemic lupus erythematosus.

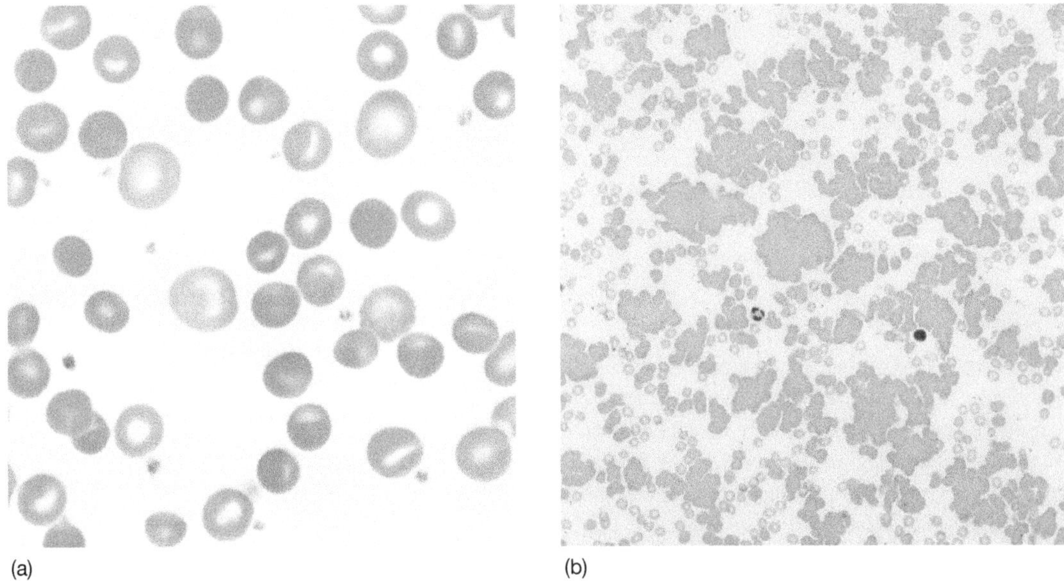

Figure 6.9 (a) Blood film in warm autoimmune haemolytic anaemia. Numerous microspherocytes are present and larger polychromatic cells (reticulocytes). **(b)** Blood film in cold autoimmune haemolytic anaemia. Marked red cell agglutination is present in films made at room temperature. The background is caused by the raised plasma protein concentration.

Laboratory findings

The haematological and biochemical findings are typical of an extravascular haemolytic anaemia. The blood film shows the presence of micro-spherocytes, polychromasia due to the reticulocytosis (Fig. 6.9a) and in some nucleated red cells. In severe cases, there are also features of intravascular haemolysis. The serum LDH may be raised and can be used to monitor response to therapy.

The DAT is positive as a result of IgG, IgG and complement (C3d), IgA or even more rarely complement (C3d) alone on the cells. In some cases, the autoantibody shows specificity within the Rh system. The antibodies both on the cell surface and free in serum are best detected at 37°C. Rare cases are DAT negative, e.g. if the surface antibody titre is too low to be detected by the assay. On the other hand, about 5% of patients in hospital show a weakly positive DAT test, usually due to complement only on the surface of red cells, without any evidence of haemolysis.

Treatment

1 **Remove the underlying cause** if one is present, e.g. drug. If an underlying disease is present, e.g. chronic lymphocytic leukaemia or lymphoma, it may be necessary to treat the underlying condition to adequately control the haemolysis.
2 **Corticosteroids**. Prednisolone is the usual first-line treatment; 1–2 mg/kg/day is a typical starting dose in adults and should then be tapered down with monitoring of the blood count and serum LDH. Those with predominantly IgG on red cells do best, whereas those with complement often respond poorly to both corticosteroids and splenectomy. While high-dose dexamethasone has been effective in ITP, it is less well tested and not established in AIHA. Antacid therapy with e.g. a proton pump inhibitor should be given. If steroid therapy is prolonged for over 3 months, especially for those over 40 years, prophylaxis against fractures is considered with vitamin D and calcium supplements and possibly with an oral bisphosphonate.
3 **Monoclonal antibody**. Anti-CD20 (rituximab) has produced prolonged remissions in a proportion of cases and may be used with steroids as first-line therapy. Prolonged use leads to immunosuppression with susceptibility to infection.
4 **Splenectomy** may be of value in those who fail to respond well or fail to maintain a satisfactory haemoglobin level on an acceptably small, e.g. <15 mg daily steroid dosage or rituximab maintenance
5 **Immunosuppression** may be tried after the above measures have failed or even before splenectomy. Azathioprine, bortezomib, cyclophosphamide, chlorambucil, ciclosporin and mycophenolate mofetil have all been tried with varying success. The three drug combination of low-dose rituximab with dexamethasone and the proteasome inhibitor bortezomib has also been used. Anti-CD52 (alemtuzumab) may be tried third line or later.
6 **Folic acid** is essential in severe and chronic cases.
7 **Blood transfusion** may be needed if anaemia is severe and causing symptoms. The blood should be the least

incompatible and, if the specificity of the autoantibody is known, donor blood is chosen that lacks the relevant antigen(s). The patients also readily make alloantibodies against donor red cells, so donor red cells phenotypically matched as far possible to the recipient are used. It may be challenging for the blood bank to match blood cells.

8 **High-dose immunoglobulin** has been used but with less success than in ITP.

9 **Venous thrombosis prophylaxis** is usually indicated.

Cold autoimmune haemolytic anaemias

In these syndromes, the IgM autoantibody attaches to red cells, mainly in the peripheral circulation where the blood temperature is cooled (Table 6.5). The autoantibody may be **monoclonal**, as in primary cold haemagglutinin syndrome or associated with lymphoproliferative disorders, or may be a transient **polyclonal** response following infections such as infectious mononucleosis or *Mycoplasma* pneumonia. The IgM antibodies, which bind to red cells optimally at 4°C, are highly efficient at fixing complement such that intravascular and extravascular haemolysis can occur. The clinical severity reflects the thermal amplitude of the specific antibody; antibodies that continue to bind at higher temperatures are more dangerous than those that only bind at colder temperatures. Only complement can be detected on red cells in laboratory tests, as the IgM antibody is eluted off as cells flow through warmer parts of the circulation.

The cold agglutinin titre is usually high, typically >1: 512. Low-titre cold agglutinins are widespread and of no clinical significance. In nearly all these cold AIHA syndromes, the antibody is directed against the 'I' antigen on the red cell surface. In infectious mononucleosis, it is anti-i. Underlying lymphoma should be excluded in all 'idiopathic' cases.

Primary cold agglutinin disease

In this disease, the patient has a chronic haemolytic anaemia aggravated by the cold and often associated with intravascular haemolysis. Mild jaundice and splenomegaly may be present. The patient may develop acrocyanosis (purplish skin discoloration) at the tip of the nose, ears, fingers and toes caused by the agglutination of red cells in small vessels.

Laboratory findings are similar to those of warm AIHA, except that spherocytosis is less marked, red cells agglutinate in the cold (Fig. 6.9b) and the DAT reveals complement (C3d) only on the red cell surface. In most patients, nodules of a monoclonal population of B lymphocytes are present in the bone marrow. Their morphology and immunophenotype differ from those in lympho-plasmacytic lymphoma, also associated with an IgM paraprotein; the *MYD88* mutation characteristic of that disease is absent. Serum protein electrophoresis reveals the presence of a monoclonal IgM kappa protein unless the level is too low to be detected. Cold agglutinin disease is indolent but may transform to an aggressive lymphoma.

Treatment involves keeping the patient warm. Plasmapheresis may be needed initially to treat hyperviscosity. Rituximab is the best first-line therapy alone. With bendamustine it gives longer term remission but, because of concern about infection, the combination is avoided in the elderly. Bortezomib-based therapy is also used. Alkylating drugs, e.g. chlorambucil or cyclophosphamide, are given as second-line therapy. Inhibition of complement C5 with eculizumab (monoclonal antibody) or pegcetacoplan (pegylated peptide) which inhibits complement C3 (both also used to treat paroxysmal nocturnal haemoglobinuria) may also be effective (Chapter 24). Sutimlimab, which inhibits complement C1s (p. 124), is an alternative second line therapy. Splenectomy is not indicated unless massive splenomegaly is present. Corticosteroids are of less value than in warm antibody AIHA.

Paroxysmal cold haemoglobinuria is a rare syndrome of acute intravascular haemolysis after exposure to the cold. It is caused by the Donath–Landsteiner antibody, an IgG antibody with specificity for the P blood group antigens, which binds to red cells in the cold but causes lysis with complement in warm conditions. Viral infections are predisposing causes and the condition is usually self-limiting. In the past this condition was associated with advanced syphilis.

Alloimmune haemolytic anaemias

In these anaemias, antibody produced by one individual reacts with red cells of another. Three important situations are transfusion of ABO-incompatible blood (Chapter 33), Rh disease of the newborn (Chapter 34) and after allogeneic transplantation (Chapter 25). The increased use of allogeneic transplantation for renal, hepatic, cardiac and bone diseases has led to the recognition of alloimmune haemolytic anaemia, resulting from the destruction of red cells of the recipient by antibodies produced by donor lymphocytes. This occurs with haemopoietic stem cell transplantation before the blood group of the recipient becomes that of the donor (Chapter 25).

Some batches of anti-D immunoglobulin used to treat immune thrombocytopenia have caused intravascular haemolysis within 24 hours in RhD-positive recipients. The doses are much higher than those used to prevent Rh sensitization which are safe from this side effect.

Drug-induced immune haemolytic anaemias

Drugs may cause immune haemolytic anaemias via three mechanisms (Fig. 6.10):

1 Antibody directed against a drug–red cell membrane complex, e.g. penicillin, ampicillin; this only occurs with massive doses of these antibiotics.

2 Deposition of complement via a drug–protein (antigen) – antibody complex onto the red cell surface, e.g. quinidine, rifampicin.

3 A true autoimmune haemolytic anaemia in which the role of the drug is unclear, e.g. fludarabine.

In each case, the haemolytic anaemia gradually disappears when the drug is discontinued.

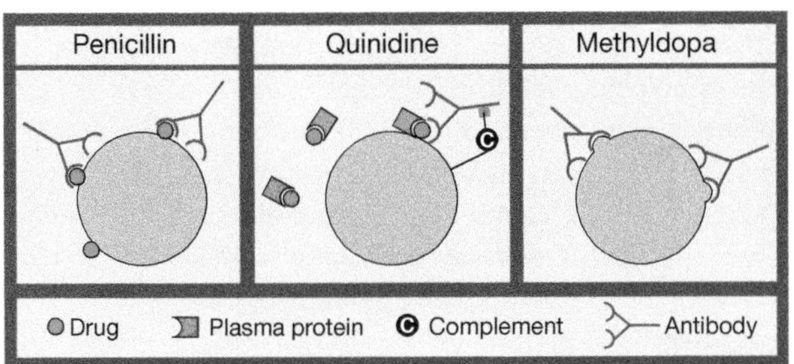

Figure 6.10 Three different mechanisms of drug-induced immune haemolytic anaemia. In each case the coated (opsonized) cells are destroyed in the reticuloendothelial system.

Table 6.6 Red cell fragmentation syndromes.

Cardiac haemolysis	Prosthetic heart valves Patches, grafts Perivalvular leaks
Arteriovenous malformations	Kasabach–Merritt syndrome, giant haemangiomas and others
Microangiopathic	TTP-HUS Disseminated intravascular coagulation Malignant disease Vasculitis, e.g. polyarteritis nodosa, systemic lupus erythematosus Malignant hypertension Pre-eclampsia/HELLP syndrome Renal vascular disorders Ciclosporin Homograft rejection

HELLP, haemolysis with elevated liver function tests and low platelets; HUS, haemolytic-uraemic syndrome; TTP, thrombotic thrombocytopenic purpura.

Red cell fragmentation syndromes

These arise through physical damage to red cells either on abnormal surfaces, e.g. artificial heart valves or arterial grafts, arteriovenous malformations or by red cells passing through abnormal small vessels, **microangiopathic haemolytic anaemia (MAHA)**. The abnormality may be caused by deposition of fibrin strands, often associated with disseminated intravascular coagulation (DIC), or platelet adherence, as in thrombotic thrombocytopenic purpura (TTP; Chapter 29), or vasculitis, e.g. polyarteritis nodosa (Table 6.6).Mucin secreting carcinomas and acute leukaemia (especially promyelocytic) are particularly associated with a MAHA. The peripheral blood contains many deeply staining red cell fragments (Fig. 6.11). When DIC underlies the haemolysis, clotting abnormalities and a low platelet count are also present. TTP is discussed in detail in Chapter 29.

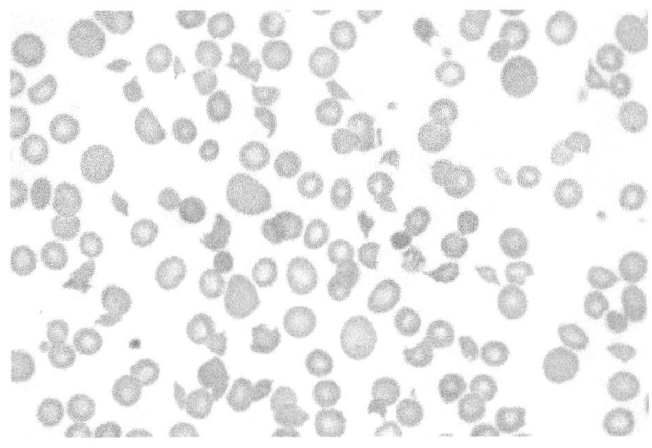

Figure 6.11 Blood film in microangiopathic haemolytic anaemia (in this patient Gram-negative septicaemia). Numerous contracted and deeply staining cells and cell fragments are present.

March haemoglobinuria

This is caused by damage to red cells between the small bones of the feet, usually during prolonged marching or running. It can be prevented by using soft shoes and running on soft ground. The blood film does not show fragments but haemoglobinuria may occur.

Infections

Infections can cause haemolysis in a variety of ways. They may precipitate an acute haemolytic crisis in G6PD deficiency or cause intravascular thrombosis and microangiopathic haemolytic anaemia, e.g. with meningococcal or pneumococcal septicaemia. Malaria causes haemolysis by extravascular destruction of parasitized red cells as well as by direct intravascular lysis. Blackwater fever is an acute intravascular haemolysis accompanied by acute renal failure caused by *Falciparum* malaria. *Clostridium perfringens* septicaemia can cause intravascular haemolysis with marked microspherocytosis. Tick-borne illnesses such as babesiosis can also enter red cells and cause haemolysis, which is usually not as severe as in malaria.

Chemical and physical agents

Certain drugs, e.g. dapsone and sulfasalazine, in high doses cause oxidative intravascular haemolysis with Heinz body formation in normal subjects. In Wilson disease, an acute haemolytic anaemia can occur as a result of high levels of copper in the blood. Chemical poisoning, e.g. with lead, chlorate or arsine, can cause severe haemolysis. Severe burns damage red cells, causing acanthocytosis or spherocytosis.

Secondary haemolytic anaemias

In many systemic disorders, such as inflammatory bowel disease or rheumatological syndromes, red cell survival is modestly shortened. This may contribute to anaemia (Chapter 32).

SUMMARY

- Haemolytic anaemia is caused by shortening of the red cell life. The red cells may break down in the reticuloendothelial system (extravascular) or in the circulation (intravascular).
- Haemolytic anaemia may be caused by inherited red cell defects, which are usually intrinsic to the red cell, or to acquired causes, which are usually caused by an abnormality of the red cell environment.
- Features of extravascular haemolysis include jaundice, gallstones and splenomegaly with raised reticulocytes, unconjugated serum bilirubin and absent haptoglobins. In intravascular haemolysis, e.g. caused by ABO mismatched blood transfusion, there is haemoglobinaemia, methaemalbuminaemia, haemoglobinuria and haemosiderinuria.
- Genetic defects include those of the red cell membrane, e.g. hereditary spherocytosis or elliptocytosis; enzyme deficiencies, e.g. glucose-6-phosphate dehydrogenase or pyruvate kinase deficiency; or haemoglobin defects, e.g. sickle cell disease.
- Acquired causes of haemolytic anaemia include warm or cold, auto- or allo-antibodies to red cells, red cell fragmentation syndromes, infections, toxins and paroxysmal nocturnal haemoglobinuria (Chapter 24).

Now visit **www.wiley.com/go/haematology9e** to test yourself on this chapter.

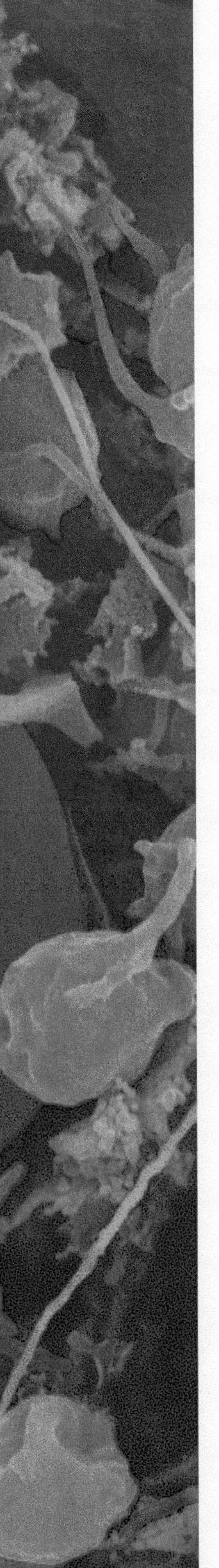

CHAPTER 7

Genetic disorders of haemoglobin

Key topics

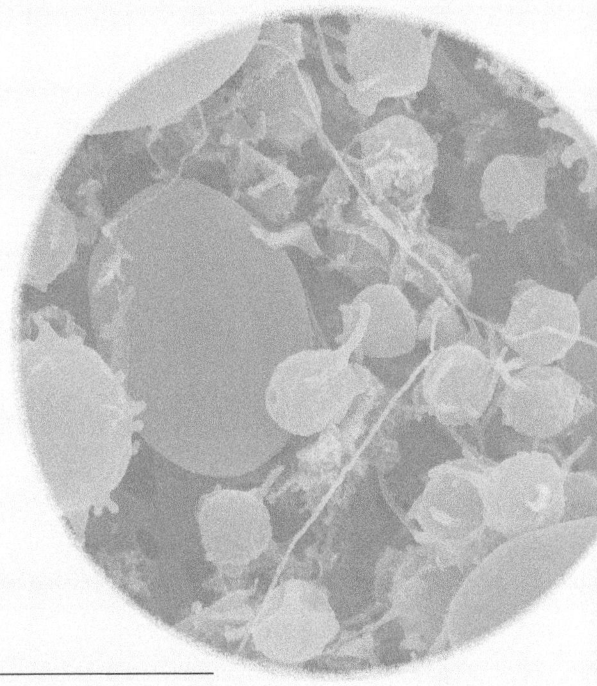

Hoffbrand's Essential Haematology, Ninth Edition. A. Victor Hoffbrand, Pratima Chowdary, Graham P. Collins, and Justin Loke.

© 2024 John Wiley & Sons Ltd. Published 2024 by John Wiley & Sons Ltd.

Companion website: www.wiley.com/go/haematology9e

This chapter discusses inherited diseases caused by reduced or abnormal synthesis of globin, the protein component of the haemoglobin molecule. Mutations in globin genes are the most prevalent monogenic disorders worldwide and affect approximately 7% of the world's population.

Haemoglobin synthesis during human development

Normal adult blood contains three types of haemoglobin (Hb), (Table 2.3). The major component is Hb A, with the molecular structure $\alpha_2\beta_2$, i.e. two α and two β globin chains forming a tetramer. The minor haemoglobins in adult blood are foetal Hb (HbF), $(\alpha_2\gamma_2)$ and Hb $A_2(\alpha_2\delta_2)$. Hb A_2 normally represents 1.5–3.5% of total adult haemoglobin and Hb F about 0.5%.

In the embryo and foetus, Hb Gower 1 (the primary embryonic haemoglobin) and Hb F dominate at different stages (Fig 7.1). Minor haemoglobins detectable at early stages of gestation include Hb Portland and Hb Gower 2. These haemoglobins include ζ- and e-globins instead of α- and β-globins.

Molecular aspects of haemoglobin synthesis

The genes for the globin chains and their regulatory elements occur in two clusters: e, γ, δ and β (the 'β-globin cluster') located on chromosome 11q, and ζ and α (the 'α-globin cluster') on chromosome 16p. Several inactive globin pseudogenes also form part of these globin gene clusters. Two types of γ-globin occur, Gγ and Aγ, which are interchangeable and differ by having either a glycine or an alanine amino acid at position

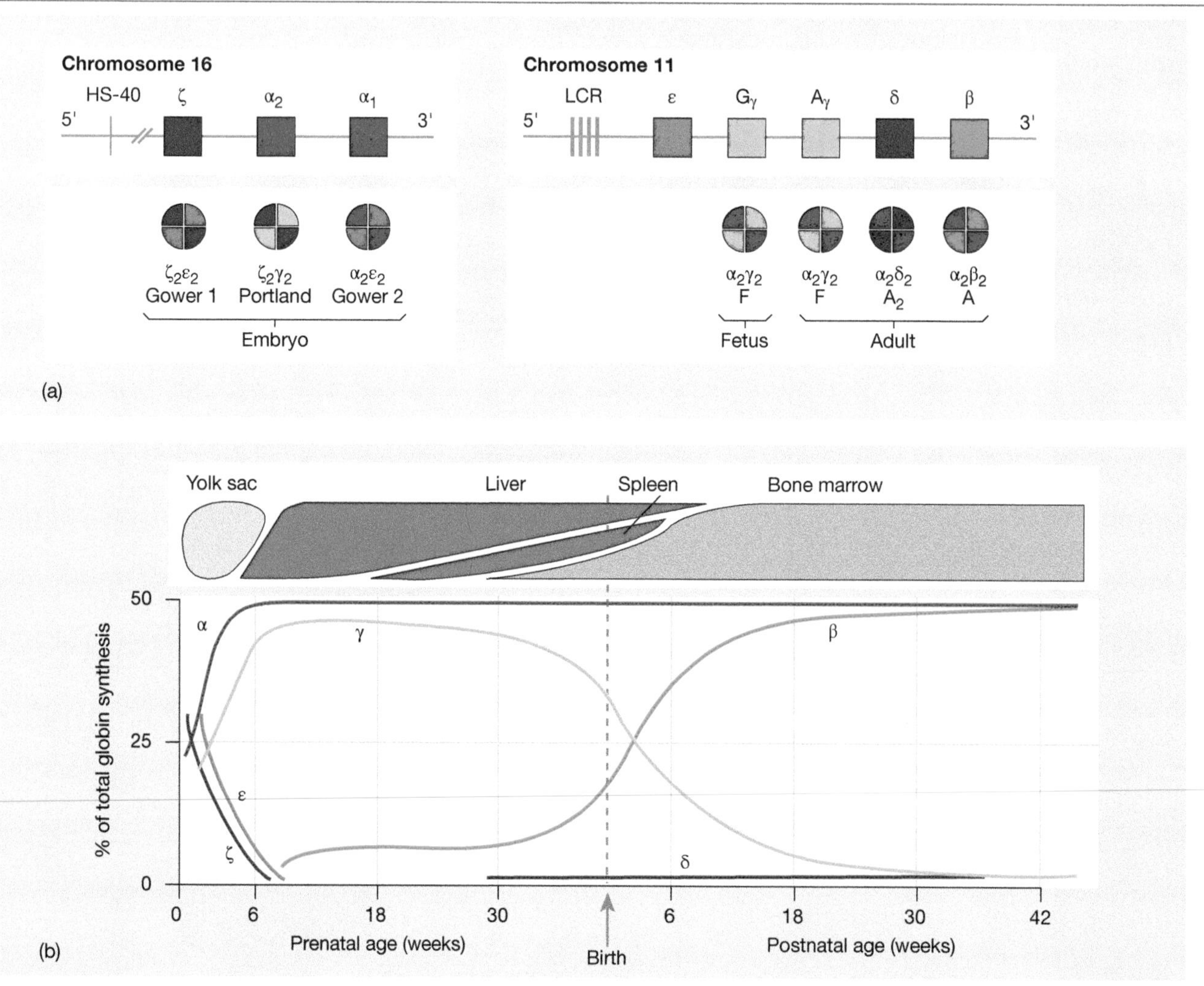

Figure 7.1 (a) The globin gene clusters on chromosomes 16p and 11q. In embryonic, foetal and adult life, different genes are activated or suppressed. The different globin chains are synthesized independently and then combine with each other to produce the different haemoglobins. The γ gene may have two sequences, which code for either a glutamic acid or alanine residue at position 136 (Gγ or Aγ, respectively). LCR, locus control region; HS-40, see text for description. **(b)** Synthesis of individual globin chains in prenatal and postnatal life.

136 in the polypeptide chain. The α-globin gene is duplicated, and both α genes (α_1 and α_2) on each chromosome 16 are active. Thus, in health there are four α-globin genes and two β-globin genes (Fig. 7.1); the cell regulates expression of these genes such that α- and β-globin protein synthesis is balanced.

All the globin genes have three exons (coding regions) and two introns (non-coding regions whose DNA is not represented in the finished protein). An initial globin RNA is transcribed from both introns and exons, and from this transcript the RNA derived from introns is removed by splicing (Fig. 7.2). Introns almost always begin with a G-T dinucleotide and end with an A-G dinucleotide; the introns in the globin genes are typical in this regard. The pre-mRNA splicing machinery recognizes these sequences as well as neighbouring conserved sequences and excises the introns from the newly formed transcript. The subsequent mature mRNA resulting from transcription is polyadenylated at the 3′ end (Fig. 7.2) and this stabilizes it. Thalassaemia may arise from mutations or deletions of any of these sequences.

A number of other conserved regulatory sequences are important in globin synthesis, and mutations at these sites may also give rise to thalassaemia by reducing synthesis of one or other of the globin chains. These regulatory sequences influence gene transcription, ensure its fidelity, specify sites for the initiation and termination of transcription, and ensure the stability of newly synthesized mRNA.

Promoters are found 5′ of the gene. Enhancers occur either 5′ or 3′ to the gene and are important in the tissue-specific regulation of globin gene expression and in regulation of the synthesis

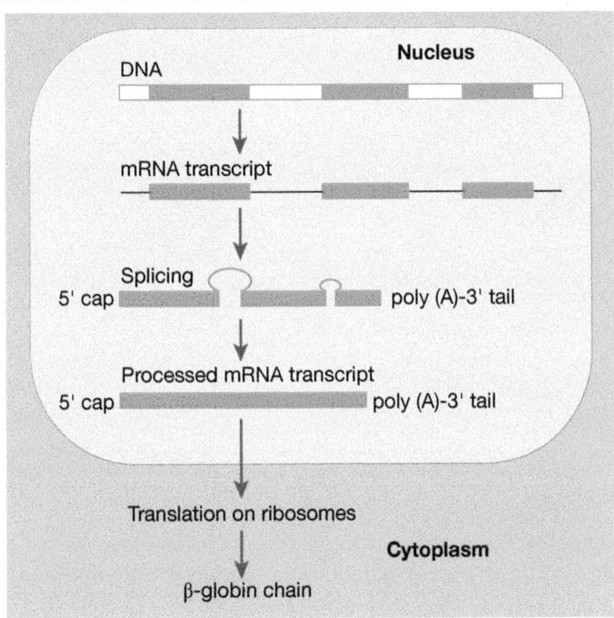

Figure 7.2 The expression of a human β-globin gene from transcription, excision of introns, splicing of exons, and translation to ribosomes. The primary transcript is 'capped' at the 5′ end and a poly-A tail is then added.

of the various globin chains during foetal and postnatal life. The locus control region (LCR) is a genetic regulatory element situated upstream of the β-globin cluster, which controls genetic activity at this cluster by opening up the chromatin to allow several key transcription factors to bind (Fig. 7.1). A similar region, called HS-40 approximately 40 kilobases 5′ to the α- gene cluster regulates α-globin synthesis. Four multispecies conserved regions (MCS-Rs) 1, 2, 3 and 4 in this region are the upstream erythroid-specific enhancers of the α-globin cluster, comparable to the LCR for the globin cluster. In addition, transcription factors such as GATA1 that bind to α– and β-globin gene regulatory sequences but are encoded on other chromosomes are important in globin synthesis and mutations of them can cause altered globin synthesis and a thalassaemia syndrome.

Switch from foetal to adult haemoglobin

The globin genes are arranged on chromosomes 11 and 16 in the order in which they are expressed in development (Fig. 7.1). Embryonic haemoglobins are usually only expressed in yolk sac erythroblasts. **The β-globin gene is expressed at a low level in early foetal life, but the main switch to adult haemoglobin occurs 3–6 months after birth, when synthesis of the γ chain is largely replaced by β chains.** This explains why clinical defects in β-globin synthesis may not be detected at birth but are usually manifest by the end of the first year of life. The switch from γ- to β-gene expression involves both silencing of the γ-genes and competition between the γ- and β-genes for the β-globin LCR. Expression of the adult β-globin gene depends on lack of competition from the upstream γ gene for the LCR sequences. Failure of silencing of the γ gene due to point mutations in their promoter causes persistence of foetal haemoglobin production, with downregulation of expression of the β gene.

BCL11A is a major transcriptional regulator of this switch. It is activated by the transcription factor KFL1 which plays key role in binding to the LCR not only indirectly switching off γ-globin synthesis but also activating β-globin synthesis. Other nuclear transcriptional factors are involved. The methylation state of cytosine bases (expressed genes are associated with hypomethylated cytosine bases in the promoter regions, non-expressed with hypermethylated cytosine bases), the state of the chromosome packaging, i.e. status of histone proteins and of DNA enhancer sequences all play a part in determining whether a particular gene will be transcribed.

Haemoglobin abnormalities

These result from the following:

1 **Synthesis of an abnormal haemoglobin with an altered amino acid sequence.**
2 **Reduced rate of synthesis of normal α- or β-globin chains (the α- and β-thalassaemias, Fig. 7.3), leading to a globin deficit and imbalance.**

Table 7.1 shows some of the abnormal haemoglobins that arise from synthesis of an α- or β-globin chain with an amino acid substitution. Clinically the most important is sickle cell disease,

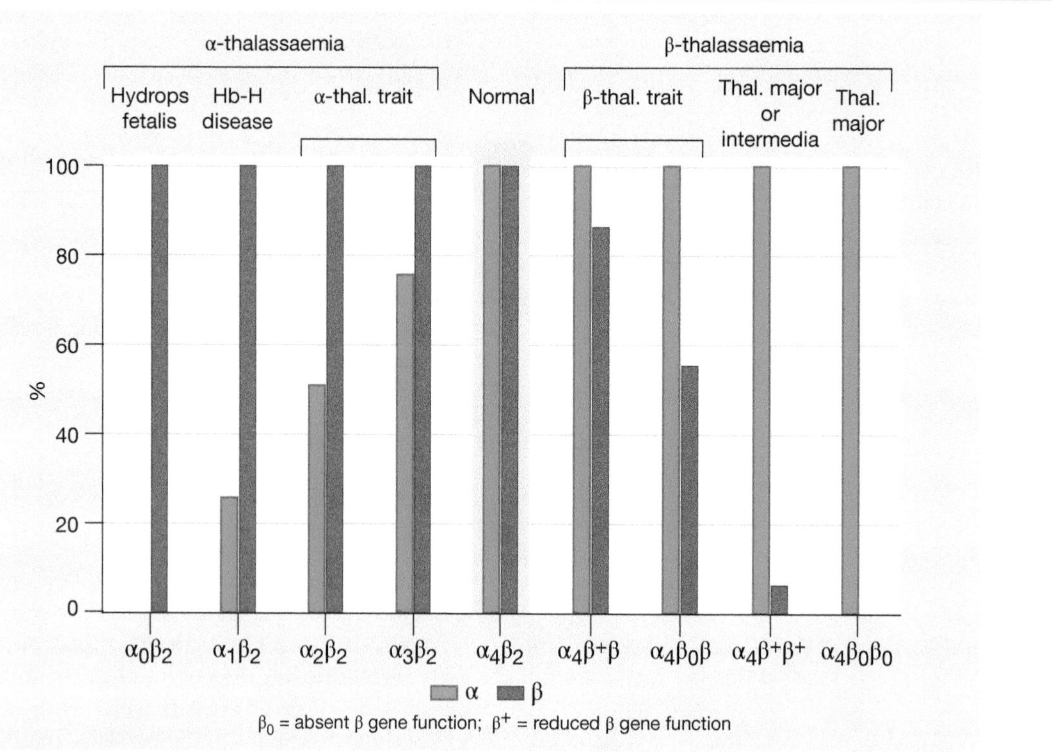

Figure 7.3 The ratio of α- : β-globin chain synthesis (*y*-axis) depending on the number of functioning α- and β-chain genes (*x*-axis). Source: A.B. Mehta, A.V. Hoffbrand (2014) *Haematology at a Glance*, 4th edn. Reproduced with permission of John Wiley & Sons.

Table 7.1 The clinical syndromes produced by haemoglobin abnormalities.

Syndrome	Abnormality
Haemolysis	Crystalline haemoglobins (Hb S, C, D, E, etc.) Unstable haemoglobins, e.g. Hb Köln, Hb Zurich resulting in 'Heinz body' congenital haemolytic anaemias
Thalassaemia	α- or β-thalassaemia, resulting from reduced and imbalanced globin synthesis
Familial polycythaemia (erythrocytosis)	Altered oxygen affinity, e.g. Hb Chesapeake, Hb Montefiore
Methaemoglobinaemia	Failure of reduction (various types of Hb M)

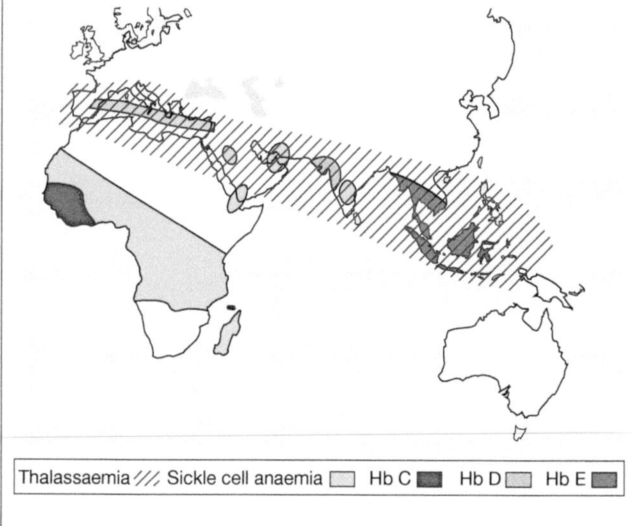

Figure 7.4 The geographical distribution of the thalassaemias and the more common, inherited, structural haemoglobin abnormalities.

resulting most commonly from homozygous Hb S, described further below. Hb C, D and E are also common and, like Hb S, result from DNA sequence variants leading to amino acid changes in the β chain and altered physicochemical properties. Hb C is found most commonly in persons of sub-Saharan African origin, while HbD Punjab (Los Angeles), the most frequent type of HbD, is detected frequently in western China and South Asia, Hb E in South-East Asia (Fig. 7.4).

Unstable haemoglobins are a rare cause of a chronic haemolytic anaemia of varying severity with intravascular haemolysis

(Table 6.2). Heinz bodies represent denatured haemoglobin resulting from the instability and can be detected in blood films with use of special stains. Abnormal haemoglobins may also cause (familial) polycythaemia or erythrocytosis (Chapter 15) or congenital methaemoglobinaemia (Chapter 2). Many amino acid substitutions in haemoglobin are of no clinical consequence.

The genetic defects of haemoglobin are the most common genetic disorders worldwide. They occur primarily in tropical and sub-tropical areas (Fig. 7.4) and most appear to have been selected because the carrier state affords some protection against malaria.

Thalassaemias

These are a heterogeneous group of genetic disorders that result from a reduced rate of synthesis of α- or β-globin chains (Fig. 7.3, Table 7.2). β-Thalassaemia is more common in the Mediterranean region, while α-thalassaemia is more common in South and South-East Asia (Fig. 7.4).

Clinically the three main syndromes are transfusion-dependent **thalassaemia major**, non-transfusion-dependent thalassaemia (**thalassaemia intermedia**) with a moderate degree of anaemia due to a variety of genetic defects (Table **7.3**) and **thalassaemia minor**, usually due to a carrier state for α- or β-thalassaemia and characterized by erythrocyte microcytosis and mild or no anaemia.

α-Thalassaemia syndromes

These are caused by α-globin gene deletions or less frequently mutations (Table 7.2). The clinical severity is related to the number of the four α-globin genes missing or inactive. Loss of all four genes completely suppresses α chain synthesis (Fig. 7.5) and because the α chain is essential for foetal as well as adult haemoglobin, this is incompatible with life and leads to death usually *in utero* as **hydrops fetalis** (Fig. 7.6).

Hb H disease is due to deletion of three of the four α genes. There is a moderately severe (haemoglobin 70–110 g/L) microcytic, hypochromic anaemia (Fig. 7.7) with splenomegaly. Erythropoiesis is effective and iron loading is not a problem. Haemoglobin H is a tetramer of self-associating β-globin chains (β_4) which can be detected in red cells of these patients by electrophoresis (Fig. 7.12) or in reticulocyte preparations (Fig. 7.7). In foetal and early infant life, before β-globin chains are produced at high levels, **Hb Bart's** (γ_4) occurs.

The α-**thalassaemia traits** are caused by loss of one or two α-globin genes and are usually not associated with anaemia. The mean corpuscular volume (MCV) and mean corpuscular haemoglobin (MCH) are low and the red cell count is over 5.5×10^{12}/L. Haemoglobin electrophoresis is usually normal so DNA analysis is needed to be certain of the diagnosis. Uncommon non-deletional forms of α-thalassaemia are caused by point mutations causing dysfunction of the genes, or rarely by

Table 7.2 Classification of thalassaemia*

Clinical syndromes

Hydrops fetalis
- Four-gene-deletion α-thalassaemia

Thalassaemia major
- Transfusion dependent; resulting from homozygous β0-thalassaemia or other combinations of β-thalassaemia trait

Thalassaemia intermedia (non-transfusion-dependent thalassaemia)
- Many potential genetic mechanisms; see Table 7.3

Thalassaemia minor
- β^0-thalassaemia trait
- β^+-thalassaemia trait
- α^0-thalassaemia trait
- α^+ thalassaemia trait

Genetic type	Haplotype	Heterozygous thalassaemia trait (minor)**	Homozygous
α-Thalassaemias†			
α^0	– –/	MCV, MCH low	Hydrops fetalis
α^+	–α/	MCV, MCH minimally reduced	As heterozygous α^0-thalassaemia
			Compound heterozygote $\alpha^0\alpha^+$ (– –/–α) is haemoglobin H disease
β-Thalassaemias			
β^0		MCV, MCH low (Hb A_2 >3.5%)	Thalassaemia major (Hb F 98%, Hb A_2 2%)
β^+		MCV, MCH low (Hb A_2 >3.5%)	Thalassaemia major or intermedia (Hb F 70–80%, Hb A 10–20%, Hb A_2 variable)

* See text for the less common diseases: δβ-thalassaemia, Hb Lepore and dominant β-thalassaemia trait.
** α^0 = 2 α genes deleted or mutated, α^+ = one α gene deleted or mutated.

Table 7.3 Thalassaemia intermedia: (non-transfusion dependent thalassaemia) – a clinical syndrome resulting from many genotypes.

With homozygous β-thalassaemia
Homozygous or compound heterozygotes with mild (β+) thalassaemia. Coinheritance of α-thalassaemia
Enhanced ability to make foetal haemoglobin (γ chain production)
With heterozygous β-thalassaemia
Coinheritance of additional α-globin genes (ααα/αα or ααα/ααα) increasing globin imbalance. Dominant β-thalassaemia trait
δβ-thalassaemia and hereditary persistence of foetal haemoglobin
Homozygous δβ-thalassaemia
Heterozygous δβ-thalassaemia/β-thalassaemia. Homozygous Hb Lepore (some cases)
Haemoglobin E/β-thalassaemia compound heterozygote (some cases)
Haemoglobin H disease

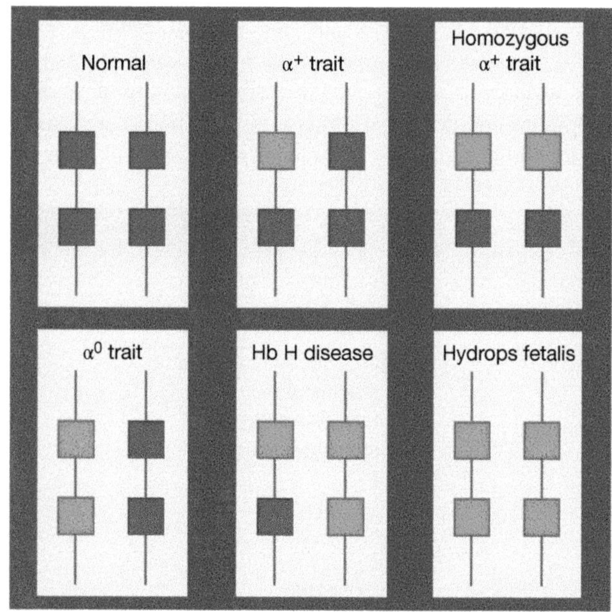

Figure 7.5 The genetics of α-thalassaemia. Each α gene may be deleted or (less frequently) dysfunctional. The orange boxes represent normal genes, and the blue boxes represent gene deletions or dysfunctional genes.

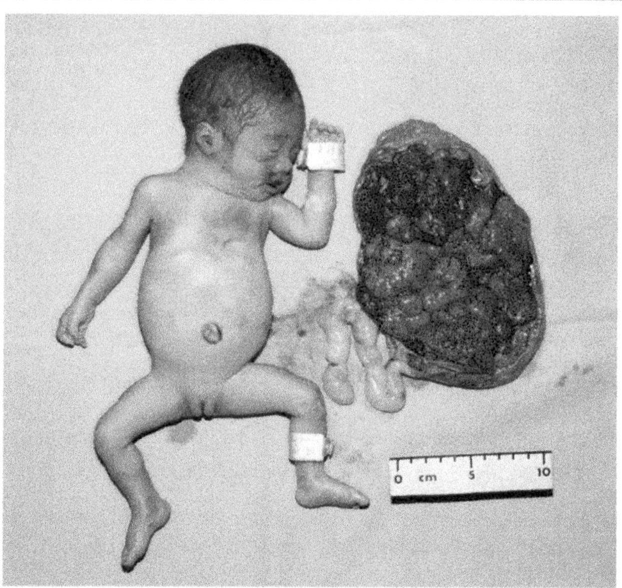

Figure 7.6 α-Thalassaemia: hydrops fetalis, the result of the deletion of all four α-globin genes (homozygous α^0-thalassaemia). The main haemoglobin present is Hb Bart's (γ_4). The condition is incompatible with life beyond the foetal stage. Source: Courtesy of Professor D. Todd.

mutations affecting termination of translation, which give rise to an elongated but unstable chain, e.g. Hb Constant Spring.

Two rare forms of α-thalassaemia are associated with developmental neurological abnormalities. They are caused by small germline chromosomal deletions resulting in a loss of a group of genes on chromosome 16, including the α-globin cluster (ATR-16 syndrome), or by mutation of a gene on chromosome X (*ATRX*) that controls the transcription of globin and other genes; the latter only affects males. α-Thalassaemia has also been described in myelodysplastic syndromes due to an acquired mutation in the *ATRX* gene.

β-Thalassaemia syndromes

β-Thalassaemia major

This condition occurs on average in one in four offspring if both parents are carriers of the β-thalassaemia trait. Either no β chain (β^0) or small amounts (β^+) are synthesized

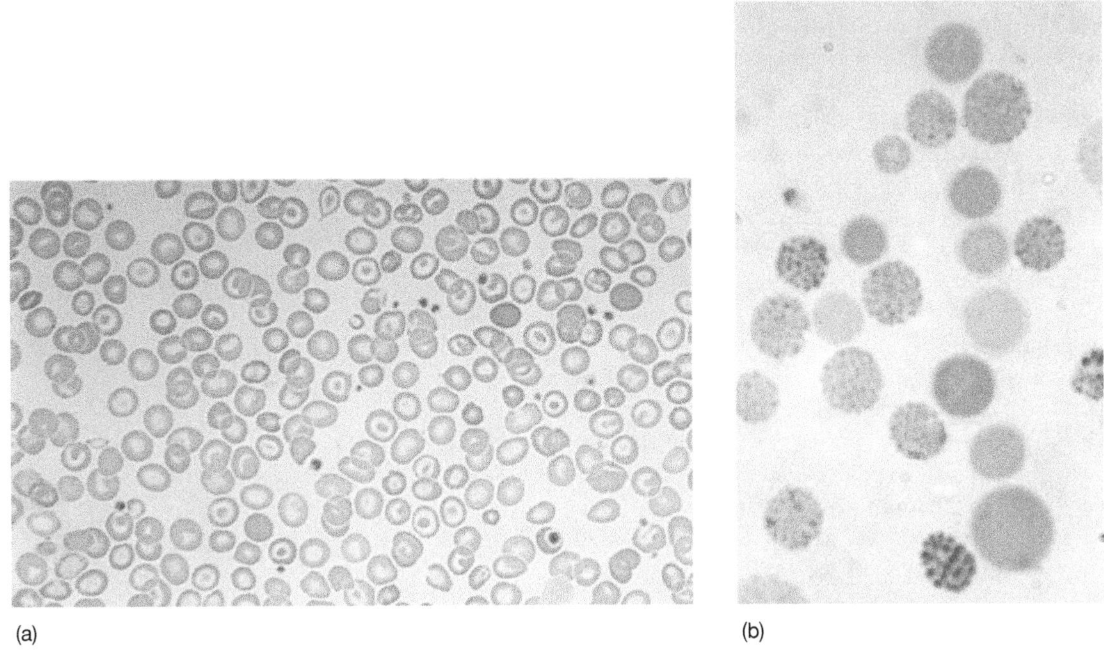

Figure 7.7 **(a)** α-Thalassaemia: Hb H disease (three α-globin gene deletion). The blood film shows marked hypochromic, microcytic cells with target cells and poikilocytosis. **(b)** α-Thalassaemia: Hb H disease. Supravital staining with brilliant cresyl blue or methylene blue reveals multiple fine, deeply stained deposits ('golf ball' cells) caused by precipitation of aggregates of β-globin chains. Hb H can also be detected as a fast-moving band on haemoglobin electrophoresis (see Fig. 7.12).

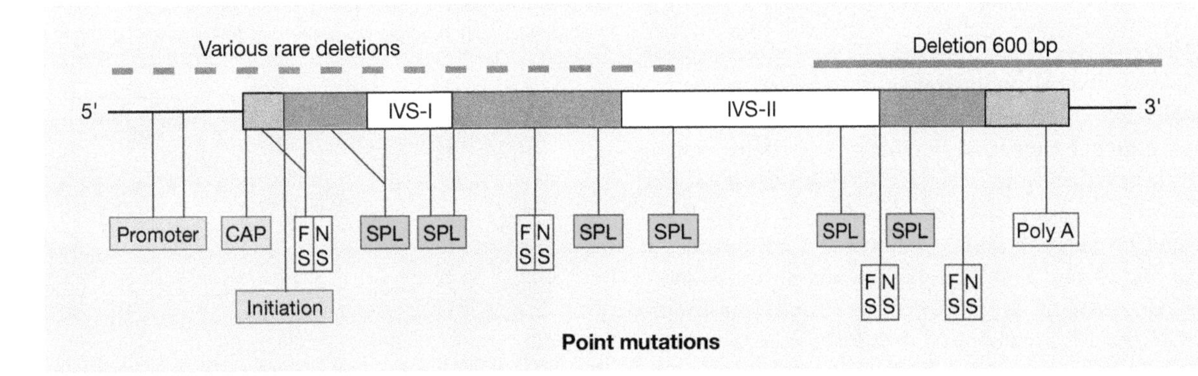

Figure 7.8 Examples of mutations that produce β-thalassaemia. These include single base changes, small deletions and insertions of one or two bases affecting introns, exons or the flanking regions of the β-globin gene. FS, 'frameshifts': deletion of nucleotide(s) that places the reading frame out of phase downstream of the lesion; NS, 'nonsense': premature chain termination as a result of a new translational stop codon, e.g. UAA; SPL, 'splicing': inactivation of splicing or new splice sites generated (aberrant splicing) in exons or introns; promoter, CAP, initiation: reduction of transcription or translation as a result of lesion in promoter, CAP or initiation regions; Poly A, mutations on the polyadenylation addition signal resulting in failure of poly A addition and an unstable mRNA.

(Fig. 7.3). Excess unpaired α chains precipitate in erythroblasts and in mature red cells and generate reactive cytotoxic oxidant species causing severe ineffective erythropoiesis and chronic haemolysis that are typical of this disease. The greater the α chain excess, the more severe the anaemia. Production of γ chains helps to 'mop up' some excess α chains and to ameliorate the condition. Also a protein in red cells, α-haemoglobin stabilizing protein (AHSP), cleared by autophagy helps to clear excess α-globin chains.

Unlike α-thalassaemia, the majority of genetic lesions in β-thalassaemia are point mutations rather than gene deletions. These mutations may be within the gene complex itself or in promoter or enhancer regions. Over 300 different genetic defects have been detected (Fig. 7.8). Population studies indicate that probably only 20 β-thalassaemia alleles account for more than 80% of the β-thalassaemia mutations in the whole world since certain mutations are particularly frequent in some ethnic communities. This simplifies in many countries detection of the mutations in foetal DNA for antenatal diagnosis.

Thalassaemia major is often a result of inheritance of two different mutations, each affecting β-globin synthesis (compound heterozygotes). In some cases, deletion of the β gene, δ and β genes or even δ, β and γ genes occurs. In others, unequal chromosome crossing-over has produced δβ fusion genes (so called Lepore syndrome, named after the Italian-American family in which this was first diagnosed).

Secondary modifiers of the β-thalassaemia phenotype are those that reduce the degree of imbalance of the globin chains. They include the co-inheritance of α-thalassaemia and a variety of genetic modifiers of γ-chain production in adult life such as *Xmn*1-^{G} γ and *BCL11A* – have been mapped. It seems likely that the genetic variance may also be due to variations in many other alleles each with small effects on the trait, i.e. a polygenic component.

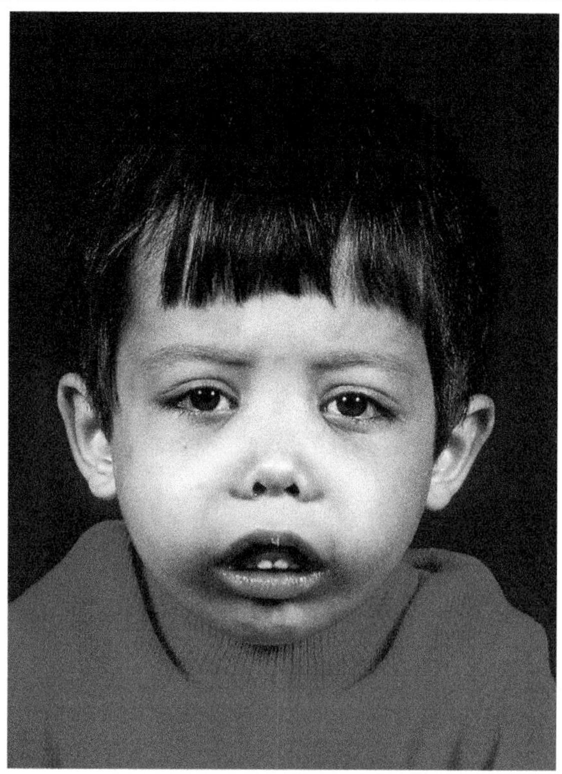

Figure 7.9 The facial appearance of a child with β-thalassaemia major. The skull is bossed with prominent frontal and parietal bones; the maxilla is also enlarged. This is a result of chronic anaemia and compensatory expansion (hyperplasia) of the marrow.

Clinical features

1 **Severe anaemia** becomes apparent at 3–6 months after birth when the switch from γ to β chain production should take place. Typically the infant presents in the first year with failure to thrive, pallor and a swollen abdomen.
2 **Enlargement of the liver and spleen** occurs as a result of excessive red cell destruction, extramedullary haemopoiesis and later because of iron overload. The large spleen increases blood requirements by increasing red cell destruction and pooling, and by causing expansion of the plasma volume.
3 **Expansion of bones** caused by intense marrow hyperplasia leads to a thalassaemic facies (Fig. 7.9) and to thinning of the cortex of many bones, with a tendency to fractures and bossing of the skull with a 'hair-on-end' appearance on X-ray (Fig. 7.10). This is seen less commonly in the modern era, since it is prevented by blood transfusion. Extramedullary haemopoiesis may form 'pseudotumours' especially in the para-spinal region (Fig. 7.14).
4 **Thalassaemia major is the disease that most frequently underlies transfusional iron overload.** Regular transfusions are usually commenced in the first year of life and, unless the disease is cured by stem cell transplantation or sufficiently improved by gene therapy, are continued for life. Every 500 mL of blood transfused contains 200–250 mg iron. Iron absorption is increased despite iron overload because of low serum hepcidin levels due to release of proteins such as erythroferrone from the increased numbers of early red cell precursors in the marrow.

   In children, excess iron causes failure of growth and delayed puberty. Without iron chelation, death from cardiac damage usually occurs in teenage. In both children and adults, diabetes mellitus, hypothyroidism, hypoparathyroidism pituitary and sex hormone damage are frequent. With

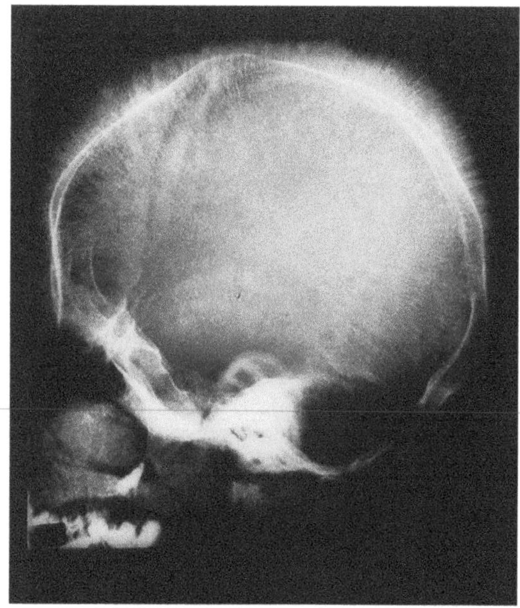

Figure 7.10 Skull X-ray in β-thalassaemia major without chronic transfusion support. There is a 'hair-on-end' appearance as a result of expansion of the bone marrow into cortical bone.

increasing age, long-term complications of iron overload on the liver, endocrine system and heart may become apparent and cancers of both haematological and solid organs are more frequent than in the general population. The clinical features of iron overload, its diagnosis and management are further discussed in Chapter 4.

5 **Infections** occur frequently. In infancy, without adequate transfusion, anaemia predisposes to bacterial infections. Pneumococcal, *Haemophilus* and meningococcal infections are likely if splenectomy has been carried out. *Yersinia enterocolitica* occurs, particularly in iron-loaded patients being treated with deferoxamine; it may cause severe gastroenteritis. Iron overload itself also predisposes to other bacterial infections, e.g. *Klebsiella,* and to fungal infections. Transmission of viruses by blood transfusion is now rare. Improved chelation therapy has reduced deaths from cardiac iron overload so infections account for an increasing proportion of deaths in thalassaemia major.
6 **Liver disease** in thalassaemia major is most frequently a result of hepatitis C, but hepatitis B is also common where the virus is endemic. Human immunodeficiency virus (HIV) has been transmitted to some patients by blood transfusion. Iron overload may also cause liver damage.
7 **Hepatocellular carcinoma** incidence is increased in those with iron overload resulting in hepatic fibrosis or cirrhosis and with chronic hepatitis B or C. Ultrasound and measurement of serum alphafetoprotein every 6–12 months are advisable in such patients.
8 **Osteopenia** may occur even in well-transfused patients. It is more common in diabetic patients with endocrine abnormalities, including those resulting from iron-related damage to the pituitary gland. Expansion of the marrow may cause brittle bones. Polymorphisms of genes controlling collagen formation, the vitamin D and oestrogen receptors and transforming growth factors influence the degree of bone damage.,
9 **Prothrombotic state** results from a variety of causes. Haemolysis causes red cells to express prothrombotic molecules; activated platelets (especially after splenectomy) and other coagulation abnormalities due to liver disease also cause an increased risk of venous and arterial thrombosis, pulmonary hypertension, cardiac events and strokes. Vascular disease can also result from direct damage to the endothelium caused by iron.

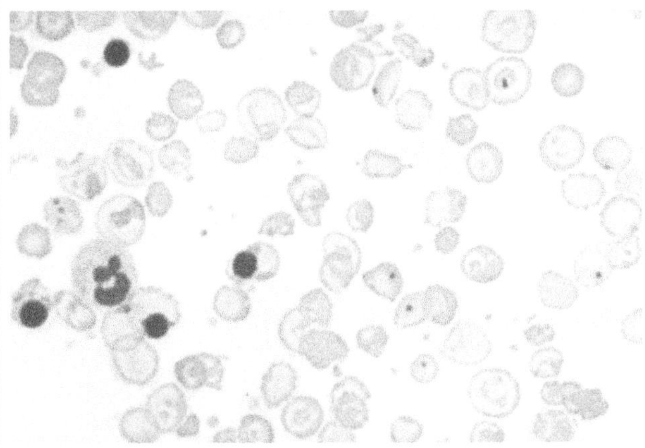

Figure 7.11 Blood film in β-thalassaemia major post-splenectomy. There are hypochromic cells, target cells and many nucleated red cells (normoblasts). Howell–Jolly bodies are seen in the same red cells.

Laboratory diagnosis

1 There is a severe hypochromic, microcytic anaemia with normoblasts, target cells and basophilic stippling in the blood film (Fig. 7.11).
2 High-performance liquid chromatography (HPLC) is now usually used as the first-line method to diagnose haemoglobin disorders (Fig. 7.12a). HPLC or haemoglobin electrophoresis (Fig. 7.12b) reveals the absence or almost complete absence of Hb A, with nearly all the circulating haemoglobin being Hb F. The Hb A_2 percentage is normal, low or slightly raised. DNA analysis is used to identify the defect on each allele, important for antenatal diagnosis.
3 The assessment of the degree of iron overload and of the consequent organ damage is described in Chapter 4.

Treatment

1 **Regular blood transfusions** are needed to maintain the haemoglobin over 95–100 g/L. This usually requires 2–3 units every 3–4 weeks. Fresh blood, filtered to remove white cells, gives the best red cell survival with the fewest reactions. The patients should be genotyped at the start of the transfusion programme in case red cell antibodies against transfused red cells develop. Transfusions prevent complications, including skeletal deformation.
2 As a result of chronic transfusions, **thalassaemia major is the dominant disease worldwide for which iron chelation is essential**. The three available drugs, deferiprone, deferasirox and deferoxamine, have considerably improved quality of life and life expectancy for thalassemia patients. The two oral drugs are preferred as compliance with infusions of deferoxamine is particularly difficult for SCD patients. The drugs and their use are described in Chapter 4.
3 Regular **folic acid**, e.g. 5 mg weekly or 0.4–1 mg daily, is given due to the ongoing haemolysis with risk for folate deficiency, especially if the diet is poor.
4 **Endocrine therapy** is given either as replacement because of end-organ failure or to stimulate the pituitary if puberty is delayed. Diabetes will require insulin therapy.
5 **Osteopenia** incidence is increased in children and adults with thalassaemia major, and bone density should be monitored regularly from the age of about 10 years. Vitamin D levels should be measured regularly, and oral supplements of vitamin D and calcium given if needed.

(a)

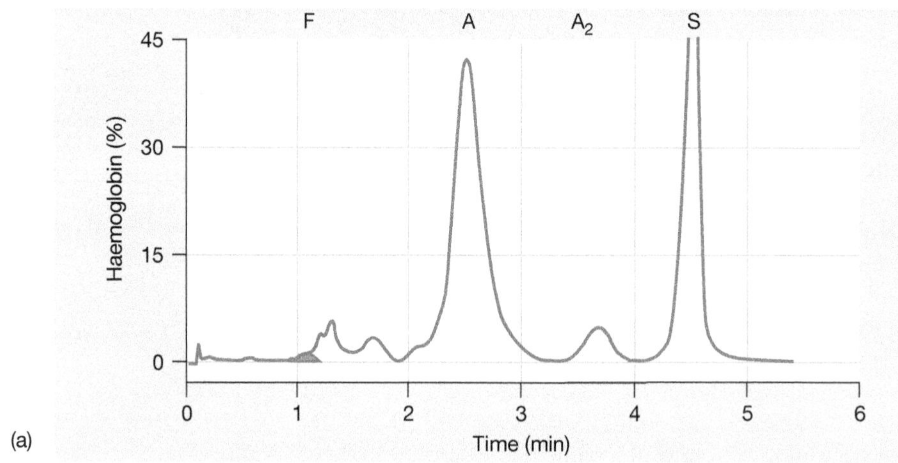

(b)

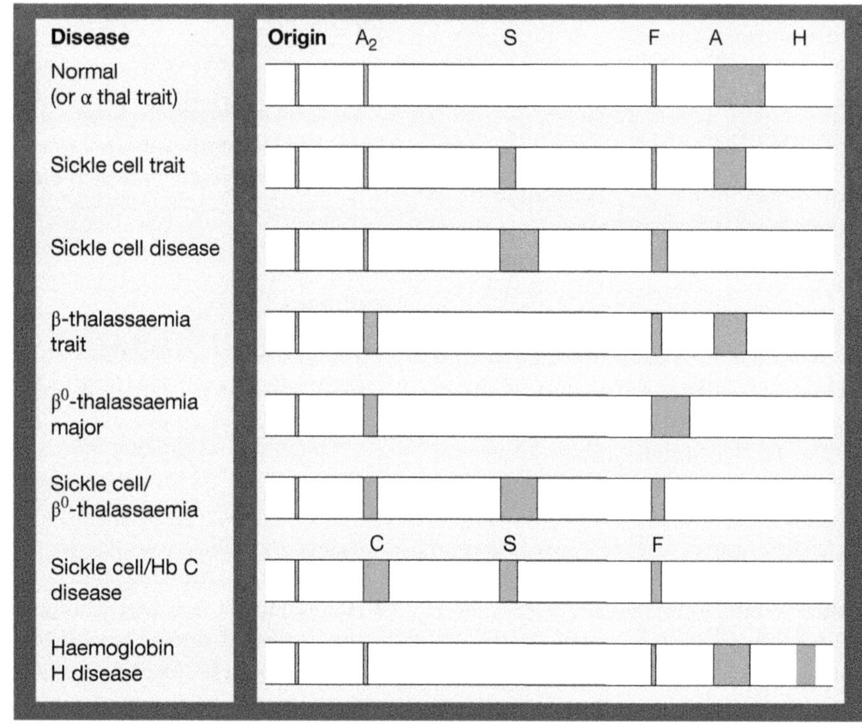

Figure 7.12 **(a)** High-performance liquid chromatography. The different haemoglobins elute at different times from the column and their concentrations are read automatically. In this example, the patient is a carrier of sickle cell disease. **(b)** Haemoglobin electrophoretic patterns in normal adult human blood and in subjects with sickle cell (Hb S) trait or disease, β-thalassaemia trait, β-thalassaemia major, Hb S/β-thalassaemia or Hb S/Hb C disease and Hb H disease.

Bisphosphonates may also be effective in preventing and treating osteopenia in adults with thalassaemia, although their role in children is less established, with concern about their effects on growth.

6 **Luspatercept** is a recombinant fusion protein comprising the modified extracellular domain of the human activin receptor fused to the Fc domain of IgG1. It binds to transforming growth factor β-superfamily ligands and so blocks signalling from them. It enhances erythroid maturation. Given as a subcutaneous injection once every three weeks, it reduces transfusion requirements. It is associated with transient bone pains, arthralgias and headache. It is expensive.

7 **Splenectomy** may be needed to reduce blood transfusion requirements. If possible, this should be delayed until the patient is over 6 years old because of the high risk of

dangerous infections post-splenectomy. The vaccinations and antibiotics to be given are described in Chapter 10. With improvements in blood transfusion and iron chelation, splenectomy is now performed much less frequently than in earlier decades.

8 **Immunization** against hepatitis B should be carried out in all non-immune patients. Treatment for transfusion-transmitted hepatitis C is given if viral genomes are detected in plasma.

9 **Allogeneic stem cell transplantation** offers the prospect of permanent cure. The success rate (long-term thalassaemia major-free survival) is over 80% in well-chelated younger patients without liver fibrosis or hepatomegaly. HLA antigen-matching siblings or matching unrelated volunteers are the usual donors but haplo-identical related donors are being increasingly used. Failure is mainly a result of recurrence of thalassaemia or death, e.g. from infection or severe chronic graft-versus-host disease.

10 **Gene therapy trials** for treating the thalassaemia major phenotype are in progress. These aim either to introduce a normal β-globin gene or to enhance Hb F production to reduce haemolysis. An autologous stem cell transplantation technique is employed. In one technique, patient stem cells are harvested from bone marrow or peripheral blood, and a lentiviral vector used to introduce a β-globin gene construct or a modified beta-globin gene β -A-T87Q *in vitro* into these stem cells. The construct is designed to enhance synthesis of normal β-globin. The 'corrected' stem cells are reinfused into the patient, who has been treated with myeloablative conditioning, e.g. with busulphan to eliminate the faulty stem cells. This approach has reduced or eliminated the need for long-term red cell transfusions in most treated transfusion-dependent patients with a non-β^o/β^o genotype. There is approval for this therapy in Europe but the costs are high and the need for myeloablative chemotherapy a concern. Long-term studies are in progress to determine the durability and freedom from leukaemia of this gene therapy.

The alternative technique is aimed at enhancing foetal haemoglobin synthesis by editing the *BCL11A* gene, which normally suppresses γ-globin chain synthesis, or by editing the γ-globin chain enhancers or promoters. In some of these techniques, the CRISPR/Cas9 technique for gene editing is employed (Fig. 7.13). Some of these gene therapy techniques are approved for clinical use.

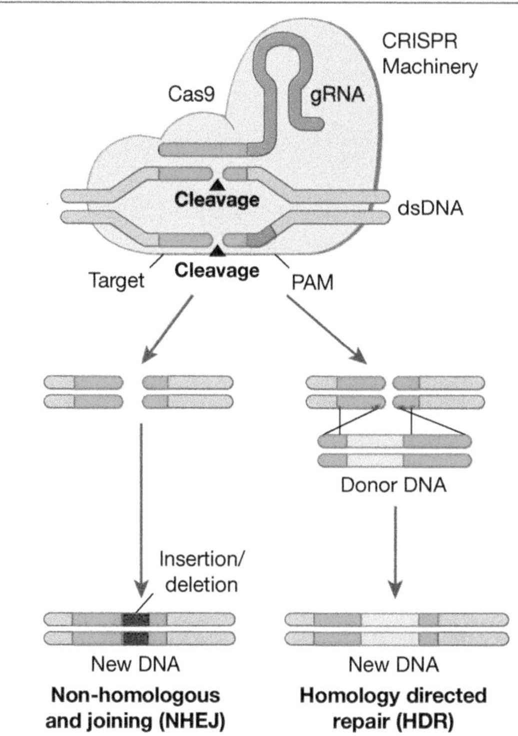

Figure 7.13 CRISPR/Cas9 gene editing. CRISPR, pronounced 'crisper,' is commonly used in biotechnology as a shorthand term for CRISPR/Cas9 gene editing. CRISPR (clusters of regularly interspaced short palindromic repeats) is a specialized region of DNA consisting of nucleotide repeats and 'spacers,' DNA elements that are interspersed among these repeated sequences and that in bacteria usually represent integrated viral genetic elements, and for which cells have evolved protective machinery to excise and repair DNA. In CRISPR/Cas9 gene editing, a short RNA template is created that matches a target sequence in the genome DNA. This guide RNA directs the CRISPR machinery to the target DNA. Associated Cas9 nuclease then site-specifically cleaves double-stranded DNA, activating the endogenous double-strand break DNA repair machinery, which includes homology-directed repair and non-homologous end joining. In the absence of a homologous repair template, non-homologous end joining can result in insertions and deletions (indels), disrupting the target sequence. Alternatively, precise mutations and knock-ins can be made by providing a homologous repair template with the new sequence of interest and exploiting the homology directed repair pathway. Source: New England Bio Labs Inc.

β-Thalassaemia trait (minor)

This is a common, usually symptomless abnormality characterized, like α-thalassaemia trait, by a hypochromic, microcytic blood picture (MCV and MCH low) but high red cell count (>5.5 × 10^{12}/L) and mild anaemia (haemoglobin 100–120 g/L). It is usually more severe than α-thalassaemia trait but with some genotypes, the MCV may be just below normal or even normal.

A raised level of Hb A_2 (>3.5%) confirms the diagnosis. Since iron deficiency lowers the Hb A_2 level, a falsely normal result may be found in the presence of concomitant iron deficiency or rarely even without iron deficiency.

The diagnosis of β-thalassaemia trait allows the possibility of prenatal counselling, which is legally mandated in some regions of the world with a high incidence of thalassaemia major, such as Cyprus. If the partner also has β-thalassaemia trait, there is a 25% risk of a child with thalassaemia major so antenatal diagnosis with, if positive, therapeutic abortion is offered.

Thalassaemia intermedia (non-transfusion dependent thalassaemia (NTDT): a clinical syndrome

This is thalassaemia of moderate severity (haemoglobin 70–100 g/L) without the need for regular transfusions (Table 7.3). Transfusion may occasionally be required, for example during an acute illness with temporary suppression of erythropoiesis or during pregnancy. **Thalassaemia intermedia is caused by a variety of genetic defects**, such as homozygous β-thalassaemia with production of more Hb F than usual, e.g. due to mutations of the *BCL11A* gene, or with mild defects in β chain synthesis. The syndrome may also result from β-thalassaemia trait alone of unusual severity ('dominant' β-thalassaemia trait), by β-thalassaemia trait in association with another mild globin abnormality such as Hb Lepore.

The coexistence of α-thalassaemia trait improves the haemoglobin level in homozygous β-thalassaemia by reducing the degree of α-/β-globin chain imbalance and thus of α chain precipitation and ineffective erythropoiesis. This may result in an intermedia syndrome rather than thalassaemia major. Conversely, patients with β-thalassaemia trait who also have excess (five or six) α-globin genes tend to be more anaemic than usual for the trait due to the greater chain imbalance.

The patient with thalassaemia intermedia may show liver fibrosis and cirrhosis, endocrine abnormalities, bone deformity and extramedullary erythropoiesis (Fig. 7.14), leg ulcers, gallstones, osteoporosis, pulmonary hypertension and venous thrombosis. The lower the haemoglobin level below 100 g/L, the greater the incidence of these clinical problems. They are all more frequent with increasing age. Iron overload, dominantly in the liver, is caused by increased iron absorption (due to low erythroferrone levels caused by ineffective erythropoiesis) and by transfusions, e.g. during pregnancy or infections or given to reduce bone deformity.

Iron chelation, usually with oral drugs, may be needed, e.g. if the serum ferritin is greater than 800 μg/L or liver iron is greater than 5 mg/g dry weight. Splenectomy may be required to avoid the need for transfusions. **Luspatercept** (see above) enhances effective erythropoiesis and can reduce the level of anaemia, the extent of organ damage and iron overload.

Hb H disease (three-gene-deletion α-thalassaemia) is a type of thalassaemia intermedia without iron overload or extramedullary haemopoiesis.

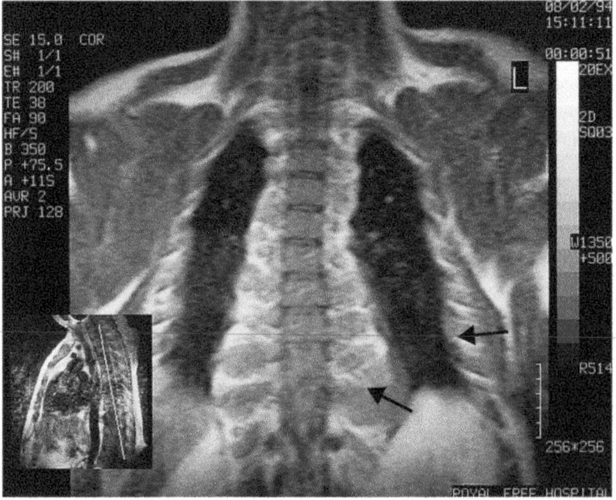

Figure 7.14 β-Thalassaemia intermedia (non-transfusion-dependent thalassaemia): magnetic resonance imaging (MRI) scan showing masses of extramedullary haemopoietic tissue arising from the ribs and in the paravertebral region without encroachment of the spinal cord.

δβ-Thalassaemia

This involves failure of production of both β and δ chains. Hb F production is increased to 5–20% in the heterozygous state, which resembles thalassaemia minor haematologically. In the homozygous state, only Hb F is present and haematologically the picture is one of thalassaemia intermedia.

Haemoglobin Lepore

This is an abnormal haemoglobin caused by unequal crossing-over of the β and δ genes to produce a polypeptide chain consisting of the δ chain at its amino end and β chain at its carboxyl end. The δβ-fusion chain is synthesized inefficiently and normal δ and β chain production is abolished. The Hb Lepore homozygotes show thalassaemia intermedia and the heterozygotes thalassaemia trait.

Hereditary persistence of foetal haemoglobin

Hereditary persistence of foetal haemoglobin (HPFH) is a heterogeneous group of genetic conditions caused by deletions or cross-overs affecting the production of β and γ chains; in non-deletion forms, by point mutations upstream from the γ-globin genes or in the *BCL11A* and other genes.

Association of β-thalassaemia trait with other genetic disorders of haemoglobin

The combination of β-thalassaemia trait with Hb E trait usually causes a transfusion-dependent thalassaemia major syndrome, but some cases are intermediate. β-thalassaemia trait co-inherited with Hb S trait produces the clinical picture of sickle cell disease rather than of thalassaemia. β-thalassaemia trait with Hb D trait causes a hypochromic, microcytic anaemia of varying severity.

Sickle cell disease

Sickle cell disease is a group of haemoglobin disorders resulting from the inheritance of the sickle β-globin gene (Hb S). The sickle β-globin abnormality is caused by

Normal β-chain	Amino acid	pro	glu	glu
	Base composition	CCT	GAG	GAG
Sickle β-chain	Base composition	CCT	GTG	GAG
	Amino acid	pro	val	glu

Figure 7.15 Molecular pathology of sickle cell anaemia. There is a single base change in the DNA coding for the amino acid in the sixth position in the β-globin chain (adenine is replaced by thymine). This leads to an amino acid change from glutamic acid to valine. A, adenine; C, cytosine; G, guanine; glu, glutamic acid; pro, proline; T, thymine; val, valine.

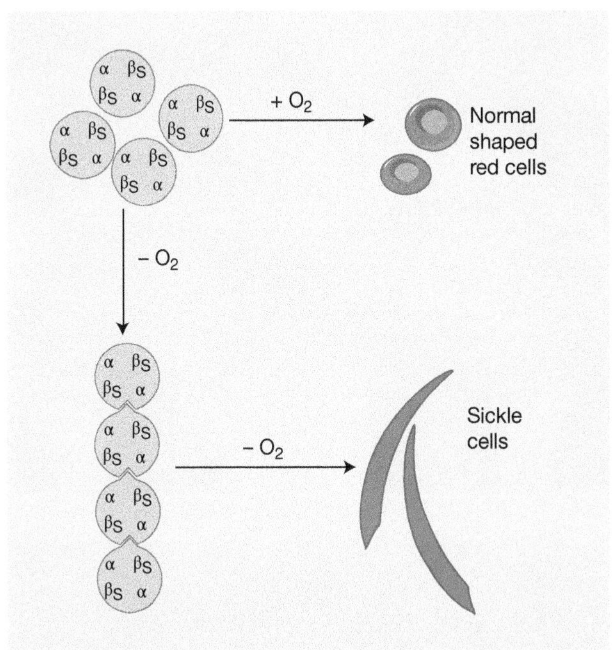

Figure 7.16 The formation of the sickle polymer. Source: Adapted from H.F. Bunn, J.C. Aster (2011) *Hematologic Pathophysiology*. New York: McGraw Hill.

substitution of valine for glutamic acid in position 6 in the β-globin chain (Fig. 7.15). Homozygous sickle cell anaemia (Hb S/S) is the most common severe sickle cell syndrome. The doubly heterozygote conditions of Hb S/C, Hb S/β-thalassaemia, Hb S/D, HbS/Lepore also cause sickling disease that varies in severity.

Hb S (Hb $\alpha_2\beta_2$S) is insoluble and forms crystals when exposed to low oxygen tension (Fig. 7.16). Deoxygenated sickle haemoglobin polymerizes into long fibres, each consisting of seven intertwined double strands with cross-linking (Fig. 7.16). The red cells containing this denatured fibrous haemoglobin experience membrane damage and form sickle shapes, and may block different areas of the microcirculation or large vessels, causing infarcts of various organs. The carrier state is widespread (Fig. 7.4) and is found in up to 30% of West African people, maintained at this level because of the protection afforded by the carrier state against severe Falciparum malaria but against no other type of malaria. Different ethnic groups in Africa and Asia carry the sickle gene within different β-globin haplotypes showing multiple origins of the mutation.

Homozygous disease

Clinical features

Clinical features are of a severe haemolytic anaemia punctuated by crises. The symptoms of anaemia are often mild in relation to the severity of the anaemia because Hb S gives up oxygen (O_2) to tissues relatively easily compared with Hb A (Fig. 2.10). The clinical expression of Hb SS is very variable; some patients have an almost normal quality of life, free of crises, while others develop severe crises even as infants and may die in early childhood or as young adults. Disease modifiers include the co-inheritance of α-thalassaemia trait, increased haemoglobin F synthesis and β-globin haplotype. Crises may be vaso-occlusive (painful or visceral), aplastic or haemolytic. There may be serious damage to many organs. The co-inheritance of a raised Hb F production with Hb SS results in a milder clinical course. Co-inheritance of α-thalassaemia also leads to milder anaemia but no amelioration of clinical course.

Vaso-occlusive crises

Painful

These are the most frequent type of crisis in sickle cell disease. They may be sporadic and unpredictable or precipitated by infection, acidosis, dehydration or deoxygenation, (e.g. altitude, operations, obstetric delivery), stasis of the circulation, exposure to cold, strenuous exercise. For adults with recurrent painful vaso-occlusive crises, there is a 50% unemployment rate. Infarcts causing severe pain occur in the bones (hips, shoulders and vertebrae are commonly affected). Avascular necrosis of bones, especially of the femoral head, causes long-term problems (Fig. 7.17). The 'hand–foot' syndrome (painful dactylitis caused by infarcts of the small bones) is frequently the first presentation of the disease, typically before age 5, and may lead to digits of varying lengths (Fig. 7.18).

Visceral

These are caused by sickling within organs causing infarction and sequestration of blood, often with a severe exacerbation of anaemia. The **acute sickle chest syndrome** is the most common cause of death in both children and adults. It

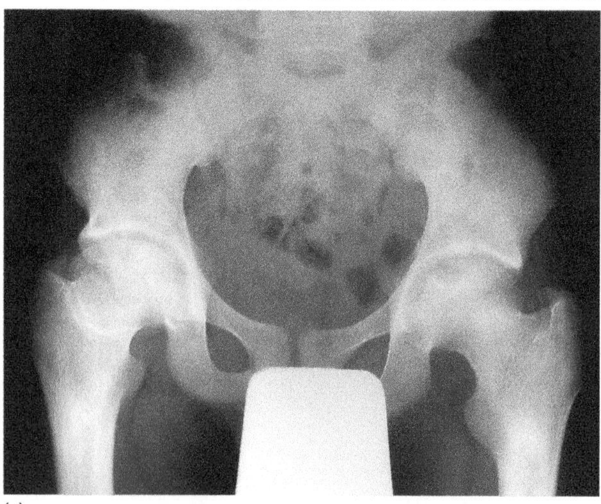

(a)

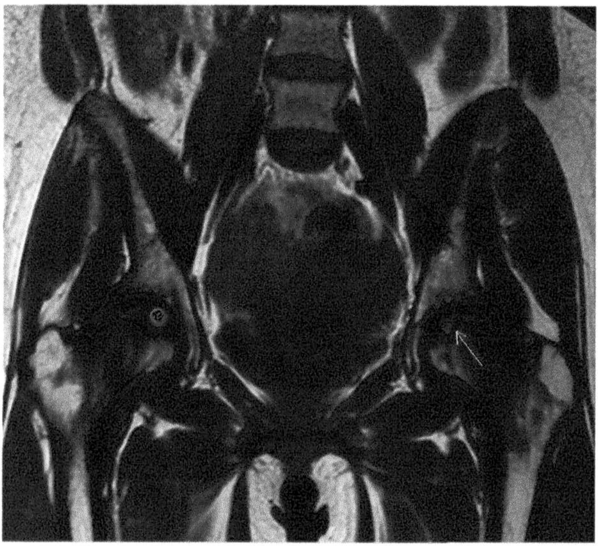

(b)

Figure 7.17 Sickle cell anaemia. **(a)** Radiograph of the pelvis of a young man of West Indian origin which shows avascular necrosis with flattening of the femoral heads, more marked on the right, coarsening of the bone architecture and cystic areas in the right femoral neck caused by previous infarcts. **(b)** Coronal hip magnetic resonance image (MRI) revealing established osteonecrosis of femoral heads bilaterally (yellow arrow) with crescent sclerotic margin (blue dot) as a consequence of sickle cell. Source: Courtesy of Dr A. Malhotra.

presents with dyspnoea, falling arterial PO_2, chest pain and pulmonary infiltrates on chest X-ray. It must be distinguished from a chest infection or pulmonary embolus. Treatment is with analgesia, oxygen, exchange transfusion and ventilatory support if necessary. Hepatic and girdle sequestration crises may lead to severe illness requiring exchange transfusions.

Splenic sequestration is typically seen in infants and presents with an enlarging spleen, falling haemoglobin and abdominal pain. Treatment is with transfusion. Splenic crises tend to be recurrent and splenectomy may be needed.

Aplastic crises

These occur as a result of infection with parvovirus or from folate deficiency and are characterized by a sudden fall in haemoglobin (the existing red cells having a short life-span) and reticulocytes, usually requiring transfusion (Fig. 22.7).

Haemolytic crises

These are characterized by an increased rate of haemolysis and fall in haemoglobin but rise in reticulocytes and usually accompany a painful crisis.

Other organ damage

Almost every organ in the body may be damaged. The most serious is of the brain or spinal cord. **A stroke, either infarction or haemorrhage, occurs in 7% of all patients. Up to a third of children have had a silent cerebral infarct by the age of 6 years (Fig. 7.19)**. The risk is greater in those with HbSS compared with other sickle syndromes, and in those with the lowest haemoglobin (and lowest haemoglobin F) levels, highest white cell counts and systolic blood pressure. Transient ischemic attacks or seizures may be the presenting features. Transcranial Doppler ultrasonography (TCD) detects increased blood flow (>200 cm/s) indicative of arterial stenosis. This occurs mainly in the circle of Willis and the internal carotids. TCD should be carried out annually from early childhood and if abnormal, stroke can be prevented by regular blood transfusions; hydroxyurea (hydroxycarbamide) therapy is also beneficial but transfusions are the preferred option for both primary and secondary prevention. Cognitive impairment may also result from cerebral vascular disease and is also an indication for transfusion therapy.

Ulcers of the lower legs are common, as a result of vascular stasis and local ischemia (Fig. 7.20). Ulcers are always colonized with pathogenic bacteria (*Pseudomonas aeruginosa*, *S. aureus* and *Streptococcus* spp.) and acute infection can occur. The ulcers are painful and resistant to healing.

Pulmonary hypertension, detected by Doppler echocardiography, progressive loss of lung function and an increased tricuspid regurgitant velocity are common and increase the risk of death. **Left ventricular failure** due to myocardial fibrosis is also a frequent major problem. **Proliferative retinopathy**, a serious complication which may cause blindness, is caused by neo-vascularization with potential for vitreous haemorrhage and retinal detachment. **Priapism** is an unwanted painful and sustained for more than 3 hours, erection of the penis. It is another common clinical complication which if repeated can lead to fibrosis and impotence. **Chronic damage to the liver** may occur through microinfarcts. **Pigment (bilirubin) gallstones** are frequent. The spleen is enlarged in infancy and early

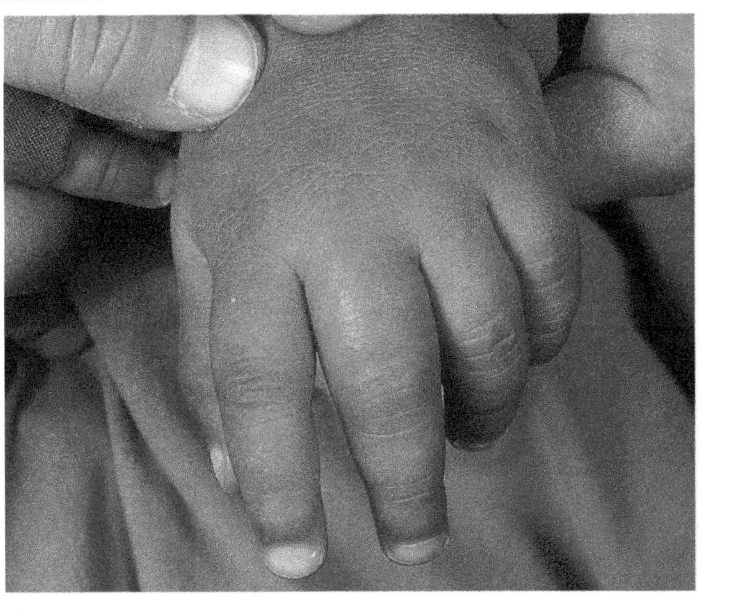

(a)

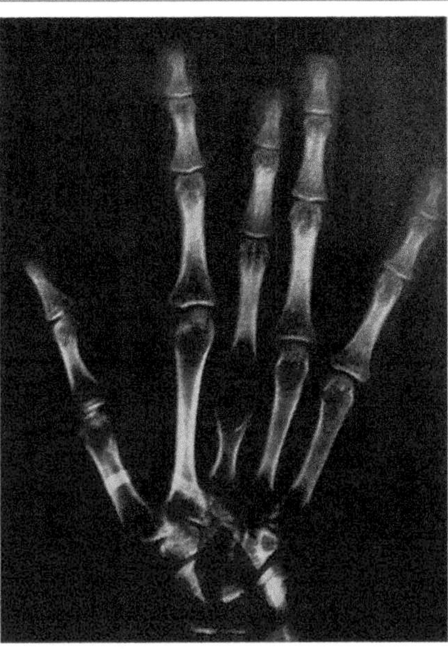

(b)

Figure 7.18 Sickle cell anaemia: **(a)** painful swollen fingers (dactylitis) in a child and **(b)** the hand of an 18-year-old Nigerian boy with previous 'hand–foot' syndrome. There is marked shortening of the right middle finger because of dactylitis in childhood affecting the growth of previous epiphysis.

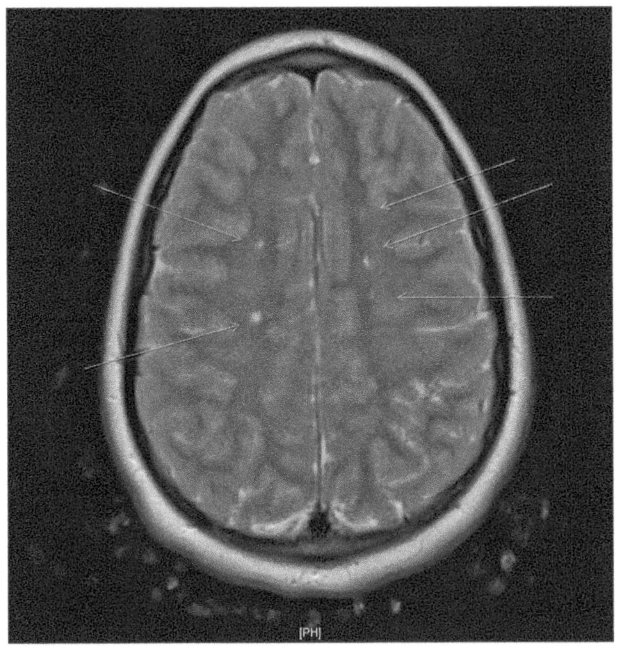

Figure 7.19 T2-weighted magnetic resonance image (MRI) of a 9-year-old girl with sickle cell anaemia, showing five hyperintensities in the deep white matter (arrows), which are silent cerebral infarcts. Source: Courtesy of Professor David Rees, Kings College Hospital.

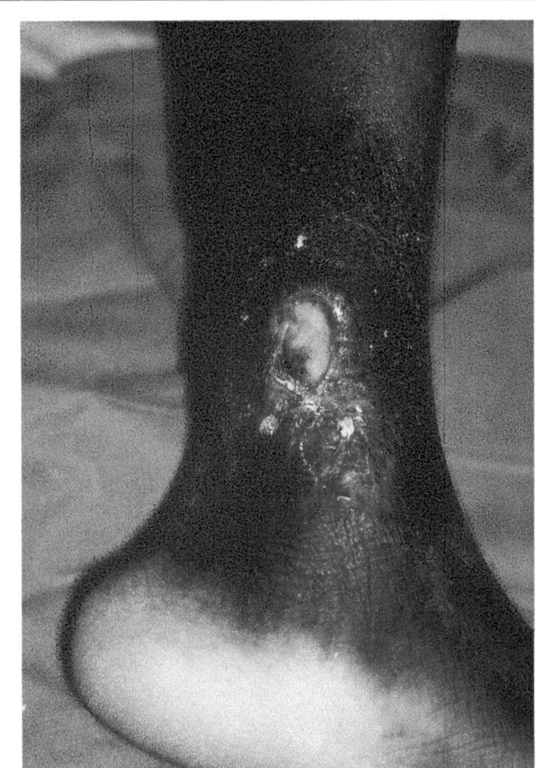

Figure 7.20 Sickle cell anaemia: medial aspect of the ankle of a 15-year-old Nigerian boy showing necrosis and ulceration.

childhood, but later is often reduced in size as a result of infarcts (**autosplenectomy**).

The kidneys are vulnerable to infarctions of the medulla with papillary necrosis. There may be acute deterioration in renal function. Failure to concentrate urine aggravates the tendency to dehydration and crisis, and nocturnal enuresis may develop. Renal tract infections may accelerate deterioration of kidney function. **Chronic renal insufficiency** is a common complication in adulthood.

Infections are a major cause of illness and death. They often precipitate crises. Loss of splenic function in early childhood leads to *Pneumococcal* infections with risk of fulminant sepsis and meningitis. *Haemophilus* infections are the next most frequent in childhood. Pneumonia and urinary tract infections are common. In Africa, *Salmonella*, *Klebsiella*, *Staphylococcal* and *Escherichia coli* infections are particularly frequent. Osteomyelitis may occur, usually from *Salmonella* species. Vaccination against coronavirus infection is given to both children and adults. Remdesivir or related drug antiviral therapy is indicated if infection occurs (p. 161).

There is also an increased incidence of **venous thrombosis** and this tends to recur, so long-term anticoagulation may be needed.

Laboratory findings

1 The haemoglobin is usually 60–90 g/L – low in comparison to mild or no symptoms of anaemia.
2 Sickle cells and target cells occur in the blood (Fig. 7.21). Features of splenic atrophy, e.g. Howell–Jolly bodies may also be present.
3 Screening tests for sickling are positive when the blood is deoxygenated, e.g. with dithionate and disodium phosphate, $NaHPO_4$.
4 HPLC or haemoglobin electrophoresis (Fig. 7.12). In Hb SS, no Hb A is detected. The amount of Hb F is usually 5–15%; higher levels are associated with a milder disorder.

Treatment

1 General

(a) Prophylactic – avoid those factors known to precipitate crises, especially dehydration, anoxia, e.g. high altitudes, infections, stasis of the circulation and cooling of the skin surface.
(b) Folic acid e.g. 1 mg daily or 5 mg weekly.
(c) Good general nutrition and hygiene.
(d) Oral penicillin should start at diagnosis and continue at least until the age of 5 if no pneumococcal infections have occurred.
(e) *Pneumococcal*, *Haemophilus* and *meningococcal* vaccination is effective at reducing the infection rate with these organisms. Influenza and hepatitis B vaccination are also given, as transfusions may be needed and malarial prophylaxis is required in countries where malaria is prevalent. Covid vaccination is imperative as patients with sickle cell anaemia are vulnerable to severe, potentially fatal disease.
(f) Transcranial Doppler studies should be performed annually on all children older than two years to detect those at risk of stroke. In older children and adults, annual retinal examination is needed.

2 Special situations

(a) *Acute crises*

1 Treat by rest, warmth, rehydration by oral fluids and/or intravenous normal saline (3 L in 24 hours) and antibiotics if infection is present.
2 Analgesia at the appropriate level should be given. Suitable drugs are paracetamol, a non-steroidal anti-inflammatory agent and opiates, depending on the severity of pain.
3 Blood transfusion is given if there is very severe anaemia with symptoms or with impending critical organ complications. For hepatic or splenic sequestration and for aplastic crisis, blood transfusion is essential and may be life-saving.

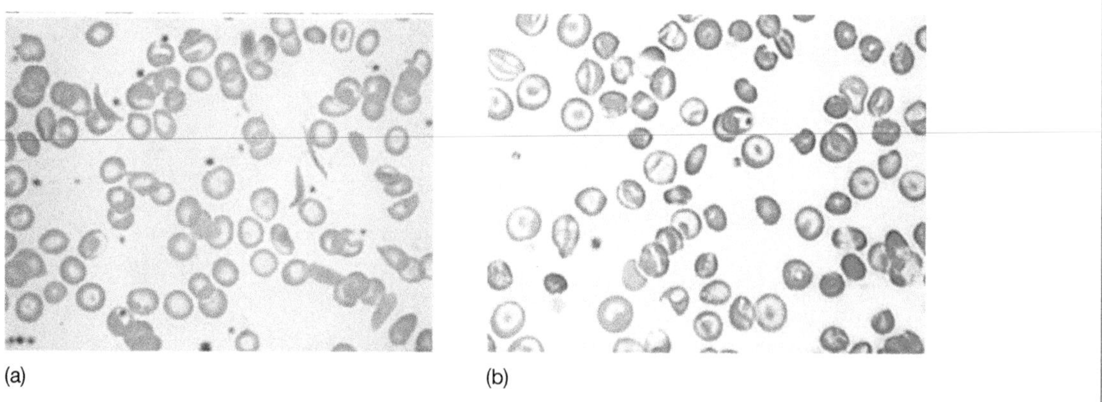

Figure 7.21 **(a)** Sickle cell anaemia: peripheral blood film showing deeply staining sickle cells, target cells and polychromasia. **(b)** Homozygous Hb C disease: peripheral blood film showing many target cells, deeply staining rhomboidal and irregularly contracted cells.

4 *Exchange transfusion* may be indicated, particularly if there is neurological damage or repeated painful crises. This exchange is aimed at achieving an Hb S percentage of less than 30% and, after a stroke, is continued for at least one year with subsequent hydroxyurea.

(b) *Pregnancy* Particular care is needed in pregnancy. There is debate about whether or not all patients need transfusions to reduce Hb S levels during pregnancy or before delivery or for minor operations. Transfusions throughout pregnancy are definitely recommended for those with a poor obstetric history, a multiple pregnancy, a history of frequent crises, previously receiving hydroxyurea (discontinued because of the pregnancy), worsening anaemia, previous or current chest syndrome, stroke or other major complication. Low-dose aspirin is given from 12 weeks (and stopped before delivery) to reduce the risk of pre-eclampsia. Low-molecular-weight heparin is given from 28 weeks to 6 weeks post-partum if there is a previous history of venous thrombosis.

(c) *Surgery*. Careful anaesthetic and recovery techniques must be used to avoid hypoxaemia or acidosis. Preoperative transfusions are indicated before medium-risk, e.g. abdominal or orthopaedic, or high-risk surgery, e.g. brain or cardiovascular procedures.

(d) *Proliferative retinopathy*. The patients are treated with laser photocoagulation or vitrectomy. The incidence of proliferative changes is substantially higher in HbS/C and HbS/β^{+} thalassemia patients than in HbS/S. Patients with SCD should have annual ophthalmological evaluation, beginning in the second decade.

(e) *Leg ulcers* are treated with bed rest and elevation of the leg. Debridement, elastic dressings, zinc sulphate and, in some cases, red cell transfusions and skin grafting may be needed. Voxelotor has been found to help in some cases.

(f) *Priapism*. At the onset of priapism, patients should drink extra fluids and try to urinate. An oral dose of anti-adrenergic agonists pseudoephedrine or terbutaline may help. Persistent priapism requires intravenous hydration and opioid analgesia and aspiration and irrigation of the corpora with dilute phenylephrine or etilefrine solution or intracavernosal injection of these drugs. For patients with recurrent episodes, daily sildenafil or daily alpha-adrenergic agonist may help.

3 Treatment aimed at prevention of crises

(a) Blood transfusions Their use in acute crises has been described above. The choice between simple transfusion and exchange transfusion (usually performed with a cell separator as a single procedure) depends on clinical judgement in each case, depending on the indication, avoidance of hyperviscosity and iron overload and on venous access and availability of a cell separator. Transfusions are sometimes given repeatedly as prophylaxis to patients having frequent crises or who have had major organ damage, e.g. of the brain or show abnormal transcranial Doppler studies. The aim is to suppress Hb S production over a period of several months or even years, with a target haemoglobin S of <30%.

Sickle cell patients have the highest incidence of alloimmunization against donated blood. This may be partly due to the frequency of transfusions and partly due to the large number of variants in the Rh system which occur in individuals of African descent. Delayed haemolytic transfusion reactions caused by these antibodies in which both the transfused and the patient's own red cells are destroyed are particularly dangerous. Recommended treatment is with eculizumab, an inhibitor of C5 convertase in the complement pathway (see p. xxx). High doses of steroids or gamma globulin may also be helpful.

Iron overload due to blood transfusions is best assessed by the total number of units transfused and by liver iron estimated by magnetic resonance imaging (MRI). Sickle cell patients tend not to adhere to burdensome subcutaneous deferoxamine infusions, so if iron chelation is needed, oral iron chelating drugs, most often deferasirox; deferiprone is also approved in this setting,.

(b) Hydroxyurea (hydroxycarbamide) This increases Hb F levels and improves the clinical course of children or adults. It is now recommended for all infants and children with HbS/S over the age of 9 months. In adults it is given to those with severe or moderately severe disease, e.g. who are having three or more painful crises each year. It should not be used during pregnancy. It can be used in primary prevention of stroke or to replace blood transfusions when they have been given for a year to prevent recurrence of stroke. In sub-Saharan Africa, it reduces malarial infections in childhood among Hb SS patients. Careful monitoring is needed to avoid severe neutropenia. There is no evidence that prolonged administration of hydroxyurea over many years to children or adults predisposes to any form of neoplastic disease. Research into other drugs, e.g. decitabine or butyrates, which enhance Hb F synthesis or increase the solubility of Hb S, is taking place.

(c) Crizanlizumab is an antibody directed against P-selectin, an adhesion molecule that mediates adhesion of sickle cells to blood vessel walls. Given intravenously it reduces the time to first and second crises and the incidence of vaso-occlusive crises, including priapism. It is approved for those aged 16 years or more. It is avoided in pregnancy.

(d) Voxelotor is a small molecule that binds to the α globin chain and stabilizes deoxygenated haemoglobin in a relaxed state preventing polymerization. It increases the lifespan of sickle red cells by reducing haemolysis but it can make crises worse. Hopefully in the long term, it will reduce complications of SCD such as pulmonary hypertension, renal and neurological disease. It is approved for those aged 12 years or more and can be given in conjunction with hydroxyurea.

(e) **L-glutamine** is a precursor of glutathione which protects cells from oxidative damage. Supplementation with L-glutamine in some studies has reduced the frequency and severity of painful crises. A powdered form of the amino acid is approved for treatment of sickle cell anaemia for those aged 5 or more. It should not be used in pregnancy or lactation or in those with severe renal or liver disease.

4 **Treatments aimed at curing sickle cell disease**

(a) **Allogeneic stem cell transplantation.** This can cure sickle cell anaemia, with a 90–100% survival rate from the transplant and 73–100% of patients disease free after the procedure. As for thalassaemia major, haplo-identical family members as well as HLA matched siblings and unrelated individuals are chosen as donors. The mortality rate is less than 10% if patients and donors are carefully selected but the side effects of the myeloablative chemotherapy can include infertility, impaired renal and cardiac function, a small increased risk of a haematological malignancy and other early and late side effects. Reduced intensity transplants have been used often producing beneficial mixed donor chimerism, but these transplants have been associated with more graft failure and infections consequent on prolonged immunosuppressive treatment. Outcomes of haplo-identical transplants are improving. Transplantation is only indicated in the severest of cases whose quality of life or life expectancy is substantially impaired. Ongoing debate concern the exact indications and optimum age for allogeneic transplantation.

(b) **Gene therapy** Clinical trials are in progress using an autologous marrow stem cell transplant procedure, as described for thalassaemia major (p. XX). Stem cells are mobilized with plerixafor rather than G-CSF, which can cause severe complications in sickle cell anaemia. A lentiviral vector is used to introduce a β-globin gene construct or a modified beta-globin gene βA (T87Q) *in vitro* into these stem cells. Other trials are aimed at increasing Hb F production in harvested stem cells before they are reinfused. These include using a lentiviral vector to embed a γ- globin coding sequence into the β-globin gene or an RNA, which silences *BCL11A* and so enhances foetal haemoglobin synthesis. Gene editing techniques to replace the faulty codon in the sickle gene or to knock out the *BCL11A* gene are also being developed. Some gene editing techniques to replace the faulty codon in the sickle gene or to knock out the *BCL11A* gene are now approved.

Sickle cell trait

This is a benign condition with no anaemia and normal appearance of red cells in a blood film. Life expectancy is normal. Haematuria is the most common symptom and is thought to be caused by minor infarcts of the renal papillae. There is also an increased risk of exertional rhabdomyolysis, chronic kidney disease, venous thrombosis including pulmonary embolus and splenic infarction. Hb S varies from 25% to 45% of the total haemoglobin (Fig. 7.12). Care must be taken to avoid constriction of the circulation or de-oxygenation with anaesthesia, pregnancy and at high altitudes.

Combination of haemoglobin S with other genetic defects of haemoglobin

The most common of these are Hb S/β-thalassaemia and HbS/C disease. In Hb S/β-thalassaemia, the MCV and MCH are lower than in homozygous Hb SS and splenomegaly is usual. The clinical picture is of sickle cell anaemia. Patients with Hb S/C disease have a particular tendency to thrombosis and pulmonary embolism, especially in pregnancy. Compared with Hb SS disease, they have a higher incidence of retinal abnormalities including a proliferative retinopathy (see above), milder anaemia, splenomegaly and generally a longer life expectancy. Diagnosis is made by haemoglobin electrophoresis or HPLC, particularly with family studies.

Co-inheritance of hereditary persistence of foetal haemoglobin ameliorates sickle cell disease as for thalassaemia major since the haemoglobin γ-globin gene promoter then outcompetes the β-globin promoter for interaction with the LCR.

Haemoglobin C disease

This genetic defect of haemoglobin is frequent in West Africa and is caused by substitution of lysine for glutamic acid in the β-globin chain at the same point as the substitution in Hb S. Hb C tends to form rhomboidal crystals and in the homozygous state there is a mild haemolytic anaemia with marked target cell formation, cells irregularly contracted and with a rhomboidal shape (Fig. 7.21b). The spleen is enlarged. The carriers show a few target cells only.

Haemoglobin D disease

This is a group of variants all with the same electrophoretic mobility. Heterozygotes show no haematological abnormality, while homozygotes have a mild haemolytic anaemia. When HbD Punjab (Los Angeles) is co-inherited with Hb S, the resulting sickling disease may be severe.

Haemoglobin E disease

This is the most common haemoglobin variant in South-East Asia. In the homozygous state, there is a mild microcytic, hypochromic anaemia. Haemoglobin E/β^0-thalassaemia, however, resembles homozygous β^0-thalassaemia both clinically and haematologically.

Prenatal diagnosis of genetic haemoglobin disorders

It is important to give genetic counselling to couples at risk of having a child with a major haemoglobin defect. If a pregnant woman is found to have a haemoglobin abnormality, her partner should be tested to determine whether he also carries a defect. When both partners show an abnormality and there is a risk of a serious defect in the offspring, particularly of β-thalassaemia major, it is important to offer antenatal diagnosis. Several techniques are available, the choice depending on the stage of pregnancy and the potential nature of the defect.

DNA diagnosis

The majority of samples are obtained by chorionic villus biopsy, although amniotic fluid cells are sometimes used. Techniques to sample maternal blood for foetal cells or foetal DNA are being developed. Foetal blood may be sampled directly in the mid-trimester. The DNA is then analysed after amplification by the polymerase chain reaction (PCR). It may be performed by using primer pairs that only amplify individual alleles ('allele-specific priming') or by using consensus primers that amplify all the alleles, followed by restriction digestion to detect a particular allele. This is best illustrated by Hb S, in which the bacterially derived enzyme Dde I detects the A-T change (Fig. 7.22).

Pre-implantation genetic diagnosis which avoids the need for pregnancy termination involves performing conventional *in vitro* fertilization, followed by removing one or two cells from the blastomeres on day 3. PCR is used to detect thalassaemia mutations so that unaffected blastomeres can be selected for implantation. HLA typing can also be used to select a blastomere HLA matching a previous thalassaemia major child, so that the new baby could potentially act as a donor for stem cell transplantation into its older sibling. Ethical considerations are important in deciding to use these applications.

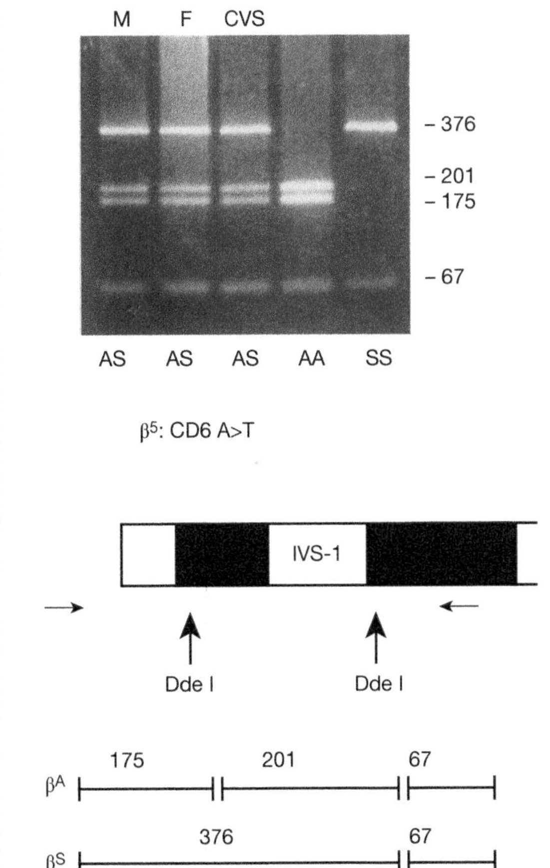

Figure 7.22 Sickle cell anaemia: antenatal diagnosis by Dde I-polymerase chain reaction (PCR) analysis. The DNA is amplified by two primers that span the sickle cell gene mutation site and produce a product of 473 base pairs (bp) in size. The product is digested with the restriction enzyme Dde I and the resulting fragments analysed by agarose gel electrophoresis. The replacement of an adenine base in the normal β-globin gene by thymine results in Hb S and removes a normal restriction site for Dde I, producing a larger 376 bp fragment than the normal 175 and 201 bp fragments in the digested amplified product. In this case, the CVS DNA shows both the normal fragments and the larger sickle cell product and so is AS. The gel shows DNA from the mother (M), father (F), foetal DNA from a chorionic villus sample (CVS), a normal DNA control (AA) and a homozygous sickle cell DNA control (SS). Source: Courtesy of Dr J. Old.

SUMMARY

- Genetic disorders of haemoglobin fall into two main groups:
  1 The thalassaemias in which synthesis of the α- or β-globin chain is reduced.
  2 Structural disorders such as sickle cell anaemia in which an abnormal haemoglobin is produced.
- The α- or β-thalassaemias occur clinically as minor forms with microcytic hypochromic red cells and a raised red cell count with or without anaemia.
- Total absence of function of all four α-globin genes causes fatal hydrops fetalis.
- Absence of function of both β-globin genes causes β-thalassaemia major, a transfusion-dependent anaemia associated with iron overload with liver, endocrine and cardiac damage. Iron chelation therapy has greatly improved life expectancy.
- Thalassaemia intermedia (non-transfusion dependent thalassaemia) is a clinical term for a group of disorders showing mild to moderate anaemia and is usually caused by variants of β-thalassaemia. In the more severe forms, there are bone deformities, enlargement of the liver and spleen, extramedullary haemopoiesis and iron overload due to increased iron absorption.
- The most frequent structural defect of haemoglobin is caused by the sickle mutation in the β-globin chain. In the homozygous form, there is a range of clinical courses. Severe cases are characterized by a severe haemolytic anaemia, associated with vaso-occlusive crises. These may be painful, affecting bone or involve soft tissues, e.g. chest, spleen or central nervous system.
- Crises may also be haemolytic or aplastic.
- Management of sickle cell anaemia involves prevention and treatment of infections and, for acute crises, pain relief and hydration. Blood transfusions are given to prevent organ, especially brain, damage.
- Hydroxyurea is valuable in reducing the frequency and severity of acute crises.
- Allogeneic stem cell transplantation offers possible cure for both thalassaemia major and sickle cell anaemia but is expensive and carries short and long term risks.
- Gene transfer therapy is proving beneficial in some cases in both thalassaemia major and sickle cell anaemia.
- Antenatal diagnosis using PCR technology to amplify chorionic villous DNA is used to detect severe genetic defects of haemoglobin production, with termination of the pregnancy offered if appropriate.

Now visit **www.wiley.com/go/haematology9e** to test yourself on this chapter.

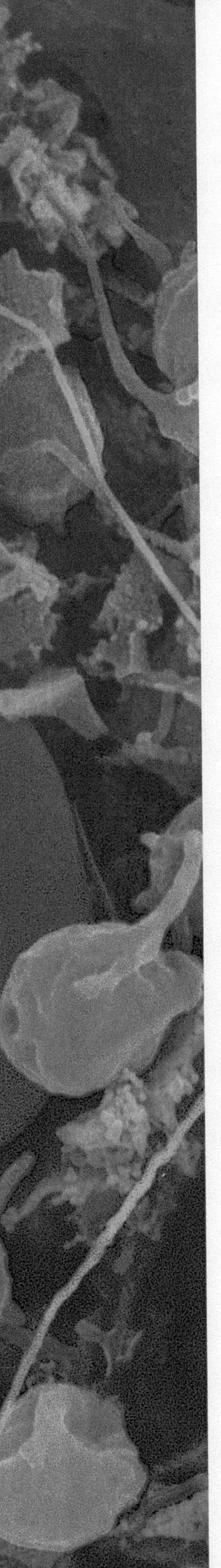

CHAPTER 8

The white cells, part 1: granulocytes, monocytes and their benign disorders

Key topics

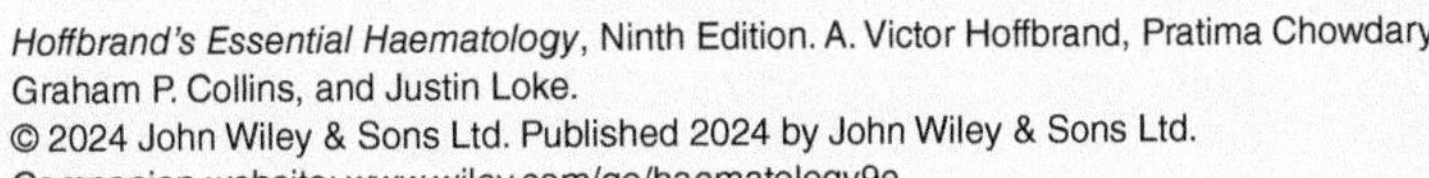

Hoffbrand's Essential Haematology, Ninth Edition. A. Victor Hoffbrand, Pratima Chowdary, Graham P. Collins, and Justin Loke.

© 2024 John Wiley & Sons Ltd. Published 2024 by John Wiley & Sons Ltd.

Companion website: www.wiley.com/go/haematology9e

The white blood cells (leucocytes) divide into two broad groups: the **phagocytes** and the **lymphocytes.** Phagocytes comprise cells of the **innate** immune system, which can act very quickly after an infection, whereas lymphocytes mediate the **adaptive immune response,** which can develop immunological memory, for example after vaccination. Certain lymphocyte subtypes such as natural killer (NK) cells lack memory capacity and are considered part of the innate immune system.

Phagocytes subdivide into granulocytes (which include neutrophils, eosinophils and basophils) and monocytes. Their normal development, function and benign disorders are dealt with in this chapter (Table 8.1; Fig. 8.1). Lymphocytes are considered in Chapter 9.

The function of phagocytes and lymphocytes in protecting the body against infection is closely connected with two soluble protein systems of the body: immunoglobulins and **complement.** These proteins which are involved in blood cell destruction in a number of diseases are discussed with the lymphocytes in Chapter 9.

Granulocytes

Neutrophil (polymorph)

This cell has a characteristic dense nucleus of between two and five lobes, and a pale cytoplasm with an irregular outline containing many fine dark pink–blue (azurophilic) or grey–blue

Table 8.1 White cells: normal blood counts.

Adults	Blood count	Children	Blood count
Total leucocytes	$4.0–11.0 \times 10^9/L$		*Total leucocytes*
Neutrophils	$1.8–7.5 \times 10^9/L$ $1.5–7.5 \times 10^9/L$*	Neonates	$10.0–25.0 \times 10^9/L$
Eosinophils	$0.04–0.4 \times 10^9/L$	1 year	$6.0–18.0 \times 10^9/L$
Monocytes	$0.2–0.8 \times 10^9/L$	4–7 years	$6.0–15.0 \times 10^9/L$
Basophils	$0.01–0.1 \times 10^9/L$	8–12 years	$4.5–13.5 \times 10^9/L$
Lymphocytes	$1.5–3.5 \times 10^9/L$		

* The lower limit of normal is $1.8 \times 10^9/L$ in Caucasians and $1.5 \times 10^9/L$ in people of African and Middle–East descent.
In normal pregnancy the upper limits are total leucocytes $14.5 \times 10^9/L$, neutrophils $11 \times 10^9/L$. Minor variations in the 'normal' range may be present from laboratory to laboratory.

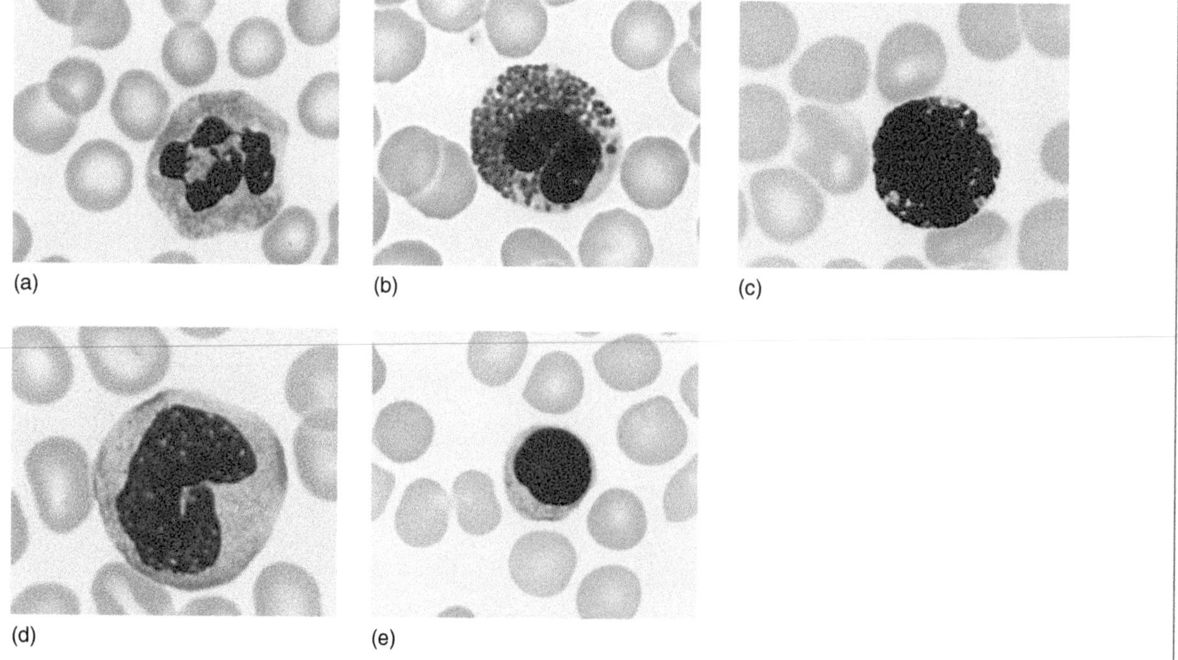

Figure 8.1 White blood cells (leucocytes): **(a)** neutrophil (polymorph); **(b)** eosinophil; **(c)** basophil; **(d)** monocyte; **(e)** lymphocyte.

staining granules (Fig. 8.1a). The granules are divided into primary, which appear at the promyelocyte stage, and secondary (specific), which appear at the myelocyte stage and predominate in the mature neutrophil (Fig. 8.7). Both types of granule are lysosomal in origin: the primary contains myeloperoxidase and other acid hydrolases; the secondary contains lactoferrin, lysozyme and other enzymes.

Neutrophil precursors

These do not usually appear in normal peripheral blood but are present in the marrow (Fig. 8.2). The earliest recognizable precursor is the **myeloblast**, a cell of variable size which has a large nucleus with fine chromatin and usually two to five nucleoli (Fig. 8.2b). The cytoplasm is basophilic and no granules are present. The normal bone marrow contains up to 5% of myeloblasts.

Myeloblasts give rise to promyelocytes, slightly larger cells which retain nucleoli but have developed primary cytoplasmic granules (Fig. 8.2a). Promyelocytes give rise to myelocytes, which have specific or secondary granules. The nuclear chromatin is more condensed and nucleoli are not visible. Separate myelocytes of the neutrophil, eosinophil and basophil series can be identified. The myelocytes give rise to **metamyelocytes**, non-dividing cells, which have an indented or horseshoe-shaped nucleus and a cytoplasm filled with primary and secondary granules.

Neutrophil forms between the metamyelocyte and fully mature neutrophil are termed '**band**', 'stab' or 'juvenile'. These may occur in normal peripheral blood. They do not contain the clear, fine filamentous distinction between nuclear lobes that is seen in mature neutrophils.

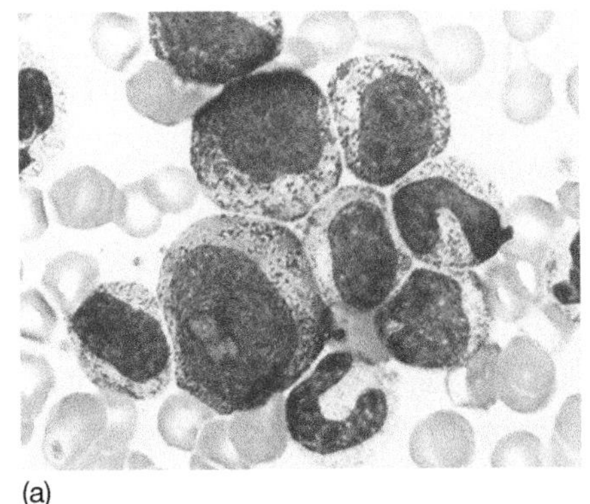

(a)

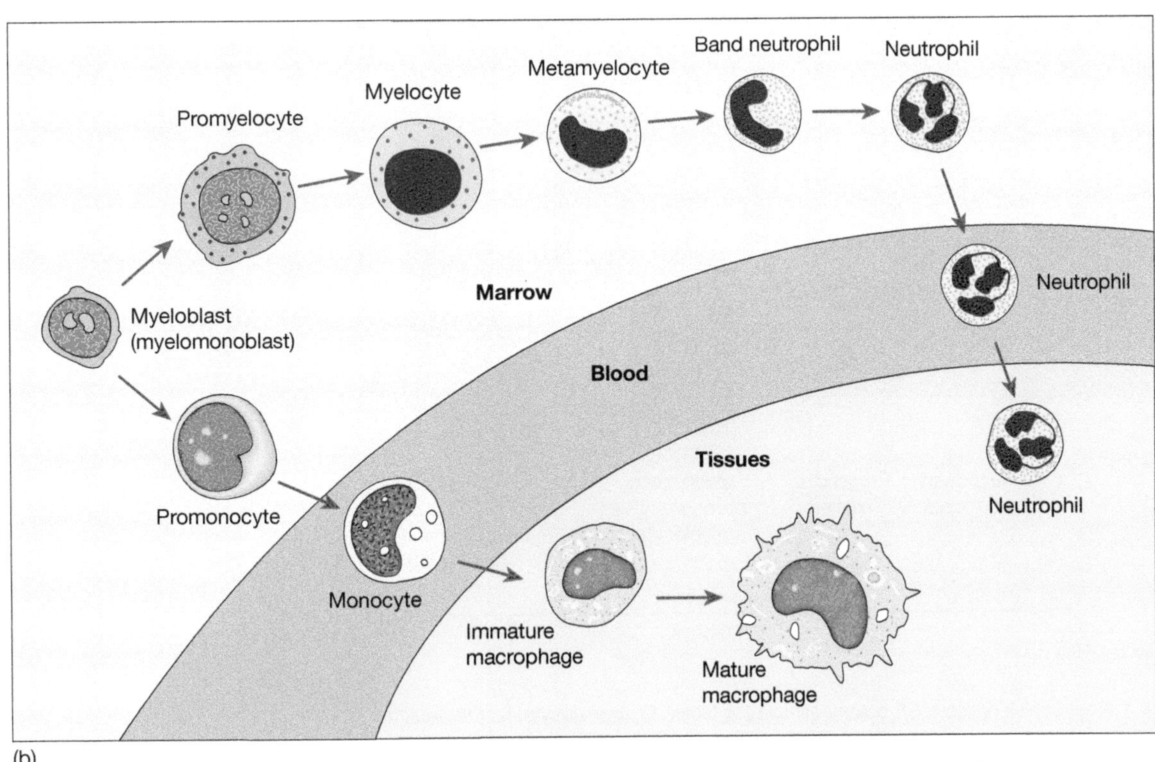

(b)

Figure 8.2 **(a)** Granulopoiesis. A promyelocyte, myelocytes, and metamyelocytes. Source: A.V. Hoffbrand *et al*. (2019) *Color Atlas of Clinical Hematology.* Reproduced with permission of John Wiley & Sons. **(b)** The formation of the neutrophil and monocyte phagocytes. Eosinophils and basophils are also formed in the marrow in a process similar to that for neutrophils.

Normal neutrophil count

The lower limit of the normal neutrophil count is 1.8×10^9/ in Caucasians and in people of African and Middle Eastern descent 1.5×10^9/L (Table 8.1). Lower normal values are also found from 2 to 3 weeks after birth for the first few months of life (Table 34.1).

Up to 98% of people of West African origin carry a polymorphism in the Duffy antigen chemokine receptor gene *DARC* which leads to loss of DARC expression on red cells. This has been selected for during evolution because the malaria parasite *Plasmodium vivax* uses DARC as a receptor to enter the red cell. DARC is a chemokine receptor and the loss of its expression affords some protection from malaria. Loss on leucocytes is associated with lowering of the median neutrophil count by around $0.3–0.5 \times 10^9$/L. A similar effect is seen in some populations in the Middle East. The reduction in the neutrophil count may result from increased neutrophil margination. This occurs in other ethnic groups without significant clinical consequences.

Eosinophils

These cells are similar to neutrophils, except that the cytoplasmic granules are coarser and more deeply red staining, and there are rarely more than three nuclear lobes (Fig. 8.1b). Eosinophil myelocytes can be recognized, but earlier stages are indistinguishable from neutrophil precursors. The blood transit time for eosinophils is longer than for neutrophils. They enter inflammatory exudates and have a special role in allergic responses, defence against parasites and removal of fibrin formed during inflammation. Thus they play a role in local immunity and tissue repair.

Basophils

These are only occasionally seen in normal peripheral blood. They have many dark cytoplasmic granules which overlie the nucleus; they contain heparin and histamine (Fig. 8.1c). They resemble tissue mast cells which have the same cell of origin.

Granulopoiesis

Granulocytes and monocytes are formed in the bone marrow from a common precursor cell (Fig. 1.2). In the granulopoietic series, progenitor cells, myeloblasts, promyelocytes and myelocytes form a proliferative or mitotic pool of cells, while the metamyelocytes, band and segmented granulocytes make up a post-mitotic maturation compartment (Fig. 8.3).

Large numbers of band and segmented neutrophils (10–15 times more than in the blood) are held in the normal marrow as a 'reserve pool'. **The bone marrow normally contains more myeloid cells than erythroid cells in the ratio of 2 : 1 to 12 : 1, the largest proportion being neutrophils and metamyelocytes.** Following their release from the marrow, granulocytes spend only 6–10 hours in the circulation before entering tissues, where they perform their phagocytic function. Under the influence of selectin adhesion molecules, they first tether to the endothelium. They then roll along it before, under the influence of integrins adhering to and then transmigrating through the vascular wall. After average 4–5 days in the tissues, they are destroyed during defensive action or as the result of senescence. In the bloodstream there are two pools normally of about equal size: the circulating pool (included in the blood count) and a marginating pool (not included in the blood count) attached to the vascular wall.

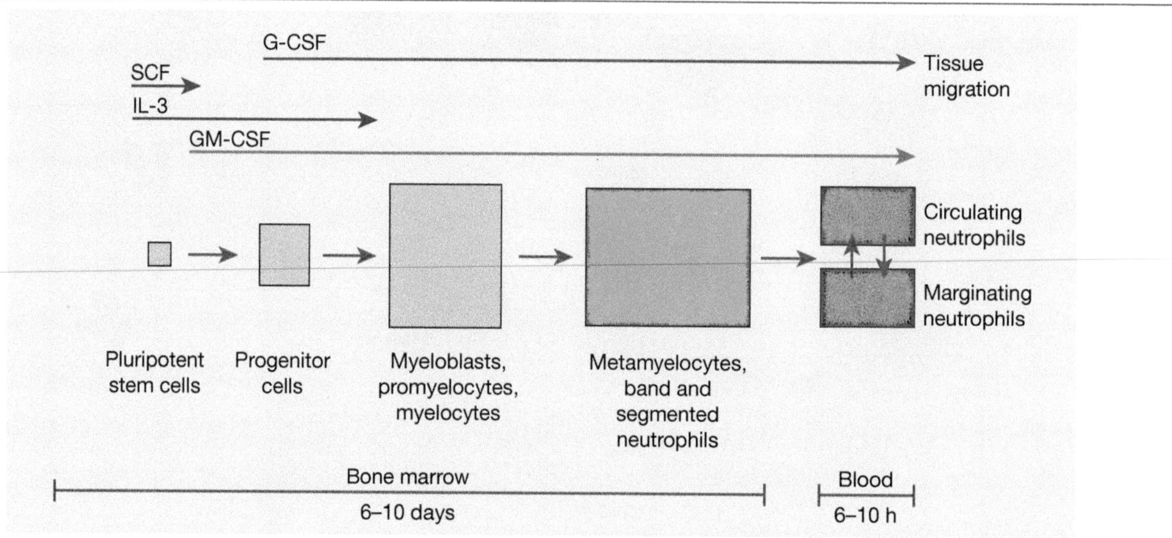

Figure 8.3 Neutrophil kinetics. CSF, colony-stimulating factor; G, granulocyte; IL, interleukin; M, monocyte; SCF, stem cell factor.

Control of granulopoiesis: myeloid growth factors

Many growth factors are involved in granulopoiesis including interleukin-1 (IL-1), IL-3, IL-5 (for eosinophils), IL-6, IL-11, granulocyte–macrophage colony-stimulating factor (GM-CSF), granulocyte CSF (G-CSF) and monocyte CSF (M-CSF) (Fig. 1.6). The growth factors stimulate proliferation and differentiation and also affect the function of the mature cells on which they act, e.g. phagocytosis, superoxide generation and cytotoxicity in the case of neutrophils (Fig. 1.5). They also inhibit apoptosis.

Increased granulocyte and monocyte production in response to an infection is induced by increased production of growth factors and cytokines such as IL-1. IL-6 or tumour necrosis factor (TNF) from stromal cells. Monocytes and T lymphocytes, stimulated by endotoxin (Fig. 8.4).

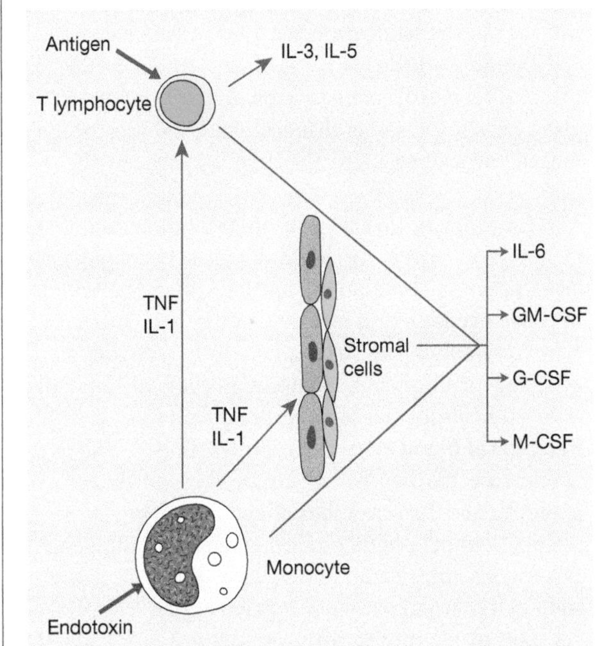

Figure 8.4 Regulation of haemopoiesis; pathways of stimulation of leucopoiesis by endotoxin, for example from infection. It is likely that endothelial and fibroblast cells release basal quantities of granulocyte–macrophage colony-stimulating factor (GM-CSF) and granulocyte colony-stimulating factor (G-CSF) in the normal resting state and that this is enhanced substantially by tumour necrosis factor (TNF) and interleukin-1 (IL-1).

Clinical applications of G-CSF

Clinical administration of G-CSF (such as filgrastim) subcutaneously produces a rise in neutrophils. Short-acting G-CSF is given daily. Longer acting PEGylated G-CSF, pegfilgrastim and eflapegrastim, can be given once in 7–14 days. Indications are:

- **Post-chemotherapy and post-allogeneic or autologous stem -cell transplantation (SCT)** to accelerate neutrophil recovery and shorten the period of neutropenia (Fig. 8.5). Post-chemotherapy G-CSF is usually given if the risk of febrile neutropenia is considered >20%. G-CSF administration may translate into a reduction of length of time in

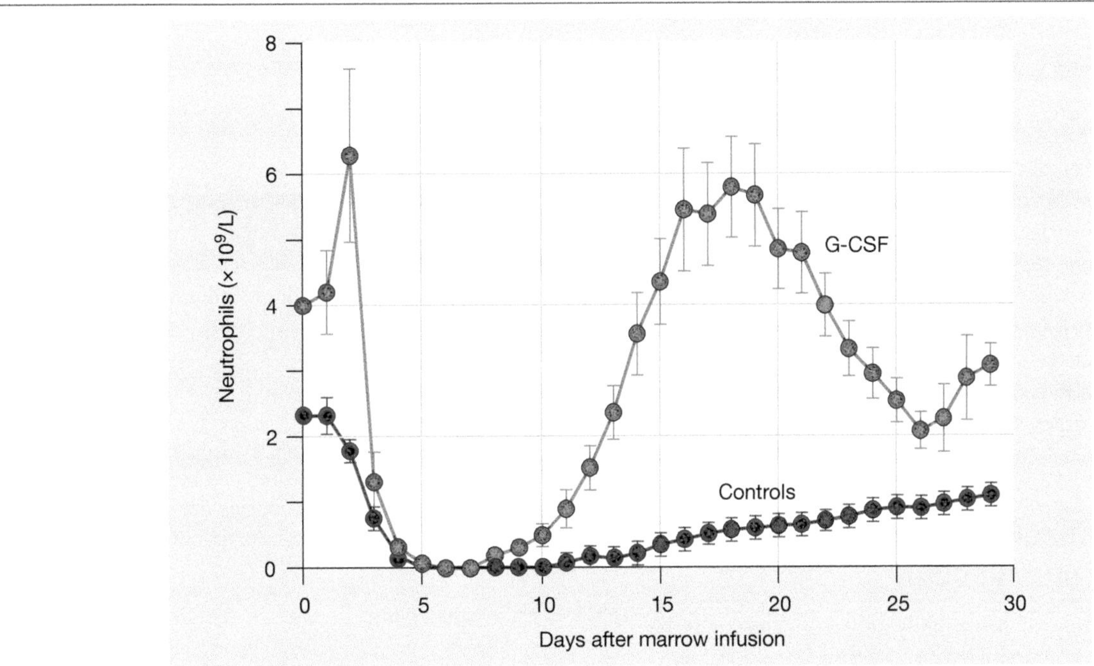

Figure 8.5 Typical effect of granulocyte colony-stimulating factor (G-CSF) on recovery of neutrophils.

hospital, antibiotic usage and frequency of infection, but periods of extreme neutropenia after intensive chemotherapy cannot be prevented. The injections may also allow repeated courses of chemotherapy, e.g. for lymphoma, to be given on schedule rather than being delayed because of prolonged neutropenia, particularly a problem in older patients.

- **Myelodysplasia (MDS) and aplastic anaemia.** G-CSF is not given alone for MDS but has been given with erythropoiesis-stimulating agents in an attempt to improve haemoglobin level and neutrophil count.
- **Severe benign neutropenia** Both congenital and acquired neutropenia, including cyclical and drug-induced neutropenia, often respond well to G-CSF.
- **Peripheral blood stem cell mobilization** G-CSF is used to increase the number of circulating multipotent progenitors from donors or the patient, improving the harvest of sufficient peripheral blood stem cells for allogeneic or autologous transplantation. It is avoided in sickle cell stem cell transplantation as it may cause a 'crisis'.
- **As part of chemotherapy regimens, e.g. FLAG-IDA, p. xxx.** May induce cell cycling in quiescent cancer cells.

Monocytes

These are usually larger than other peripheral blood leucocytes and possess a large central oval or indented nucleus with clumped chromatin (Fig. 8.1d). The abundant cytoplasm stains blue and contains many fine vacuoles, giving a ground-glass appearance. Cytoplasmic granules are also often present. The monocyte precursors in the marrow (monoblasts and promonocytes) are difficult to distinguish from myeloblasts and monocytes.

Monocytes spend only a short time in the marrow and, after circulating for 20–40 hours, leave the blood to enter the tissues, where they mature and carry out their principal functions. Their extravascular life span after their transformation to **macrophages (histiocytes)** may be as long as several months or even years. In tissues the macrophages become self-replicating without replenishment from the blood. They assume specific functions in different tissues, e.g. lymph nodes, brain and liver (Fig. 8.6). GM-CSF and M-CSF are involved in monocyte production and activation. When activated by inflammation, monocytes/macrophages secrete cytokines which massively attract more blood monocytes and other leucocytes to the tissue.

Disorders of neutrophil and monocyte morphology and function

The normal function of neutrophils and monocytes may be divided into three phases. Defects resulting in clinical syndromes can occur in each of these phases (Table 8.2).

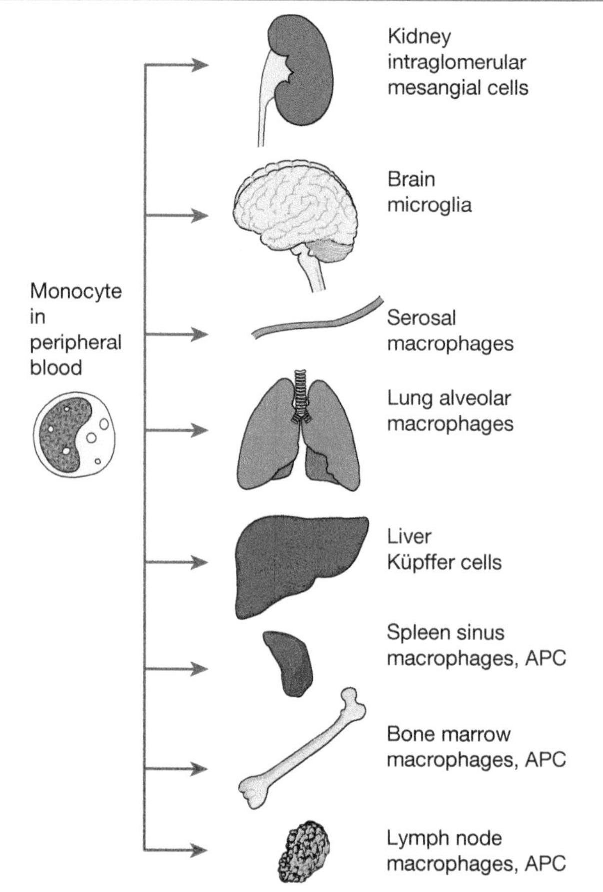

Figure 8.6 Reticuloendothelial system: distribution of macrophages. Other tissues, e.g. skin and intestine, also are rich in macrophages. APC, antigen presenting cells

Table 8.2 Congenital disorders of neutrophil morphology and function.

Clinical features	Abnormality/disease
None or minimal	Pelger–Huët Neutrophil hypersegmentation Alder-Reilly May-Hegglin Myeloperoxidase deficiency
Recurrent infections due to adherence/chemotaxis defects	Leucocyte adhesion deficiency, Specific granule deficiency
Recurrent infections due to killing defects	Chronic granulomatous disease Chediak-Higashi syndrome (defects also of chemotaxis)

Chemotaxis (cell mobilization and migration)

The phagocyte is attracted to bacteria or the site of inflammation by chemotactic substances released from damaged tissues, by complement components and by the interaction of **leucocyte adhesion molecules** with ligands on the damaged tissues. The leucocyte adhesion molecules also mediate recruitment and interaction with other immune cells and with platelets (Chapter 29). They are also variously expressed on endothelial cells and platelets (Chapter 1).

Phagocytosis

The foreign material, e.g. bacteria, fungi or dead or damaged cells of the host are phagocytosed (Fig. 8.7). Recognition of a foreign particle is aided by opsonization with immunoglobulin or complement, because both neutrophils and monocytes have Fc and C3b receptors (Chapter 9).

Macrophages have a central role in processing and presenting foreign antigens on human leucocyte antigen (HLA) molecules to the immune system (Chapter 9, Chapter 25). They also secrete a large number of growth factors and chemokines, which regulate haemopoiesis, inflammation and immune responses.

Chemokines are chemotactic cytokines which may be produced constitutively and control lymphocyte traffic under physiological conditions. Inflammatory chemokines are induced or up-regulated by inflammatory stimuli. They bind to and activate cells via chemokine receptors and play an important part in recruiting appropriate cells to the sites of inflammation.

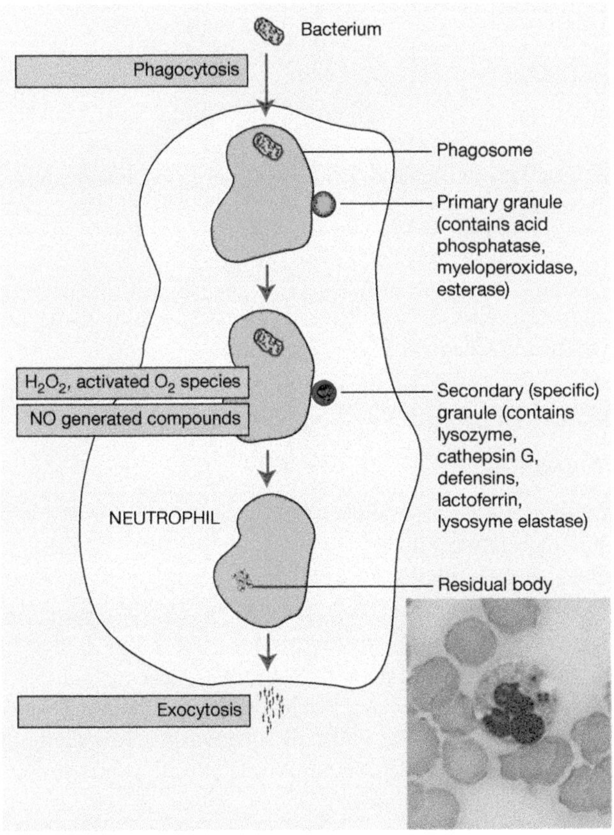

Figure 8.7 Phagocytosis and bacterial destruction. On entering the neutrophil, the bacterium is surrounded by an invaginated surface membrane and fuses with a primary lysosome to form a phagosome. Enzymes from the lysosome attack the bacterium. Secondary granules also fuse with the phagosomes, and additional enzymes from these granules including lactoferrin attack the organism. Various types of activated oxygen, generated by glucose metabolism, also help to kill bacteria. Undigested residual bacterial products are excreted by exocytosis. Inset: Neutrophil ingesting meningococci. Source (inset): A.V. Hoffbrand *et al.* (2019) *Color Atlas of Clinical Hematology: Molecular and Cellular Basis of Disease*, 5th edn. Reproduced with permission of John Wiley & Sons.

Killing and digestion

These occur by **oxygen-dependent** and **oxygen-independent** pathways. In the oxygen-dependent reactions, superoxide (O_2–), hydrogen peroxide (H_2O_2) and other activated oxygen (O_2) species are generated from O_2 and reduced nicotinamide adenine dinucleotide phosphate (NADPH). In neutrophils, H_2O_2 reacts with myeloperoxidase and intracellular halide to kill bacteria; activated oxygen may also be involved (Fig. 8.7). Nitric oxide (NO), generated through NO synthase from L-arginine, is an oxygen-independent mechanism by which phagocytes also kill microbes.

Another non-oxidative microbicidal mechanism involves microbicidal proteins. These may act alone, e.g. cathepsin G, or in conjunction with H_2O_2, e.g. lysozyme, elastase. They may also act with a fall in pH within phagocytic vacuoles into which lysosomal enzymes are released. Lactoferrin, an iron-binding protein, is bacteriostatic by depriving bacteria of iron and by generating free radicals (Fig. 8.7).

Finally they are part of another more recently recognized microbicidal killing mechanism called NETosis. Neutrophil extracellular traps (NETs) consist of a network of extracellular strings of DNA associated with modified histones and granular enzymes which together kill microbes (Fig. 8.8). NETosis may result from nuclear and cytoplasmic material associated with disintegration and death of the cell. It may also occur from extrusion of DNA, histones and granules from viable cells (Fig. 8.8). Antibodies, immune complexes, cytokines and chemokines can all induce NETosis. The importance of NETosis in inflammation and thrombosis is discussed further in Chapter 29.

Morphological abnormalities

Congenital

A number of hereditary conditions may give rise to changes in granulocyte morphology (Table 8.2, Fig. 8.9). The **Barr body** (Fig. 8.9h) appears as a 'drumstick' attached to a nuclear lobe of female neutrophils. It is due to the presence of two X-chromosomes. Congenital **hypersegmentation of the**

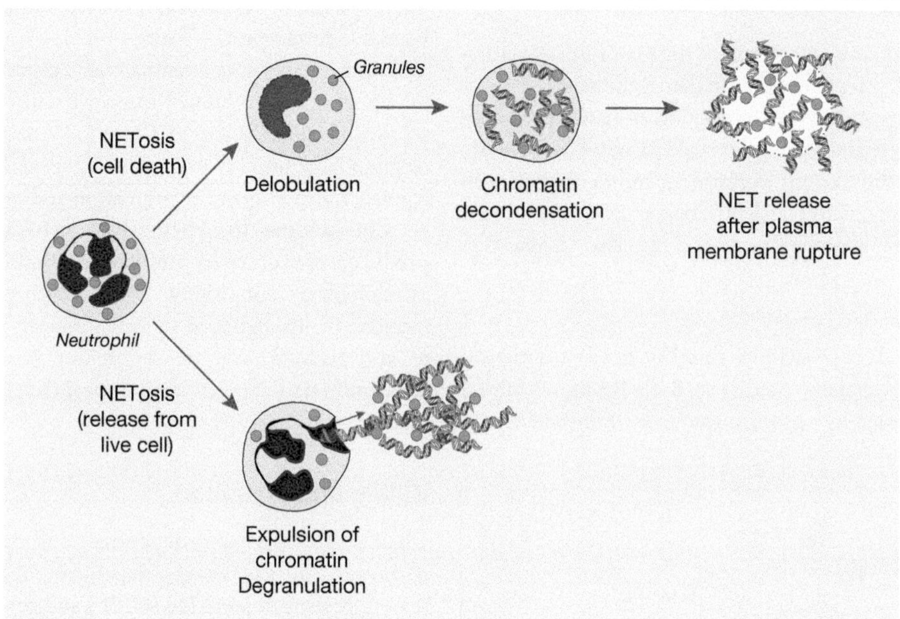

Figure 8.8 The formation of extracellular neutrophil extracellular traps (NETs) by cell disintegration and death (upper panel) or from viable cells (lower panel). The NETS kill microbes by a process termed NETosis (see text).

neutrophils, the Alder-Reilly abnormality (large coarse purple granules in the neutrophils, monocytes and lymphocytes associated with mucopolysaccharidosis) are not associated with clinical problems. **Myeloperoxidase deficiency** is one of the most frequent of the congenital abnormalities of neutrophils but surprisingly is either symptomless or associated with a relatively mild increase in fungal infections.

The **Pelger–Huët anomaly** with bi-lobed neutrophils in the peripheral blood is an uncommon symptomless condition, most common in Northern Europeans. Occasional unsegmented neutrophils are also seen. Inheritance is autosomal dominant, usually due to mutations in the gene *LBR* encoding the lamin B receptor, which is important for cholesterol synthesis. In myelodysplastic neoplasias 'pseudo'-Pelger–Huët cells occur in the blood. They lack the *LBR* mutations.

The **May–Hegglin anomaly** is a rare condition in which the neutrophils contain basophilic inclusions of RNA (resembling morphologically Döhle bodies) in the cytoplasm. There is an associated mild thrombocytopenia with giant platelets. Inheritance is autosomal dominant and usually due to mutations in the *MYH9* gene, which encodes a myosin heavy chain.

Acquired

Döhle bodies (light blue/grey staining whorls of endoplasmic reticulum at the periphery of the cytoplasm) and toxic changes (cytoplasmic vacuoles and intense staining of granules) are found in infection. Hypersegmentation (more than 5 lobes) of the nucleus is characteristic of megaloblastic anaemia; hypersegmented neutrophils occur more rarely as a congenital anomaly and from other causes (Chapter 5). Morphological changes, frequent in acute myeloid leukaemia and in myelodysplasia, are described in Chapters 13 and 16.

Defects of phagocytic cell function

Congenital

Chemotaxis

These defects occur in rare congenital abnormalities. **Leucocyte adhesion deficiencies** are usually due to autosomal recessive inheritance of mutations of surface adhesion proteins such as integrins. **Neutrophil-specific granule deficiency** is due to mutation of a myeloid transcription factor. The neutrophils are bi-lobed, lack cytoplasmic granules and there is reduced bactericidal activity as well as impaired chemotaxis. Clinically both these congenital deficiencies are associated with recurrent bacterial and fungal infections.

Phagocytosis

These defects usually arise because of a lack of opsonization, which may be caused by congenital or acquired causes of hypogammaglobulinaemia or lack of complement components.

Killing

The rare X-linked or autosomal recessive **chronic granulomatous disease** illustrates faulty killing by phagocytes. It results from abnormal leucocyte oxidative metabolism. There is an abnormality affecting different elements of the respiratory burst oxidase or its activating mechanism resulting in failure of superoxide generation. Most cases are due to mutations of a

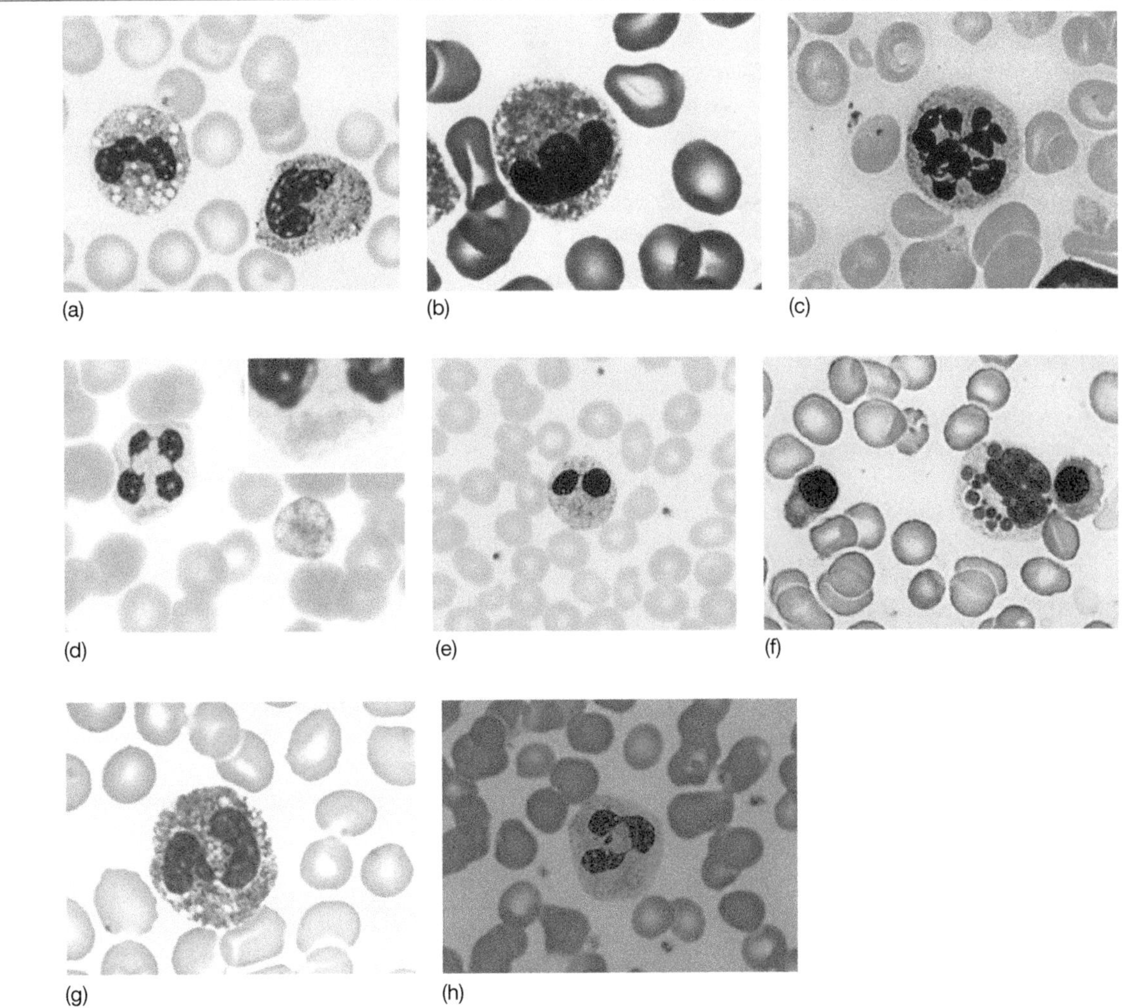

Figure 8.9 Abnormal morphology of neutrophils: **(a)** Neutrophil leucocytosis due to infection: toxic changes shown by the presence of vacuoles and red–purple granules in the band form neutrophils. **(b)** Neutrophil leukocytosis due to infection: a Döhle body (see text) and toxic changes (vacuoles and intense staining of granules) in the cytoplasm. **(c)** Hypersegmented neutrophil in peripheral blood of a patient with megaloblastic anaemia. **(d)** May–Hegglin anomaly: the neutrophils contain basophilic inclusions 2–5 mm in diameter; there is an associated mild thrombocytopenia with giant platelets. **(e)** Pelger–Huët anomaly: coarse clumping of the chromatin in pince-nez configuration. **(f)** Chédiak–Higashi syndrome: bizarre giant granules in the cytoplasm of a monocyte. **(g)** Alder-Reilly anomaly: coarse violet granules in the cytoplasm of a neutrophil. **(h)** Barr body, a 'drumstick' attached to one of the lobes of the neutrophil nucleus. Source: Courtesy of Professor Barbara Bain.

cytochrome b gene located on the X-chromosome but 30% are due to mutations of autosomal genes. The patients have recurring infections, usually bacterial but sometimes fungal, which start in infancy or early childhood. Failure to switch off the inflammatory response leads to the characteristic granuloma formation.

Chediak-Higashi syndrome includes albinism, recurrent infections, a mild bleeding disorder and peripheral neuropathy. There are giant granules in the neutrophils, eosinophils, monocytes and lymphocytes, accompanied by neutropenia, thrombocytopenia and marked hepatosplenomegaly. It is due to mutations in the *CHS1 (LYST)* gene, which encodes a lysosomal trafficking regulator.

Acquired

These may be faults in the neutrophils or in their environment. Diseases causing reduced chemotaxis, phagocytosis and killing include acute or chronic myeloid leukaemia and myelodysplastic neoplasms. Renal failure, diabetes, malnutrition, corticosteroids and other drugs impair various aspects of neutrophil function.

VEXAS syndrome

VEXAS (vacuoles, E1 enzyme, X-linked, auto-inflammatory, somatic) syndrome is a newly recognized adult-onset disease characterized by acquired somatic mutation of the *UBA1* gene in haemopoietic progenitor cells. *UBA1* located on the X chromosome encodes the major E1 enzyme that initiates ubiquitylation. The male patients have a macrocytic anaemia and various inflammatory disorders including relapsing polychondritis, Sweet syndrome and vasculitides. Most are thrombocytopenic. There is prominent vacuolization of early myeloid and erythroid precursors. Treatment is symptomatic control with corticosteroids and the JAK2 inhibitor ruxolitinib which reduces inflammation. Allogeneic stem cell transplantation is a potentially curative option but so far there has been limited experience.

Causes of neutrophil leucocytosis

An increase in circulating neutrophils to levels greater than 7.5×10^9/L is one of the most frequently observed blood count changes (Table 8.3). Neutrophil leucocytosis is sometimes accompanied by fever as a result of the release of leucocyte pyrogens. Other characteristic features of reactive neutrophilia may include (a) a 'shift to the left' in the differential white cell count, an increase in the number of band forms and the occasional presence of more primitive cells such as metamyelocytes and myelocytes in peripheral blood; and (b) the presence of cytoplasmic toxic granulation and Döhle bodies (Fig. 8.9a, b).

The leukaemoid reaction

The leukaemoid reaction is an excessive reactive leucocytosis usually characterized by the presence of immature cells, e.g. myeloblasts, promyelocytes and myelocytes in the peripheral blood.

Table 8.3 Causes of neutrophil leucocytosis.
Bacterial infections (especially pyogenic bacterial, localized or generalized)
Inflammation and tissue necrosis, e.g. myositis, vasculitis, cardiac infarct, trauma
Metabolic disorders, e.g. uraemia, eclampsia, acidosis, gout
Pregnancy
Neoplasms of all types, e.g. carcinoma, lymphoma, melanoma
Acute haemorrhage or haemolysis
Drugs, e.g. corticosteroids which inhibit margination; lithium, tetracycline
Chronic myeloid leukaemia, myeloproliferative neoplasms Non-haematological neoplasms
Treatment with G-CSF (granulocyte colony-stimulating factor)
Asplenia
Rare inherited disorders

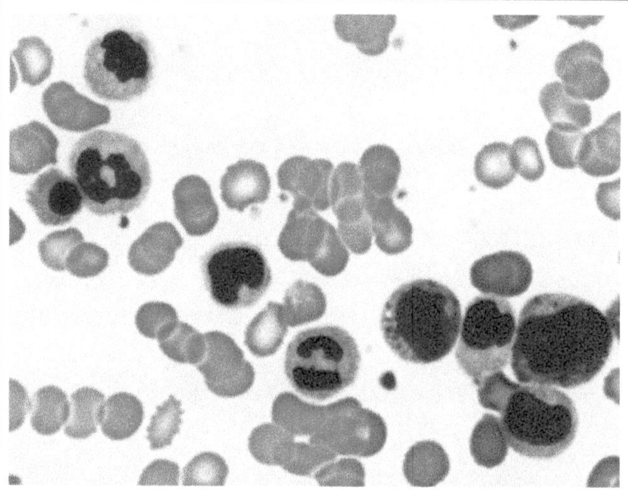

Figure 8.10 Leuco-erythroblastic blood film. This shows an erythroblast, promyelocyte, myelocyte and metamyelocytes in a patient with metastatic breast carcinoma in the bone marrow.

Table 8.4 Causes of leuco-erythroblastic blood film.
Metastatic neoplasm in the marrow
Primary myelofibrosis
Acute and chronic myeloid leukaemias
Myeloma, lymphoma
Miliary tuberculosis
Severe megaloblastic anaemia
Severe haemolysis
Osteopetrosis
Secondary marrow fibrosis e.g. due to rheumatological syndromes

Underlying disorders include severe or chronic infections, severe haemolysis or metastatic cancer. Leukaemoid reactions are often particularly marked in children.

Leuco-erythroblastic reaction

This is characterized by the presence of erythroblast and granulocyte precursors in the blood (Fig. 8.10). It is due to metastatic infiltration of the marrow or certain benign or neoplastic blood disorders (Table 8.4).

Neutropenia

Neutropenia may be selective (Table 8.5) or part of a general pancytopenia (Chapter 24). It may also be acute or chronic (lasting >3 months). Neutropenia due to peripheral destruction or

Table 8.5 Causes of neutropenia.

Selective neutropenia
Congenital

Acquired
Drug-induced
Anti-inflammatory (aminopyrene, gold, levamisole, penicillamine)
Antibacterial (cephalosporins, co-trimoxazole, meropenem, metronidazole, penicillins, sulfasalazine, tobramycin, vancomycin)
Anticonvulsants (carbamazepine, valproate) Antithyroids (carbimazole, methimazole) Hypoglycaemics (tolbutamide)
Phenothiazines (chlorpromazine, thioridazine)
Psychotropics and antidepressants (clozapine, olanzapine, imipramine)
Miscellaneous (deferiprone, furosemide, mepacrine, rituximab, ticlopidine)

Cyclical
Idiopathic and clonal neutropenia of uncertain significance (Chapter 16)

Autoimmune
Associated with chronic autoimmune diseases, e.g. systemic lupus erythematosus, Sjogren's syndrome
Rheumatoid arthritis (Felty syndrome), hypersensitivity and anaphylaxis

Large granular lymphocytic leukaemia (p. xxx)

Infections
Viral, e.g. hepatitis, influenza, HIV
Fulminant bacterial infection, e.g. typhoid, military tuberculosis

Part of general pancytopenia (Table 24.1)

HIV, human immunodeficiency virus.

margination (see below) is associated with a bone marrow showing normal or even increased neutrophils and/or their precursors. The much more serious failure of neutrophil production is associated with a marrow showing reduced numbers of neutrophils and their precursors. When the absolute neutrophil level falls $<0.5 \times 10^9$/L due to failure of production, recurrent infections are likely, and if $<0.2 \times 10^9$/L the risks are particularly serious, especially if there is also a functional defect of neutrophils.

Congenital neutropenia

Severe congenital neutropenia (previously called Kostmann syndrome) usually presents in the first year of life with life-threatening infections. Most cases are dominantly inherited, caused by mutations of the gene *ELANE2*, coding for neutrophil elastase. Other types are autosomal recessive; underlying mutations of more than 10 genes have been described. Monocytosis, eosinophilia and hypergammaglobulinaemia may be present. In some cases, the neutropenia occurs as part of other syndromes with non-haematological manifestations, e.g. Wiskott–Aldrich (p. 364, Shwachman–Diamond (p. 317) or Chédiak–Higashi (p. 107). G-CSF produces a clinical response in most patients. Some of the forms predispose to myelodysplastic neoplasias or acute myeloid leukaemia.

Acquired neutropenia

Drug-induced

Drugs are the most likely cause of an isolated acquired neutropenia. A large number of drugs other than those used in chemotherapy have been implicated (Table 8.5). They may induce neutropenia either by direct toxicity or immune-mediated damage, the drug acting as a hapten. For many the mechanism remains obscure. The onset of neutropenia is often within 1–2 weeks of starting the drug but it may develop later only after weeks or months or only after a second exposure.

Cyclical

This is a rare syndrome with 2- to 4-week periodicity. Severe but temporary neutropenia occurs. Monocytes tend to rise as the neutrophils fall. Germline mutations of *ELANE2*, the gene for neutrophil elastase, underlie some cases.

Idiopathic and clonal neutropenia of uncertain significance

In these conditions, there is neutropenia without morphological features in the blood or marrow cells of myelodysplasia or another haematological neoplasm. They are defined and discussed under the general descriptions of idiopathic and clonal cytopenias in Chapter 16.

In the idiopathic form (benign chronic neutropenia, idiopathic cytopenia of undetermined significance, ICUS) no dysplasia or clonal genetic mutations are detected. This is the most common type of chronic neutropenia in both children and adults. It is more common in females and thought to be brought about in some cases by immune cells causing inhibition of myelopoiesis in the bone marrow. In the clonal form (CCUS, Chapter 16), clonal genetic mutations are found in the blood and bone marrow cells similar to those found in clonal haemopoiesis of indeterminate prognosis (CHIP, Chapter 16).

Autoimmune neutropenia

In some cases of chronic neutropenia an autoimmune mechanism can be demonstrated. The antibody may be directed against one of the neutrophil-specific antigens. The detection of neutrophil antibodies requires difficult laboratory procedures and test characteristics (sensitivity and specificity) are poor, so the tests are not performed routinely.

Clinical features

Severe neutropenia is particularly associated with infections of the mouth and throat. Painful and often intractable ulceration may occur at these sites (Fig. 8.11), in the skin or

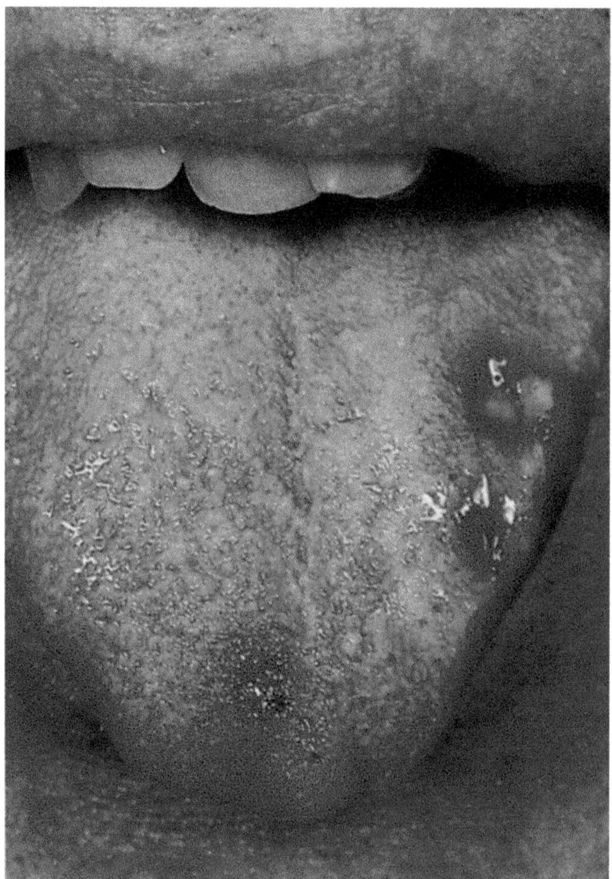

Figure 8.11 Ulceration of the tongue in severe neutropenia.

at the anus. Septicaemia rapidly supervenes. Organisms carried as negative organisms in the bowel may become pathogens. Other features of infections associated with severe neutropenia are described in Chapter 12.

Diagnosis

Bone marrow examination is useful in determining the cause of the neutropenia, i.e. whether there is reduction in early precursors or whether there is reduction only of circulating and marrow neutrophils, with late precursors present in the marrow. Marrow aspiration (with cytogenetic and molecular genetic tests) and trephine biopsy may also provide evidence of leukaemia, myelodysplasia or other infiltration.

Management

The treatment of patients with acute severe neutropenia is described on Chapter 12. In many patients with drug-induced neutropenia, spontaneous recovery occurs within 1–2 weeks after stopping the drug. Patients with chronic neutropenia have recurrent infections which are mainly bacterial in origin, although fungal and viral infections (especially herpes) also occur. **Early recognition and vigorous treatment with antibiotics, antifungal or antiviral agents, as appropriate, are essential**. Prophylactic antifungal agents, e.g. fluconazole, are often given and antibacterial agents, e.g. ciprofloxacin, may reduce the risk, but resistance is of concern (Chapter 12). G-CSF or its PEGylated form is effective at raising the neutrophil count in a variety of benign chronic neutropenic states. Corticosteroid therapy or splenectomy has been associated with good results in some patients with autoimmune neutropenia. Corticosteroids impair neutrophil function, however, and should not be used indiscriminately in patients with neutropenia. Rituximab (anti-CD20) may also be effective, although it may itself be a cause of neutropenia. Haemopoietic stem cell transplantation may be indicated if clonal evolution to myelodysplasia or leukaemia occurs.

Causes of monocytosis, eosinophil and basophil leucocytosis

Monocytosis

A rise in blood monocyte count above 0.8×10^9/L is infrequent. The conditions causing monocytosis are listed in Table 8.6.

Eosinophilic leucocytosis (eosinophilia)

The causes of an increase in blood eosinophils (Fig. 8.12) above 0.4×10^9/L are listed in Table 8.7. **It is most frequently due to allergic diseases, parasites, skin diseases or drugs**. If a cause such as asthma or severe atopy is not obvious, a diligent search for precipitants must be undertaken, including testing for *Strongyloides*, stool ova and parasites. Sometimes no underlying cause is found, and no clonal marker can be detected. If the eosinophil count is elevated above 1.5×10^9/L for over 6 months and associated with tissue damage for which no other cause can be detected, the **hypereosinophilic syndrome (HES)** is diagnosed. In the HES, the heart valves, central nervous system (CNS), skin and lungs may be affected. In 25% of cases a clonal T-cell population is driving the eosinophilia.

Table 8.6 Causes of monocytosis.

Chronic bacterial infections: tuberculosis, brucellosis, bacterial endocarditis, typhoid
Connective tissue diseases: SLE, temporal arteritis, rheumatoid arthritis
Protozoan infections
Chronic neutropenia
Hodgkin lymphoma, AML and other malignancies
Chronic myelomonocytic leukaemia (CMML)

AML, acute myeloid leukaemia; SLE, systemic lupus erythematosus.

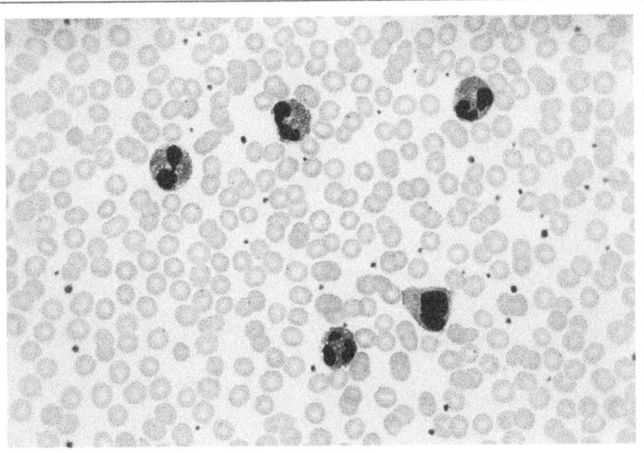

Figure 8.12 Blood film showing eosinophilia.

Table 8.7 Causes of eosinophilia.

Allergic diseases, especially hypersensitivity of the atopic type, e.g. bronchial asthma, hay fever and food sensitivity
Parasitic diseases, e.g. amoebiasis, hookworm, ascariasis, tapeworm infestation, filariasis, schistosomiasis, strongyloidiasis and trichinosis
Recovery from acute infection
Certain skin diseases, e.g. psoriasis, pemphigus and dermatitis herpetiformis, urticaria and angioedema, atopic dermatitis and skin parasites, e.g. scabies, myiasis
Drug sensitivity
Polyarteritis nodosa, vasculitis, serum sickness Autoimmune, e.g. inflammatory bowel disease, sarcoidosis
Graft-versus-host disease
Hodgkin lymphoma and some other lymphoid neoplasias, especially clonal T-cell disorders, adenocarcinoma
Metastatic malignancy with tumour necrosis
Hypereosinophilic syndrome (idiopathic)
Pulmonary syndromes Eosinophilic pneumonia, transient pulmonary infiltrates (Loeffler's syndrome), allergic granulomatosis (Churg–Strauss syndrome), tropical pulmonary eosinophilia
Myeloid/lymphoid neoplasias with clonal rearrangement of *PDGFRA* or *B or of other tyrosine kinases*
Other myeloproliferative neoplasms, including systemic mastocytosis

Treatment is usually first with high-dose corticosteroids and second-line with cytotoxic drugs, e.g. imatinib, hydroxycarbamide, methotrexate, immunosuppressants, ciclosporin or α-interferon. Mepolizumab a humanized antibody to IL-5, is a promising new treatment for the hypereosinophilic syndromes.

Loeffler syndrome is a transient reactive form affecting the lungs and the Churg–Strauss syndrome consists of a vasculitis with eosinophilic granulomas of the respiratory tract.

In other cases of chronic eosinophilia, often with similar clinical features to idiopathic cases, a clonal cytogenetic or molecular abnormality is present such as a mutation or rearrangement in *PDGFRA* or *B*. Chronic eosinophilic leukaemia is then diagnosed (p. xxx). These cases sometimes respond to tyrosine kinase inhibitors such as imatinib.

Basophil leucocytosis (basophilia)

An increase in blood basophils above 0.1×10^9/L is uncommon. The usual cause is a myeloproliferative disorder such as chronic myeloid leukaemia or polycythaemia vera. Basophil increases are sometimes also seen in myxoedema, during chickenpox infection and in ulcerative colitis.

Histiocytic and dendritic cell disorders

Histiocytes are myeloid-derived tissue macrophages. The neoplastic disorders are listed in Table 8.8.

Dendritic cells

These mainly derive from a separate lineage from monocytes and are specialized antigen-presenting cells found mainly in the skin, lymph nodes, spleen and thymus (Chapter 9). They continuously travel through tissues to the draining lymph nodes where they survive for days or a few weeks. There are two subsets (Fig. 1.6):

1 Myeloid-derived dendritic cells, including Langerhans' cells, which are present in skin and mucosae and are characterized by the presence of tennis racquet-shaped Birbeck

Table 8.8 Classification of the histiocytic and dendritic cell neoplasms WHO (2022).

Plasmacytoid dendritic cell neoplasms
Mature plammacytoid dendritic cell proliferation associated with myeloid neoplasm
Blastic plasmacytoid dendritic cell neoplasm (Chapter 13)
Langerhans cell and other dendritic neoplasms
Langerhans cells neoplasms
Langerhans cell histiocytosis
Langerhans cell sarcoma
Other dendritic neoplasms
Histiocytic neoplasms
Juvenile xanthogranuloma
Erdheim–Chester disease
Rosai–Dorfman disease
ALK-positive histiocytosis
Histiocytic sarcoma

granules, seen in electron-microscopy sections in neutrophils, eosinophils, macrophages and lymphocytes. They are positive for the myeloid antigens CD33, CD13, CD11b and CD11c.

2 Plasmacytoid dendritic cells which lack these myeloid antigens have a plasma cell appearance but express early T-cell markers including CD4. They are found in lymphoid tissues.

The primary role of dendritic cells is antigen presentation to T and B lymphocytes (Chapter 9).

Haemophagocytic lymphohistiocytosis

Haemophagocytic lymphohistiocytosis (HLH, haemophagocytic syndrome) is a rare, recessively inherited or more frequently acquired disease, defined by overwhelming activation of macrophages and T lymphocytes causing a 'cytokine storm'. HLH is usually precipitated by a viral (especially Epstein–Barr), bacterial (such as TB) or fungal infection or occurs in association with autoimmune diseases or neoplasms, most commonly non-Hodgkin lymphoma.

In the familial form, various genes involved in the regulation of macrophage function such as perforin and *UNC13D* have been shown to be mutated. Severely damaging mutations may result in presentation in childhood and 'milder' variants may only present in adulthood when a trigger such as a neoplasm develops.

Patients present with fever and pancytopenia, often with splenomegaly and liver dysfunction. **There are increased numbers of histiocytes in the bone marrow which ingest red cells, white cells and platelets (Fig. 8.13).** Clinical features often also include lymphadenopathy, hepatic and splenic enlargement, coagulopathy and central nervous system signs. The condition may be confused with severe sepsis. Common laboratory anomalies include very elevated serum ferritin and C-reactive protein, reduced albumin and fibrinogen, low or absent NK cell activity, and elevated CD25 level (soluble IL-2 receptor).

Treatment is of the underlying infection or neoplasm, if known, with support care, and with anti-macrophage and immunomodulatory drugs. Chemotherapy with daunorubicin, etoposide, corticosteroids, ciclosporin, ruxolitinib, rituximab (anti-CD20) or anti-thymocyte globulin may be tried. Targeted therapy, including blockade of specific cytokines such as IL-1, IL-6, and IFNγ, and inhibition of the JAK–STAT pathways, improves outcome for some patients. The condition is, however, often fatal.

Dendritic and histiocytic neoplasms

These neoplasms frequently show mutations in the MAPK pathway (Fig. 1.8) of genes *BRAF, ARAF, MAP2K1, NRAS and KRAS*. CD163 is positive and so a useful marker. Treatments have been developed that target the MAPK pathway such as BRAF and MEK inhibitors.

Langerhans cell histiocytosis

Langerhans cell histiocytosis (LCH) is the commonest histiocytic disorder. It is associated with the formation of granulomatous-like lesions containing langerin (CD207) positive histiocytes which also stain for CD1a and S100. There is usually a brisk inflammatory infiltrate. It can occur in any organ but has a predilection for skin, lungs, bone and the pituitary gland. The BRAF V600E mutation is present in a majority of cases with other mutations involving the MAPK pathway in a significant number of BRAF mutation negative cases.

A number of clinical patterns of LCH have been described:

- Multisystem, high-risk disease occurring in children usually in the first 3 years of life. They present with hepatosplenomegaly, lymphadenopathy, cytopenias and eczematous skin lesions.

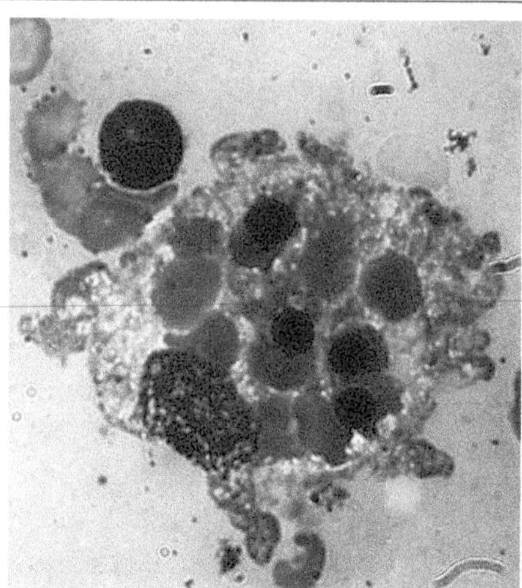

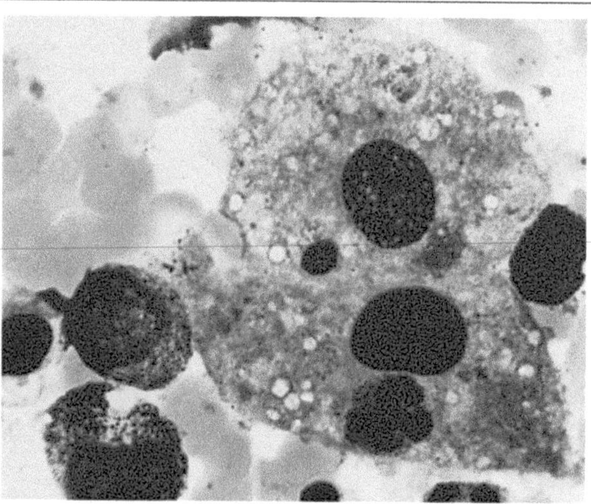

Figure 8.13 Haemophagocytic lymphohistiocytosis: bone marrow aspirates showing histiocytes that have ingested red cells, erythroblasts and neutrophils.

- Pulmonary LCH. This is seen in adult patients who smoke. Smoking cessation maybe enough to lead to disease resolution.
- CNS involvement: this can range from mass lesion in the meninges or parenchyma to anterior pituitary involvement presenting with diabetes insipidus (especially seen in patient with multisystem disease) to neurodegenerative LCH.

When treatment is required, a number of agents can be used. These include steroids, chemotherapy, e.g. cladribine, cytarabine, methotrexate, vinblastine, and targeted inhibitors such as the BRAF inhibitor vemurafenib and the MEK inhibitor cobimetinib.

Other histiocytic neoplasms (all rare)

Juvenile xanthogranuloma: caused by mutations of the receptor for M-CSF, this very rare disease usually present as a solitary skin lump with histology showing foamy histiocytes and giant cells. It usually resolves spontaneously.

Erdheim–Chester disease (ECD): a multisystem disease of adults with accumulation of lipid laden histiocytes which are CD68 positive and CD1a negative. Long bone involvement and a 'hairy kidney' appearance are often seen. It has similar molecular drivers to LCH and can co-exist with this disease in a significant number of cases.

Rosai-Dorfman disease: presenting with painless lymphadenopathy, this condition is associated with the accumulation of foamy macrophages with accompanying emperipoiesis (the presence of one intact cell inside another).

ALK-positive histiocytosis: a multisystem disease occurring especially in infants unified by the presence of *ALK* gene translocation.

Histiocytic sarcoma: An extranodal malignancy of mature tissue histiocytes which may be associated with other haematological neoplasms. Outcomes are generally very poor.

Lysosomal storage diseases

Gaucher, Tay-Sachs and Niemann–Pick diseases all result from hereditary deficiency of the enzymes required for glycolipid breakdown.

Gaucher disease

Gaucher disease is an uncommon autosomal recessive disorder characterized by an accumulation of glucosylceramide in the lysosomes of reticuloendothelial cells as a result of deficiency of glucocerebrosidase (Fig. 8.14).

Three types occur: a chronic adult (type I), acute infantile neuronopathic (type II) and subacute neuronopathic with onset in childhood or adolescence (type III). It is caused by mutations in the glucocerebrosidase gene. Over 300 mutations have been described. One (a single base pair substitution in codon 370) is particularly common in Ashkenazi Jews where 1 in 15–20 subjects may be carriers. This explains the high incidence of type 1 disease in this ethnic group. **The clinical manifestations of the most frequent Type 1 disease are caused by the accumulation of sphingolipid-laden macrophages in the spleen, liver and bone marrow (Fig. 8.15).** The outstanding physical sign is splenomegaly. Moderate liver enlargement and pingueculae (conjunctival deposits) are other characteristics. Gaucher disease is commonly associated with marked anaemia, leucopenia and thrombocytopenia, occurring singly or in combination. Often the presenting symptom is easy bruising due to thrombocytopenia with abnormal platelet function and coagulation defects. In many untreated cases, bone deposits cause osteonecrosis with bone pain and pathological fractures. Osteoporosis is also frequent. Expansion of the lower end of the femur may produce the 'Erlenmeyer flask deformity' (Fig. 8.15).

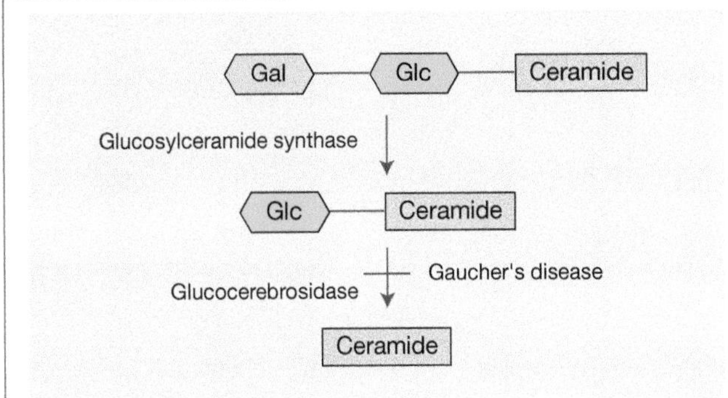

Figure 8.14 Gaucher disease results from a deficiency of glucocerebrosidase. Gal, galactose; Glc, glucose.

Gaucher cells are not inert lipid storage containers but are metabolically active, secreting cytokines and enzymes into plasma that cause secondary pathology. Polyclonal hypergammaglobulinaemia is frequent due to activation of B lymphocytes by NK cells, themselves activated by macrophages laden with glycolipids. Monoclonal gammopathy of underdetermined significance, MGUS, is also frequent and there is an increased risk of myeloma, myelodysplasia and of malignancies generally. Pulmonary hypertension, alveolar fibrosis and cholesterol gallstones are other consequences of macrophage activation. Carriers of a Gaucher mutation also have an increased incidence and earlier onset of Parkinson's disease, possibly due to excess deposition of α-synuclein in basal ganglia.

Diagnosis is made by assay of white cell glucocerebrosidase and DNA analysis. Serum levels of lysosomal enyzmes chitotriosidase and PARC (pulmonary-activation- regulated cytokine) are raised and useful in monitoring therapy. The levels of angiotensin-converting enzyme (ACE), and ferritin are also elevated.

Enzyme replacement therapy (ERT) with glucocerebrosidase as imiglucerase (Cerezyme), velaglucerase or taliglucerase, made by recombinant technology using mammalian or plant cell lines and given intravenously once every 2 weeks, is effective in shrinking the spleen, raising blood counts and

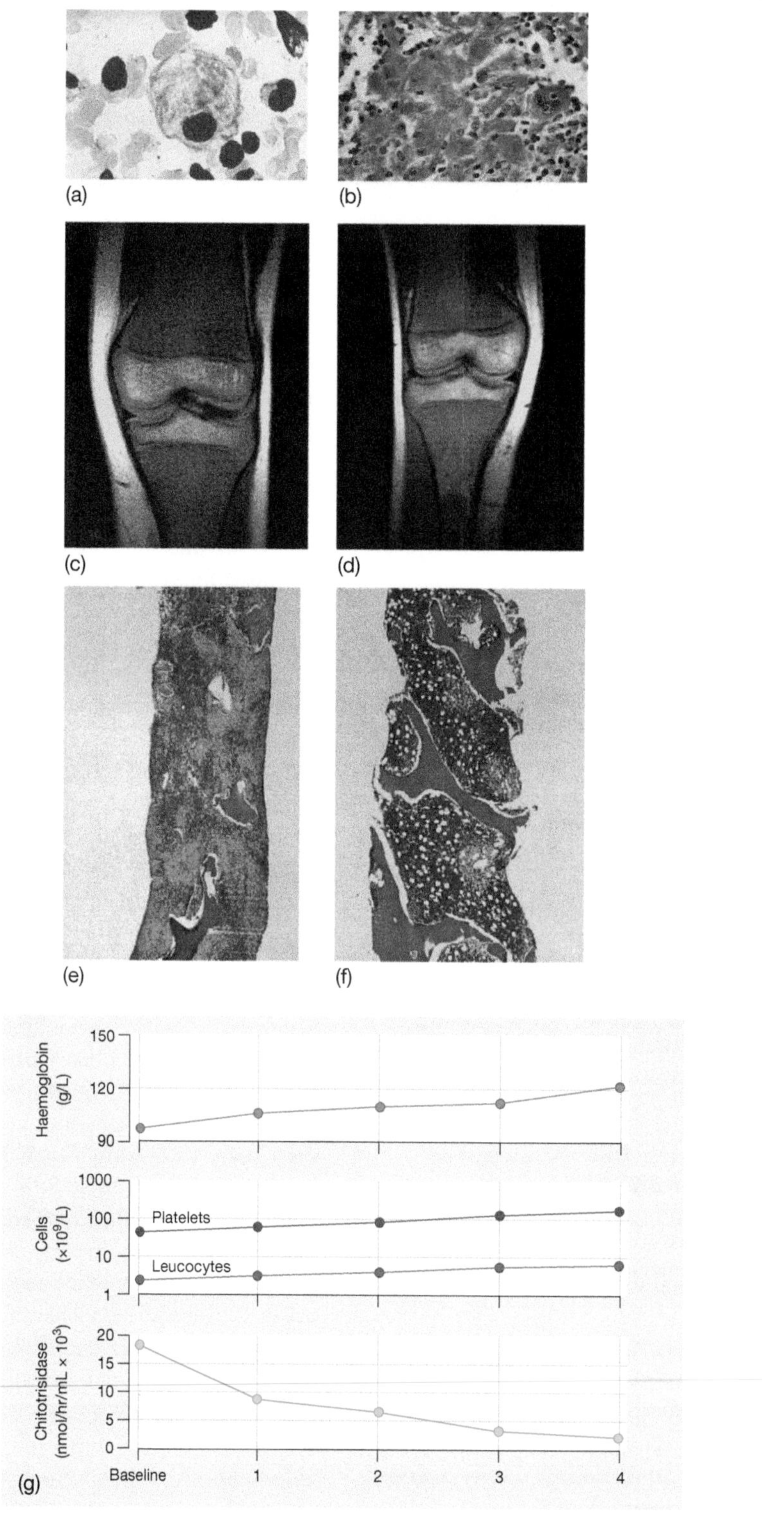

Figure 8.15 Gaucher disease: **(a)** bone marrow aspirate – a Gaucher cell with 'fibrillar' cytoplasmic pattern; **(b)** spleen histology – pale clusters of Gaucher cells in the reticuloendothelial cord; **(c)** magnetic resonance imaging (MRI) scan of the left knee of a patient before treatment showing Erlenmeyer flask deformity with expansion of the marrow and thinning of the cortical bone; **(d)** following a year of glucocerebrosidase therapy with subsequent remodelling of bone; and bone marrow trephine biopsy before **(e)** and after **(f)** 2 years of glucocerebrosidase therapy. **(g)** Improvement in blood counts and chitotriosidase levels with glucocerebrosidase therapy.
Source: (g) A.B. Mehta, D.A. Hughes. In A.V. Hoffbrand *et al.* (eds) (2016) *Postgraduate Haematology*, 7th edn. Reproduced with permission of John Wiley & Sons.

improving bone structure (Fig. 8.15). Oral drugs miglustat or eliglustat are useful alone in mild disease or in combination with the intravenous enzyme. They inhibit glucosylceramide synthase (Fig. 8.14) and so reduce the amount of substrate being produced in lysosomes. The use of ERT has virtually eliminated the need for splenectomy, which is avoided as far as possible as it leads to infiltration of other organs, e.g. bones. ERT cannot reverse established osteonecrosis, bone deformation, or hepatic, splenic or marrow fibrosis. Enzyme replacement has no impact on CNS disease in types II and III disease. Stem cell transplantation has been carried out successfully in severely affected patients, usually with type II or III disease.

Niemann–Pick disease

Niemann–Pick (N-P) disease shows certain clinical and pathological similarities to Gaucher disease. It is caused by sphingomyelinase deficiency due to mutations in the genes for lysosomal and cholesterol trafficking proteins. Sphingomyelin and cholesterol accumulate in macrophages causing massive hepatosplenomegaly. This is often fatal due to neurogeneration or lung involvement. Occasional patients live into adult life. Physical and mental development is commonly affected. A 'cherry-red' spot is commonly seen in the retina of affected infants. Pancytopenia is a regular feature and in marrow aspirates 'foam cells' of similar size to Gaucher cells are seen.

SUMMARY

- Phagocytes (granulocytes and monocytes) are the body's main defence against bacterial infection.
- Granulocytes include neutrophils (polymorphs), eosinophils and basophils. They are made in the bone marrow under the control of a variety of growth factors and have a short life span in the bloodstream before entering tissues.
- Neutrophil leucocytosis occurs in bacterial infection and in other types of inflammation.
- Neutropenia, if severe, predisposes to infections. It may be caused by bone marrow failure, chemotherapy, radiotherapy or drugs, or may be selective caused by immune, drug or other mechanisms or occur congenitally. G-CSF may be given to raise the neutrophil count.
- Eosinophilia is most frequently caused by allergic diseases, including skin diseases, parasitic infections or drugs. It can also be caused by a clonal increase in eosinophils, termed chronic eosinophilic leukaemia, or by an idiopathic condition, the hypereosinophilic syndrome, which is associated with damage to the lungs, heart, skin or other tissues.
- Mutations of a wide variety of genes cause rare congenital diseases of neutrophils and monocytes characterized by defects of chemotaxis, phagocytosis or killing.
- Histiocytes and dendritic cells are tissue macrophages derived from circulation monocytes. They may form clonal neoplastic diseases including Langerhans' cell histiocytosis, and other rare syndromes which affect single or multiple organs.
- The haemophagocytic lymphohistiocytosis syndrome (HLH) may be congenital or acquired especially after a viral or other infection or associated with malignancy. It involves destruction of red cells, granulocytes and platelets by tissue macrophages and may prove fatal. It is treated with support care, chemotherapy or immune modulating drugs.
- Histiocytic and dendritic cell neoplasms are clonal disorders usually with mutations in the MAP kinase pathway. They include Langerhan cell histiocytosis, Erdheim–Chester and Rosai–Dorfman diseases as well as other rare conditions.
- Lysosomal storage diseases are caused by inherited defects in the enzymes responsible for breakdown of glycolipids. Gaucher disease, the most frequent to affect haemopoiesis, is caused by glucocerebrosidase deficiency and is associated with accumulation of glycolipids in the macrophages of the reticuloendothelial system. Splenomegaly, pancytopenia and bone lesions cause the main clinical manifestations. Treatment is with enzyme replacement or substrate reduction therapy.

Now visit **www.wileyessential.com/haematology9e** to test yourself on this chapter.

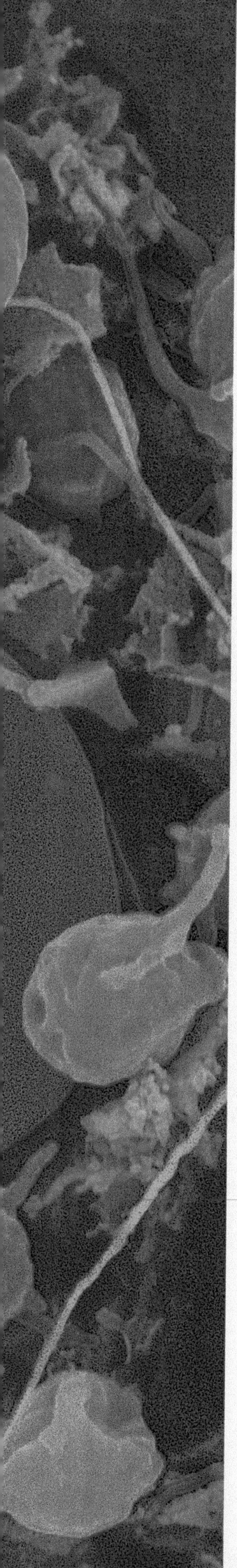

CHAPTER 9

The white cells, part 2: lymphocytes and their benign disorders

Key topics

Hoffbrand's Essential Haematology, Ninth Edition. A. Victor Hoffbrand, Pratima Chowdary, Graham P. Collins, and Justin Loke.
© 2024 John Wiley & Sons Ltd. Published 2024 by John Wiley & Sons Ltd.
Companion website: www.wiley.com/go/haematology9e

Lymphocytes are the immunologically competent cells that assist phagocytes in defence of the body against infection and other foreign invasions, including protection from neoplastic cells (Fig. 9.1). Two unique features of lymphocytes are their ability to generate antigenic specificity and the phenomenon of immunological memory. A complete description of the functions of lymphocytes is beyond the scope of this book, but information essential to an understanding of the diseases of the lymphoid system, and of the role of lymphocytes in other haematological diseases, is included here.

Lymphocytes

In postnatal life, the bone marrow and thymus are the primary lymphoid organs in which lymphocytes develop (Fig. 9.2). The secondary lymphoid organs in which specific immune responses are generated are the lymph nodes, spleen and lymphoid tissues of the alimentary and respiratory tracts and of other organs. In the bone marrow, lymphocytes derive from haemopoietic stem cells through a common myeloid/lymphoid progenitor (Fig. 1.2).

B lymphocytes

The immune response depends upon two types of lymphocytes, B and T cells (Table 9.1). They both derive from the haemopoietic stem cell through myeloid/lymphoid and then lymphoid progenitor cells. Interleukins 4 and 7 are involved (Fig. 1.7). B cells are named after the avian organ (bursa) in which they were first identified, and T cells are named after the thymus.

B cells mature in the bone marrow and circulate in the peripheral blood until they undergo recognition of antigen

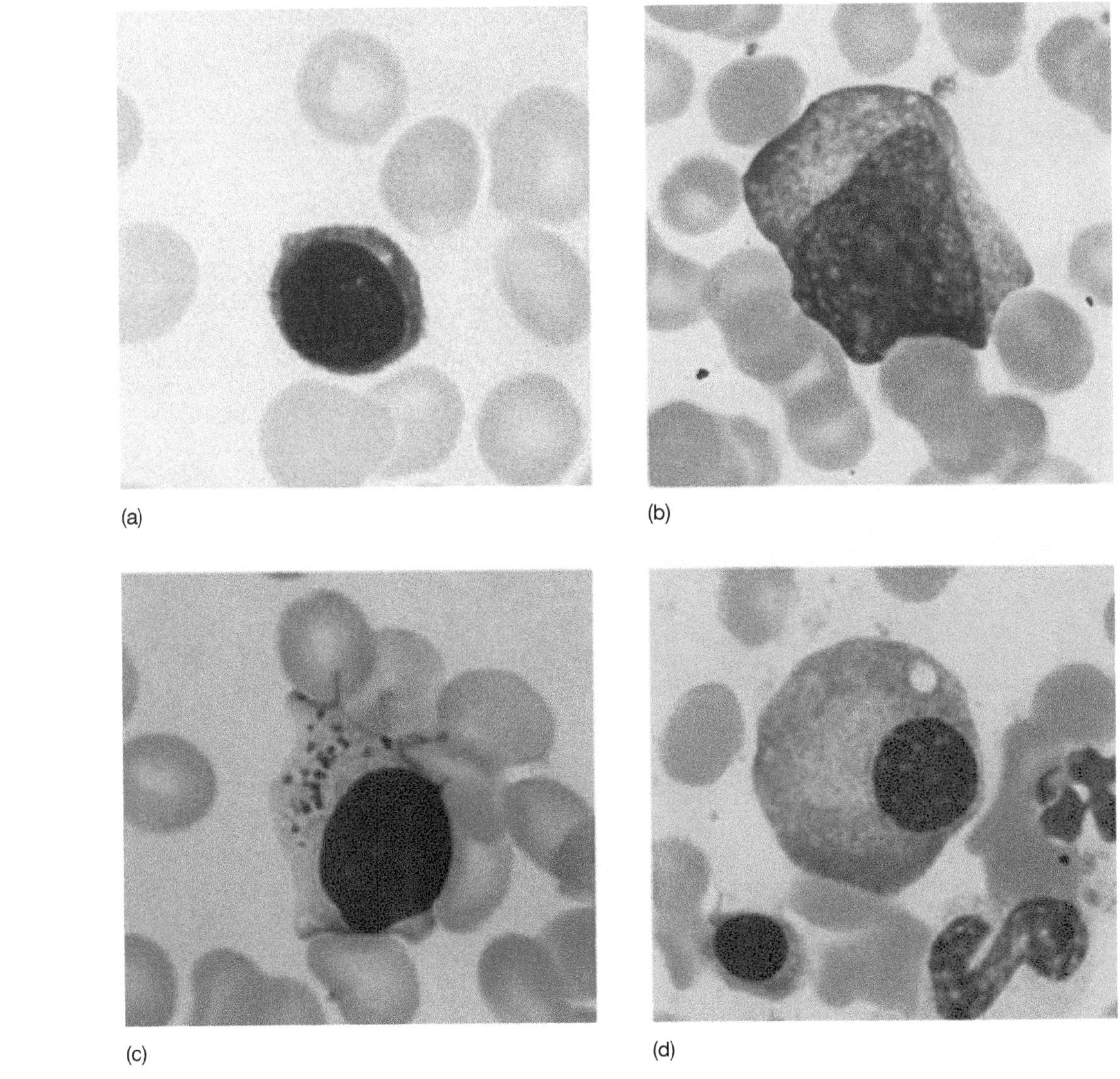

Figure 9.1 Lymphocytes: **(a)** small lymphocyte; **(b)** activated lymphocyte; **(c)** large granular lymphocyte; **(d)** plasma cell.

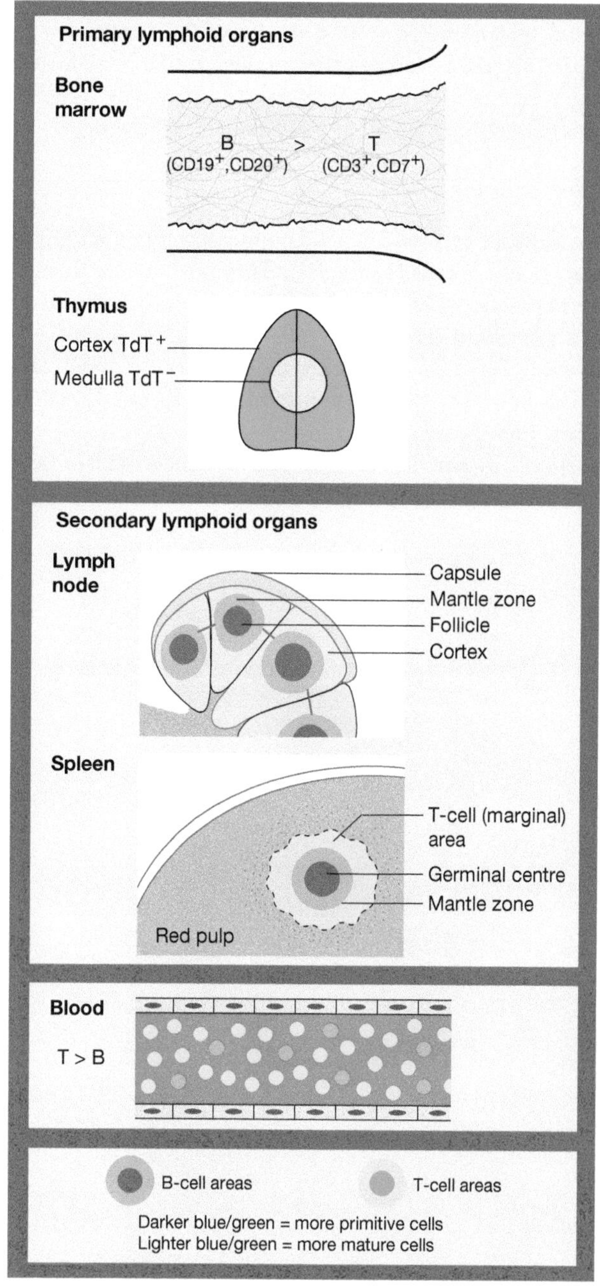

Figure 9.2 Primary and secondary lymphoid organs and blood. TdT, terminal deoxytidyl transferase.

Table 9.1 Functional aspects of T and B cells.

	T cells	B cells
Origin	Thymus	Bone marrow
Tissue distribution	Parafollicular areas of cortex in nodes, periarteriolar in spleen	Germinal centres of lymph nodes, spleen, gut, respiratory tract; also subcapsular and medullary cords of lymph nodes
Blood	80% of lymphocytes; CD4 > CD8	20% of lymphocytes
Membrane receptors	TCR for antigen	BCR (= immunoglobulin) for antigen
Function	CD8+: CMI against intracellular organisms CD4+: T-cell help for antibody production and generation of CMI	Humoral immunity by generation of antibodies
Characteristic Surface Markers	CD1 CD2 CD3 CD4 or 8 CD5 CD6 CD7 HLA class I HLA class II when activated	CD19 CD20 CD22 CD9 (pre-B cells) CD10 (precursor B cells) CD79 a and b HLA class I and II
Genes rearranged	TCR α, β, γ, δ	IgH, Igk, Igl

BCR, B-cell receptor; C, complement; CMI, cell-mediated immunity; HLA, human leucocyte antigen; Ig, immunoglobulin; TCR, T-cell receptor.

(Fig. 20.3). The **B-cell receptor (BCR)** is membrane-bound immunoglobulin (Fig. 9.3) which binds to a specific antigen. This leads to activation of phosphoinositide 3-kinase (PI3K), which produces a second messenger phosphatidylinositol (3,4,5)-trisphosphate (PIP3; Fig. 9.4). This activates Bruton tyrosine kinase (BTK), which phosphorylates further downstream enzymes. The overall effect is to induce expression of AKT, which is an anti-apoptotic pro-survival kinase. Effective drugs for treating the B-cell neoplasms, chronic lymphocytic leukaemia and non-Hodgkin lymphoma inhibit BTK (ibrutinib, acalabrutinib, zanabrutinib, pirtobrutinib) and PI3K, e.g. idelalisib, Chapter 18. The B-cell receptor itself is secreted as free soluble immunoglobulin (Fig. 9.5).

The B cell can mature into a memory B cell or plasma cell. Plasma cells home to the bone marrow and have a characteristic morphology with an eccentric round nucleus, a 'clock-face' chromatin pattern, and strongly basophilic cytoplasm (Fig. 9.1d). They express intracellular but not surface immunoglobulin and produce large amounts of antibody.

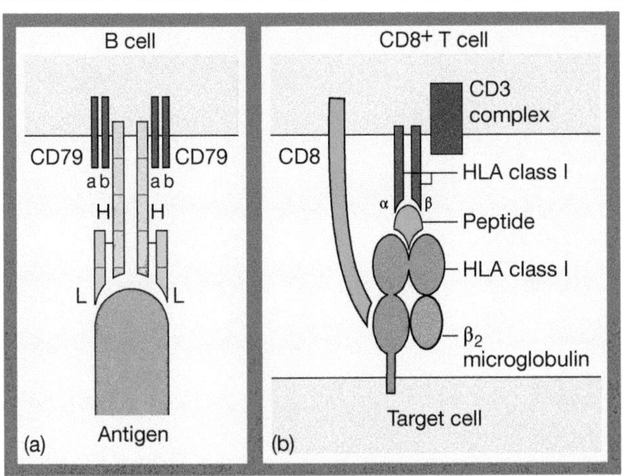

Figure 9.3 Antigen receptors on lymphocytes and their interaction with antigen. **(a)** The B-cell antigen receptor is membrane-bound immunoglobulin (Fig. 9.4). The antigen-binding immunoglobulin molecule is associated with the CD79a,b heterodimer, which acts as a signal transduction unit. **(b)** The T-cell receptor consists of a number of components that together constitute the CD3 complex. Two antigen-binding chains (α, β) are associated with several proteins (γ, δ, e, ζ) that mediate signal transduction. Antigen is recognized in the form of short peptides held on the surface of human leucocyte antigen (HLA) molecules. CD8⁺ T cells interact with peptide on a class I HLA molecule and the CD8 heterodimer interacts with the α_3 domain of the class I protein.

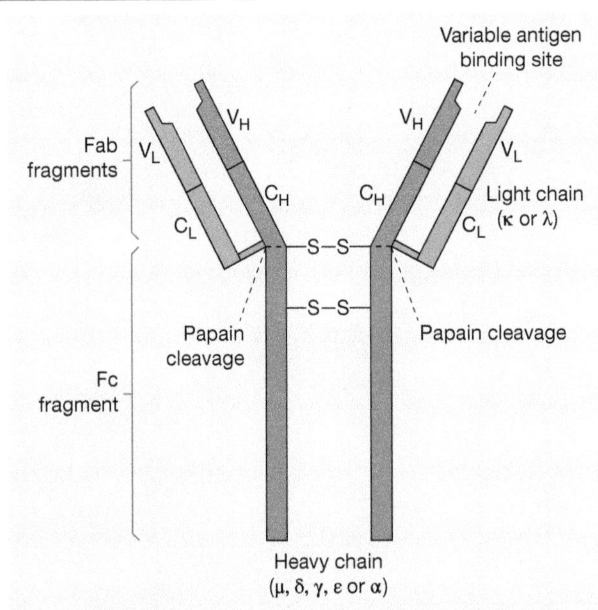

Figure 9.5 Basic structure of an immunoglobulin (Ig) molecule. Each molecule is made up of two light (**K** or **I**; blue areas) and two heavy (purple) chains, and each chain is made up of variable (V) and constant (C) portions, the V portions including the antigen-binding site. The heavy chain (m, δ, γ, ε or α) varies according to the immunoglobulin class. IgA molecules form dimers, while IgM forms a ring of five molecules. Papain cleaves the molecules into an Fc fragment and two Fab fragments.

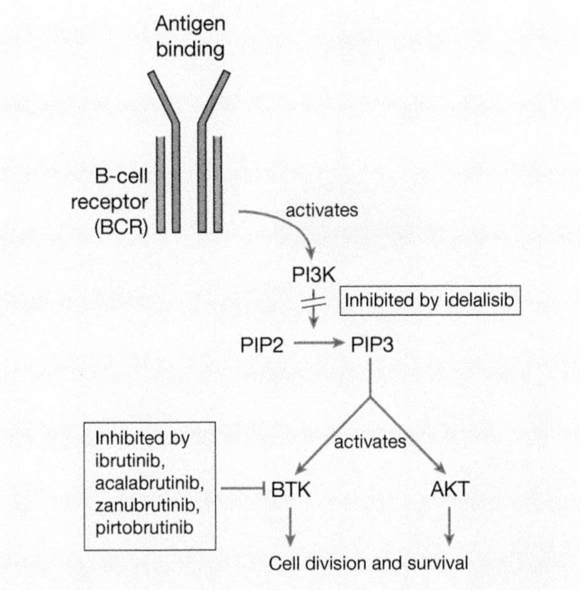

Figure 9.4 Signalling from the B-cell receptor after antigen binding occurs through phosphoinositide-3-kinase (PI3K), which produces a second messenger phosphatidyl triphosphate (PIP3), which activates Bruton tyrosine kinase (BTK) and AKT. Idelalisib inhibits PI3K and ibrutinib, acalabrutinib, zanabrutinib (covalent) and pirtobrutinib (non-covalent) inhibit BTK.

T lymphocytes

T lymphocytes develop from cells that have migrated to the thymus, where they differentiate into mature T cells during passage from the cortex to the medulla. During this process, self-reactive T cells are deleted (negative selection), whereas T cells with some specificity for host human leucocyte antigen (HLA) molecules are selected (positive selection). The mature helper cells express CD4 and cytotoxic cells express CD8 (Table 9.1). The cells also express one of two T-cell antigen receptor heterodimers, αβ (>90%) or γδ (<10%). They recognize antigen only when it is presented at a cell surface (see below and Fig. 9.11).

Engineering of T lymphocytes for therapy, including chimeric antigen receptor T cells

The immunological capacity of T cells is being harnessed for different types of therapeutic uses:

1 T lymphocytes can be harvested from patients, manipulated *in vitro* and reinfused to treat haematological and other neoplasias (Fig. 9.6). **Chimeric antigen receptor T cells (CAR-T cells)** are T lymphocytes that have been genetically engineered to express a construct that includes both an antigen-specific receptor and various co-stimulatory

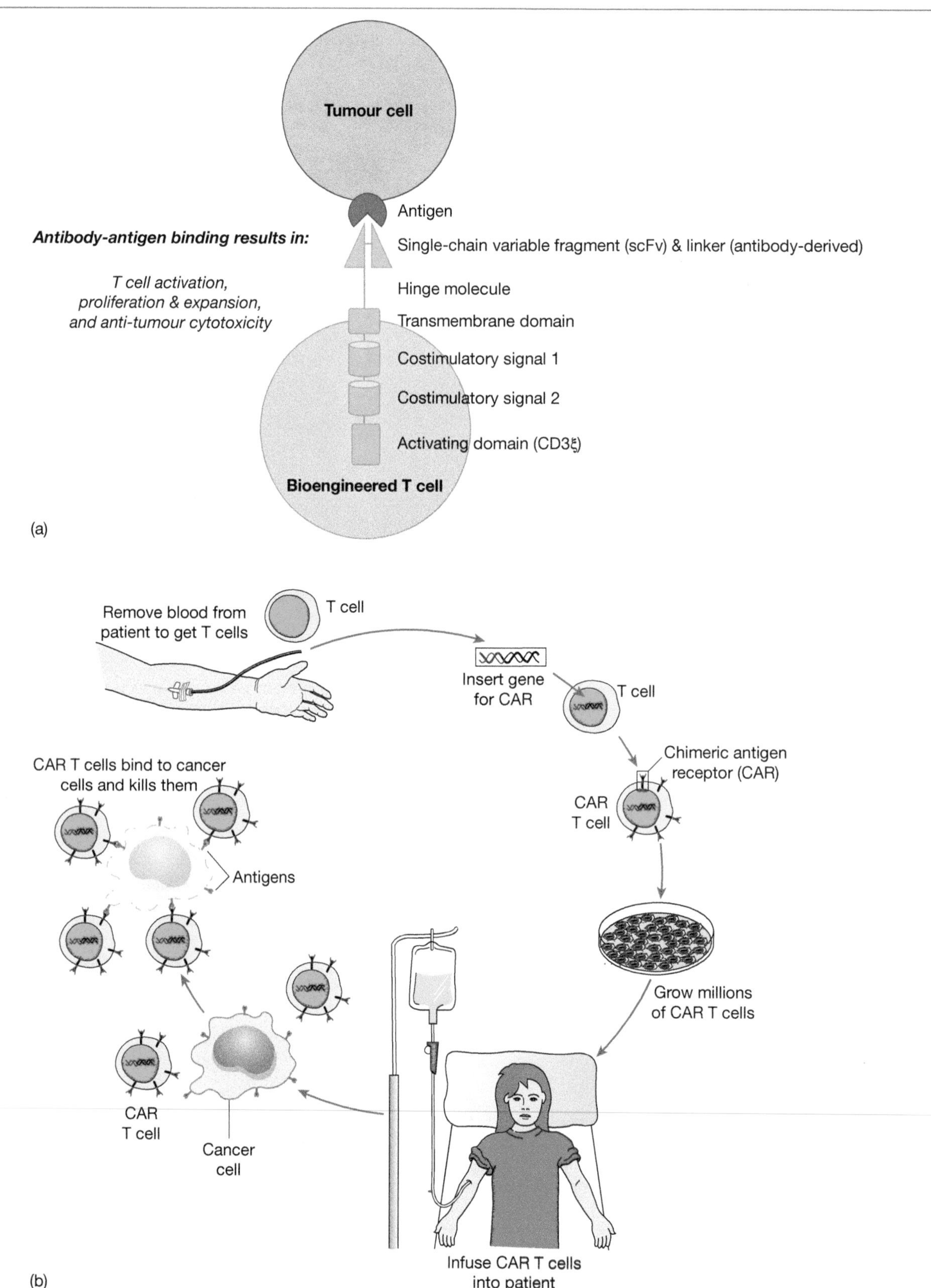

Figure 9.6 Chimeric antigen receptor (CAR)-T cells. **(a)** These T cells are engineered to express a gene construct with immune costimulatory and activating signals, and a T-cell receptor with antigen specificity relevant to the tumour target, e.g. CD19 in B-cell lymphoid neoplasms. **(b)** T lymphocytes are harvested from the patient, genetically engineered *in vitro* to become CAR-T cells, expanded *in vitro* and reinfused. Expansion *in vivo* is being explored to speed up the process. Source: https://visualsonline.cancer.gov/details.cfm?imageid=11776. Reproduced with permission of Terese Winslow.

molecules (Fig. 9.6a). The effectiveness largely depends on which co-stimulatory molecules are chosen. Effective CAR-T cells have been developed against CD19 and CD20, antigens expressed by B-ALL cells and the cells of most B-cell lymphomas. Other CAR-T cells have been developed against antigens expressed on multiple myeloma cells, e.g. B-cell maturation antigen (BCMA). Some are approved especially for young patients with refractory or second or later relapse of B-acute lymphoblastic leukaemia. Third- and fourth-generation T cells with improved intracellular domains are more effective and persistent in antitumour activity.

2 T cells with particular antigen specificity can be harvested from a healthy donor and infused into a patient to control an infection. This is being used to treat difficult post-allogeneic stem cell transplant viral infections, such as cytomegalovirus and Epstein–Barr virus (EBV). Similar procedures have been introduced for treating post-transplantation EBV positive lymphoid malignancies.

Natural killer cells

Natural killer (NK) cells are cytotoxic lymphocytes that lack the T-cell receptor (TCR) and are considered part of the innate rather than the adaptive immune system. They are large cells with cytoplasmic granules (Fig. 9.1c) and typically express surface molecules CD16 (Fc receptor), CD56 and CD57.

NK cells are designed to kill target cells that have a low level of expression of HLA class I molecules, such as may occur during viral infection or on a malignant cell. NK cells do this by displaying a number of receptors for HLA molecules on their surface. When HLA is expressed on the target cell, these deliver an inhibitory signal into the NK cell. When HLA molecules are absent on the target cell, this inhibitory signal is lost and the NK cell can then kill its target.

In addition, NK cells display antibody-dependent cell-mediated cytotoxicity (ADCC). In this, antibody binds to antigen on the surface of the target cell and then NK cells bind to the Fc portion of the bound antibody and kill the target cell.

CAR-NK cells are being developed. These have the advantage over CAR-T cells that they do not need to be autologous and therefore can be used 'off the shelf'.

Lymphocyte circulation

Lymphocytes in the peripheral blood migrate through **post-capillary venules** into the substance of the lymph nodes or into the spleen or bone marrow (Fig. 20.3). T cells home to the perifollicular zones of the cortical areas of lymph nodes (paracortical areas; Fig. 9.2) and to the periarteriolar sheaths surrounding the central arterioles of the spleen. B cells selectively accumulate in follicles of the lymph nodes and spleen. Lymphocytes return to the peripheral blood via the efferent lymphatic stream and the thoracic duct.

Immunoglobulins

Immunoglobulins are a family of proteins produced by plasma cells and B lymphocytes that bind to antigen. They are divided into five subclasses or isotypes: immunoglobulin G (IgG), IgA, IgM, IgD and IgE. IgG, the most abundant, contributes approximately 80% of normal serum immunoglobulin. It is further subdivided into four subclasses: IgG_1, IgG_2, IgG_3 and IgG_4. IgA is subdivided into two types.

IgM is usually produced first in response to antigen, IgG subsequently and for a more prolonged period. The same cell can switch from IgM to IgG, IgA or IgE synthesis. IgA is the main immunoglobulin in secretions, particularly of the gastro-intestinal tract. IgD and IgE (involved in delayed hypersensitivity reactions) are minor immunoglobulin fractions. Biochemical and biological properties of the three main immunoglobulin subclasses are summarized in Table 9.2.

The immunoglobulins are all made up of the same basic structure (Fig. 9.5). This consists of **two heavy chains** which are called gamma (γ) in IgG, alpha (α) in IgA, μ in IgM, delta (δ) in IgD and epsilon (ε) in IgE, and **two light chains** – kappa (k) or lambda (λ) – which are common to all five immunoglobulins. The heavy and light chains each have

Table 9.2 Some properties of the three main classes of immunoglobulin (Ig).

	IgG	IgA	IgM
Molecular weight	140 000	140 000	900 000
Normal serum level (g/L)	6.0–16.0	1.5–4.5	0.5–1.5
Present in	Serum and extracellular fluid	Serum and other body fluids, e.g. of bronchi and gut	Serum only
Complement fixation	Usual	Yes (alternative pathway)	Usual and very efficient
Placental transfer	Yes	No	No
Heavy chain	(γ_{1-4})	α (α_1 or α_2)	μ

highly variable regions, which give the immunoglobulin specificity, and constant regions, in which there is virtual complete correspondence in amino acid sequence in all antibodies of a given isotype, e.g. IgG, IgA, or isotype subclass, e.g. IgG_1, IgG_2. IgG antibody can be broken into a constant Fc fragment and two highly variable Fab fragments (Fig. 9.5). IgM molecules are much larger because they consist of five subunits.

Immunoglobulins and albumin constitute more than 90% of serum proteins, and their plasma concentration is a function of the rate of synthesis and rate of degradation; also on recycling pathways involving the neonatal Fc receptor (FcRn) on endothelial cells. In this pathway, internalized IgG and albumin captured by FcRn under acidic endosomal conditions are recycled to the cell surface, where exocytosis and a shift to neutral pH promote their extracellular release.

The main role of immunoglobulins is defence of the body against foreign organisms. They are also important in the pathogenesis of a number of haematological disorders. For example, secretion of a specific immunoglobulin from a monoclonal population of lymphocytes or plasma cells causes **paraproteinaemia** (Chapter 22). Bence–Jones protein in the urine in some cases of myeloma consists of a monoclonal secretion of light chains (either κ or λ) or light-chain fragments. Immunoglobulins may bind to blood cells in a variety of immune disorders and cause their agglutination, e.g. in cold agglutinin disease (Chapter 6), their destruction following direct complement lysis or opsonization with elimination by the reticuloendothelial (RE) system, as in autoimmune haemolytic anaemia and immune thrombocytopenia.

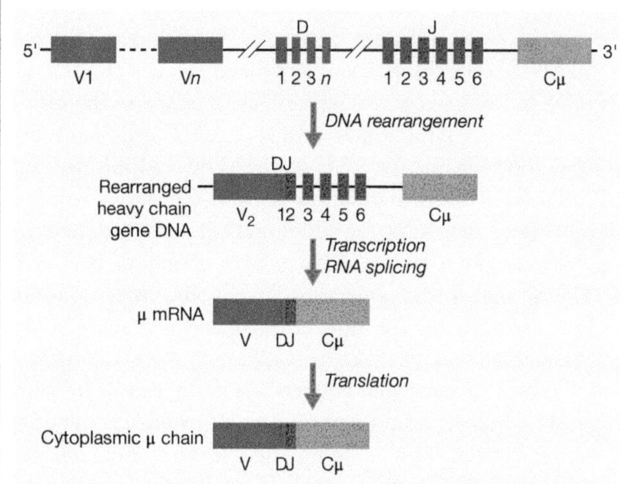

Figure 9.7 Rearrangement of a heavy-chain immunoglobulin gene. One of the V segments is brought into contact with a D, a J and a C (in this case Cm) segment, forming an active transcriptional gene from which the corresponding mRNA is produced. The DJ rearrangement precedes VDJ joining. The class of immunoglobulin depends on which of the nine constant regions (1μ, 1δ, 4γ, 2α, 1e) is used.

Antigen–receptor gene rearrangements

Immunoglobulin gene rearrangements

The immunoglobulin heavy-chain and κ and λ light-chain genes occur on chromosomes 14, 2 and 22, respectively. **In the germline state, the heavy-chain gene consists of separate segments for variable (V), diversity (D), joining (J) and constant (C) regions. Each of the V, D and J regions contains a number (*n*) of different gene segments (Fig. 9.7).** In cells not committed to immunoglobulin synthesis, these gene segments remain in their separate germline state. During early differentiation of B cells, there is rearrangement of heavy-chain genes so that one of the V heavy-chain segments combines with one of the D segments, which has itself already combined with one of the J segments. Thus, they form a transcriptionally active gene for the heavy chain. The protein coding segments of the constant region mRNA are joined to the variable region after splicing out intervening RNA. The class of immunoglobulin that is secreted depends on which of the nine (4γ, 2α, 1μ, 1δ and 1e) constant regions is used. Diversity is introduced by the variability of which V segment joins with which D and with which J segment. In the arbitrary example shown in Fig. 9.7, V_2 joins with D_1 and J_2. Additional diversity is generated by the enzyme terminal deoxynucleotidyl transferase (TdT), which inserts a variable number of new bases into the DNA of the D region at the time of gene rearrangement. Further mutation of the V region genes occurs in the germinal centres of secondary lymphoid tissues (called somatic mutation; see below).

Similar rearrangements occur during generation of the light-chain gene (Fig. 9.8). **Recombinase enzymes** coded for by recombinase activating genes (RAGs) are needed both in B and T cells to join up the adjacent pieces of DNA after excision of intervening sequences. These recognize certain heptamer and nonamer-conserved sequences flanking the various gene segments. Mistakes in recombinase activity play an important part in the chromosome translocations of B- or T-cell malignancy.

T-cell receptor gene rearrangements

The vast majority of T cells contain a TCR composed of a heterodimer of α and β chains (Fig. 9.3). In a minority of T cells, the TCR is composed of γ and δ chains. The α, β, γ and δ genes of the TCRs each include V, D, J and C regions. During T-cell ontogeny, rearrangements of these gene segments occur in a similar fashion to those for immunoglobulin genes, thus creating T cells expressing a wide variety (10^8 or more) of TCR structures (Figs. 9.3 and 9.9). TdT is involved in creating additional diversity, and the same recombinase enzymes used in B cells are involved in joining up TCR gene segments.

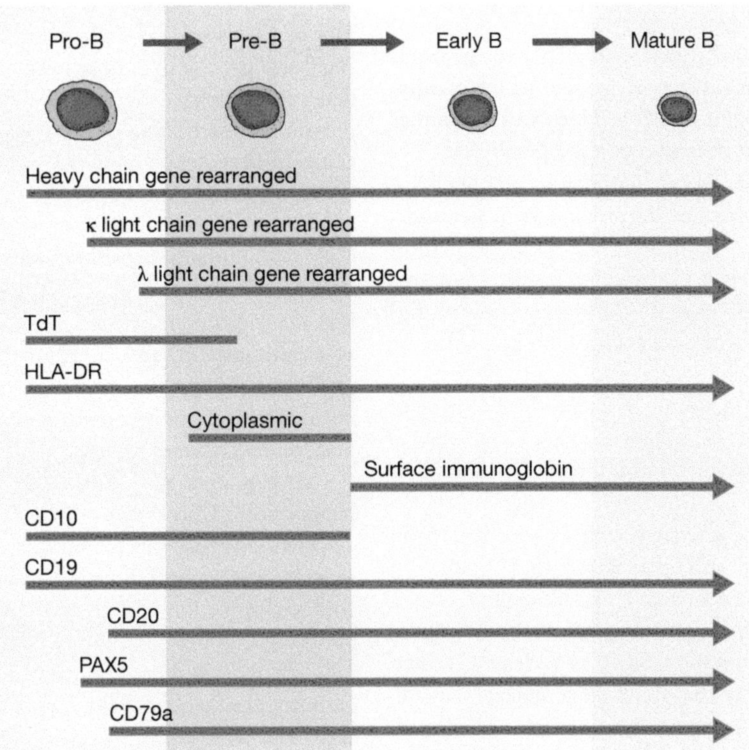

Figure 9.8 The sequence of immunoglobulin gene rearrangement, antigen and immunoglobulin expression during early B-cell development. Intracytoplasmic CD22 is not depicted, but is also a feature of very early B cells. HLA, human leucocyte antigen; TdT, terminal deoxynucleotidyl transferase.

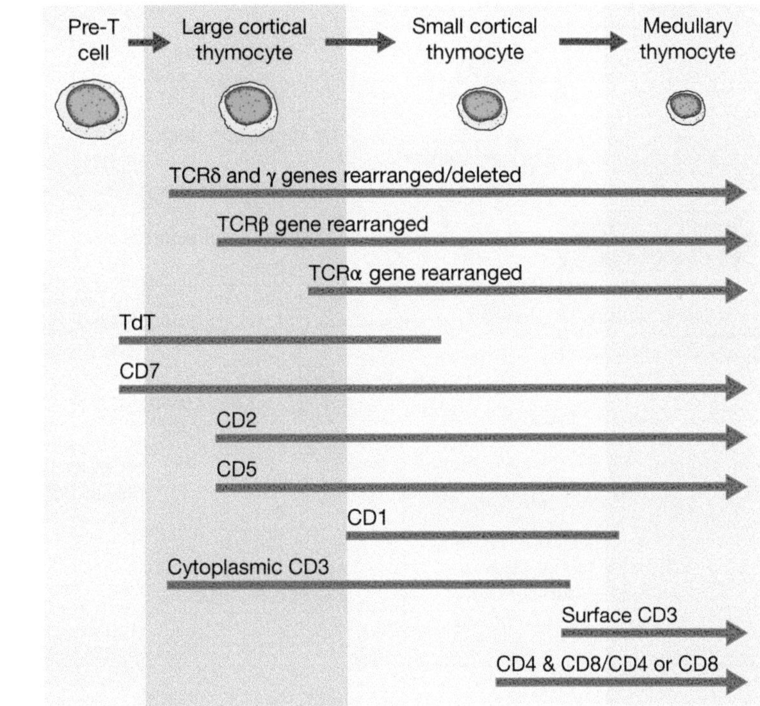

Figure 9.9 The sequence of events during early T-cell development. The earliest events appear to be the expression of surface CD7, intranuclear terminal deoxynucleotidyl transferase (TdT) and intracytoplasmic CD3, followed by T-cell receptor (TCR) gene rearrangement. Early medullary thymocytes express both CD4 and CD8, but they then lose one or other of these structures.

Complement

The complement system includes a series of plasma proteins constituting an amplification enzyme system which is capable of lysis of bacteria (or of blood cells) or can 'opsonize' (coat) bacteria or cells so that they are phagocytosed. The complement sequence consists of nine major components – C1, C2, etc. – which are activated in turn and form a cascade, resembling the coagulation sequence (Fig. 9.10). The most abundant and pivotal protein is C3, which is present in plasma at a level of approximately 1.2 g/L. The early (opsonizing) stages leading to coating of the cells with C3b can occur by three different pathways:

1 The **classical pathway**, activated by IgG or IgM coating of cells
2 The **lectin pathway,** activated by binding to lectin residues on a pathogen
3 The **alternate pathway**, activated by IgA, endotoxin (from Gram-negative bacteria) and other factors (Fig. 9.10).

The classical pathway is initiated by the binding of C1q, a component of C1 complex, to the Fc domain of an antigen-bound antibody. This binding stimulates C1s to cleave C4, then C2 to form active (denoted by a bar above the complex) C2bC4b, which functions as the enzyme C3 convertase. The lectin (mannose-binding lectin, MBL) pathway is initiated when host MBL binds to mannose and fucose residues on a suitable surface such as a pathogen. The alternate pathway is constitutively activated at a low rate by endogenously generated C3b and is amplified by additional C3b. C3b forms a complex with a plasma protein Bb which forms a C3 convertase. Protein Bb is itself generated from protein B bound to C3b, by the action of protein D.

All three pathways converge at C3. C3 is cleaved by C3 convertase into C3a and C3b. C3b converts C5 to C5a and C5b. C5b initiates formation with C6, C7, C8, C9, the membrane attack complex. The complement cascade can be inhibited at various points by a C1 esterase inhibitor, CD55 (decay accelerating factor) and CD59 (membrane inhibitor of reactive lysis) and by antibodies, e.g. eculizumab and ravulizumab, humanized antibodies against complement C5 and pegcetacoplan which targets complement C3 (Chapter 24).

Macrophages and neutrophils have C3b receptors. They phagocytose C3b-coated cells. C3b is degraded to C3d, detected in the direct antiglobulin test using an anti-complement agent (Chapter 25). If the complement sequence goes to completion (C9), there is generation of an active phospholipase that punches holes in the cell membrane, e.g. of the red cell or bacterium, causing direct lysis. The complement pathway also generates the biologically active fragments C3a and C5a, which act directly on phagocytes to stimulate the respiratory burst enhancing their ability to kill phagocytosed

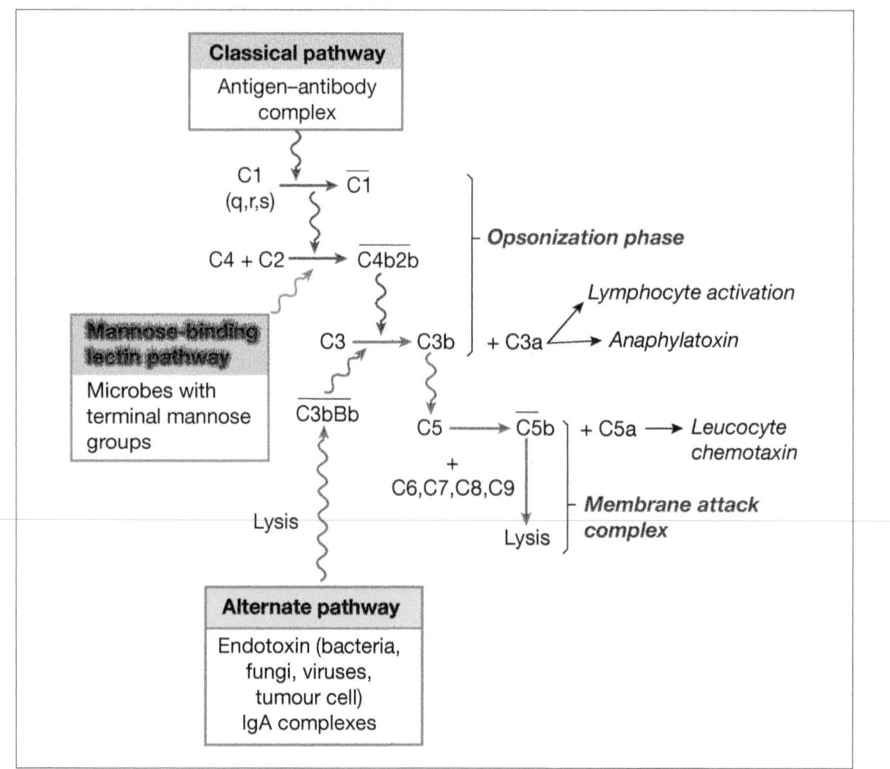

Figure 9.10 The complement (C) cascade comprises three distinct pathways: the classical, the lectin (mannose-binding lectin, MBL) and the alternate pathways. All three pathways generate C3 convertase, an enzyme that converts C3 to active fragments C3a and C3b.

cells. Both may trigger anaphylaxis by release of mediators from tissue mast cells and basophils, which cause vasodilatation and increased permeability.

The immune response

One of the most striking features of the immune system is its capacity to produce a highly *specific* response. For both T and B cells, this specificity is achieved by the presence of a particular receptor on the lymphocyte surface (Fig. 9.3). Naïve (or virgin) B and T lymphocytes which leave the bone marrow and thymus are resting cells that are not in cell division. They recirculate in the lymphatic system. Specialized macrophages called dendritic cells (DCs; Chapter 8) process antigens before presenting them to B and T lymphocytes – they are therefore known as **antigen-presenting cells** (APCs) (Fig. 9.11).

The immune system contains millions of different lymphocytes. Each of these lymphocytes is unique as it has a receptor that shows differences in structure from that of any other lymphocyte. Consequently, each lymphocyte will bind to only a restricted number of antigens. T and B cells undergo clonal expansion if they meet an APC that is presenting an antigen that can trigger their antigen receptor molecules. At this stage, lymphocytes may develop into effector cells (plasma cells or cytotoxic T cells) or into memory cells.

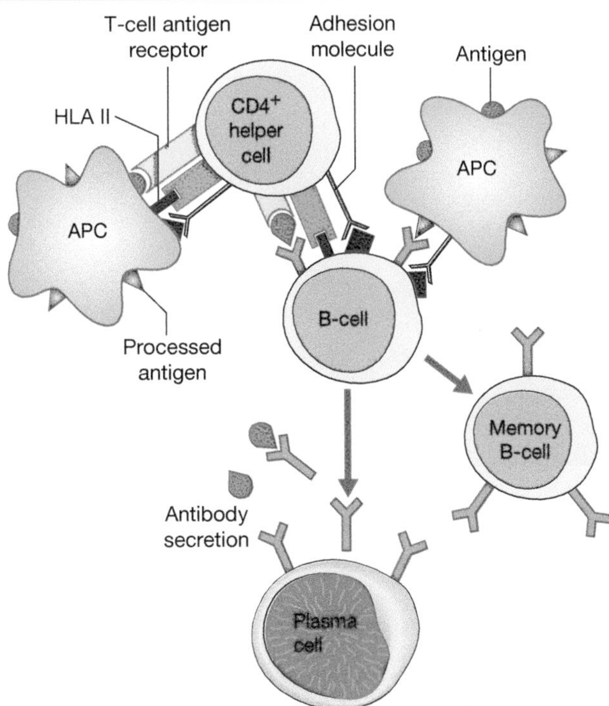

Figure 9.11 The immune response. Interaction between an antigen-presenting cell (APC) with processed antigen on its surface presented together with HLA Class II and a CD4+ T cell with a T-cell receptor which recognizes that antigen. Both cells interact with a B cell with recognition between its surface receptor (Ig) and the antigen. T cells and B cells react with different epitopes on the antigen. Clones of B and T cells are stimulated to proliferate. The B cells become plasma cells or memory B cells.

Dendritic cell precursors constitutively migrate at low levels from blood into tissues, but their rate of migration is increased at the site of inflammation. Immature DCs are efficient at micro-pinocytosis, which allows them to capture antigens from the environment.

T cells are unable to bind antigen free in solution and require it to be presented on APCs in the form of peptides held on the surface of HLA molecules (Figs. 9.3b and 9.11). T cells recognize the antigen only when it is presented with 'self' HLA molecules and so are known as **HLA-restricted**. The CD4 molecule on helper cells recognizes class II (HLA-DP, -DQ and -DR) molecules, whereas the CD8 molecule recognizes class I (HLA-A, -B and -C) molecules (Chapter 25). The antigen recognition site of the TCR is joined to several other subunits in the CD3 complex, which together mediate signal transduction. Depending on their cytokine production, $CD4^+$ T cells can be broadly subdivided into two sub-types, T helper type 1 (Th1) and T helper type 2 (Th2). Th1 cells produce mainly IL-2, TNF-β and γ-interferon (IFN-γ) and are important in boosting cell-mediated immunity (and granuloma formation), whereas Th2 cells produce IL-4 and IL-10 and are mainly responsible for providing help for antibody production.

Antigen-specific immune responses are generated in **secondary lymphoid organs** and commence when antigen is carried into a lymph node on dendritic cells (Fig. 9.12). B cells recognize antigen through their surface immunoglobulin and, although most antibody responses require help from antigen-specific T cells, some antigens such as polysaccharides can lead to T-cell-independent B-cell antibody production. In the follicle, germinal centres arise as a result of continuing response to antigenic stimulation (Fig. 9.13). These consist of follicular dendritic cells (FDCs), which are loaded with antigen, B cells and activated T cells which have migrated up from the T zone. Proliferating B cells move to the dark zone of the germinal centre as **centroblasts**, where they undergo somatic mutation of their immunoglobulin variable-region genes (Fig. 9.13). Their progeny are known as **centrocytes** and these must be selected for survival by antigen on FDCs, otherwise they undergo apoptosis. If selected they become memory B cells or plasma cells (Fig. 9.13). Plasma cells migrate to the bone marrow and other sites in the RE system and produce high-affinity antibody.

Lymphocytosis

Lymphocytosis often occurs in infants and young children in response to infections that would produce a neutrophil reaction in adults. Conditions particularly associated with lymphocytosis are listed in Table 9.3.

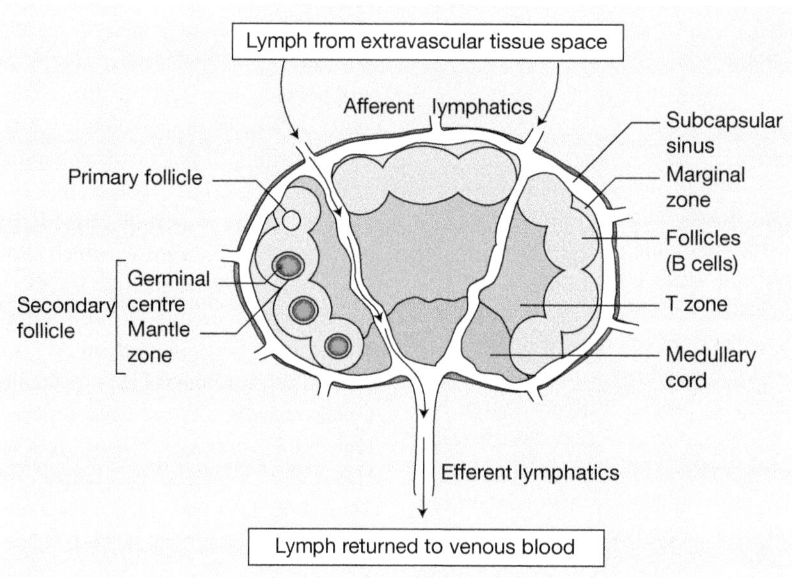

(a)

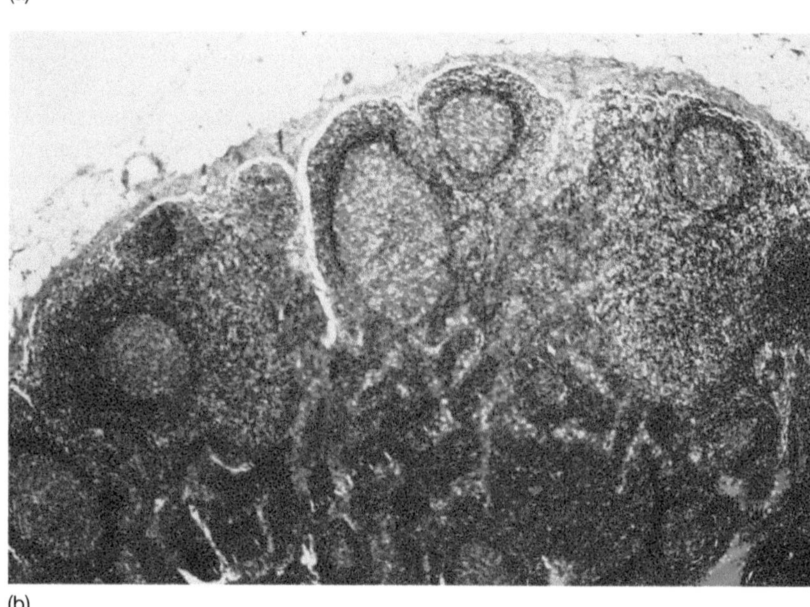

(b)

Figure 9.12 **(a)** Structure of a lymph node. **(b)** Lymph node showing germinal follicles surrounded by a darker mantle zone rim and lighter, more diffuse marginal and T-zone areas.

Infectious mononucleosis

Infectious mononucleosis is caused by primary infection with Epstein–Barr virus (EBV) and characterized by fever, sore throat, lymphadenopathy and atypical lymphocytes in the blood. A similar clinical picture and blood film appearance may be caused less frequently by cytomegalovirus (CMV), human immunodeficiency virus (HIV) and other viral infections and by toxoplasmosis.

In most cases, primary infection with EBV is subclinical. The disease is characterized by a lymphocytosis caused by clonal expansions of T cells reacting against B lymphocytes infected with EBV. The disease is associated with a high titre of heterophile ('reacting with cells of another species') antibodies which react with sheep, horse or ox red cells.

Clinical features

The majority of patients are between the ages of 15 and 40 years. A prodromal period of a few days occurs with lethargy, malaise, headaches, stiff neck and a dry cough. In established disease, the following features may be found:

1 Bilateral cervical lymphadenopathy in 75% of cases. Symmetrical generalized lymphadenopathy occurs in 50% of cases. The nodes are discrete and may be tender.

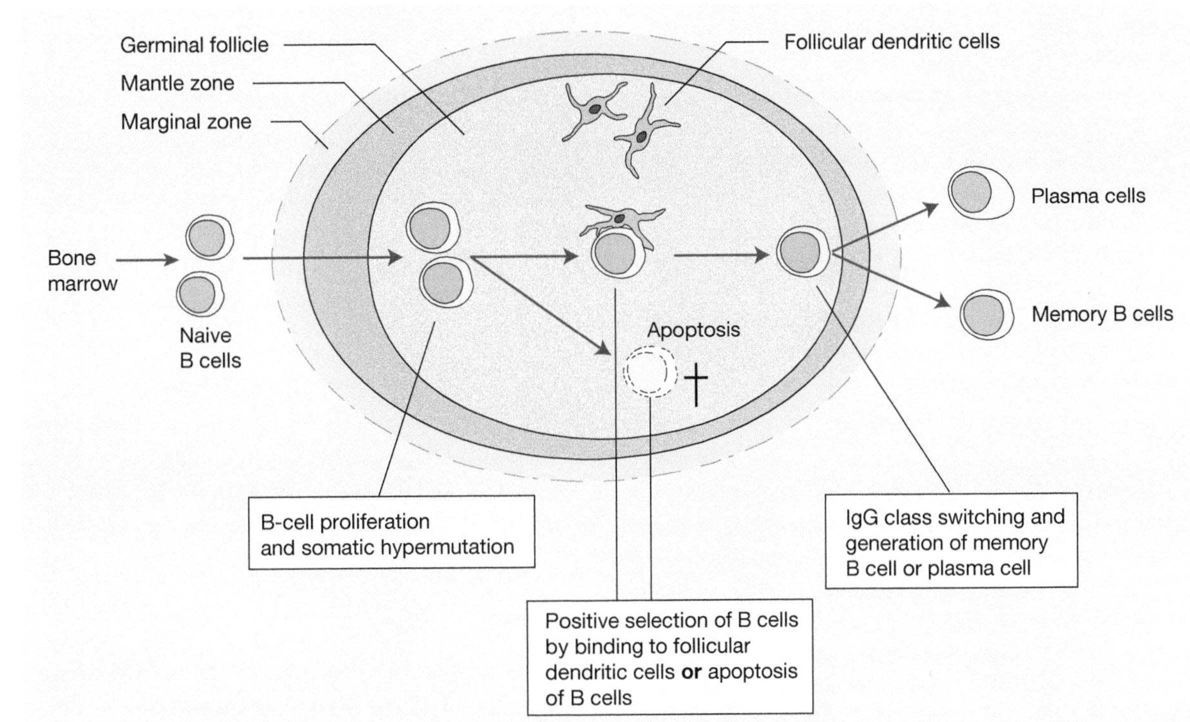

Figure 9.13 Generation of a germinal centre. B cells activated by antigen migrate from the T outer mantle zone to the follicle, where they undergo massive proliferation. Cells enter the dark zone as centroblasts and accumulate mutations in their immunoglobulin V genes. Cells then pass back into the light zone (Fig. 9.11) as centrocytes. Only those cells that can interact with antigen on follicular dendritic cells and receive signals from antigen-specific T cells (Fig. 9.10) are selected and migrate out as plasma cells and memory cells. Cells not selected die by apoptosis.

Table 9.3 Causes of lymphocytosis.

Infections

Acute

- Bacterial: pertussis, bordetella
- Viral: infectious mononucleosis, rubella, mumps, acute infectious lymphocytosis, infectious hepatitis, cytomegalovirus, human immunodeficiency virus (HIV), herpes simplex or zoster

Chronic

- Tuberculosis, toxoplasmosis, brucellosis, leishmaniasis, syphilis

Other non-neoplastic disorders

- Physiological stress (trauma, major surgery, septic shock, myocardial infarction)
- Hyposplenism
- Hypersensitivity, e.g. insect bites, drug reaction
- Stress, e.g. trauma, major surgery, myocardial infarct, septic shock
- Chronic polyclonal (idiopathic; cigarette smoking, associated with cancer but polyclonal)
- Thyrotoxicosis

Neoplastic

- Chronic lymphoid leukaemias and monoclonal B lymphocytosis (Chapter 18)
- Acute lymphoblastic leukaemia (Chapter 17)
- Non-Hodgkin lymphoma (Chapter 20)

2 Over half of patients have a sore throat with inflamed oral and pharyngeal surfaces. Follicular tonsillitis is frequently seen.
3 Fever may be mild or severe.
4 A morbilliform rash, severe headache and eye signs, e.g. photophobia, conjunctivitis and periorbital oedema, are not uncommon. The rash may follow therapy with amoxicillin or ampicillin.
5 Palpable splenomegaly occurs in over half of patients and hepatomegaly in approximately 15%. Approximately 5% of patients are jaundiced.
6 Peripheral neuropathy, severe anaemia caused by autoimmune haemolysis or purpura caused by thrombocytopenia are less frequent complications.

Diagnosis

Pleomorphic atypical lymphocytosis

A moderate rise in white cell count, e.g. $10–20 \times 10^9$/L, with an absolute lymphocytosis is usual, and some patients have even higher counts. Large numbers of atypical lymphocytes are seen in the peripheral blood film (Fig. 9.14). These T cells are variable in appearance, but most have nuclear and cytoplasmic features similar to those seen during reactive lymphocyte transformation. The greatest number of atypical lymphocytes are usually found between the seventh and tenth days of the illness.

Heterophile antibodies

Heterophile antibodies against sheep or horse red cells may be found in the serum at high titres. Slide screening tests, such as the **Monospot test**, use formalinized horse red cells to test for the IgM antibodies which agglutinate the cells. Highest titres occur during the second and third weeks and the antibody persists in most patients for 6 weeks.

EBV antibody

A rise in the titre of IgM antibody against the EBV capsid antigen (VCA) may be demonstrated during the first 2–3 weeks. Specific IgG antibody to the EBV nuclear antigen (EBNA) and IgG VCA antibodies develop later and persist for life. A polymerase chain reaction (PCR) assay is also available.

Haematological abnormalities

Haematological abnormalities other than the atypical lymphocytosis are frequent. Occasional patients develop an autoimmune haemolytic anaemia. The IgM autoantibody is typically of the 'cold'-reactive type and usually shows 'i' blood group specificity. Thrombocytopenia is frequent due to an autoimmune thrombocytopenic purpura in a small proportion of patients.

Differential diagnosis

The differential diagnosis of infectious mononucleosis includes cytomegalovirus, HIV, toxoplasmosis, influenza, rubella, infectious hepatitis and other infections; bacterial tonsillitis and acute lymphoblastic leukaemia.

Treatment

In the great majority of patients only symptomatic treatment is required. Corticosteroids are sometimes given to those with severe systemic symptoms. Patients characteristically develop an erythematous rash if given amoxicillin or ampicillin therapy. Most patients recover fully 4–6 weeks after initial symptoms. However, convalescence may be slow and associated with severe malaise and lethargy.

Lymphopenia

Lymphopenia may occur in severe bone marrow failure, with corticosteroid and other immunosuppressive therapy, in Hodgkin lymphoma and with widespread irradiation. It also occurs during treatment with the monoclonal antibody alemtuzumab (anti-CD52), after CAR-T cell therapy and in a variety of immunodeficiency syndromes, the most important of which is HIV infection (see Chapter 32).

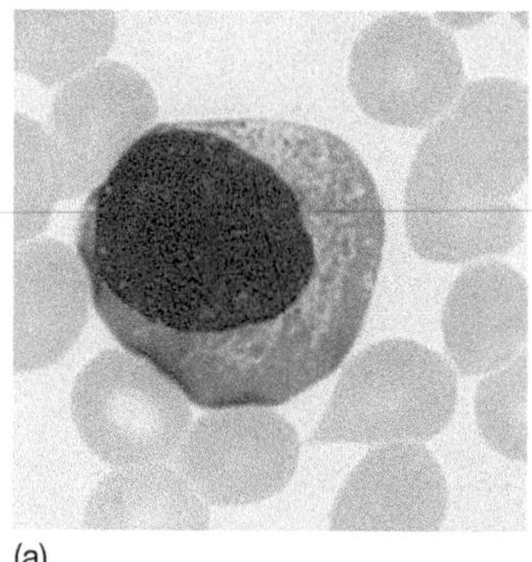
(a)

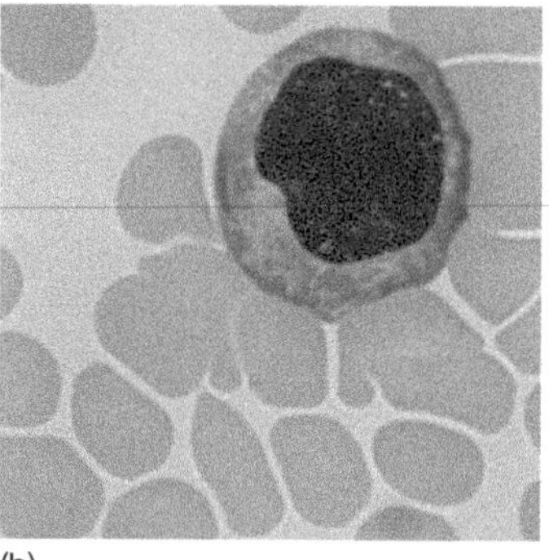
(b)

Figure 9.14 (a and b) Infectious mononucleosis: representative 'reactive' T lymphocytes in the peripheral blood film of a 21-year-old man (see also Fig. 9.1b).

Immunodeficiency

A large number of inherited or acquired deficits in any of the components of the immune system can cause an impaired immune response with increased susceptibility to infection (Table 9.4). If the principal lack is T cells (as in HIV infection), this leads not only to bacterial infections but also to viral, protozoal, fungal and mycobacterial infections. In some cases, however, lack of specific subsets of T cells which control B-cell maturation may lead to a secondary lack of B-cell function, as in many cases of common variable immunodeficiency. This may develop in children or adults of either sex. In others, a primary defect of B cells or of APCs is present. X-linked agammaglobulinaemia is due to an inherited defect of the enzyme Bruton tyrosine kinase and is characterized by failure of B-cell development; pyogenic bacterial infections dominate the clinical course. Immunoglobulin replacement therapy can be given by monthly courses of intravenous immunoglobulin.

Rare syndromes include aplasia of the thymus, severe combined (T and B) immunodeficiency as a result of adenosine deaminase deficiency and selective deficiencies of IgA or IgM. Acquired immune deficiency occurs after cytotoxic chemotherapy, CAR-T cell therapy or radiotherapy and is particularly pronounced after allogeneic stem cell transplantation, where dysregulation of the immune system persists for 1 year or more. Autoimmune lymphoproliferative syndrome (ALPS) is a rare immunodeficiency caused by mutations in genes affecting the extrinsic apoptotic pathway (*FAS*, *FASL* and *CASP10*). New syndromes include severe B-cell deficiency after CAR-T cell therapy aimed at B-cell malignancies and T-cell depletion through use of bi-specific antibodies including anti-CD3. Immunodeficiency is frequently associated with lymphoid and plasma cell neoplasms such as chronic lymphocytic leukaemia and myeloma. Blood transfusions can cause a temporary immunodeficiency.

Table 9.4 Classification of immunodeficiencies.

Primary	*Examples:*
B cell (antibody deficiency)	X-linked agammaglobulinaemia, acquired common variable hypogammaglobulinaemia, selective IgA, IgM or IgG subclass deficiencies
T cell	Thymic aplasia (DiGeorge's syndrome)
Mixed B and T cell	Severe combined immune deficiency (as a result of ADA or PNP or MHC class II deficiency or other causes); multisystem disorders: ataxiatelangiectasia; Wiskott–Aldrich and polyendocrinopathy syndromes
Secondary	*Examples:*
B cell (antibody deficiency)	Myeloma, nephrotic syndrome, protein-losing enteropathy, drugs, e.g. ibrutinib CAR-T cells
T cell	AIDS, bi-specific antibodies including anti-CD3 specificity
T and B cell	Hodgkin lymphoma Non-Hodgkin lymphoma Drugs: steroids, ciclosporin, azathioprine, fludarabine, etc. Radiation therapy Chronic lymphocytic leukaemia Post-stem cell transplantation AntiCD52 (alemtuzumab), other chemotherapy Post-transfusion

ADA, adenosine deaminase; AIDS, acquired immune deficiency syndrome; Ig, immunoglobulin; MHC, major histocompatibility complex; PNP, purine nucleoside phosphorylase.

Differential diagnosis of lymphadenopathy

The principal causes of lymphadenopathy are listed in Fig. 9.15. The clinical history and examination give essential information. **The age of the patient, length of history, associated symptoms of possible infectious or malignant disease, whether the nodes are painful or tender, consistency of the nodes and whether there is generalized or local lymphadenopathy are all important.** The size of the liver and spleen are assessed. In the case of local node enlargement, it is important to look for inflammatory or malignant disease in the associated lymphatic drainage area.

Further investigations will depend on the initial clinical diagnosis, but it is usual to include a full blood count, blood film and erythrocyte sedimentation rate (ESR). Chest X-ray, Monospot test or other EBV assay, cytomegalovirus and *Toxoplasma* titres or PCR, anti-HIV and Mantoux tests are frequently needed. In many cases, it will be essential to make a histological diagnosis by node biopsy, usually core biopsy, e.g. with a Trucut needle, in which a core of node is removed under radiological control. Fine needle aspirates give less material, destroy the architecture and so are less reliable in diagnosis (Chapter 20). **Computed tomography (CT) scanning is valuable in determining the presence and extent of deep node enlargement. Appearances that suggest a 'normal' node include:**

1 **Short axis diameter <1 cm.**
2 **Normal architecture (elongated, fatty hilum, not round or indistinct).**
3 **Normal enhancement (no necrosis or hypervascularity).**
4 **Normal number of nodes (no increase defined as a cluster of ≥3 nodes in a single nodal station or ≥2 nodes in ≥2 node regions.**

In cases of deep node enlargement, where enlarged superficial nodes are not available for biopsy, bone marrow or liver biopsy, CT- or ultrasound-guided Trucut deep node biopsy is needed in an attempt to reach a histological diagnosis. Biopsy of the spleen is not performed, as it may cause splenic rupture requiring splenectomy. Follow-up CT scan after 3–6 months is recommended if nodes are suspicious and biopsy has been performed, and there is no underlying disorder. FDG-PET (fluorodeoxyglucose-positron emission tomography) scanning is not recommended, as it is non-specific, more expensive and less effective. It may be negative in some low-grade lymphomas and positive in inflammatory and autoimmune disorders.

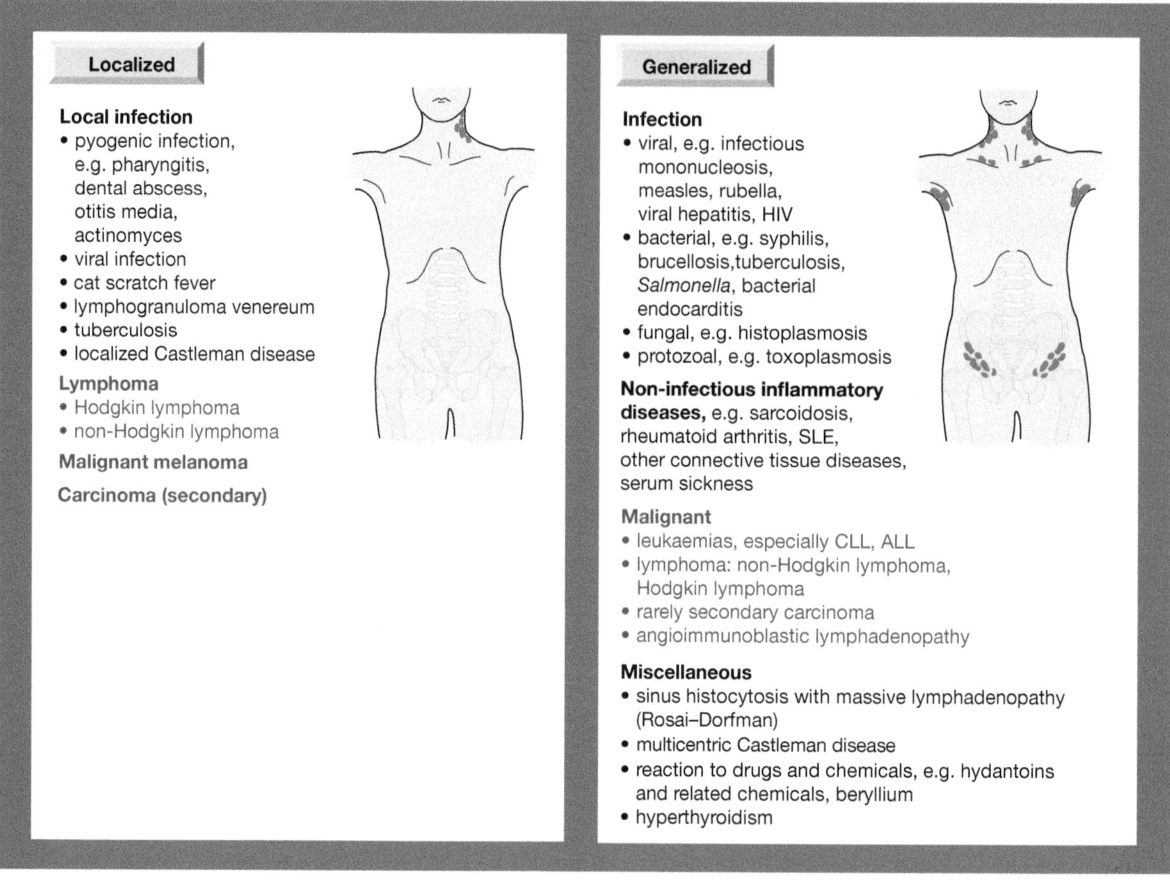

Figure 9.15 Causes of lymphadenopathy. HIV, human immunodeficiency virus; ALL, acute lymphoblastic leukaemia; CLL, chronic lymphocytic leukaemia; SLE, systemic lupus erythematosus. Malignancies are listed in red.

SUMMARY

- Lymphocytes are immunologically competent white cells that are involved in antibody production (B cells) and with the body's defence against viral infection or other foreign invasion (T cells).
- They arise from haemopoietic stem cells in the marrow, T cells being subsequently processed in the thymus.
- B cells secrete antibodies specific to individual antigens. They do this for antigens presented to them by T cells or independently of T cells.
- T lymphocytes are further subdivided into helper ($CD4^+$) and cytotoxic ($CD8^+$) cells. They recognize peptides on HLA antigens.
- Natural killer cells are cytotoxic $CD8^+$ cells that kill target cells with low expression of HLA molecules.
- Specialized macrophages called dendritic cells process antigens before presenting them to B and T lymphocytes. They are called antigen-presenting cells.
- The immune response occurs in the germinal centre of lymph nodes and involves B-cell and T-cell interaction. It results in B-cell proliferation, somatic mutation, selection of cells by recognition of antigen on antigen-presenting cells and formation of plasma cells which secrete immunoglobulin or become memory B cells.
- Immunoglobulins include five subclasses or isotypes, IgG, IgA, IgM, IgD and IgG, all made up of two heavy chains and two light chains (κ or λ).
- Complement is a cascade of plasma proteins that can either lyse cells or coat (opsonize) them so they are phagocytosed.
- Lymphocytosis is usually caused by acute or chronic infections or by lymphoid leukaemias or lymphomas.
- Lymphadenopathy may be localized (because of local infection or malignancy) or generalized because of infection, non-infectious inflammatory diseases, malignancy or drugs.

Now visit **www.wiley.com/go/haematology9e** to test yourself on this chapter.

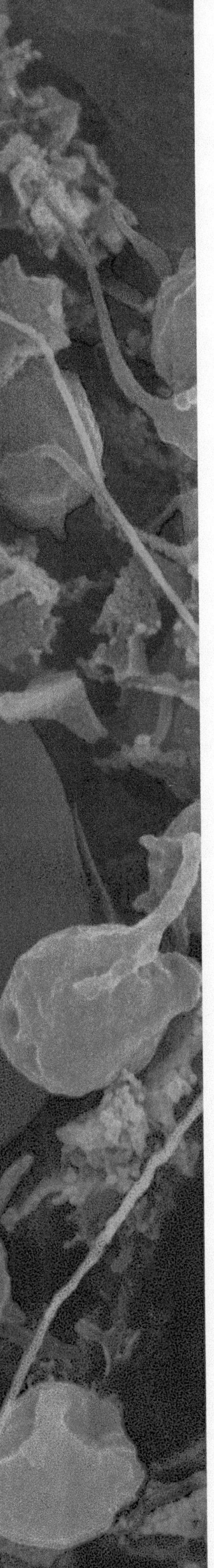

CHAPTER 10

The spleen

Key topics

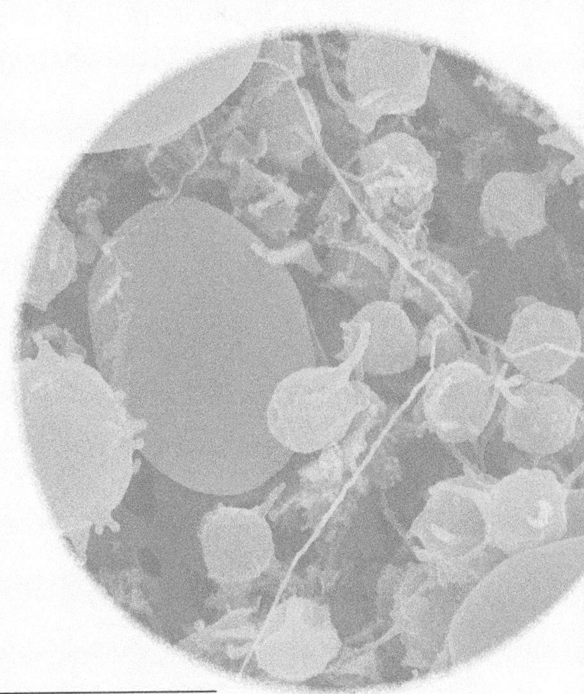

Hoffbrand's Essential Haematology, Ninth Edition. A. Victor Hoffbrand, Pratima Chowdary, Graham P. Collins, and Justin Loke.

© 2024 John Wiley & Sons Ltd. Published 2024 by John Wiley & Sons Ltd.

Companion website: www.wiley.com/go/haematology9e

The spleen has an important and unique role in the function of the haemopoietic and immune systems. As well as being directly involved in many diseases of these systems, a number of important clinical features are associated with hypersplenic and hyposplenic states.

The anatomy and circulation of the spleen

The spleen lies under the left costal margin, has a normal weight of 150–250 g and a length of between 5 and 13 cm. It is normally not palpable, but becomes palpable when the size is increased to over 14 cm.

Blood enters the spleen through the splenic artery, which then divides into **trabecular arteries**, which permeate the organ and give rise to **central arterioles** (Fig. 10.1). The majority of the arterioles end in **cords**, which lack an endothelial lining and form an open blood system unique to the spleen, with a loose reticular connective tissue network lined by fibroblasts and many macrophages. The blood re-enters the circulation by passing across the endothelium of venous **sinuses**. Blood then passes into the splenic vein and back into the general circulation. The cords and sinuses form the **red pulp**, which is 75% of the spleen and has an essential role in monitoring the integrity of red blood cells (see below). With its neutrophils, macrophages, dendritic cells and T lymphocytes, it has an important innate immune function. A minority of the splenic vasculature is closed, in which the arterial and venous systems are connected by capillaries with a continuous endothelial layer.

The central arterioles are surrounded by a core of lymphatic tissue known as **white pulp**, which has an organization similar to lymph nodes (Fig. 10.1). The **periarteriolar lymphatic sheath** (PALS) lies directly around the arteriole and is equivalent to the T zone of the lymph node (p. 118). B-cell follicles are found adjacent to the PALS and these are surrounded by the **marginal** and **perifollicular zones**, which are rich in macrophages and dendritic cells. Lymphocytes migrate into white pulp from the sinuses of the red pulp or from vessels that end directly in the marginal and perifollicular zones.

There are both rapid (1–2 min) in the closed system and slow (30–60 min) in the open-system blood circulations through the spleen. The slow circulation becomes increasingly important in splenomegaly.

The functions of the spleen

The spleen is the largest filter of the blood in the body and several of its functions are derived from this.

Control of red cell integrity

The spleen has an essential role in the 'quality control' of red cells by filtering, 'culling and pitting'. Excess DNA, nuclear remnants (**Howell–Jolly bodies**), **siderotic granules and Heinz bodies** are removed (Fig. 10.2). In the relatively hypoxic environment of the red pulp, and because of plasma skimming in the cords, the membrane flexibility of aged and abnormal red cells is impaired and they are trapped within the sinus, where they are ingested by macrophages. This process in increased if there is a fault in red cell metabolism or they are coated with antibody, if they are misshapen or rigid. Reticulocytes spend time in the spleen losing their RNA and reducing in size. Aged red cells are removed generally by macrophages of the reticuloendothelial system.

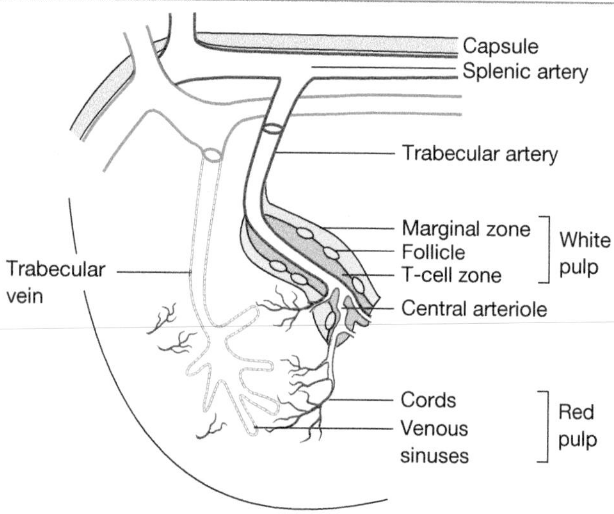

Figure 10.1 Schematic representation of the blood circulation in the spleen. Most blood flows in an 'open' circulation through splenic cords and regains entry into the circulation through the venous sinuses.

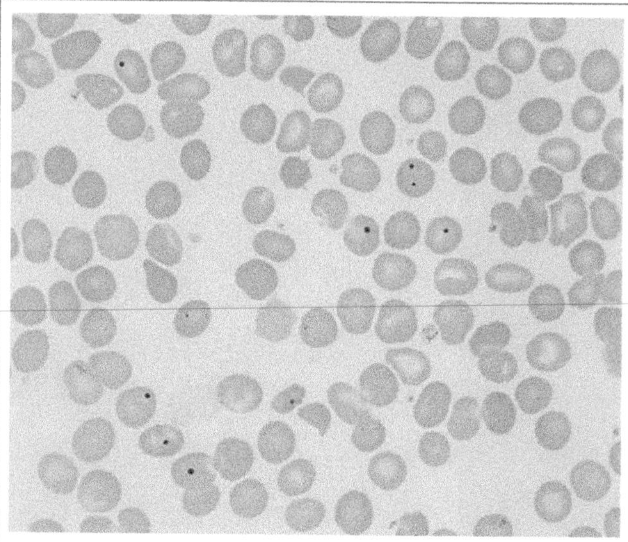

Figure 10.2 Splenic atrophy: peripheral blood film showing Howell–Jolly bodies, Pappenheimer bodies (siderotic granules; see p. xx) and misshapen cells.

Immune function

The lymphoid tissue in the spleen is in a unique position to respond to antigens filtered from the blood and entering the white pulp. Macrophages and dendritic cells in the marginal zone initiate an immune response and then present antigen to B and T cells to start adaptive immune responses. A unique set of B cells are able to produce an IgM response to bacterial pathogens without the help of T cells. This arrangement is particularly efficient at mounting an immune response to encapsulated bacteria.

Extramedullary haemopoiesis

The spleen, like the liver, undergoes a transient period of haemopoiesis at around 3–7 months of foetal life, but is not a site of erythropoiesis in the normal infant, child or adult. However, haemopoiesis may be present from birth in both organs in certain genetic disorders of haemoglobin synthesis such as thalassaemia major, haemoglobin C/C or E/E or be re-established as **extramedullary haemopoiesis**, in disorders such as primary myelofibrosis or in chronic severe haemolytic and megaloblastic anaemias. Extramedullary haemopoiesis may result either from reactivation of dormant stem cells within the spleen or homing of stem cells from the bone marrow to the spleen.

Imaging the spleen

Ultrasound is the most frequently used technique to image the spleen (Fig. 10.3). This can also detect whether or not blood flow in the splenic, portal and hepatic veins is normal, as well as assessing liver size and consistency. Focussed abdominal ultrasound for trauma (FAST) is particularly useful for patients who are unstable as with a ruptured spleen.

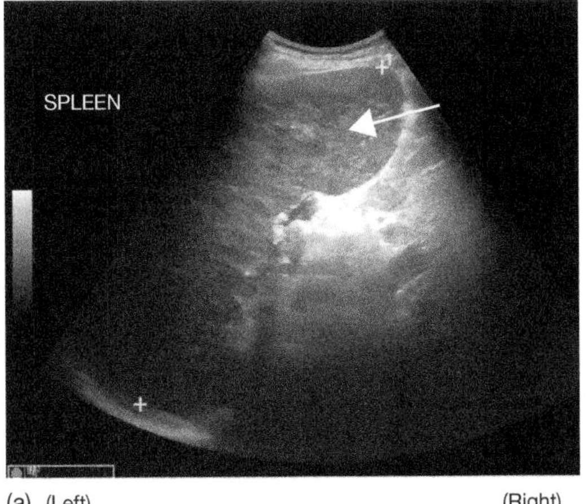

(a) (Left) (Right)

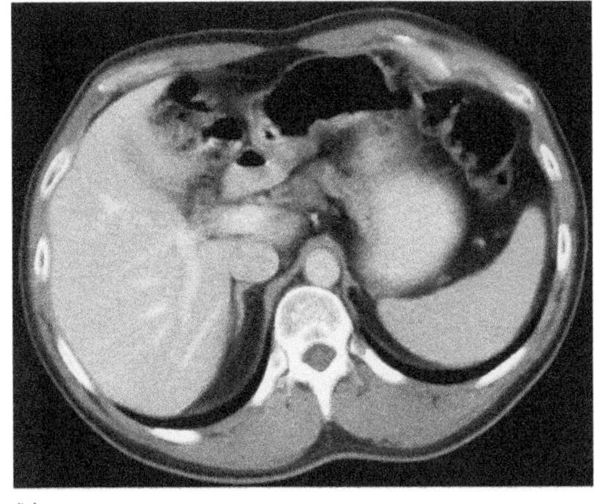

(b)

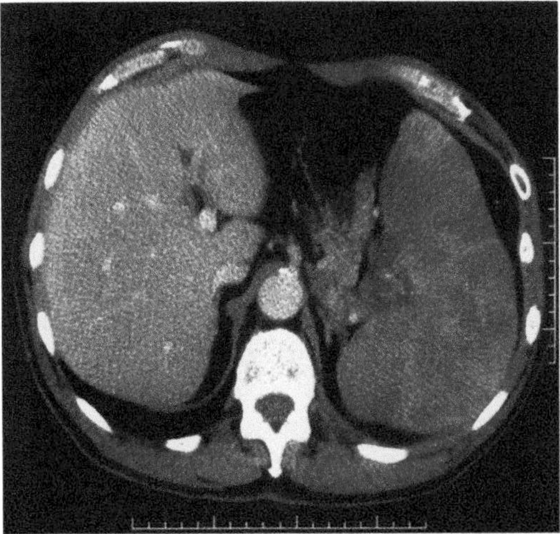

(c)

Figure 10.3 Imaging the spleen. **(a)** Ultrasound of spleen showing splenomegaly (15.3 cm). **(b)** Normal spleen (10 cm) on computed tomography (CT) scan. **(c)** CT scan: the spleen is enlarged and shows multiple low-density areas. A diagnosis of diffuse large B-cell lymphoma was made histologically after splenectomy. Source: Courtesy of Dr T. Ogunremi.

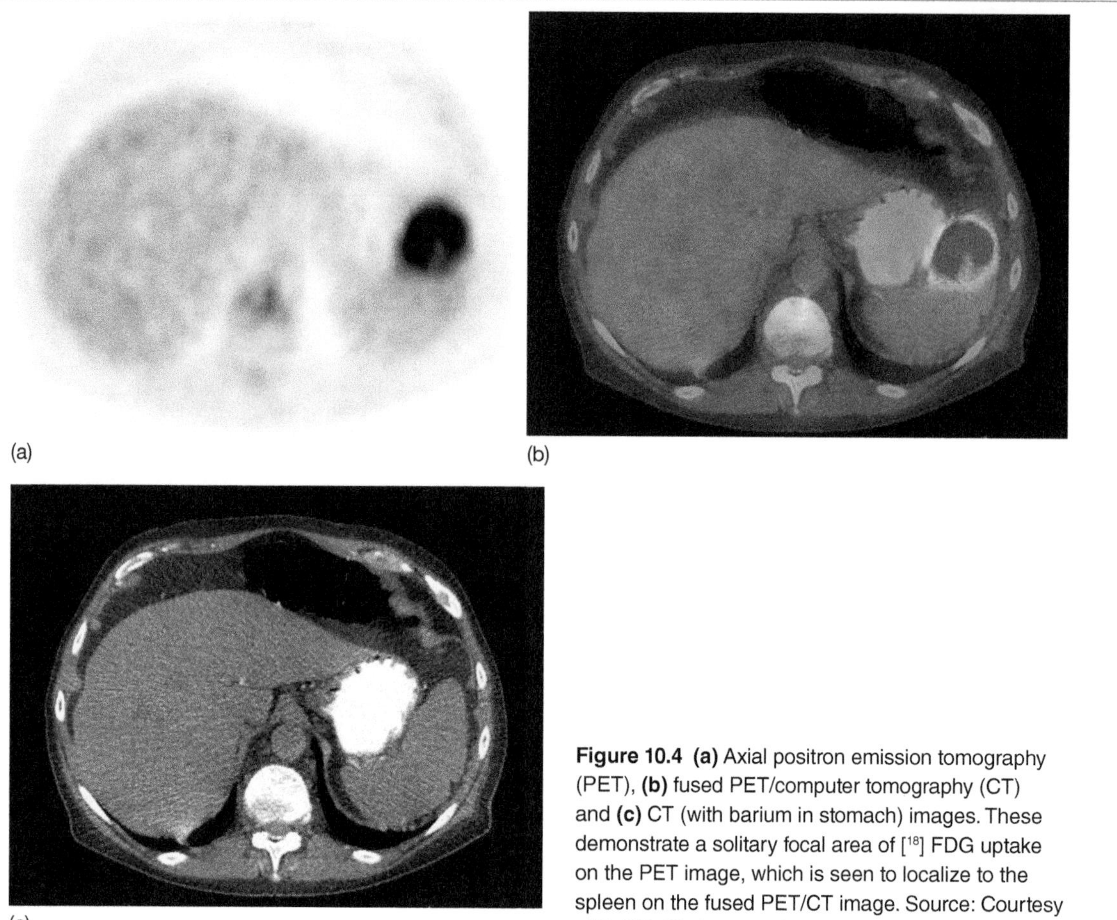

Figure 10.4 **(a)** Axial positron emission tomography (PET), **(b)** fused PET/computer tomography (CT) and **(c)** CT (with barium in stomach) images. These demonstrate a solitary focal area of [18] FDG uptake on the PET image, which is seen to localize to the spleen on the fused PET/CT image. Source: Courtesy of Dr V.S. Warbey and Professor G.J.R. Cook.

Computed tomography (CT) is preferable for detecting structural detail and any associated lymphadenopathy, e.g. for lymphoma staging. Magnetic resonance imaging (MRI) also gives improved fine detail structure. Positron emission tomography (PET) is used particularly for initial staging and for detecting residual disease after treatment of lymphoma (Fig. 10.4).

Splenomegaly

Splenic size is increased in a wide range of conditions (Table 10.1). Splenomegaly is usually felt under the left costal margin, but massive splenomegaly may be felt as far as the right iliac fossa (Fig. 15.11). The spleen moves with respiration and a medial splenic notch may be palpable in some cases. **In developed countries the most common causes of splenomegaly are infectious mononucleosis, haematological malignancy and portal hypertension, whereas malaria and schistosomiasis are more prevalent causes on a global scale (Table 10.1).** Chronic myeloid leukaemia, primary myelofibrosis, lymphoma, Gaucher disease, malaria, leishmaniasis and schistosomiasis are potential causes of massive splenomegaly.

Tropical splenomegaly syndrome

A syndrome of massive splenomegaly of uncertain aetiology has been found frequently in many malarious zones of the tropics, including Uganda, Nigeria, New Guinea and the Congo. Smaller numbers of patients with this disorder are seen in southern Arabia, Sudan and Zambia. Previously, such terms as 'big spleen disease', 'cryptogenic splenomegaly' and 'African macroglobulinaemia' have been used to describe this syndrome.

While it seems probable that malaria is the fundamental cause of the tropical splenomegaly syndrome, this disease is not the result of active malarial infection, as parasitaemia is usually scanty and malarial pigment is not found in biopsy material from the liver and spleen. An abnormal host response to the continual presence of malarial antigen, which results in a reactive and relatively benign lymphoproliferative

Table 10.1 Causes of splenomegaly.

Haematological Chronic myeloid leukaemia*, chronic lymphocytic leukaemia, acute leukaemia, malignant lymphoma*, hairy cell leukaemia Langerhans cell histiocytosis, primary myelofibrosis*, polycythaemia vera, essential thrombocythaemia (some cases), systemic mastocytosis, Thalassaemia major or intermedia* Sickle cell anaemia (before splenic infarction) Haemolytic anaemias Megaloblastic anaemia (if severe)
Portal hypertension Cirrhosis Congestive heart failure Hepatic, portal, splenic vein thrombosis
Storage diseases Gaucher disease* Niemann–Pick disease Histiocytosis X
Systemic diseases Sarcoidosis Amyloidosis Collagen diseases – systemic lupus erythematosus, rheumatoid arthritis
Infections Acute: septicaemia, bacterial endocarditis, typhoid, infectious mononucleosis, cytomegalovirus Chronic: tuberculosis, brucellosis, syphilis
Tropical Tropical splenomegaly (possibly caused by malaria)*, malaria, leishmaniasis,* schistosomiasis*, trypanosomiasis

* Possible causes of massive (>20 cm) splenomegaly.

disorder that predominantly affects the liver and spleen, seems more likely.

Splenomegaly is usually gross and the liver is also enlarged. Portal hypertension may be a feature. The anaemia is often severe and leucopenia is usual; some patients develop a marked lymphocytosis. Serum immunoglobulin (Ig) M levels are high and there are high titres of malarial antibody.

Although splenectomy corrects the pancytopenia, there is an increased risk of fulminant malarial infection. Antimalarial therapy has proved successful in the management of many affected patients.

Hypersplenism

Normally, only approximately 5% (30–70 mL) of the total red cell mass is present in the spleen, although 30–50% of the total marginating neutrophil pool and 20–40% of the platelet mass are located there. As the spleen enlarges, the proportion of haemopoietic cells within the organ increases such that up to 40% of the red cell mass, and 90% of platelets (Fig. 27.5), may be pooled in an enlarged spleen.

Table 10.2 Causes of hyposplenism.

Splenectomy and splenic embolization *Irradiation*
Haematological disorders Sickle cell disease Essential thrombocythaemia
Circulatory Splenic arterial/venous thrombosis
Auto-immune disease Systemic lupus erythematosus Rheumatoid arthritis
Chronic graft-versus-host disease
Gastrointestinal Gluten-induced enteropathy Dermatitis herpetiformis Inflammatory bowel diseases
Infiltrations Lymphomas Sézary syndrome Myeloma Amyloidosis Secondary carcinomas, especially breast Cysts, e.g. hydatid
Nephrotic syndrome
Congenital aplasia syndrome

Hypersplenism is a clinical syndrome that can be seen in any form of splenomegaly. It is characterized by:

- Enlargement of the spleen.
- Reduction of at least one cell line in the blood in the presence of normal bone marrow function.

Depending on the underlying cause, splenectomy may be indicated if the hypersplenism is symptomatic. It is followed by a rapid improvement in the peripheral blood count.

Hyposplenism

The most frequent cause is surgical removal of the spleen, e.g. after traumatic rupture, but hyposplenism can also occur in sickle cell anaemia, gluten-induced enteropathy, amyloidosis and many other conditions (Table 10.2).

Functional hyposplenism is revealed by the blood film findings of Howell–Jolly bodies or Pappenheimer bodies (siderotic granules on iron staining; Fig. 10.3) and by other abnormalities of blood cells (Table 10.3).

Splenectomy

Surgical removal of the spleen may be indicated for treatment of haematological disorders but now much more frequently after splenic rupture (Table 10.4). It is indicated rarely for

Table 10.3 The blood film appearances of hyposplenism.

Blood film features
Red cells Target cells Acanthocytes Irregularly contracted or crenated cells Howell–Jolly bodies (DNA remnants) Siderotic (iron) granules (Pappenheimer bodies)
White cells ± Mild lymphocytosis, monocytosis
Platelets ± Thrombocytosis

Table 10.4 Indications for splenectomy.

Splenic rupture
Some cases of:
Chronic autoimmune thrombocytopenia
Haemolytic anaemia, e.g. hereditary spherocytosis, autoimmune haemolytic anaemia, thalassaemia major or intermedia
Chronic lymphocytic leukaemia and lymphomas
Primary myelofibrosis
Tropical splenomegaly

splenic tumours or cysts (Table 10.4). With advances in drug treatment of immune thrombocytopenia, chemotherapy and immunotherapy for lymphomas and chronic lymphocytic leukaemia, and the introduction of JAK2 inhibitors for treatment of primary myelofibrosis, splenectomy for these conditions is now much less frequently indicated than previously. Splenectomy can be performed by open abdominal laparotomy or by laparoscopic surgery. Angio-embolization can be used in selected cases of rupture to control haemorrhage with preservation of splenic function.

The platelet count can often rise dramatically in the early postoperative period, reaching levels of up to 1000×10^9/L and peaking at 1–2 weeks. Thrombotic complications are seen in some patients and prophylactic aspirin or heparin is often required during this period. Long-term alterations in the peripheral blood cell count may also be seen, including a persistent thrombocytosis, lymphocytosis or monocytosis.

Prevention of infection in hyposplenic patients

Patients with hyposplenism are at lifelong increased risk of infection from a variety of organisms. This is seen particularly in children under the age of 5 years and those with sickle cell anaemia. The most characteristic susceptibility is to the encapsulated bacteriae *Streptococcus pneumoniae*, *Haemophilus influenzae* type B and *Neisseria meningitidis*. *Streptococcus pneumoniae* is a particular concern and can cause a rapid and fulminant disease. Malaria and infection caused by animal bites tend to be more severe in splenectomized individuals.

Measures to reduce the risk of serious infection include the following:

1. Patients should be informed about their increased susceptibility to infection and advised to carry a card about their condition. They should be counselled about the increased risk of infection on foreign travel, including that from malaria and tick and animal bites.
2. Prophylactic oral penicillin 250mg bd is recommended, usually for life. High-risk groups include those aged under 16 years or older than 50 years, splenectomy for a haematological malignancy or a history of previous invasive pneumococcal disease. Low-risk adults, if they choose to discontinue penicillin, must be warned to seek immediate medical advice if they develop a high fever. Erythromycin 250mg bd may be prescribed for patients allergic to penicillin. A supply of appropriate antibiotics should also be given for patients to take in the event of onset of fever before medical care is available.
3. Vaccination against pneumococcus, haemophilus, meningococcus and influenza infection is recommended (Table 10.5). All types of vaccine, including live vaccines, can be given safely to hyposplenic individuals, although the immune response to vaccination may be impaired.

Vaccination

When splenectomy is being planned the patient should be considered for immunization against pneumococcus, *H. influenzae* type B (Hib) and meningococcal infection (Table 10.4). Vaccines, including live inoculations, can be given safely after splenectomy and appropriate vaccines that were not administered before splenectomy should be given 14 days post splenectomy.

Table 10.5 Suggested schedule for vaccine immunization in individuals with asplenia or splenic hypofunction.

Age at which asplenia or splenic dysfunction acquired	Vaccination schedule* Month 0	Month 1	Later
Under 2 years	Complete according to national routine childhood schedule, including booster doses of Hib/MenC and PCV13	A dose of MenACWY conjugate vaccine should be given at least 1 month after the Hib/MenC and PCV13 booster doses	After the second birthday, one additional dose of Hib/MenC and a dose of PPV should be given
Over 2 years and under 5 years (previously completed routine childhood vaccinations with PCV7)	HibMenC booster PCV13	MenACWY conjugate vaccine	PPV (at least 2 months after PCV13)
Over 2 years and under 5 years (previously completed routine childhood vaccinations with PCV13)	HibMenC booster PPV	MenACWY conjugate vaccine	
Over 2 years and under 5 years (unvaccinated or previously partially vaccinated with PCV7)	HibMenC vaccine First dose of PCV13	MenACWY conjugate vaccine	Second dose of PCV13 and then PPV (at least 2 months after PCV13)
Over 5 years (regardless of vaccination history)	HibMenC vaccine PVV	MenACWY conjugate vaccine (boosters every 5 years)	

*Where possible, vaccination course should ideally be started at least 2 weeks before surgery or commencement of immunosuppressive treatment PCV, pneumococcal conjugate vaccine; PPV, pneumococcal polysaccharide vaccine.
Source: J.M. Davies *et al.* (2011) *Br. J. Haematol.* 155: 308–17. Reproduced with permission of John Wiley & Sons.

SUMMARY

- The normal adult spleen weighs 150–250 g and is 5–13 cm in diameter. It has a specialized circulation because the majority of arterioles end in 'cords' which lack an endothelial lining. The blood re-enters the circulation via venous sinuses. The cords and sinuses form the red pulp, which monitors the integrity of red blood cells.
- The central arterioles are surrounded by lymphoid tissue called white pulp, which is similar in structure to a lymph node.
- The spleen removes aged or abnormal red cells, and excess DNA and siderotic granules, from intact red cells. It also has a specialized immune function against capsulated bacteria, *Pneumococcus*, *Haemophilus influenzae* and *Meningococcus*, against which splenectomized patients are immunized.
- Splenectomy is needed for splenic rupture and in some haematological diseases.
- Enlargement of the spleen (splenomegaly) occurs in many malignant and benign haematological diseases, in portal hypertension and with systemic diseases, including acute and chronic infections.
- Hyposplenism occurs in sickle cell anaemia, gluten-induced enteropathy, amyloidosis and rarely in other diseases.
- Vaccination against capsulated organisms and prolonged antibiotic prophylaxis is needed for patients with absent splenic function.

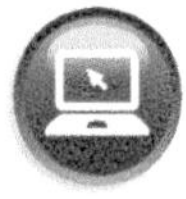

Now visit **www.wiley.com/go/haematology9e** to test yourself on this chapter.

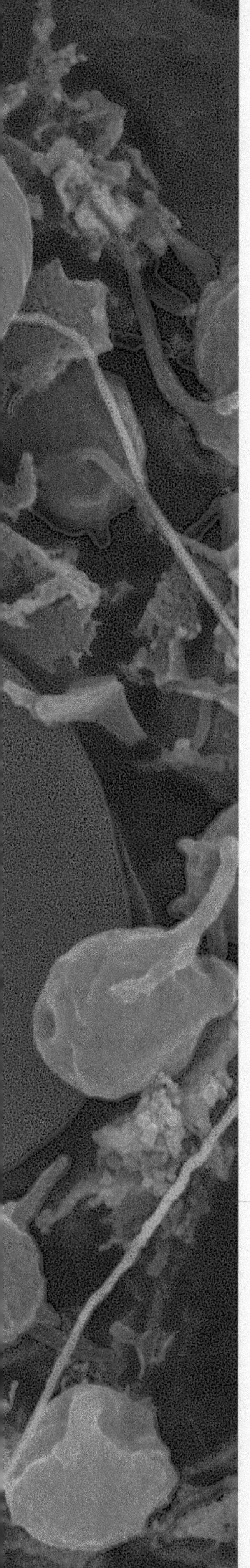

CHAPTER 11

The aetiology and genetics of haematological neoplasia

Key topics

Hoffbrand's Essential Haematology, Ninth Edition. A. Victor Hoffbrand, Pratima Chowdary, Graham P. Collins, and Justin Loke.

© 2024 John Wiley & Sons Ltd. Published 2024 by John Wiley & Sons Ltd.

Companion website: www.wiley.com/go/haematology9e

Table 11.1 Glossary.

Acquired mutation: see 'somatic mutation'
Allele burden: The fraction of alleles with a specific sequence in relation to the total number of alleles for the same region of the genome. For example, a heterozygous mutation in a pure population of leukaemia cells has an allele burden of 0.5. If 70% of cells are leukaemic and 30% of cells are normal, the mutant allele burden of the heterozygous mutation would be $0.7 \times 0.5 = 0.35$.
Amplification: A genetic modification producing an increased number of copies of a genomic region.
Autosomal dominant: Inherited mutation affecting one allele on a non-sex chromosome is sufficient to confer the disease.
Autosomal recessive: Inherited mutation must affect both alleles on the respective non-sex chromosomes to confer the disease.
Branching evolution (of cancer): A form of clonal evolution of cancer which leads to the generation of more than one clone of cells characterized by distinct somatic mutations, but which share at least one mutation traceable back to a single ancestral cell.
Cancer genome: The genome of a cancer cell, which differs from the germline genome as a result of somatic mutations.
Chromosomal translocation: See 'genomic rearrangements'.
Chromothripsis: A single catastrophic event by which hundreds to thousands of chromosomal rearrangements occur in confined genomic regions of one or a few chromosomes (from Greek θρύΨις = shattering into small pieces).
Clonal evolution (of cancer): The stepwise acquisition of mutations in a founder cell and its progeny leading towards the development of a cancer.
Clonal mutation: A mutation present in a population of related cells derived from a single cell.
Constraint hypothesis: A hypothesis about clonal evolution proposing that the observed order of acquisition of somatic mutations during cancer evolution reflects a requirement for a specific mutation to occur before another for a growth advantage to be gained by the host cell(s).
Co-occurrence (of cancer mutations): The occurrence of two or more mutations in the same type cancer more often than would be expected by chance.
Convergent evolution (of cancer): A pattern of cancer evolution during which independent clones expand after acquiring the same or very similar mutation. This is likely to reflect the fact that such a mutation is particularly advantageous to the specific cancer cell, giving a marked growth advantage when acquired by chance.
Deletion: A genetic modification leading to the loss of a genomic region.
Dominant negative mutation: A heterozygous mutation that leads to marked or complete loss of function of the coded protein and of the normal protein coded by the other (wild-type) copy of the gene.
Driver gene or driver mutation: A mutated gene that confers a selective growth advantage to a cancer cell.
Epigenetics: The study of changes to DNA and chromatin, other than those that alter the DNA nucleotide sequence, that alter the transcriptional potential of a cell and are usually heritable.
Exome: The collection of all exons in a genome.
Exome sequencing: Sequencing of all exons in a genome. This has referred to exons of protein-coding genes, but increasingly non-protein-coding genes are included (e.g. long non-coding RNAs).
Gain-of-function mutation: A mutation that gives the coded protein a novel or markedly enhanced function.
Genome-wide association studies (GWAS): studies of many common and uncommon genetic variants in different individuals to determine if any variant is associated with a disease or trait. The primary outcome of these studies is the identification of variants such as SNPs which are *associated* with, but do not necessarily cause the disease in question.
Genomic instability: Increased frequency of mutations in the genome caused by either increased DNA damage or deficient DNA repair.
Genomic rearrangement: A mutation that juxtaposes nucleotides that are normally distant from each other, such as a chromosomal translocation, inversion or deletion.
Genotoxin: Chemical or other agent that modifies DNA and generates mutations.
Germline genome: An individual's genome as formed at the time of conception (fertilized oocyte). This genome is shared by all cells in the body.
Germline mutation: Mutations present in the germline genome. Sporadic mutations acquired in the germ cells of parents are also included in this category.
Germline variants: Variations in sequences or copy number of DNA segments observed between different individuals that are responsible of the phenotypic variation between people. Two unrelated individuals differ by approximately 3 million such variants.
Haplotype: A contiguous region of the genome containing a set of tightly linked genes that are usually inherited as a block.
Indel: A mutation that results in insertion or deletion of one or a few nucleotides to DNA.
Kataegis: Localized hypermutation of a region of the genome, thought to be mediated by APOBEC enzymes (from Greek καταιγίς = storm).
Linear evolution (of cancer): A form of clonal evolution of cancer that generates a single final clone of cancer cells which harbours all mutations that ever arose during its evolution.
Loss-of-function mutation: A mutation that leads to marked or complete loss of function of the coded protein.
Loss-of-heterozygosity (LOH): A genetic modification leading to the loss of the maternally or paternally derived copy of a genomic region. This can happen as a result of deletion or uniparental disomy (uPD).

Methylation: Covalent addition of a methyl group to a DNA, RNA, protein or other molecule.
Missense mutation: A nucleotide substitution, e.g. G to T, that results in an amino acid change, e.g. valine to phenylalanine.
Mutational signature: A recurrent pattern of DNA mutations attributable to a particular type of mutagen or mutational process, characterized by certain nucleotide mutations in a specific 5′ and 3′ nucleotidic context.
Mutual exclusivity: The occurrence of two or more mutations in the same cancer type less often than would be expected by chance.
Next-generation sequencing (NGS): DNA sequencing using one of the methodologies developed since 2005 and which allow massively parallel sequencing of thousands or millions of fragments of DNA simultaneously.
Nonsense mutation: A nucleotide substitution that results in the generation of a stop codon, i.e. TAA, TGA or TAG.
Non-synonymous mutation: A mutation that alters the encoded amino acid sequence of a protein. These include missense, nonsense, splice site, gain of translation start, loss of translation stop and indel mutations.
Oncogene: A gene that confers growth advantage to a cell and contributes to its progression/transformation to cancer.
Opportunity hypothesis: A hypothesis proposing that the observed order of acquisition of somatic mutations during cancer evolution reflects the statistical likelihood that mutations are acquired in this order. This likelihood is determined by the earlier mutation influencing the opportunity for acquiring the next. Implicit in this hypothesis is that the reverse order can also be observed, albeit less often.
Passenger mutation: A mutation that does not give a selective growth advantage to its host cell.
Proto-oncogene: A gene that when activated by mutations becomes an **oncogene** and imparts a growth advantage of its host cell.
Satellite DNA consists of large arrays of tandemly repeating, non-coding DNA. It is the main component of centromeres and forms the main structural component of heterochromatin. With its repetitive DNA, it has a different density compared to the rest of the genome.
Single nucleotide polymorphism (SNP): A DNA sequence variation occurring commonly within a population, e.g. 1%, in which a single nucleotide in the genome differs between individuals.
Somatic mutation: A mutation that occurs in any cell of the body after conception. Sometimes called *acquired mutation*.
Substitution (or nucleotide substitution): A DNA mutation leading to the replacement of a native nucleotide with another.
Splice sites: DNA sequences flanking exons which are important for mRNA splicing.
Subclonal mutation: A mutation that exists in only a subset of the neoplastic cells within a tumour.
Transition (mutation): Change of a nucleotide to another of the same group such as C >T (both pyrimidines) or G >A (both purines).
Transversion (mutation): Change of a nucleotide to another of the opposite group such as A >C (purine to pyrimidine).
Tumour-suppressor gene: A gene that inhibits the development of cancer, commonly by limiting cell proliferation. These genes are frequently inactivated in cancer cells.
Uniparental disomy (uPD): A genetic modification leading to the loss of the maternally or paternally derived copy of a genomic region as a result of replacement of this sequence with the equivalent sequence derived from the other parent.
Untranslated region (UTR): An exonic region located before the start (5' UTR) or after the stop (3'UTR) codon of a gene and which does not code for any amino acids.
Whole genome sequencing: Sequencing of the entire sequence of an individual genome using germline DNA, tumour-derived DNA or DNA from another cellular source such as cell lines, single cells etc.
Whole exome sequencing: Sequencing of all the exons of all the genes in an individual genome (there are approximately 30,000 coding genes in a mammalian genome). As with whole genome sequencing this could be done using germline DNA, tumour-derived DNA or DNA from another cellular source.
X-linked gene: Any gene located on the X chromosome.

Source: Adapted from M. Wang *et al.* In A. Mead *et al.* (eds) (2024) *Hoffbrand's Postgraduate Haematology*, 8th edn (2025, in press).

Haemopoietic malignancies (neoplasms) are **clonal diseases** that derive from a single cell in the marrow or peripheral lymphoid tissue that has undergone genetic alteration (Fig. 11.1). In this chapter, we discuss the aetiology and genetic basis of haematological malignancies. Table 11.1 provides a glossary of the specialised terms used. Subsequent chapters discuss general aspects of management of these diseases and then the aetiology, diagnosis and management of the individual conditions.

The incidence of haematological neoplasms

Cancer is an important cause of morbidity and mortality, as approximately 50% of, for example, the UK and US population will develop cancer in their lifetime. The majority of cancers are epithelial neoplasms; haematological cancers represent approximately 7% of all malignant disease, if non-melanomatous skin

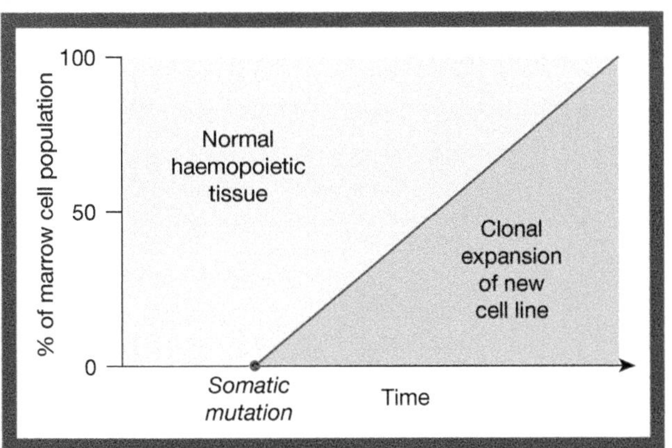

Figure 11.1 Theoretical graph to show the replacement of normal bone marrow cells by a clonal population of malignant cells arising by successive mitotic divisions from a single cell with an acquired genetic alteration.

cancer is excluded (Fig. 11.2). There are major geographical variations in the occurrence of some haematological cancers, most notably chronic lymphocytic leukaemia (CLL), which is common in Europe and North America but rare in the Far East (Chapter 18).

The aetiology of haemopoietic neoplasia

Cancer results from the accumulation of genetic mutations within a cell. The number of DNA mutations varies widely from over 100 in some cancers to about 10 in most haematological malignancies (Fig. 11.3). Factors such as genetic inheritance and environmental lifestyle will influence the risk of developing a malignancy, but most cases of leukaemia and lymphoma appear to result simply as a result of the chance acquisition of critical genetic changes. Mutations accumulate with age but some mutations can be acquired as early as in utero.

Inherited factors (germline predisposition)

The incidence of leukaemia is greatly increased in some genetic diseases such as Down syndrome, where a transient myeloproliferative disorder develops in 10% and acute leukaemia occurs with a 20- to 30-fold increased frequency. Additional leukaemia-predisposing disorders include Bloom syndrome (biallelic mutations of the gene *BLM* leading to genomic instability), Fanconi anaemia, Shwachman–Diamond syndrome, severe congenital neutropenia, ataxia telangiectasia, Type1 neurofibromatosis, Li-Fraumeni, and Noonan syndrome. Non-syndromic-inherited gene mutations can also predispose to myelodysplastic syndromes (MDS) and acute myeloid leukaemia (AML); these include germline mutations of *GATA2*, *CEBPA*, *DDX41*, *RUNX1* or *ETV6* (Appendix Table 10). *RUNX1* heterozygous mutations cause a familial platelet disorder.

There is also a weak familial tendency in the diseases CLL, Hodgkin lymphoma, non-Hodgkin lymphoma (NHL) and myeloma with certain haplotypes and alleles associated with increased risk, although the genes predisposing to this higher risk are largely unknown. Increasingly it is recognized that germline predispositions to haematological neoplasia may not be detected until adulthood or may be found in patients with no family history of neoplasia.

Certain haplotypes may predispose to neoplastic transformation. The *JAK2V617F* mutation is more frequent in the 25% of the population who have inherited the haplotype called 46/1 and these 25% have a 3–4 increased risk of developing myeloproliferative disease.

Environmental influences

Chemicals

Chronic exposure to industrial solvents or chemicals such as benzene is a known but now fortunately rare cause of MDS or AML.

Drugs

DNA alkylating agents, such as chlorambucil or melphalan, predispose to later development of MDS or AML, especially if combined with radiotherapy. The karyotype in such cases is almost always complex with *TP53* mutations usually present. Etoposide and other topoisomerase inhibitors including anthracyclines are associated with a risk of the development of secondary leukaemia associated with balanced translocations including that of the *KTM2A (MLL)* gene at 11q23. Topoisomerases create double-strand breaks, relaxing over-wound DNA. The inhibitors of the enzyme increase the chances of these free ends participating in translocations. The majority of MDS/AML cases post-cytotoxic chemotherapy are associated with *TP53* mutations.

Radiation

Radiation, especially to the marrow, is leukaemogenic. This is illustrated by a dose-dependent increased incidence of leukaemia in survivors of the 1945 atom bomb explosions in Japan.

Infection

The World Health Organization estimated in 2002 that infections are responsible for 18% of all cancers. Infectious agents contribute to a range of haematological malignancies.

Viruses

Viral infection is associated especially different subtypes of lymphoma (Table 20.3). The retrovirus human T-lymphotropic virus type 1 (HTLV-1) is the cause of adult T-cell leukaemia/lymphoma (ATLL, Chapter 18), although most people infected with the HTLV-1 virus do not develop a neoplasm. Epstein–Barr virus (EBV) is associated with almost all cases of endemic

Estimated new cases

Males			Females		
Prostate	268,490	27%	Breast	287,850	31%
Lung & bronchus	117,910	12%	Lung & bronchus	118,830	13%
Colon & rectum	80,690	8%	Colon & rectum	70,340	8%
Urinary bladder	61,700	6%	Uterine corpus	65,950	7%
Melanoma of the skin	57,180	6%	Melanoma of the skin	42,600	5%
Kidney & renal pelvis	50,290	5%	Non-Hodgkin lymphoma	36,350	4%
Non-Hodgkin lymphoma	44,120	4%	Thyroid	31,940	3%
Oral cavity & pharynx	38,700	4%	Pancreas	29,240	3%
Leukemia	35,810	4%	Kidney & renal pelvis	28,710	3%
Pancreas	32,970	3%	Leukemia	24,840	3%
All Sites	**983,160**	**100%**	**All Sites**	**934,870**	**100%**

Estimated deaths

Males			Females		
Lung & bronchus	68,820	21%	Lung & bronchus	61,360	21%
Prostate	34,500	11%	Breast	43,250	15%
Colon & rectum	28,400	9%	Colon & rectum	24,180	8%
Pancreas	25,970	8%	Pancreas	23,860	8%
Liver & intrahepatic bile duct	20,420	6%	Ovary	12,810	4%
Leukemia	14,020	4%	Uterine corpus	12,550	4%
Esophagus	13,250	4%	Liver & intrahepatic bile duct	10,100	4%
Urinary bladder	12,120	4%	Leukemia	9,980	3%
Non-Hodgkin lymphoma	11,700	4%	Non-Hodgkin lymphoma	8,550	3%
Brain & other nervous system	10,710	3%	Brain & other nervous system	7,570	3%
All Sites	**322,090**	**100%**	**All Sites**	**287,270**	**100%**

Figure 11.2 Ten Leading Cancer Types for the Estimated New Cancer Cases and Deaths by Sex, United States, 2022. Estimates are rounded to the nearest 10 and exclude basal cell and squamous cell skin cancers and *in situ* carcinoma except urinary bladder. Source: S. Siegel *et al.* (2020) *CA Cancer J. Clin.* 72: 7–33. Reproduced with permission of John Wiley & Sons.

(African) Burkitt lymphoma, post-transplant lymphoproliferative disease (p. 334) and a proportion of patients with Hodgkin lymphoma and diffuse large B-cell lymphoma. The latent virus expresses certain genes to maintain itself but this gene expression may drive B-cell proliferation. This is held in check by EBV-specific T-cells but immunosuppressed subjects, e.g. after organ transplantation, are unable to mount a T-cell response and a B-cell lymphoproliferative disease results. Human herpes virus 8 infection (KSHV/HHV8) causes primary effusion lymphoma (Table 20.3). Chronic hepatitis C increases the risk of B-cell lymphomas.

Human immunodeficiency virus (HIV) infection is associated with an increased incidence of lymphomas at unusual sites such as the central nervous system. These HIV-associated lymphomas are usually of B-cell origin and of high-grade histology. The risk of developing lymphoma increases with lower CD4 lymphocyte counts.

Bacteria

Helicobacter pylori infection has been implicated in the pathogenesis of gastric mucosa B-cell (MALT) lymphoma (Chapter 21) and antibiotic treatment may even bring about disease remission without the need for chemotherapy. Chronic *Chlamydia trachomatis* infection predisposes to ocular adnexal lymphoma.

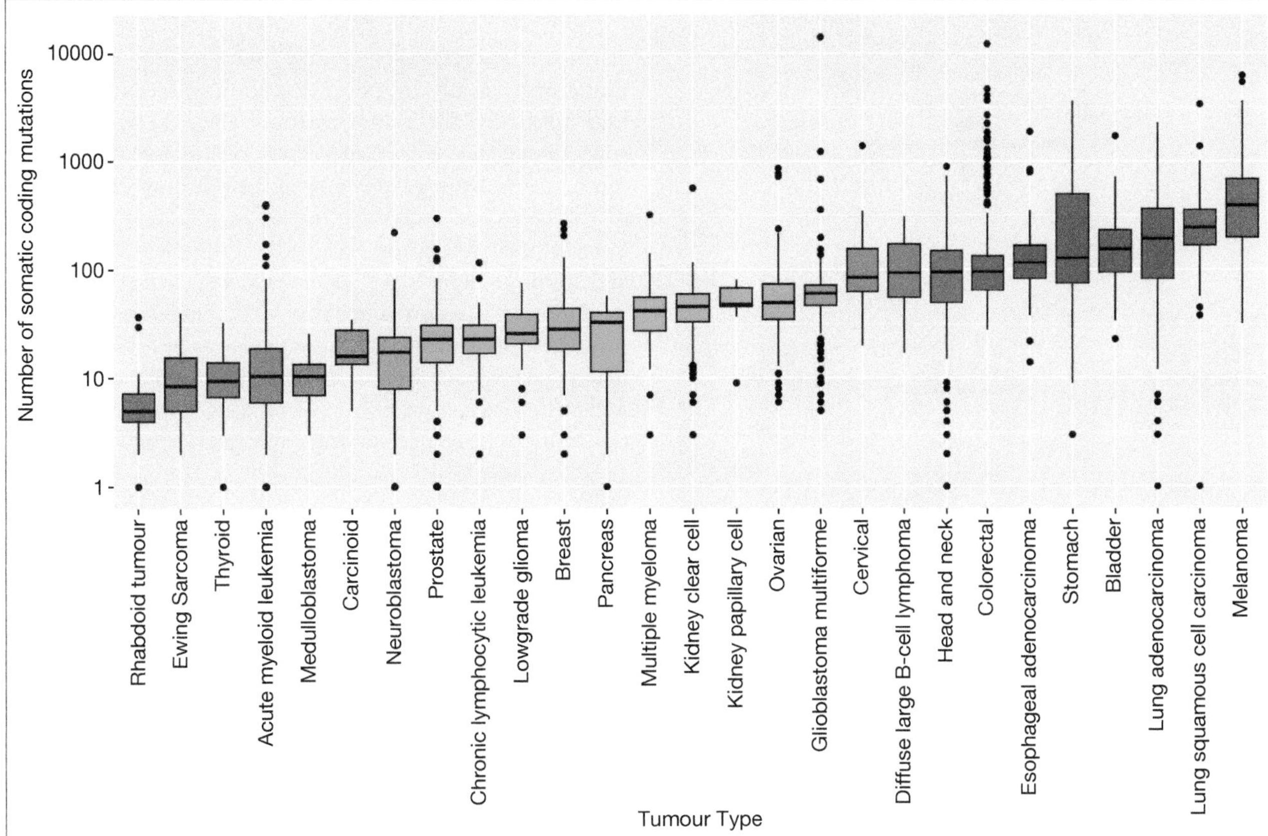

Figure 11.3 Frequency of somatic coding mutations by tumour type. Source: Data from M.S. Lawrence *et al.* (2013) *Nature* 449: 214–8.

Protozoa

Endemic Burkitt lymphoma occurs in the tropics, particularly in malarial areas. It is thought that malaria may alter host immunity and predispose to tumour formation as a result of EBV infection.

Endogenous mutations

An important albeit slow mechanism of background mutation is the spontaneous deamination of methylated cytosines especially at CpG islands (particular parts of the genome rich in cytosine-guanine dinucleotides), which if not repaired leads to cytosine to thymine transition. Off-target mutational activity of a variety of enzymes may also cause C>T transition.

Aberrant activity of the recombinase activating gene enzymes (RAG-recombinases) which mediate VDJ recombination during B-cell development underlies oncogenesis in B-ALL (Chapter 17).

The genetics of haemopoietic neoplasia

The genes that are involved in the development of cancer can be divided broadly into two groups: **oncogenes** and **tumour-suppressor genes**.

Oncogenes

Oncogenes arise because of gain-of-function mutations or inappropriate expression pattern in normal cellular genes called **proto-oncogenes** (Fig. 11.4). Oncogenic versions are generated when the activity of proto-oncogenes is increased or they acquire a novel function. This can occur in a number of ways, including translocation, mutation or duplication. In general, these mutations affect the processes of cell signalling, cell differentiation and cell survival. One of the striking features of haematological malignancies, in contrast to most solid tumours, is their high frequency of chromosomal translocations. Several oncogenes involved in haematological malignancies are involved in the suppression of apoptosis, of which the best example is *BCL2*, which is overexpressed in follicular lymphoma (Chapter 21).

The types of mutations that are detected in the neoplastic cells of a patient with cancer fall into two broad groups.

Driver mutations are those that confer a selective growth advantage to a cancer cell, also defined as mutations that are found in the cancer more often than would be expected by chance. Certain driver mutations occur together, e.g. of *NPM1* and *FLT3* in AML where they cooperate to drive malignant transformation, whereas others are mutually exclusive such as

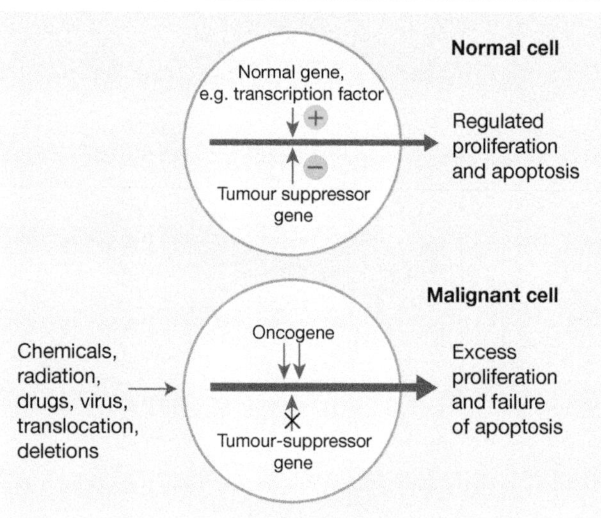

Figure 11.4 Proliferation of normal cells depends on a balance between the action of proto-oncogenes and tumour-suppressor genes. In a malignant cell, this balance is disturbed, leading to uncontrolled cell division.

JAK2 and *CALR* where one of these mutations alone is sufficient to cause transformation. The sequence in which different driver mutations occur in a tumour may affect the clinical features of the resulting disease.

Passenger mutations do not confer a growth advantage and may have already been coincidentally present in the cell from which the cancer arose, or may subsequently arise as a neutral genetic change in the proliferating cell. It is important that targeted drug treatments are directed against the activity of driver mutations.

Tyrosine kinases

Tyrosine kinases are enzymes which phosphorylate proteins on tyrosine residues. They exist on cell surfaces as receptors, e.g. KIT, PDGFRA or PDGFRB, or as free cytoplasmic enzymes which are important mediators of intracellular signalling, e.g. JAK2 and ABL1. They therefore regulate such core activities as proliferation, transcription, translation, energy metabolism and differentiation. Mutations, alteration of expression of tyrosine kinases leading to unregulated activation of the kinase and so of downstream signalling pathways, underlie a large number of haematological malignancies. Tyrosine kinases are the targets of many extremely effective drugs called **tyrosine kinase inhibitors (TKIs)**. Common examples of TKIs discussed in the relevant disease-specific chapters are of **ABL1** in chronic myeloid leukaemia (CML), **JAK2** in myeloproliferative neoplasms, **FLT3** in AML, **KIT** in both systemic mastocytosis and AML, **PDGFRA** in eosinophilic myeloproliferative disorders and **Bruton tyrosine kinase (BTK)** in chronic lymphocytic leukaemia and other B-cell lymphoproliferative disorders.

Tumour-suppressor genes

Tumour-suppressor genes may acquire loss-of-function mutations, usually by point mutation or deletion, which lead to malignant transformation (Fig. 11.4). Tumour-suppressor genes commonly act as components of control mechanisms that regulate entry of the cell from the G_1 phase of the cell cycle into the S phase or passage through the S phase to G_2 and mitosis (Fig. 1.8). Examples of oncogenes and tumour-suppressor genes involved in haemopoietic malignancies are shown in Table 11.2. The most significant tumour-suppressor gene in human cancer is ***TP53***, which is inactivated by mutation or deletion in over 50% of cases of malignant disease, including many haemopoietic neoplasias, especially those related to prior exposure to alkylating agents or radiation.

Clonal progression

Malignant cells arise as a multistep process with the acquisition of mutations in different intracellular pathways. This may occur by a **linear evolution**, in which the final clone harbours all the mutations that arose during evolution of the malignancy (Fig. 11.5a), or by **branching evolution**, in which there is more than one clone of cells characterized by different somatic mutations, but which share at least one mutation traceable back to a single ancestral cell (Fig. 11.5b). During this progression of the disease, one sub-clone may gradually acquire a growth advantage. Selection of sub-clones may also occur during anti-cancer treatment, which may selectively kill some subclones but allow others to survive and new clones to appear (Fig. 11.6). The presence of certain mutations that confer resistance to chemotherapy allows some neoplastic sub-clones to persist and expand, even as other clonal cells are eliminated. The most frequent of these mutations found in haematological neoplasms are of *TP53* and of *PPMID*, which encodes a protein phosphatase involved in the regulation of DNA damage responses.

Progression of subclinical clonal haematological mutations to clinical disease

The use of sensitive immunological and molecular tests has shown that many healthy individuals harbour clones of cells with acquired somatic mutations, from which overt haematological clinical disease may arise (Table 11.3). This is particularly frequent in the elderly. Clones of cells identical to those of chronic lymphocytic leukaemia can be present in the blood of individuals with a normal lymphocyte count. Progression of monoclonal gammopathy of undetermined significance (MGUS) to myeloma has been well recognized for many decades (Chapter 22). Clones of blood cells with somatic mutations increase in frequency with age (clonal haemopoiesis of indeterminate potential (CHIP), Chapter 16) and may predispose to myeloid and lymphoid malignancies.

Table 11.2 Some of the more frequent genetic abnormalities within haematological neoplasms (see also individual disease-specific chapters).

Disease	Genetic abnormality	Genes involved
AML (*de novo*)	t(8;21) translocation t(15;17) translocation Nucleotide insertion Mutation	*RUNX1::RUNX1T1* (*CBFα*) *PML::RARA* *NPM1*, *FLT3* *FLT3*, *DNMT3A*, *IDH1*, *IDH2*, *CEBBPA*
MDS/AML post-cytotoxic therapy	Chromosome 11q23 translocation Chromosome 17p deletion or mutation	*KMT2A(MLL) TP53*
MDS	Loss of chromosome 5 (-5, del (5q)) Mutation	*RPS14*, *CSKN1A* *SF3B1* or other splicing genes, *TET2*, *DNMT3A*, *ASXL1*, *EZH2*
CML	t(9;22) translocation	*BCR::ABL1*
Myeloproliferative neoplasms	Point mutation Insertion-deletion	*JAK2, MPL CALR*
Systemic mastocytosis	Point mutation	*KIT*
B-ALL	t(12;21) translocation t(9;22) translocation 11q23 translocations	*ETV6::RUNX1* *BCR::ABL1 AF4/KMT2A(MLL)*
T-ALL	Mutation	*NOTCH1*
Non-Hodgkin lymphomas		
Follicular lymphoma	t(14;18) translocation	*BCL2*
Lymphoplasmacytic lymphoma	Mutation	*MYD88, CXCR4*
Burkitt lymphoma	t(8;14) translocation	*MYC*
Hairy cell leukaemia	Mutation	*BRAF*
Large granular lymphocyte leukaemia	Mutation	*STAT3*
CLL	Chromosome 13p,11q, 17p deletion;trisomy12 Mutations	*TP53* *NOTCH1*, *SF3B1*, *ATM*
Mantle cell lymphoma	t(11;14)	CCND1/IgH

AML, acute myeloid leukaemia; B-ALL, B-acute lymphoblastic leukaemia; CLL, chronic lymphocytic leukaemia; CML, chronic myeloid leukaemia; MDS, myelodysplastic syndromes; T-ALL, T-acute lymphoblastic leukaemia.

Chromosome nomenclature

The normal somatic cell has 46 chromosomes and is called **diploid**; ova or sperm have 23 chromosomes and are called **haploid**. The chromosomes occur in pairs and are numbered 1–22 in approximately decreasing size order (for historical reasons, chromosome 20 is slightly larger than chromosome 19). There are two sex chromosomes, XX in females, XY in males.

Karyogram is the term used to describe the chromosomes derived from a mitotic cell which have been set out in numerical order (Fig. 11.7). A somatic cell with more or fewer than 46 chromosomes is termed **aneuploid**; more than 46 is **hyperdiploid**, fewer than 46 **hypodiploid**; 46 but with chromosome rearrangements, **pseudodiploid**. About 30% of patients with B-ALL have 50–67 chromosomes, which is termed **high hyperdiploid**; less commonly patients with B-ALL have 31–39 chromosomes (**low hypodiploid**).

Each chromosome has two arms: the shorter called 'p', the longer called 'q'. These meet at the **centromere** and the distal ends of the chromosomes are called **telomeres**. On staining

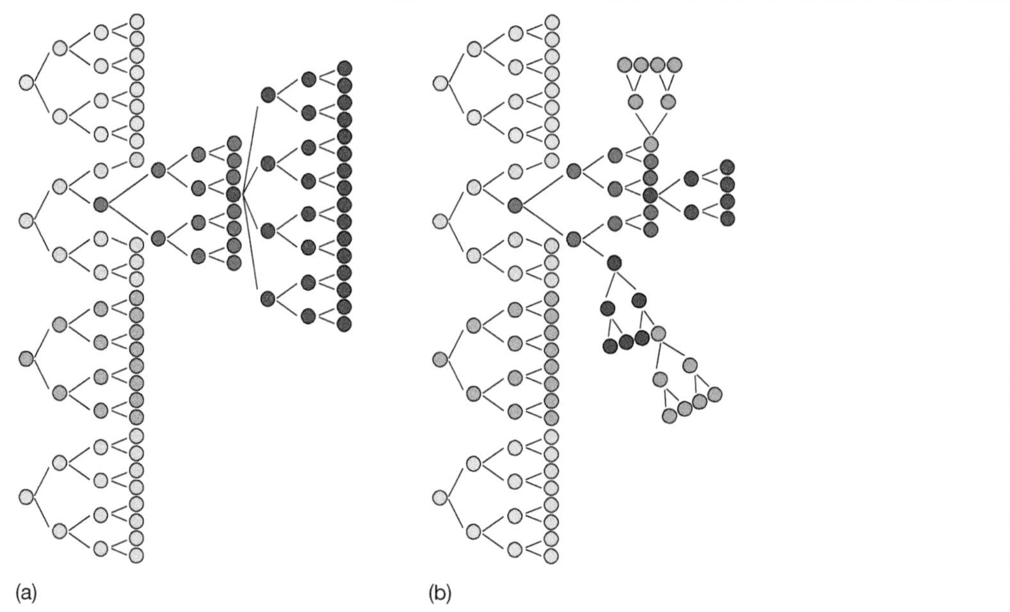

Figure 11.5 Multistep origin of a malignant tumour. **(a)** Linear evolution: successive mutations lead to growth advantage of one clone. **(b)** Branching evolution: sub-clones arise at different stages of the tumour evolution. These sub-clones share at least one common founder mutation. Green, brown and pink cells are all overtly malignant but may have different phenotypes and behaviour.

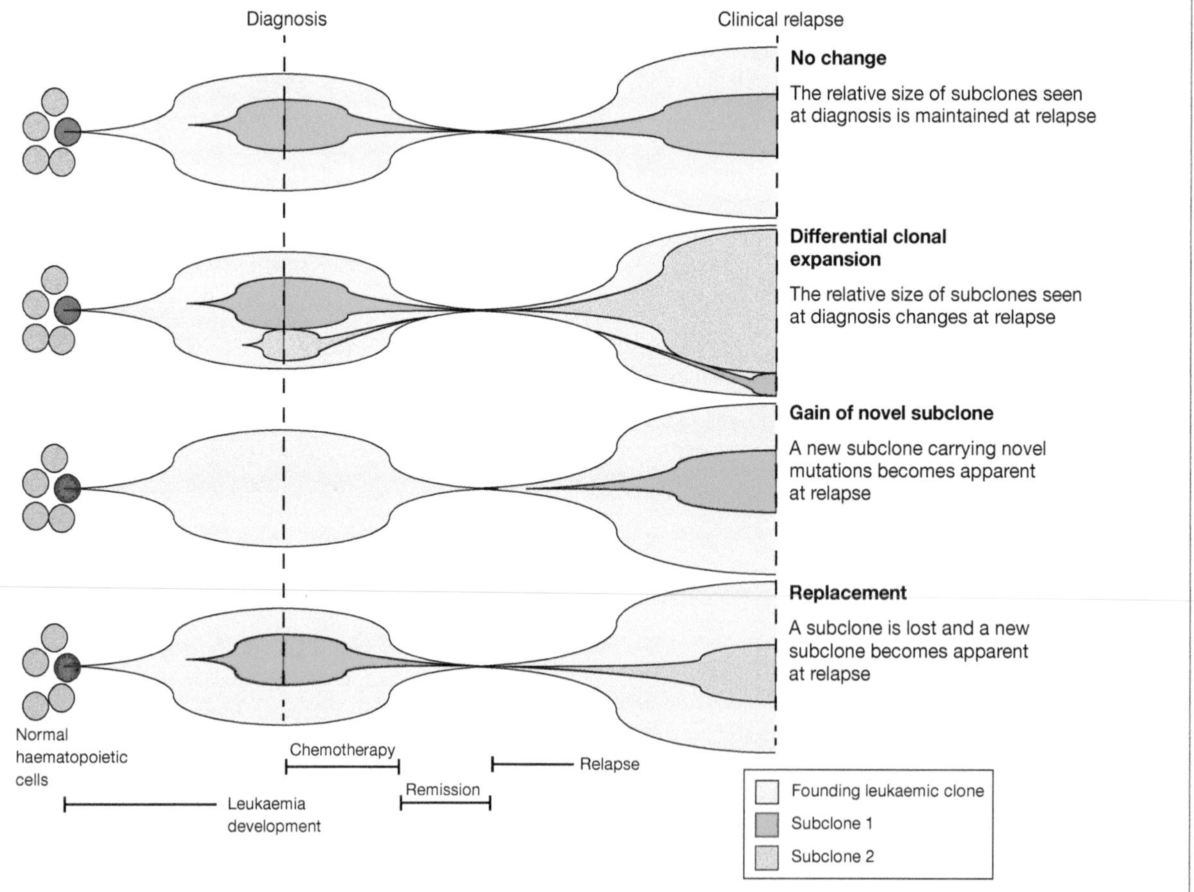

Figure 11.6 Examples of different potential patterns of clonal progression between the development, treatment and relapse of leukaemia. Source: Adapted from N. Bolli, G. Vassiliou. In A.V. Hoffbrand *et al.* (eds) (2016) *Postgraduate Haematology*, 7th edn. Reproduced with permission of John Wiley & Sons.

Table 11.3 Examples of clonal abnormalities which may be detected in otherwise healthy individuals and which may or may not progress to overt clinical disease.

Clonal abnormality	Disease(s)
Monoclonal B lymphocytosis	Chronic lymphocytic leukaemia and non-Hodgkin lymphoma
IgM paraprotein (MGUS)	Waldenstrom macroglobulinaemia
IgG paraprotein (MGUS)	Multiple myeloma
In situ follicular neoplasia	Follicular lymphoma
Mutation in foetal bone marrow, e.g. *ETV6::RUNX1*	Childhood acute lymphoblastic leukaemia
CHIP (clonal haemopoiesis of indeterminate potential (Chapter 16). Stem or progenitor cell clone in bone marrow, e.g. mutation of *TET2*, *DNMT3*, *ASXL1*, less frequently of 'lymphoid' genes.	Myelodysplastic syndromes, acute myeloid leukaemia; less commonly lymphoid neoplasms

MGUS, Monoclonal gammopathy of uncertain significance.

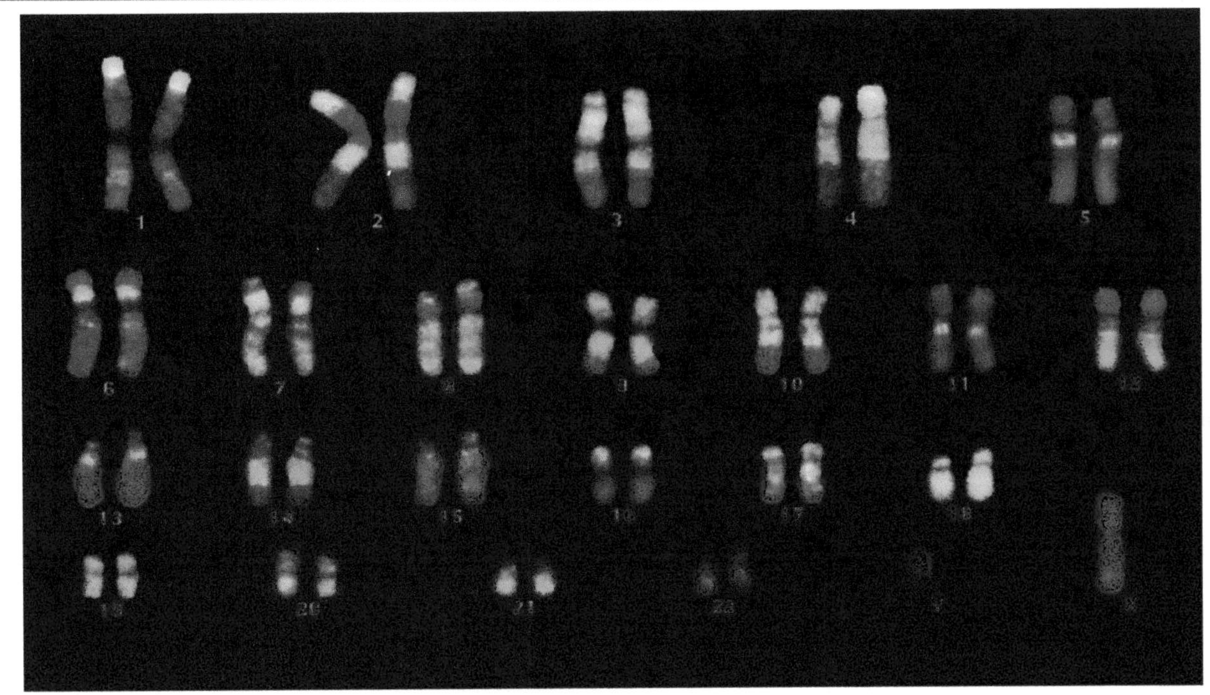

Figure 11.7 A colour-banded karyogram from a normal male. Each chromosome pair shows an individual colour-banding pattern. This involves a cross-species multiple-colour chromosome banding technique. Probe sets developed from the chromosomes of gibbons are combinatorially labelled and hybridized to human chromosomes. The success of cross-species colour banding depends on a close homology between host and human conserved DNA, divergence of repetitive DNA and a high degree of chromosomal rearrangement in the host relative to the human karyotype. Source: Courtesy of Professor C.J. Harrison.

with Giemsa (G-banding) or quinacrine (Q-banding), each arm divides into regions numbered outwards from the centromere and each region divides into bands (Fig. 11.8).

When a whole chromosome is lost or gained, a – or + is put in front of the chromosome number. If only part of the chromosome is lost, it is prefixed with **del** (for deletion). If there is extra material replacing part of a chromosome, the prefix **add** (for additional material) is used. Chromosome translocations are denoted by **t**, the chromosomes involved placed in brackets with the lower numbered chromosome first. The prefix **inv** describes an inversion where part of the chromosome has been inverted to run in the opposite direction. An **isochromosome**,

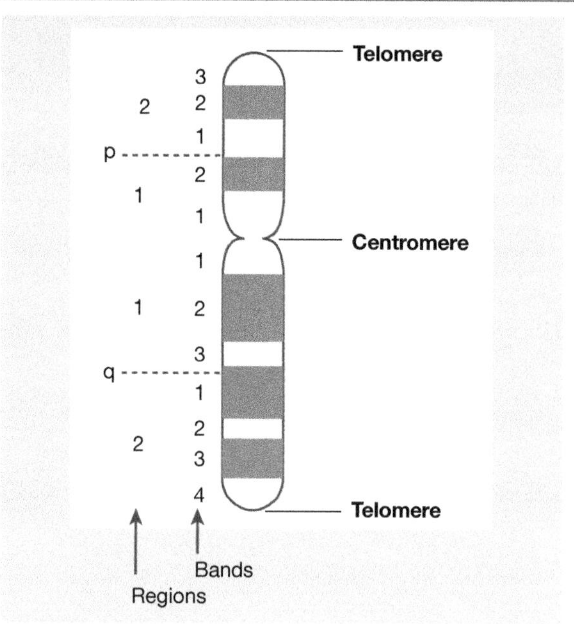

Figure 11.8 A schematic representation of a chromosome. The bands may be divided into sub-bands according to staining pattern. Loci are described orally by noting region and then band, e.g. 'q12' is 'q one-two' rather than 'q twelve'.

denoted by **i**, describes a chromosome with identical chromosome arms at each end; for example, i(17q) would consist of two copies of 17q joined at the centromere.

Telomeres

Telomeres are repetitive sequences at the ends of chromosomes. They decrease by approximately 200 base pairs of DNA with every round of cell replication. When they decrease to a critical length, the cell exits from the cell cycle.

Germ cells and stem cells, which need to self-renew and maintain a high proliferative potential, contain the enzyme **telomerase,** which can add extensions to the telomeric repeats and compensate for loss at replication, and so enable the cells to continue proliferation. Telomerase is also often expressed in malignant cells, but this is probably a consequence of the malignant transformation rather than an initiating factor. Germline mutations in components of the telomere complex cause dyskeratosis congenita (Chapter 24), which predisposes to haematological neoplasms. Patients with dyskeratosis typically have telomere lengths in both lymphocytes and granulocytes that are less than the second percentile for age.

Genetic abnormalities in haematological neoplasms

The genetic abnormalities underlying the different types of leukaemia and lymphoma are described with the diseases, which are themselves increasingly classified according to genetic change rather than morphology. The types of gene abnormality include the following (Fig. 11.9).

Point mutation

These may be *substitutions* or *indels* (*insertions* or *deletions*). When substitutions affect coding exons they can be *synonymous* (no change in the coded amino acid), *missense* (change in the coding to that for another amino acid) or *nonsense* (change in the amino acid to a stop codon). If *indels* are not a multiple of three nucleotides they cause a *frameshift* leading to aberrant sequence of amino acids until a stop codon is reached. Point mutations outside coding sequences may affect splicing with reduced (or zero) incorporation of an exon in the final mRNA or affect gene regulatory sequences (see also Fig. 7.8).

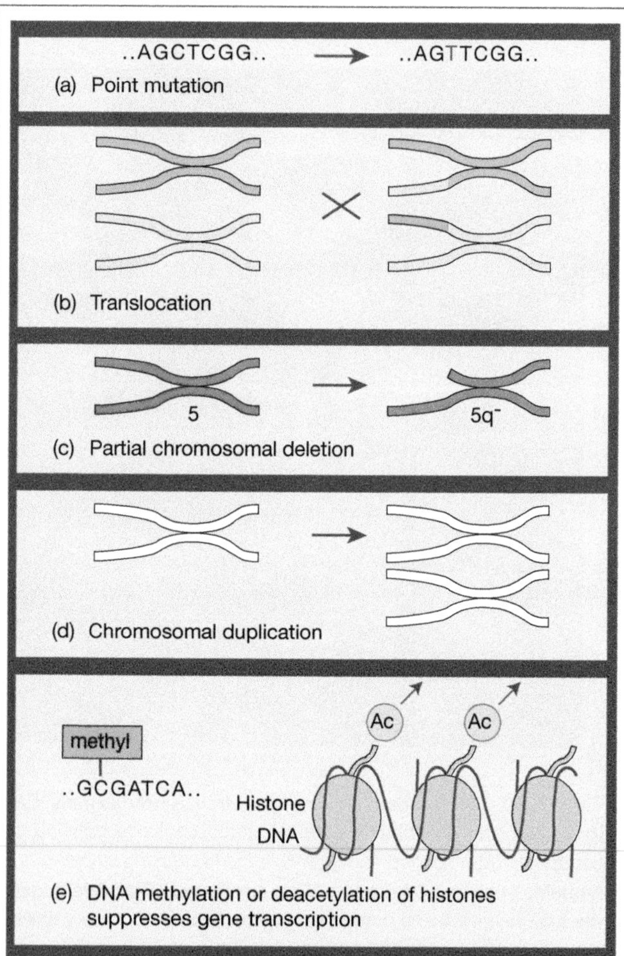

Figure 11.9 Types of genetic abnormality which may lead to haemopoietic malignancy. **(a)** Point mutation; **(b)** chromosomal translocation; **(c)** chromosomal deletion or loss; **(d)** chromosomal duplication; **(e)** epigenetic changes: DNA methylation or deacetylation of histone tails suppresses gene transcription (see also Fig. 16.1).

Substitutions are illustrated by the single-nucleotide variant 1849 G>T in the *JAK2* gene resulting in the Val617Phe (V617F) mutation in the JAK2 protein. This leads to constitutive activation of the protein and uncontrolled cell proliferation. *JAK2 V617F* is present in most cases of myeloproliferative neoplasia (Chapter 15). Point mutations within the *RAS* oncogenes leading to activation or within the *TP53* tumour-suppressor gene leading to inactivation are common in haemopoietic malignancies.

A point mutation involving several base pairs is illustrated in 35% of cases of AML with a normal karyotype by the mutated **nucleophosmin** (*NPM1*) gene showing an insertion of four base pairs, resulting in a frameshift change. Internal tandem duplications with varying lengths (ranging from three to hundreds of nucleotides, median 39 base pairs) or single-base pair point mutations in the tyrosine kinase domain occur in the *FLT3* gene in 30% of cases of AML. Most cases of MDS with ring sideroblasts have point mutations in the *SF3B1* gene, which alters RNA splicing.

Chromosomal translocations and inversions

These are a characteristic feature of haematological malignancies, and there are two main mechanisms whereby they may contribute to malignant change (Fig. 11.10):

1 **Juxtaposition of parts of two genes normally far away from each other to generate a chimeric fusion gene** that is dysfunctional or encodes a novel '**fusion protein**', e.g. *BCR::ABL1* in t(9;22) in CML (Fig. 14.1), *RARA::PML* in t(15,17) in acute promyelocytic leukaemia (Fig. 13.7) or *ETV6::RUNX1* in t(12;21) in B-ALL (Chapter 17).

2 **Overexpression of a normal cellular gene**, e.g. overexpression of *BCL2* in the t(14;18) translocation of follicular lymphoma or of *MYC* in Burkitt lymphoma (Fig. 11.11). Interestingly, this class of translocation nearly always involves an immunoglobulin gene or T-cell receptor (TCR) locus, presumably as a result of aberrant activity of the recombinase enzymes which are involved in immunoglobulin or TCR gene rearrangement in immature B or T cells. Since the immunoglobulin and TCR genes are actively transcribed in B and T lymphocytes, respectively, the translocated gene that is moved adjacent to these promoters is typically expressed at high levels.

Deletions

Chromosomal deletions may involve a small part of a chromosome, e.g. 5q-, the entire short or long arm or the whole chromosome, e.g. monosomy 7. The critical event is probably loss of a tumour-suppressor gene or of a microRNA, as in the 13q14 deletion in CLL (see below). The critical gene or genes in many recurrent deletions associated with haematological malignancies are not understood, in part because these large regions may contain dozens of genes.

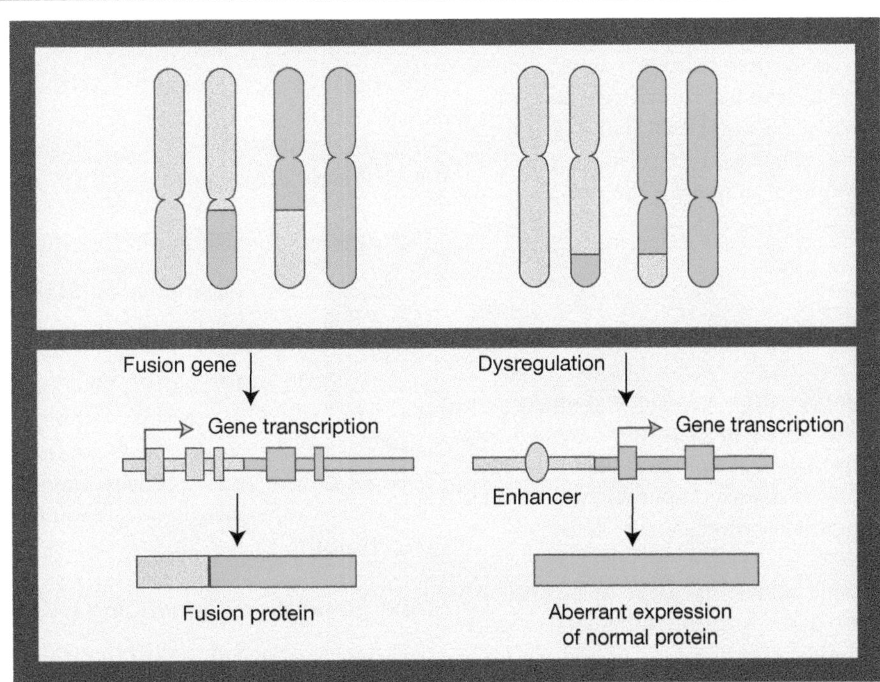

Figure 11.10 The two possible mechanisms by which chromosomal translocations can lead to dysregulated expression of an oncogene.

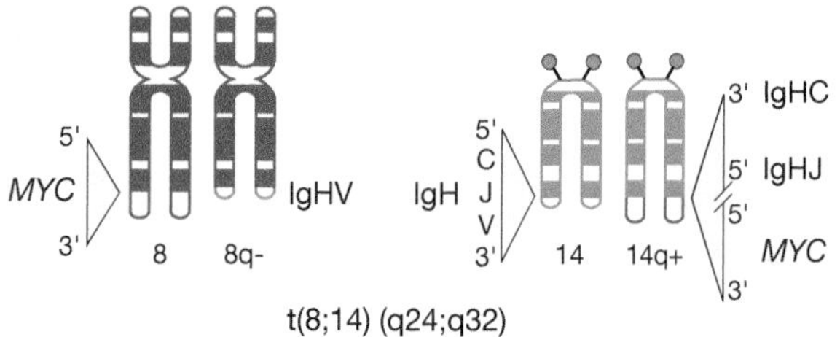

Figure 11.11 The genetic events in one of the three translocations found in Burkitt lymphoma and B-cell acute lymphoblastic leukaemia. The oncogene *MYC* is normally located on the long arm (q) of chromosome 8. In the t(8;14) translocation, *MYC* is translocated into proximity to the immunoglobulin heavy-chain gene on the long arm of chromosome 14. Part of the heavy-chain gene (the V region) is reciprocally translocated to chromosome 8. C, constant region; IgH, immunoglobulin heavy-chain gene; J, joining region; V, variable region.

Duplication or amplification

In chromosomal duplication, e.g. trisomy 12 in CLL or gene amplification, gains are common, especially in chromosomes 8, 12, 19, 21 and Y. Gene amplification is increasingly recognized within haemopoietic malignancy and an example is that involving the *KMT2A (MLL)* gene.

Loss of heterozygosity (LOH)

For each gene we have alleles inherited from both parents. This is called heterozygosity. In cancers, including the haematological malignancies, cells may display only one allele in areas of the genome, one allele being lost either by deletion or by replacement by the other allele which is duplicated, a situation termed *acquired uniparental disomy* (aUPD). This is a result of crossing over between two homologous chromosomes at mitosis (*mitotic recombination*). *FLT3* internal tandem duplications in AML are often duplicated by aUPD.

Epigenetic alterations

Gene expression in cancer may be dysregulated not only by structural changes to the genes themselves, but also by alterations in the mechanism by which specialized proteins gain access to genomic DNA genes to transcribe them. These changes are called **epigenetic** and are stably inherited with each cell division, so they are passed on as the malignant cell divides. The most important mechanisms (illustrated in Fig. 16.1) are:

1 Methylation of cytosine residues (mediated by DNMT3A) in DNA. This methylation is usually inhibitory to gene transcription. The products of genes *TET2* and *IDH1/2,* genes are involved in the demethylation of cytosine residues and like *DNMT3A* are often mutated in the myeloid malignancies.
2 Alterations to histones. Genomic DNA is wrapped around histones like beads on a string which, with further folding and compacting, form chromatin. Access to DNA is controlled by modification of histones such as methylation, acetylation and phosphorylation. Abnormalities of these processes, particularly important in the myeloid malignancies, lead to aberrant gene transcription.

A common mutation among the haematological malignancies is of the *KMT2A* (previously called MLL) gene. The protein product methylates specific lysine residues in histone tails allowing increased gene expression. *KMT2A* is involved in over 80 different chromosomal translocations leading to many fusion partnerships. The resulting aberrant methylation of histones increases self-renewal of haemopoietic progenitors. Demethylating agents such as azacitidine and decitabine which alter gene transcription are valuable in treating MDS and AML.

MicroRNAs

Chromosomal abnormalities, both deletions and amplifications, can result in loss or gain of short (micro) RNA sequences. These sequences are normally transcribed but not translated. MicroRNAs (miRNAs) control expression of adjacent or distally located genes. Deletion of the miR15a/miR16-1 locus may be relevant to CLL development with the common 13q14 deletion, and deletions of other microRNAs have been described in AML and other haematological neoplasms.

Diagnostic methods used to study neoplastic haemopoietic cells

Karyotype analysis

Karyotype analysis involves direct morphological analysis of chromosomes from neoplastic cells under the microscope (Fig. 14.1). This requires neoplastic cells to be in metaphase and so cells are cultured to encourage cell division prior to chromosomal preparation.

Fluorescence *in situ* hybridization analysis

Fluorescence *in situ* hybridization (FISH) analysis involves the use of fluorescent-labelled genetic probes which hybridize to specific parts of the genome. It is possible to label each chromosome with a different combination of fluorescent labels (Fig. 11.12). This is a sensitive technique that has the advantage of detecting extra or fewer copies of genetic material in both metaphase and interphase (non-dividing) cells or, by using two different probes, chromosomal translocations (Fig. 14.1e).

Next generation sequencing (NGS)

Gene sequence analysis is used to detect the genetic mutations that can cause neoplastic disease. **Next generation sequencing (NGS)** is used to study individual genes of interest; sequencing of the whole exome (3×10^7 base pairs) or genome (3×10^9 base

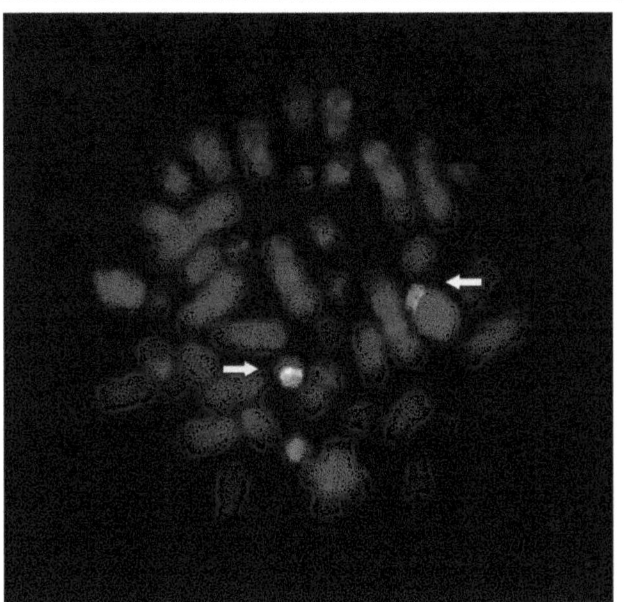

Figure 11.12 An example of fluorescence *in situ* hybridization (FISH) analysis showing the t(12;21) translocation. The green probe hybridizes to the region of the *ETV6* gene on chromosome 12 and the red probe hybridizes to the region of the *RUNX1* gene on chromosome 21. The arrows point to the two derived chromosomes resulting from the reciprocal translocation. Source: Courtesy of Professor C.J. Harrison.

pairs) of the tumour or a specific panel of genes can be performed for moderate cost. Tumour-specific panels targeting known mutational "hotspots" are the most widely applied. Whole genome sequencing may also give important information on chromosomal rearrangements and is increasingly widely used. NGS analysis of the transcriptome is performed by RNA-seq. This gives information on the expression levels of different genes. The results are then compared to the germline sequence of the patient or a reference sequence to identify the mutations in the tumour. Increasingly, cancer treatment is based on assessment of the patient's germline genome and the genome of their tumour. Gene sequencing identifies point mutations such as of *FLT3* in AML (Chapter 13), of *JAK2* in the myeloproliferative neoplasms and of *KIT* in systemic mastocytosis (Chapter 15).

Flow cytometry

In this technique, antibodies labelled with different fluorochromes recognize the pattern and intensity of expression of different antigens on the surface of normal and neoplastic cells (Fig. 11.13). Normal cells each have a characteristic profile, but neoplastic cells often express an aberrant phenotype that can be useful in allowing their detection (Figs 11.14 and 17.8). In the case of B-cell malignancies such as CLL, expression of only one light chain, κ or λ, by the neoplastic cells distinguishes them from a normal polyclonal population which expresses both κ and λ chains, usually in a κ : λ ratio of 2 : 1 (Fig. 20.5).

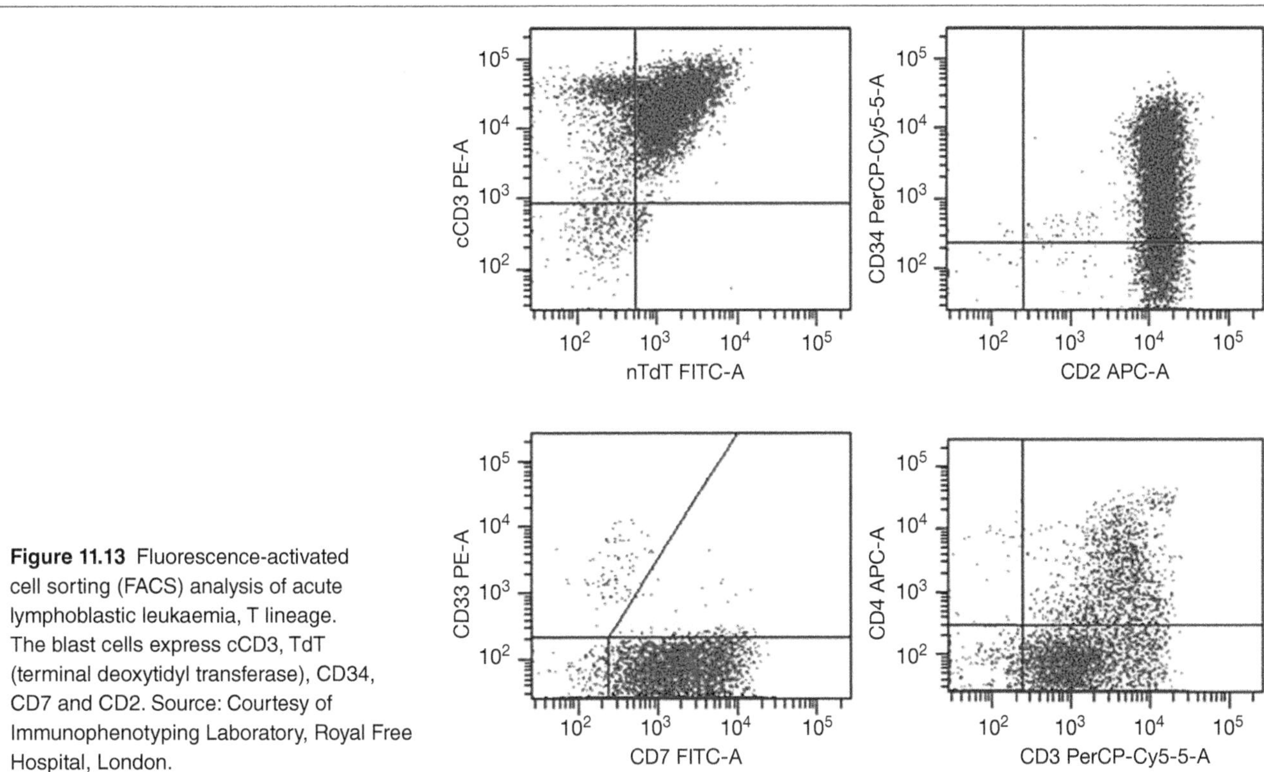

Figure 11.13 Fluorescence-activated cell sorting (FACS) analysis of acute lymphoblastic leukaemia, T lineage. The blast cells express cCD3, TdT (terminal deoxytidyl transferase), CD34, CD7 and CD2. Source: Courtesy of Immunophenotyping Laboratory, Royal Free Hospital, London.

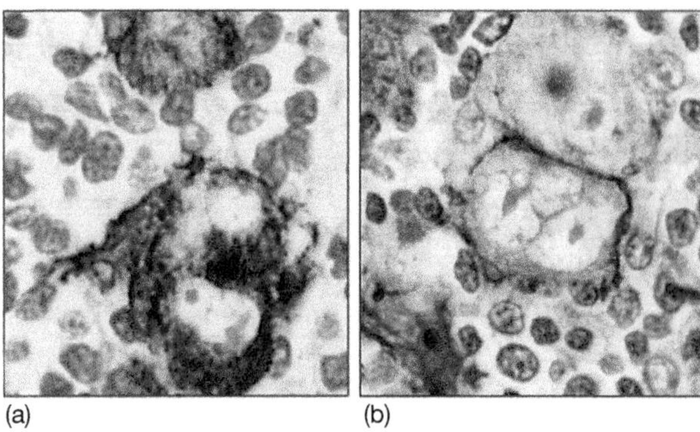

Figure 11.14 Immunohistological identification of Reed–Sternberg cells in Hodgkin lymphoma. The binucleate cells stain positively for **(a)** CD15 and **(b)** CD30.

The commonly used markers for the diagnosis of the neoplastic haematological diseases are listed in the relevant chapters.

Immunohistology (immunohistochemistry)

Antibodies can also be used to stain tissue sections. The fixed sections are incubated with an antibody, washed and incubated with a second antibody linked to an enzyme, usually peroxidase. A substrate is added that the enzyme converts to a coloured precipitate, usually brown. The presence and architecture of neoplastic cells can be identified by visualization of stained tissue sections under the microscope (Fig. 11.14). The clonal nature of B-cell malignancies can be shown in tissue sections by staining for κ or λ chains. A malignant clonal population, e.g. in B-cell NHL, will express one or other light chain but not both (Fig. 20.5).

Circulating neoplastic DNA

Cell-free DNA derived from the bone marrow neoplastic cells or from lymphoma cells situated outside the marrow may be found in peripheral blood. This circulating DNA has genomic changes similar to those of the neoplastic disease, can be used to track karyotype and mutations during therapy and is able to detect emerging new clones.

Value of genetic markers in the management of haematological neoplasia

The detection of genetic abnormalities is important in several aspects of the management of patients with leukaemia or lymphoma.

Initial diagnosis

Many genetic abnormalities are so specific for a particular disease that their presence determines that diagnosis. An example is the t(11;14) translocation, which defines mantle cell lymphoma. Clonal immunoglobulin or *TCR* gene rearrangements are useful in establishing clonality and determining the lineage of a lymphoid malignancy.

For establishing a treatment protocol

Each major type of haematological malignancy can be further subdivided on the basis of detailed genetic information. For instance, AML is a diverse group of disorders with characteristic genotypes. Individual subtypes respond differently to standard treatment. The *RUNX1::RUNX1T1* (t(8;21)) and *CBF8::MYH11* (inv(16)) subgroups have a favourable prognosis, whereas monosomy 7 carries a poor prognosis. In those with normal cytogenetics, molecular analysis may show *FLT3* internal tandem duplication, an unfavourable marker, or *NPM1* mutation, which is generally favourable. The pattern of genetic changes detected by molecular studies in a new case of AML may distinguish those cases with preceding MDS (and an unfavourable prognosis) from those without MDS (p. xxx). Treatment strategies are now tailored for the individual and in some instances knowledge of the underlying genetic abnormality can lead to more rational treatment, e.g. the use of all-*trans* retinoic acid in acute promyelocytic leukaemia with t(15;17) (p. 180).

Genetic information is also valuable for giving a prognosis. For instance, hyperdiploidy in ALL is a favourable finding, whereas for most haematological neoplasias *TP53* mutations or deletions predict for poor prognosis and lack of responsiveness to chemotherapy.

Monitoring the response to therapy: minimal residual disease

The detection of minimal residual disease (MRD, also called measurable residual disease, i.e. persistent clonal cells that cannot be seen by conventional microscopy of the blood or bone marrow) when the patient is in remission after chemotherapy or stem cell transplantation is possible using the following techniques (in increasing order of sensitivity, Fig. 11.15):

1. Cytogenetic analysis by FISH analysis.
2. Fluorescence-activated cell sorting to detect tumour cells using immunological markers that detect 'leukaemia-specific' combinations of antigens (Figs 11.13 and 17.8). The benefits of this technique is its wide applicability.
3. PCR and/or sequence analysis to detect tumour-specific translocations or mutations specific to the original clone (Fig. 11.16). PCR use for MRD often utilizes quantitative techniques (qPCR, including real-time qPCR) based frequently on the use of DNA intercalating fluorescent dyes. This technique often requires a diagnostic/pre-treatment sample. Templates include cDNA from reverse transcription of fusion RNA transcripts, e.g. *MLL::AF4,* or mutant genes (*NPM1*) (also known as RT-PCR or RT-qPCR) (Fig. 11.16). PCR-based techniques also include allele-specific oligonucleotide (ASO-PCR), such as that used in

10^0
10^1
Morphology
10^2
Cytogenetics by FISH
10^3
Flow cytometry
10^4
PCR, NGS
10^5
10^6

Figure 11.15 Sensitivity of detection of leukaemic cells in bone marrow using four different techniques. 10^1 to 10^6 = 1 cell in 10 to 1 cell in 10^6 detected. PCR and NGS techniques include a number of different methodologies (see text). FISH; fluorescent *in situ* hybridization, PCR; polymerase chain reaction; NGS; next generation sequencing.

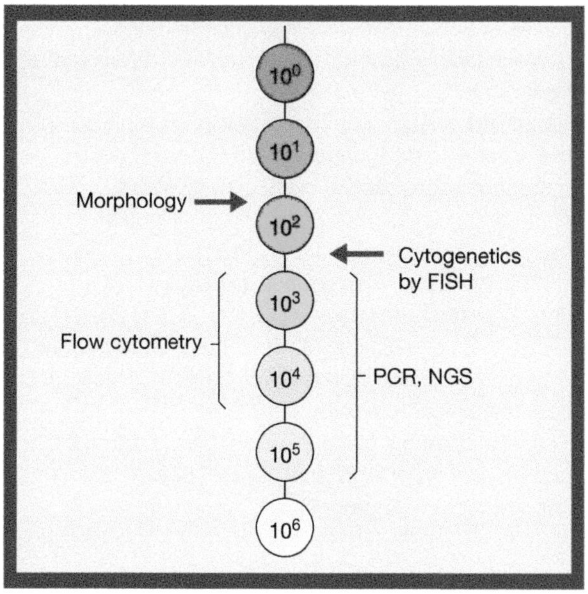

tracking immunoglobulin or T-cell receptor clonal rearrangements in ALL (Chapter 17).

4 NGS can also be used to detect and quantify whether mutations found at diagnosis are still present in the bone marrow in clinical remission (Fig. 13.12). Use of NGS-based MRD techniques can be found in both AML and ALL. Use of NGS for MRD requires different techniques to diagnostic NGS, e.g. in targeted amplicon sequencing (see above), which has limited sensitivity. Methods to increase sensitivity of NGS for MRD include both bioinformatic modifications to the analysis pathway and physical modifications to the DNA sample prepared for readout on the NGS analyser (the "library"). For example, early in the preparation of NGS libraries, the incorporation of unique molecular identifiers (barcodes) identifies individual DNA molecules, which can improve confidence in identifying mutations found at low frequencies.

Collectively, these approaches have an important role in planning the treatment of many forms of neoplastic haemopoietic disease. Sensitivity of these tests depend on the assay used. Improvements in technical efficiency have improved techniques to 1 in 10^6 cells.

Intensity of fluorescence
5
4
3
2
1
0
10^{-1}
10^{-2}
10^{-3}
10^{-4}
FU1
FU2
0 4 8 12 16 20 24 28 32 36 40 44
Cycle number

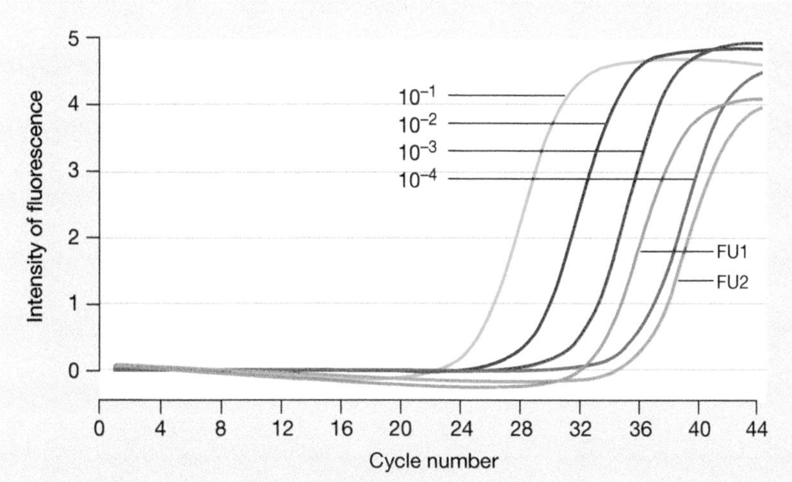

Figure 11.16 Real-time quantitative polymerase chain reaction (PCR) in acute B-lineage lymphoblastic leukaemia for minimal residual disease using the immunoglobulin heavy chain as target. Primers are designed based on DNA from sequence analysis of the presenting leukaemic clone. Bone marrow samples taken in clinical remission are amplified by PCR using these primers and fluorescent-labelled using Sybergreen. The intensity of the signal measures the total DNA molecules amplified in successive cycles. In this example, the intensities of amplification of DNA from two follow-up bone marrow samples (FU1 and FU2) are compared with serial dilutions of (10^{-1} to 10^{-4}) of the DNA from the presentation bone marrow. FU1 shows a level of residual disease of approximately 1 in 5000 (0.02%) and FU2 of 1 in 12 000 (0.008%). Source: Courtesy of Dr L. Foroni.

SUMMARY

- The haemopoietic neoplasms are clonal diseases that derive from a single cell in the marrow or peripheral lymphoid tissue which has undergone genetic alteration.
- They represent approximately 7% of all malignant disease.
- Inherited and environmental factors predispose to neoplastic development, but the relative contribution of these is usually unclear.
- Infections (viral and bacterial), drugs, radiation and chemicals can all increase the risk of developing a haemopoietic malignancy.
- Haematological neoplasia occurs because of genetic alterations that lead to increased activation of oncogenes or decreased activity of tumour-suppressor genes. They usually show about 10 acquired genetic mutations and progress in a linear or branching manner.
- These genetic alterations may occur through a variety of mechanisms such as point mutation, chromosomal translocation or gene deletion.
- Epigenetic changes are important in the aetiology of many myeloid malignancies.
- Important investigations include study of the chromosomes (karyotype analysis), molecular genetics, fluorescent *in situ* hybridization (FISH), mutation analysis, flow cytometry and immunohistochemistry.
- These tests allow detection in blood or bone marrow of minimal residual disease in patients in clinical and haematological remission.
- The investigations guide the diagnosis, treatment and monitoring of individual cases. They are also an important guide to prognosis.

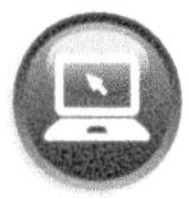

Now visit **www.wiley.com/go/haematology9e** to test yourself on this chapter.

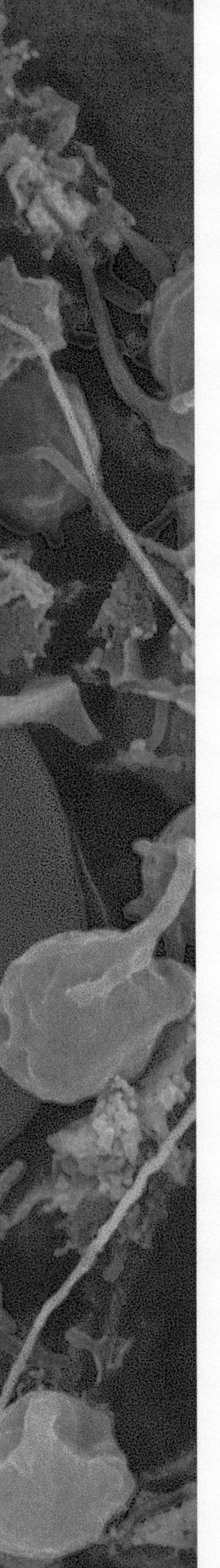

CHAPTER 12

Management of haematological malignancy

Key topics

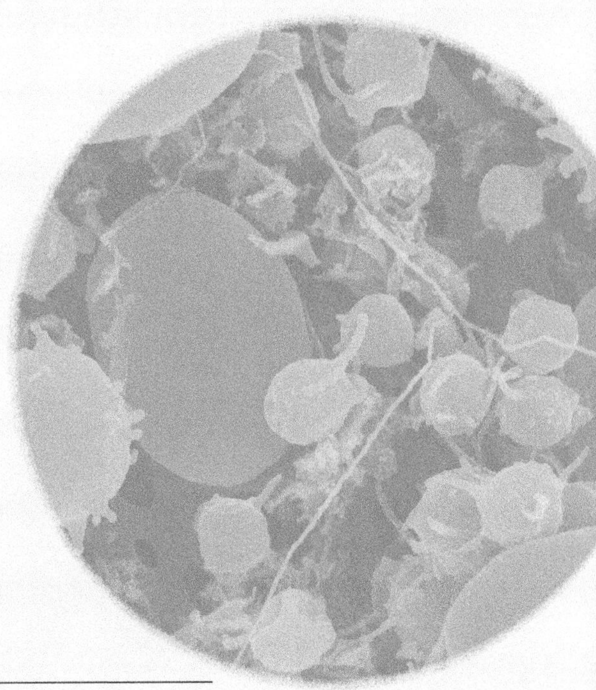

Hoffbrand's Essential Haematology, Ninth Edition. A. Victor Hoffbrand, Pratima Chowdary, Graham P. Collins, and Justin Loke.

© 2024 John Wiley & Sons Ltd. Published 2024 by John Wiley & Sons Ltd.

Companion website: www.wiley.com/go/haematology9e

Details of specific treatment of individual diseases are given in the appropriate chapter. Supportive care and general aspects of the agents used in the treatment of haematological malignancy are described here.

General supportive therapy

When considering treatment, it is valuable to assess the normal daily living abilities of the patient, using assessments such as the ECOG (Eastern Cooperative Oncology Group) performance status (Table 12.1). When formulating a treatment plan, it is also important to consider co-morbid conditions such as cardiac, pulmonary and renal disease.

Patients with haematological malignancies often present with clinical problems related to suppression of normal haemopoiesis by bone marrow disease. Bone marrow failure may also result from chemotherapy or radiotherapy given to treat the disease. Prevention or treatment of bone marrow failure is a major component of support therapy in the treatment of the haematological malignancies. These aspects and the other components of support therapy are discussed next.

Table 12.1 Eastern Cooperative Oncology Group (ECOG) performance status.

Grade	Description
0	Fully active, able to carry on all pre-disease performance without restriction
1	Restricted in physically strenuous activity, but ambulatory and able to carry out work of a light or sedentary nature, e.g. light housework, office work
2	Ambulatory and capable of all self-care, but unable to carry out any work activities. Up and about more than 50% of waking hours
3	Capable of only limited self-care, confined to bed or chair more than 50% of waking hours
4	Completely disabled. Cannot carry on any self-care. Totally confined to bed or chair
5	Dead

Insertion of central venous catheter

A central venous catheter is usually inserted for those patients who will need intensive treatment, especially with chemotherapy drugs ('vesicants') that can cause damage to the soft tissue if they extravasate from peripheral blood vessels. The central venous catheter commonly used in clinical practice are:

Hickman- or Broviac-style catheters are placed in the operating theatre or interventional radiology suite via a skin tunnel from the chest into the jugular vein, with the catheter tip terminating in the superior vena cava or at the cavo-atrial junction (Fig. 12.1).

A totally implantable venous access device, sometimes called **Port-a-cath or Mediport**, is similar to a Hickman catheter, but these devices also include a reservoir (port) with a silicone membrane (septum) through which a needle can be inserted. The reservoir and membrane are buried under the skin of the patient's chest wall so that the patient does not have catheter components protruding from the body. This makes it easier for the patient to bathe or swim, but it is more difficult

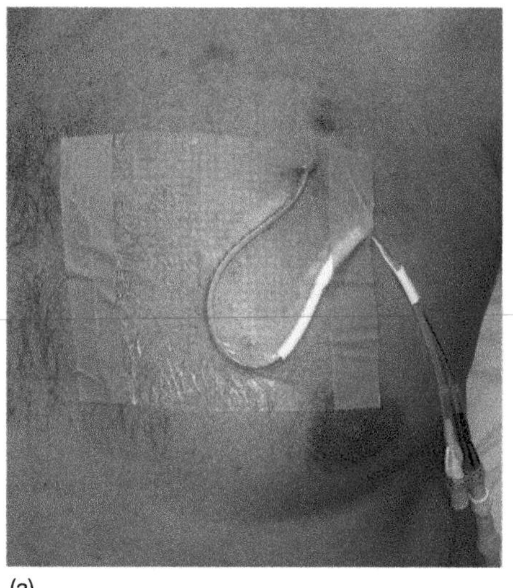
(a)

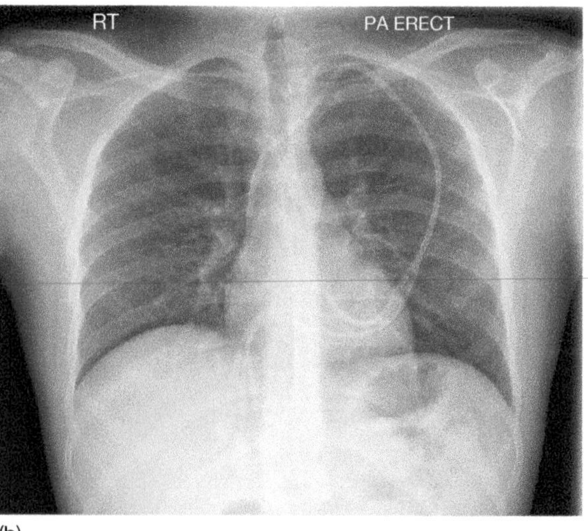

(b)

Figure 12.1 (a) A central venous line in a patient undergoing intensive chemotherapy. **(b)** Chest X-ray showing correct placement of a central venous line, in this case a tunnelled triple lumen left internal jugular line. Source: Courtesy of Dr P. Wylie.

to remove a totally implantable device than a Hickman-style catheter.

Finally, **peripherally inserted central catheters (PICC lines)** are placed in the arm, usually in a cephalic or brachial vein, and then extended up via the axillary and subclavian veins to the superior vena cava. PICC lines have the advantage that they can be placed at the bedside, often by a nurse rather than a surgeon or radiologist, but they typically do not last as long as the other catheter types.

These lines give ease of access for administering chemotherapy, blood products, antibiotics and intravenous feeding. Blood may also be taken for laboratory tests through the catheter. However, they require site and line care and are a risk factor for venous thrombosis and infection.

Blood component support (Chapter 33)

Red cell and platelet transfusions are used to treat anaemia and thrombocytopenia. A number of particular issues apply to the support of patients with haematological malignancy:

1 **The threshold haemoglobin (Hb) for transfusion will depend on clinical factors such as symptoms and speed of onset of anaemia, but many units give red cell support for an Hb < 70 g/L, with a higher threshold in older patients or those with ischemia at any site**. Red cell transfusions should be avoided if at all possible in patients with a very high white cell count (> 100 × 10^9/L) because of hyperviscosity and so the risk of precipitating thrombotic episodes as a result of white cell stasis.

2 **Additional care is required in the management of patients undergoing allogeneic stem cell transplants (SCTs) with ABO mismatch with the donor stem cells**. ABO incompatibility can be defined as major, minor, or bidirectional (Table 12.2). Potential complications include haemolysis and delayed red cell engraftment. In the early post-transplant period, blood component ABO requirements depend on donor-recipient ABO compatibility.

3 **Awareness of transfusion associated circulatory overload (TACO) is important.** This is pulmonary oedema/respiratory compromise secondary to volume overload. Volume required to precipitate TACO is dependent on patient risk factors, which can be assessed, e.g. pre-existing cardiac, respiratory or renal impairment, concurrent fluid balance issues. Close monitoring, transfusion of single units of red cells at a time and use of prophylactic diuretics may reduce the risk of TACO.

4 **The trigger for platelet transfusion is typically a platelet count below 10 × 10^9/L, but the threshold should be increased in the presence of active bleeding or fever.**

5 Fresh frozen plasma (FFP) or cryoprecipitate may be needed to reverse coagulation defects.

6 All potential SCT patients should have CMV IgG serostatus determined prior to red cell transfusion as transfusion of plasma-containing components from CMV unscreened donors may lead to false positive results.

7 Febrile reactions with blood products are not uncommon and should be assessed and managed accordingly.

8 Granulocyte transfusions are rarely given for severely neutropenic patients with serious infection not responding to antibiotics as a bridge to endogenous recovery of haemopoiesis. Their efficacy is not proven.

9 **Blood products given to patients with severely impaired T-cell function (such as those who have received fludarabine, with aplastic anaemia, Hodgkin lymphoma or post-allogeneic SCT) should be irradiated prior to administration to prevent transfusion-associated graft-versus-host disease (p. 461).**

10 The use of recombinant erythropoiesis-stimulating agents (ESAs) to reduce the need for blood transfusion, e.g. in myelodysplastic neoplasias, is discussed on p. 217.

11 Granulocyte colony-stimulating factor (G-CSF) may be given to accelerate neutrophil recovery after intensive chemotherapy regimens.

Table 12.2 Definition of major, minor and bidirectional ABO incompatibility in ABO incompatible allogeneic SCT.

Major ABO incompatibility	Recipient's plasma antibodies (anti-A and/or B) incompatible with donor red cells, e.g. group A donor and group O recipient
Minor ABO incompatibility	Donor's plasma contains antibodies (anti-A and/or B) react with the recipient's red cells, e.g. donor group O and recipient group A
Bidirectional ABO incompatibility	Both the donor and recipient's plasma antibodies (anti-A and/or B) are reactive with recipient and donor red cells respectively, e.g. donor group A and recipient group B

Source: Adapted from Joint United Kingdom (UK) Blood Transfusion and Tissue Transplantation Services Professional Advisory Committee (https://www.transfusionguidelines.org/).

Haemostasis support

Support with vitamin K or FFP may be required. Cryoprecipitate or antithrombin concentrates may be needed for certain coagulation factor deficiency, such as that precipitated by asparaginase in the management of acute lymphoblastic leukaemia. Special measures are required in the management of coagulopathies induced by the disease, e.g. acute promyelocytic leukaemia (Chapter 13). Antiplatelet drugs such as aspirin or clopidogrel are usually discontinued in patients undergoing intensive chemotherapy. Patients on long-term warfarin or direct-acting oral anticoagulants will need a coagulation plan to be in place, depending on history of clots and patient risk factors; for example, some patient may be switched to low-molecular-weight heparin, which can then itself be stopped if the platelet count falls below 50×10^9/L. Progesterones are given to premenopausal women undergoing intensive chemotherapy to prevent menstruation. Tranexamic acid or aminocaproic acid can be given to reduce haemorrhage in patients with chronic low-grade blood loss despite platelet transfusion.

Anti-emetic therapy

Nausea and vomiting are common side effects of chemotherapy. A key objective is to prevent nausea occurring early in the treatment, as it is difficult to control once the symptom has already arisen. The 5-HT$_3$ (serotonin) receptor antagonists, such as ondansetron, granisetron and palonosetron, can control nausea from intensive chemotherapy in over 60% of cases. The addition of dexamethasone can increase this by approximately 20%. Metoclopramide, prochlorperazine or cyclizine, benzodiazepines, e.g. lorazepam; domperidone, neurokinin-1 receptor antagonists, e.g. aprepitant, fosaprepitant or cannabinoids, e.g. nabilone, dronabinol, can all have a role.

Tumour lysis syndrome

Chemotherapy may trigger an acute rise in plasma uric acid, potassium and phosphate and cause hypocalcaemia because of rapid lysis of tumour cells. Patients should be assessed for risk of TLS prior to receiving chemotherapy to decide whether prevention or treatment of TLS is required. Established criteria are categorized as either laboratory or clinically based (Table 12.3). This syndrome is seen most commonly with rapidly dividing neoplasias and can cause acute renal failure with life-threatening electrolyte disturbances. The highest risk conditions are:

1. Acute leukaemia with high WBC counts, e.g. over 100×10^9/L.
2. Burkitt lymphoma or lymphoblastic lymphoma.
3. Bulky high grade lymphoma.

Patient-specific risk factors include age and pre-existing renal impairment.

Allopurinol, intravenous fluids and electrolyte replacement are the mainstay of prevention. Close monitoring of blood tests to measure electrolytes may be required multiple times a day. Rasburicase, an enzyme that oxidizes uric acid to allantoin, is highly effective in controlling hyperuricaemia. Patients should be tested for G6PD deficiency prior to use of rasburicase. Allopurinol and rasburicase may counteract each other's effectiveness (Fig. 12.2).

Table 12.3 Definition of tumour lysis syndrome.

Laboratory tumour lysis syndrome
The presence of two or more of the following abnormalities in a patient with cancer or undergoing treatment for cancer within 3 days prior to and up to 7 days after initiation of treatment
Uric acid ≥476 μmol/L or 25% increase from baseline
Potassium ≥6·0 mmol/L or 25% increase from baseline
Phosphate ≥2·1 mmol/L or 25% increase from baseline (children)
Phosphate ≥1·45 mmol/L or 25% increase from baseline (adults)
Calcium ≤1·75 mmol/L or 25% decrease from baseline
Clinical tumour lysis syndrome
A patient with laboratory tumour lysis syndrome and at least one of
Creatinine ≥ 1·5 × ULN* (age >12 years or age-adjusted)
Cardiac arrhythmia
Sudden death
Seizure

*ULN, upper limit of normal
Source: Adapted from M.S. Cairo, M. Bishop (2004) *Br. J. Haematol.* 127: 3–11.

Psychological support

Patients with a diagnosis of malignant disease commonly feel concerns about such issues as the discomfort of treatment, finance, sexuality and fear of mortality. Even when patients achieve a clinical remission, there is understandable concern about the chance of disease relapse. **Psychological support should be an integral part of the relationship between physician and patient, and patients should be allowed to express their fears and concerns at the earliest opportunity.** Most patients value the opportunity to read more about their disorder and many excellent booklets or websites are now available.

Teamwork is also crucial, and the nursing staff and trained counsellors have a vital role in offering support and information during inpatient and outpatient care. Many units have specialist input from clinical psychologists and psychiatric help may occasionally be required. Inadequate communication is perhaps the most common failing of medical teams. The immediate family should be kept informed of the patient's progress whenever possible and appropriate.

Reproductive issues

Men who are to receive cytotoxic drugs should be offered sperm storage, ideally before treatment commences or, if impossible, within a short period of time thereafter. Ethical issues relating to storage or potential usage of tissue in the event of treatment failure will need to be addressed. Permanent infertility in women is less common after chemotherapy, although premature menopause may occur, and menopause is inevitable with myeloablative allogeneic SCT. **Storage of**

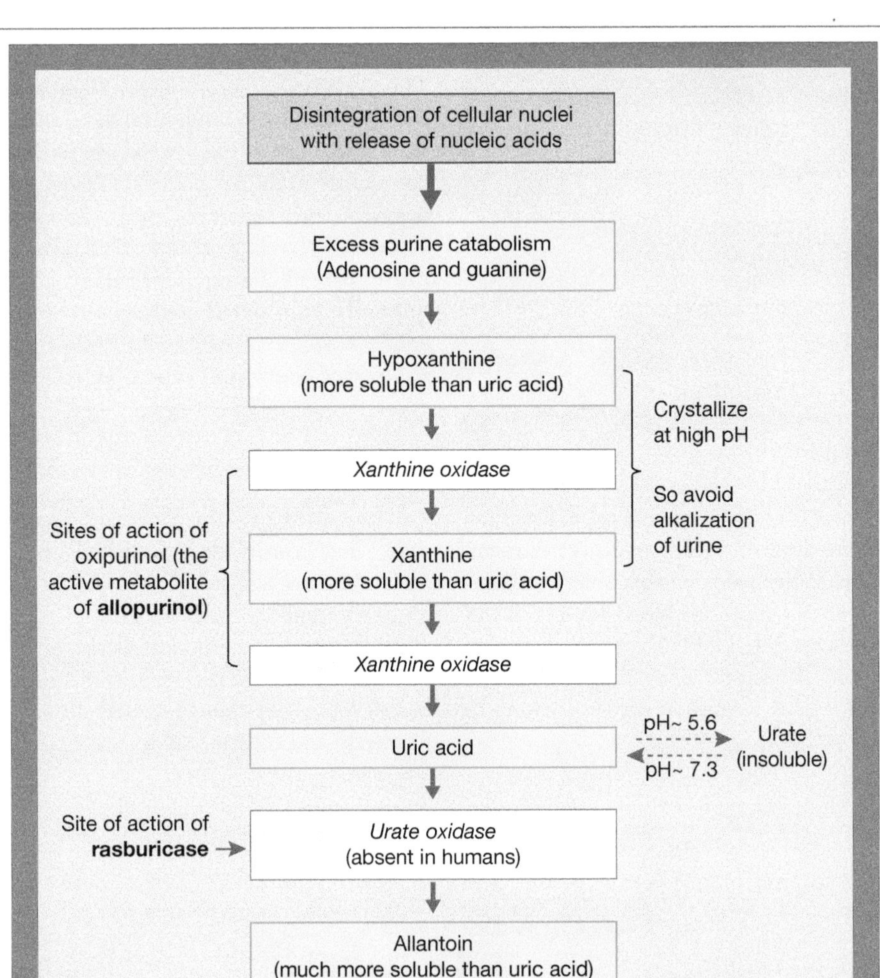

Figure 12.2 Mechanisms of action of xanthine oxidase inhibitor (allopurinol) and exogenous urate oxidase (rasburicase). Source: G.L. Jones *et al*. (2015) *Br. J. Haematol*.169: 661–7. Reproduced with permission of John Wiley & Sons.

fertilized ova is often impractical and specialist advice should be obtained in relation to storage of eggs.

Nutritional support

Some degree of weight loss is virtually inevitable in patients undergoing inpatient chemotherapy because of the combination of a poor nutritional intake, mucositis affecting oral intake, malabsorption caused by drugs and a catabolic disease state. If a weight loss of more than 10% occurs, nutritional support is often given, either enterally via a nasogastric tube or parenterally through a central venous catheter.

Pain

Pain directly due to the malignancy is rarely a major problem in haematological malignancies except for myeloma. Pain is a frequent issue in patients with multiple myeloma and can be managed by a combination of analgesia and chemotherapy/radiotherapy. Advice from palliative care teams or specialist pain management practitioners should be sought when required. Bone pain can also be a presenting feature for other diseases with extensive marrow involvement such as the acute leukaemias. Occasionally, lymph nodes in patients with lymphoma are painful; lymphomas sometimes also involve bone. **The mucositis, graded by the WHO (Table 12.4), that follows intensive chemotherapy can cause substantial discomfort and pain. Continuous infusions of opiate analgesia are often required**. Mucositis with ulceration can also lead to septicaemia. Palifermin, a recombinant human keratinocyte growth factor, is approved for patients with severe grades of mucositis resulting from chemotherapy.

Prophylaxis and treatment of infection

Patients with haematological malignancy are at great risk of infection, which is the major cause of morbidity and mortality. Immunosuppression may result from neutropenia,

Table 12.4 The World Health Organisation (WHO) Oral Mucositis Grading Scale.

Grade	Clinical features
0 (none)	None
I (mild)	Oral soreness, erythema
II (moderate)	Oral erythema, ulcers, solid diet tolerated
III (severe)	Oral ulcers, liquid diet only
IV (life-threatening)	Oral alimentation impossible

hypogammaglobulinaemia and impaired cellular function. These can be secondary to the primary disease or its treatment. Neutropenia is a particular concern and in many patients neutrophils are totally absent from the blood for periods of 2 weeks or more. The use of G-CSF to reduce periods of neutropenia is discussed in Chapter 8. A protocol for the management of infection in an immunosuppressed patient is illustrated in Fig. 12.3.

Bacterial infection

This is the most common problem and usually arises from the patient's own commensal bacterial flora. Gram-positive skin organisms, e.g. *Staphylococcus* and *Streptococcus*, commonly colonize central venous lines, whereas Gram-negative gut bacteria, e.g. *Pseudomonas aeruginosa*, *Escherichia coli*, *Proteus*, *Klebsiella* and anaerobes, can cause overwhelming septicaemia. Even organisms not normally considered pathogenic, such as *Staphylococcus epidermidis*, may cause life-threatening infection. In the absence of neutrophils, local superficial lesions can rapidly cause severe septicaemia.

Prophylaxis of bacterial infection

Protocols used to limit bacterial infection vary from unit to unit. They usually do not include the use of prophylactic antibiotics because of the danger of resistance developing. During periods of neutropenia, topical antiseptics for bathing and chlorhexidine mouthwashes and a 'clean diet' are recommended. The patient is sometimes nursed in a reverse-barrier room. Oral non-absorbed antimicrobial agents, such as neomycin and colistin, reduce gut commensal flora, but many

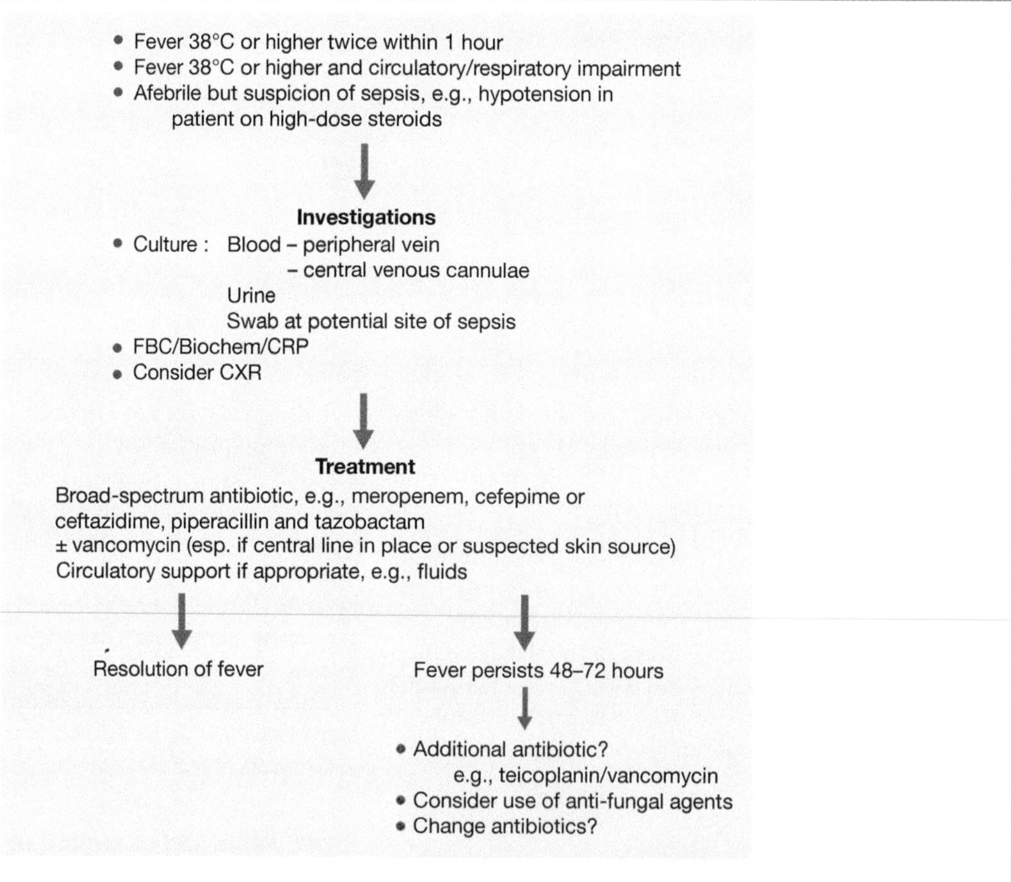

Figure 12.3 A protocol for the management of fever in the neutropenic patient. CRP, C-reactive protein; CXR, chest X-ray; FBC, full blood count.

units do not use them in order to avoid bacterial resistance. Regular surveillance cultures can be taken to document the patient's bacterial flora and its sensitivity.

Treatment of bacterial infection

Fever is the main indication that infection is present, because if neutropenia is present pus will not be formed and infections are often not localized. Fever may be caused by blood products or drugs, but infection is the most common cause and fever of >38°C in neutropenic patients should be investigated and treated very quickly. Cultures are taken from any likely focus of infection, including from central venous lines and peripheral veins, from urine and from mouth swabs. The mouth and throat, intravenous catheter site and perineal and perianal areas are particularly likely foci. A chest X-ray is indicated as chest infections are frequent.

Antibiotic therapy must be started immediately after blood and other cultures have been taken; in many febrile episodes no organisms are isolated. There are different antibiotic regimes in use and a close link with the microbiology team is essential. A typical regimen might be based on a single agent, such as a broad-spectrum penicillin, e.g. piperacillin/tazobactam, meropenem or a broad-spectrum cephalosporin with anti-*Pseudomonal* activity. *Staphylococcus epidermidis* is a common source of fever in patients with intravenous lines and an agent such as teicoplanin, vancomycin or linezolid may be needed. If an infective agent and its antibiotic sensitivities become known, appropriate changes in the regimen are made. If no response occurs within 48–72 hours, changing the antibiotics or adding antifungal therapy is considered.

Viral infection

Prophylaxis and treatment of viral infection

Herpes viruses such as herpes simplex, varicella zoster, CMV and Epstein–Barr virus (EBV) undergo latency following primary infection and are never eradicated from the host. Most patients with haematological malignancy have already been infected with these viruses so viral reactivation is a common problem. Aciclovir or valaciclovir is frequently given prophylactically. Herpes simplex is a common cause of oral ulcers, but is usually controlled easily by aciclovir. Varicella zoster frequently reactivates in patients with lymphoproliferative diseases to cause shingles (Fig. 18.2), which requires treatment with high doses of aciclovir or valaciclovir. Primary infection, usually in children, can be very serious and immunoglobulin is used to prevent infection following recent exposure. While the live attenuated varicella vaccine (Zostavax®) is contraindicated for many patients with haematological malignancy, the non-live recombinant adjuvant-enhanced vaccine (Shingrix®) represents a safer and more effective alternative. Reactivation of CMV infection is particularly common following SCT (Chapter 25), but may also occur following intensive chemotherapy. Failure of immune control of EBV following allogeneic transplantation can lead to outgrowth of a B-cell tumour known as post-transplant lymphoproliferative disease (Chapter 25).

Coronavirus infection is a particular danger to patients immunosuppressed either because of their haematological disease or because of its treatment with chemotherapy, immunotherapy, radiotherapy or by stem cell therapy. They may produce poor responses to vaccination especially if therapy has been within the preceding year. Remdesivir, molnupiravir, nirmatreivir plus ritonavir and sotrovimab are antivirals approved for treatment in this setting.

Fungal infection

Prophylaxis and treatment of fungal infection

Because of the intensity of current chemotherapy, fungal infections are a major cause of morbidity and mortality. The two major subtypes are yeasts, such as *Candida* species, and moulds, of which *Aspergillus fumigatus* is the most common.

Invasive aspergillosis is an important cause of infectious death in intensively immunocompromised patients (Fig. 12.4). Infection occurs through inhalation of *Aspergillus* spores (conidia) and air filtration systems are used in many haematology wards. The major risk factor is neutropenia – nearly 70% of patients become infected if they are neutropenic for over 34 days. Steroid use is also important, as is age, chemotherapy and antimicrobial history.

The diagnosis of invasive aspergillosis can be difficult. Definitive diagnosis requires demonstration of invasive growth on a biopsy specimen, but such evidence is rarely available. Polymerase chain reaction for fungal DNA or enzyme-linked immunosorbent assay (ELISA) for *Aspergillus* galactomannan or β1–3 d-glucan is useful. High-resolution computed tomography (HRCT) chest scan is valuable and early features are nodular lesions with a 'ground glass' halo appearance. Later on, wedge lesions and the air crescent sign are seen (Fig. 12.5). A high index of suspicion for fungal infection should be maintained,

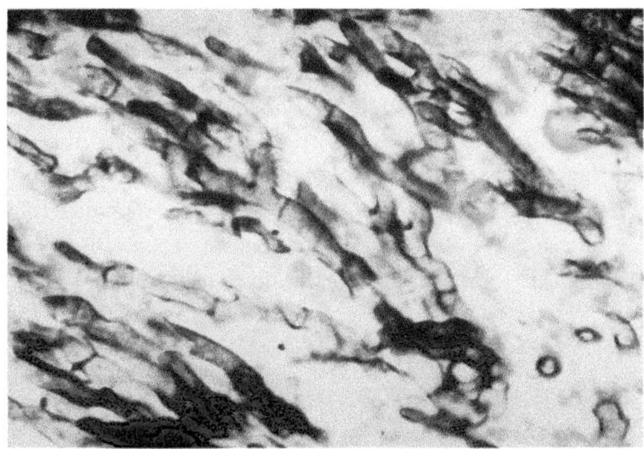

Figure 12.4 Cytology of sputum illustrates the branching septate hyphae of *Aspergillus* (methenamine silver stain).

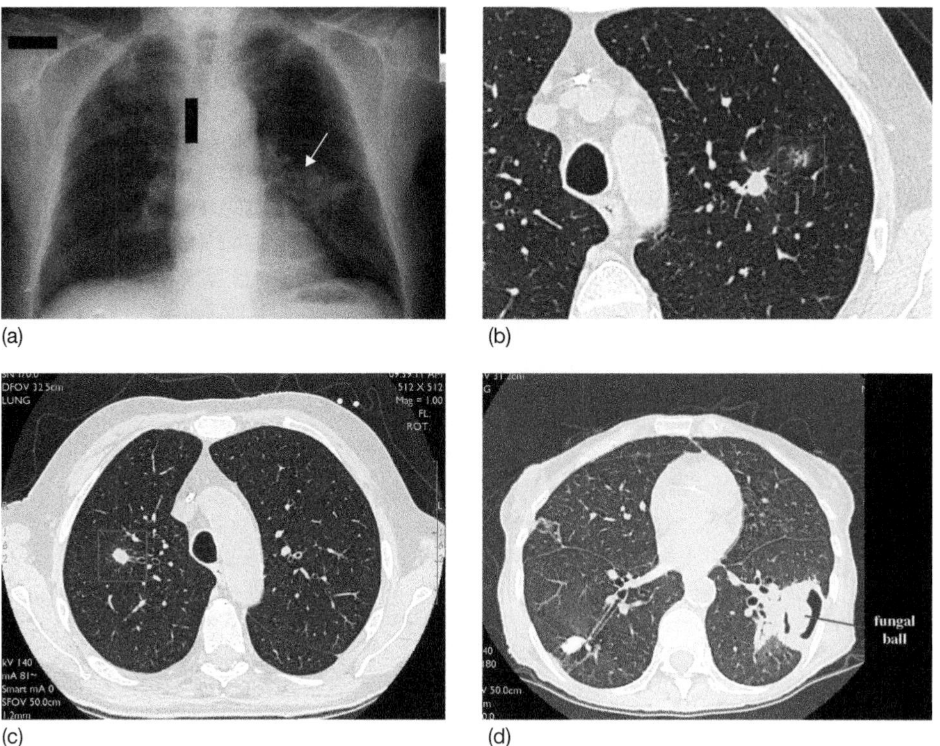

Figure 12.5 **(a)** Chest X-ray of patient with pulmonary aspergillosis which shows an area of cavitation containing a central fungal ball (arrow), leading to the typical 'air-crescent' sign. **(b)** and **(c)** Computed tomography (CT) scans in *aspergillosis* show hazy ground-glass shadowing with bronchiolar dilatation. **(d)** Nodules are seen in early aspergillosis, whereas a fungal ball with surrounding air is typical of more advanced disease.

and treatment is often started empirically for a fever that has failed to resolve after 2–4 days of antibiotic treatment.

Prophylaxis or treatment for patients at risk of *Aspergillus* infection is usually performed with itraconazole, caspogfungin, micafungin, voriconazole, posaconazole, isavuconazole or lipid formulation amphotericin. Surgery to remove lung lesions may be needed.

Candida species are a common hospital pathogen and frequently cause oral infection. *Candida* is significant when isolated from normally sterile body fluids such as blood or urine. Prophylaxis or treatment is usually with fluconazole, itraconazole or caspofungin. Anidulafungin and micafungin are also licensed. *Pneumocystis jirovecii (carinii)* is an important cause of pneumonitis. Prophylaxis is with co-trimoxazole or atovaquone (highly effective) or with nebulized pentamidine (less effective) and is given to those who have received intensive (combination) chemotherapy or fludarabine. Treatment is with high-dose co-trimoxazole.

Drugs used in the treatment of haemopoietic malignancies

Specific therapy is aimed at reducing the neoplastic cell burden by the use of drugs or radiotherapy. The hope in some diseases is to eradicate the neoplasia completely, and cure rates for haematological malignancy are gradually improving. However, cure is often not achievable, so palliation can also be an important aim.

A wide variety of drugs is used in the management of haemopoietic malignancies. Drugs acting at different sites (Fig. 12.6) are often combined in regimens that minimize the potential for resistance to occur against a single agent. Many act specifically on dividing cells and their selectivity is dependent on the high proliferation rate within the tumour. It is unusual for all neoplastic cells to be killed by a single course of treatment so several courses of treatment, which gradually eradicate the neoplastic cell burden are usual. This 'log kill' hypothesis also gives the residual normal haemopoietic cells the opportunity to recover between treatment courses.

Cytotoxic drugs (Table 12.5)

Alkylating agents, such as chlorambucil, cyclophosphamide, melphalan and bendamustine, are activated to expose reactive alkyl groups which make covalent bonds to molecules within the cell. These have a particular affinity for purines and are thus able to crosslink DNA strands and impair DNA replication, resulting in a block at G_2 and death of the cell by apoptosis (Fig. 1.9). Bendamustine is a unique drug in this class, as it also appears to have activity associated with purine analogue function.

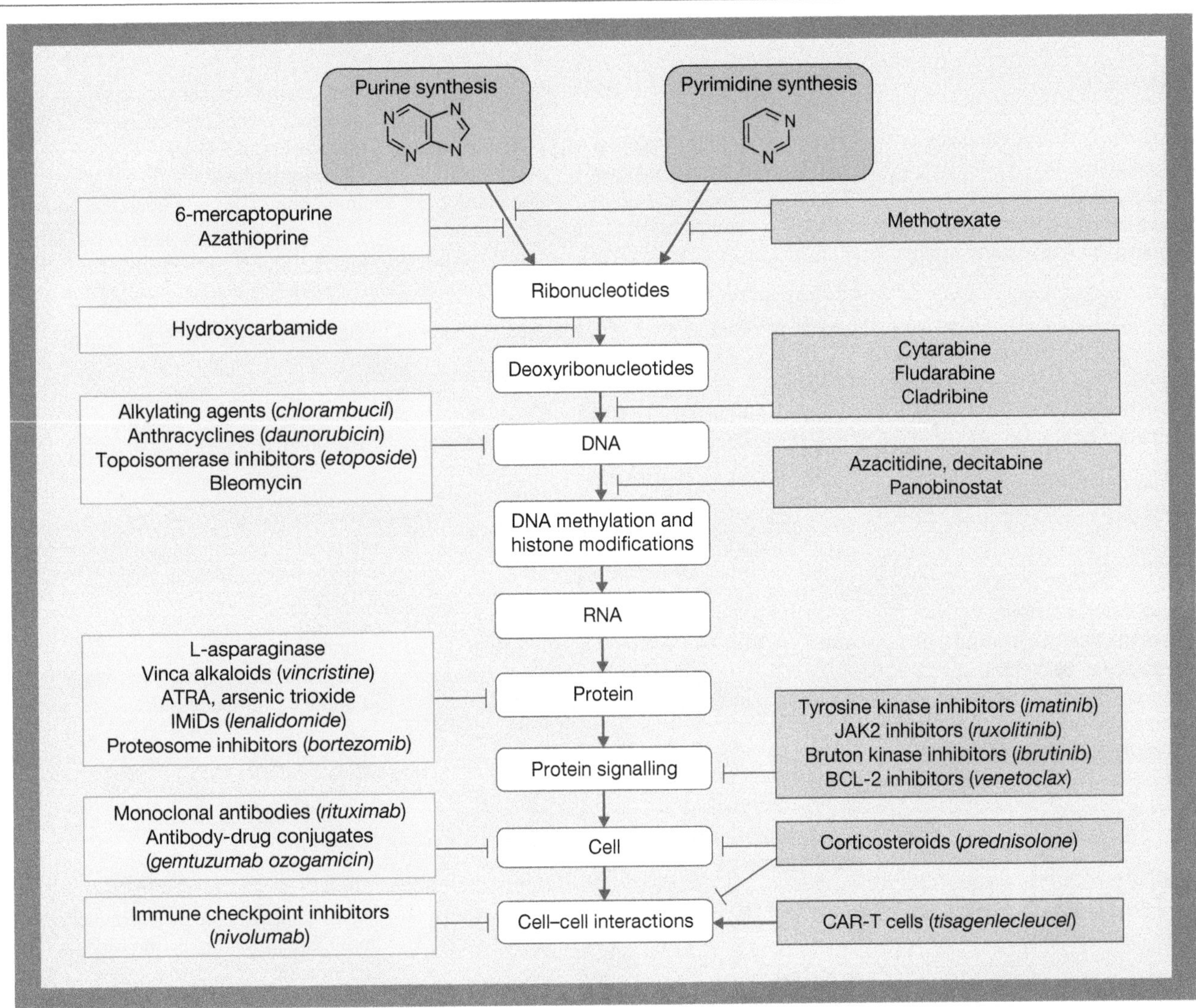

Figure 12.6 The site of action of some drugs used in the treatment of haemopoietic malignancies. One example of the drugs in each of the different major classes is given. ATRA, all-*trans* retinoic acid; CAR, chimeric antigen receptor, IMiDs, immunomodulatory imide drugs.

Table 12.5 Drugs used in the treatment of leukaemia and lymphoma.

Drug/drug class	Mechanism of action	Particular side effects*
Alkylating agents		
Cyclophosphamide	Cross-link DNA, impede RNA formation	Marrow aplasia, haemorrhagic cystitis, cardiomyopathy, loss of hair
Chlorambucil		Marrow aplasia, hepatic toxicity, dermatitis, alopecia
Busulphan		Marrow aplasia, pulmonary fibrosis, hyperpigmentation, seizures, hepatic toxicity, alopecia
Melphalan		Marrow aplasia, alopecia
Bendamustine	Cross-link DNA as for other alkylating agents, and also purine nucleoside analogue	Myelosuppression
Antimetabolites		
Hydroxycarbamide (hydroxyurea)	Inhibit ribonucleotide reductase	Pigmentation, nail dystrophy, skin keratosis, epitheliomas
Methotrexate	Inhibit pyrimidine or purine synthesis or incorporation into DNA	Mouth ulcers, gut toxicity

Cytarabine (Ara-C)	Inhibits DNA synthesis	CNS, especially cerebellar toxicity and conjunctivitis at high doses
Mercaptopurine**, thioguanine**	Purine analogue	Jaundice, gut toxicity
Clofarabine	Purine analogue	Myelosuppression
Fludarabine, Cladribine (2-chlorodeoxyadenosine, 2-CDA) pentostatin (deoxycoformycin)	Purine analogues; inhibit adenosine deaminase or other purine pathways	Immunosuppression (low CD4 counts); renal and neurotoxicity (at high doses)
Cytotoxic antibiotics		
Anthracyclines, e.g. daunorubicin, idarubicin; mitoxantrone, CPX-351 (liposomal combination of anthracycline and cytarabine)	Bind to DNA and interfere with mitosis	Cardiac toxicity, hair loss
Bleomycin	Induce DNA breaks	Pulmonary fibrosis, skin pigmentation
Amasacrine (m-AMSA)	Topoisomerase inhibitor	Hair loss, mucositis
Plant derivatives		
Vincristine (Oncovin®), vinblastine	Spindle damage	Neuropathy (peripheral or bladder or gut)
Etoposide	Mitotic inhibitor	Hair loss, oral ulceration
Epigenetic modifiers		
Demethylating (hypomethylating) agents: azacitidine, decitabine	Inhibit DNA methlytransferase	Myelosuppression, injection site reactions (for subcutaneous azacytidine)
Histone deacetylase inhibitors (panobinostat, romidepsin)	Inhibit histone deacetylase	Fatigue, thrombocytopenia
Ivosidenib (IDH1inhibitor) Enasidenib (IDH/2 inhibitor)	IDH inhibitor	Differentiation syndrome
Revumenib	Menin inhibitor	QT prolongation, differentiation syndrome
Signal transduction inhibitors		
Imatinib, dasatinib, nilotinib, bosutinib, ponatinib, asciminib	Inhibit ABL tyrosine kinase	Myelosuppression, fluid retention, pancreatitis, GI upset, thrombosis (ponatinib)
Midostaurin, gilteritinib, crenolanib, quizartinib, sorafenib	Inhibit FLT3 kinase	Myelosuppression, GI upset
Ibrutinib, acalbrutinib, zanabrutinib Pirtobrutinib	Inhibit BTK protein (covalent) (non-covalent)	Bleeding, disease flare, atrial fibrillation
Idelalisib, duvelisib, copanlisib	Inhibit PI3K delta	Colitis, atrial dysrhythmia
Ruxolitinib, pacritinib, fedratinib, momelitinib	Inhibit JAK2	Marrow suppression
Crizotinib	Inhibit ALK	Visual disturbance, hepatic enzyme elevation, GI effects
Gladesgib	Inhibit Hedgehog pathway	Marrow suppression, myalgias, nausea, embryo-foetal toxicity
Miscellaneous		
Corticosteroids	Lymphoblast lysis	Diabetes, osteoporosis, psychosis
All-trans-retinoic acid (tretinoin)	Induces differentiation	Skin hyperkeratosis, leucocytosis and pleural effusion
Arsenic trioxide	Induces differentiation or apoptosis	Hyperleucocytosis, prolonged QTc interval, neuropathy
α-Interferon	Activation of RNAase and natural killer activity	Flu-like symptoms, thrombocytopenia, leucopenia, weight loss
Venetoclax	Inhibit BCL-2 signalling	Tumour lysis
Omacetaxine	Inhibits protein translation	Injection site reactions, GI effects, myelosuppression
Bortezomib, ixazomib, carfilzomib	Proteasome inhibition	Neuropathy
L-asparaginase, PEG-asparaginase	Deprive cells of asparagine	Hypersensitivity, low albumin and coagulation factors, pancreatitis
Thalidomide, lenalidomide, pomalidomide	Immunomodulation, alteration of protein degradation	Neuropathy, constipation, thrombosis

Monoclonal antibodies		
Rituximab, ofatumumab, obinutuzumab (all anti-CD20)	Induction of apoptosis	Infusion reactions, immunosuppression
Alemtuzumab (anti-CD52)	Lysis of target cell by complement fixation	Infusion reactions, immunosuppression
Ibritumomab (Zevalin®) (anti-CD20 with ^{90}Y radioisotope)	Toxicity to bound cell	Myelosuppression, nausea
Gemtuzumab ozogamicin (Mylotarg®) (anti-CD33 with calicheamicin cytotoxin)	Kill myeloid cells	Myelosuppression, hepatic sinusoidal occlusive syndrome
Inotuzumab ozogamicin (Besponsa®) (anti-CD22 with calicheamicin cytotoxin)	Kill neoplastic B cells	Cytokine release syndrome, hepatic sinusoidal occlusive syndrome
Tagraxofusp (Elzonristm®) (anti-CD123 with diphtheria toxin)	Kill myeloid cells or blastic plasmacytoid dendritic cells	Oedema and capillary leak syndrome, nausea, fever, hepatotoxicity, hypoalbuminemia, myelosuppression
Blinatumomab (Blincyto®) (bispecific CD20/CD3)	Recruit cytotoxic T cells to neoplastic B cells	Neurotoxicity, cytokine release syndrome
Brentuximab (Adcetris®) (anti-CD30)	Kill CD30$^+$ lymphocytes	Myelosuppression, neuropathy
Daratumumab (Darzalex®) (anti-CD38)	Kill malignant plasma cells	Infusion reactions, myelosuppression, difficulty matching for transfusion
Elotuzumab (Empliciti®) (anti-SLAMF7)	Kill malignant plasma cells	Fatigue, GI effects, neuropathy, myelosuppression
Belantamab mafodotin (Blenrep®) (anti-BCMA)	Kill malignant plasma cells	Ocular, GI side effects
Polotuzumab vedotin ((Polivy®) (anti-CD79b)	Kills malignant B cells	Hepatotoxity, neuropathy
Magrolimab (anti-CD47)	Macrophage checkpoint inhibitor	Myelosuppression, electrolyte disturbance
Immune checkpoint inhibitors		
Nivolumab, pembrolizumab, ipilimumab	Inhibit PD-1, PDL-1 or CTLA4 signalling and activate cytotoxic T cells	Autoimmune manifestations (myocarditis, colitis, thyroid disease, iridocyclitis, hepatic injury, kidney dysfunction), infection
Chimeric antigen receptor T cells		
Tisagenlecleucel, axicabtagene ciloleucel	Kill CD19$^+$ cells directly	Cytokine release syndrome, neurotoxicity

*Many of the drugs cause nausea, vomiting, mucositis and bone marrow toxicity, and in large doses infertility. Tissue necrosis is a problem if the drugs are extravasated during infusion.
**Allopurinol potentiates the action and side effects of mercaptopurine. CNS, central nervous system; GI, gastrointestinal.

Antimetabolites block metabolic pathways used in DNA synthesis. There are four major groups:

1 **Inhibitors of *de novo* DNA synthesis**. Hydroxycarbamide (hydroxyurea) is used widely in the treatment of myeloproliferative disorders. It inhibits the enzyme ribonucleotide reductase, which converts ribonucleotides to deoxyribonucleotides. It is not thought to permanently damage DNA and is also used in non-malignant disorders such as sickle cell anaemia (Chapter 7).
2 **Folate antagonists**, such as methotrexate (p. xx). Methotrexate is widely used alone or in combination with cytarabine as intrathecal prophylaxis of central nervous system (CNS) disease in patients with ALL, AML or high-grade non-Hodgkin lymphoma. High systemic doses may also penetrate the CNS. Folinic acid (formyl THF) is able to overcome the activity of methotrexate and is sometimes administered to 'rescue' normal cells after high-dose methotrexate therapy.
3 **Pyrimidine analogues** include cytarabine (ara-C), which is an analogue of 2′-deoxycytidine. It is incorporated into DNA, where it inhibits DNA polymerase and blocks replication.
4 **Purine analogues** include fludarabine (which inhibits DNA synthesis in a manner similar to ara-C), mercaptopurine, azathioprine, bendamustine, clofarabine and pentostatin.

Cytotoxic antibiotic drugs include the anthracyclines, such as doxorubicin, daunorubicin, idarubicin and the chemically similar mitoxantrone. These are able to intercalate into DNA and then bind strongly to topoisomerases, which are critical for relieving torsional stress in replicating DNA by nicking and resealing DNA strands. If topoisomerase activity is blocked, DNA replication cannot take place.

Bleomycin is a metal chelating antibiotic that generates superoxide radicals within cells that degrade preformed DNA. It is active on non-cycling cells.

Plant derivatives include the vinca alkaloids, e.g. vincristine, which is derived from the periwinkle plant. It binds to tubulin and prevents its polymerization to microtubules. This blocks cell division in metaphase. Etoposide inhibits topisomerase action.

Targeted drugs

A wide range of targeted drugs which block specific proteins are now in use and are likely to eventually replace the cytotoxic agents described above.

ABL1 inhibitors such as imatinib, dasatinib and nilotinib bind to the BCR::ABL1 fusion protein. They block binding of adenosine triphosphate (ATP) and thus prevent the overactive tyrosine kinase from phosphorylating substrate proteins, leading to apoptosis of the cell. **Asciminib** blocks BCR::ABL1 at a different site (Fig. 14.5). They are used in chronic myeloid leukaemia (CML) and *BCR::ABL1*$^+$ ALL.

Covalent inhibitors of Bruton kinase (BTK) in the B-cell signalling pathways include ibrutinib, acalabrutinib and zanabrutinib widely used in B-cell malignancies. Non-covalent pirtobrutinib is approved for resistant CLL and mantle cell lymphoma. Idelalisib or duvelisib, which inhibit the delta isoenzyme of PI3 kinase, is now rarely used for B-cell disorders.

A wide range of additional kinase inhibitors include JAK2 inhibitors, e.g. ruxolitinib effective in primary myelofibrosis and polycythaemia vera; crizotinib, which blocks ALK activity; and **inhibitors of the FLT3 kinase such as midostaurin, gilteritinib and crenolanib used for *FLT3* mutated AML**. Glasdegib inhibits Hedgehog signalling, an important survival pathway for neoplastic cells.

Ivosidenib and enasidenib inhibit mutant isocitrate dehydrogenase (IDH) 1 and 2, respectively, and are useful in the ~25% of AML cases that have one of these mutations.

Bortezomib, ixazomib and carfilzomib are proteasome inhibitors used widely in the treatment of myeloma and some lymphomas.

Monoclonal antibodies are highly effective and are particularly employed against B-cell malignancies. Rituximab binds to CD20 on B cells and mediates cell death, primarily through direct induction of apoptosis and opsonization. Other anti-CD20 antibodies, e.g. obinutuzumab and ofatumumab, are available. Alemtuzumab binds to CD52 and is highly efficient at fixing complement, which lyses the target B and T cells. Anti-CD30 (brentuximab) is effective in Hodgkin lymphoma. Antibodies may also carry attached toxins, e.g. gemtuzumab, anti-CD33, inotuzumab, anti-CD22, or tagraxofusp, anti-CD123, or radioactive isotopes, e.g. ibritumomab, anti-CD20. Bispecific antibodies, e.g. blinatumomab, recruit CD3$^+$ T cells to B-cell tumour cells (Fig 17.10).

Other agents

Corticosteroids have a potent lymphocytotoxic activity and have an important role in many chemotherapeutic regimens in the treatment of lymphoid malignancy and myeloma.

All-trans retinoic acid (ATRA) is a vitamin A derivative that acts as a differentiation agent in acute promyelocytic leukaemia (APML). Tumour cells in APML are arrested at the promyelocyte stage as a result of transcriptional repression resulting from the PML::RARα fusion protein (p. 176). ATRA relieves this block and may lead to a brisk neutrophilia within a few days of treatment, with other side effects known as the 'ATRA' or 'differentiation' syndrome (p. 180).

Arsenic is also useful in treatment of acute promyelocytic leukaemia. It induces differentiation and apoptosis.

Demethylation agents, e.g. azacytidine, decitabine, act to increase transcription by reducing methylation on cytosine residues within DNA. However, the precise mechanism of their clinical activity is unclear.

Interferon-α is an antiviral and antimitotic substance produced in response to viral infection and inflammation. It has proven useful in treatment of CML, myeloma and myeloproliferative neoplasms.

Immunomodulatory drugs include thalidomide, lenalidomide and pomalidomide. They are effective in myeloma and in some types of myelodysplasia.

Asparaginase is an enzyme derived from bacteria that breaks down the amino acid asparagine within the circulation. ALL cells lack asparagine synthase and thus need a supply of exogenous asparagine for protein synthesis. Intramuscular asparaginase is an important agent in the treatment of ALL, although hypersensitivity reactions are not uncommon and blood clotting may be disturbed. PEGylation of asparaginase increases half-life and decreases frequency of required injection.

Platinum derivatives, e.g. cisplatin, are used in combinations for treating lymphoma.

Immune checkpoint inhibitors are antibodies designed to overcome T-cell self-tolerance to neoplastic cells. Approved check-point inhibitors block PD-1, PD-L1 or CTLA4 molecules that mediate self-tolerance. They can be useful in some cases of relapsed Hodgkin lymphoma or in leukaemias relapsed after allogeneic SCT.

Chimeric antigen receptor (CAR)-T cells

Chimeric antigen receptors are T-cell receptors that are bioengineered using retroviral vectors to give T cells the antigen specificity of a monoclonal antibody (Chapter 9). The receptors are called 'chimeric' because the components of the engineered T-cell receptor construct include both tumour antigen-reactive and T-cell-activating functions. CAR-T cells can be derived either from the patient's own immune cells (autologous) or a donor (allogeneic). The latter offers the possibility of an off-the-shelf product. Autologous CAR-T cells targeting CD19 are approved for treatment of B-cell ALL (Chapter 17) and for relapsed/refractory B-cell large cell lymphoma (Chapter 21), and are proving effective also in refractory multiple myeloma (Chapter 22) and refractory acute myeloid leukaemia (Chapter 13). NK cells harvested from cord blood are in clinical trials also aimed at 'off the shelf' treatment.

Myelosuppression is the most common adverse event after CAR-T cell infusion. **Two major CAR-T specific complications include cytokine release syndrome (CRS) and immune cell-associated neurotoxicity syndrome (ICANS).** Cardinal features of CRS are fever, hypotension, and hypoxia, by which the severity of CRS can be assessed. Other associated toxicities include cough, vomiting, diarrhoea, skin rashes, renal failure, tremor, confusion, aphasia, fits, and delirium due to encephalitis. The cytokines released from the neoplastic and normal cells include tumour necrosis factor, interferon-gamma and many interleukins (ILs). The plasma levels of some of these interleukins may be measured to assess the severity and progress. Treatment is with corticosteroids and with anti-IL6 receptor antibodies such as toclizumab. Monitoring in a critical care setting may be required.

The other important adverse effect is neurotoxicity (ICANS). Symptoms can be vague, ranging from confusion to agitation and seizures. A feature of ICANS include problems with speech, and handwriting. This usually occurs early post infusion (within a week); monitoring for severity is undertaken using the Immune Effector Cell Encephalopathy (ICE) score. Supportive care is the mainstay of management. Finally, as CAR-T cells also destroy normal B cells, treated patients require lifelong immunoglobulin infusions.

SUMMARY

- Progress in the treatment of haemopoietic malignancies has been the result of improvements in both supportive therapy and specific tumour treatments.
- Initial assessment includes a performance score and tests for co-morbidities.
- Supportive treatments often include insertion of a central venous catheter; appropriate use of red cell, platelet transfusions; growth factors, early administration of drugs to treat infection; optimization of the blood coagulation system; drugs to reduce side effects of the disease or its treatment such as nausea or pain; psychological support.
- Tumour lysis syndrome is a potentially life-threatening complication of chemotherapy in certain haematological malignancies, especially leukaemias with a very high white cell count or rapidly proliferating lymphomas
- Gram-positive skin organisms such as *Staphylococcus epidermidis* are common infections and often colonize central venous catheters.
- Gram-negative bacteria are usually derived from the gut and can cause severe septicaemia.
- The use of air filters, handwashing and prophylactic antibiotics can reduce infection rates.
- Neutropenic patients who develop a fever should be treated urgently with broad-spectrum antibiotics.
- Herpes viruses are a common cause of infection in patients who are significantly immunosuppressed.
- Fungal infections are a major clinical problem for patients undergoing chemotherapy. Oral and intravenous antifungal drugs may be used for either prevention or treatment.
- A wide range of drugs is now available for the treatment of haemopoietic malignancy: alkylating agents, antimetabolites, anthracyclines, signal transduction inhibitors, including tyrosine kinase, Bruton kinase and JAK2 inhibitors, mono- and bi-specific monoclonal antibodies, antibodies linked to a toxin, immune modulators, e.g. thalidomide, lenalidomide, proteasome inhibitors; others, e.g. corticosteroids, ATRA, arsenic, demethylating agents, interferon, asparaginase, platinum derivatives.
- CAR-T cells have entered clinical practice for therapy of resistant B-lymphoid and plasma cell malignancies. They may cause a cytokine release syndrome including neurotoxicity.

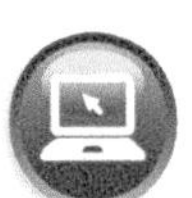

Now visit **www.wiley.com/go/haematology9e** to test yourself on this chapter.

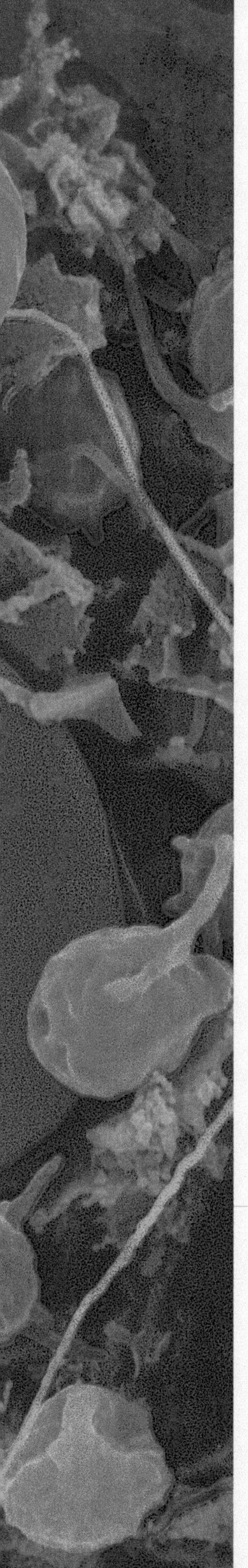

CHAPTER 13

Acute myeloid leukaemia

Key topics

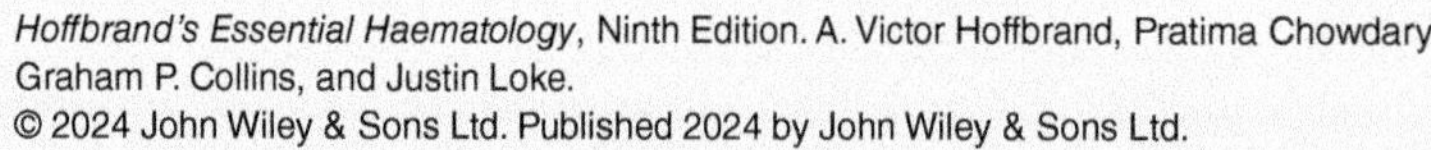

Hoffbrand's Essential Haematology, Ninth Edition. A. Victor Hoffbrand, Pratima Chowdary, Graham P. Collins, and Justin Loke.

© 2024 John Wiley & Sons Ltd. Published 2024 by John Wiley & Sons Ltd.

Companion website: www.wiley.com/go/haematology9e

The leukaemias are a group of disorders characterized by the accumulation of malignant white cells in the bone marrow and blood. These abnormal cells cause symptoms because of (i) bone marrow failure, e.g. anaemia, neutropenia, thrombocytopenia; and, less commonly, (ii) infiltration of organs, e.g. liver, spleen, lymph nodes, meninges, brain, skin or testes.

Classification of leukaemia

The main classification is into four types: **acute or chronic leukaemias,** which are further subdivided into **lymphoid or myeloid leukaemias**. Acute leukaemias are usually aggressive diseases in which malignant transformation occurs in a haemopoietic stem cell or early progenitor. Acquired genetic damage results in an increased rate of proliferation, reduced apoptosis and a block in cellular differentiation. Together these events cause accumulation in the bone marrow of early haemopoietic cells known as **blast cells**. The dominant clinical feature of acute leukaemia is usually bone marrow failure caused by accumulation of blast cells, although organ infiltration also can occur. If untreated, acute leukaemias are usually rapidly fatal, although with modern treatments most younger patients are ultimately cured of their disease.

Diagnosis of acute leukaemia

Acute leukaemia is normally defined as the presence of at least 20% of blast cells in the bone marrow or blood at clinical presentation. However, it can be diagnosed with less than 20% blasts if certain leukaemia-specific cytogenetic or molecular genetic abnormalities are present (Table 13.1 and Table 17.1).

The **lineage of the blast cells** is defined by microscopic examination (morphology; Fig. 13.5 and Fig. 17.3), immunophenotypic (flow cytometry; Fig. 13.1), cytogenetic and molecular analysis (Table 13.4 and Table 11.1). These assessments define whether the blasts are of myeloid or lymphoid lineage and also localize the stage of cellular differentiation (Table 13.2). A typical 'myeloid' immunophenotype is CD13$^+$, CD33$^+$, CD117$^+$, TdT$^-$ (Table 13.2; Fig. 13.1). Special antibodies

Table 13.1 Classification of acute myeloid leukaemia (AML) according to the World Health Organization (WHO) (2022).

Acute myeloid leukaemia with defining genetic abnormalities
Acute promyelocytic leukaemia (APL) with *PML::RARα* fusion
AML with *RUNX1::RUNX1T1 fusion*
AML with *CBFB::MYH11* fusion
AML with *DEK::NUP214* fusion
AML with *RBM15::MRTFA* fusion
AML with *BCR::ABL1* fusion (require blast count of ≥20%)
AML with *KMT2A* rearrangement
AML with *MECOM* rearrangement
AML with *NUP98* rearrangement
AML with *NPM1* mutation
AML with *CEBPA* mutation (require blast count of ≥20%)
AML, myelodysplasia-related (see Table 13.2)
AML with other defined genetic alterations
Acute myeloid leukaemia, defined by differentiation
AML with minimal differentiation
AML without maturation
AML with maturation
Acute basophilic leukaemia
Acute myelomonocytic leukaemia
Acute monocytic leukaemia
Acute erythroid leukaemia
Acute megakaryoblastic leukaemia
Myeloid sarcoma
Secondary AML (myeloid neoplasm)

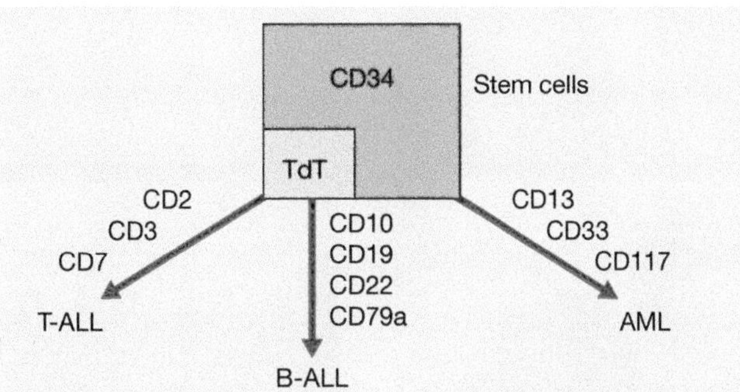

Figure 13.1 Development of three cell lineages from pluripotential stem cells giving rise to the three main immunological subclasses of acute leukaemia. CD34 is expressed on most stem cells, whereas TdT expression is characteristic of a lymphoid lineage. Examples of surface markers which are seen characteristically in T-ALL, B-ALL and AML are shown; others are described in the relevant sections of this chapter and Chapter 17. AML, acute myeloid leukaemia; B-ALL, B-cell acute lymphoblastic leukaemia; CD, cluster of differentiation; HLA, human leucocyte antigen; T-ALL, T-cell acute lymphoblastic leukaemia; TdT, terminal deoxynucleotidyl transferase.

Table 13.2 Cytogenetic and molecular abnormalities defining acute myeloid leukaemia, myelodysplasia related (WHO, 2022).

Defining cytogenetic abnormalities
Complex karyotype (>3 abnormalities)
5q deletion or loss*
Monosomy 7, 7q deletion, or loss of 7q*
11q deletion
12p deletion or loss*
Monosomy 13 or 13q deletion
17p deletion or loss*
Isochromosome 17q
idic(X)(q13)
Defining somatic mutations
ASXL1, BCOR, EZH2, SF3B1, SRSF2, STAG2, U2AF1, ZRSR2

* Loss due to unbalanced translocation.
Idic = Isodicentric, contains mirror–image segments of genetic material.

are helpful in the diagnosis of the rare undifferentiated, erythroid or megakaryoblastic subtypes (Table 13.3). Acute lymphoblastic leukaemia is discussed in Chapter 17. Occasionally, a case of leukaemia will express both myeloid and lymphoid markers. **Acute leukaemias of ambiguous lineage (mixed phenotype acute leukaemias)** are rare cases that express markers for both myeloid and lymphoid differentiation, either on the same blast cells or on two different cell populations in the same patient.

Cytogenetic and **molecular** analysis is essential and is usually performed on marrow cells, although blood may be used if the circulating blast cell count is high. Cytochemistry can also be useful in determining the blast cell lineage (Fig. 13.2) but is no longer performed in centres where the newer and more definitive tests are available.

Acute myeloid leukaemia (AML)

Pathogenesis

The AML genome contains an average of about 10 mutations within protein-coding genes in each case, among the smallest number of any adult cancer (Fig. 11.3). Many AML 'driver mutations' promoting clonal expansion have been identified, with the most common being within *FLT3*, *NPM1* and *DNMT3A* (Fig. 13.3). Some other mutations, e.g. of *ASXL1* or mutations in splicing-associated genes, are frequent in myelodysplastic neoplasias (MDS) and when found in AML suggest that it is secondary to MDS, which may not have been recognized clinically. This has resulted in a list of cytogenetic and somatic mutations which are associated with MDS, and as such, the presence of which suggests a preceding MDS phase (Table 13.2). These secondary AML are often associated with chemotherapy resistance and a poor prognosis.

The mutations usually occur on only one of the two alleles for the gene and, depending on the gene, may be 'loss of function', 'gain of function' or 'neomorphic', i.e. conferring a novel function. Some AML cases are characterized by a gene-fusion event, which usually arises from translocations, with the most common being *PML::RARA*, *CBF::MYH11* and *RUNX1::RUNX1T1* (Table 11.1), which are found in around 15%, 12% and 8% of cases, respectively. The wide variety of cytogenetic abnormalities and molecular mutations is such that there are hundreds of patterns of mutations. However, molecular cooperativity of mutations result in recurring patterns of mutations, for example *NPM1*, *FLT3*-ITD and

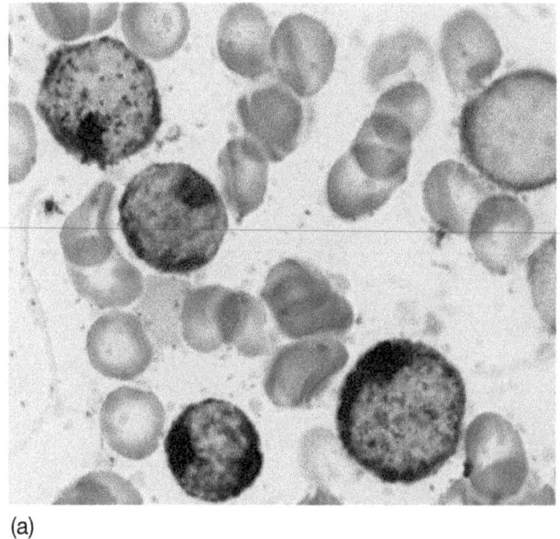
(a)

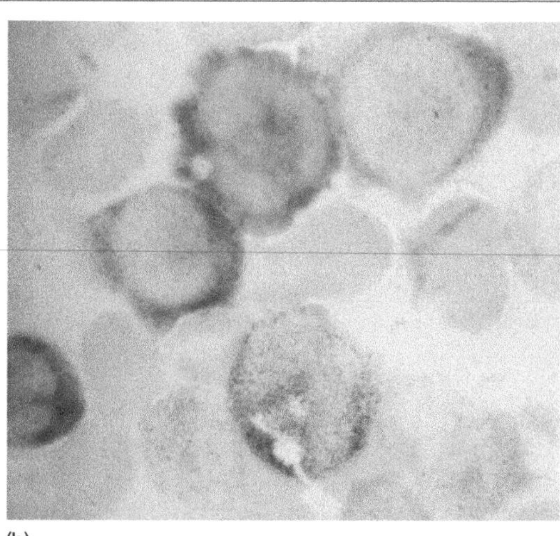
(b)

Figure 13.2 Cytochemical staining in acute myeloid leukaemia. (a) Sudan black B shows black staining in the cytoplasm. (b) Myelomonocytic: non-specific esterase/chloracetate staining shows orange-staining monoblast cytoplasm and blue-staining (myeloblast) cytoplasm.

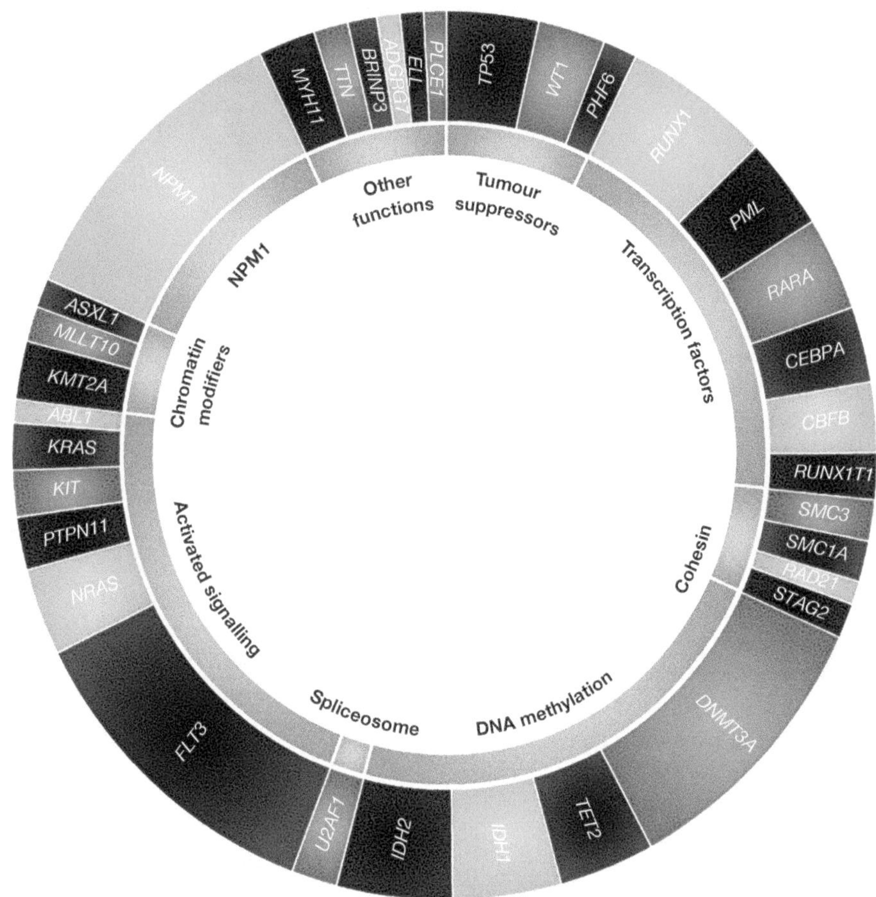

Figure 13.3 The genetic landscape in adult AML. Data drawn from TCGA data set, showing all the genes mutated in at least 2% of the 200 patients sequenced, and the distribution of mutations between these genes. Source: From S. Charrot *et al.* (2019) *Br. J. Haematol.* 188: 49–62. Reproduced with permission of John Wiley & Sons.

DNMT3A mutations frequently co-occur in the same patient. Mutations of genes *DNMT3A*, *TET2*, *ASXL1* and less commonly *IDH1*, *IDH2*, *TP53* or spliceosome genes may be found in the blood cells of healthy subjects, especially after age 60 years (age-related clonal haemopoiesis or clonal haemopoiesis of indeterminate potential, Chapter 16). Patients with these mutations can develop AML, which may present many years later. The likelihood of AML development is higher in those with *IDH1*, *IDH2*, *TP53* or spliceosome gene mutations, more than one mutation, high mutation allele burden, or an elevated red cell distribution width.

Incidence

AML is the most common form of acute leukaemia in adults and becomes increasingly common with age, with a median onset of 65 years. It forms only a minor fraction (10–15%) of the leukaemias in childhood. Cytogenetic and molecular abnormalities and response to initial treatment have a major influence on prognosis (Table 13.5).

Classification

AML is classified according to the World Health Organization (WHO; 2022) scheme (Table 13.1). There is an increasing focus on the genetic abnormalities within the malignant cells, and it is likely that ultimately all AML cases will be classified by specific genetic subtype. Currently this is not yet possible, but many genetic subtypes have been determined. Approximately 60% of AML cases exhibit karyotypic abnormalities on cytogenetic analysis and most cases with a normal karyotype carry mutations in genes such as *FLT3*, *NPM1*, *CEBPA* or *DNMT3A*, detected only by molecular methods (see below).

Five main groups of AML are recognized (Table 13.1):

1 **AML with defining genetic abnormalities.** The detection of these abnormalities defines the neoplasm as AML, and so the diagnostic criteria for this subgroup are relaxed in that the bone marrow blast cell count does not need to exceed 20% in order to make a diagnosis (with the exception of AML with *BCR::ABL1* fusion and AML with *CEBPA* mutation).

2 **AML defined by differentiation.** These include cases lacking a defining genetic abnormality.
3 **AML, myelodysplasia-related.** In this group the AML is defined by the presence of cytogenetic or molecular abnormalities related to myelodysplasia, and/or a history of MDS (or MDS/MPN) (Table 13.2).
4 **Myeloid sarcoma** is rare, but refers to a disease that resembles a solid tumour but is composed of clustered myeloid blast cells. This is often called 'extramedullary leukaemia', 'granulocytic sarcoma' or 'chloroma'. Bone marrow involvement often occurs concurrently.
5 **Secondary myeloid neoplasms** include those that arise in patients
   - with germline predisposition (Appendix, Table 1). Genetic counselling and family history is an important part of the assessment of these patients. This subtype of AML also include myeloid leukaemia of Down syndrome (ML-DS). This usually occurs before the age of 5 years and may follow an episode of transient abnormal myelopoiesis (TAM). TAM occurs as a multi-step process provoked by trisomy 21-associated abnormal foetal haemopoiesis. There are acquired mutations of GATA1. TAM begins *in utero* and often presents in newborns, about 10% of those with Down syndrome, as a self-limiting leukaemic syndrome which resolves spontaneously in the majority of patients. Patients with TAM which proceed to ML-DS have megakaryoblastic features, but often respond to chemotherapy alone.
   - following exposure to radiation or cytotoxic drugs such as etoposide or alkylating agents. AML secondary to cytotoxic drugs or radiation commonly exhibit mutations in the *TP53* or *KMT2A (MLL)* gene. The clinical response is usually poor.
   - AML arising in patients with myeloproliferative diseases is categorized as MPN while that arising as transformation of MDS is categorized as myelodysplasia related.

Other subtypes of AML:

Acute leukaemias of mixed or ambiguous lineage

These acute leukaemias are grouped together in WHO (2022) (Appendix, Table 2). They are separated into those with defining genetic abnormalities and those defined on immunophenotyping alone. The assignment of lineage by immunophenotyping depends on the strength and pattern of antigen expression as well as the coordinated expression of more than one antigen of the same lineage (Appendix, Table 3). They usually have a poor prognosis. There are no clear evidence for optimal treatment strategies, but use of ALL style chemotherapy schedules, or if not responsive, to use AML directed regimens are reasonable. In the case of *BCR::ABL1* mutated leukaemia, use of TKI should be considered. Menin inhibitors are promising treatments for MLL fusion-driven acute leukaemias.

Blastic Plasmacytoid Dendritic Cell Neoplasm (BPDCN)

This is a rare but aggressive neoplasia, characterized by skin and heterogeneous systemic manifestations. These include blood, bone marrow, lymph node and CNS infiltration. It is often placed in the myeloid disorders category (with "myeloid" pattern of genetic mutations) though the cell of origin is unclear. It is important to differentiate BPDCN from AML with leukaemia cutis, and BPDCN immunophenotypically expresses CD123, CD4, CD56 and TCL1, but is negative for lineage markers such as MPO. Treatments include intensive AML or ALL protocols including SCT. Novel CD123-targeting treatments have an emerging role.

Clinical features

The clinical features of AML are dominated by the pattern of bone marrow failure caused by the accumulation of malignant cells within marrow (Fig. 13.4). Infections are frequent, and anaemia and thrombocytopenia are often profound. A bleeding tendency caused by thrombocytopenia and disseminated intravascular coagulation (DIC) is characteristic of the promyelocytic variant of AML. Tumour cells can infiltrate a variety of tissues. Gum hypertrophy and infiltration (Fig. 13.5), skin involvement (leukaemia cutis) and central nervous system (CNS) disease are characteristic of the myelomonocytic and monocytic subtypes.

Investigations

Table 13.4 lists the initial clinical and laboratory tests to be performed in newly diagnosed cases of AML; similar work-up is needed for all new haematological malignancies.

Haematological investigations reveal a normochromic normocytic anaemia with thrombocytopenia in most cases. The total white cell count is usually increased, and blood film examination typically shows a variable numbers of blast cells. The bone marrow is hypercellular and typically contains many leukaemic blasts (Fig. 13.6). Blast cells are characterized by morphology, immunological (flow cytometric) (Table 13.3), cytogenetic and molecular genetic analysis for confirming the diagnosis, determining prognosis and developing a treatment plan (Tables 13.4 and 13.5).

Tests for DIC are often positive in patients with the promyelocytic variant of AML, and in some cases with monocytic differentiation (see below). Biochemical tests are performed as a baseline before treatment begins and may reveal raised uric acid and lactate dehydrogenase.

Cytogenetics and molecular genetics

Cytogenetics and molecular genetics have two roles: initial diagnostic classification (Table 13.1) and accompanying prognostication (Table 13.5) but following treatment a number of

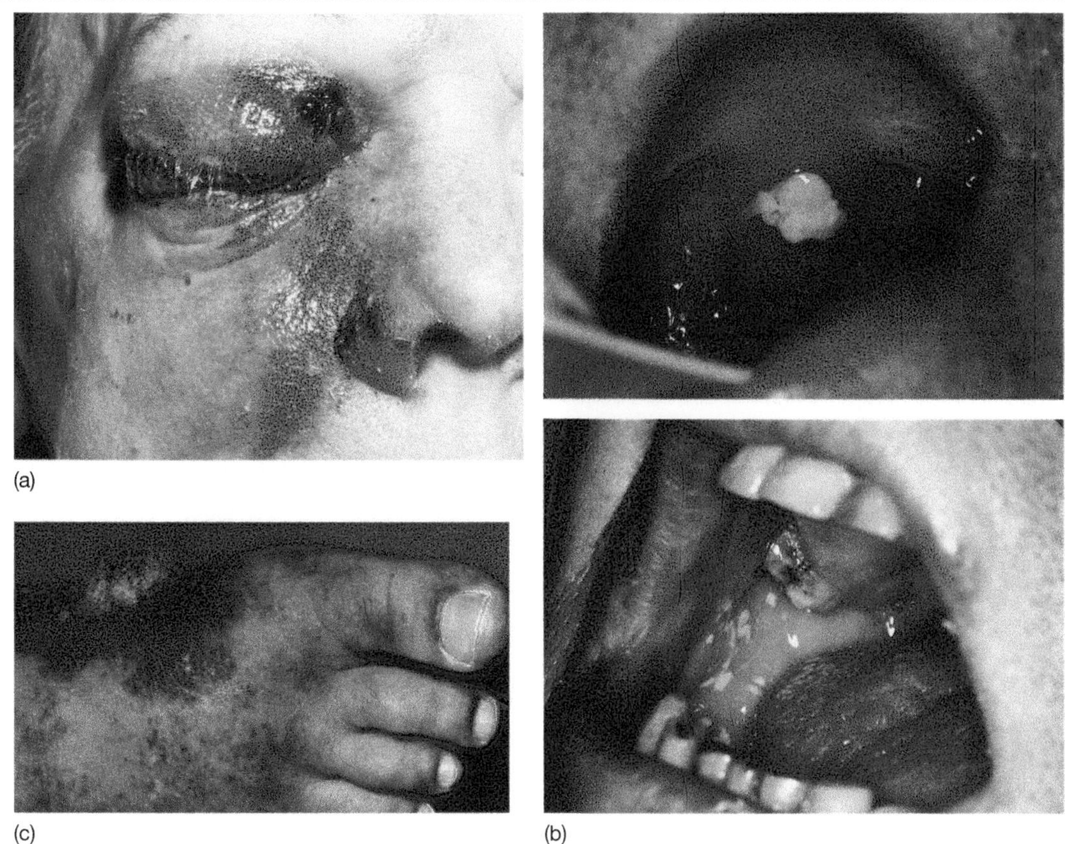

Figure 13.4 **(a)** An orbital infection in a female patient (aged 68 years) with acute myeloid leukaemia and severe neutropenia (haemoglobin 83 g/L, white cells 15.3×10^9/L, blasts 96%, neutrophils 1%, platelets 30×10^9/L). **(b)** Acute myeloid leukaemia: top: plaque *Candida albicans* on soft palate; lower: plaque *Candida albicans* in the mouth, with lesion of herpes simplex on the upper lip. **(c)** Skin infection (*Pseudomonas aeruginosa*) in a female patient (aged 33 years) with acute lymphoblastic leukaemia receiving chemotherapy and with severe neutropenia (haemoglobin 101 g/L, white cells 0.7×10^9/L, neutrophils $<0.1 \times 10^9$/L, lymphocytes 0.6×10^9/L, platelets 20×10^9/L).

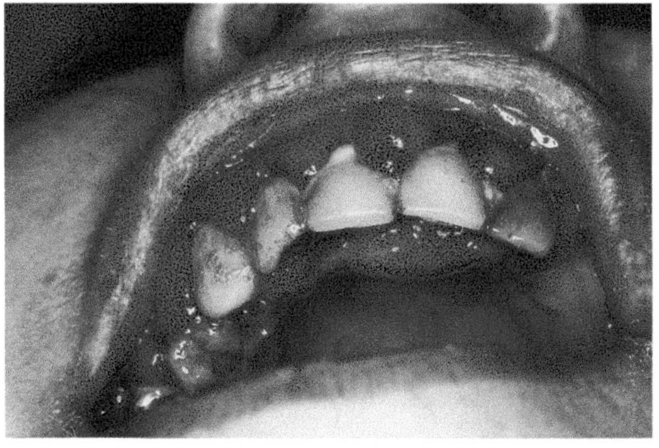

Figure 13.5 Monocytic acute myeloid leukaemia: the gums are swollen and haemorrhagic because of infiltration by leukaemic cells.

translocations and mutations can be used as markers of measurable/minimal residual disease, e.g. t(8;21) or *NPM1* mutations.

Two of the most common – t(8;21) and inv(16) – are associated with a good prognosis. **Acute promyelocytic leukaemia** (APML) is a variant of AML that contains the t(15;17) translocation in which the gene *PML* on chromosome 15 is fused to the retinoic acid receptor α gene, *RARA*, on chromosome 17 (Fig. 13.7). The resultant PML::RARα fusion protein functions as a transcriptional repressor, whereas normal (wild-type) RARα is an activator. Normally, the PML protein forms homodimers with itself, whereas the RARα protein forms heterodimers with the retinoid X receptor protein, RXR. The PML::RARα fusion protein binds to PML and RXR, preventing them from linking with their natural partners. This results in the cellular phenotype of arrested differentiation.

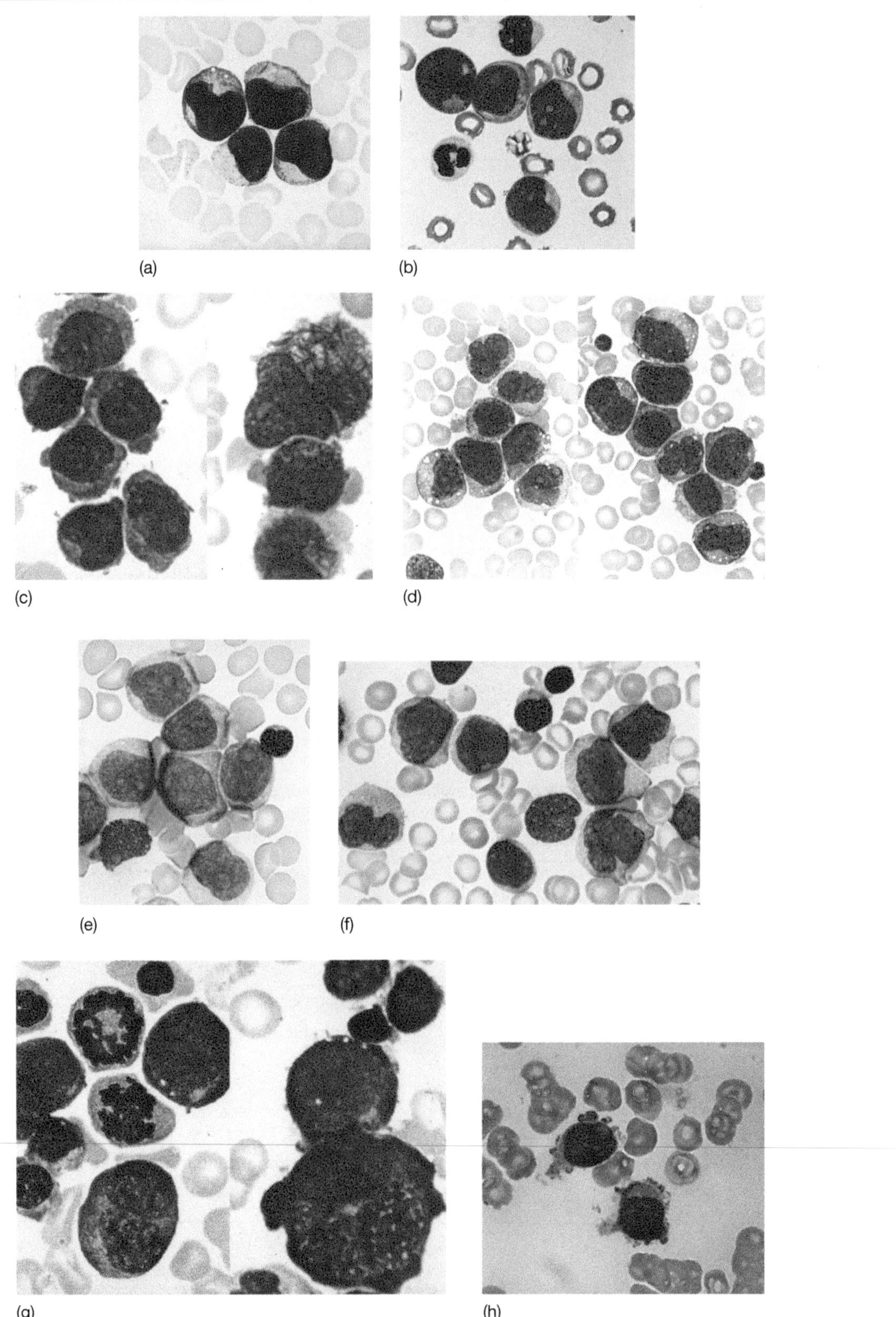

Figure 13.6 Morphological examples of acute myeloid leukaemia. **(a)** Blast cells without differentiation show few granules but may show Auer rods, as in this case; **(b)** cells in differentiation show multiple cytoplasmic granules; **(c)** acute promyelocytic leukaemia blast cells contain prominent granules or multiple Auer rods; **(d)** myelomonocytic blasts have some monocytoid differentiation; **(e)** monoblastic leukaemia in which >80% of blasts are monoblasts; **(f)** monocytic with <80% of blasts monoblasts; **(g)** erythroid showing preponderance of erythroblasts; **(h)** megakaryoblastic showing cytoplasmic blebs on blasts.

Table 13.3 Specialized tests for acute myeloid leukaemia (AML).

Immunological markers (flow cytometry)	Indicates
CD13, CD33, CD34, CD117	Usually positive in AML
CD11c, CD14, CD64	Monocytic differentiation
Glycophorin (CD235a), CD36	Erythroid differentiation
CD41, CD61	Megakaryoblastic differentiation
Myeloperoxidase, CD65	Granulocytic differentiation
Chromosome and genetic analysis (see Tables 13.1 and 13.4)	
Cytochemistry	
Myeloperoxidase	Myeloid differentiation (usually bright in Auer rods)
Sudan black	Myeloid differentiation (usually bright in Auer rods)
Non-specific esterase	Monocytic differentiation

Table 13.4 The initial evaluation of a new patient with suspected acute myeloid leukaemia.

Assessment of medical history, examination and performance status; analysis for co-morbidities (Chapter 12)
Full blood count and differential with blood film
Bone marrow aspirate and trephine biopsy
Immunophenotyping of bone marrow (and/or blood if blast cells present)
Cytogenetic analysis by karyotype
Mutation analysis
Cytochemical analysis (performed in some countries instead of immunophenotyping)
Biochemistry (liver, renal, uric acid, calcium, phosphate, LDH, CRP)
Coagulation - PT, APTT, Fibrinogen, D dimer
Pregnancy test
Information on oocyte or sperm storage
Early tissue typing and donor search
CMV serology, Hepatitis B, C and HIV test
CXR with ECG and ECHO

CXR, chest X-ray; ECG, electrocardiography; ECHO, echocardiography; HIV, human immunodeficiency virus; LDH, lactate dehydrogenase.

Point mutations affecting the genes *FLT3*, *NPM1*, *DNMT3A*, *IDH1*, *IDH2 TET2*, *RUNX1*, *TP53* and others are frequent in AML, especially in those cases without a cytogenetic abnormality (Fig. 13.3). They may be used to subclassify the disease (Table 11.1) and have prognostic significance (Table 13.5). Some of these genes are involved in DNA methylation or histone methylation or acetylation (Fig. 16.1) and are also mutated in cases of myelodysplasia and myeloproliferative neoplasms (Chapters 15 and 16). The presence in *de novo* AML of an MDS-associated mutation, e.g. *ASXL1* or *SF3B1*, is unfavourable.

Table 13.5 Examples of prognostic factors in acute myeloid leukaemia.

	Favourable	Intermediate	Unfavourable
Cytogenetics	t(15;17) t(8;21) inv(16)	Normal t(9;11) Other changes neither unfavourable or favourable	Deletions of chromosome 5 or 7 or 17p, Inv(3) or t(3;3) t(6;9), t(v;11q23); *KTM2A* rearranged Complex rearrangements (≥3 unrelated abnormalities) t(9;22) *BCR::ABL1*
Molecular genetics	*NPM1* mutation *CEBPA* mutation	Wild type/Mutated *NPM1* and *FLT3-ITD*	Mutations of *TP53*, *RUNX1*, *ASXL1* and spliceosome mutations;
Bone marrow response to remission induction	<5% blasts after first course		>20% blasts after first course
Age	Child	<60 years	>60 years
Performance status	Good		Bad
Co-morbidities	Absent		Present
White cell count	<10 × 10⁹/L		>100 × 10⁹/L
Post-cytotoxic therapy (based on medical history) or transformation of MDS or MPN			Unfavourable
Minimal residual disease in remission	Absent	Absent	Present

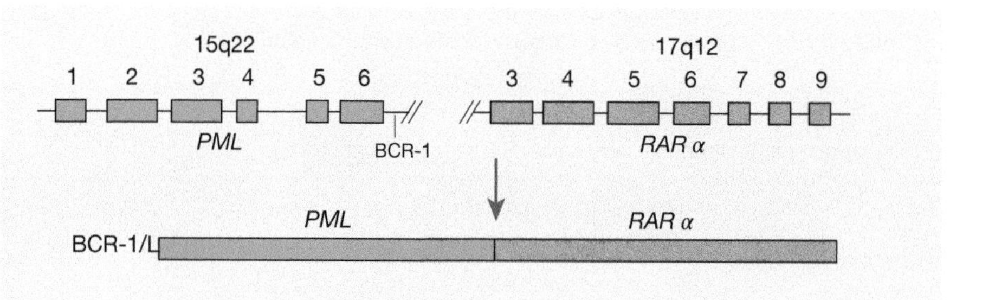

Figure 13.7 Generation of the t(15;17) translocation. The *PML* gene at 15q22 may break at one of three different breakpoint cluster regions (BCR-1, -2 and -3) and joins with exons 3–9 of the *RARα* gene at 17q12. Three different fusion mRNAs are generated – termed long (L), variable (V) or short (S) – and these give rise to fusion proteins of different size. In this diagram only the long version resulting from a break at BCR-1 is shown.

Treatment

Management is both supportive and specific. APML has its own management protocol (next section).

1 **General supportive therapy** for bone marrow failure is described in Chapter 12 and includes the insertion of a central venous cannula, blood product support and prevention of tumour lysis syndrome. The platelet count is generally maintained above 10×10^9/L and the haemoglobin above 80 g/L (except for acute promyelocytic leukaemia, see below). Any episode of fever must be treated promptly. The drugs are myelotoxic with limited selectivity between leukaemic and normal marrow cells, so marrow

failure resulting from the chemotherapy is severe and prolonged, and intensive supportive care is required. Local antifungal policies may recommend use of posaconazole or liposomal amphotericin as invasive fungal infections pose a challenge to this patient group at risk of prolonged neutropenia. Irradiated blood products are required for patients given fludarabine containing regimens. Prednisolone eye drops for patients using high/intermediate dose cytarabine are required to prevent keratoconjunctivitis. Pre-treatment echocardiogram may be warranted for patients with history of heart disease/older patients prior to anthracycline use.

2 The **aim of treatment** in acute leukaemia in fit patients is to induce complete remission (less than 5% blasts in the bone marrow, with recovery of normal blood counts and improved clinical status), which occurs after one or two courses in up to 80% of younger patients and 60% of those over 60 and fit for intensive therapy (Table 13.7). Then to consolidate this with intensive therapy, hopefully eliminating the disease (Fig. 13.8). Depending on whether stem cell transplantation (SCT) is planned and on patient recovery, one to four courses of consolidation with, e.g. high-dose cytarabine, are given. A typical good response in AML is shown in Fig. 13.11. CNS prophylaxis is not usually given.

3 Allogeneic SCT is considered in first remission in patients with poor or intermediate risk disease (Table 13.5). This is based on a balance of the risk of relapse versus transplant-related mortality (Table 13.6). As intermediate and adverse risk disease constitutes the majority of patients over the age of 40, patients deemed fit should have CMV serology recorded, and tissue typing with an unrelated / sibling donor search initiated at diagnosis (Chapter 25). Allogeneic SCT is not used for patients in the favourable risk group unless they have disease relapse or poor response via MRD monitoring.

4 Reduced-intensity conditioning regimens have raised the age at which patients may be considered for SCT. Potential donors are discussed in Chapter 25, but due to results with

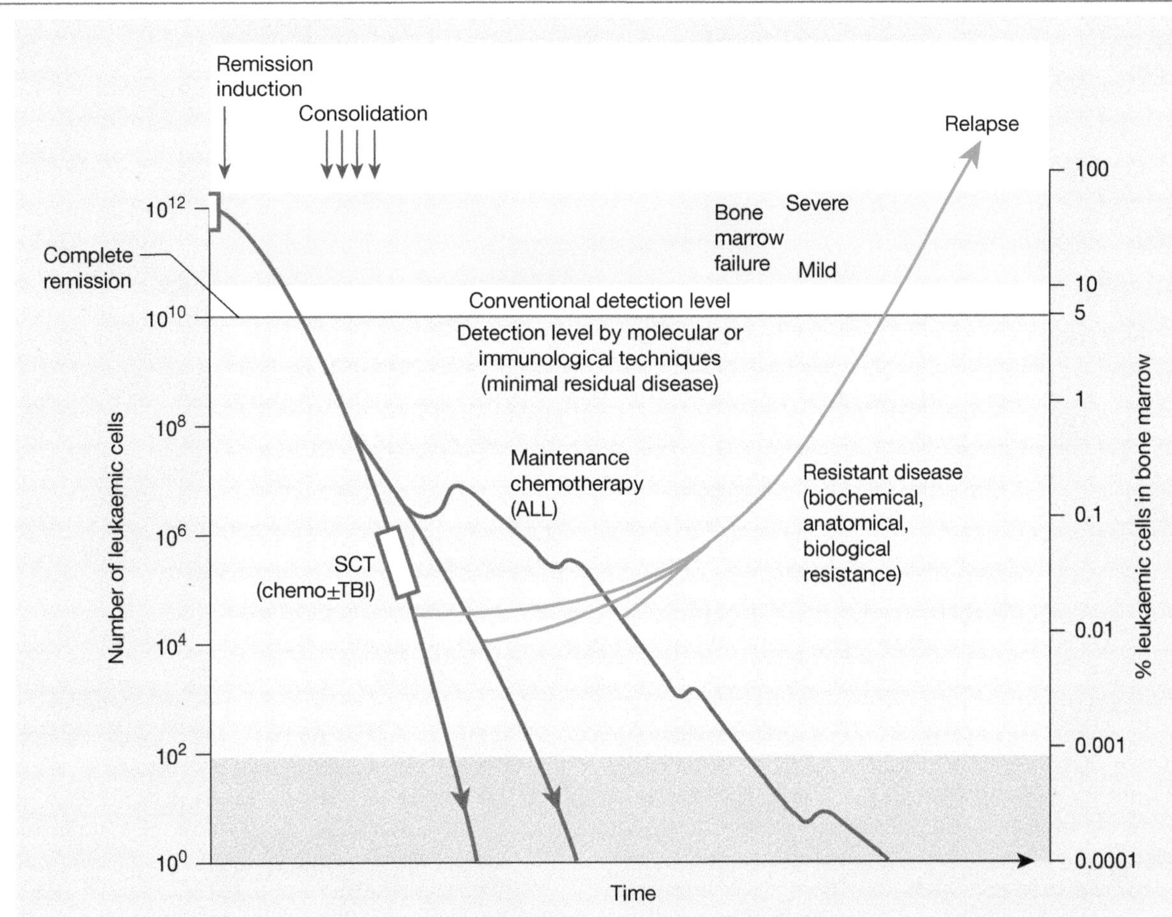

Figure 13.8 Acute leukaemia: principles of therapy for acute myeloid leukaemia or acute lymphoid leukaemia (ALL). The decision for stem cell transplantation (SCT) in remission is based on prognostic factors as well as tests for minimal residual disease (Table 13.5). TBI, total body irradiation.

Table 13.6 A table to demonstrate selection of patients for allogenic-SCT (Allo-SCT) with estimated relapse risk with and without transplant and estimate of incidence of non-relapse mortality (NRM) following allo-SCT.

		Estimated risk of relapse following consolidation with:		Maximal tolerated NRM prognostic scores for allo-SCT to be considered:	
2022 ELN risk stratification	**MRD after cycle 2 chemotherapy**	**Chemotherapy alone (%)**	**Allo- SCT (%)**	**HCT-CI score**	**NRM risk (%)**
Favourable	Negative	30	15–20	N/A (not advisable to proceed)	
	Positive	75	30–40	≤3–4	<30
Intermediate	Negative	55	25–30	≤2	<20
	Positive	75	35	≤3–4	<30
Adverse	N/A	>90	50	≤5	<35

HCT-CI, Hematopoietic Cell Transplantation-Comorbidity Index; MRD, measurable residual disease.
Source: Adapted from J. Loke *et al.* (2020) *Br. J. Haematol.* 188: 129–46.

Table 13.7 Drugs used for treatment of acute myeloid leukaemia (AML) or acute promyelocytic leukaemia (APML).

Class	Examples
Anti-metabolites/nucleoside analogues	Cytarabine (Ara-C), methotrexate, hydroxycarbamide
Cytotoxics	Daunorubicin, idarubicin, mitoxantrone, CPX-351 (Vyxeos®)
Topoisomerase inhibitors	Etoposide, daunorubicin, idarubicin
DNA hypomethylating agents	Azacitidine, decitabine
Epigenetic therapies	Ivosidenib (IDH1), enasidenib (IDH2), Menin inhibitors
Signalling inhibitors	Midostaurin, gilteritinib (targets multiple tyrosine kinases including FLT3), venetoclax (BCL-2), glasdegib (Hedgehog pathway)
Differentiating agents	All-*trans* retinoic acid (ATRA), arsenic trioxide
Monoclonal antibodies	Gemtuzumab ozogamicin (anti-CD33 conjugated to calicheamicin cytotoxin), tagraxofusp (anti-CD123 conjugated to toxin)

alternative donors including haploidentical donors or umbilical stem cell source, patients should rarely be without a stem cell source. Autologous transplantation confers no benefit above that of post-remission chemotherapy.

5 **Specific therapy of AML** is determined by the age and performance status of the patient, as well as the genetic lesions within the tumour. In younger patients, intensive chemotherapy is usual. This is given in several blocks, each of approximately one week. The most frequently used drugs are cytarabine and daunorubicin (Fig. 13.9). Standard induction regimens include:
   (a) Daunorubicin and cytarabine, e.g. DA 3 + 7; 3 + 10.
   (b) Liposomal nanoparticle preparation of a fixed 5: 1 ratio of cytarabine and daunorubicin, CPX-351 (Vyxeos), in patients with secondary AML or AML with myelodysplasia-related changes.
   (c) FLAG-IDA (fludarabine, high-dose cytarabine, G-CSF and idarubicin) may be used in high-risk patients including, those with relapsed disease.
   (d) The monoclonal immune-conjugate targeted against CD33, gemtuzumab-ozogamicin (GO) provides an additional therapeutic option in combination with, e.g. DA chemotherapy for initial or consolidation AML therapy, particularly in patients with favourable risk features including t(8;21) and inv(16), where it has become standard of care.
   (e) FLT3 inhibitor, e.g. midostaurin, is given with front line DA chemotherapy in patients with *FLT3* mutated AML.

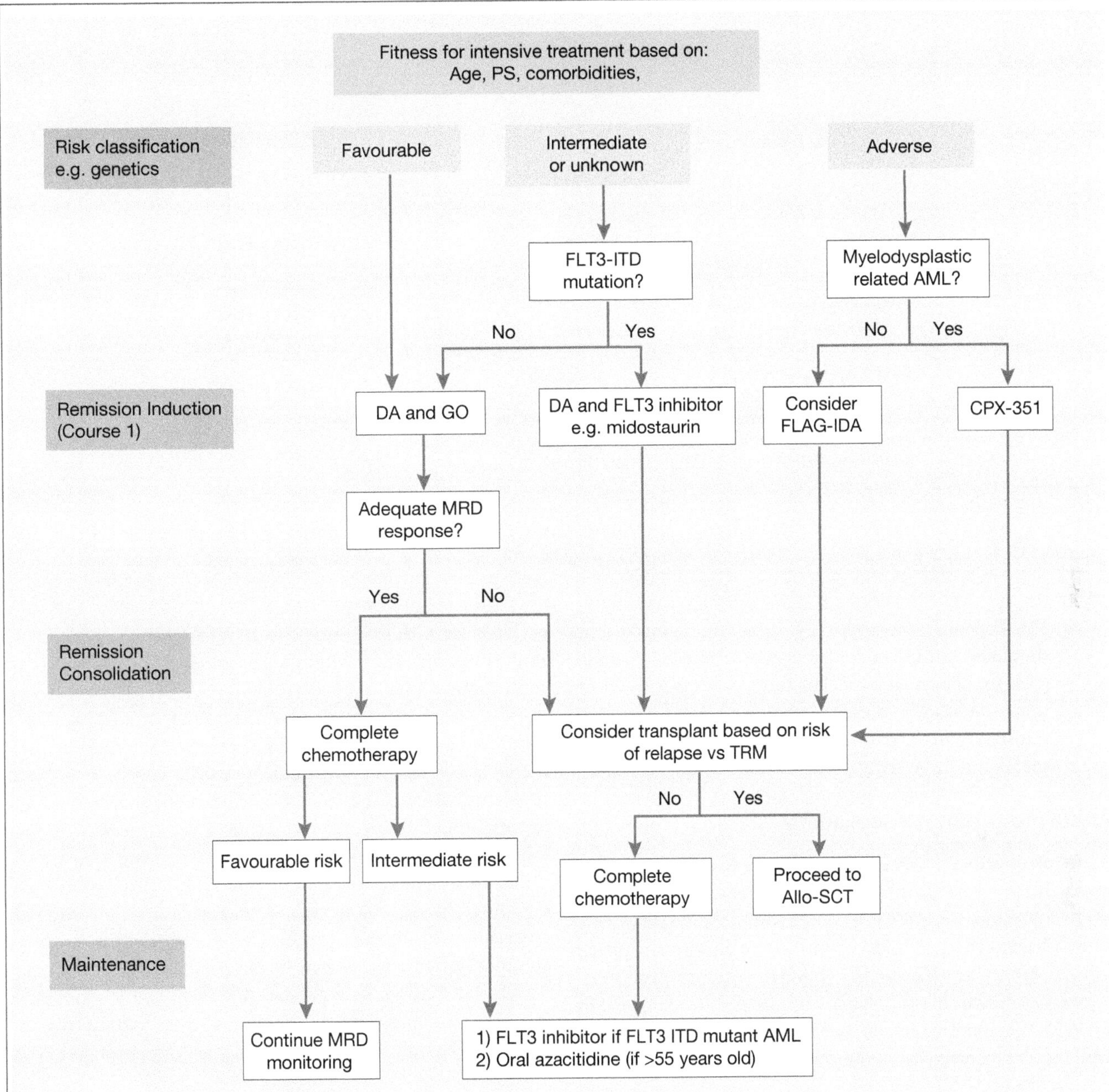

Figure 13.9 Acute myeloid leukaemia: flow chart illustrating treatment regimens for fit patients who can tolerate intensive induction. Incorporating MRD monitoring (not available in all centres). Remission consolidation for patients who achieve CR. Patients who do not achieve a CR after course 1 a further course of treatment may induce a remission. Conditioning for allogeneic stem cell transplant may be reduced intensity or myeloablative, depending on patient factors. Allo-SCT, allogeneic stem cell transplant; DA, daunorubicin and cytarabine; GO, gemtuzumab ozogamicin; MRD, measurable residual disease; PS, performance status; SCT, stem cell transplantation; TRM, transplant related mortality.

(f) In patients unfit for intensive treatment due to age or comorbidities, venetoclax with an hypomethylating agent (HMA), azacitidine or decitabine, is the standard of care (Fig. 13.10). Commencement of this regimen requires WBC $<25 \times 10^9$/L. Monitoring of tumour lysis syndrome remains important. Targeted therapies such as ivosidenib (for *IDH1* mutated AML), together with HMA have a role. Less intensive therapy includes single-agent HMA, low-dose subcutaneous cytarabine or *IDH1* or *IDH2* inhibitors. Omitting venetoclax reduces the risk of severe neutropenia with infection, but these single-drug therapies are less likely to achieve remission or prolong survival. They may be of some benefit, especially in the context of low blast count AML.

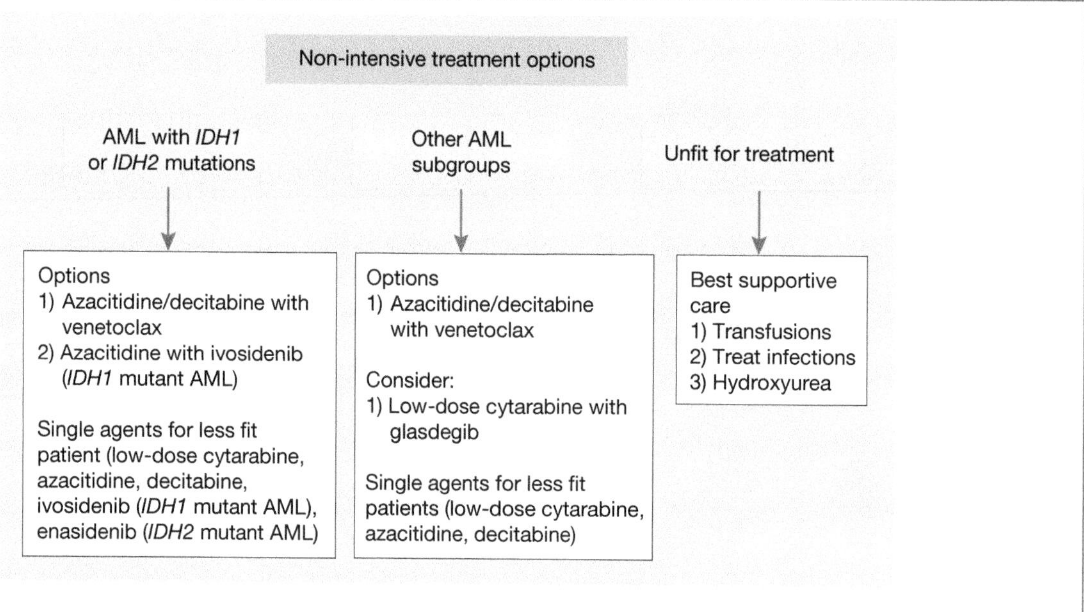

Figure 13.10 Non-intensive treatment pathways for treatment of patients with AML. Not all treatments are available internationally.

(g) Maintenance chemotherapy with oral azacitidine should be considered for patients over 55 who are ineligible for allogeneic SCT. For those patients with *FLT3* mutant AML who do not receive an allogeneic stem cell transplant, maintenance therapy with an FLT3 inhibitor should be given.

Acute promyelocytic leukaemia

Acute promyelocytic leukaemia (APML) is a clinical emergency. It requires urgent treatment with induction ATRA and of the associated coagulopathy. Suspicion of APML may arise from a haemorrhagic clinical phenotype or abnormal clotting profile. Alongside characteristic bilobed hypergranular morphology of APML blasts diagnosis can be confirmed by FISH for t(15;17) abnormality on bone marrow. The presence of PML bodies by immunostain may also be useful. A hypogranular variant of APML also exists.

APML has its own treatment protocol. A haemorrhagic syndrome can lead to catastrophic haemorrhage and may be present either at diagnosis or develop in the first few days of treatment and is the major cause of early mortality. Treatment must take place as an emergency both to treat the coagulopathy and the underlying leukaemia. APML is treated as for disseminated intravascular coagulation (DIC) with multiple platelet transfusions and replacement of clotting factors with cryoprecipitate or fresh frozen plasma (Chapter 29) with close monitoring of coagulation profile, keeping platelet count >30–50 × 10^9/L, fibrinogen >1.5 g/L with cryoprecipitate and correct APTT ratio and INR to <1.5.

In addition, ATRA therapy is given for this disease subtype and is combined initially with either arsenic trioxide (ATO) or an anthracycline. The arsenic combination gives a better clinical response with fewer side effects. ATRA should be available as an emergency stock within the hospital and be given prior to confirmatory tests.

Differentiation syndrome (also known as ATRA syndrome though it can occur with arsenic and other agents) is a complication that may arise during APML treatment. Clinical problems, which result from the neutrophilia that follows differentiation of promyelocytes, include fever, hypoxia with pulmonary infiltrates and fluid overload (presenting with weight gain). Treatment is with steroids and ATRA/ATO is only discontinued in very severe cases. **Leucocytosis** is also observed, especially with the use of ATO. Use of anthracycline or, more commonly, hydroxyurea may be of benefit.

Overall outlook for patients following initial induction is extremely positive. Molecular disease monitoring by *PML::RARA* transcripts in bone marrow aspirates following induction should be undertaken.

Prognosis and treatment stratification

The outcome for an individual patient with AML will depend on a number of factors, including age and white cell count at presentation (Table 13.5) and importantly genetic stratification. Following treatment, MRD monitoring is particularly important for patients with favourable and intermediate risk disease. Notably, results of cytogenetic and NGS results may occur at different timescales but should be available at the end of induction, particularly for patients treated as an emergency.

The initial goal is to achieve a complete remission defined as less than 5% marrow blasts without Auer rods, neutrophil count greater than 1.0 × 10^9/L, platelets greater than 100 × 10^9/L, independence of red cell transfusions and no extramedullary disease. In some patients, blast clearance may occur without bone marrow recovery. These patients with aplasia require special management.

AML therapy is selected according to the individual patient's **risk group**. Favourable cytogenetics and remission after one course of chemotherapy both predict for a better prognosis. In contrast, chromosome 5 or 7 abnormalities, blast cells with the *FLT3* internal tandem duplication mutation or other mutations including *TP53*, or poorly responsive disease places patients in poor-risk groups which need more intensive treatments (Table 13.5).

Minimal residual disease

Monitoring of minimal (measurable) residual disease (MRD) during and after chemotherapy is important in monitoring response to treatment and prognosis especially in patients with favourable or intermediate risk disease (Fig. 13.12).

Methodologies include:

(a) Molecular tests (Fig. 13.11) are highly sensitive but restricted to certain genetic subtypes, e.g. quantitative-PCR of fusion transcripts *RUNX1::RUNX1T1*, *CBFB::MYH11* and mutant *NPM1*.

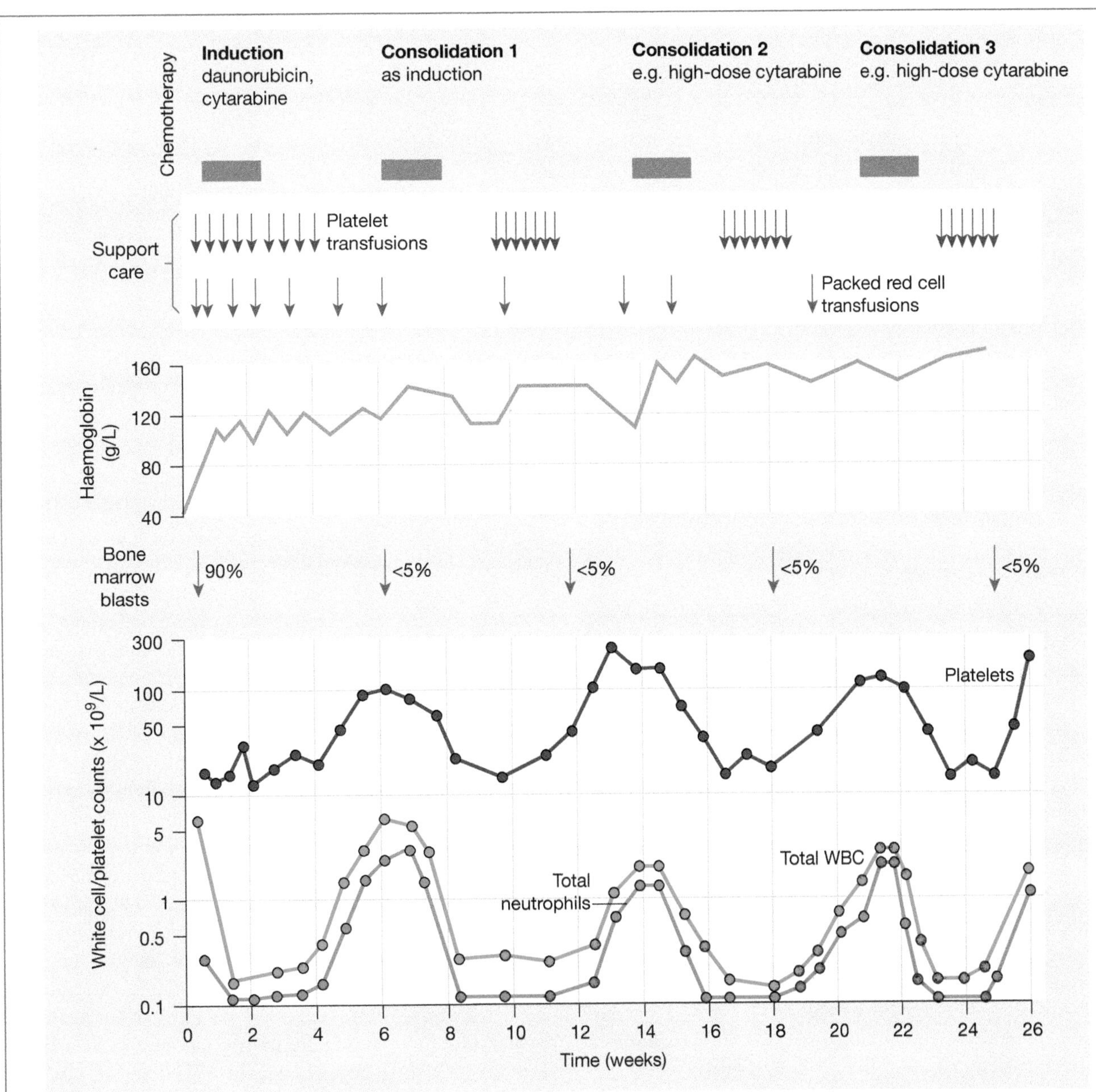

Figure 13.11 Typical flow chart for the management with chemotherapy of acute myeloid leukaemia. WBC, white blood cells.

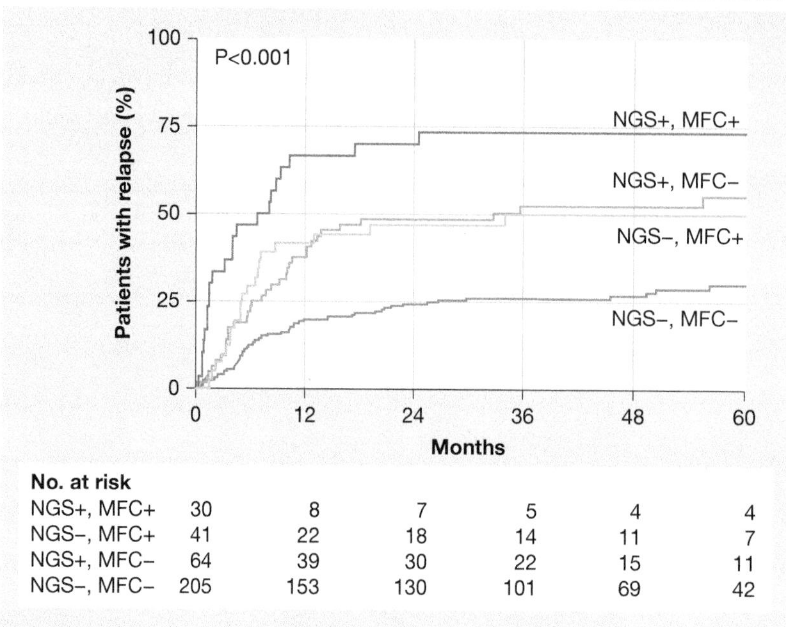

Figure 13.12 Minimal residual disease is a risk factor for relapse in AML. Depicted here is the cumulative incidence of relapse for patients in clinical complete remission, stratified by positive (+) or negative (−) results for persistent non-*DTA* (*DNMT3A*, *TET2*, *ASXL1*) mutations on next-generation sequencing (NGS) and multiparameter flow cytometry (MFC). Source: M. Jongen-Lavrencic *et al.* (2018) *N. Engl. J. Med.* 378: 1189–99. Reproduced with permission of Massachusetts Medical Society.

(b) Multiparametric flow cytometry of the abnormal immunophenotype is widely applicable and seen in over 90% of cases (Fig. 13.12).

(c) Emerging use of error corrected NGS is limited by the detection of residual mutations seen in clonal haemopoesis of indeterminate potential (CHIP, Chapter 16).

Treatment of relapse

Relapse is the major cause of treatment failure in patients with AML. The outlook following relapse from first remission depends on age, FLT3-ITD status, the duration of the first remission, the cytogenetic risk group and the availability of a suitable donor. For some patients with a suitable donor, immediate resort to allogeneic SCT without chemotherapy aimed at obtaining a second remission may be the best route. Traditionally further chemotherapy to try to obtain a second remission, allogeneic SCT with either standard or reduced-intensity conditioning has been performed for those patients who can tolerate these procedures. Regimens not used prior to relapse, such as FLAG-IDA, may be an option for fit patients. For patients with *FLT3* mutations, gilteritinib may induce a second remission prior to transplantation. Exactly which patients should receive second-line 'salvage' therapy before SCT and which should be offered SCT without re-induction therapy requires further clinical trials. Other "targeted" treatment (also used for front line treatment in elderly, see below) may have a role, e.g. for patients with mutations of *IDH1* or *IDH2*.

Patients unfit for intensive chemotherapy

The decision to opt for non-intensive chemotherapy is based on an assessment of patient's age, comorbidities, and performance status. The median age for presentation of AML is approximately 65 years and treatment outcomes in the elderly are poor because of primary disease resistance and reduced tolerability of intensive treatment protocols. Death from haemorrhage, infection or failure of the heart, kidneys or other organs is more frequent than in younger patients. However, some patients older than 70 may still remain fit for intensive chemotherapy and SCT. In elderly patients with serious disease of other organs, the decision may be made to use supportive care alone. As mentioned above the combination of azacitidine or decitabine with venetoclax gives more frequent remissions and longer overall survival than azacitidine, decitabine or low-dose subcutaneous cytarabine or supportive care alone. This has made venetoclax with hypomethylating agents (HMAs) an option even in younger patients with reduced performance status or other comorbidities. Indeed, the increased survival and remission rates may allow patients who were unfit for intensive chemotherapy to subsequently undergo a reduced intensity conditioned allogeneic stem cell transplant. The combination of venetoclax and HMA does cause more episodes of neutropenia and infection and need for transfusion support than HMA alone. Specific drugs targeted against IDH1 may also be used front line in combination with HMA in those patients with the corresponding mutation. Single-agent HMA, low dose cytarabine, or targeted treatment, e.g. IDH1 or 2 inhibitors, retain a role for less fit patients. The availability of many of these targeted agents vary internationally. FLT3 inhibitor use in association with HMA continues to undergo development.

Paediatric AML

AML is less common in children than ALL. In paediatric AML, the spectrum of genetic mutation drivers differs from adults (Fig. 13.13). Within the paediatric population mutations differ according to age, for example there is an increased prevalence of *KMT2A* fusion mutations in infancy as compared to adolescence. Overall survival is superior to that in adults (~75% at 5 years). Treatment schedules follow similar principles, but with fewer children requiring allogeneic stem cell transplant and fewer novel agents currently licensed for the paediatric population.

Outcome

The prognosis for patients with AML has been improving steadily, particularly for those under 60 years of age, and approximately one-third of this group can expect to achieve long-term cure (Fig. 13.14a). For those unfit for intensive therapy, the situation is poorer, and less than 20% of those over 70 years of age achieve long-term remission (Fig. 13.14b).

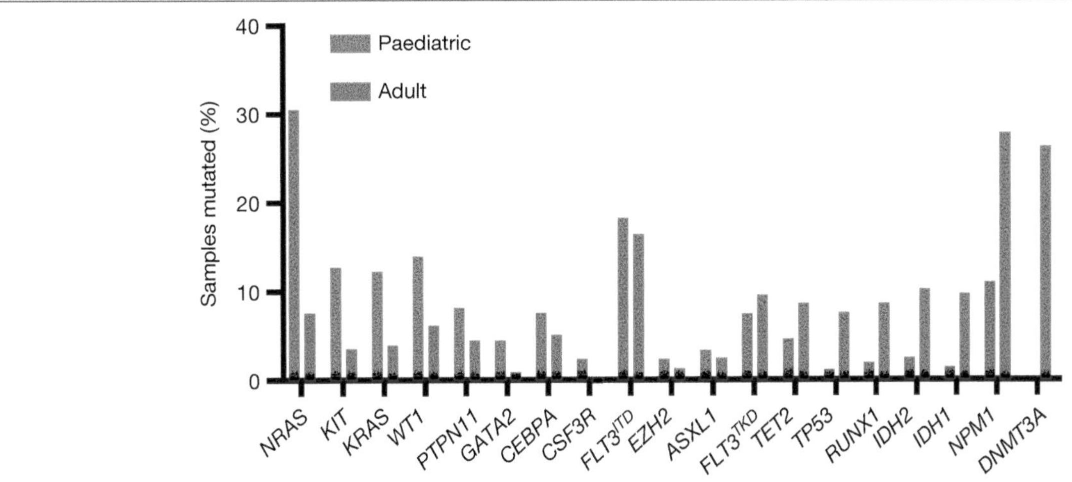

Figure 13.13 Prevalence of somatic mutations in paediatric versus adult cases of AML. Source: Adapted from H. Bolouri *et al.* (2018) *Nature Medicine* 24: 103–12. S. Charrot *et al.* (2019) *Br. J. Haematol.* 188: 49–62.

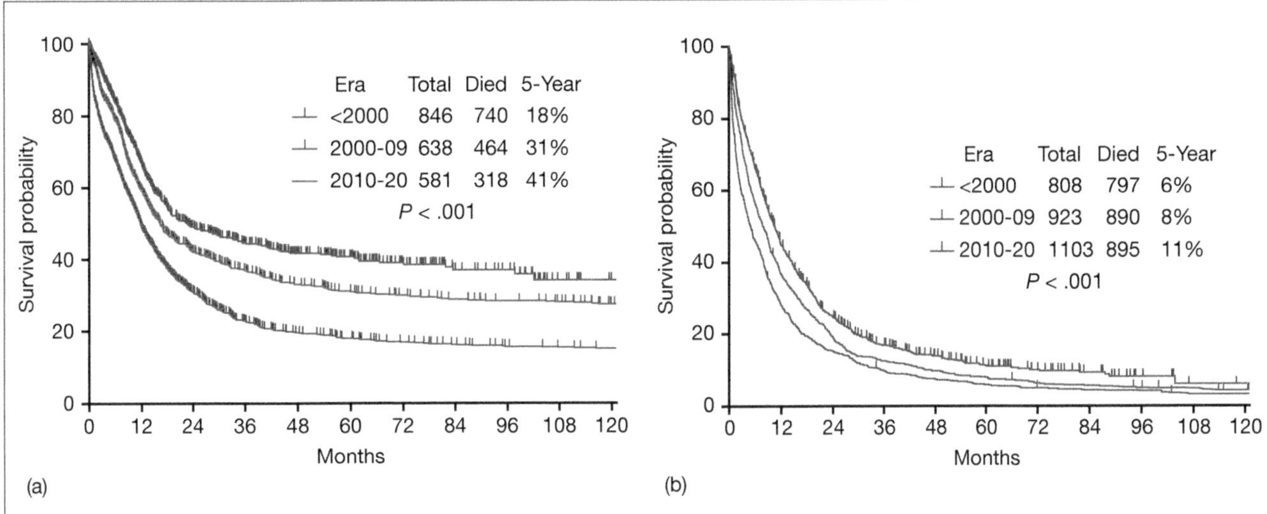

Figure 13.14 Survival of **(a)** younger patients (<60 years old) and **(b)** older patients (≥60 years old) with *de novo* acute myeloid leukemia treated at MD Anderson over five decades. Source: H.M. Kantarjian *et al.* (2021) *Cancer* 127: 1186–207. Reproduced with permission of John Wiley & Sons.

SUMMARY

- The leukaemias are a group of disorders characterized by the accumulation of malignant white cells in the bone marrow and blood. They can be classified into four subtypes on the basis of being either *acute* or *chronic*, and *myeloid* or *lymphoid*.
- Acute leukaemias are aggressive diseases in which transformation of a haemopoietic stem cell leads to accumulation of blast cells in the bone marrow.
- The clinical features of acute leukaemia mainly result from bone marrow failure and include anaemia, infection and bleeding. Tissue infiltration can also occur.
- Acute myeloid leukaemia (AML) is rare in childhood, but becomes increasingly common with age, with a median onset of 65 years.
- The disease may arise *de novo* or result from transformation of a previous bone marrow neoplastic disease, e.g. myelodysplasia, myeloproliferative disease.
- The diagnosis is made by analysis of blood and bone marrow using microscopic examination (morphology) as well as immunophenotypic, cytogenetic and molecular studies.
- Cytogenetic and molecular abnormalities are used to classify and indicate prognosis in the majority of cases of AML.
- In younger patients treatment is primarily with intensive chemotherapy. This is usually given in three or four blocks, each of approximately one week using drugs such as cytarabine and daunorubicin. The blood count must be given time to recover before the next block of therapy can be given and this can typically take 4–6 weeks.
- Acute promyelocytic leukaemia is a variant of AML that carries a t(15;17) chromosomal translocation. It commonly presents with disseminated intravascular coagulation with life-threatening bleeding and is treated with retinoic acid (ATRA) and arsenic or chemotherapy.
- Minimal/measurable residual disease after chemotherapy or stem cell transplantation is detected by molecular genetic or multi-parameter flow cytometry. It is important for indicating prognosis and whether further treatment is needed.
- The prognosis for patients with AML has been improving steadily, particularly for those under 60 years of age, and approximately one-third of this group can expect to achieve long-term cure.
- The outcome for elderly people remains disappointing but has improved for selected patients who receive initial therapy with azacitidine or decitabine and venetoclax, with the introduction of targeted drugs to specific mutations if present, and with azacitidine maintenance.
- Children have an improved 5-year survival (75%) and overall cure rate compared to adults.
- New drugs targeting specific signal transduction pathways and other gene mutations have been introduced for treating relapsed disease and for front line therapy.
- Allogeneic stem cell transplantation is useful in treating some subsets of patients in first remission after initial courses of chemotherapy and may also be curative for patients with relapsed disease.

Now visit **www.wiley.com/go/haematology9e** to test yourself on this chapter.

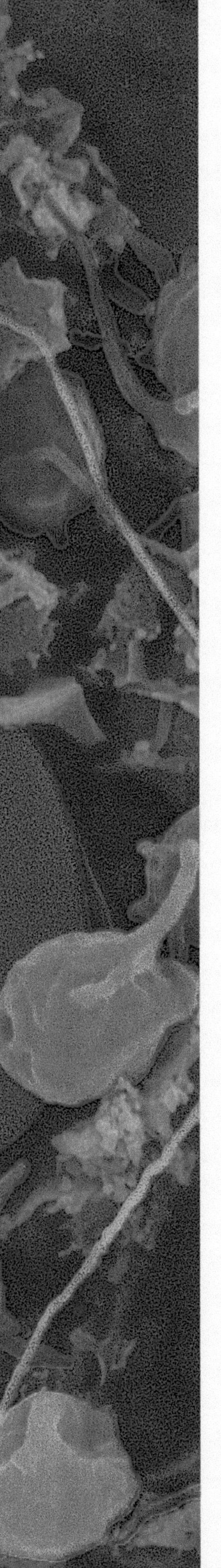

CHAPTER 14

Chronic myeloid leukaemia

Key topics

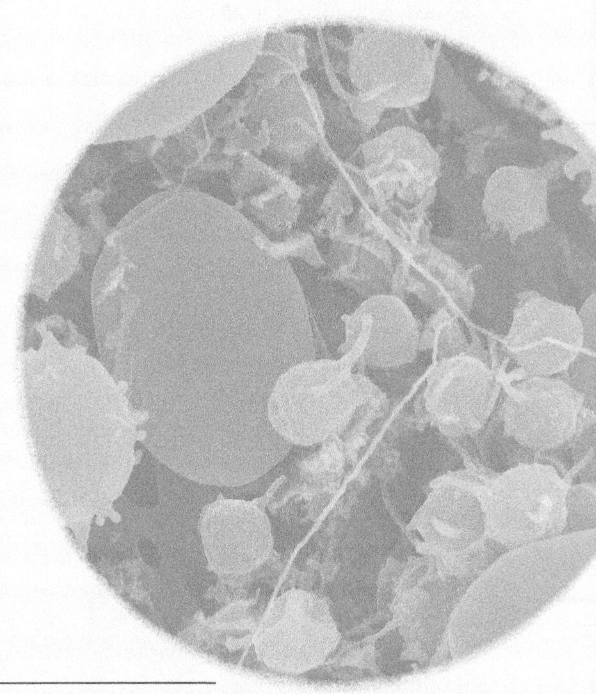

Hoffbrand's Essential Haematology, Ninth Edition. A. Victor Hoffbrand, Pratima Chowdary, Graham P. Collins, and Justin Loke.

© 2024 John Wiley & Sons Ltd. Published 2024 by John Wiley & Sons Ltd.

Companion website: www.wiley.com/go/haematology9e

The chronic leukaemias are distinguished from acute leukaemias by their slower progression; with currently available treatments, most patients with chronic leukaemias will live many years. The World Health Organization (WHO) 2022 classification of the myeloproliferative neoplasms (Table 15.1) includes chronic myeloid leukaemia *BCR::ABL1* positive (CML), discussed here, the non-leukaemic myeloproliferative neoplasms, rare chronic neutrophilic, eosinophilic and juvenile myelo-monocytic leukaemias, described in Chapter 15.

Chronic myeloid leukaemia

Chronic myeloid leukaemia, *BCR::ABL1* rearrangement positive (CML) is a clonal disorder of a pluripotent stem cell. The disease accounts for around 15% of leukaemias and may occur at any age. The diagnosis of CML is rarely difficult and is assisted by the characteristic presence of the **Philadelphia (Ph) chromosome**. This results from the t(9,22)(q34;q11) translocation between chromosomes 9 and 22, as a result of which part of the oncogene *ABL1* is moved to the *BCR* gene on chromosome 22 (Fig. 14.1a) and part of chromosome 22 moves to chromosome 9. The abnormal chromosome 22 is the Ph chromosome; the variant chromosome 9 does not have a specific name. In the Ph translocation 5′ exons of *BCR* are fused to the 3′ exons of *ABL1* (Fig. 14.1b, c).

The resulting chimeric *BCR::ABL1* gene usually codes for a fusion protein of size 210 kDa (p210). This has constitutively active tyrosine kinase activity in excess of the normal 145 kDa ABL1 product, resulting in uncontrolled cell proliferation.

The Ph translocation is also seen in a minority of cases of acute lymphoblastic leukaemia (ALL), and in some of these the breakpoint in *BCR* occurs in the same region as in CML (Chapter 17). However, in other cases of ALL, the breakpoint in *BCR* is further upstream, in the intron between the first and second exons, leaving only the first *BCR* exon intact. This chimeric *BCR::ABL1* gene is expressed as a p190 protein which, like p210, has enhanced tyrosine kinase activity. The p190 protein is not seen in CML. Rarely, other fusion proteins occur from different fusions, such as a p230 variant, but many clinical laboratories are unable to test for these.

In most patients the Ph chromosome is seen by karyotypic examination of neoplastic cells (Fig. 14.1d), but in a few the Ph abnormality cannot be seen under the microscope, although the same molecular rearrangement is detectable by more sensitive techniques: fluorescence *in situ* hybridization (FISH; Fig. 14.1e) or reverse transcriptase PCR (RT–PCR) for *BCR::ABL1* transcripts. This Ph-negative *BCR::ABL1*-positive CML behaves clinically like Ph-positive CML, since the molecular driver is identical. *BCR::ABL1*-negative atypical chronic myeloid leukaemia is a distinct disease, classified with the myelodysplastic/myeloproliferative syndromes (Chapter 16).

The Ph chromosome is an acquired abnormality of haemopoietic stem cells, so it is typically found in cells of both the myeloid (granulocytic, erythroid and megakaryocytic) and lymphoid (B and T cell) lineages. The main cause of death in CML is transformation to a blast phase, which may have myeloid or lymphoid markers, and may be preceded by an accelerated phase. These are discussed later in this chapter. The prognosis for patients with CML has been vastly improved with introduction of tyrosine kinase inhibitors (TKIs) which have improved overall survival of patients to near normal levels.

Clinical features

CML occurs in either sex (male : female ratio of 1.4 : 1), most frequently between the ages of 40 and 60 years. However, it may occur in children and neonates, as well as in the very old. In up to 50% of cases the diagnosis is made incidentally from a routine blood count. In those cases where the disease presents clinically, the following features may be seen:

1 Symptoms related to hypermetabolism, e.g. weight loss, lassitude, anorexia or night sweats.
2 Splenomegaly is nearly always present and may be massive. In some patients, splenic enlargement is associated with considerable abdominal discomfort, pain or indigestion.
3 Features of anaemia may include pallor, dyspnoea and tachycardia.
4 Bruising, epistaxis, menorrhagia or haemorrhage from other sites because of abnormal platelet function.
5 Gout or renal impairment caused by hyperuricaemia from excessive purine breakdown may be a problem.
6 Rare symptoms include visual disturbances and priapism.

Laboratory findings

1 Leucocytosis is the main feature and may reach levels greater than 200×10^9/L (Fig. 14.2). A complete spectrum of myeloid cells is seen in the peripheral blood film. The levels of neutrophils and myelocytes exceed those of blast cells and promyelocytes (Fig. 14.3). An important differential is a leukaemoid reaction resulting in high white blood cell counts, but with different neutrophil morphology and spectrum of leucocytes.
2 Increased circulating basophils is a characteristic feature.
3 Normochromic normocytic anaemia is usual.
4 Platelet count may be increased (most frequently), normal or decreased.
5 Bone marrow is hypercellular with granulocytic predominance.
6 Presence of the *BCR::ABL1* gene fusion detected by RT–PCR analysis; in 98% of cases Ph chromosome on cytogenetic analysis (Fig. 14.1d).
7 Serum uric acid is usually raised.

Bone marrow examination may not be essential to make a diagnosis but is frequently performed as it provides a full karyotype analysis and is important in confirming the disease phase (differentiating chronic phase from blast or accelerated phase). Other initial assessment should include cardiovascular tests (ECG, lipid and glucose

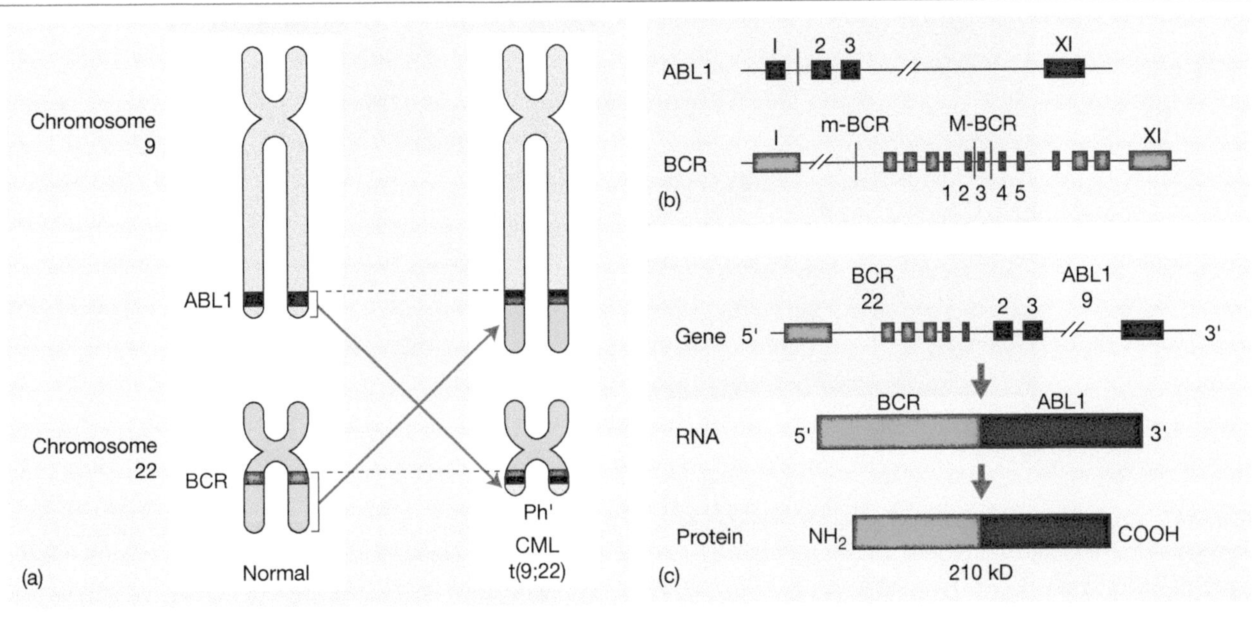

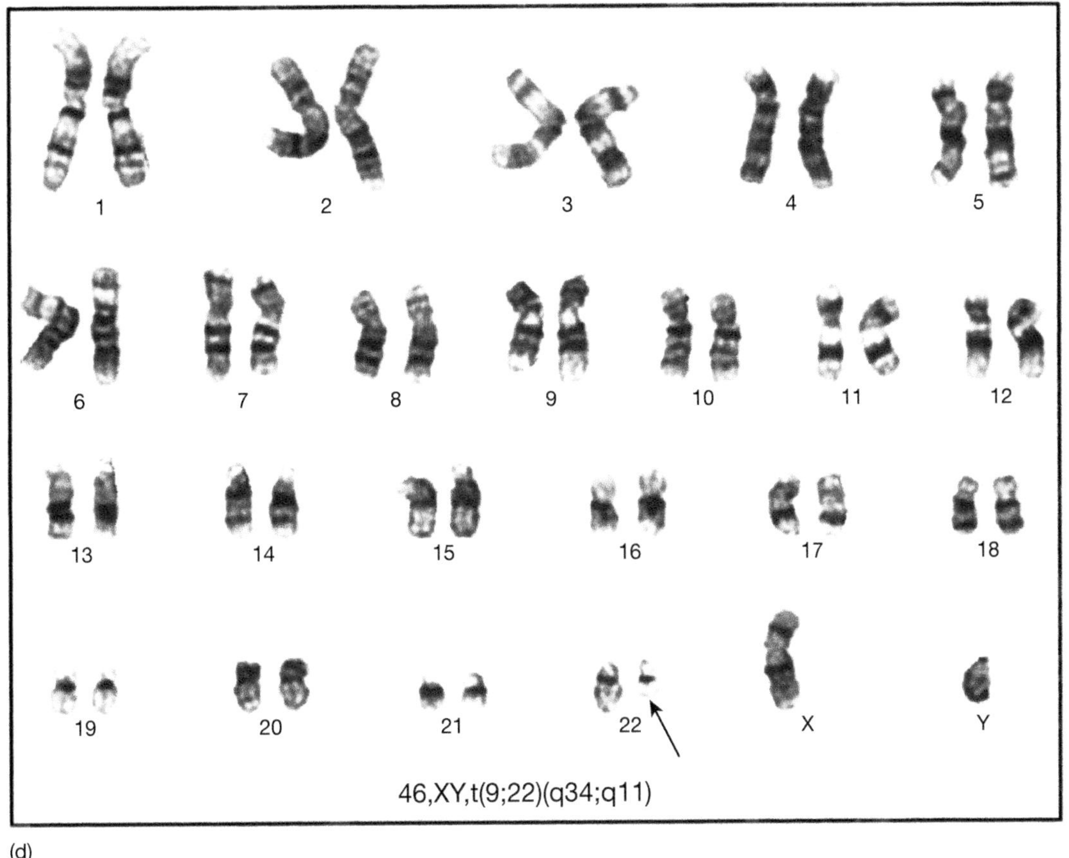

Figure 14.1 The Philadelphia chromosome. **(a)** There is translocation of part of the long arm of chromosome 22 to the long arm of chromosome 9 and reciprocal translocation of part of the long arm of chromosome 9 to chromosome 22 (the Philadelphia chromosome). This reciprocal translocation brings most of the *ABL1*-gene into the *BCR* region on chromosome 22 (and part of the *BCR* gene into juxtaposition with the remaining portion of *ABL* on chromosome 9). **(b)** The breakpoint in *ABL1* is between exons 1 and 2. The breakpoint in *BCR* is at one of the two points in the major breakpoint cluster region (*M-BCR*) in chronic myeloid leukaemia (CML) or in some cases of Ph+ acute lymphoblastic leukaemia (ALL). **(c)** This results in a 210-kDa fusion protein product derived from the *BCR::ABL1* fusion gene. In other cases of Ph+ ALL, the breakpoint in *BCR* is at a minor breakpoint cluster region *(m-BCR)*, resulting in a smaller *BCR::ABL1* fusion gene and a 190 kDa protein. **(d)** Karyotype showing the t(9,22) (q34;q11) translocation. The Ph chromosome is arrowed.

(Continued)

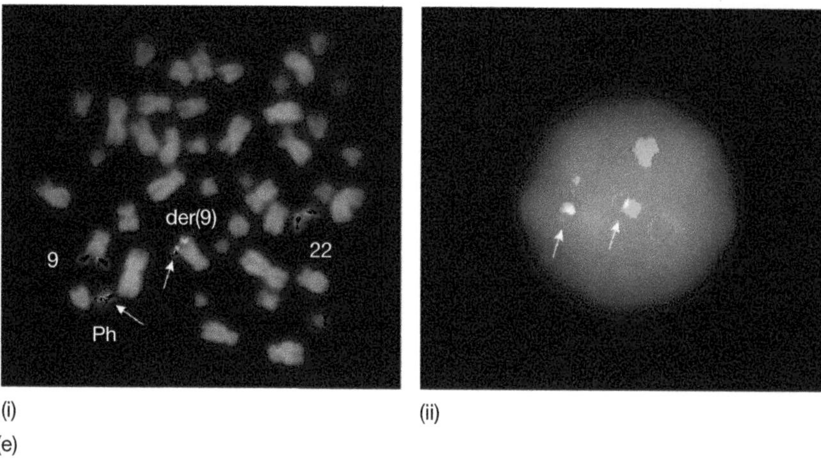

Figure 14.1 *(Continued)* **(e)** Visualization of the Ph chromosome on (i) dividing (metaphase); and (ii) quiescent (interphase) cells by fluorescence *in situ* hybridization (FISH) analysis (ABL probe in red and BCR probe in green) with fusion signals (red/green which shows as yellow) on the Ph (*BCR::ABL1*) and der(9) (*ABL1::BCR*) chromosomes. Source: Courtesy of Dr Ellie Nacheva.

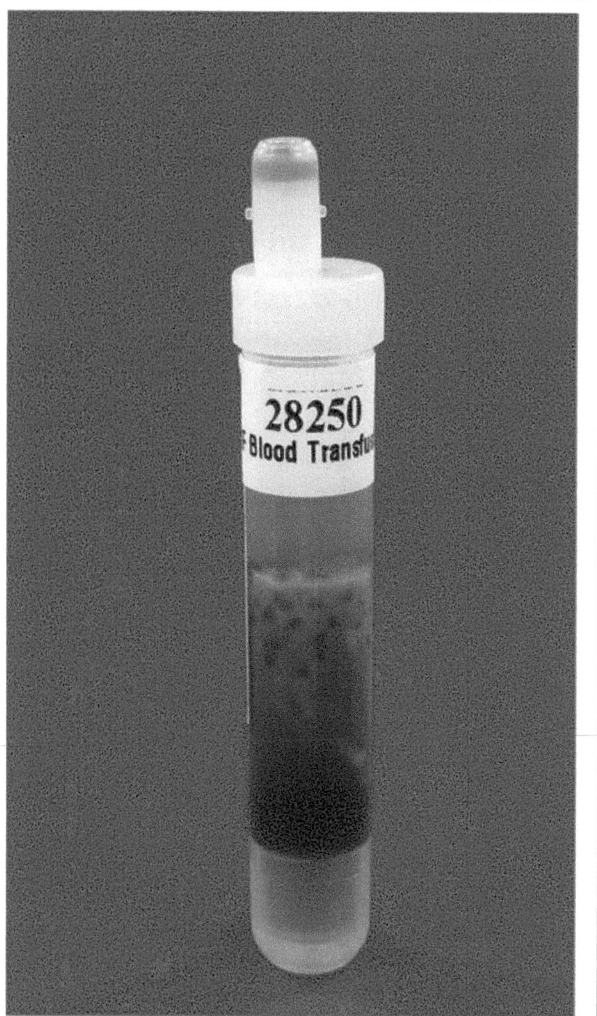

Figure 14.2 Chronic myeloid leukaemia: peripheral blood film showing a vast increase in buffy coat. The white cell count was 532×10^9/L.

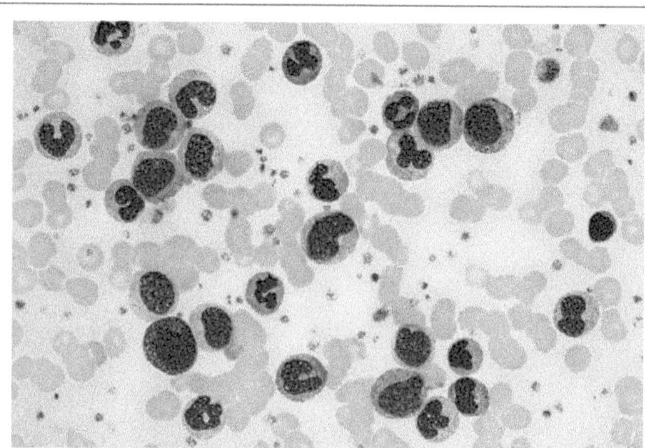

Figure 14.3 Chronic myeloid leukaemia: peripheral blood film showing various stages of granulopoiesis including promyelocytes, myelocytes, metamyelocytes and band and segmented neutrophils.

measurement) alongside hepatitis B and C test, with a view to TKI choice and initiation.

Accelerated phase disease and blast transformation

In an accelerated phase there may be an increase in blood basophils to greater than 20% or marrow/peripheral blood blast cells to 10–19% (Table 14.1). New clonal chromosomal or molecular abnormalities may appear, known as additional chromosomal abnormalities (ACA). Patients may present in this state or progress to accelerated phase whilst on therapy. The spleen may be enlarged despite control of the blood count and the marrow fibrotic. Patients in this phase are likely to have a suboptimal response to first generation TKIs alone, although a sustained response to a TKI is possible.

Table 14.1 WHO (2022) definition of advanced phase CML disease.

Accelerated phase
PB or BM blast 10–19%
PB basophils ≥20%
Increasing spleen size and increasing WBC count unresponsive to therapy
Clonal evolution on treatment
Platelets ≤100 × 10⁹/L unrelated to therapy
Platelets >1000 × 10⁹/L unresponsive to therapy
Blast crisis
PB or BM blast 20%
Extramedullary blast proliferation, apart from spleen
Large foci or clusters of blasts in the bone marrow biopsy
BM, bone marrow; PB, peripheral blood.

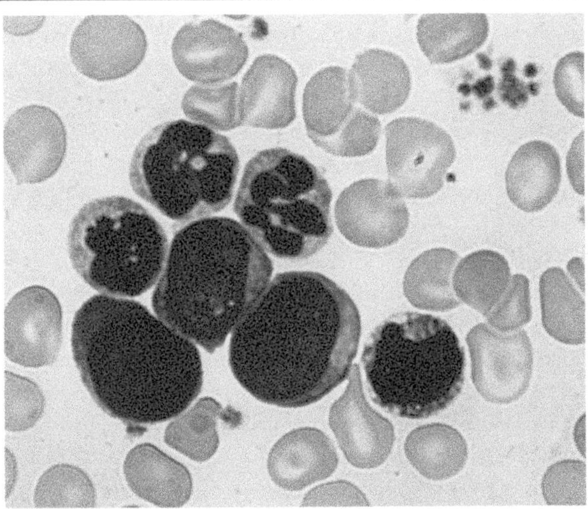

Figure 14.4 Chronic myeloid leukaemia: acute myeloblastic transformation. Peripheral blood film showing frequent myeloblasts.

Acute transformation (greater than 20% blasts in blood or marrow, either lymphoblasts or myeloblasts) may occur rapidly over days or weeks (Fig. **14.4**), this is known as blast crisis.

The presence of additional genetic mutations such as in *ASXL1, RUNX1* or *TP53* may be associated with increased risk of transformation. In approximately one-fifth of cases of acute transformation, this is lymphoblastic and patients may be treated in a similar way to ALL, with a number of patients returning to the chronic phase for months or even a year or two. In the majority, transformation is into acute myeloid leukaemia or mixed types. These are more difficult to treat and survival is rare beyond 1 year without SCT. TKIs are used in the management of blast transformation, but resistance usually occurs within a few weeks. Allogeneic SCT where possible is a valuable option.

Prognostic scores (stages)

Attempts have been made to stage CML at presentation in order to predict prognosis. In the past, the most frequently used were the Sokal, Hasford and EUTOS long-term survival scores, which took into account factors such as age, blast cell percentage, spleen size and platelet count. Scoring systems may be useful in providing guidance for initial TKI choice by identifying patients with more aggressive disease.

Treatment

Treatment of chronic phase

Tyrosine kinase inhibitors

TKIs that block the ATP binding site (Fig 14.5) are the mainstay of the treatment of CML and several different drugs are now available (Table 14.2). These have revolutionized the management of CML. Choice of initial TKI is a patient-specific decision. This is usually based on combination of disease, e.g. prognostic score, phase, and patient factors, e.g. age, comorbidities, parenthood plans. This allows a selection of initial TKI based on the side effect profile of each TKI (Table 14.2).

First-line therapy for patients with chronic phase CML is usually imatinib, nilotinib or dasatinib. Bosutinib is also available. Most experience exists with imatinib (Fig. 14.6), which is also the cheapest. Overall around 60% of patients given imatinib achieve an excellent response and remain on the drug long-term, whereas 40% proceed to a second-line agent due to intolerance or inadequate response.

Nilotinib and dasatinib achieve more rapid responses as first-line therapy and are therefore used first in some centres, although side effects are somewhat more common. They are also used as second-line therapy after imatinib (Fig. 14.7). Bosutinib is also an effective therapy, but alongside nilotinib is associated with QT prolongation. Ponatinib has the unique advantage that it is effective against CML that carries the T315I mutation within *ABL1*, but ponatinib is associated with the highest risk of thrombotic events.

Monitoring of response to tyrosine kinase inhibitors

TKIs are highly effective at reducing the number of neoplastic cells in the bone marrow and should be monitored by RT–PCR analysis for *BCR::ABL1* transcripts in marrow or blood, typically at 3, 6 and 12 months. Molecular response is assessed as the ratio of *BCR::ABL1* transcripts to *ABL1* transcripts and it is expressed as *BCR::ABL1*% on a log scale, where 10%, 1%, 0.1%, 0.01% and 0.001% correspond to a decrease of 1, 2, 3, 4 and 5 logs, respectively, below the standard baseline (Fig. 14.6).

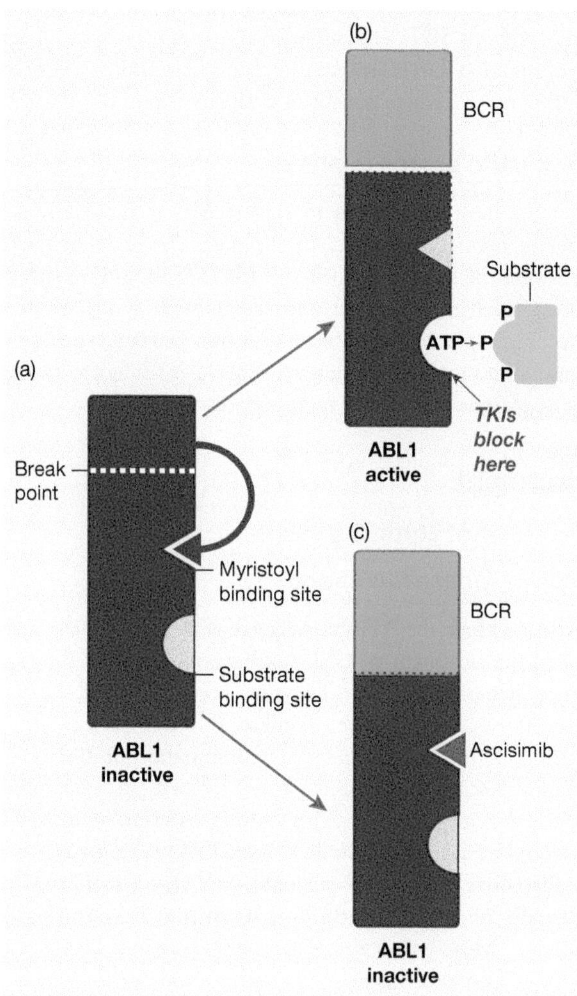

Figure 14.5 Mode of action of tyrosine kinase inhibitors (TKIs: imatinib, nilotinib, dasatinib, ponatinib, bosutinib) and of asciminib. **(a)** In the unmutated *ABL1*, the myristoyl binding site can be engaged by the myristoylated N terminal (shown as a purple arrow), inhibiting ABL1 kinase activity. **(b)** Translocation loss of N-terminus of ABL1, results in constitutive activation of the tyrosine kinase activity. TKIs block the adenosine triphosphate (ATP) binding site of ABL1, preventing phosphorylation of substrates. **(c)** Asciminib binds the myristoyl binding site, restoring auto-inhibition of ABL1 kinase function.

A major goal of therapy is achievement of a 'major molecular remission', defined as 3-log reduction (<0.1%) or better. Following a stable major molecular response (MMR) (*BCR::ABL1* ≤0.1%) monitoring intervals may be lengthened.

A complete cytogenetic response (CCyR) is defined as the absence of Ph-positive metaphases within bone marrow. Cytogenetic monitoring maintains a role in patients with uncommon transcripts/fusions which preclude molecular monitoring.

Treatment responses can be defined as **optimal** or **failure**, with an intermediate area termed **warning** (Table 14.3). Patients with optimal responses continue their original treatment, whereas those with treatment failure are treated with second-generation TKI therapy or stem cell transplantation (SCT). Patients in the warning zone should be monitored more regularly and might be considered for an early change in therapy or increase in the dose of first-line therapy. Patients who fail to achieve a *BCR::ABL1* transcript level of <10% (normalized to the International Standard) at the 3-month time point, so-called early molecular response (EMR), have a less favourable outlook.

BCR::ABL1 mutation screening

One mechanism of disease resistance to TKI therapy is selection for clones carrying mutations within the *BCR::ABL1* fusion gene, e.g. T315I. These mutations may be detected by sequencing the *ABL1* gene. The pattern of mutation can be useful for determining which treatment to choose as second-line therapy, since certain mutations confer specific resistance to one TKI while sensitivity to other TKIs persists. Indications for testing including treatment failure or warning during disease monitoring.

Response to TKI therapy and stopping therapy

TKI therapy is highly effective and after 5 years of treatment the progression-free survival is 85–90%, with overall survival over 90%. For patients becoming *BCR::ABL1* transcript negative, about 60% will remain negative on stopping TKI therapy or remain in remission with a stable low level of the transcripts. These patients are likely to be cured. Patients are selected based on previous disease history and a prolonged period of response to a TKI. Patients who stop TKI are closely monitored for loss of molecular response. For those who do become *BCR::ABL1* positive again with a rising level of transcripts, treatment with the TKI will usually result in restoration of disease control. This may have particular implications for female patients of child bearing age who may wish to discontinue TKI during pregnancy.

Additional forms of treatment for CML

Chemotherapy

Asciminib is a first-in-class drug that inhibits the enzyme activity of BCR::ABL1 by engaging its myristoyl binding site, rather than the ATP binding site (Fig 14.5). This leads to a conformational change in ABL1 so it no longer binds to substrate, e.g. downstream signalling pathway. Normally, the myristoyl binding site on ABL1 is blocked but this 'auto-blocking' is lost when *ABL1* is translocated: this results in a constitutive activation of ABL1 kinase activity. Asciminib is approved for patients who have failed two or more lines of treatment or have the T315I mutation. It is undergoing trials for earlier use or in combination with the TKIs that block the ATP binding site.

Hydroxycarbamide (hydroxyurea) treatment can control and maintain the white cell count in the chronic phase, but

Table 14.2 The tyrosine kinase inhibitors (TKIs) used for treatment of chronic myeloid leukaemia (CML).

	Action	Side effects	Role in clinical therapy
Imatinib	The first TKI, designed as a specific inhibitor of the BCR::ABL1 fusion protein. It blocks tyrosine kinase activity by competing with adenosine triphosphate (ATP) binding (Fig. 14.4).	Rash, nausea, myelosuppression, fluid retention, muscle cramps	First-line therapy. Occasional use in resistance/intolerance to other TKIs
Nilotinib	Second-generation inhibitor that has increased affinity for BCR::ABL1. Achieves molecular remission more rapidly than imatinib	Myelosuppression, peripheral vascular disease, headache, nausea, prolonged QT interval	First-line or resistance/ intolerance to first-line TKI
Dasatinib	Inhibits BCR::ABL and SRC family kinases, which play a role in driving CML progression	Headache, pleural effusion, pulmonary hypertension, cough, prolonged QT interval	First-line or resistance/ intolerance to first-line TKI
Bosutinib	BCR::ABL1 inhibitor with additional inhibitory effect on SRC family kinases	Diarrhoea, liver test abnormalities, nausea, low platelet count. Prolonged QT interval	First-line or resistance/ intolerance to first-line TKI
Ponatinib	Multitargeted TKI inhibitor	Low platelets, rash, dry skin, arterial and venous thrombosis	Resistance/intolerance to first-line TKI. The only TKI able to treat CML with the T315I mutation
Asciminib (ABL-001)	TKI inhibitor that, unlike others which bind to the ATPase site of ABL kinase, binds to the myristoyl site and thus may be active in treatment of patients with resistance to other TKIs	Rash, gastrointestinal upset, low counts	Resistance to other TKIs; may be used in combination with other TKIs

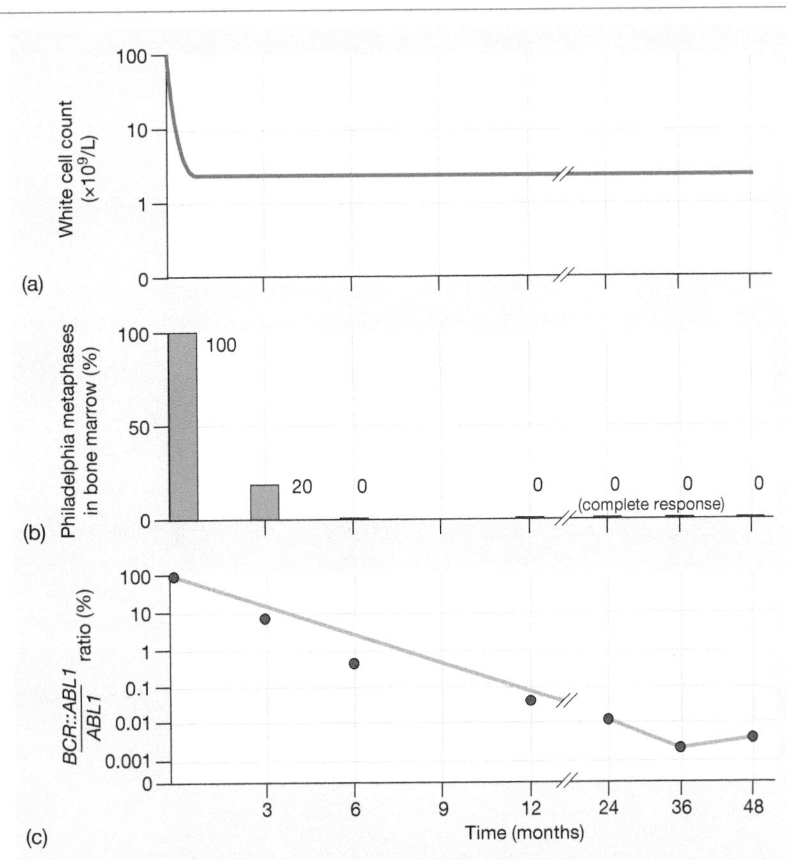

Figure 14.6 Example of an optimal haematological and cytogenetic response in a patient with chronic myeloid leukaemia who achieves complete remission with imatinib therapy. **(a)** The white cell count returns to normal within days. **(b)** Karyotypic examination of the bone marrow reveals a gradual reduction in the number of Ph+ chromosomes over the 6 months. **(c)** Polymerase chain reaction analysis of the bone marrow or blood shows a reduction in the number of *BCR::ABL1* transcripts in comparison with the normal *ABL1* transcript. *BCR::ABL1* transcripts continue to be detected at a very low level, but can become negative in some patients. In this case analysis was performed on bone marrow for the first 6 months and on peripheral blood thereafter.

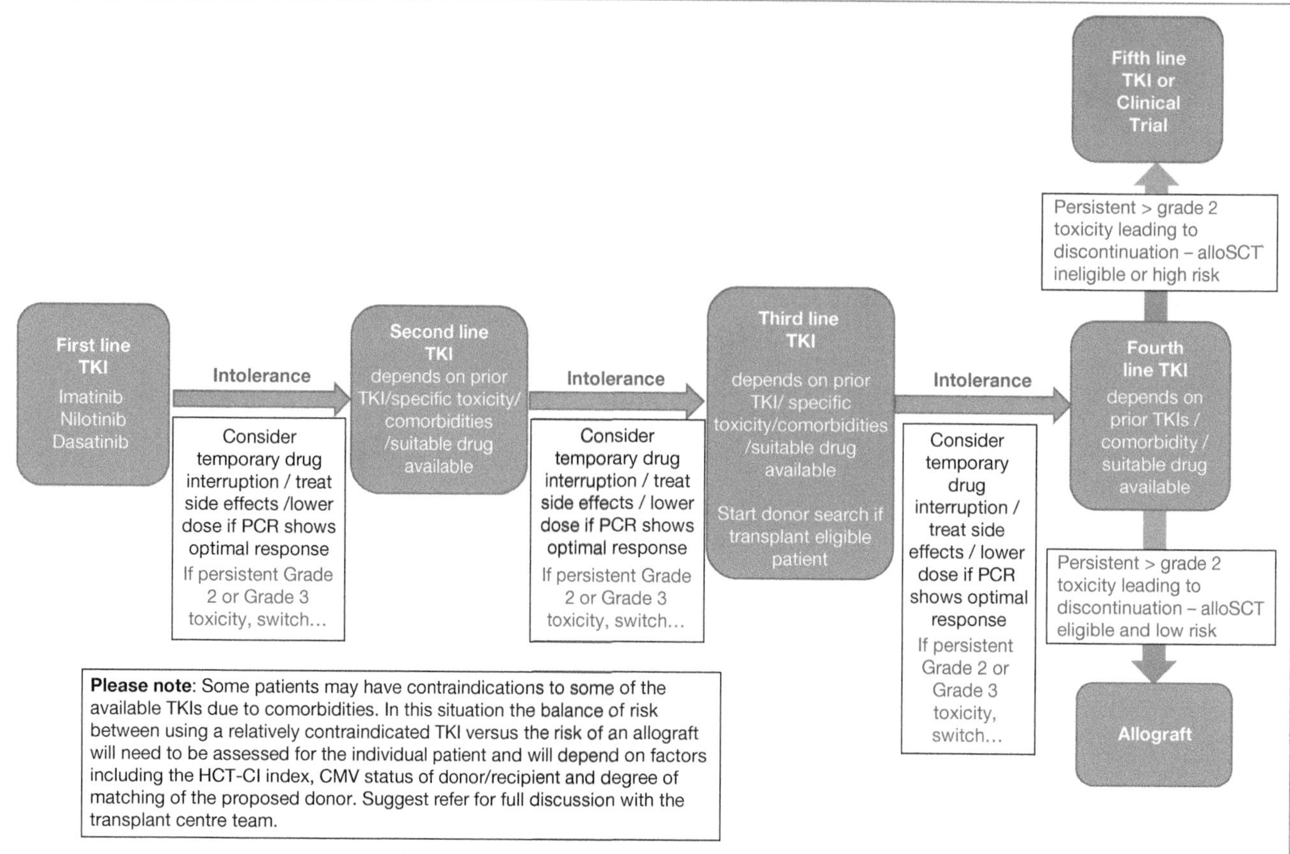

Figure 14.7 A British Society for Haematology Guideline on the diagnosis and management of chronic myeloid leukaemia. Source: G. Smith *et al.* (2020) *Br. J. Haematol.* 191: 171–93. Reproduced with permission of John Wiley & Sons.

does not reduce the percentage of *BCR::ABL1*-positive cells. TKIs have now largely replaced its use and that of DNA alkylating drugs such as busulfan. Omacetaxine is a subcutaneously administered inhibitor of protein translation that has achieved regulatory approval for relapsed/refractory CML in several countries.

α-Interferon

Formerly, this was used after the white cell count had been controlled by hydroxyurea, often in combination with the nucleoside analogue cytarabine, but has now been replaced by imatinib and other TKIs. It is still used in pregnant patients, however, since TKIs are not known to be safe in pregnancy and hydroxycarbamide is teratogenic. Almost all patients treated with interferon have symptoms of a 'flu-like' illness in the first few days of treatment. A minority (approximately 15%) of patients may achieve long-term remission with loss of the Ph chromosome on cytogenetic analysis, although the *BCR::ABL1* fusion gene can usually still be detected by PCR.

Stem cell transplantation

Allogeneic SCT is a potentially curative treatment for CML, but because of the risks associated with the procedure, it is usually reserved for TKI failures (Fig. 14.7) or patients presenting in accelerated or acute phase. The results are, however, better when it is performed in chronic rather than these later phases. The 5-year survival is over 80%. Relapse of CML after the transplant is a significant problem, but donor leucocyte infusions are highly effective in CML (Chapter 25), particularly if relapse is diagnosed early by molecular detection of the *BCR::ABL1* transcript.

Table 14.3 Milestones for monitoring BCR::ABL1 on the international scale, in response to CML treatment.

	Optimal	Warning	Failure
3 months	*BCR::ABL1* ≤10%	*BCR::ABL1* >10%	*BCR::ABL1* >10% if confirmed within 1-3 months
6 months	*BCR::ABL1* ≤1%	*BCR::ABL1* > 1–10%	*BCR::ABL1* >10%
12 months	*BCR::ABL1* ≤0.1%	*BCR::ABL1* >0.1–1%	*BCR::ABL1* >1%
Then, and at any time	*BCR::ABL1* ≤0.1%	>0.1–1%, or loss of ≤0.1% in patients discontinued TKI	>1%, resistance mutations, high-risk additional chromosome abnormalities in Ph+ cells

Source: Adapted from A. Hochhaus *et al.* (2020) European LeukemiaNet 2020 recommendations for treating chronic myeloid leukemia. *Leukemia* 34: 966–84.

SUMMARY

- Chronic myeloid leukaemia is a clonal disorder of a pluripotent stem cell. The disease accounts for around 15% of leukaemias and may occur at any age.
- All cases of CML have a translocation between chromosomes 9 and 22. This leads to the oncogene *ABL1* being moved to the *BCR* gene on chromosome 22 and generates the Philadelphia (Ph) chromosome.
- The resulting chimeric *BCR::ABL1* gene codes for a fusion protein with increased tyrosine kinase activity.
- In most patients the Ph chromosome is seen by karyotypic examination of blood or bone marrow cells, but the molecular rearrangement may rarely only be detected by FISH or PCR.
- The disease can occur at any age, but is most common between the ages of 40 and 60 years.
- The clinical features include loss of weight, sweating, anaemia, bleeding and splenomegaly. There is usually a marked neutrophilia, with myelocytes and basophils seen in the blood film.
- Transformation to an accelerated phase or acute leukaemia may occur.
- Treatment is with tyrosine kinase inhibitors such as imatinib, dasatinib, nilotinib or bosutinib. Neoplastic cells can acquire resistance to treatment and drug therapy is tailored in response to this.
- Ponatinib is a TKI inhibitor that is effective in resistant disease. Asciminib is a newer drug that inhibits the enzyme activity of BCR::ABL1 and is also used in resistant patients.
- Alpha-interferon is an effective therapy that is now mainly used in pregnancy.
- Stem cell transplantation can be curative and may be useful for advanced disease.
- The clinical outlook is now very good for patients diagnosed in chronic phase and more than 90% of patients can expect long-term control of disease and normal life expectancy.

Now visit **www.wiley.com/go/haematology9e** to test yourself on this chapter.

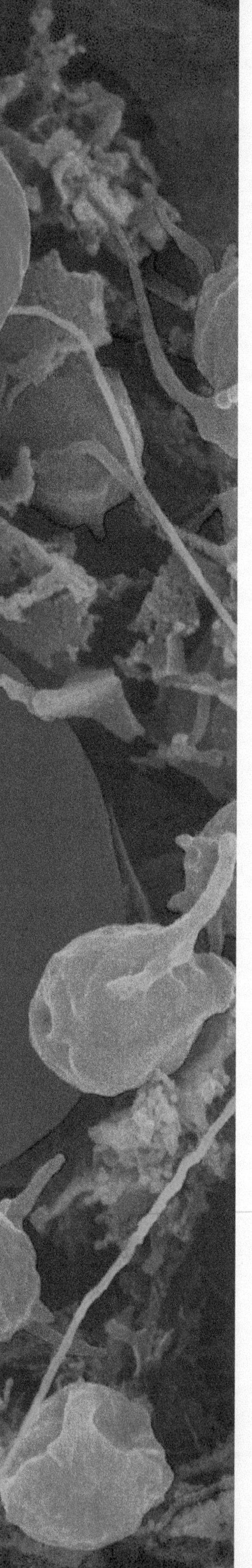

CHAPTER 15

Myeloproliferative neoplasms

Key topics

Hoffbrand's Essential Haematology, Ninth Edition. A. Victor Hoffbrand, Pratima Chowdary, Graham P. Collins, and Justin Loke.

© 2024 John Wiley & Sons Ltd. Published 2024 by John Wiley & Sons Ltd.

Companion website: www.wiley.com/go/haematology9e

The term myeloproliferative neoplasms (MPNs) describes a group of clonal disorders of haemopoiesis which result in an increase in red cells, neutrophils and/or platelets in the circulation. WHO (2022) lists eight subtypes (Table 15.1).

Mastocytosis though not included by WHO 2022 as a myeloproliferative neoplasm is also discussed in this chapter.

Table 15.1 Myeloproliferative neoplasms.
Chronic myeloid leukaemia (Chapter 14)
Polycythaemia vera
Essential thrombocythaemia
Primary myelofibrosis
Chronic neutrophilic leukaemia
Chronic eosinophilic leukaemia
Juvenile myelomonocytic leukaemia
Myeloproliferative neoplasm, not otherwise specified

BCR::ABL1-positive chronic myeloid leukaemia (CML) is an important myeloproliferative disease but since the discovery of the Ph chromosome has been considered separately and is described in Chapter 14.
Source: J.D. Khoury *et al.* (2022) The 5th edition of the World Health Organization classification of haematolymphoid tumours: myeloid and histiocytic/dendritic neoplasms. *Leukemia* 36: 1703–19.

Genetic drivers of myeloproliferation

The three major MPN closely related disorders are polycythaemia vera (PV), essential thrombocythaemia (ET) and primary myelofibrosis (PMF). They share common clinical, laboratory and genetic features. Transitional forms occur with evolution from one entity into another during the course of the disease (Fig. 15.1). These three diseases are associated with acquired mutations of genes that encode tyrosine kinases or kinase-associated proteins, primarily Janus-associated kinase 2 (***JAK2***), calreticulin (***CALR***) or ***MPL*** (the receptor for thrombopoietin; Table 15.2). Recent studies show that these causative driver mutations of MPNs can emerge very early in life, with the earliest appearance of *JAK2* V617F *in utero* at 33 weeks gestation.

Mutation of *JAK2* (*JAK2* V617F) occurs in a heterozygous, hemizygous, i.e. loss of the normal allele or homozygous state, in the marrow and blood of almost all patients with PV and in approximately 60% of those with ET or PMF, showing the common pathogenesis of these three diseases (Fig. 15.2). The mutation occurs in a highly conserved region of the pseudokinase domain, which normally negatively regulates JAK2 signalling. JAK2 has a major role in normal myeloid development by transducing signals from cytokines and growth factors including erythropoietin, granulocyte colony-stimulating factor receptor and thrombopoietin (Fig. 1.8). Why the same

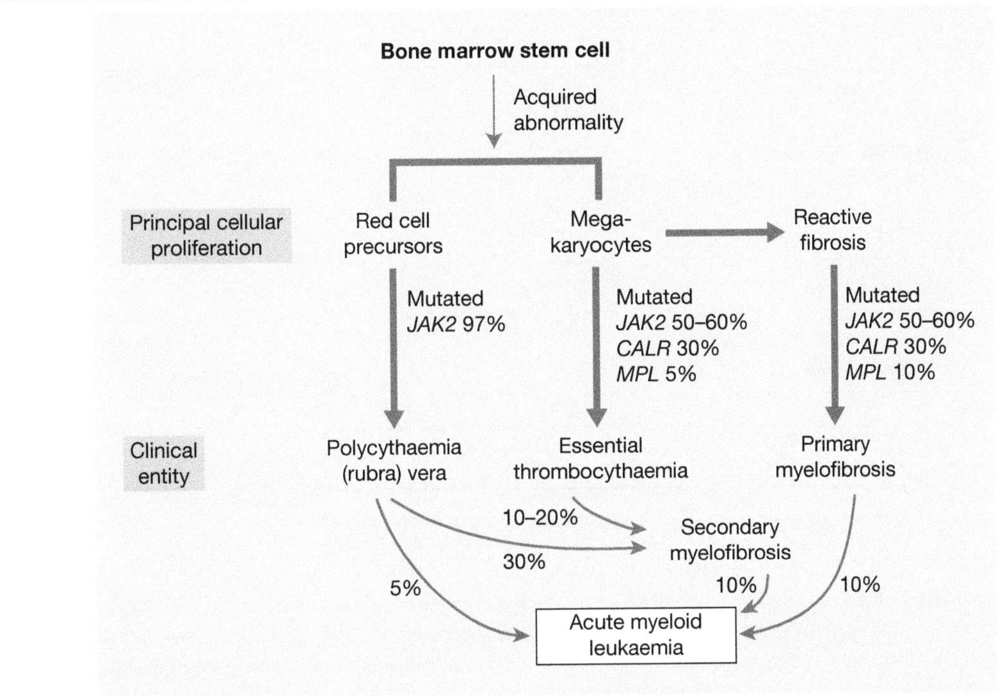

Figure 15.1 Relationship between the three myeloproliferative neoplasms. They may all arise by somatic mutation in the pluripotent stem and progenitor cells. Many transitional cases occur showing features of two conditions and, in other cases, the disease transforms during its course from one of these diseases to another or to acute myeloid leukaemia.

Table 15.2 Driver genetic mutations in myeloproliferative neoplasms.

Disease	Gene mutations or fusions
Chronic myeloid leukaemia	*ABL1* (fusion with *BCR*)
Polycythaemia vera	*JAK2*
Primary myelofibrosis	*JAK2, CALR, MPL*
Essential thrombocythaemia	*JAK2, CALR, MPL*
Mastocytosis	*KIT*
Myeloid/lymphoid neoplasm with eosinophilia and tyrosine kinase gene fusions	*PDGFRA, PDGFRB, FGFR1, JAK2,* others

mutation is associated with different myeloproliferative neoplasms is unclear, but depends partly on the dosage of the mutant allele, this being usually higher in PV than ET. Cooperating mutations and the cell differentiation stage at which the mutations developed may also influence the phenotype. A minority of PV patients show a variant *JAK2* mutation in exon 12 rather than a V617F mutation.

In those patients with ET or PMF who do not demonstrate a *JAK2* mutation, a mutation in *CALR* is present in most cases. CALR is a multifunction chaperone protein involved in the folding of immature proteins and in calcium homeostasis. The mutations typically are either a 52 base pair (bp) or 5bp deletion occur in exon 9 and result in a novel protein that interacts with the thrombopoietin receptor MPL activating its downstream signalling pathways. Constitutively activating mutations

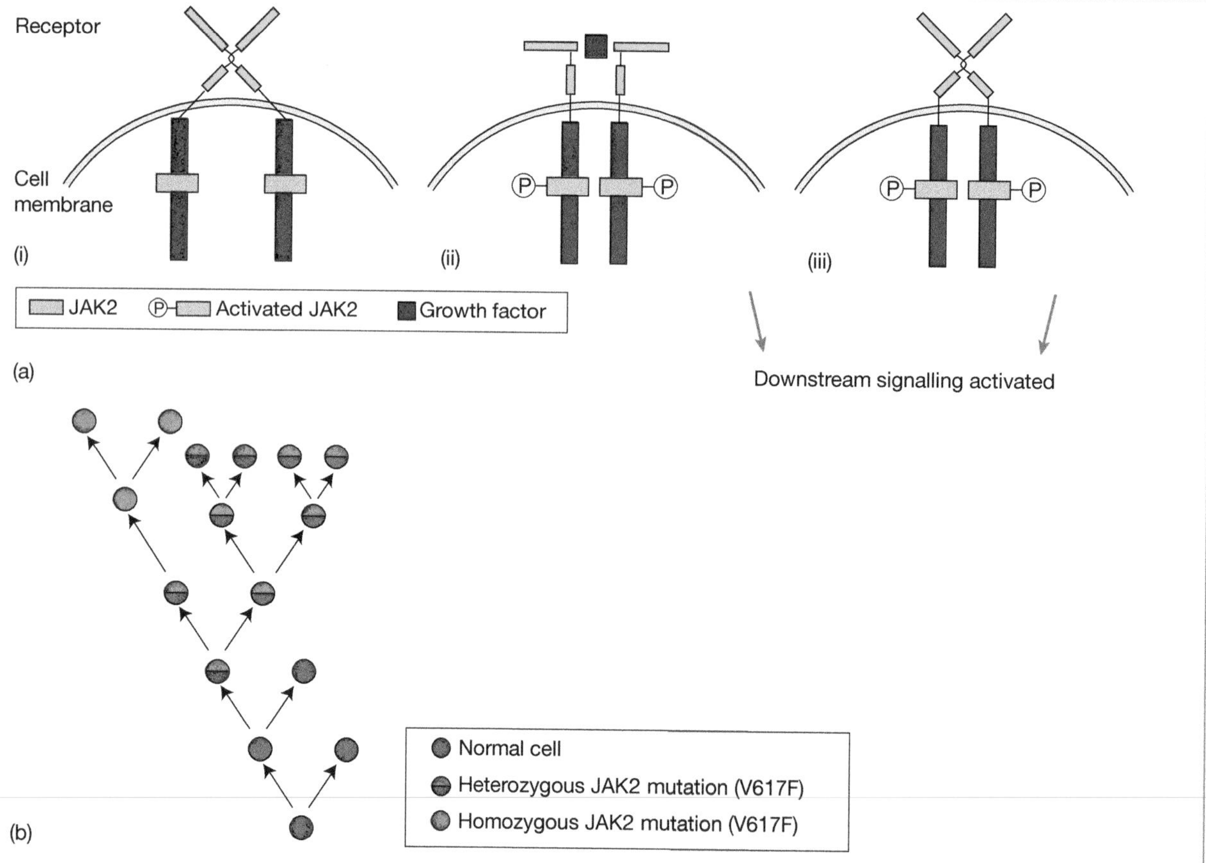

Figure 15.2 The role of *JAK2* mutation in the generation of myeloproliferative neoplasms. **(a)** (i) Most haemopoietic growth factor receptors do not have intrinsic kinase activity, but associate with a protein kinase such as JAK2 in the cytoplasm. (ii) When the receptor binds a growth factor, e.g. erythropoietin or thrombopoietin, the cytoplasmic domains move closer together and the JAK2 molecules can activate each other by phosphorylation and subsequently phosphorylate downstream proteins, e.g. STAT (signal transducer and activator of transcription) proteins (Fig. 1.7). (iii) The *JAK2* V617F and the *MPL* mutations allow the JAK protein to become activated even when no growth factor is bound. **(b)** A model for the development of myeloproliferative neoplasm following *JAK2* mutation. The primary event appears to predispose to an acquired heterozygous mutation of *JAK2* V617F. This leads to a survival advantage. In some patients, a mitotic recombination event leads to a homozygous *JAK2* mutation state.

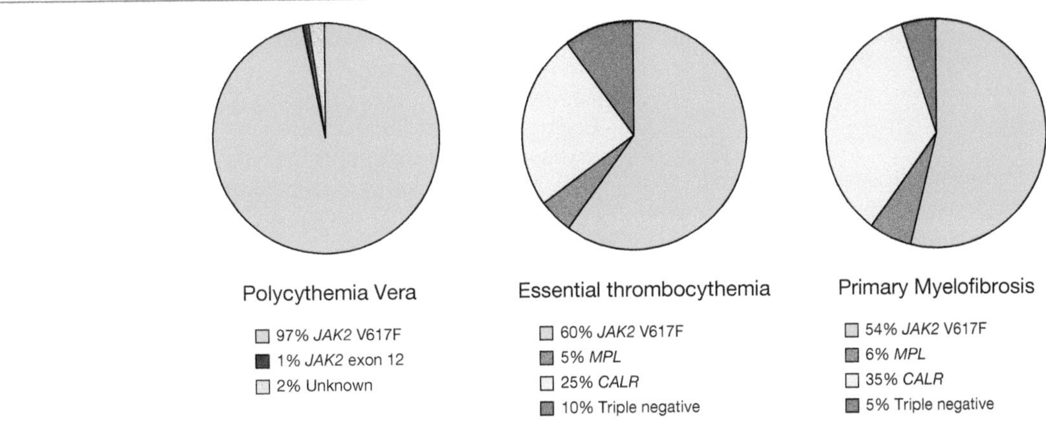

Figure 15.3 Distribution of disease driver mutations in the three major *BCR::ABL1* negative myeloproliferative neoplasms.

in the *MPL* gene encoding thrombopoietin receptor are found in about 5% of ET and 10% PMF cases. A mutation in one of these three genes is seen in 98% of cases of PV and around 90–95% of cases of ET or PMF (Fig. 15.3).

Cytogenetic and molecular genetics

Chromosome abnormalities, e.g. deletions of 9p or 20q, are found in a minority of MPN subjects. Deletions of part of 5p, trisomy 8, rearrangements of 11q23, or mutations of *TP53* and *RUNX1*, found mainly in PMF, predict for transformation to AML. Mutations in other cancer driver genes are found in over half of the patients (Fig 15.4). The commonest mutations are in *TET2, ASXL1* and *DNMT3A* with a lower prevalence in splicing regulators, e.g. *SRSF2, SF3B1*, regulators of chromatin structure, epigenetic functions and cellular signalling. These mutations synergize with *JAK2, CALR* or *MPL* mutations to increase clonal haemopoiesis. They occur in other myeloid malignancies, e.g. AML and myelodysplastic neoplasms, and especially *DNMT3A, TET2, ASXL1* in age-related clonal haemopoiesis in individuals with normal blood counts (Chapter 16). They are more frequent in older patients with MPN and are associated with more rapid

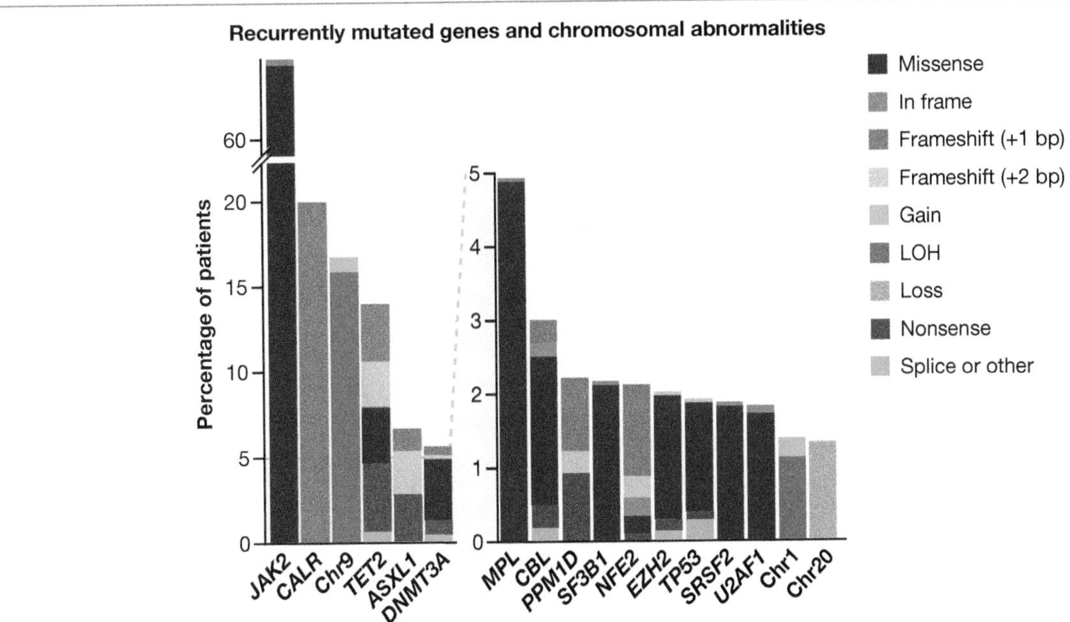

Figure 15.4 Distribution of recurrent gene mutations and chromosome (Chr) changes in myeloproliferative neoplasms. Point mutations include insertions and deletions, some of which, e.g. of calreticulin result in a frame-shift. Chromosomal changes include whole or partial gains or losses, and copy-neutral loss of heterozygosity (LOH). Source: J. Grinfield *et al.* (2018) *N. Engl. J. Med.* 379: 1416. Reproduced with permission of Massachusetts Medical Society.

progression and transformation of PV or ET to myelofibrosis. They are more frequent in primary myelofibrosis and blast phase than in PV and ET.

Germline predispositions to MPNs

There is a five to seven=fold increased incidence of myeloproliferative neoplasms in first-degree relatives of patients, implying a genetic predisposition to the diseases. A specific haplotype *JAK2 46/1*is present in 25% of the population. *JAK2* mutations occur with increased frequency in this haplotype which has a higher incidence in MPN. A number of single nucleotide polymorphisms (SNPs) in other genes have also been associated with MPNs. Family clusters of the MPNs have been associated with germline variants in various genes.

Polycythaemia

Polycythaemia is defined as an increase in the haemoglobin concentration above the upper limit of normal for the patient's age and sex.

Classification of polycythaemia

Polycythaemia is classified according to its pathophysiology, but the major subdivision is into **absolute polycythaemia** or erythrocytosis, in which the red cell mass (volume) is raised to greater than 125% of that expected for body mass and gender, and **relative** or **pseudopolycythaemia**, in which the red cell volume is normal but the plasma volume is reduced. If the haematocrit is higher than 0.60, there will always be a raised red cell mass and absolute polycythaemia. A haemoglobin (Hb) >185 g/L or haematocrit >0.52 in men, and Hb >165 g/L or haematocrit >0.48 in women, indicates that erythrocytosis is likely.

Formerly, radioisotope studies were often performed to document a raised red cell mass, but with the advent of molecular genetic testing to confirm the presence of a clonal neoplasm, these are much less commonly done today and such testing is no longer available in most regions.

Once established, absolute polycythaemia can be subdivided into **primary polycythaemia,** or **secondary polycythaemia** in which erythropoiesis is driven by an increase in erythropoietin as a result of factors such as smoking, sleep apnoea or altitude (Table 15.3). Primary polycythaemia includes both rare congenital causes of polycythaemia related to genetic changes in oxygen sensing or erythropoietin signalling, and the more common acquired myeloproliferative neoplasm **polycythaemia vera** (in which there is an intrinsic overactivity in the bone marrow).

Table 15.3 Causes of polycythaemia (erythrocytosis).

Primary erythrocytosis
Congenital
Erythropoietin receptor mutations
Erythropoietin gain of function mutation
Defects of the oxygen-sensing pathway
VHL gene mutation (Chuvash erythrocytosis)
PHD2 mutations
HIF2A mutations Other congenital defects
High oxygen-affinity haemoglobin
Acquired
Polycythaemia vera
Secondary erythrocytosis
Erythropoietin-mediated
Central hypoxia
Chronic lung disease
Right-to-left cardiopulmonary vascular shunts
Carbon monoxide poisoning
Smoking
Obstructive sleep apnoea
High altitude
Local hypoxia
Renal artery stenosis
End-stage renal disease
Hydronephrosis
Renal cysts (polycystic kidney disease)
Post-renal transplant erythrocytosis
Pathological erythropoietin production
Tumours – cerebellar haemangioblastoma, meningioma, parathyroid tumours, hepatocellular carcinoma, renal cell cancer, Wilms tumour, phaeochromocytoma, uterine leiomyoma
Drug-associated
Erythropoietin analogues, prolyl hydroxylase inhibitors, androgen administration, SGLT-2 (sodium-glucose co-transporter-2) inhibitors, gliflozins (prescribed for diabetes mellitus)

Primary polycythaemia (erythrocytosis): polycythaemia vera (PV)

In PV, the increase in red cell volume is caused by a clonal malignancy of a marrow stem cell. The disease results from somatic mutation of a single haemopoietic stem cell which gives its progeny a proliferative advantage. The *JAK2* V617F mutation is present in haemopoietic cells in about 95% of patients and a mutation in exon 12 is seen in most of the remainder. Although the increase in red cells is the diagnostic finding, in many patients there is also an overproduction of granulocytes and platelets. Some families have an inherited predisposition to MPN, but *JAK2* or *CALR* mutations are not present in the germline.

Diagnosis

Making the diagnosis of PV in a patient who presents with polycythaemia can be difficult. Current WHO criteria are listed in Table 15.4. The identification of the *JAK2* mutation has rationalized the approach to diagnosis with a three-stage approach suggested:

1 **Stage 1**
- History and examination.
- Arterial oxygen saturation (pulse oximetry).

Table 15.4 World Health Organization 2022 diagnostic criteria for polycythaemia vera (PV).

Major criteria	
1	High haematocrit (>49% in men, >48% in women) or high haemoglobin (>165 g/L in men, >160 g/L in women)
2	Bone marrow (BM) biopsy showing hypercellularity for age with trilineage growth (panmyelosis) including prominent erythroid, granulocytic and megakaryocytic proliferation with pleomorphic mature megakaryocytes
3	Presence of *JAK2 V617F* or *JAK2* exon 12 mutation
Minor criterion	
	Subnormal serum erythropoietin test

Diagnosis of PV requires meeting either all three major criteria, or the first two major criteria and the minor criterion. Criterion number 2 (BM biopsy) may not be required in cases with sustained absolute erythrocytosis: haemoglobin levels 185 g/L in men (haematocrit 55.5%) or 165 g/L in women (haematocrit 49.5%) if major criterion 3 and the minor criterion are present. However, initial myelofibrosis (present in up to 20% of patients) can only be detected by performing a BM biopsy; this finding may predict a more rapid progression to overt myelofibrosis (post-PV MF).

- Full blood count/film.
- *JAK2* V617F mutation.
- Serum erythropoietin level.
- Serum ferritin.
- Renal and liver function tests.

If JAK2 V617F *is negative and there is no clear secondary cause, consider investigations in stage 2.*

2 Stage 2

- Abdominal ultrasound.
- Bone marrow aspirate and trephine biopsy.
- Cytogenetic analysis.

Specialized tests may then be required.

3 Stage 3

- Arterial oxygen dissociation (high oxygen-affinity haemoglobin).
- Sleep study.
- Lung function studies.
- Gene mutations found in congenital polycythaemia, e.g. *EPOR, VHL, PHD2, HIF2A*.

NB. The *JAK2* V617F mutation occurs rarely in other haematological neoplasms including AML, MDS and chronic myelomonocytic leukaemia without polycythaemia.

Clinical features

PV is usually a disease of older people (median age at presentation 55-60 years) and has a slight male preponderance. Clinical features result from hyperviscosity, hypervolaemia, hypermetabolism or thrombosis.

1. Headaches, dyspnoea, blurred vision and night sweats.
2. Generalized pruritus, characteristically after a hot bath or shower, can be a severe problem.
3. Plethoric appearance: ruddy cyanosis (Fig. 15.5), conjunctival suffusion and retinal venous engorgement.
4. Splenomegaly in 75% of patients, usually not massive (Fig. 15.6).

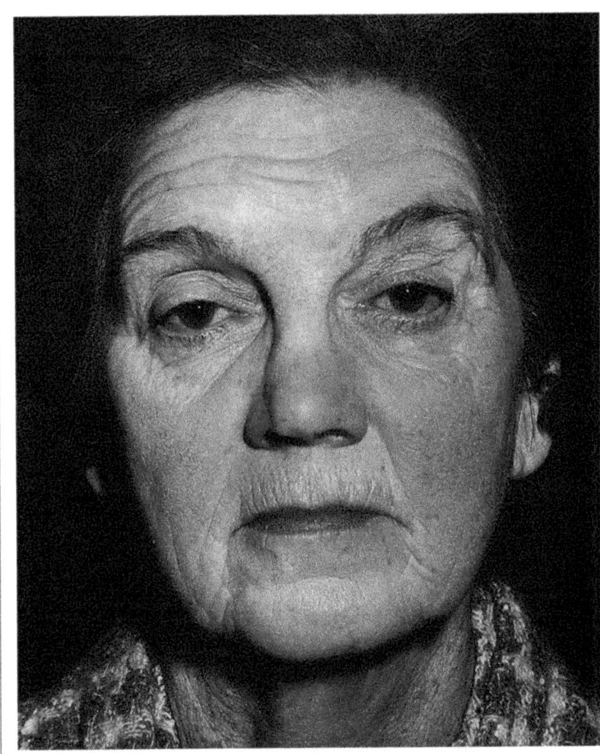

Figure 15.5 Polycythaemia vera: facial plethora and conjunctival suffusion in a 63-year-old woman. Haemoglobin 180 g/L; total red cell volume 45 mL/kg.

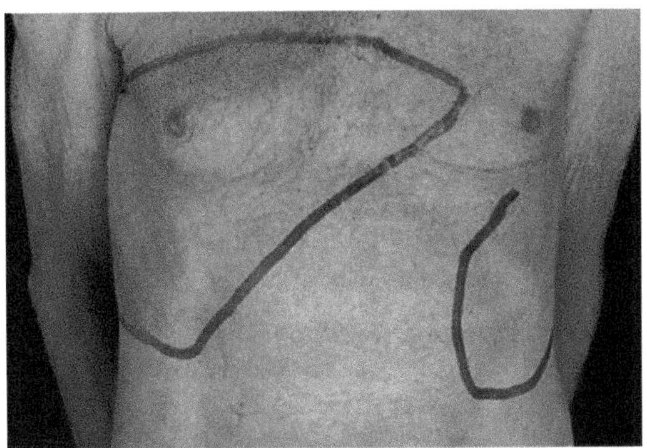

Figure 15.6 Splenomegaly: enlarged liver and spleen in a patient with polycythaemia vera.

5 Haemorrhage or thrombosis, either arterial or venous, may be seen. Raised haematocrit, white cells and platelets and older age predict for thrombosis. Arterial thrombosis may cause myocardial infarct, stroke, transient ischemic attacks, mesenteric or limb ischemia. Splanchnic venous thrombosis including the Budd–Chiari syndrome is a particular feature of *JAK2* mutated disease even in the absence of an overt MPN.
6 Gout as a result of raised uric acid production (Fig. 15.7).

Laboratory findings

1 **The haemoglobin, haematocrit and red cell count are increased. A neutrophil leucocytosis is seen in >50% of patients and some have increased basophils.**
2 A raised platelet count is present in about 50% of patients.
3 A *JAK2* mutation is present in the bone marrow and peripheral blood granulocytes in over 95% of patients. Cytogenetic and molecular genetic tests reveal additional mutations described above in a minority of patients. These may have prognostic significance.
4 The bone marrow is hypercellular with trilineage growth, as assessed by trephine biopsy (Fig. 15.10).
5 Serum erythropoietin is low.

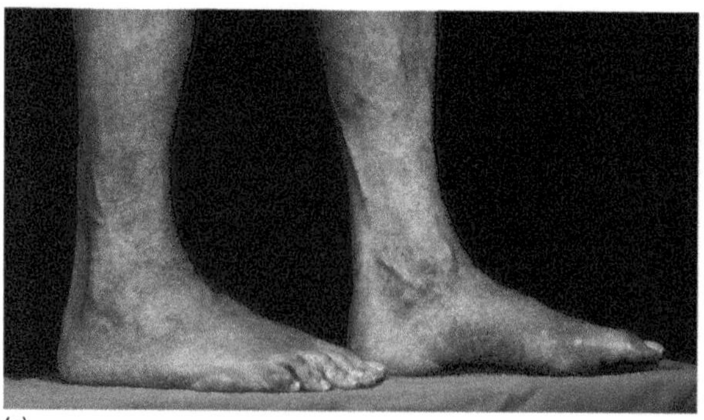

(a)

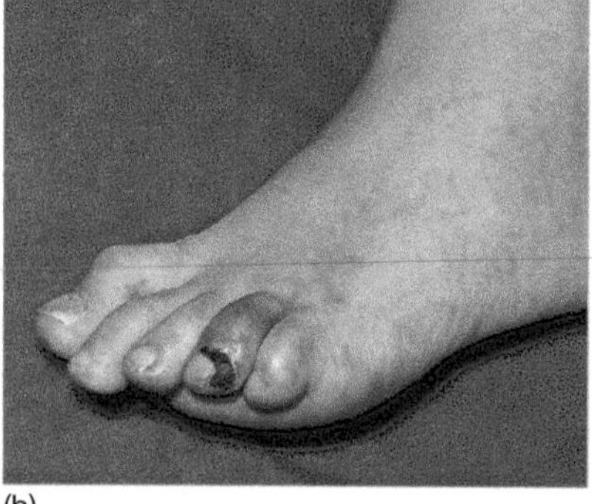

(b)

Figure 15.7 (a) The feet of a 72-year-old man with polycythaemia vera. There is inflammation of the right metatarsophalangeal and other joints (gout) caused by uric acid deposits. **(b)** Gangrene of the left fourth toe in essential thrombocythaemia.

6 Plasma urate is often increased; the serum lactate dehydrogenase (LDH) is normal or slightly raised.
7 Circulating erythroid progenitors (erythroid colony-forming unit, CFU-E, and erythroid burst-forming unit, BFU_E; p. 2) are increased compared to normal and grow *in vitro* independently of added erythropoietin (endogenous erythroid colonies).

Course and prognosis

Typically, the prognosis is good, with a median survival over 10 years. Thrombosis and haemorrhage are the major clinical problems. Increased viscosity, vascular stasis and high platelet levels and altered platelet function may all contribute to thrombosis, whereas defective platelet function may promote haemorrhage. Transition from PV to myelofibrosis occurs in approximately 6–20% of patients, especially those with a *JAK2* mutation allele burden >50%. Approximately 2% of patients progress to acute myeloid leukaemia (AML) at 10 years, more if radioactive phosphorous (rarely used nowadays) has been given. Cooperating mutations of myeloid genes also predict for these outcomes.

Treatment

Treatment is aimed at reducing the risk of complications and managing symptoms. The major complications to prevent are thromboses and haemorrhage. In all patients aspirin should be offered and haematocrit should be reduced to <0.50. Cardiovascular risk factors such as hypertension, diabetes mellitus and hyperlipidaemia should also be controlled and are indications for a lower haematocrit of <0.45.

Risk-adapted approaches have been suggested to tailor treatment to individuals. Patients considered to be at higher risk of thrombosis are those aged 65 years and over, and those with prior PV associated thrombosis (both venous and arterial). They should be offered cytoreduction, e.g. hydroxyurea. "Lower risk" patients may still benefit from cytoreduction in the presence of other risk factors such as those with cardiovascular risk factors or with leukocytosis or very high thrombocytosis.

Venesection

Venesection to reduce the haematocrit is particularly useful when a rapid reduction of red cell volume is required, e.g. at the start of therapy. It is indicated for long term treatment especially in younger patients and those with mild disease. The resulting iron deficiency may limit erythropoiesis. Venesection does not control the platelet count and with iron deficiency the platelet count may even increase. Clinical trials of hepcidin mimetics to reduce the haematocrit are in progress.

Aspirin

Low-dose aspirin 75 mg daily reduces thrombotic complications without significant increased risk of major haemorrhage and is used in almost all patients. For those considered high risk of thrombosis (age, previous thrombosis, high haematocrit, high platelet or white cell count), the dose of aspirin could be doubled.

Hydroxycarbamide (hydroxyurea)

Hydroxycarbamides or interferons are used in patients who are at high risk, i.e. over age 65 and/or prior history of thrombosis, arterial hypertension, ischemic heart disease or diabetes mellitus. Also if there is poor control or intolerance of venesection, progressive splenomegaly, extreme thrombocytosis or progressive leukocytosis. Daily treatment can control the blood count and may need to be continued for many years (Fig. 15.8). The *JAK2* mutation affects platelet function, leading to thrombosis or haemorrhage, and it is therefore necessary to control both the platelet count and haematocrit to reduce the risk. Side effects of hydroxycarbamide include myelosuppression, nausea and toxicity to the skin, especially in areas exposed to ultraviolet light. Precancerous or cancerous squamous cell skin lesions may develop. There is no evidence that hydroxycarbamide predisposes to AML. It should be avoided in pregnancy, due to teratogenicity. Therefore, it should be stopped prior to conception.

Interferon

Injectable α-interferon suppresses excess proliferation in the marrow and has produced good haematological and in some cases molecular responses. It is less convenient and more expensive than the oral agents and side effects, e.g. flu-like symptoms are frequent. The long acting pegylated – interferon Ropeginterferon is now preferred as it reduces the frequency of injections and gives better control. Interferon may be particularly valuable in controlling itching and is often used for younger patients to avoid early exposure to other drugs, and for those who might become pregnant, since JAK2 inhibitors (see below) are not known to be safe in pregnancy and hydroxycarbamide is teratogenic.

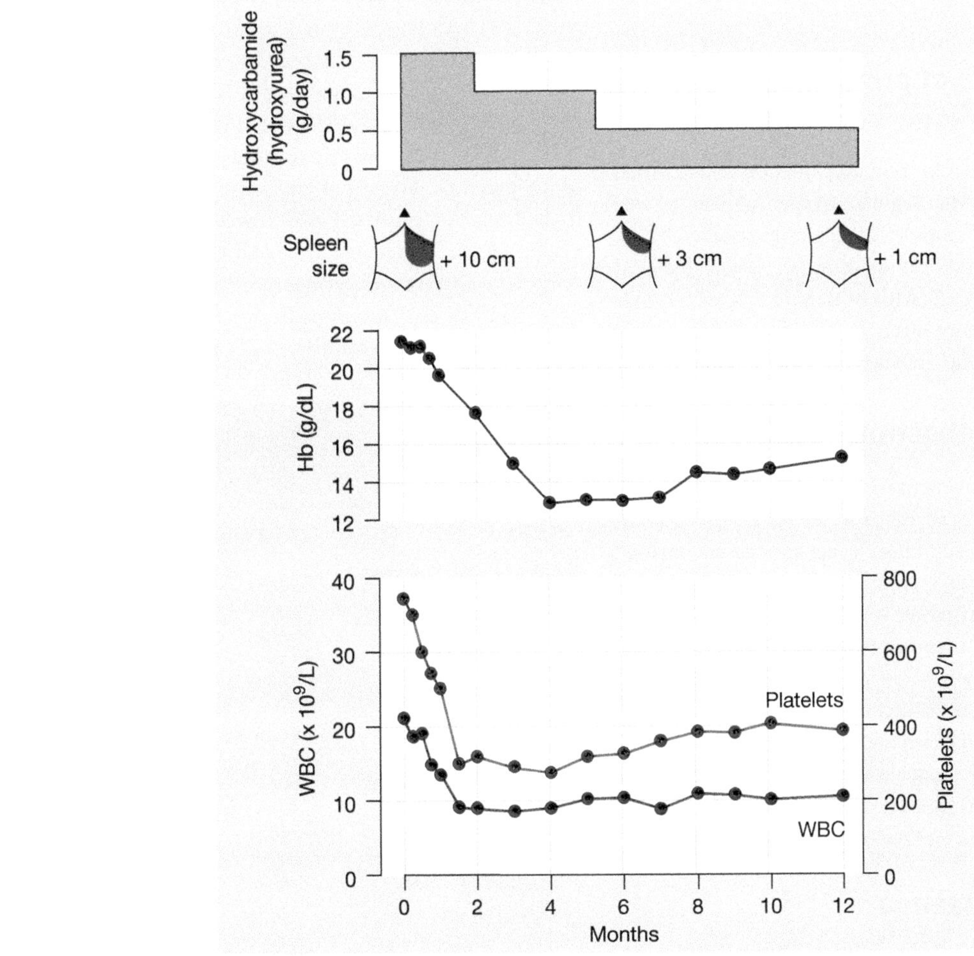

Figure 15.8 Haematological response to therapy with hydroxycarbamide (hydroxyurea) in polycythaemia vera. Hb, haemoglobin; WBC, white blood cells.

JAK inhibitors

Ruxolitinib inhibits JAK2 activity. It is used in patients who are not controlled adequately or have side effects with hydroxycarbamide therapy, or those with severe constitutional symptoms that hydroxycarbamide does not adequately treat. Reduction in the proportion of cells showing the *JAK2* mutation (VAF) correlates with the clinical response and with reduction of transformation to myelofibrosis. Fedratinib has also been approved for treatment of MPNs. Other JAK2 inhibitors at various stages of development and approval include fedratinib, pacritininib and momelotinib.

Treatment of pruritus

Pruritus often settles when the haematocrit is lowered to normal. For resistant itching antihistamines, aspirin and the protein kinase inhibitor paroxetine are effective in some cases.

Other drugs

Busulfan, radioactive phosphorous (^{32}P), and anagrelide (to control the platelet count) are used in a small minority of patients.

Congenital causes of primary polycythaemia

Congenital causes are relatively rare and include cases caused by mutations in the genes that regulate oxygen sensing as well as mutations of the erythropoietin receptor gene (*EPOR*), erythopoietin gene itself and haemoglobin mutations that lead to high oxygen-affinity variants with subsequent tissue hypoxia (Table 15.3). These patients often have a family history of polycythaemia and present at a young age.

Secondary polycythaemia

The causes of secondary polycythaemia are listed in Table 15.3. Acquired causes are due to an increase in the erythropoietin level. Hypoxia caused by smoking, sleep apnoea or chronic obstructive airway disease is a common cause, and measurement of arterial oxygen saturation is a valuable test. Renal and various tumour causes of inappropriate erythropoietin secretion are less common.

There is little evidence on which to guide a treatment plan, but one approach is to advise venesection if the haematocrit is above 0.54, with the aim of reducing to a target of around 0.50. A lower target for venesection is used if there is hypertension, diabetes, dyspnoea, angina or a previous thrombotic episode.

Apparent polycythaemia

Apparent polycythaemia, also known as pseudopolycythaemia, is the result of plasma volume contraction. By definition, the red cell mass is normal. Diuretic therapy, extreme volume loss, e.g. severe diarrhoea, anasarca, smoking, hypertension, obesity and alcohol consumption are frequent associations. Management includes volume replacement and correction of the underlying cause. Phlebotomy is not of benefit.

Essential thrombocythaemia

In this condition there is a sustained increase in the platelet count due to megakaryocyte proliferation and overproduction of platelets. The haematocrit is normal and the Philadelphia chromosome or *BCR::ABL1* rearrangement is absent. The bone marrow shows no collagen fibrosis. A persisting platelet count of greater than 450×10^9/L is the central diagnostic feature, but other causes of a raised platelet count (particularly iron deficiency, inflammatory or malignant disorder and myelodysplasia) need to be fully excluded before the diagnosis can be made.

Fifty to sixty percent of patients show the *JAK2* V617F mutation and these cases tend to resemble more closely PV with higher haemoglobin and white cell counts than *JAK2*-negative cases (Table 15.5). The *JAK2* mutation also affects platelet and neutrophil function (including increasing production of neutrophil extracellular traps, NETs, structures formed from DNA expelled by activated neutrophils), leading to a pro-thrombotic state (Chapter 8). *JAK2 exon 12* mutation is associated with erythrocytosis and is not seen in ET.

Mutations in the *CALR* gene are seen in around 60–75% of *JAK2*-negative ET patients, in total representing about a third of all patients. These patients tend to be younger and have higher platelet counts, but a lower incidence of thrombosis (Table 15.5). The higher the VAF of the mutation, the more severe the disease. Mutations within the *MPL* gene are seen in ~5% of cases. Mutations in other driver genes described in MPN occur in a minority of cases of ET with similar

Table 15.5 Typical clinical and laboratory features of essential thrombocythaemia associated with *JAK2* or *CALR* mutation.

Feature	*JAK2* mutated	*CALR* mutated
Age	Older	Younger
Haemoglobin	Higher	Lower
White cell count	Higher	Lower
Platelet count	Lower	Higher
Serum erythropoietin	Lower	Higher
Thrombosis risk	Higher	Lower
Transformation to polycythaemia vera	Yes	No
Risk of transformation to myelofibrosis	Equal	Equal
Approximate survival	17 years	>25 years

Table 15.6 World Health Organization 2022 diagnostic criteria for essential thrombocythaemia.

	Major criteria
1	Sustained platelet count above 450×10^9/L
2	Bone marrow biopsy showing proliferation mainly of the megakaryocyte lineage with increased numbers of enlarged, mature megakaryocytes with hyperlobulated nuclei. No significant increase or left shift in neutrophil granulopoiesis or erythropoiesis and very rarely minor (grade 1) increase in reticulin fibre
3	No other myeloid malignancy, polycythaemia vera, primary myelofibrosis, chronic myeloid leukaemia *BCR::ABL1* positive or myelodysplastic syndrome
4	Presence of an acquired pathogenetic mutation in *JAK2*, *CALR* or *MPL*
	Minor criteria
1	Presence of a clonal marker, e.g. abnormal karyotype.
2	Absence of evidence for reactive thrombocytosis

Diagnosis of essential thrombocythaemia requires meeting all four major criteria or the first three major criteria and both the minor criteria.

prognostic implications (see below and Fig. 15.4). Rare primary familial cases in children have been associated with germline mutations in the genes for thrombopoietin or its receptor MPL.

Diagnosis

This used to be based on the exclusion of other causes of chronic thrombocytosis, but now that specific genetic lesions have been identified, a positive diagnosis can be made in most cases (Table 15.6).

Clinical and laboratory findings

The dominant clinical features are thrombosis and haemorrhage. Most cases are asymptomatic and are diagnosed on a routine blood count. Thrombosis may occur in the venous or arterial systems (Fig. 15.7), whereas haemorrhage, as a result of abnormal platelet function, may cause either chronic or acute bleeding. Some patients, particularly those with the *JAK2* mutation, present with Budd–Chiari syndrome, when the platelet count may be normal because of splenomegaly. A characteristic symptom is erythromelalgia, a burning sensation felt in the hands or feet and promptly relieved by aspirin. Up to 40% of patients will have palpable splenomegaly, whereas in others there may be splenic atrophy because of infarction.

Abnormal large platelets and megakaryocyte fragments may be seen on the blood film (Fig. 15.9). The bone marrow is similar to that in PV, but an excess of abnormal megakaryocytes is typical. Cytogenetics and molecular analysis are performed to exclude *BCR::ABL1*-positive CML and to detect the underlying mutation of *JAK2*, *CALR* or *MPL* or any additional mutations (Fig. 15.7) which, as for PV, have prognostic significance. The condition must be distinguished from other causes of a raised platelet count (Table 15.7). Platelet function tests are rarely needed, but are consistently abnormal, with failure of aggregation with adrenaline being particularly characteristic.

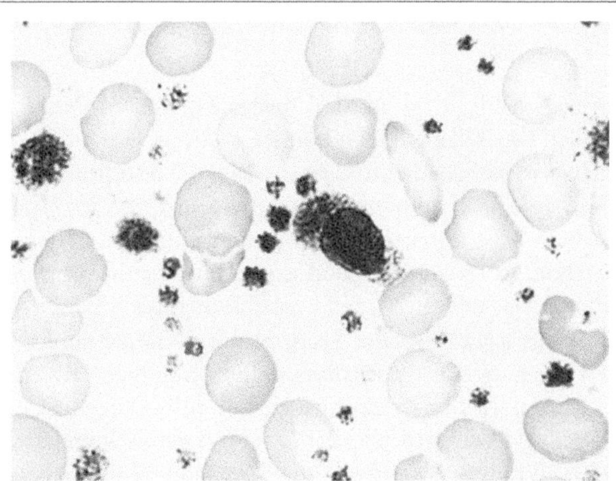

Figure 15.9 Peripheral blood film in essential thrombocythaemia showing increased numbers of platelets and a nucleated megakaryocytic fragment.

Prognosis and treatment

The principle is to reduce the risk of the major clinical problems of thrombosis (14% at 10 years) or haemorrhage. Standard cardiovascular risk factors, such as raised cholesterol, smoking, diabetes, obesity and hypertension, should be identified and treated. Low-dose aspirin at 75 mg/day is generally recommended in all cases.

Patients at **high risk** include those over 60 years of age, and/or with previous thrombosis and/or with platelet count $>1500 \times 10^9$/L, and this group should be treated with hydroxycarbamide or another cytoreductive agent to reduce the platelet count. **Low-risk** patients are those aged below 60 years without a history of thrombosis or extreme thrombocytosis, and here aspirin alone is sufficient. Very high platelet counts can be

Table 15.7 Causes of a raised platelet count.

Reactive
Haemorrhage, trauma, post-operative
Chronic iron deficiency
Malignancy
Chronic infections
Connective tissue diseases, e.g. rheumatoid arthritis
Post-splenectomy
Endogenous
Essential thrombocythaemia (*JAK2* mutation + or −)
Some cases of polycythaemia vera, primary myelofibrosis, *BCR::ABL1*-positive chronic myeloid leukaemia, myelodysplastic syndromes (5q− syndrome or myelodysplastic syndromes/ myeloproliferative neoplasms with ring sideroblasts and thrombocytosis)

Table 15.8 Diagnostic criteria for PMF.

Primary myelofibrosis (overtly fibrotic)	
All three major and one minor criteria must be met	
Major criteria	Typical megakaryocyte changes accompanied by ≥ grade 2 fibrosis
	Presence of *JAK2*, *CALR* or *MPL* mutations or presence of other clonal markers, or absence of evidence for reactive BM fibrosis
	Not meeting WHO criteria for other myeloid neoplasms
Minor criteria	Anaemia not otherwise specified
	Leucocytosis > 11×10^9/L
	Palpable splenomegaly
	Increased serum lactate dehydrogenase (LDH)
	A leuco-erythroblastic blood film

associated with a paradoxical increased risk of bleeding (acquired von Wllebrand syndrome).

Hydroxycarbamide is the most widely used treatment and is well tolerated, although after prolonged therapy some patients develop skin keratosis, epitheliomas, ulceration or pigmentation. Anagrelide is a good second-line treatment but has cardiovascular side effects, and a possible increased risk of myelofibrosis is also of concern. These two drugs can be combined at low doses to reduce side effects. α-Interferon is also effective and is often used in younger patients or during pregnancy. A long-acting PEGylated preparation of interferon is preferred, since it allows once-weekly dosing. JAK2 inhibitors are being assessed. A monoclonal antibody that binds to mutant but not wild type CALR and inhibits disease clones in culture is in clinical trials.

Course

Often the disease is stationary for 10–20 years or more. The disease may transform after a number of years to myelofibrosis (less than 10%), but the risk of transformation to AML is relatively low (less than 5%).

Primary myelofibrosis

The predominant feature of PMF is a progressive generalized reactive fibrosis of the bone marrow in association with megakaryocyte atypia and proliferation (Fig. 15.10, Table 15.8), and with the development of haemopoiesis in the spleen and liver (myeloid metaplasia or extra-medullary haemopoiesis). Clinically this leads to anaemia and massive splenomegaly (Fig. 15.11). In some patients there is osteosclerosis. The fibrosis of the bone marrow is secondary to the hyperplasia of abnormal megakaryocytes. Fibroblasts are stimulated by platelet-derived growth factor, TNF and other cytokines secreted by megakaryocytes and platelets.

Prefibrotic myelofibrosis

Up to 50% of PMF present in a **prefibrotic/early stage** with no significant increase in reticulin or collagen, but markedly abnormal megakaryocytes in a hypercellular marrow (Table 15.9). The subjects with prefibrotic PMF tend to be younger, include more females, to have smaller spleens, fewer cytopenias and fewer additional mutations (other than of *JAK2*, *CALR* or *MPL*) and more thrombocytosis than those with overt PMF. For prefibrotic disease, if there are no symptoms a watch-and-wait approach may be taken, but if symptoms are present, vascular complications, marked thrombocytosis or splenomegaly, therapy is needed.

When myelofibrosis evolves after polycythaemia vera or essential thrombocythaemia, it is termed 'post-polycythaemic' or 'post-thrombocythaemic' myelofibrosis, respectively, and behaves similarly to primary myelofibrosis.

Other causes of marrow fibrosis include chronic myeloid leukaemia, myelodysplasia, systemic mastocytosis, hairy cell leukaemia, lymphomas and other cancers, infections, e.g. tuberculosis, leishmaniasis, other inflammatory diseases, drugs, e.g. benzene, irradiation.

The *JAK2*, *CALR* and *MPL* mutations occur in approximately 55%, 25–35% and 5–10% of patients, respectively (Fig. 15.3). One-third of patients with similar features have a previous history of PV or ET and some patients present with clinical and laboratory features of both disorders.

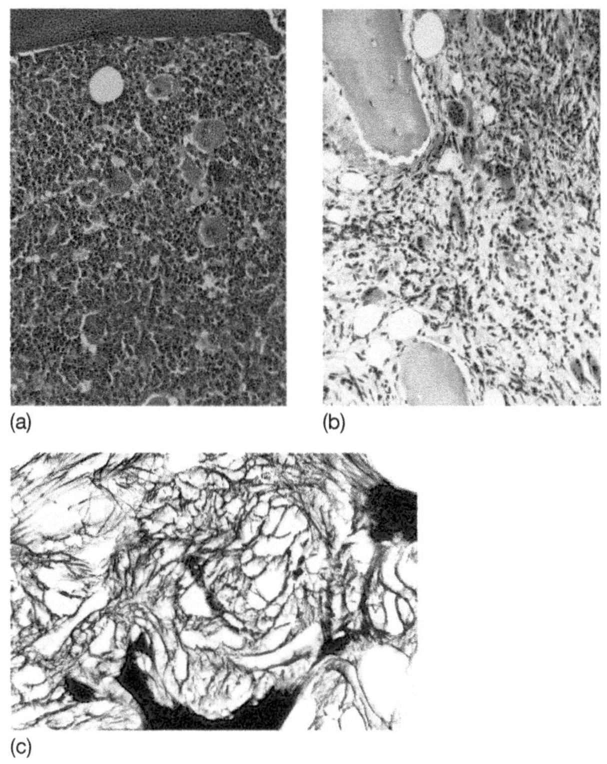

Figure 15.10 Iliac crest trephine biopsies. **(a)** Polycythaemia vera: fat spaces are almost completely replaced by hyperplastic haemopoietic tissue. All haemopoietic cell lines are increased, with megakaryocytes particularly prominent. **(b)** Primary myelofibrosis: normal marrow architecture is lost and haemopoietic cells are surrounded by increased fibrous tissue and intercellular substance. Atypical megakaryocytes are prominent. **(c)** Primary myelofibrosis: Silver staining shows a dense reticulin network. Source: A.V. Hoffbrand *et al.* (2019) *Color Atlas of Clinical Hematology*, 5th edn. Reproduced with permission of John Wiley & Sons.

Table 15.9 Diagnostic criteria of prefibrotic myelofibrosis.

Prefibrotic myelofibrosis	
All three major and one minor criteria must be met	
Major criteria	Typical megakaryocyte changes accompanied by ≤ grade 1 fibrosis
	Presence of *JAK2*, *CALR* or *MPL* mutations or presence of other clonal markers, or absence of evidence for reactive BM fibrosis
	Not meeting WHO criteria for other myeloid neoplasms
Minor criteria	Anaemia not otherwise specified
	Leucocytosis ≥ 11 × 10⁹/L
	Palpable splenomegaly
	Increased serum lactate dehydrogenase (LDH)
	Leucocytosis > 11 × 10⁹/L
	Palpable splenomegaly
	Increased serum lactate dehydrogenase (LDH)
	A leuco-erythroblastic blood film

Clinical features

1 **An insidious onset in older people is usual with symptoms of anaemia.**
2 Symptoms resulting from massive splenomegaly are frequent and include abdominal discomfort, pain or indigestion. Splenomegaly is the main physical finding (Fig. 15.5b).

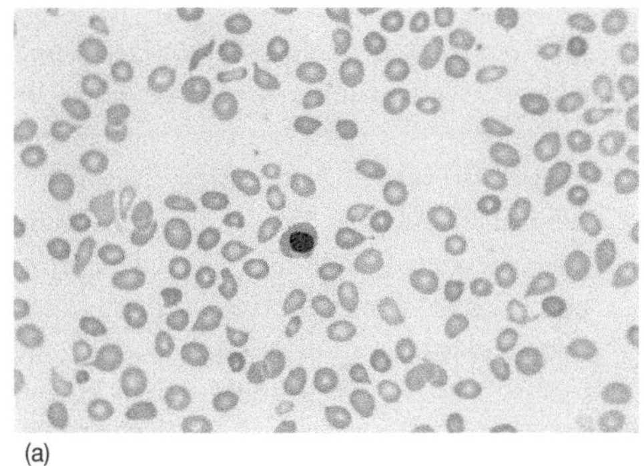

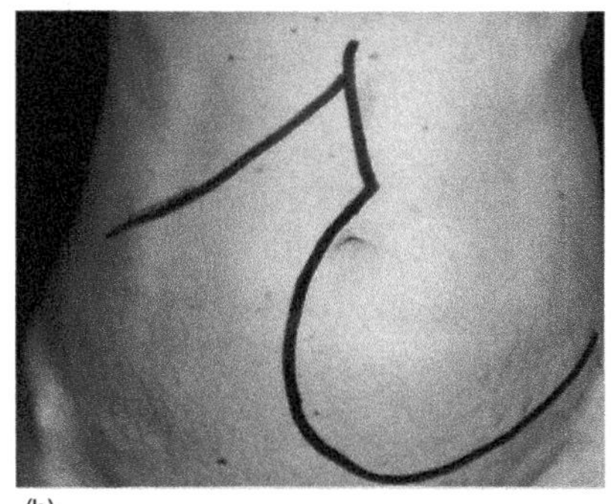

Figure 15.11 **(a)** Peripheral blood film in primary myelofibrosis. Leuco-erythroblastic change with 'tear-drop' cells and an erythroblast. **(b)** Massive splenomegaly in a patient with myelofibrosis.

3 Hypermetabolic symptoms such as loss of weight, anorexia, fever and night sweats are common.
4 Bleeding problems, bone pain or gout occur in a minority of patients. Thrombosis is also a risk in those with previous thrombosis, the *JAK2* mutation and high risk disease.

Laboratory findings

1 **Anaemia is usual, but a normal or increased haemoglobin level may be found in some patients.**
2 The white cell and platelet counts are frequently high at the time of presentation. Later in the disease leucopenia and thrombocytopenia are common. In the prefibrotic disease, leukocytosis and thrombocytosis tend to be more marked and anaemia less than in overt disease.
3 A leuco-erythroblastic blood film is found. The red cells show characteristic 'tear-drop' poikilocytes (Fig. 15.11).
4 Bone marrow is usually unobtainable by aspiration. Trephine biopsy (Fig. 15.10b) shows a fibrotic, hypercellular marrow. Silver staining shows a dense reticulin network (Fig 15.10c), except in prefibrotic PMF. The degree of fibrosis can be semi-quantitatively divided into three or four grades according to defined histological criteria. Increased megakaryocytes are frequently seen. In 10% of cases there is increased bone formation (osteosclerosis) with increased bone density on X-ray.
5 *JAK2* is mutated in approximately 60% of cases, *CALR* in ~25% and *MPL* in ~10%. The *CALR*-mutated patients have lower white cell and higher platelet counts and longest survival, while triple-negative patients have the shortest survival.
6 High serum urate and LDH levels reflect increased, although ineffective, haemopoiesis.

Outcomes

The median survival is 3–5 years and causes of death include heart failure, infection and leukaemic transformation. Transformation to AML occurs in 10–20% of patients. Prediction of survival can be undertaken using a number of prognostic models (Table 15.10). All of these models are based on clinical parameters. However, certain chromosome and molecular genetic abnormalities (Fig. 15.4) also predict for progression of myelofibrosis. These varying factors are incorporated in some prognostic models, e.g. MIPSS-70; http://www.mipss70score.it. The MYSEC-PM (http://www.mysec-pm.eu) allows for prediction of survival for patients with myelofibrosis secondary to PV and ET. Understanding prediction of survival is important in selecting subsequent treatment.

Treatment

Therapy for PMF is aimed at reducing the effects of anaemia and splenomegaly. Blood transfusions and regular folic acid therapy (especially in those with poor nutrition) are useful in severely anaemic patients.

Hydroxycarbamide may reduce splenomegaly and hypermetabolic symptoms. Androgens, e.g. danazol, improve anaemia in some cases. Erythropoiesis-stimulating agents can be tried, but may cause splenic enlargement. Splenectomy, considered for patients with severe symptomatic splenomegaly, is associated with a high morbidity and mortality, even with experienced surgeons and is with the availability of JAK2 inhibitors now rarely undertaken. Allopurinol is indicated to prevent gout and urate nephropathy from hyperuricaemia.

Ruxolitinib is an oral JAK2 inhibitor that can reduce spleen size, improve constitutional symptoms such as night sweats, pruritus and cachexia and quality of life and increase survival. It should be started in the first year from diagnosis in intermediate- and high-risk patients. Side effects include anaemia, thrombocytopenia and prolonged immunosuppression. Other JAK2 inhibitors, e.g. fedratinib, pacritinib and momelotinib, may be useful either in treatment naïve patients; or in those who have become refractory to a first line JAK inhibitor. The different target specificity of various JAK inhibitors results in different efficacy and side effect profiles. For example, momelotinib may have a beneficial effect on anaemia symptoms as compared to the other agents. Novel combinations of JAK2 inhibitors with other agents are undergoing investigation. For example, navitoclax, a BCL-2 inhibitor may improve the response to ruxolitinib monotherapy. Other novel agents at advanced stage of clinical trials include luspatercept (activin receptor ligand trap), parsaclisib (PI3Kδ inhibitor) and pelabresib (BET inhibitor).

Allogeneic stem cell transplantation (SCT) may be a curative option based on careful patient selection. Assessment of patient fitness based on comorbidity assessments, and performance status informs likely risk of transplant related mortality. Decision to proceed to transplantation rests on a balance between likely survival with SCT (based on disease relapse and treatment related mortality) compared to PMF related life expectancy from prognostic scores.

Mastocytosis

Mastocytosis is a clonal neoplastic proliferation of mast cells that accumulate in one or more organ systems. Mast cells survive for months or years in vascular tissues and most organs. WHO 2022 recognizes three disease types: cutaneous, systemic and mast cell sarcoma. **Cutaneous mastocytosis** with the skin lesions of urticarial pigmentosa (Fig. 15.12) is much more common than systemic forms of mastocytosis and tends to run an indolent course. As well as the diffuse forms, lesions may form as either isolated or multilocalized mastocytomas,

Systemic mastocytosis is a clonal myeloproliferative neoplasm with diverse presentations involving bone marrow, heart, spleen, lymph nodes and skin. The bone marrow or other organs than skin show multifocal dense (>15 cells per aggregate)

Table 15.10 A comparison of categories used between widely used prognostic models to predict survival in primary myelofibrosis. Scoring results in allocation of patients to different risk categories (see references).

Variable	DIPSS Plus	MIPSS-70+ v2.0	MYSEC-PM
Age >65 years	✓		Age (0.15× y of age)
Constitutional symptoms	✓	✓	✓
Haemoglobin (Hb) <100 g/L	✓	Hb <80 g/L in women and Hb <90 g/L in men (Severe anaemia). Hb 80–99 g/L in women and Hb 90–109 g/L in men. (Moderate anaemia).	<110 g/L
Leucocyte count >25 × 10⁹/L	✓		
Circulating blasts ≥1%	✓	≥2%	≥3%
Platelet count <100 × 10⁹/L	✓		<150 × 10⁹/L
Red blood cell transfusion need	✓		
Presence of *CALR* mutations		Absence of CALR type 1/like mutation	Absence of CALR mutation
Unfavourable karyotype	✓*	✓ (unfavourable and very high-risk categories)**	
High molecular risk mutations (*ASXL1, SRSF2, EZH2, IDH1, IDH2, U2AF1Q157*)		1 or ≥2 high molecular risk mutation categories	

DIPPS Plus (N. Gangat *et al.* (2011) *J. Clin. Oncol.* 29: 392–7).
MIPSS-70 (P. Guglielmelli *et al.* (2018) *J. Clin. Oncol.* 36: 310–8. http://www.mipss70score.it).
MYSEC-PM (F. Passamonti *et al.* (2017) *Leukemia* 31: 2726–31. http://www.mysec-pm.eu).
*Unfavourable karyotype includes +8, -7/7q-, -5,5q-, complex and others.
**Very high risk: single/multiple abnormalities of -7, i(17q), inv(3)/3q21, 12p-/12p11.2, 11q-/11q23, or other autosomal trisomies not including + 8/ + 9, e.g. +21, +19. Unfavourable indicates any abnormal karyotype not included in very high risk; or normal karyotype, sole abnormalities of 20q-, 13q-, +9, chromosome 1 translocation/duplication, -Y or sex chromosome abnormality other than –Y.

mast cell infiltrates. The cells are CD2 and/or CD25 and CD30 positive. Systemic mastocytosis is often seen in association with other haemopoietic conditions including MDS, MPN or AML. It may be indolent or smouldering The most aggressive form of systemic mastocytosis is **mast cell leukaemia**, in which large numbers of clonal, atypical mast cells circulate in the blood; median survival is only a few months. **Mast cell sarcoma** is another aggressive form.

The somatic *KIT* mutation Asp816Val (D816V) is detected in >90% of patients and is responsible for autonomous growth and enhanced survival of the neoplastic mast cells. Kit is a tyrosine kinase cell membrane receptor for the growth factor stem cell factor (SCF). In advanced cases additional point mutations, e.g. of *TET2,SRSF2, ASXL1, RUNX1* or *JAK2,* are usually present.

Symptoms are either related to organ infiltration or histamine and prostaglandin release, and include flushing, pruritus, anaphylaxis, abdominal pain, diarrhoea, bronchospasm and neurocognitive impairment such as memory loss. Symptoms may be precipitated by changes in temperature, infections and stress. The skin usually shows urticaria pigmentosa (Fig. 15.12). Serum tryptase is increased (above 20 ng/ml) and can be used to monitor treatment. Midostaurin is approved for treatment of systemic mastocytosis and avapritinib is also highly active; both inhibit the KIT tyrosine kinase. Antihistamine drugs and cromolyn are valuable in reducing mast cell mediator symptoms. The patient should have self-injection adrenaline available in case of anaphylaxis. α-Interferon or chemotherapy such as cladrabine can be helpful in resistant cases.

Chronic neutrophilic leukaemia

These patients have a persistently raised white cell count of >25 × 10^9/L with at least 80% mature neutrophils. They have no inflammatory or other causes of neutrophilia, no evidence for any other myeloproliferative neoplasm (*BCR::ABL1*

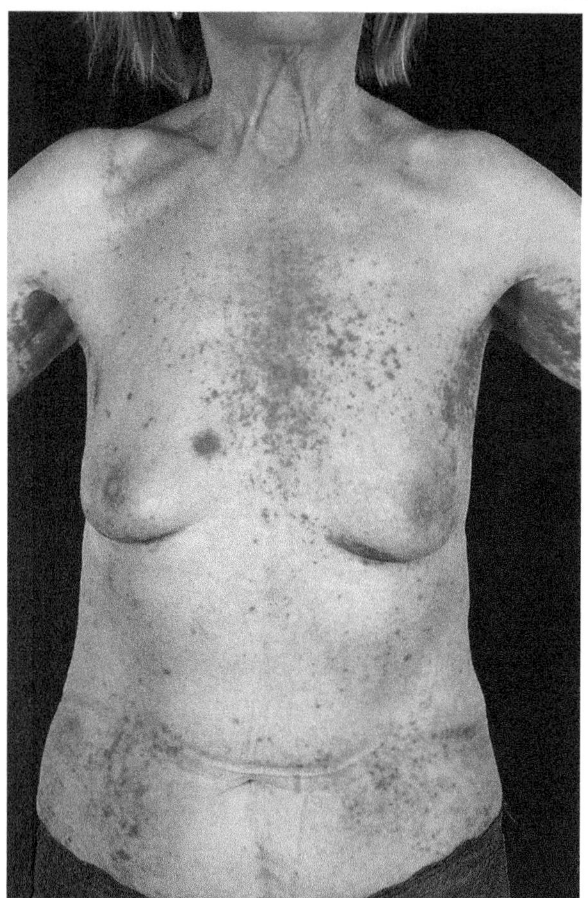

Figure 15.12 Systemic mastocytosis: female 72 years; widespread erythematous, confluent plaques of urticaria pigmentosa over chest, abdomen and upper arms. Source: Courtesy of Professor M. Rustin.

negative) and no increase in blast cells. They may have mild splenomegaly. Activating mutations in the gene encoding the receptor for colony-stimulating factor 3 (*CSF3R*) are found in most patients and kinase inhibitors may be useful. The prognosis is variable.

Chronic eosinophilic leukaemia

This is a clonal disorder with a sustained (for more than 4 weeks) proliferation of abnormal eosinophils in bone marrow and blood. Abnormal morphology of red cell precursors and/or megakaryocytes is also usually present. If clonality cannot be shown and blasts are less than 5%, the condition is diagnosed as hypereosinophilic syndrome (p. 110). The cells may infiltrate various organs, causing damage, e.g. endomyocardial fibrosis, lung fibrosis, central nervous system, skin (with pruritus) and gastrointestinal tract. Presentation with organ damage may be as an emergency, in which case high dose corticosteroids are indicated. Other treatments such as hydroxycarbamide, α-interferon and cladrabine may be tried.

Juvenile myelomonocytic leukaemia (JMML)

This disease presents most frequently in the first 6 years of life, with a median age of 2 years. JMML has features of both myelodysplasia and a myeloproliferative neoplasm. There is often an eczematous skin rash, hepatosplenomegaly and lymphadenopathy. There is monocytosis to more than 1.0×10^9/L and clonal cytogenetic change. Components of the GM-CSF receptor signalling pathway and its downstream effector the RAS/MAPK pathway (Fig. 1.8) are mutated in over 90% of patients. Children with two genetic disorders, Noonan syndrome and neurofibromatosis, are at increased risk of JMML, and mutations in the genes *PTPN11* and *NF1*, which are part of the RAS/MAPK pathway, respectively, underlie these genetic disorders.

Co-mutations in epigenetic regulatory and spliceosome genes are commonly found. The only curative treatment is allogeneic SCT. If untreated, median survival time can be as short as 12 months, often from acute transformation with leukaemic infiltration, e.g. of the lungs, although in very rare cases spontaneous resolution can occur.

Myeloid/lymphoid neoplasm with eosinophilia and tyrosine kinase gene fusions

These are myeloid or lymphoid neoplasms driven by tyrosine kinases activated by gene rearrangements. The histology ranges through myeloproliferative, myelodysplastic, acute myeloid or lymphoblastic leukaemia and mixed phenotype acute leukaemia. Extramedullary disease is common; eosinophilia is usual but not invariable. An interstitial deletion lesion in chromosome 4 resulting in *FIP1L1-PDGFRA* fusion gene if present is most common but *PDGFRA* may have other partners. Fusion genes involving *PDGFRA* and *PDGFRB* predict for a response to tyrosine kinase inhibitors. Other translocations in this category may involve *FGFR1* and *JAK2*. Pemigatinib is approved for relapsed, or refractory myeloid/lymphoid neoplasms with *FGFR1* translocations.

SUMMARY

- Myeloproliferative neoplasms are a group of conditions arising from marrow stem cells and characterized by clonal proliferation of one or more haemopoietic components in the bone marrow. The three major subtypes are polycythaemia vera (PV), essential thrombocythaemia (ET) and primary myelofibrosis (PMF).
- These subtypes are closely related to each other. Mutation of the *JAK2* gene is detected in almost all patients with PV and approximately 60% of those with ET and primary myelofibrosis. Mutations in *CALR* or *MPL* are present in most cases of ET or PMF without a *JAK2* mutation.
- Polycythaemia is defined as an increase in the haemoglobin concentration above normal for the age and sex. The major subdivision is into **absolute polycythaemia**, in which the red cell mass is raised, and **relative polycythaemia**, in which the red cell volume is normal but the plasma volume is reduced.
- Absolute polycythaemia is divided into primary or secondary polycythaemia. Primary polycythaemia includes rare congenital types and the much more frequent acquired type, polycythaemia vera (PV).
- The diagnosis of PV is made by finding polycythaemia together with a *JAK2* mutation. It occurs in older patients and the increase in blood viscosity leads to headaches, plethoric appearance, splenomegaly and thrombosis.
- Treatment of PV aims to maintain the haematocrit lower than 50% and in those at high risk of thrombosis < 45%. Usual treatments include venesection, hydroxycarbamide, *JAK2* inhibitors and aspirin. Survival is usually over 10 years, but there may be progression to AML or myelofibrosis.
- Secondary polycythaemia can arise from rare congenital causes or acquired disorders such as lung disease or tumours that secrete erythropoietin. Venesection and treatment of the underlying cause may be needed.
- Essential thrombocythaemia is diagnosed by persistent raised platelet count >450 × 10^9/L in the absence of other causes. *JAK2*, *CALR* or *MPL* genes are mutated in most cases. Low dose aspirin is given in nearly all cases. In those at high risk, the platelet count is lowered usually with hydroxycarbamide.
- The predominant feature of primary myelofibrosis is a progressive generalized reactive fibrosis of the bone marrow in association with haemopoiesis in the spleen and liver. Symptoms usually result from anaemia and a grossly enlarged spleen.
- Diagnosis of primary myelofibrosis is made on blood film, which shows a leuco-erythroblastic appearance, together with bone marrow biopsy and *JAK2*, *CALR* and *MPL* mutation screen. Treatment is mainly with red cell transfusion and JAK2 inhibition. Stem cell transplantation offers a chance of cure in fit patients.
- Systemic mastocytosis is a clonal proliferation of mast cells with involvement of bone marrow, skin (as urticaria pigmentosa) and other organs. There is usually an underlying *KIT* mutation, most commonly D816V, and the disease may respond to tyrosine kinase inhibitors.
- Chronic neutrophilic leukaemia, chronic eosinophilic leukaemia and juvenile myelomonocytic leukaemia are rare MPNs.
- Myeloid/lymphoid neoplasms with eosinophilia and tyrosine kinase fusions are clonal disorders that sometimes respond to tyrosine kinase inhibitors.

Now visit **www.wiley.com/go/haematology9e** to test yourself on this chapter.

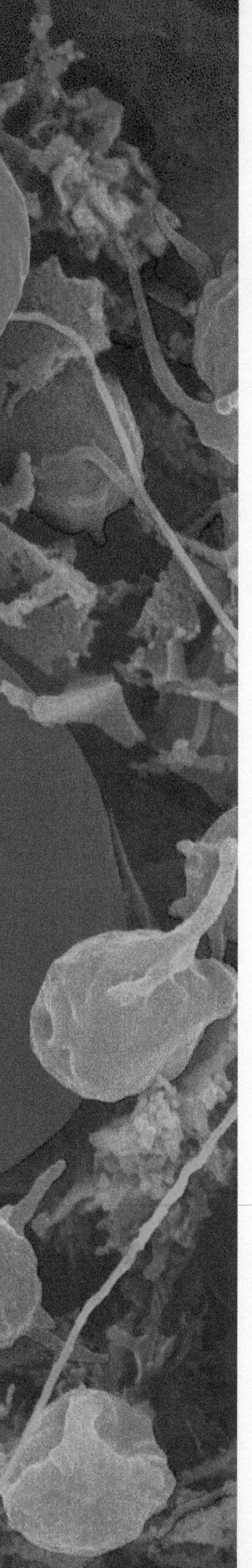

CHAPTER 16

Myelodysplastic neoplasms

Key topics

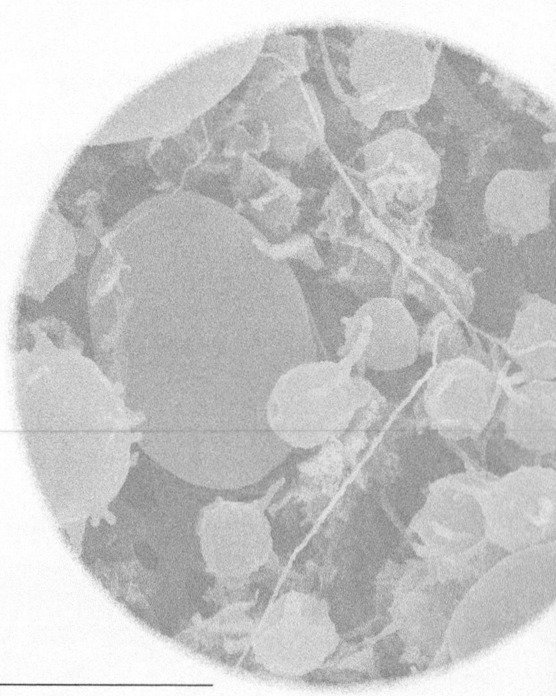

Hoffbrand's Essential Haematology, Ninth Edition. A. Victor Hoffbrand, Pratima Chowdary, Graham P. Collins, and Justin Loke.

© 2024 John Wiley & Sons Ltd. Published 2024 by John Wiley & Sons Ltd.

Companion website: www.wiley.com/go/haematology9e

Myelodysplastic neoplasms (MDS)

MDS includes a group of clonal disorders of haemopoietic stem cells characterized by bone marrow failure in association with dysplastic cell morphology in one or more cell lineages (Table 16.1).

A hallmark of these diseases is simultaneous proliferation and apoptosis of haemopoietic cells (**ineffective haemopoiesis**), leading to the paradox of a hypercellular bone marrow but pancytopenia in peripheral blood. There is a tendency for MDS to progress to acute myeloid leukaemia (AML), although death from complications of cytopenias or from unrelated causes often occurs before this develops.

In most cases, the disease is *de novo* (primary), but in a proportion of patients it is a result of chemotherapy or radiotherapy given for treatment of another disorder. This latter type is termed therapy-related MDS (t-MDS) and is now classified together with therapy-related AML, since the marrow blast proportion has little influence on outcome in this poor-prognosis form of myeloid neoplasm (Chapter 13). Secondary MDS describes MDS arising from germline mutations or inherited marrow failure syndromes.

Pathogenesis

The pathogenesis of the MDS begins with genetic changes in a multipotent haemopoietic progenitor cell. The immune system may have a role in suppressing bone marrow function once an abnormal clone is present and immunosuppression is sometimes used in treatment (see below). The marrow microenviroment (stromal cells) probably also contributes to abnormal haemopoiesis, though the microenvironmental defects are not yet well defined.

Table 16.1 The World Health Organization (2022) classification of myelodysplastic syndromes (MDS). Therapy-related myeloid neoplasms and MDS arising as a consequence of a germline mutation are classified separately.

	Blasts	Cytogenetics	Mutations
MDS with defining genetic abnormalities			
MDS with low blasts and isolated 5q deletion (MDS-5q)	<5% BM and <2% PB	5q deletion alone, or with 1 other abnormality other than monosomy 7 or 7q deletion	
MDS with low blasts and *SF3B1* mutation* (MDS-*SF3B1*)		Absence of 5q deletion, monosomy 7 or complex karyotype	*SF3B1*
MDS with biallelic *TP53* inactivation (MDS-bi*TP53*)	<20% BM and PB	Usually complex	Two or more *TP53* mutations, or 1 mutation with evidence of *TP53* copy number loss or cnLOH
MDS, morphologically defined			
MDS with low blasts (MDS-LB)	<5% BM and <2% PB		
MDS, hypoplastic** (MDS-h)			
MDS with increased blasts (MDS-IB)			
MDS-IB1	5–9% BM or 2–4% PB		
MDS-IB2	10–19% BM or 5–19% PB or Auer rods		
MDS with fibrosis (MDS-f)	5–19% BM; 2–19% PB		

*Detection of ≥15% ring sideroblasts may substitute for SF3B1 mutation. Acceptable related terminology: MDS with low blasts and ring sideroblasts.
**By definition, ≤25% bone marrow cellularity, age adjusted.
BM, bone marrow; cnLOH, copy neutral loss of heterozygosity; PB, peripheral blood.

Table 16.2 Examples of recurrent cytogenetic abnormalities in MDS and their prognostic implications.

Prognosis	Cytogenetic abnormality
Very good	–Y or del(11q)
Good	Normal or del(5q)
Intermediate	del(7q) or double-independent clones
Poor	inv(3) or double including –7 or del(7q)
Very poor	Complex: >3 abnormalities

Source: Based on P.L. Greenberg *et al.* (2012) *Blood* 120: 2454–65.

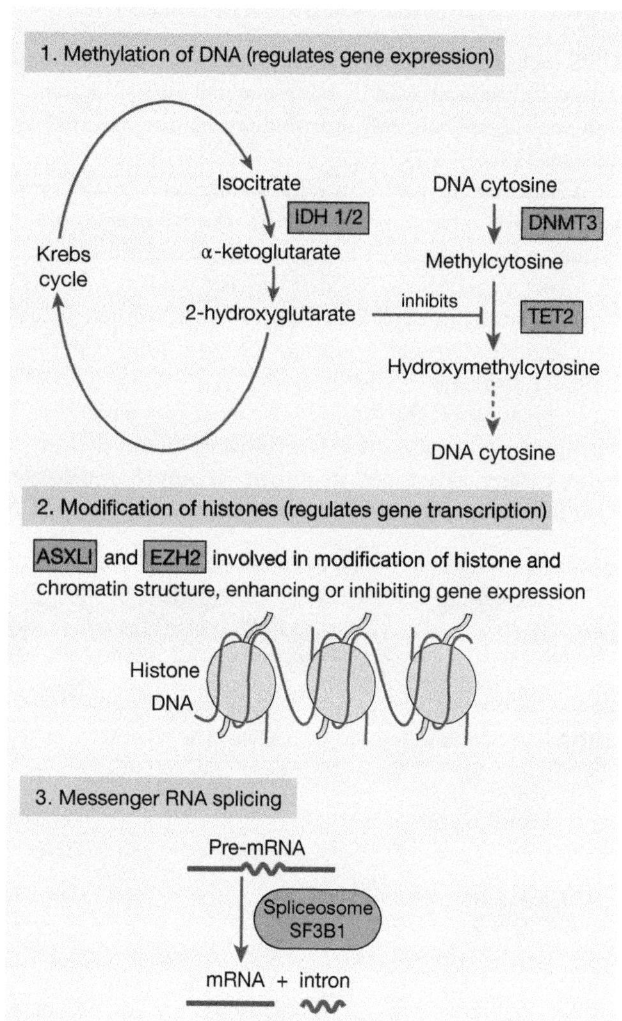

Figure 16.1 Genes involved in DNA methylation, histone modification and in mRNA splicing are frequently mutated (loss of function or gain in function) in myelodysplastic syndromes, acute myeloid leukaemia or myeloproliferative neoplasms.

Germline predisposition to MDS is present in a proportion of cases of all ages most frequently in those presenting before 30 years old but even in 6% of those at all decades in the elderly. The genes involved have been listed in Table 13.2. Often other organ systems are affected by these gene mutations.

Acquired chromosome abnormalities in marrow cells are frequent, detectable in more than half of cases (Table 16.2). Most of these are numerical abnormalities or segmental chromosomal deletions, rather than the balanced translocations that are common in AML.

In addition, molecular analysis shows that clonally derived cells in MDS typically carry several point mutations. More than 40 different driver mutations have been identified in MDS and usually involve genes involved in epigenetic processes such as DNA methylation (*TET2* and *DNMT3A*) and chromatin modification (*ASXL1* and *EZH2*), as well as in RNA splicing (*SF3B1*, *SRSF2*, *U2AF1*) (Figs. 16.1 and 16.2). Most of these gene mutations, e.g. of *TET2*, may be found in other myeloid malignancies, including AML and the myeloproliferative neoplasms (MPN). However, in MDS, common AML-associated mutations including *FLT3* or *NPM1* are rare, probably because these are strong leukaemia drivers that result when they are acquired in rapid progression to AML. The molecular mutations have prognostic significance. At the time MDS progresses to AML, additional mutations are often acquired.

A striking example of genotype–phenotype correlation is mutation in the *SF3B1* gene, which encodes a component of the RNA spliceosome. *SF3B1* mutations are seen in almost all cases of MDS with ring sideroblasts (ring sideroblasts are abnormal erythroid precursors, discussed in Chapter 3 and further below). *TP53* mutations are detected most commonly in patients with t-MDS and are often associated with complex chromosome rearrangements, chemotherapy resistance and a poor prognosis.

Classification

MDS are classified on the basis of three defined genetic abnormalities with cytogenetic and molecular genetic analysis (Table 16.1) or morphologically according to the proportion of blast cells in the blood or bone marrow (Table 16.1). Hypoplastic MDS and MDS with fibrosis are two separate sub-types.

Cell morphological abnormalities (dysplasia) may be present in a single myeloid lineage (**'single-lineage dysplasia'**) – red cells, neutrophils or platelets – or present in two or more myeloid lineages (**'multilineage dysplasia'**).

- Erythroid dysplasia can also be associated with **ring sideroblasts.** The definition of a pathological ring sideroblast is an erythroid precursor with five or more iron granules encircling at least one-third of the nucleus. Nearly all of these patients have mutations in *SF3B1*. In the absence of this mutation and the presence of ≥15% ring sideroblasts, they can be classed as MDS with low blasts and ring sideroblasts.

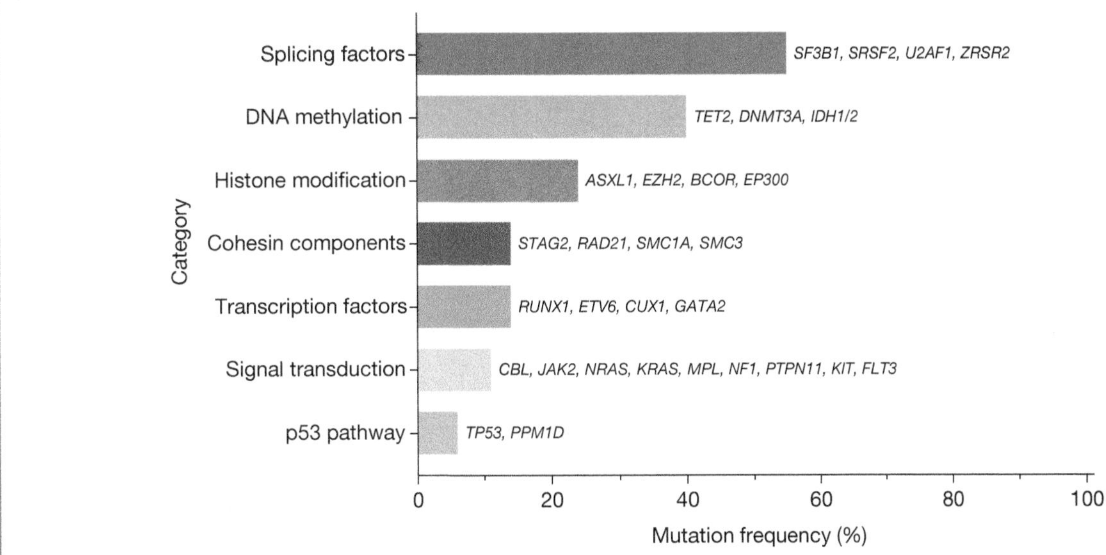

Figure 16.2 Recurrently mutated genes in MDS can be organized into biological categories. Estimated mutation frequencies and examples of commonly implicated genes in each category are depicted. The most frequently mutated genes are *TET2, SF3B1, ASXL1, SRSF2, DNMT3A and RUNX1*. Source: J.A. Kennedy, B.L. Ebert (2017) *J. Clin. Oncol.* 35: 968–74. Reproduced with permission of American Society of Clinical Oncology. Data also from E. Papaemmanuil *et al.* (2013) *Blood* 122: 3616–27. T. Haferlach *et al.* (2014) *Leukemia* 28: 241–7.

- If the blast cell count is increased in the bone marrow, the diagnosis is made of **MDS with increased blasts (MDS-IB)**. IB1 or IB2 is defined according to the % blasts (Table 16.1).
- **5q– syndrome,** also called **MDS with isolated del(5q), is a distinct entity**. A key gene that is deleted is *RPS14*, encoding a ribosomal protein (Fig. 24.7). This subtype is more common in women and typically there is a macrocytic anaemia with thrombocytosis in 50% of cases. This subtype has a favourable prognosis and responds well to lenalidomide therapy (Tables 16.2 and 16.3).
- **Childhood MDS** is classified by WHO 2022 into those with low blasts (<2%in PB, <5% in BM), hypoplastic or not otherwise specified and those with increased blasts (2–19% in peripheral blood, 5–19% in bone marrow). They differ biologically from adult MDS. Clinically, hypoplastic variants are more common, and there is a need to exclude other causes of dysplasia such as non-neoplastic causes, e.g. metabolic diseases.

Clinical features

The disease has an incidence of at least 1 in 10 000 persons per year and a slight male predominance. The median age is 70 years and fewer than 5% of patients are under 50 years of age. The evolution is often slow and the disease may be found by chance when a patient has a blood count for some unrelated reason. The symptoms, if present, are those of anaemia, infections from neutropenia or functional neutrophil defects, or of easy bruising or bleeding from thrombocytopenia or functional platelet defects (Fig. 16.3).

In some patients, transfusion-dependent anaemia dominates the course, while in others recurring infections or spontaneous bruising and bleeding are the major clinical problems. The function of the neutrophils, monocytes and platelets is often impaired, so that infections and bleeding may occur out of proportion to the severity of the cytopenia. The spleen is not usually enlarged.

Dysplastic cell morphology features in bone marrow may be seen in a wide range of conditions, such as excess alcohol intake, megaloblastic anaemia, parvovirus or HIV infection, recovery from cytotoxic chemotherapy, other myeloid neoplasms, and granulocyte colony-stimulating factor (G-CSF) therapy. These alternative conditions must be ruled out before making a diagnosis of MDS, and diagnostic tests may need to be repeated over time in some patients.

Laboratory findings

Peripheral blood

Pancytopenia is a frequent finding. The red cells are usually macrocytic but occasionally microcytic; normoblasts may be present. The reticulocyte count is low. Neutrophils are often reduced in number and frequently show lack of granulation (Fig. 16.4). Their chemotactic, phagocytic and adhesive functions are impaired. The pseudo-Pelger abnormality, i.e. single

Table 16.3 Revised International Prognostic Scoring System (IPSS-R) prognostic risk categories/scores and clinical outcomes. Inclusion of mutations from NGS profiling (IPSS-M) is available from 'clinical calculators', present online (https://mds-risk-model.com).

Prognostic variable	**0**	**0.5**	**1**	**1.5**	**2**	**3**	**4**
Cytogenetics (Table 16.2)	Very good		Good		Intermediate	Poor	Very poor
Bone marrow blast %	≤2		>2–<5		5–10	>10	
Haemoglobin (Hb) concentration (g/L)	≥100		80–<100	<80			
Platelet count	≥100	50–<100	<50				
Neutrophil count (×10^9/L)	≥0.8	<0.8					

Time taken for 25% of cases to evolve to acute myeloid leukaemia (AML)

Risk category	**Risk score**	**Survival (median in years)**	**Median time to evolution of AML in 25% + of cases (years)**
Very low	≤1.5	8.8	Not reached
Low	>1.5–3	5.3	10.8
Intermediate	>3–4.5	3.0	3.2
High	>4.5–6	1.6	1.4
Very high	>6	0.8	0.73

Source: Based on P.L. Greenberg *et al.* (2012) *Blood* 120: 2454–65.

Table 16.4 Acronyms describing clonal haemopoiesis and related states.

Acronym	**State**	**Description**
CHIP	Clonal haemopoiesis of indeterminate potential	Somatic mutation of myeloid malignancy-associated genes in blood or bone marrow at ≥2% variant allele frequency in people without a haematological neoplasm. Conveys a risk of subsequent haematological neoplasm diagnosis or acute vascular events
ARCH	Ageing-related clonal haemopoiesis	Clonal haemopoiesis defined by presence of somatic mutations in blood and marrow and an expanded haemopoietic clone, with or without a leukaemia-associated driver mutation. Incidence increases with age. No specific variant allele frequency
ICUS	Idiopathic cytopenia(s) of undetermined significance	Patient with one or more cytopenias but no evidence of myelodysplastic syndromes or another haematological neoplasm or specific disorder. Either no somatic mutation is detected or a mutation has not been sought
CCUS	Clonal cytopenia(s) of undetermined significance	As ICUS but with a clonal mutation present
IDUS	Idiopathic dysplasia of undetermined significance	Unexplained morphological dysplasia of blood or marrow cells with normal blood count

or bilobed nucleus of neutrophils, is often present. The platelets may be unduly large or small and are usually decreased in number, but in ~10% of cases are elevated. In poor-prognosis cases, variable numbers of myeloblasts (<20%) are present in the blood.

Bone marrow

The cellularity is usually increased. A small number of dysplastic cells may be seen in marrow from healthy elderly individuals, so at least 10% of the cells in a lineage should be dysplastic in

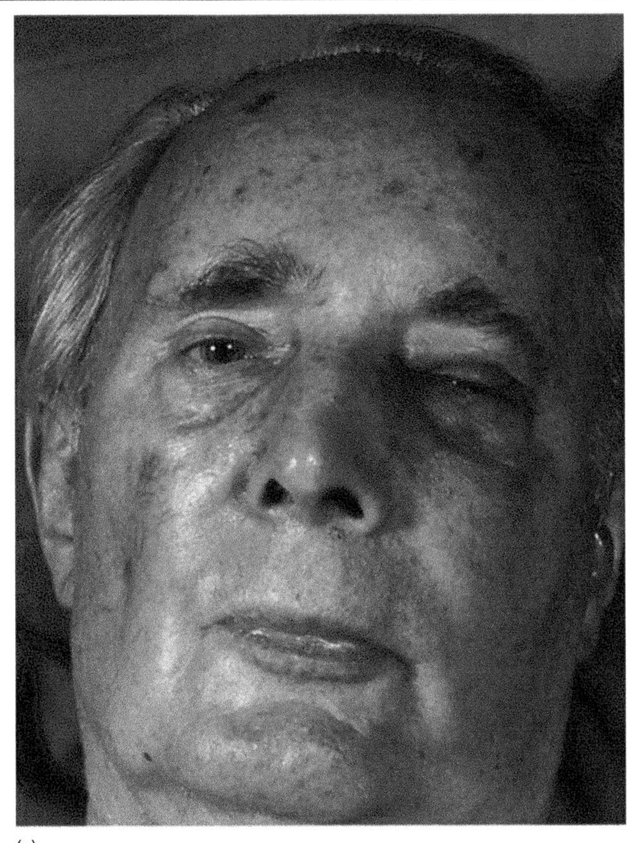

(a)

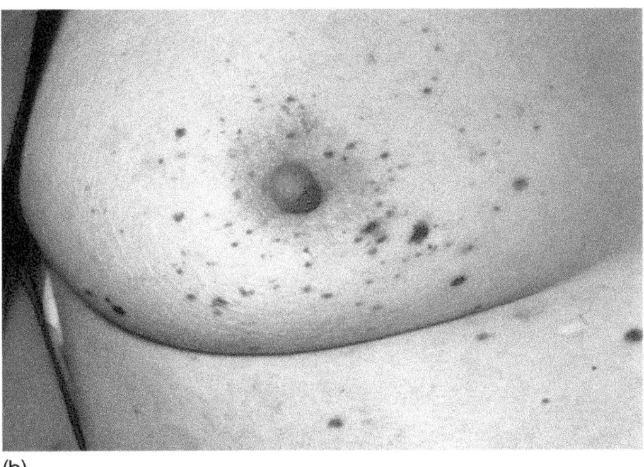

(b)

Figure 16.3 Physical signs seen in myelodysplastic neoplasias (MDS). **(a)** A 78-year-old male patient with MDS with multilineage dysplasia (MDS-MLD) had recurring infections of the face and maxillary sinuses associated with neutropenia (haemoglobin 98 g/L; white cells 1.3×10^9/L; neutrophils 0.3×10^9/L; platelets 38×10^9/L). **(b)** Purpura of the skin of the breast in a 58-year-old female with MDS-MLD (haemoglobin 105 g/L; white cells 2.3×10^9/L; platelets 8×10^9/L).

order to consider the diagnosis of MDS. Typical dysplastic features are:

- ***Erythroid*** Multinucleate normoblasts, internuclear bridges and nuclear budding (Fig. 16.4). Ring sideroblasts are seen in a specific subset of MDS and are caused by iron deposition in the mitochondria of erythroblasts.
- ***Myeloid*** The granulocyte precursors often show defective granulation and may be difficult to distinguish from monocytes.
- ***Megakaryocytes*** Dysplastic megakaryocytes may show micronuclear, small binuclear or polynuclear forms (Fig. 16.4).

In a minority of cases (about 10%), the marrow is hypocellular and may resemble aplastic anaemia; in others there is fibrosis that may cause confusion with primary myelofibrosis.

Genetic abnormalities

Cytogenetic analysis is essential in cases of unexplained cytopenias or suspected MDS. Common abnormalities include 5q–, partial or total loss of chromosomes 5 or 7, or trisomy 8 (Table 16.2). Several cytogenetic abnormalities such as 5q– are considered so diagnostic of MDS that they allow diagnosis of MDS even in the absence of morphological abnormalities within cells.

The mutations that may be found by molecular testing have been described above and summarized in Fig. 16.2, while Fig. 16.1 illustrates those involved in epigenetic processes.

Treatment

A key subdivision for considering treatment of MDS is stratifying into patients with lower-risk or higher-risk disease. 'Risk' here describes risk of progression to leukaemia or death from complications of cytopenias.

The Revised International Prognostic Scoring System (IPSS-R) classifies patients according to the proportion of marrow blasts, the type of karyotype abnormality, and the number and severity of cytopenias (Table 16.3). For example, patients with less than 5% blasts in the marrow, only one cytopenia and favourable cytogenetics generally will have lower-risk MDS. Lower-risk MDS includes patients whose

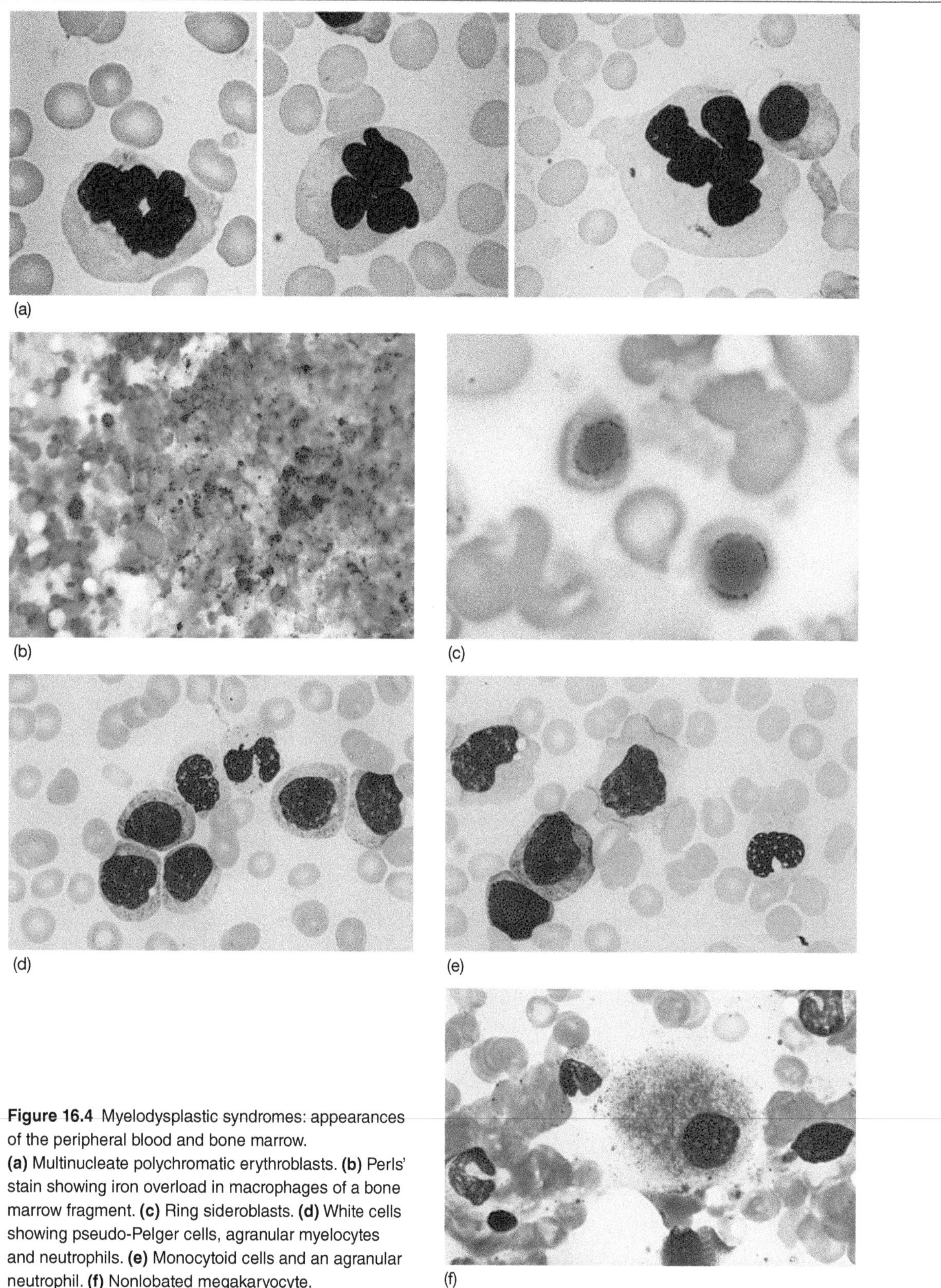

Figure 16.4 Myelodysplastic syndromes: appearances of the peripheral blood and bone marrow.
(a) Multinucleate polychromatic erythroblasts. **(b)** Perls' stain showing iron overload in macrophages of a bone marrow fragment. **(c)** Ring sideroblasts. **(d)** White cells showing pseudo-Pelger cells, agranular myelocytes and neutrophils. **(e)** Monocytoid cells and an agranular neutrophil. **(f)** Nonlobated megakaryocyte.

IPSS-R score equals 3.5 or lower, i.e. very low, low and part of intermediate risk. The rest (IPSS-R ≥ 4) defines a higher risk MDS group. Clinically, patients behave heterogeneously, with these additional clinical risk factors, e.g. bleeding history, co-morbidities, important in interpreting the results from prognostic models, especially for those with an intermediate score. A further refinement to this prognosis model is now available through the inclusion of mutations from NGS profiling (IPSS-M) (Table 16.3).

Lower-risk myelodysplastic syndromes

The treatment aim in this group of patients is to manage the effect of cytopenias (Fig. 16.5). Those with mild cytopenias and minimal symptoms can often be observed with serial blood counts or, if necessary improving marrow function with haemopoietic growth factors, either singly or in combination. **Erythropoiesis-stimulating agents (ESAs)** (Chapter 2) may improve anaemia in 40–50% of cases with an endogenous erythropoietin level <500 U/L, although the haemoglobin should not be raised above 120 g/L. Patients with a low red cell transfusion requirements are more likely to respond to ESAs. G-CSF shows synergy with ESAs and may increase the erythroid response rate.

Luspatercept (Chapter 7) raises haemoglobin levels in MDS by improving effective erythropoiesis. It is well established as effective in patients with ring sideroblasts and trials in other types of MDS suggest it is also, for many patients, more effective than ESAs. Luspatercept may replace ESAs as first-line treatment of anaemia in all low-risk patients. Trials

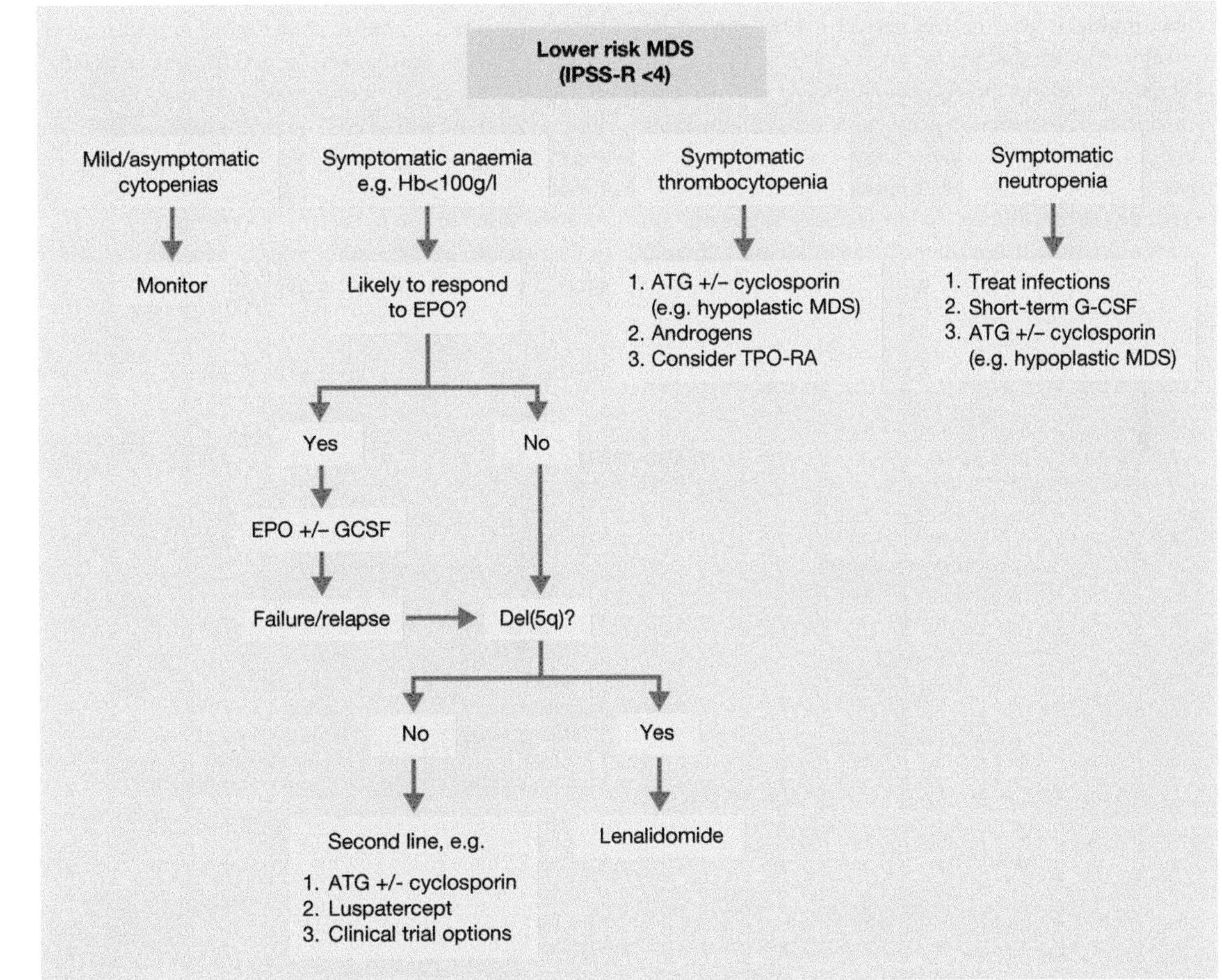

Figure 16.5 Management of lower-risk MDS. Availability of options limited by local licensing. Allogeneic stem cell transplant is an option for a sub-set of patients with lower-risk MDS. Source: Adapted from P. Fenaux *et al.* (2021) *Ann. Oncol.* 32: 142–56. ATG, antithymocyte globulin; EPO, erythropoietin; G-CSF, granulocyte colony-stimulating factor; Hb, haemoglobin; IPSS-R, revised international prognostic scoring system; TPO-RA, thrombopoietin receptor agonist.

of treating the anaemia with prolyl hydroxylase inhibitors (Chapter 2) are also in progress.

Thrombomimetics, such as **eltrombopag or romiplostim**, can be given for severe thrombocytopenia or bleeding, but may stimulate blast growth, and are not currently approved for use in MDS in Europe. Ciclosporin or anti-thymocyte globulin occasionally helps, particularly for those with a hypocellular bone marrow and normal karyotype.

Long-term transfusion support with red cells or platelets is often needed. For example, after prolonged used of ESAs, patients may become refractory to these agents. Antibiotics may be required either prophylactically or to treat infections. In the long term, iron overload may be a problem after multiple transfusion. In patients with lower risk MDS, iron chelation therapy e.g. with deferasirox should be considered after 20–50 units have been transfused or if the ferritin rises above 1000 μg/L. Measurement of liver and cardiac iron by magnetic resonance imaging (MRI) is helpful in deciding whether or not chelation therapy is indicated.

Lenalidomide is particularly effective for anaemia in MDS associated with del(5q), where it can often reduce the size of the del(5q) clone and reduce transfusion requirements in the majority of patients. Patients with del(5q) and more than one additional cytogenetic abnormality or a *TP53* mutation are less likely to respond to lenalidomide. Lenalidomide's mechanism of action includes augmentation of ubiquitin-mediated degradation of casein kinase 1. Casein kinase 1, a serine/threonine kinase involved in regulation of signal transduction pathways, is encoded on chromosome 5q. It is haploinsufficient in del5q cells, so del5q cells exposed to lenalidomide experience a greater reduction in casein kinase 1 compared to healthy cells, and del5q cells are selectively killed.

In selected patients standard or more frequently reduced-intensity allogeneic stem cell transplantation (SCT) offers the chance of a permanent cure. For example, younger patients not responding to conventional therapy with severe symptomatic cytopenias.

Higher-risk myelodysplastic syndromes

In these patients, a variety of treatments has been attempted to improve the overall prognosis, with varying degrees of success. Treatment is aimed at preventing the progression of MDS to AML (Fig. 16.6).

Stem cell transplantation

SCT offers the prospect of a complete cure for MDS, and the advent of reduced-intensity conditioning is increasing the age range of patients who may be treated. Patients who lack *TP53* mutations have a >50% chance of long-term disease-free survival, while those with *TP53* mutations have a <20% chance of a favourable outcome. Myeloablative conditioning should be considered in young and fit patients. Chemotherapy should be given prior to the transplant in patients with >10% blasts in the marrow. Iron chelation prior to allograft is considered in patients with evidence of systemic iron overload.

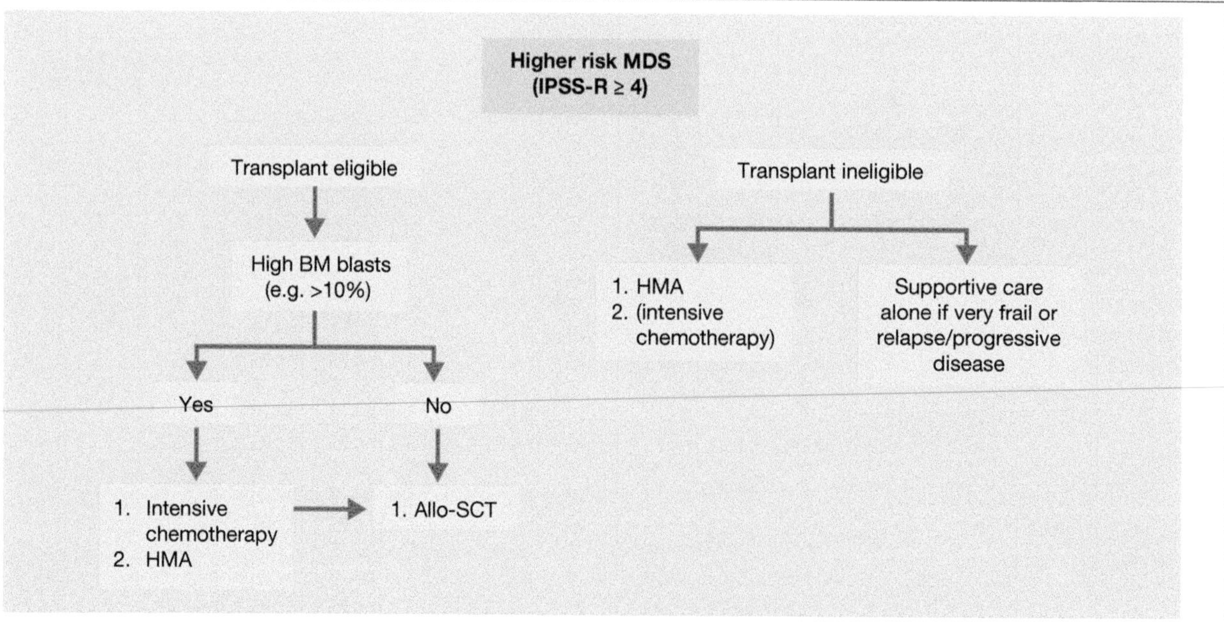

Figure 16.6 Management of higher-risk MDS. Source: Adapted from P. Fenaux *et al.* (2021) *Ann. Oncol.* 32: 142–56. Allo-SCT, allogeneic stem cell transplant; BM, bone maroow; HMA, hypomethylating agent; MDS, myelodysplastic syndrome.

Intensive chemotherapy

Chemotherapy as given in AML (Chapter 13) is occasionally tried in higher-risk patients, usually as a bridge to SCT. Although the majority may obtain a remission, relapse is likely and frequently occurs within a few months. The risks of intensive chemotherapy are great because prolonged pancytopenia may occur in some cases without normal haemopoietic cell regeneration, presumably because normal stem cells are much reduced. For patients who are not transplant eligible, intensive chemotherapy maybe considered in fit patients without adverse cytogenetic features (more likely to respond to chemotherapy).

Hypomethylating agents

Azacitidine and decitabine are DNA methyltransferase inhibitors which inhibit methylation of newly formed DNA. They are nucleoside analogues that irreversibly bind to DNA methyltransferase and also are incorporated into DNA and RNA, causing DNA double-strand breaks. They improve blood counts in 40–50% of higher-risk MDS patients. Azacitidine is given for 7 days every month and is continued for as long as the patient is responding. It can improve survival by approximately 9 months compared to supportive care alone. Decitabine is typically given for 5 days per month and can delay progression to AML. The exact mechanism of the clinical activity of these drugs in MDS is unknown. Oral, longer form of hypomethylating agents are currently in development.

General supportive care only

This is most suitable in elderly patients with other major medical problems. Transfusions of red cells and platelets, and therapy with antibiotics and antifungals, are given as needed (Chapter 12).

Clonal haemopoiesis of indeterminate potential (CHIP)

By age 65, at least 10% of the population have acquired a clone of haemopoietic cells with a single acquired mutation in a leukaemia driver gene at a variant allele frequency (VAF) (mutation allele burden) of ≥2% (≥4% for X-linked genes), but without evidence of a haematological malignancy or unexplained cytopenia. This is akin to other precursor conditions of overt haematological malignancies, such as monoclonal B lymphocytosis (MBL) (Chapter 18) and monoclonal gammopathy of uncertain significance (MGUS) (Chapter 22). These age-associated mutations are primarily mutations in *DNMT3A*, *TET2* and *ASXL1* (Table 11.2). This phenomenon has been termed clonal haemopoiesis of indeterminate potential (CHIP, Table 16.4). CHIP becomes more frequent with age, affecting >30% of the population over age 85 years. Because of the association with ageing, some investigators use the term 'ageing-related clonal haemopoiesis' (ARCH).

CHIP carries a ~1% risk per year of development of an overt haematological neoplasm meeting World Health Organization (WHO) diagnostic criteria. Different mutations drive substantially different growth rates, mutations in *DNMT3A* displaying the slowest average annual growth rates of ~5%. Clones with mutations in the other common driver genes (*TET2, ASXL1, PPM1D* and *SF3B1*), expand at roughly twice this rate, i.e. ~10%/year. Variations in expression levels of certain genes, e.g.TCL1A (T-cell leukaemia/lymphoma protein 1A), may also determine the incidence and rate of expansion of the clone. The risk of transformation is higher in those with larger clone size, multiple mutations, mutations of *TP53*, or of genes for splicing factors, e.g. *SRSF2, SF3B1*. More importantly from a public health standpoint, CHIP is associated with an increased risk of non-haematological diseases including atherosclerosis, e.g. myocardial infarction and stroke, venous thrombosis, chronic obstructive pulmonary disease, gout and chronic liver disease resulting in an increase in the overall mortality. This is often as a result of dysregulated inflammation. A protective effect against Alzheimer's disease has also been reported. A lymphoid variation of CHIP is associated with lymphoid malignancy, immune deficiency and autoimmunity. Understanding the presence of CHIP has important implications in the interpretation of genetic results at diagnosis and following treatment of other diseases. For example, awareness of CHIP is important in interpreting NGS results performed for different indications. Subjects with CHIP are not excluded from being donors for stem cell transplantation.

Some patients have blood cytopenias (haemoglobin < 130 g/L in males, < 120 g/L in females, absolute neutrophil count < 1.8×10^9/L, platelets < 150×10^9/L) but no specific diagnosis is apparent even after extensive evaluation. There is insufficient dysplasia in blood or marrow cells to warrant a diagnosis of MDS. These patients' haematological abnormalities are termed **idiopathic cytopenias of undetermined significance (ICUS).** In time the diagnosis often becomes clear in people with ICUS. Some will evolve to overt MDS. If a clonal mutation is present, the term **CCUS (clonal cytopenias of undetermined significance)** is used. These patients have a risk of developing MDS or AML exceeding 75% by 4 years. Finally, dysplastic cells are rarely seen in a peripheral blood film even though the blood counts are normal and there is no evidence of MDS. This state has been termed **idiopathic dysplasia of undetermined significance (IDUS).**

Myelodysplastic/myeloproliferative (MDS/MPN) neoplasms

These disorders are classified distinctly by WHO 2022 as they show the presence of dysplastic features and usually at least one cytopenia similar to MDS, but also an increased number of circulating cells in one or more lineages similar to myeloproliferative neoplasms (MPN; Table 16.5). They share common

Table 16.5 World Health Organization 2022 classification of myelodysplastic/myeloproliferative neoplasms (MDS/MPN).

Subtype	Diagnostic features
Chronic myelomonocytic leukaemia (CMML) (myelodysplastic and myeloproliferative sub-types)	***Pre-requisite criteria (present in all cases)*** Monocytosis > 0.5 × 10⁹/L and monocytes represent ≥10% of circulating white cells Blasts constitute <20% of the cells in the peripheral blood and bone marrow Not meet CML or MPN criteria, or myeloid/lymphoid neoplasms with tyrosine kinase fusions ***Supporting criteria*** 1. Dysplasia affecting 1 or more myeloid lineages 2. Acquired clonal abnormality (cytogenetic or molecular, e.g. *RAS*, *TET2* mutations 3. Abnormal partitioning of peripheral blood monocyte subsets 1 and 2 required in monocytosis ≥0.5 × 10⁹/L but <1.0 × 10⁹/L 1, or 2, or 3 required if monocytosis ≥1.0 × 10⁹/L
MDS/MPN with neutrophilia (previously known as atypical chronic myeloid leukaemia)	Peripheral blood leukocytosis; *BCR::ABL1* absent; *SETBP1* mutations in 30%
MDS/MPN with *SF3B1* mutation and thrombocytosis If ≥15% ring sideroblasts but wild –type *SF3B1*, the term MDS/MPN with ring sideroblasts and thrombocytosis is used	Platelet count ≥450 × 10⁹/L Large atypical megakaryocytes. *SF3B1* mutation
MDS/MPN, not otherwise specified	MDS and MPN features without specific findings of other disorders in this group

clinical and genetic features, such as mutations of the *TET2* tumour-suppressor gene in about 20% of cases and of *JAK2* in a smaller proportion of patients.

Chronic myelomonocytic leukaemia (CMML)

This is defined by a persistent monocytosis of $\geq 0.5 \times 10^9$/L with blasts <20% in the marrow, dysplasia in other lineages and negative for the *BCR::ABL1* translocation. The total white cell count (WBC) is usually raised and may exceed 100×10^9/L. CMML may be separated into 'dysplastic' and 'proliferative' subtypes depending on WBC < or $\geq 13 \times 10^9$/L, respectively. Proliferative sybtypes are associated with RAS pathway mutations. Patients may develop skin rashes and around half have splenomegaly. Bruising is frequent and gum hypertrophy and lymphadenopathy may also be present. *TET2*, *ASXL1*, *SRSF2*, *JAK2*, RAS pathway and other mutations (Fig. 16.1) are frequent and the pattern of mutations differs from the pattern seen in MDS without proliferative features. Treatment is difficult, although azacitidine or decitabine, hydroxycarbamide, ruxolitinib and etoposide may be useful in shrinking spleen size and alleviating disease-related symptoms. SCT may be tried in younger patients. Median survival is approximately 2 years, with transfusion dependency, white cells $>13.0 \times 10^9$/L, increased marrow blasts, complex cytogenetics and mutation status predictors of poor outcome.

MDS/MPN neoplasm with neutrophilia

These patients with what was previously termed atypical chronic myeloid leukaemia have an increased white cell count with mainly granulocytes and granulocyte precursors in the blood and hypercellular bone marrow, but the *BCR::ABL1* fusion genes are not present. There are usually some morphological features in the blood or bone marrow of MDS. Treatment is difficult and the outlook is poor.

MDS/MPN with *SF3B1* mutation and thrombocytosis

This rare syndrome resembles MDS with single-lineage dysplasia with ring sideroblasts, but the anaemia is accompanied by a platelet count $>450 \times 10^9$/L, mutations of *SF3B1* are present, often accompanied by those of *JAK2* or *MPL*.

SUMMARY

- MDS includes a group of clonal disorders of haemopoietic stem cells that lead to bone marrow failure and low blood cell counts. A hallmark of the disease is increased proliferation and apoptosis of haemopoietic cells, leading to the paradox of a hypercellular bone marrow with pancytopenia. There is a tendency to progress to AML.
- In most cases the disease is *primary (de novo)*, but it may be *therapy-related* due to chemotherapy or radiotherapy given for treatment of another malignancy.
- The main clinical features of anaemia, infection and bleeding are caused by a reduction in the blood count. Most patients are over 70 years of age.
- Diagnosis is made by examination of the blood and bone marrow together with cytogenetic and molecular genetic studies of the neoplastic cells. They are classified into six major subtypes.
- Scoring systems can divide patients into those with low-grade or high-grade disease. These include mutations detected by NGS.
- Lower-risk MDS may not need treatment. Haemopoietic growth factors, lenalidomide or blood product support are useful when required. Luspatercept is a promising new agent to treat the anaemia in some patients.
- Higher-risk MDS may be treated by intensive chemotherapy, demethylating drugs or stem cell transplantation. Allogeneic transplantation is the only curative procedure.
- Clonal haemopoiesis of indeterminate potential (CHIP) is an age-related condition that may progress to an overt haematological neoplasm. It is associated with disease of other systems including cardiovascular.
- Other subjects have a single lineage cytopenia with no evidence of dysplasia, with or without a clonal mutation or have dysplasia in blood cells without cytopenia or mutation.
- MDS/MPN are a group of disorders classified between myelodysplasia and myeloproliferative neoplasms and show the presence of dysplastic features, but also an increased number of circulating white cells or platelets.

Now visit **www.wiley.com/go/haematology9e** to test yourself on this chapter.

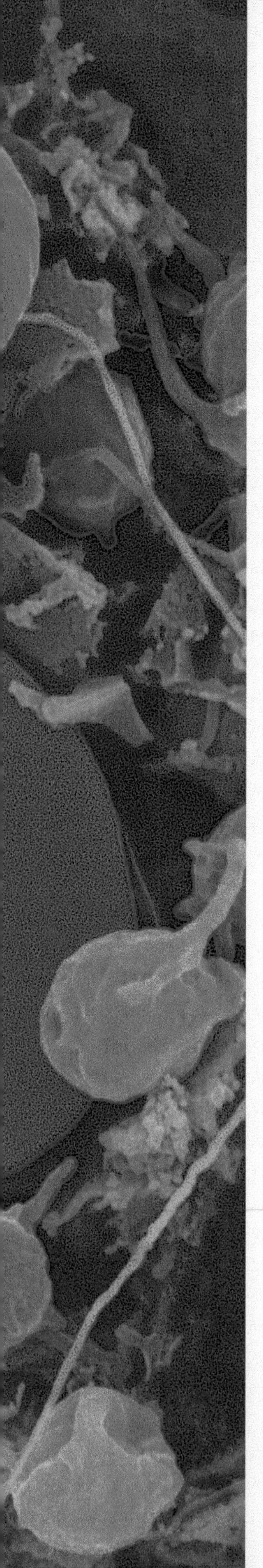

CHAPTER 17

Acute lymphoblastic leukaemia

(Written with Dr Connor Sweeney)

Key topics

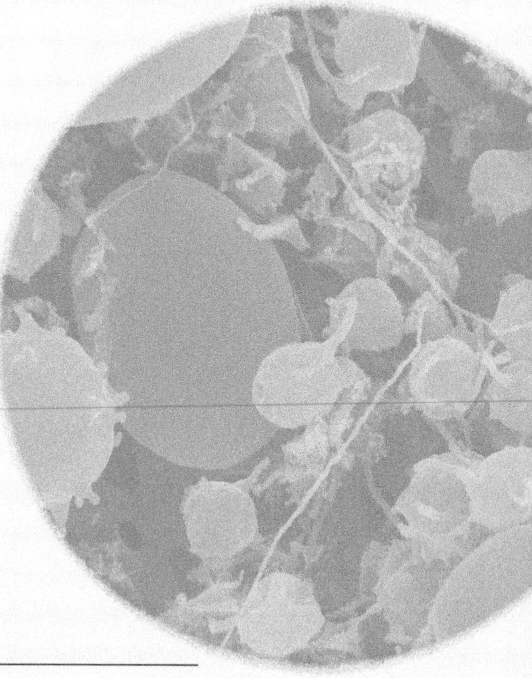

Hoffbrand's Essential Haematology, Ninth Edition. A. Victor Hoffbrand, Pratima Chowdary, Graham P. Collins, and Justin Loke.

© 2024 John Wiley & Sons Ltd. Published 2024 by John Wiley & Sons Ltd.

Companion website: www.wiley.com/go/haematology9e

Acute lymphoblastic leukaemia (ALL) is caused by an accumulation of lymphoblasts in the bone marrow and is the most common malignancy of childhood, though it can occur at any age. The definition of acute leukaemia and distinguishing ALL from acute myeloid leukaemia are described in Chapter 13.

Incidence and pathogenesis

The incidence of ALL is highest at 3–7 years, with 75% of cases occurring before the age of 6. There is a secondary rise in incidence after the age of 40 years. B-cell lineage represents 85% of cases and these have an equal sex incidence; there is a male predominance for the 15% of T-cell ALL (T-ALL).

The pathogenesis is varied. **A proportion of cases of childhood ALL are initiated by genetic mutations that occur during development in utero** (Fig. 17.1). Studies in identical twins have shown that both may be born with the same chromosomal abnormality, e.g. the t(12;21), *ETV6-RUNX1* translocation. This has presumably arisen spontaneously in a haemopoietic progenitor cell that has passed from one twin to the other as a result of shared placental circulation. Massive expansion of the lymphoid system in the foetus predisposes to somatic mutations. Also, the process of VDJ recombination to generate antigen receptor diversity (Chapter 9) is prone to generation of 'off target' genomic abnormalities. Environmental exposure during pregnancy may be important for this first event. One twin may develop ALL early, e.g. at age 5 because of a second transforming event affecting the copy numbers of several genes, including those in B-cell development (see below). The other may remain well or develop ALL later, perhaps as a result of a different transforming event. The *ETV6-RUNX1* translocation is present in the blood of approximately 10% of newborn infants, but only 1 in 100 of these go on to develop ALL at a later date. The mechanism of the 'second genetic hit' within the neoplastic cell is unclear, but an abnormal response of the immune system to infection is suggested by epidemiological studies. In other cases, the disease seems to arise as a postnatal mutation in an early lymphoid progenitor cell.

Children with a high level of social activity, notably those attending early nursery daycare or those with older siblings, have a reduced incidence of ALL, whereas those living in more isolated communities and who have a reduced exposure to common infections in the first years of life have a higher risk.

Certain germline polymorphisms in a group of genes mainly involved in B-cell development (e.g. *IKZF1*) appear to predispose to ALL, since they are more frequent in children with B-cell ALL (B-ALL) than controls. *IKZF1* is also deleted in the leukaemic cells in 30% of high-risk B-ALL and 95% of ALL *BCR::ABL1* positive cases. Children with constitutional trisomy 21 (Down syndrome) have a remarkably increased risk of B-ALL and AML compared with other children. There is a 33-fold increase in B-ALL and 150-fold increase in AML in young children with Down syndrome.

In general, the genomic landscape in ALL is characterized by primary chromosomal abnormalities and a wide

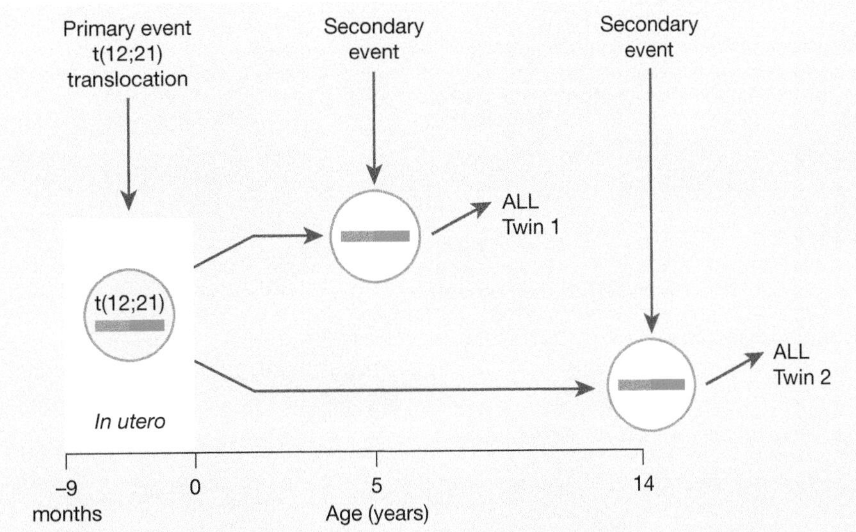

Figure 17.1 Prenatal origin of acute lymphoblastic leukaemia (ALL) in a pair of identical twins. Both tumours had an identical t(12;21) translocation. ALL was diagnosed in the first twin at age 5 years and in the second at age 14 years, indicating probable origin of the leukaemic clone *in utero* and dissemination to both twins via a shared placental blood supply. Due to the prolonged latency of the ALL, it is presumed that a secondary event is required to initiate the development of overt leukaemia. At the time of the diagnosis of ALL in Twin 1, the t(12;21) translocation could be detected in the bone marrow of Twin 2. It is likely that such a 'foetal origin' of childhood ALL occurs in a significant number of sporadic ALL cases. Source: Adapted from J.L. Wiemels *et al.* (1999) *Blood* 94: 1057–62.

range of secondary deletions and mutations involving key pathways implicated in leukaemogenesis. These are described in more detail below. For childhood ALL, an average of 11 somatically acquired structural variations are present (Fig. 11.1).

Classification

Acute lymphoblastic leukaemia, B cell or T cell, is subclassified by the World Health Organization (WHO 2016) according to the underlying genetic defect (Table 17.1). Within B-ALL there are several specific genetic subtypes, such as those with the t(9;22) [*BCR::ABL1*] or t(12;21) [*ETV6-RUNX1*] translocations, rearrangements of the *KMT2A(MLL)* gene or alteration in chromosome number (aneuploidy; Table 17.1). The subtype in both B-ALL and T-ALL is an important guide to the optimal treatment protocol and to prognosis.

Among *BCR::ABL1* (Philadelphia chromosome) negative cases, some patients have a gene expression signature similar to *BCR::ABL1* positive cases. These '*BCR::ABL1*-like' cases comprise about 15% of children with ALL (more common in Down syndrome), 20–25% of adolescents and young adults, and at least 10–15% of older adults. About 60% of patients with *BCR::ABL1*-like ALL have overexpression of *CRLF2* and 85% of these cases have JAK-STAT pathway mutations, including of *JAK2*. In *BCR::ABL1*-like ALL without *CRLF2* overexpression, fusions involving *JAK2, ABL1, ABL2* and other tyrosine kinases are common.

In T-ALL an abnormal karyotype is found in 50–70% of cases and the NOTCH signalling pathway is activated in most cases. Early T-precursor (ETP) ALL leukaemia has a unique immunophenotype. Blasts in ETP ALL express the T-cell marker CD7, but lack CD1a and CD8 that characterize more mature T cells. They also express at least one myeloid/stem-cell-associated marker. The genetic profile of ETP ALL is also distinct. Common T-cell-associated gene alterations such as of *NOTCH1* or *CDKN1/2* are rare in this subtype, but myeloid-associated gene mutations are common. The prognosis is worse than for other patients with T-ALL.

Clinical features

Clinical features are a result of the following:

Table 17.1 World Health Organization (2022) classification of acute lymphoblastic leukaemia (ALL) / lymphoblastic lymphoma. The corresponding chromosomal translocations are included in the Table. See also Appendix.

B-cell lymphoblastic leukaemias/lymphomas
B-lymphoblastic leukaemia/lymphoma NOS
B-lymphoblastic leukaemia/lymphoma with high hyperdiploidy (>50 chromosomes)
B-lymphoblastic leukaemia /lymphoma with hypodiploidy (<45 chromosomes)
B-lymphoblastic leukaemia/lymphoma with iAMP21
B-lymphoblastic leukaemia/lymphoma with *BCR::ABL1* fusion, t(9;22)
B-lymphoblastic leukaemia/lymphoma with *BCR::ABL1*-like features
B-lymphoblastic leukaemia/lymphoma with *KMT2A* rearrangement
B-lymphoblastic leukaemia/lymphoma with *ETV6::RUNX1* fusion, t(12;21)
B-lymphoblastic leukaemia/lymphoma with *ETV::RUNX1*-like features
B-lymphoblasic leukaemia/lymphoma with *TCF3::PBX1* fusion, t(17;19)
B-lymphoblastic leukaemia/lymphoma with *IGH::IL3* fusion, t(5;14)
B-lymphoblasic leukameia/lymphoma with other defined genetic abnormalities
T-cell lymphoblastic leukaemias/lymphomas
T-lymphoblastic leukaemia/lymphoma NOS
Early T-precursor lymphoblastic leukaemia/lymphoma

N.B. A minority of patients present with nodal or extranodal masses and <20% blasts in the bone marrow, which are classified as lymphoblastic lymphoma. They are treated similarly to ALL.
NOS, not otherwise specified.

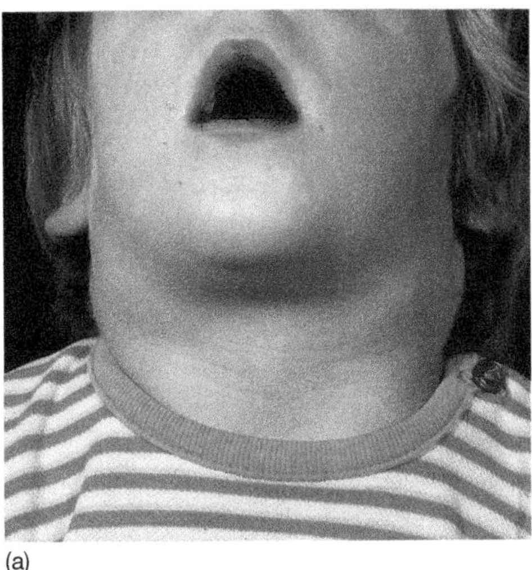

(a)

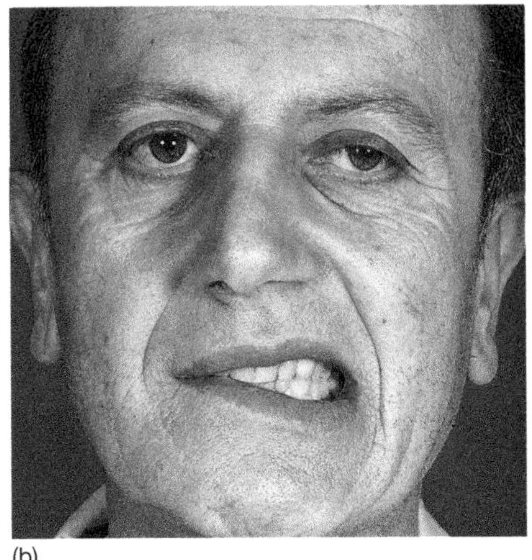

(b)

Figure 17.2 Acute lymphoblastic leukaemia. **(a)** Marked cervical lymphadenopathy in a boy. **(b)** Facial asymmetry in a 59-year-old man due to a right lower motor neurone seventh nerve palsy resulting from meningeal leukaemic infiltration. Source: A.V. Hoffbrand *et al.* (2019) *Color Atlas of Clinical Hematology*, 5th edn. Reproduced with permission of John Wiley & Sons.

Bone marrow failure

- Anaemia (pallor, lethargy and dyspnoea).
- Neutropenia (fever, malaise, features of mouth, throat, skin, respiratory, perianal or other infections).
- Thrombocytopenia (spontaneous bruises, purpura, bleeding gums and menorrhagia).

Organ infiltration

This can cause tender bones, lymphadenopathy (Fig. 17.2a), moderate splenomegaly, hepatomegaly and meningeal syndrome (headache, nausea and vomiting, blurring of vision and dipolpia) (Fig 17.2b). Fundal examination may reveal papilloedema and sometimes retinal haemorrhage. Many patients have a fever at presentation, which usually resolves after starting chemotherapy. Less common manifestations include testicular swelling or signs of mediastinal compression, which is more common in T-ALL (Fig. 17.3).

If lymph node or solid extranodal masses predominate with <20% blasts in the marrow, the disease is classified as lymphoblastic lymphoma, but is treated as ALL.

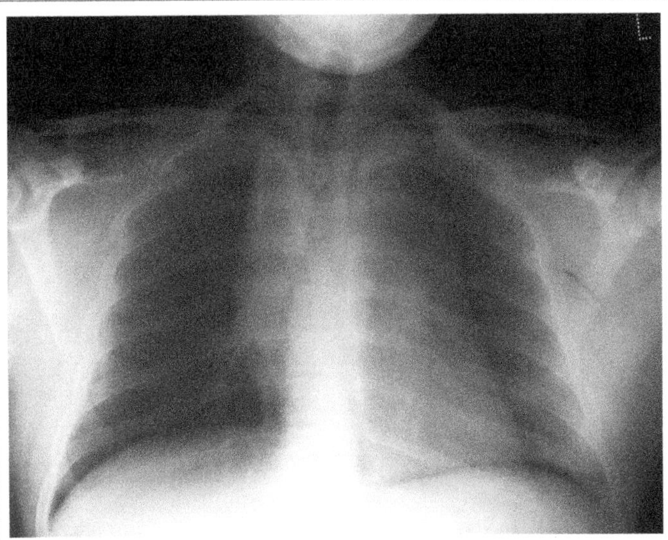

(a)

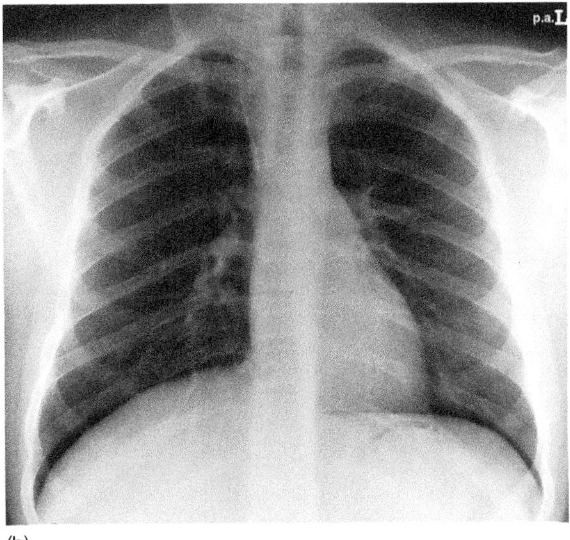

(b)

Figure 17.3 Chest X-ray of a boy aged 16 years with acute lymphoblastic leukaemia (T-ALL). **(a)** There is a large mediastinal mass caused by thymic enlargement at presentation. **(b)** After 1 week of therapy with prednisolone, vincristine and daunorubicin, the mass has resolved.

Investigations

Haematological investigations reveal a normochromic, normocytic anaemia with thrombocytopenia in most cases. The total white cell count may be decreased, normal or increased, sometimes to 200×10^9/L or more. The blood film typically shows a variable number of blast cells. The bone marrow is hypercellular with >20% leukaemic blasts. The blast cells are characterized by morphology (Fig. 17.4), immunological tests (Table 17.2), cytogenetic and molecular genetic analysis (Table 17.1). Identification of the immunoglobulin or T-cell receptor (TCR) clonal gene rearrangement (Fig. 9.7), (aberrant) immunophenotype and molecular genetics of the neoplastic cells is important to determine treatment and to detect minimal residual disease (MRD) during follow-up (Table 17.3).

Lumbar puncture for cerebrospinal fluid (CSF) examination is important in disease staging, but should be performed only by experienced physicians, as a traumatic procedure may promote the spread of neoplastic cells from blood to the central nervous system (CNS). Initial assessment of the CSF should always be combined with the concurrent administration of intrathecal chemotherapy.

Biochemical tests may reveal a raised serum uric acid, serum lactate dehydrogenase or, less commonly, hypercalcaemia. Liver and renal function tests are performed as a baseline before treatment begins. Radiography may reveal lytic bone lesions and a mediastinal mass caused by enlargement of the thymus and/or mediastinal lymph nodes, which is characteristic of T-ALL (Fig. 17.3).

The differential diagnosis includes acute myeloid leukaemia (AML), aplastic anaemia, marrow infiltration by other malignancies, e.g. rhabdomyosarcoma, neuroblastoma and Ewing sarcoma, infections such as infectious mononucleosis and pertussis, juvenile rheumatoid arthritis and immune thrombocytopenia.

Cytogenetics and molecular genetics

Cytogenetic analysis shows differing frequencies of abnormalities in infants, children and adults, which partly explains the different prognoses of these groups (Fig. 17.5). Cases are stratified according to the number of chromosomes in the neoplastic cell (**ploidy**) or by specific molecular abnormalities. The two parameters define good-and poor-prognosis disease.

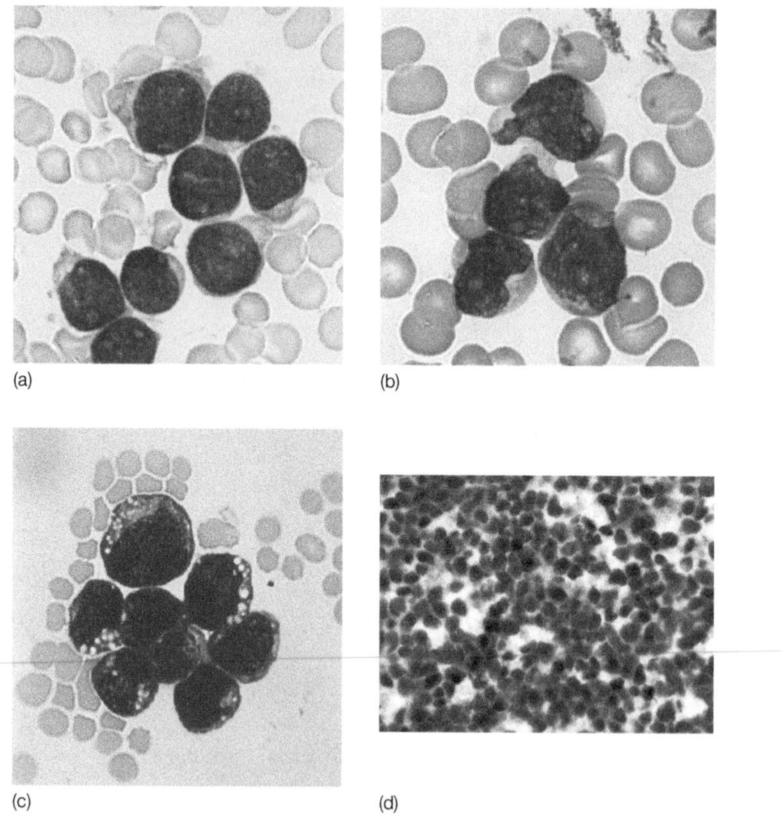

Figure 17.4 Morphology and immunophenotyping of acute lymphoblastic leukaemia. **(a)** Lymphoblasts show scanty cytoplasm without granules. **(b)** Lymphoblasts are large and heterogeneous with abundant cytoplasm. **(c)** Lymphoblasts are deeply basophilic with cytoplasmic vacuolation. **(d)** Acute lymphoblastic leukaemia: bone marrow cells staining positive for terminal deoxytidyl transferase (TdT) by immunoperoxidase. Source: A.V. Hoffbrand *et al.* (2019) *Color Atlas of Clinical Hematology*, 5th edn. Reproduced with permission of John Wiley & Sons.

Table 17.2 Immunological markers for classification of acute lymphoblastic leukaemia (ALL; see also Fig. 11.13). Markers that distinguish the early T-precursor subtype are described in the text.

	ALL	
Marker	**B**	**T**
B lineage-associated		
CD19	+	–
cCD22	+	–
cCD79a	+	–
CD10	+ or –	–
cIg	+ (pre-B)	–
sIg	–	–
TdT	+	+
T lineage-associated		
CD7	–	+
cCD3	–	+
CD2	–	+
TdT	+	+
CD1a	–	+
CD4, CD8	–	+
Myeloid or stem cell lineage-associated		
CD34, CD117, HLADR, CD13, CD33, CD11b, or CD65	Negative except in biphenotypic acute leukaemia	Negative except in early T-cell precursor subtype or biphenotypic acute leukaemia

c, cytoplasmic; s, surface; TdT, terminal deoxynucleotidyl transferase.

Table 17.3 Specialized tests for acute lymphoblastic leukaemia (ALL).

Immunological markers (flow cytometry)*	See Table 17.2; Fig. 11.13
*Immunoglobulin and TCR genes**	B-ALL: clonal rearrangement of immunoglobulin genes
	T-ALL: clonal rearrangement of TCR genes
*Chromosomes and molecular genetic analysis**	See Table 17.1

* Tests needed at diagnosis for subsequent monitoring for minimal residual disease.
B-ALL, B-cell acute lymphoblastic leukaemia; T-ALL, T-cell acute lymphoblastic leukaemia; TCR, T-cell receptor.

Hyperdiploid cells have more than 50 chromosomes and cases with this abnormality generally have a good prognosis, whereas **hypodiploid** cases (less than 45 chromosomes) carry a poor prognosis. The most common specific chromosome abnormality in childhood B-ALL is the t(12;21)(p13;q22) *ETV6::RUNX1* translocation. The RUNX1 protein plays an important part in transcriptional control of haemopoiesis and is repressed by the ETV6::RUNX1 fusion protein. The frequency of the Ph translocation t(9;22) increases with age and carried an unfavourable prognosis, though outcomes have improved significantly with the addition of BCR-ABL1 tyrosine kinase inhibitors (TKIs) to treatment regimens. ALL with *BCR::ABL1*-like features also has an unfavourable prognosis and the role of kinase inhibitors is being tested in trials. Translocations of chromosome 11q23 involve the *KMT2A* (*MLL*) gene and are seen particularly in cases of infant leukaemia.

Using more sensitive molecular genetic tests, as well as fluorescence *in situ* hybridization (FISH) analysis, some cases that have normal results from conventional cytogenetic testing are found to have fusion genes, e.g. *BCR::ABL1*. These molecular genetic changes may carry prognostic significance.

T-ALL accounts for 15% of childhood and 25% of adult ALL. The clinical presentation is often with a very high white cell count, mediastinal mass or pleural effusion. TCR genes (and in 20% the *IGH* gene) show clonal rearrangement and cytogenetic changes often involve the TCR loci with different partner genes. The majority of cases have acquired genetic abnormalities that lead to constitutive activation of the

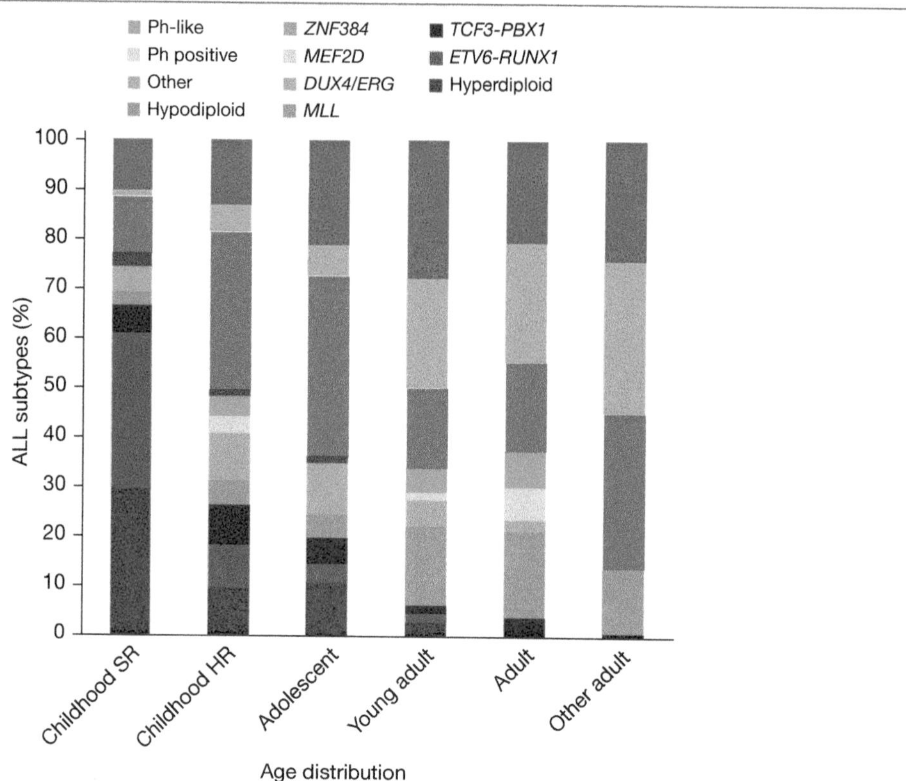

Figure 17.5 Age distribution of cytogenetically or molecularly defined acute lymphoblastic leukaemia (ALL) subtypes. The prevalence of ALL subtypes varies in children with standard-risk (SR)_ALL (age 1–9 years and WBC count < 50×10^9/L), children with high-risk (HR) ALL (age 10–15 years and/or WBC count > 50×10^9/L), and adolescents (age 16–20 years), young adults (age 21–39 years), adults (age 40–59 years), and older adults (age 60–86 years) with ALL. The incidence of Ph-positive and Ph-like increases with ageing; *ETV6::RUNX1* and hyperdiploid genotypes dominate in childhood standard-risk disease. *MLL(KMT2A)*, *ZN384*, *MEF2D* and *DUX4/ERG* indicate rearrangements of these genes. In the WHO (2022) classification, Ph is replaced by *BCR::ABL1. MLL is now termed KTM2A*. Source: I. Iacobucci, C.G. Mullighan (2017) *J. Clin. Oncol*. 35: 975–83. Reproduced with permission of American Society of Clinical Oncology.

NOTCH signalling pathway and drugs that target these abnormalities are being developed (Fig. 17.6). *KMT2A* fusion, *ABL*-class fusions and *CDKN2A/B* deletions may also be present as in B-ALL.

Treatment

General supportive therapy

General supportive therapy for bone marrow failure is described in Chapter 12 and includes the insertion of a central venous cannula, blood product support and prevention of tumour lysis syndrome. The risk of tumour lysis syndrome is highest in children with a high white cell count, T-cell disease or concurrent renal impairment at presentation. Any episode of fever must be treated promptly.

Specific therapy for ALL in children

Specific therapy for ALL is with chemotherapy and sometimes radiotherapy (Fig. 17.7) and treatment protocols are complex. There are several phases in a treatment course, which usually has four components (Fig. 17.7). The protocols are **risk adjusted** to reduce the treatment given to patients with good prognosis. The factors that guide treatment include age, gender, white cell count at presentation and baseline cytogenetic and molecular genetic findings. The initial response to therapy is also important, as slow clearance of blood or marrow blasts after a week or two of induction therapy or persistence of minimal residual disease (MRD, see below) is associated with a relatively high risk of relapse. ALL in infants (<1 year) has a poor clinical outcome, with cure rates of only 20–50%. The disease is associated with a chromosomal translocation involving the *KMT2A* gene in 80% of cases and is treated using specific protocols.

Minimal (measurable) residual disease

Even when the blood and bone marrow appear to be clear of leukaemia by light microscopy, small numbers of neoplastic cells may sometimes be detected by flow cytometry (sensitivity

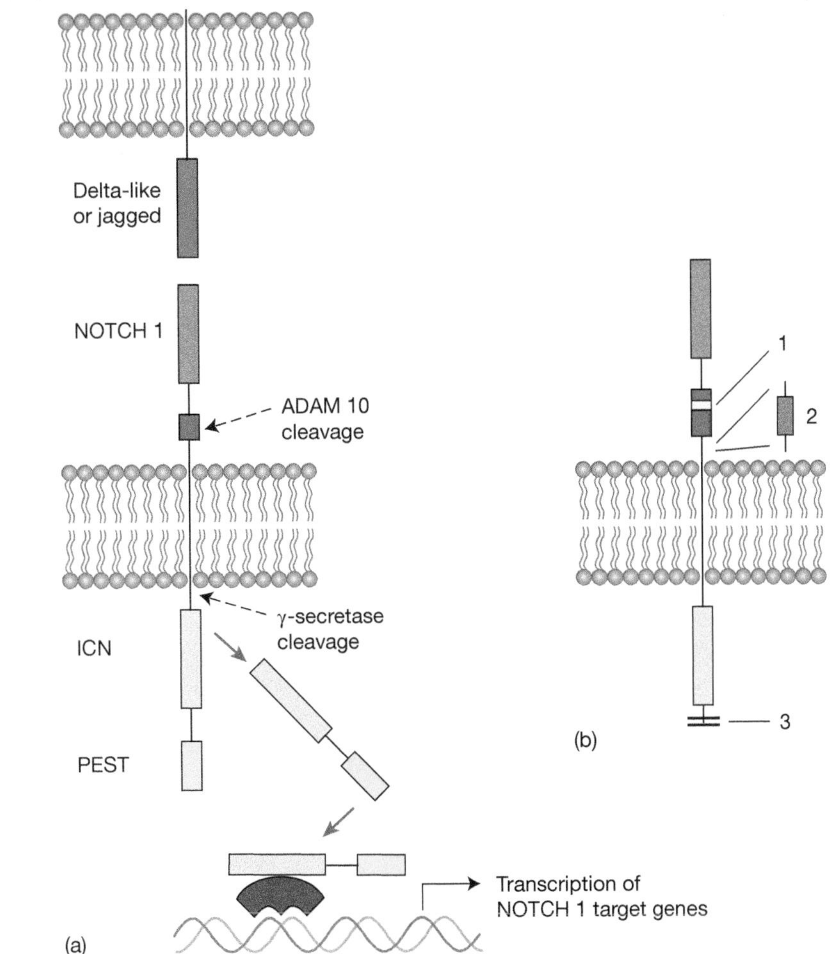

Figure 17.6 The molecular basis of activation of NOTCH1 signalling in T-cell acute lymphoblastic leukaemia (T-ALL). **(a)** The molecular basis of NOTCH signalling. NOTCH is expressed at the cell membrane and after binding to a ligand (Delta-like or Jagged) on a neighbouring cell, the protein is cleaved in two places – first by extracellular ADAM 10 and then by an intracellular γ-secretase complex. The portion of intracellular NOTCH1 (ICN) that is released is then translocated to the nucleus, where it leads to activation of NOTCH1 target genes. **(b)** Several types of genetic abnormalities are seen in the NOTCH signalling pathway in 60% of patients with T-ALL. These include (1) mutations in the extracellular cleavage site (2) insertion of an internal tandem duplications in the juxtamembrane region or (3) deletion of the intracellular PEST domain. The net result of all these mutations is to increase the rate of cleavage and nuclear translocation of the ICN domain of NOTCH1, leading to aberrant activation of target genes including *MYC*. NOTCH1 can also be activated by translocations and by inactivating mutations in the enzyme which degrades ICN.

1 in 10^4) or molecular methods (Chapter 11; Fig. 17.8). The most sensitive method is NGS of the *IGH* chain gene or TCR junctional sequence (sensitivity 1 in 10^6). There is good correlation between results of tests performed on peripheral blood and bone marrow. A positive result indicates **minimal (also called 'measurable') residual disease** and testing for the presence of MRD at day 29 in children or after 3 months of treatment in adults has prognostic significance and is now used in planning therapy (Figs. 17.7, 17.9, and 17.11). The value of tests for MRD at the end of induction or during consolidation with respect to subsequent therapy continues to be explored in trials, in which the intensity of consolidation or maintenance therapy is reduced in those who rapidly become MRD negative, whereas more intensified therapy, bi-specific antibody, CAR-T cell therapy or allogeneic stem cell transplantation (SCT), is given to those with persistent MRD. Some children become MRD negative as early as day 29 of therapy and are in a good prognostic category, whereas in adults the findings on MRD testing at 3 months have greater prognostic importance (Table 17.4). One example is the reduction in the number of intensification blocks in children with no evidence of MRD at day 29 within the UKALL 2003 trial. This reduction did not impair the excellent prognosis in these low-risk children and is now standard therapy.

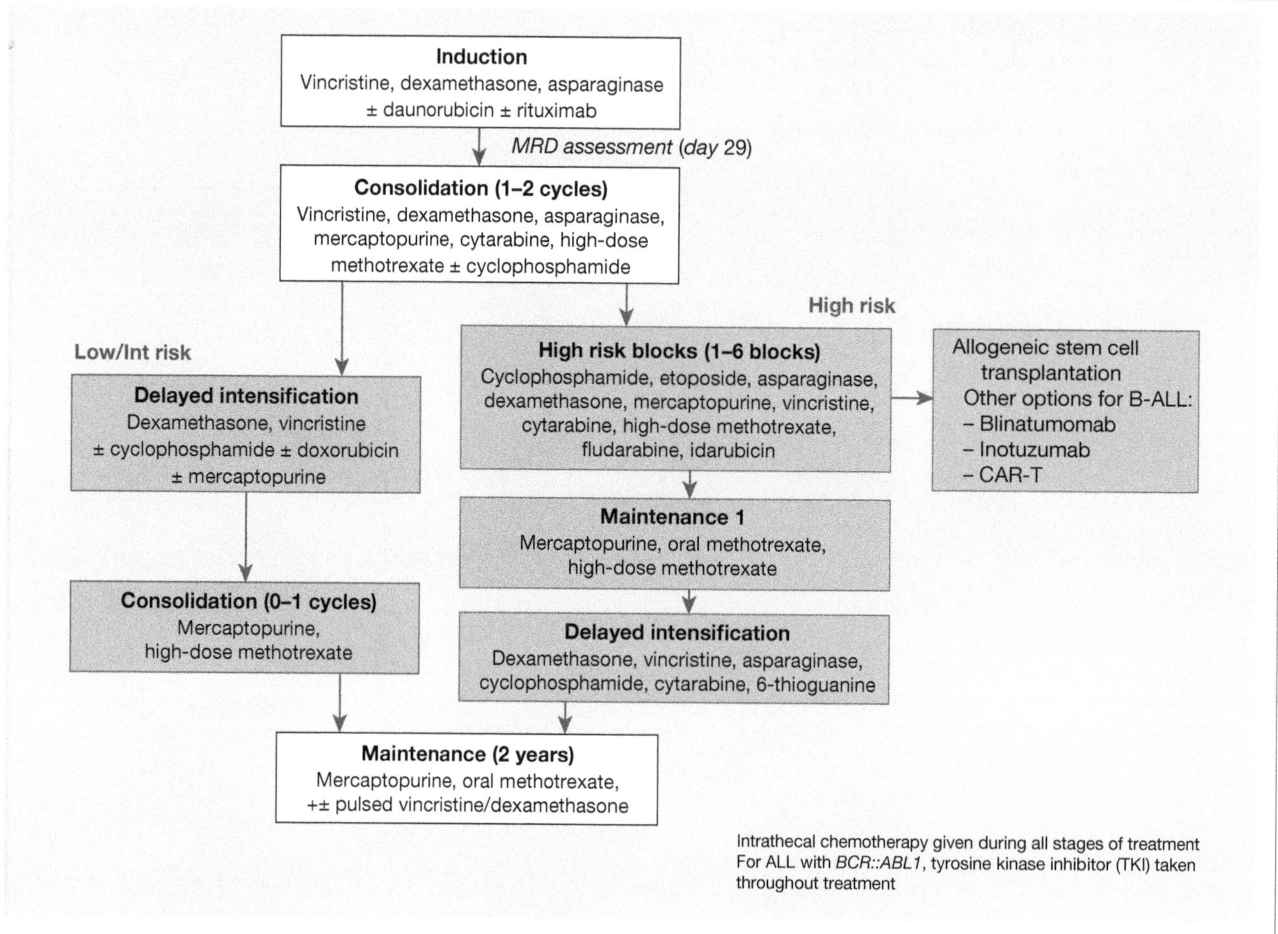

Figure 17.7 Flowchart illustrating typical treatment for children and young adults with acute lymphoblastic leukaemia. Based on the approach used in the ALLTogether trial (NCT04307576).

Remission induction

At presentation, the patient with acute leukaemia has a very high tumour burden and is at great risk from the complications of bone marrow failure and leukaemic infiltration. The aim of **remission induction** is to rapidly kill most (>99%) of the tumour cells and get the patient into remission. This is defined as less than 5% blasts in the bone marrow, with a normal or near-normal peripheral blood count and no other symptoms or signs of the disease. Dexamethasone, vincristine and pegylated-asparaginase are the most commonly used drugs, with or without rituximab are the most and are very effective – achieving remission in over 95% of children and in 80–90% of adults (in whom daunorubicin is also usually added, as in some protocols for high risk children). In some protocols rituximab is added to induction therapy. In patients with *BCR::ABL1* positive ALL, a TKI such as imatinib is incorporated into treatment regimens. After induction of remission, a patient may still be harbouring large numbers of neoplastic cells and, without further chemotherapy, virtually all patients will relapse (Fig. 13.8). Nevertheless, achievement of remission is a valuable first step in the treatment course. Patients who fail to achieve remission need to change to a more intensive protocol with the goal of reaching SCT.

Intensification (consolidation)

These courses use high doses of multidrug chemotherapy in order to eliminate the disease or reduce the tumour burden to very low levels. The doses of chemotherapy are near the limit of patient tolerability and during intensification blocks patients may need substantial support. Typical protocols involve the use of vincristine, cyclophosphamide, cytarabine, daunorubicin, etoposide or mercaptopurine, given as blocks in different combinations. Rituximab and a TKI are included for those for whom these drugs were indicated in induction. The numbers of blocks given in children depends on the child's risk category and varies between one and three. Risk is assessed by initial clinical and laboratory findings, baseline cytogenetic and molecular genetic findings, and MRD status following treatment.

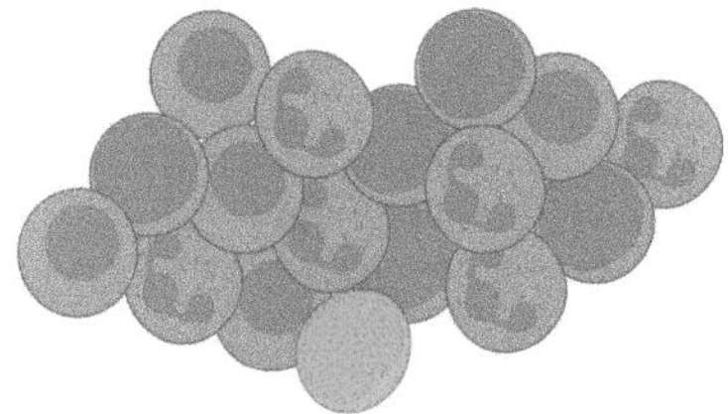

Minimal (measurable) residual disease
High sensitivity detection of rare leukaemia cells following treatment

Multi-colour flow cytometry
Fluorescent-labelled antibodies detect expression of antigens on leukaemia cells
Sensitivity 10^{-4}
Applicable in >90% *cases*

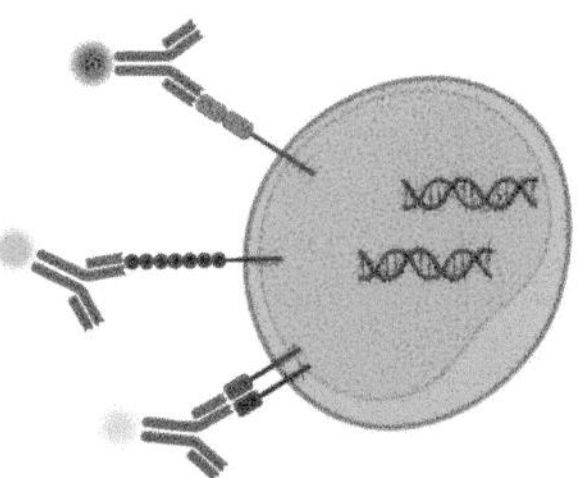

Molecular techniques
Genetic analysis to identify:
- Fusion genes (RT-qPCR)
  Applicable in 40–50% *case*
  Sensitivity 10^{-4} *to* 10^{-5}
- Immunoglobulin or T-cell receptor clonal rearrangement (ASO-PCR or next-generation sequencing)
  Applicable in >90% *cases*
  Sensitivity 10^{-4} *to* 10^{-5} *(ASO-PCR) and* 10^{-6} *(next-generation sequencing)*

Figure 17.8 Minimal (measurable) residual disease using multi-colour flow cytometry and molecular techniques can detect rare leukaemia cells, which are undetectable using conventional light microscopy. Immunophenotyping with flow cytometry uses fluorochrome-labelled antibodies to identify leukaemia cells on the basis of aberrant antigen expression. Distinct genetic techniques can also detect low levels of leukaemia. Where a recurrent gene fusion is present, fusion transcripts can be quantified using reverse transcription PCR (RT-qPCR). The rearranged V(D)J sequences of the immunoglobulin (B-ALL) or T-cell receptor (T-ALL) that are found specifically in a patient's leukaemia clone can be detected using either allele-specific oligonucleotide (ASO)-PCR or next-generation sequencing. Unlike ASO-PCR, next-generation sequencing does not require patient-specific primers, is high-throughput and offers greater sensitivity.

Central nervous system-directed therapy

Few of the drugs given systemically reach the CSF and therefore specific treatment is required to prevent or treat CNS disease. Intrathecal methotrexate is used for prophylaxis. CNS relapses still occur and present with headache, vomiting, papilloedema and blast cells in the CSF. Treatment of such relapses is with intrathecal methotrexate, cytarabine and hydrocortisone, with or without cranial irradiation, in addition to systemic chemotherapy, because bone marrow disease is often also present.

Maintenance

Maintenance therapy with daily oral mercaptopurine and once-weekly oral methotrexate is given to prevent late relapses. Intravenous vincristine with a short course (5 days) of oral corticosteroid is added at monthly or 3-monthly (in adults) intervals. There is a high risk of varicella or measles during maintenance therapy in children who lack immunity to these viruses. If exposure to these infections occurs, prophylactic immunoglobulin should be given. In addition, oral co-trimoxazole or atovaquone is given to reduce the risk of *Pneumocystis jirovecii* infection. Adults also receive antiviral and pneumocystis prophylaxis. Maintenance may in some protocols begin soon after remission induction and is interrupted by the periods of intensification chemotherapy. In typical regimens, intensive chemotherapy finishes around 38 weeks and then maintenance begins again and lasts until week 112 in girls or 164 in boys.

Treatment of relapse

If relapse, detected by MRD tests or by reappearance of ALL cells in the blood or marrow, occurs during or soon after maintenance chemotherapy, the prognosis is relatively poor. Re-induction with intensive chemotherapy with the aim of inducing a remission, followed by an allogeneic SCT is the traditional approach. However, more recently monoclonal antibody and other targeted treatments have been introduced that can induce remission in B-cell ALL whilst avoiding the need for intensive chemotherapy. These include the bi-specific T-cell engager (BiTE) **blinatumomab**, which links CD3 on the patient's T cells to CD19 on the surface of malignant B cells, enabling the T cells to exert cytotoxic activity. Adverse effects of blinatumomab include cytokine release syndrome and neurotoxicity.

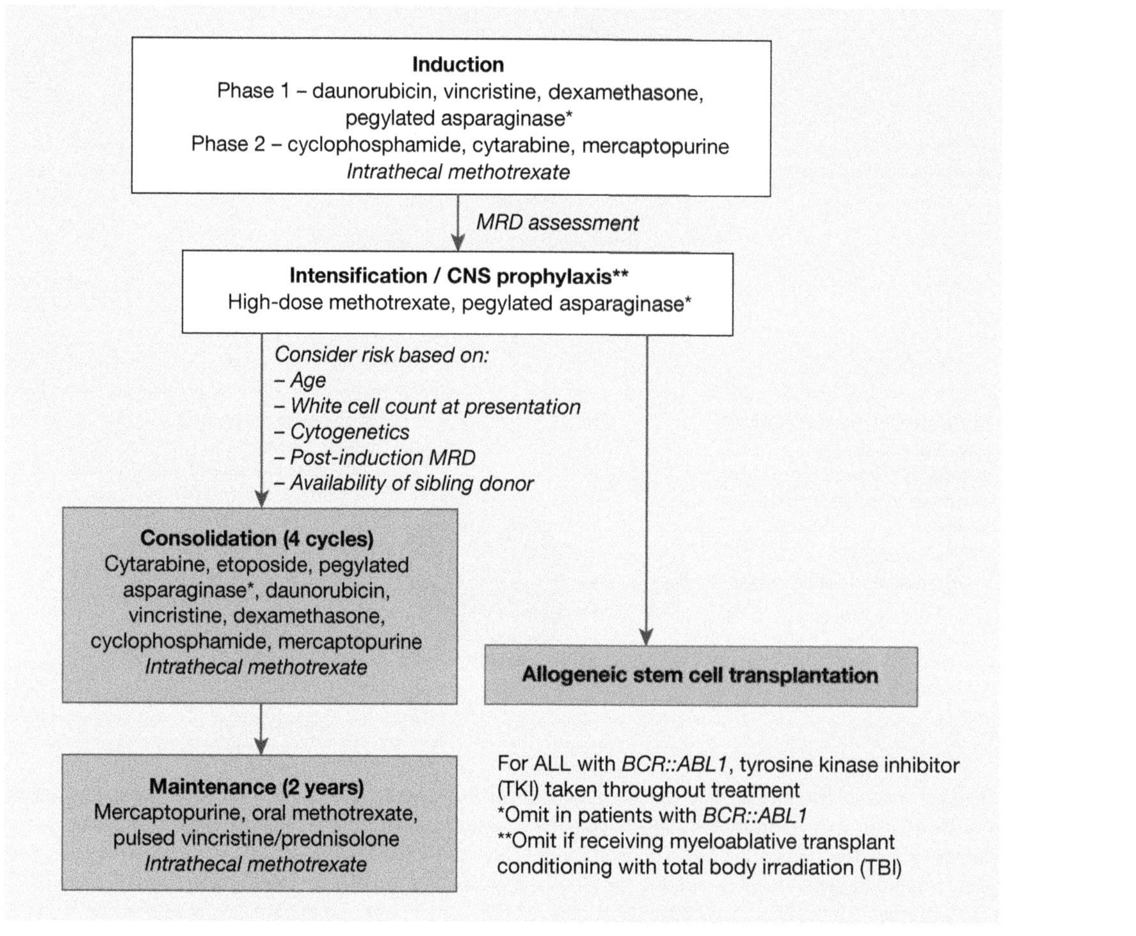

Figure 17.9 Flowchart illustrating typical treatment for adults aged 25–60 years with acute lymphoblastic leukaemia. Based on the approach used in the UKALL14 trial (NCT01085617).

Table 17.4 Prognosis in acute lymphoblastic leukaemia (ALL).

	Good	Poor
WBC	Low (<50 × 10⁹/L)	High (e.g. >50 × 10⁹/L B-ALL, >100 × 10⁹/L T-ALL)
Sex	Female	Male
Age	Child (1–10 years)	Adult (or infant <1 year)
Immunophenotype (in children)	B-cell	T-cell
Cytogenetics	Normal or hyperdiploidy; *ETV6* rearrangement	t(9;22); most translocations involving 11q23 (*KTM2A*); hypodiploidy (<45 chromosomes)
Molecular genetics	Absence of high-risk mutations	Mutations of *TP53*, *NRAS*, *NR3C1*, *BTG*; *BCR::ABL1*-like expression pattern
Time to clear blasts from blood	<1 week	>1 week
Time to remission	<4 weeks	>4 weeks
CNS disease at presentation	Absent	Present
Minimal (measurable) residual disease (MRD)	Negative or <0.01% at 1 month (children); 3 months (adults)	Still positive (>0.01%) at 3–6 months

CNS, central nervous system; WBC, white blood cell count.

Inotuzumab ozogamicin is an anti-CD22 antibody-cytotoxic drug conjugate that can be used to treat relapsed and refractory B-cell ALL that has cell surface expression of CD22. Daratumumab (anti-CD38) and the BCL-2 inhibitors venetoclax and navitoclax are being assessed in clinical trials.

Chimeric antigen receptor (CAR)-T cell therapy is another approach to targeting neoplastic B cells. B-ALL is one of the first diseases for which this treatment has been successful. The patient's own T cells are programmed to kill B cells expressing CD19 (Chapter 9). Anti-CD19 CAR-T cell therapy is approved for patients with relapsed and refractory B-ALL. The side effects of CAR-T cell therapy are described in Chapter 12. Relapses of ALL with CD19 negative blast cell subsets may occur after CAR-T cell therapy, which represents a mechanism of immune evasion by the leukaemia cells. CAR-T cells for treating B cell malignancies with different antigen specificity such as CD22 are in development.

Chemotherapy or immunotherapy including CAR-T cell therapy for relapsed disease is usually followed, where possible, by allogeneic SCT. If relapse occurs after years off all therapy, the outlook is better, but allogeneic SCT is usually also recommended in this setting.

Late toxicity

The long-term toxicity of therapy is a major concern of those treating children with ALL. Specific concerns are the high risk of avascular bone necrosis, seen in teenagers and young adults in association with high doses of dexamethasone, the potential long-term cardiac risk of even modest anthracycline doses, the impact of alkylating agents on fertility and the small risk of second tumours. New generation clinical trials in children are aimed at reducing the risk of toxicity while preserving anti-leukaemic activity. This is achieved by risk stratifying patients to reduce the intensity of treatment in patients with standard-risk disease and increasing the intensity in those with greater risk of relapse.

Targeted therapy for ALL in adults

Improving treatment outcomes for adults with ALL has proven challenging compared to the great successes that have been observed with childhood therapy. In both adults and children, the rates of remission after induction therapy are high, but the rate of disease relapse is much higher in adults (Fig. 17.11). Although cure rates in children now approach 90%, no more than 40% of adult patients remain free of leukaemia after 5 years and this rate is much lower in patients over age 50.

A significant factor is that the genetic subtypes of the ALL differ according to age. Hyperdiploidy and t(12;21) (*ETV::RUNX1*), which carry a good prognosis and together make up 50% of childhood cases, are both rare in adult patients. *BCR:: ABL1*-positive and *BCR::ABL1*-like disease are much more common with age (Fig. 17.5). The introduction of TKIs combined with either chemotherapy or blinatumomab has substantially improved the prognosis for *BCR::ABL1*-positive cases. In the majority of patients, remission can be achieved. However, relapse is common due to the appearance of resistant subclones that harbour mutations in the *BCR-ABL1* fusion gene. *BCR-ABL1*-like cases may be amenable to treatment with either TKIs such as imatinib (fusions involving *ABL1*, *ABL2*, *CSF1R*, or *PDGFRB*) or JAK inhibitors (rearrangements of *JAK2* and *EPOR*).

An additional factor that has contributed to the relatively poor outcome for ALL in adults is the lower doses of chemotherapy that have traditionally been used in adult patients. This is now being addressed in younger adult patients, who are increasingly being treated using 'childhood' protocols with higher intensity chemotherapy regimens. CNS prophylaxis in adults usually involves a combination of intrathecal chemotherapy with methotrexate, with or without cytarabine and steroids, and systemic treatment with high-dose methotrexate and cytarabine. The presence of MRD after 3 months or more of therapy in adults is an unfavourable prognostic indicator (Fig. 17.11). Many of these patients are treated by allogeneic SCT if a suitable sibling or matched unrelated donor is available (Fig 17.9)

Trials employing less intensive chemotherapy combined with inotuzumab ogogamicin and/or blinatumomab (Fig 17.10) as first-line therapy have demonstrated high rates of durable

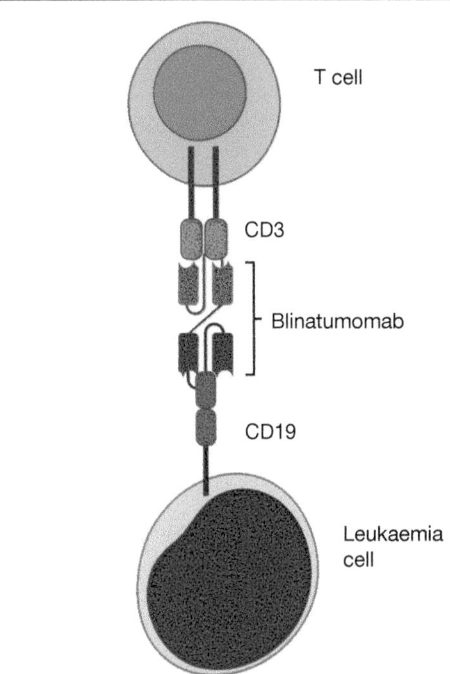

Figure 17.10 Blinatumomab is a bi-specific T-cell engager (BiTE®) construct that consists of two connected single-chain variable antibody fragments. Its mode of action is to bring CD19-expressing B cells into proximity with CD3-expressing T cells, resulting in T-cell-mediated lysis and concomitant T-cell proliferation.

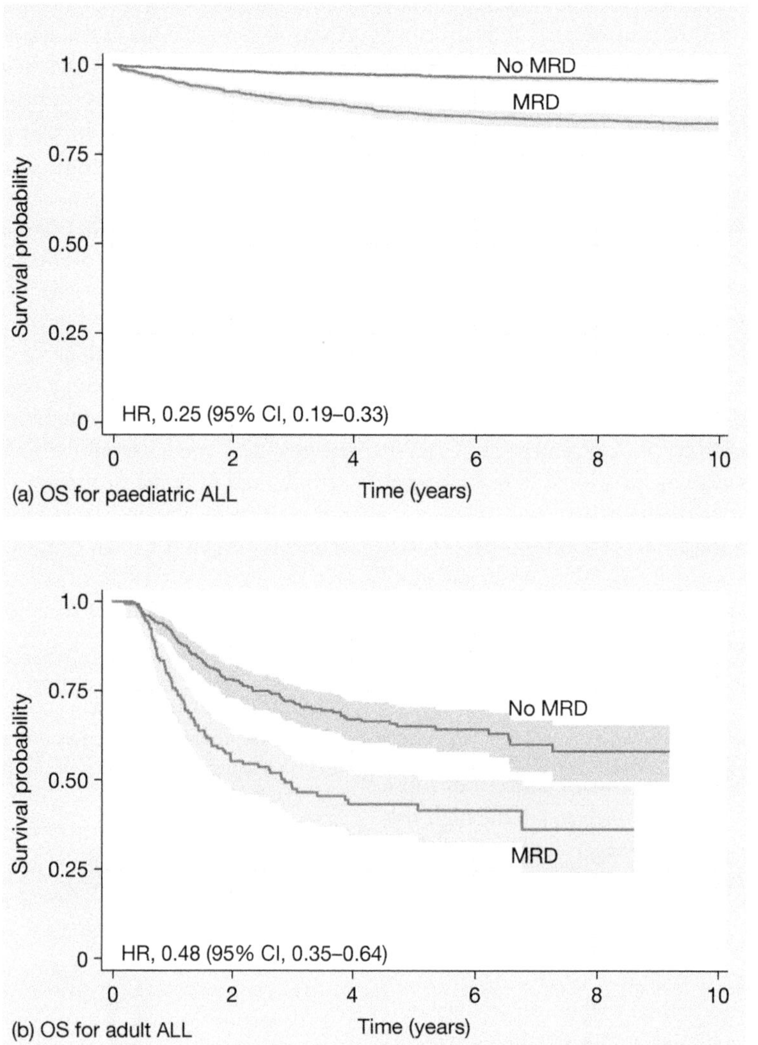

Figure 17.11 Overall survival of patients with *BCR::ABL1* negative ALL according to end of induction MRD (No MRD = <0.01%; MRD = ≥0.01%). Source: Data are derived from UKALL2003. **(a)** Data are derived from: UKALL (2003) Paediatric and young adult, and **(b)** UKALL 14 adult trials. Courtesy of Professors Ajay Vora, Adele Fielding and Anthony Moorman.

complete remission and in future may be preferable to more intensive regimens that are associated with greater toxicity.

In older adults, who are more susceptible to side effects from chemotherapy, using these monoclonal antibodies without chemotherapy in first-line and relapsed settings is likely to improve outcomes.

Prognosis

There is a great variation in the chance of individual patients achieving a long-term cure based on a number of biological variables (Table 17.4). Approximately 15–20% of children relapse after first-line therapy and need further treatment, but over 90% of children can expect to be cured (Fig. 17.11). The cure rate in adults drops significantly to less than 5% over the age of 70 years. The challenge in both adults and children over the next few years is to better define risk groups and to ascertain the optimal way of incorporating novel immunotherapies into treatment regimens for individual patients. Risk stratification may be accomplished using both existing MRD technology and also newer assessment of molecular patterns; these patterns may, for example, define subgroups with specific drug sensitivities or children at particular risk of a specific drug toxicity.

SUMMARY

- Acute lymphoblastic leukaemia is caused by an accumulation of lymphoblasts in the bone marrow. It is the most common malignant disease of childhood – 75% of cases occur before the age of 6 years; 85% of cases are of B-cell lineage with the rest of T-cell lineage.
- The first genetic mutation occurs in many cases *in utero*, with a secondary genetic event occurring later in childhood, possibly as a reaction to an infection.
- The clinical presentation is with the features of bone marrow failure (anaemia, infection and bleeding) together with symptoms of tissue infiltration by tumour cells, leading to bone pain, enlarged lymph nodes, meningeal and testicular infiltration in some cases.
- Diagnosis is by examination of blood and bone marrow. Important tests include microscopic examination of the neoplastic cells, immunophenotyping, chromosomal and molecular genetic analyses.
- ALL is subclassified according to the underlying genetic defect and a wide variety of genetic lesions are seen. The number of chromosomes in the neoplastic cell has prognostic importance: *hyperdiploid* cells have >50 chromosomes and are generally associated with a good prognosis, whereas *hypodiploid* cases (<45 chromosomes) carry a poor prognosis. Other cytogenetic abnormalities are also of prognostic significance, e.g. t(9;22), increasingly frequent with age, which is unfavourable, though it can be targeted with specific tyrosine kinase inhibitors.
- Treatment protocols for ALL are complex and usually have four components – remission induction, intensification or consolidation, CNS-directed therapy and maintenance.
- Treatment is *risk adjusted* to reduce the treatment given to patients with good prognosis. This is based on age, gender, white cell count and cytogenetics at presentation.
- Small numbers of neoplastic cells may sometimes be detected by flow cytometry or molecular analysis even when the blood and bone marrow appear to be clear of leukaemia. This *minimal residual disease* at specific time points has prognostic significance and is used in planning therapy.
- If relapse occurs during chemotherapy the outlook is poor, but if it happens after years off all treatment the outlook is better. Further chemotherapy and allogeneic SCT should be considered. CAR-T cells and bi-specific antibodies that recruit T cells are active therapies in the setting of relapsed/refractory disease.
- Overall, >90% of children can now be cured. The cure rate in adults is about 40%, but drops significantly with advancing age to less than 5% over the age of 70 years.

Now visit **www.wiley.com/go/haematology9e** to test yourself on this chapter.

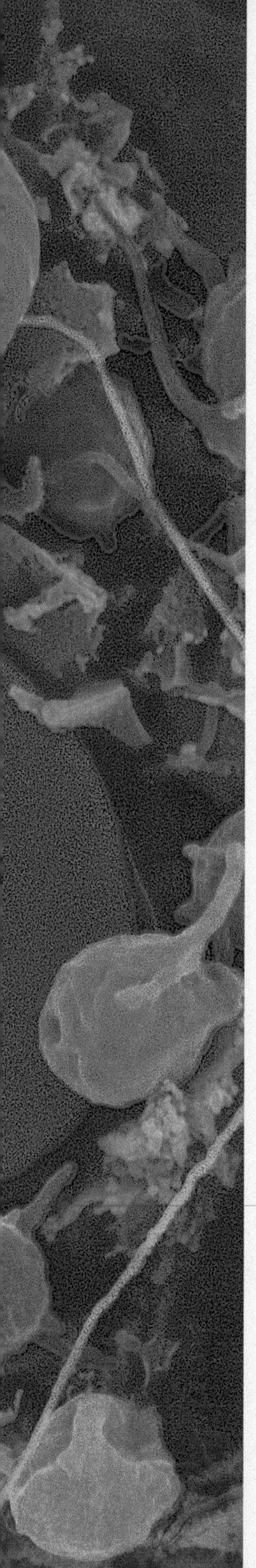

CHAPTER 18

The chronic lymphocytic leukaemias

Key topics

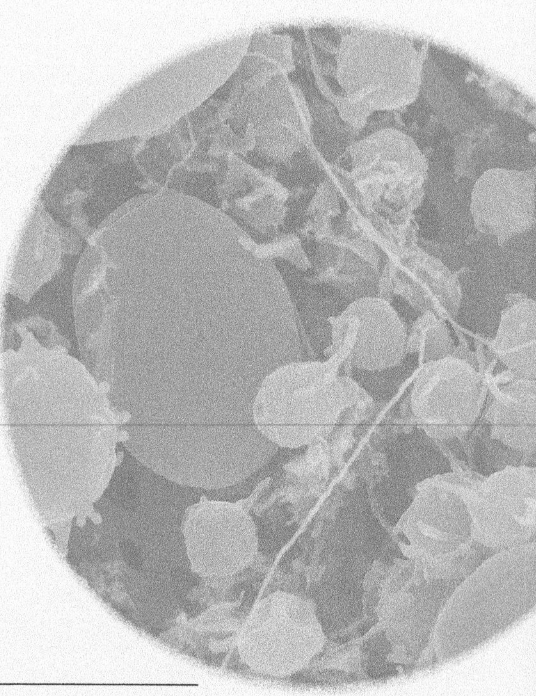

Hoffbrand's Essential Haematology, Ninth Edition. A. Victor Hoffbrand, Pratima Chowdary, Graham P. Collins, and Justin Loke.

© 2024 John Wiley & Sons Ltd. Published 2024 by John Wiley & Sons Ltd.

Companion website: www.wiley.com/go/haematology9e

Several disorders are included in the chronic lymphocytic leukaemias group. All are characterized by accumulation in the blood of mature lymphocytes of either B- or T-cell type (Table 18.1). In general, these diseases are not cured and run a chronic and fluctuating course. New treatments are, however, producing spectacular improvements in life expectancy.

Diagnosis

Patients with chronic lymphocytic leukaemias are often asymptomatic and discovered incidentally when a full blood count is performed for another clinical indication. Alternatively, they may have constitutional symptoms, or may have local signs and symptoms related to lymph node or spleen enlargement. The usual laboratory finding is chronic persistent blood lymphocytosis, in some cases accompanied by anaemia or thrombocytopenia. Reactive lymphocytosis should be ruled out (Chapter 9). The clonal nature of the lymphocytosis in the chronic lymphocytic leukaemias can be proven with flow cytometry or DNA analysis. Subtypes of chronic lymphocytic leukaemias are distinguished by morphology, immunophenotype and genetic analysis.

There is some overlap between chronic lymphocytic leukaemias and the non-Hodgkin lymphomas in which lymphoma cells may be found circulating in the blood. Moreover chronic leukaemias may involve lymph nodes and other lymphatic tissue. **In particular, distinction between chronic lymphocytic leukaemia (CLL) and small lymphocytic lymphoma (SLL) is arbitrary, depending on the relative proportion of the disease in soft tissue masses compared to blood and bone marrow.** CLL and SLL is one disease which we refer to here as CLL; the cells have an identical immunophenotype and genetic abnormalities.

Table 18.1 Classification of the chronic lymphocytic leukaemias.

B-cell	T-cell
■ Chronic lymphocytic leukaemia (CLL)/small lymphocytic lymphoma (SLL) ■ Hairy cell leukaemia (HCL) ■ Splenic B-cell lymphoma/leukaemia with prominent nucleoli	■ T-cell large granular lymphocytic leukaemia (T-LGL) ■ T-cell prolymphocytic leukaemia (T-PLL) ■ Adult T-cell leukaemia/lymphoma (ATLL) ■ Sézary syndrome (Chapter 21)

Note that this classification includes these disorders within the category of lymphoid malignancies and does not distinguish mature B-cell leukaemias separately (see Appendix).
Source: Adapted from R. Alaggio *et al.* (2022) The 5th edition of the World Health Organization classification of haematolymphoid tumours: lymphoid neoplasms. *Leukemia* 36: 1720–48.

Monoclonal B-cell lymphocytosis (MBL)

Clonal B cells with the same phenotype as CLL but accompanied by no other features diagnostic of a B-lymphoproliferative disorder are found in the blood of many older people. Indeed, monoclonal B-cell lymphocytosis (MBL) has been demonstrated in >10% of persons over the age of 50 years and becomes more frequent with advancing age. It is believed that all cases of clinical CLL progress from this precursor clonal state, which is usually undetected. Genetic changes and immune deficiencies similar to those found in CLL may be present in MBL. In WHO5 MBL is termed *'low count'* if the clonal B cells are $< 0.5 \times 10^9$/L and CLL/SLL MBL if the total B cell count is $\geq 0.5 \times 10^9$/L but $< 5 \times 10^9$/L. **If CLL is to be diagnosed, there must be a monoclonal B-cell count $\geq 5 \times 10^9$/L and/or tissue involvement outside the bone marrow.** Rare cases of MBL are non-CLL type and usually consistent with marginal zone origin.

B-cell diseases

Chronic lymphocytic leukaemia

pathogenesis

CLL is the most common of the chronic lymphocytic leukaemias and has a peak incidence between 60 and 80 years of age. There are geographical variations in incidence. It is the most common form of leukaemia within Europe and the USA, but less frequent elsewhere, especially in Asia. There is a seven-fold increased risk of CLL in the close relatives of patients, which indicates a genetic predisposition to the disease.

The CLL neoplastic cell is a mature B cell with weak surface expression of immunoglobulin (IgM or IgD). CLL cells generally have a low proliferative rate, exhibit impaired apoptosis and a prolonged lifespan. This is reflected in their accumulation in the blood, bone marrow, liver, spleen and lymph nodes. There is up-regulation of the anti-apoptotic proteins BCL-2 and MCL1 and down-regulation of pro-apoptotic proteins such as BCLX. SLL (Chapter 21) is the tissue equivalent of CLL, SLL cells having the same immunophenotype and cytogenetics as CLL. The difference is that in SLL the neoplastic cells accumulate almost exclusively in the lymph nodes, and by definition there are fewer than 5×10^9/L circulating monoclonal B cells.

Cytogenetic and molecular genetic abnormalities that may be present at diagnosis are listed below. Multiple clones from linear or branching evolution may be present at diagnosis. At later stages, after chemotherapy one or other resistant subclone may become dominant (Chapter 11).

clinical features

1 The mean age at diagnosis is 72 years, with only 15% of cases before 50 years of age. The male : female ratio is approximately 2 : 1.

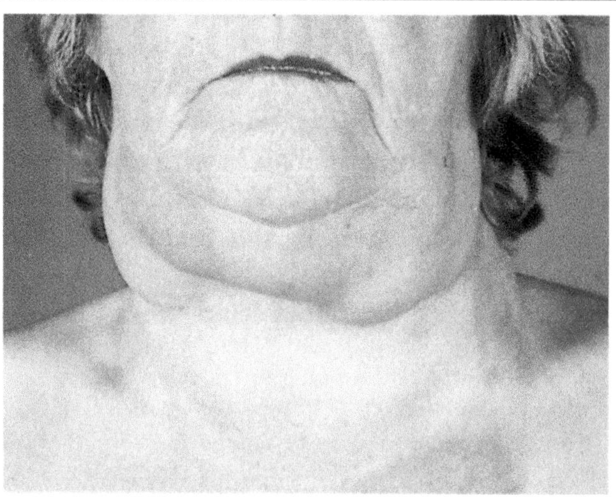

Figure 18.1 Chronic lymphocytic leukaemia: bilateral cervical lymphadenopathy in a 67-year-old woman. Haemoglobin 125 g/L; white blood count 150×10^9/L (lymphocytes 146×10^9/L); platelets 120×10^9/L.

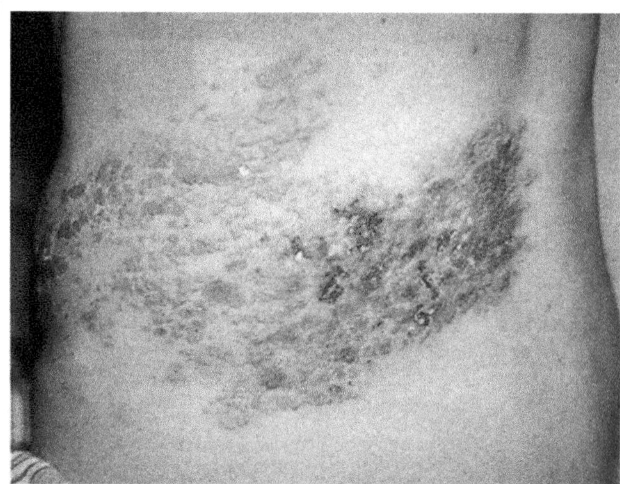

Figure 18.2 Chronic lymphocytic leukaemia: dermatomal herpes zoster infection in a 68-year-old female.

2 The majority of cases are diagnosed from the results of a routine blood test taken for another reason.
3 Enlargement of cervical, axillary or inguinal lymph nodes is the most frequent clinical sign (Fig. 18.1). The nodes are usually discrete and non-tender. Whilst CT scanning is not required for staging or formal response assessment, it is often performed to enable a thorough assessment of disease distribution. It is also required prior to certain treatments to assess the risk of the tumour lysis syndrome.
4 A rapidly enlarging lymph node or the sudden development of constitutional symptoms may indicate transformation to a high-grade lymphoma (Richter transformation).
5 Clinical features of anaemia such as pallor and dyspnoea may be present and patients with thrombocytopenia may show bruising or purpura.
6 Splenomegaly and, less commonly, hepatomegaly are often seen in later stages.
7 Immunosuppression is often a significant problem resulting from hypogammaglobulinaemia and cellular immune dysfunction. Early in the disease course, bacterial infections such as sinus and chest infections predominate, but with advanced disease, viral infections such as herpes zoster (Fig. 18.2) and fungal infections are also seen.

laboratory findings

1 Lymphocytosis. The absolute clonal B-cell lymphocyte count is $\geq 5 \times 10^9$/L and may be 300×10^9/L or more. Typically, between 70% and 99% of white cells in the blood film appear as small lymphocytes. 'Smudge' or 'smear' cells are also present (Fig. 18.3). These result from altered expression of cytoskeletal proteins such as vimentin in clonal cells, leading to fragility of the cells.

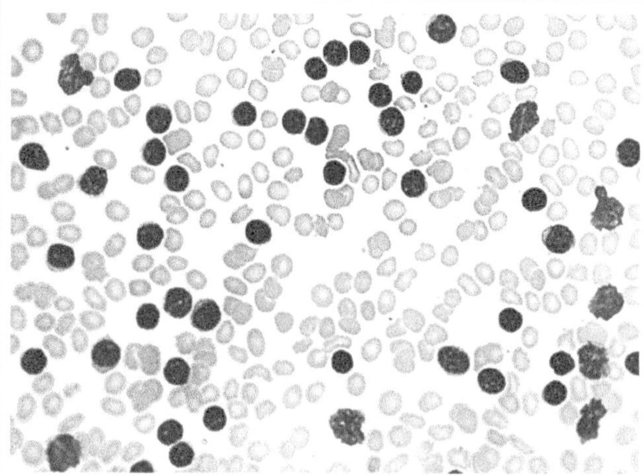

Figure 18.3 Chronic lymphocytic leukaemia: peripheral blood film showing lymphocytes with thin rims of cytoplasm, coarse condensed nuclear chromatin and rare nucleoli. Typical smudge cells are present.

2 Immunophenotyping of the lymphocytes shows them to be B cells ($CD19^+$) with expression of only one type of light chain (known as 'light chain restriction', Fig. 20.6). Characteristically, the cells are also brightly positive for CD5 and CD23, but show low levels of surface immunoglobulin, CD20, CD22 and CD79b (Table 18.2). CD10 and FMC7 are usually negative.
3 Normochromic normocytic anaemia is present in later stages as a result of marrow infiltration or hypersplenism. Usually the marrow must be at least 60–70% involved by CLL cells before cytopenias due to marrow replacement develop. Autoimmune haemolysis may also occur (see below).

Table 18.2 Immunophenotype of the chronic B-cell leukaemias/lymphomas (all CD19⁺).

	CLL	Hairy cell leukaemia	Follicular lymphoma	Mantle cell lymphoma
SIg	Weak	++	++	+
CD5	+	–	–	+
CD22/FMC7	–	+	+	++
CD23	+	–	–	–
CD79b	–	–/+	++	++
CD103*	–	+	–	–

* CD103 is positive only in classic hairy cell leukaemia (HCL); splenic B-cell lymphoma/leukaemia with prominent nucleoli (previously known as a variant form of HCL) is negative for CD103 as well as for CD25, also typically expressed in classical HCL.
CLL, chronic lymphocytic leukaemia; SIg, surface immunoglobulin.

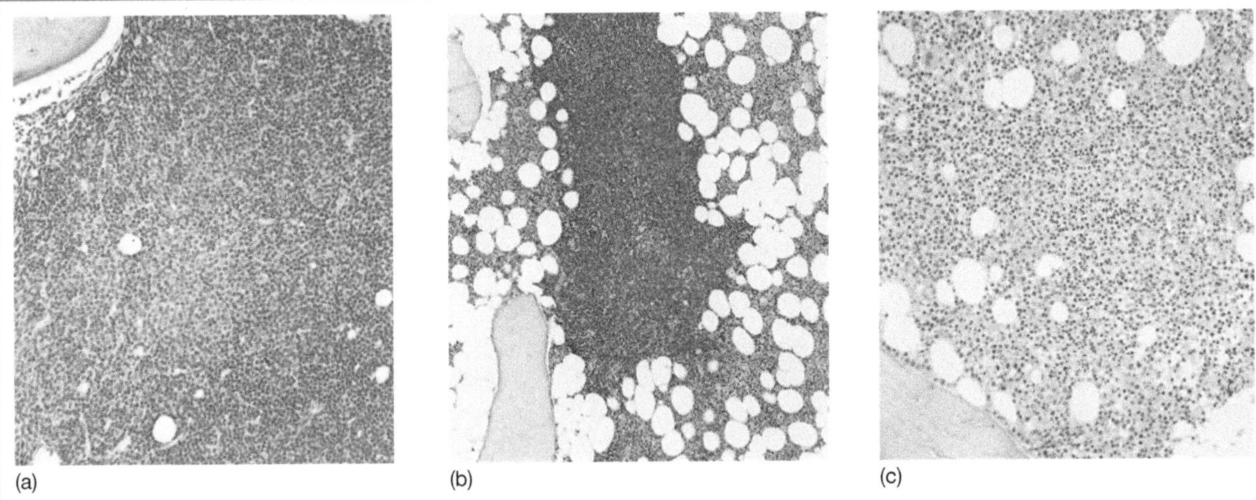

Figure 18.4 Chronic lymphocytic leukaemia: trephine biopsies showing **(a)** a marked diffuse increase in marrow lymphocytes (closely packed cells with small dense nuclei); **(b)** a nodular pattern of lymphocyte accumulation (in a different patient); and **(c)** interstitial infiltration.

Thrombocytopenia occurs in many patients and may also have an autoimmune basis.

4 Bone marrow aspiration shows lymphocytic replacement of normal marrow elements. Trephine biopsy reveals nodular, diffuse or interstitial involvement by lymphocytes (Fig. 18.4).
5 Reduced concentrations of serum immunoglobulins are present, and this becomes more marked with advanced disease. Rarely, a paraprotein is also present.
6 Autoimmunity directed against cells of the haemopoietic system is common. Autoimmune haemolytic anaemia is most frequent but immune thrombocytopenia, neutropenia and red cell aplasia also occur.

Genetics and molecular genetics

The four most common chromosomal abnormalities in CLL, listed from best prognosis to poorest, are deletion of 13q14, trisomy 12, deletion at 11q23 (involving the *ATM* gene) and 17p deletion (involving the *TP53* gene). The *TP53* gene can also be disrupted by mutations which confer a similar poor prognosis. More than 80% of patients with CLL have one of these findings. Normal karyotype has an outlook similar to trisomy 12. The 13q14 deletion leads to loss of microRNAs (p. xxx) that normally control expression of proteins that regulate B-cell survival.

The most common genetic point mutations at presentation are found in *ATM*, *NOTCH1* and *SF3B1* (all at around

Table 18.3 Staging of chronic lymphocytic leukaemia.

(a) Rai classification

Stage	
0	Absolute lymphocytosis ≥5 × 10^9/L without adenopathy, organomegaly or cytopenias due to replacement of marrow by clonal cells
I	Enlarged lymph nodes (adenopathy)
II	Enlarged liver or spleen ± adenopathy
III	Anaemia (Hb <100 g/L)* ± adenopathy ± organomegaly
IV	Thrombocytopenia (platelets <100 × 109/L)* ± adenopathy ± organomegaly

(b) International Working Party classification (Binet)

Stage	*Organ enlargement***	*Haemoglobin* (g/L)*	*Platelets* (×10^9/L)*
A (50–60% of patients)	0, 1 or 2 areas	≥100	≥100
B (30%)	3, 4 or 5 areas	≥100	≥100
C (<20%)	Not considered	<100	or <100

*Secondary causes of anaemia, e.g. iron deficiency or autoimmune haemolytic anaemia or autoimmune thrombocytopenia must be treated before staging. For example, a patient may have Stage 0 disease but be anaemic due to autoimmune haemolysis.
**One area = lymph nodes >1 cm in neck (including Waldeyer's ring), axillae, groins or spleen, or liver enlargement.
Hb, haemoglobin.
Source: (b) Adapted from J.L. Binet *et al.* (1981) *Cancer* 48: 198.

10% prevalence). In addition, point mutations in *TP53* can be seen in up to 5% of patients, and these, as well as the *NOTCH1* and *SF3B1* mutations, have negative prognostic implication and confer resistance to cytotoxic chemotherapy (Table 18.3).

Somatic hypermutation of the immunoglobulin genes

When B cells recognize antigen in the germinal centre of secondary lymphoid tissues, they undergo a process called somatic hypermutation in which random mutations occur in the immunoglobulin heavy‐chain gene (Chapter 9). In CLL the *IGVH* gene shows evidence of this hypermutation in approximately 50% of cases, whereas in the other cases the *VH* genes are unmutated. *IGVH*‐mutated cases are defined by the *IGVH* gene having < 98% homology with the germline sequence. CLL with unmutated immunoglobulin genes has an unfavourable prognosis and may respond less well to initial and subsequent therapy (Table 18.3).

Staging

It is useful to stage patients at presentation both for prognosis and for deciding on therapy. The Rai and Binet staging systems are shown in Table 18.3. Typical survival ranged historically from 12 years for Rai stage 0 to less than 4 years for stage IV, but there is considerable variation between patients, and with current therapies survival rates have improved substantially. Many patients in Rai stage 0 or Binet stage A have a normal life expectancy.

Prognosis

A number of clinical, laboratory and molecular features have been correlated with prognosis. More recently the **CLL International Prognostic Index (CLL‐IPI)** has been developed and identified five factors: age, stage, serum β2‐microglobulin, *IGVH* gene mutational status and *TP53* disruption. With appropriate weighting, four risk groups are then constructed defined as low, medium, high and very high risk (Table 18.4). Importantly the score mainly applies to patients subsequently treated with chemotherapy. Application of newer therapies changes the impact of elements within this scoring system.

treatment

The aim of treatment is to control symptoms and maintain a good quality of life for as long as possible. The only known curative treatment is allogeneic stem cell transplantation which is not appropriate for the vast majority of patients due to its high risk and the availability of alternative highly effective therapies.

Many patients will never need treatment. Treatment is given for troublesome enlarged lymph nodes or spleen, constitutional symptoms such as weight loss, or cytopenias as a

Table 18.4 The CLL International Prognostic Index (CLL-IPI).

Characteristic	Points
Rai stage ≥ 1	1
Age > 65y	1
Unmutated *IGVH* gene	2
Serum β2- microglobulin > 3.5 g/dL	2
Deletion 17p or *TP53* gene mutation	4
Total score	CLL-IPI risk group
0–1	Low
2–3	Intermediate
4–6	High
7–10	Very high

IGVH, immunoglobulin heavy chain variable. See Table 18.3 for Binet/Rai staging.

result of bone marrow suppression. The lymphocyte count alone is not a good guide to the need for treatment, but if it doubles in <6 months, treatment will usually be required soon. As a general guide, patients in Binet stage C will need treatment, as will some in stage B, and patients in Rai stages III or IV will need treatment, as will a smaller proportion of patients in stages I or II (Table 18.3).

First line treatment options (Fig 18.5)

1 **Bruton kinase inhibitor (BTKi)s.** The surface immunoglobulin on a B cell acts as the B-cell receptor (BCR) for antigen and B cells need to receive stimulatory signals through the BCR in order to remain alive (Fig. 9.4). Inherited inactivating mutations of the *BTK* gene are a cause of immunodeficiency with B-cell lymphopenia (Chapter 9). **Ibrutinib and the second generation acalabrutinib and zanabrutinib are oral drugs which covalently bind to and inactivate BTK and lead to B-cell apoptosis.** Monotherapy treatment with any of these three agents is highly effective with prolonged progression free and overall survival and is established as a first line treatment, continued to progression or intolerance. The BTK inhibitors are effective in patients with mutated or unmutated *IgVH* genes. Acalabrutinib (but not ibrutinib) is even more effective when combined with obinutuzumab than when used alone. The combination of ibrutinib with venetoclax (see below) is also extremely effective and offers a fixed duration (just over 1 year) treatment alternative for higher risk patients.

   Remarkably, the BTK inhibitors are effective for cases in which the leukaemic cells have a chromosome 17p deletion or *TP53* mutation, genetic changes which confer relative resistance to standard chemotherapy and to BCL-2 inhibition. They are also active in Richter transformation (see below). Most patients treated with BTK inhibitors do not achieve negativity for minimal residual disease (MRD) although remissions are frequently durable. Potential side effects include increased susceptibility to atrial fibrillation, hypertension, bleeding due to an anti-platelet effect, or *Aspergillus* and other infections. The side effect profiles of each agent differs with, for example, the risk of atrial fibrillation, flutter and hypertension being lower for second generation BTK inhibitors but neutropenia is more common with zanubrutinib. The drugs need to be discontinued several days before elective surgical procedures due to bleeding risk; drug interactions also need to be considered.

2 **BCL-2 inhibitors.** BCL-2 is expressed at a high level in most CLL cells and has potent anti-apoptotic effects, leading to abnormally prolonged cell survival. **Venetoclax, a direct inhibitor of BCL-2, is a highly active oral agent in CLL, inducing frequent responses and a higher rate of negativity for MRD than occurs with BTK inhibitors.** Venetoclax is less effective in those with unmutated *IGVH* genes or with the *TP53* mutation. Combination of venetoclax with the anti-CD20 antibody obinutuzumab is often the preferred first treatment for patients with mutated *IGVH* genes and no *TP53* mutation. Unusually for a targeted agent, venetoclax regimens are of fixed duration (usually one year) rather than continuous treatment until progression, as with the BTK inhibitors. This reduces expense and allows the same regimen to be re-introduced at first relapse.

   Venetoclax is generally well tolerated although neutropenia with subsequent infection risk is a frequent side effect. Baseline assessment of tumour lysis syndrome (TLS) risk is important with careful TLS prophylaxis and monitoring which includes hospitalization for high risk patients. If it is to be given in combination with ibrutinib, the BTK inhibitor is given for some weeks before starting venetoclax.

3 **Chemo-immunotherapy.** The combination of **fludarabine, cyclophosphamide and rituximab (FCR)** was considered the standard regimen for fitter patients for many years. It is an active regimen and some patients achieve long remissions, especially those with mutated *IGVH* genes among whom approximately 50% treated first line with FCR remain in remission for over 10 years. It is, however, profoundly myelosuppressive with associated infection risk. It also confers an increased risk of treatment-induced myeloid malignancies. A *TP53* mutation or deletion is associated with a poor response to FCR and chemotherapy should generally be avoided in such cases. **Bendamustine and rituximab (BR)** is an alternative approach that is better tolerated although also myelosuppressive. It was the more common regimen used in older patients but has been shown inferior to BTKi therapy. **Chlorambucil with obinutuzumb** was also a commonly used combination in the elderly but now less so. In regions of the world where targeted agents are available and reimbursed, chemo-immunotherapy is

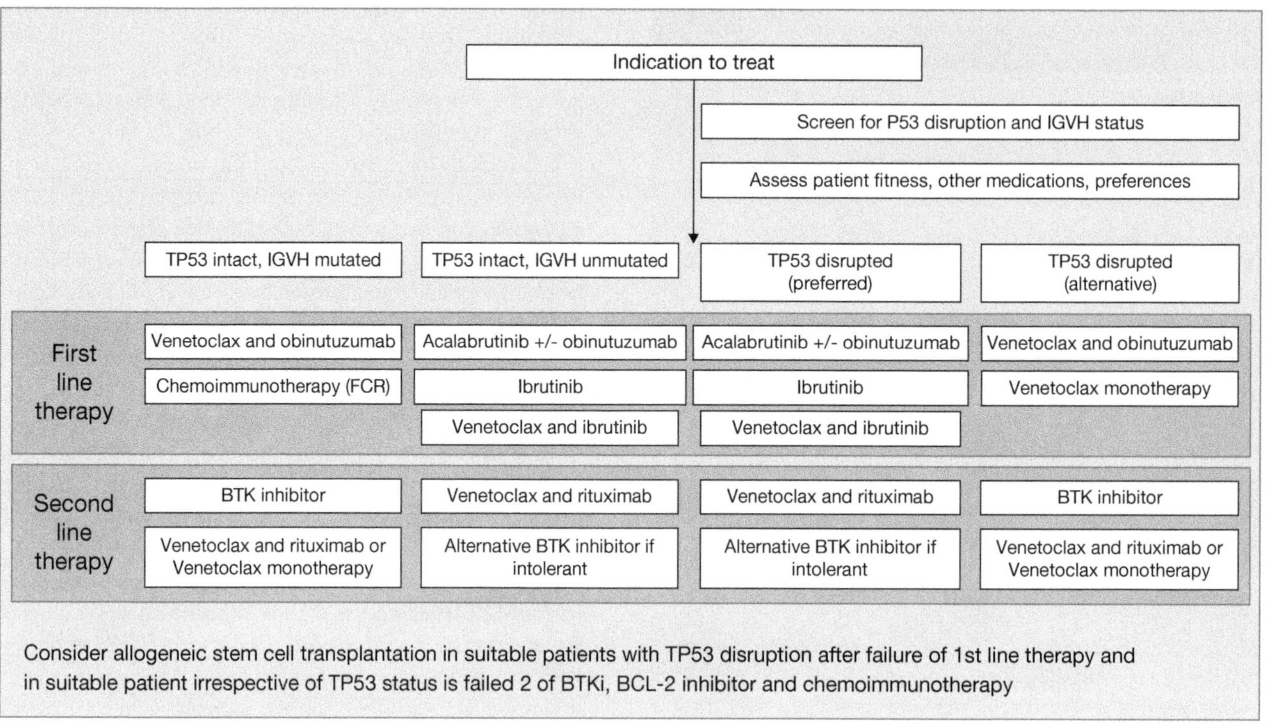

Figure 18.5 Treatment algorithm for CLL. Source: Based on British Society of Haematology Guidelines (2022) *Br. J. Haematol.* 194: 547–57. Zanabrutinib is a third effective covalent BTKi inhibitor more recently approved in some countries. Non-covalent BTK inhibitors, e.g. pirtobrutinib are in clinical trials for treatment of patients who relapse and are resistant to front-line covalent BTK inhibitors (see text).

now much less frequently used and generally reserved for later lines of therapy.

4 **Anti-CD20 monoclonal antibodies** include rituximab and the second-generation glyco-engineered antibody obinutuzumab (Chapter 12). Although CD20 expression by CLL cells is relatively weak, these agents are active although single-agent activity is modest. They are well tolerated making combination with other active agents relatively straightforward. Such combinations include obinutuzumab, more effective than rituximab, with venetoclax or acalabrutinib or chlorambucil. Whilst chemotherapy is less commonly used in CLL, the addition of anti-CD20 antibodies is standard with these drugs. Anti-CD20 antibodies can also be used as a treatment of associated autoimmune haematological conditions such as ITP or AIHA.

5 PI3 kinase inhibitors, e.g. idelalisib is an oral drug which blocks PI3Kδ activity, an isoenzyme particularly important for B-cell survival. Whilst effective in CLL, adverse events include colitis, pneumonitis and atypical infection. These toxicities have limited its use in CLL and the drug class as a whole is not being actively developed (Fig. 18.5).

Treatment at relapse

The principle of only treating a patient for symptoms of nodal enlargement, organomegaly, development of cytopenias and other complications also holds true at relapse. In the absence of these, a policy of observation (called 'watch and wait' or 'active surveillance') is appropriate. Similar agents to those discussed for front line treatment can be used at relapse. For example, progression on or after a BTKi may be treated with a BCL-2 inhibitor in combination with obinatuzumab, usually to good effect. Where available and appropriate, a PI3 kinase inhibitor may also be used. Relapse after multiple-targeted agents may be treated with chemo-immunotherapy although responses are likely to be less durable.

Third-generation, non-covalent BTK inhibitors, pirtobrutinib or nemtabrutinib are being developed aimed at circumventing resistance mechanisms such as BTK^{C481S} and *PLCG2* mutations which impair the efficacy of covalent BTK inhibitors. Agents which lead to the targeted degradation of BTK are also in clinical trials.

Other agents being actively investigated in multiply relapsed or refractory disease, include CD19-directed CAR-T cell therapy (Chapters 9, 12 and 17) and antibody-drug conjugates which target novel antigens such as ROR1.

Other forms of treatment

- ***Corticosteroids*** Prednisolone or other corticosteroids are given for autoimmune haemolytic anaemia, thrombocytopenia and red cell aplasia.

- ***Radiotherapy*** This is valuable in reducing the size of bulky lymph node groups that are unresponsive to chemotherapy.
- ***Ciclosporin*** Red cell aplasia may respond to ciclosporin or other calcineurin inhibitors.
- ***Immunoglobulin replacement*** Immunoglobulin given intravenously or subcutaneously is useful for patients with severe hypogammaglobulinaemia and recurrent infections, especially during winter months.
- ***Vaccination*** Patients should be vaccinated with a conjugated pneumococcal vaccine, with the Shingrix™ recombinant adjuvanted zoster vaccine, and should receive annual influenza vaccination and COVID vaccines on a schedule recommended for immunocompromised individuals.
- ***Allogeneic stem cell transplantation (SCT)*** SCT may be curative but has a significant mortality rate. It is typically employed only in younger patients with multiply relapsed disease.

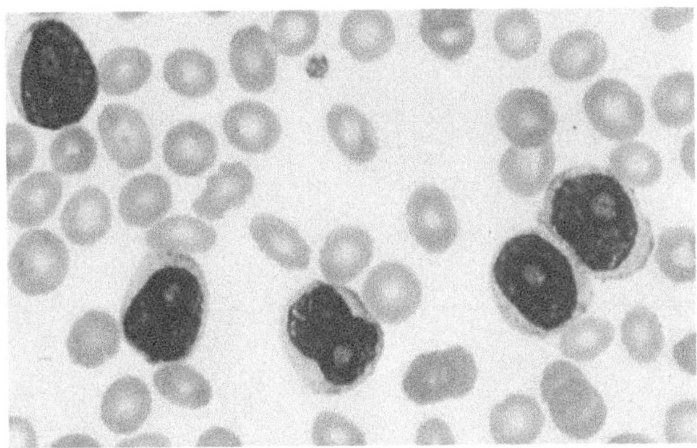

Figure 18.6 Prolymphocytic progression of CLL: blood film showing prolymphocytes that have prominent central nucleoli and an abundance of pale cytoplasm.

Course of disease

Many patients in Binet stage A or Rai stage 0 or I never need therapy, and this is particularly likely for females and those with favourable prognostic markers (Table 18.4). For those who do need treatment, a typical pattern is of response to several courses of therapy with a prolonged disease-free interval, before the gradual onset of extensive bone marrow infiltration or bulky disease. Molecular and cytogenetic tests often show that initially small subclones with genetic characteristics that confer treatment resistance, e.g. chromosome 17p deletion or *TP53* mutations, now form the bulk of the resistant disease. The new oral therapies (BTK, BCL-2 and the more rarely used PI3 kinase inhibitors) are proving effective even at these late stages and in patients with *TP53*-mutant disease.

Richter transformation. CLL, like low-grade lymphomas, may transform into a high-grade lymphoma (Richter transformation). This usually resembles a diffuse large B-cell lymphoma with mutations of *TP53*, *MYC*, *NOTCH1* and *CDKN2A* genes. Less frequently, transformation resembles Hodgkin lymphoma. Richter transformation is often signalled by a dominant node that is brighter on positron emission tomography (PET) scans than other nodes although a biopsy is required to make the diagnosis. Richter transformation is usually clonally related to the underlying CLL in patients who respond poorly to treatment usually with frequent *TP53* mutations contributing to the chemotherapy resistance. Occasional cases of clonally unrelated Richter transformation may arise (especially in untreated CLL) in which the outcomes are often better. Richter transformation requires therapy as for other high-grade B-cell lymphomas, e.g. with R-CHOP, Chapter 21. Prognosis is usually poor although BTK inhibitors appear to have activity and are being investigated in this condition together with other agents such as CAR-T cells and bispecific antibodies.

Prolymphocytic progression of CLL is diagnosed if >15% of the clonal cells show a prolymphocytic appearance. The prolymphocyte is around twice the size of a CLL lymphocyte and has a large central nucleolus (Fig. 18.6). The diagnosis of B-cell prolymphocytic leukaemia (B-PLL) is no longer recognized in WHO5 as the term included several different entities including a variant of mantle cell lymphoma, prolymphocytic progression of CD5+ CLL and other cases now classified in WHO5 as 'splenic lymphoma/leukaemia with prominent nucleoli'.

Splenic B-cell lymphomas/leukaemias

This is a new WHO 5 grouping of diseases including hairy cell leukaemia (HCL), splenic B-cell lymphoma with prominent nucleoli (SBLPN) (previously known as the hairy cell leukaemia variant), splenic diffuse red pulp small B-cell lymphoma and splenic marginal zone lymphoma. HCL and SBLPN are discussed next, the other two entities in Chapter 21.

Hairy cell leukaemia

Hairy cell leukaemia (HCL) is an uncommon B-cell lymphoproliferative disease with a male: female ratio of 4 : 1 and a peak incidence at 40–60 years. Patients typically present with infections, anaemia or splenomegaly. Lymphadenopathy is uncommon. Pancytopenia is usual at presentation and the lymphocyte count is rarely over 20×10^9/L. Monocytopenia is a distinctive feature.

The blood film reveals a variable number of unusual large lymphocytes with villous cytoplasmic projections (Fig. 18.7). Immunophenotyping shows CD11c, CD19, CD25, CD103 and CD123 positivity in most cases (Table 18.2). **A mutation in exon 15 of the gene for the protein kinase *BRAF* (V600E) underlies the disease.** The bone marrow trephine biopsy shows a characteristic appearance of mild fibrosis and a diffuse cellular infiltrate (Fig. 18.7).

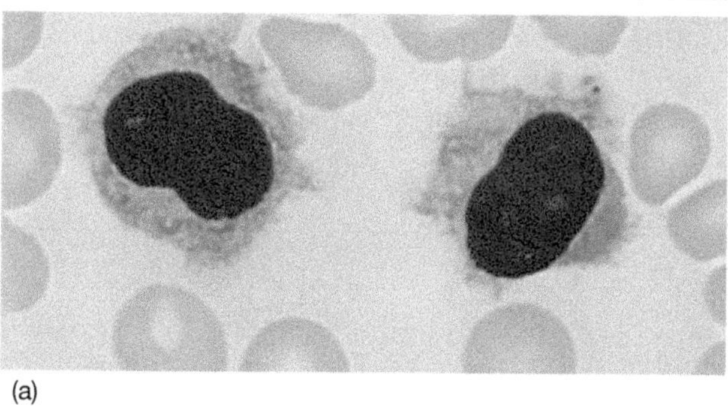

(a)

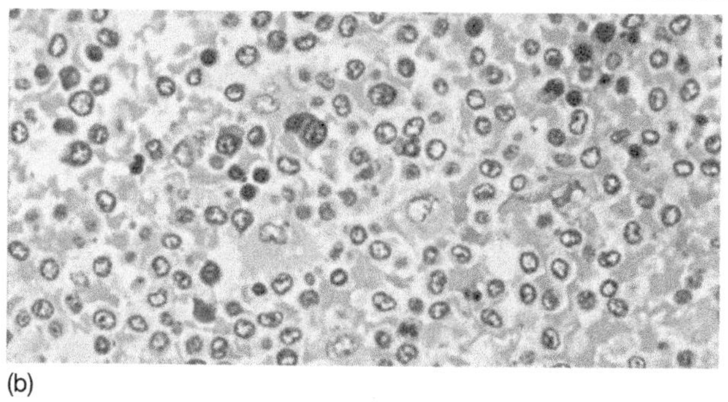

(b)

Figure 18.7 Hairy cell leukaemia: **(a)** peripheral blood film showing typical 'hairy' cells with oval nuclei and finely mottled pale grey-blue cytoplasm with an irregular edge; **(b)** bone marrow trephine biopsy.

There are several highly effective treatments for HCL and the median relapse-free survival after initial chemotherapy is more than 10 years. **The treatment of choice is cladribine (2-chlorodeoxyadenosine, CDA) or pentostatin (deoxycoformycin, DCF)**. Both agents achieve complete responses in over 80% of cases. In two-thirds of cases a long-term remission is achieved. Rituximab may be combined with chemotherapy for first-line treatment or be reserved for use at relapse. Alpha-interferon is also effective and is sometimes used first for those with severe cytopenias to improve these before the more effective drugs, which initially tend to lower further the neutrophil and platelet counts, are given. If relapse occurs after a long remission, retreatment with CDA or DCF with or without rituximab can be tried. *BRAF* inhibitors such as vemurafenib are potentially useful in refractory disease, as is moxetumomab pasudotox, an anti-CD22 antibody conjugated to a bacterial toxin.

Splenic B-cell lymphoma/leukaemia with prominent nucleoli is the designation introduced by WHO5 for what was previously known as the HCL variant. *BRAF* mutation is absent, monocytopenia less common and the immunophenotype is distinct, e.g. these cases typically lack CD123, CD25 or CD103 expression. The outlook is less favourable than for HCL. Responsiveness to chemotherapy is decreased and the disease-free interval is shorter. Splenectomy may be required in some cases. Mutations in the gene *MAP2K1,* which encodes a protein in the MAP kinase pathway (Fig. 1.8) are frequent and specific pathway inhibitors may be considered.

Lymphocytosis in non-Hodgkin lymphomas

Some cases of splenic marginal zone lymphoma show circulating monoclonal B lymphocytes with a villous cell outline and were previously termed 'splenic lymphoma with villous lymphocytes'. Lymphocytosis may also be seen in other types of non-Hodgkin lymphoma, e.g. follicular, mantle cell, diffuse large B cell, discussed further in Chapters 20 and 21.

T-cell diseases

T-cell prolymphocytic leukaemia

T-cell prolymphocytic leukaemia (T-PLL) presents with a high white cell count, lymphadenopathy is usually marked and skin lesions and serous effusions are common. Most cases express CD4. Treatment is with intravenous alemtuzumab (anti-CD52) followed by SCT in appropriate patients. There is an association with ataxia-telangiectasia syndrome due to germline mutations in *ATM* with faulty DNA repair.

Large granular lymphocytic leukaemia

Large granular lymphocytic (LGL) leukaemia is characterized by the presence of circulating lymphocytes with abundant cytoplasm and large azurophilic granules (Fig. 18.8a). Such cells may be either T or natural killer (NK) cells and show variable expression of CD16, CD56 and CD57. **Cytopenia, especially neutropenia, is the main clinical problem.** Anaemia, splenomegaly and arthropathy with positive serology for rheumatoid arthritis are also common. The median age is 50 years.

Treatment may not be needed, but if required, steroids, cyclophosphamide, ciclosporin/tacrolimus or methotrexate may relieve the cytopenia. *STAT3* mutations similar to those found in cytotoxic lymphocytes of patients with immune aplastic anaemia (Chapter 24), are present in 50% of cases and patients may respond to JAK-STAT inhibitors, including ruxolitinib or tofacitinib. Granulocyte colony-stimulating factor (G-CSF) has been used in cases associated with neutropenia.

Adult T-cell leukaemia/lymphoma

Adult T-cell leukaemia/lymphoma (ATLL) was the first malignancy to be associated with a human retrovirus, human T-cell lymphotrophic virus type 1 (HTLV-1). The virus is endemic in parts of Japan and the Caribbean and the disease is very rare in people who have not lived in these areas. ATLL lymphocytes have a bizarre morphology with a convoluted 'cloverleaf' nucleus and a consistent $CD4^+$ phenotype (Fig. 18.8b).

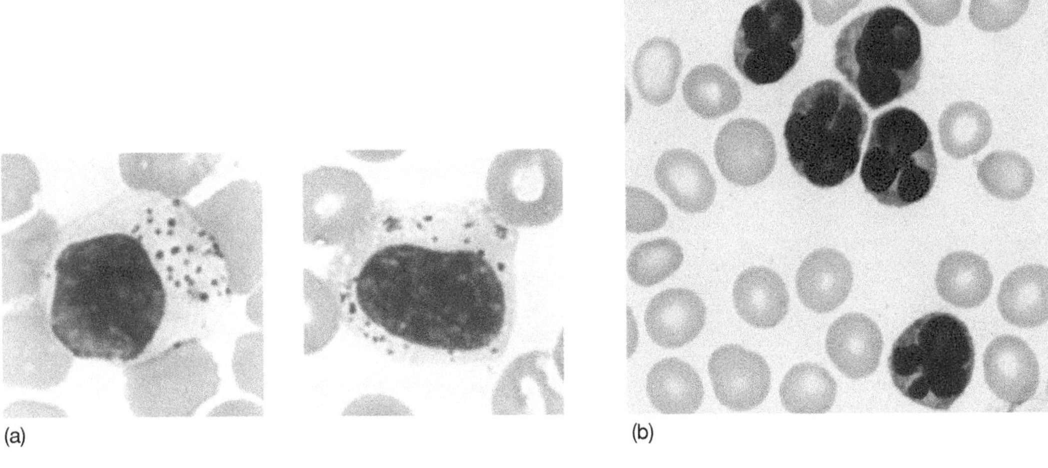

Figure 18.8 **(a)** Large granular lymphocytes in the peripheral blood. **(b)** Adult T-cell leukaemia/lymphoma. Typical convoluted lymphoid cells in peripheral blood.

Most subjects infected with the HTLV-1 virus do not develop the disease. The clinical presentation is often acute and dominated by hypercalcaemia, skin lesions, hepatosplenomegaly and lymphadenopathy. Diagnosis is by morphology and serology. Zidovudine, an anti-retroviral drug, and alpha-interferon are first-line therapy if leukaemia is dominant, but combination chemotherapy is used if the presentation is more like a lymphoma. Allogeneic SCT may be used, but the cure rate is only about 35%. The overall prognosis is poor.

SUMMARY

- Chronic lymphocytic leukaemias are characterized by the accumulation of mature B or T lymphocytes in the blood.
- Individual subtypes are distinguished on the basis of morphology, immunophenotype and cytogenetics.
- Chronic lymphocytic leukaemia (CLL, B cell) represents 90% of cases and has a peak incidence between 60 and 80 years of age. There is genetic predisposition to development of the disease. It is preceded by monoclonal B-cell lymphocytosis.
- Most cases of CLL are identified when a routine blood test is performed. As the disease progresses the patient may develop enlarged lymph nodes, splenomegaly, hepatomegaly and bone marrow failure.
- Immunosuppression is a significant problem in CLL because of hypogammaglobulinaemia and cellular immune dysfunction.
- In CLL, anaemia and thrombocytopenia may develop because of autoimmune haemolysis and thrombocytopenia as well as from bone marrow infiltration.
- Diagnosis of CLL is usually performed by immunophenotypic analysis of peripheral blood, which reveals a clonal population of $CD5^+$ $CD23^+$ light-chain restricted B cells.
- The best guide to prognosis is the stage of the disease. CLL that has acquired somatic mutations in the immunoglobulin genes has a relatively good prognosis compared to unmutated cases. Lymphocyte doubling time, immunological markers, cytogenetics and molecular genetics also provide important prognostic information.
- Treatment for CLL is usually given only when clinical symptoms develop. Many patients require no therapy.
- Drugs which block the activity of BTK (ibrutinib, acalabrutinib, zanabrutinib), or BCL-2 (venetoclax) sometimes in combination with anti-CD20 antibodies, especially obinatuzumab, are highly effective treatments which have generally replaced immuno-chemotherapy in regions where they are available. Where first-line immune-chemotherapy is used such as fludaraabine, cyclophosphamide and rituximab (FCR) or bendamustine and rituximab (BR), BTK inhibitors remain active in relapsed or refractory disease.
- Less common subtypes of B-cell chronic lymphoproliferative disorders include, hairy cell leukaemia and splenic B-cell lymphoma/leukaemia with prominent nucleoli (previously known as hairy cell variant).
- T-cell chronic leukaemias include T-cell prolymphocytic leukaemia, large granular lymphocytic leukaemia and adult T-cell leukaemia/lymphoma.

Now visit **www.wiley.com/go/haematology9e** to test yourself on this chapter.

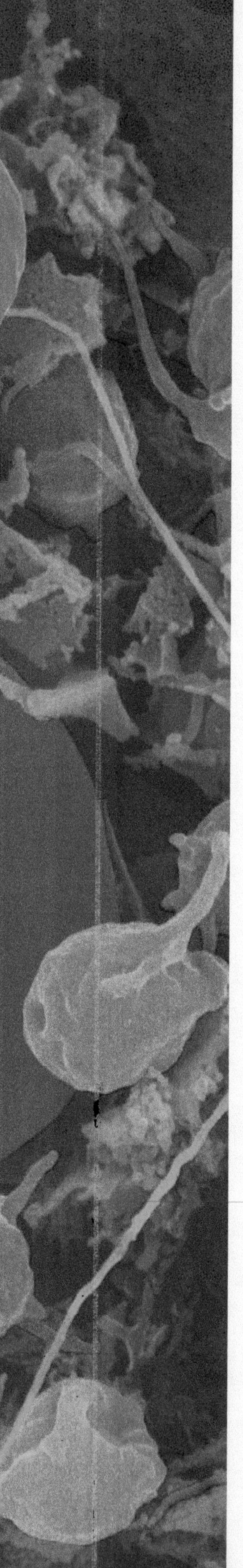

CHAPTER 19

Hodgkin lymphoma

Key topics

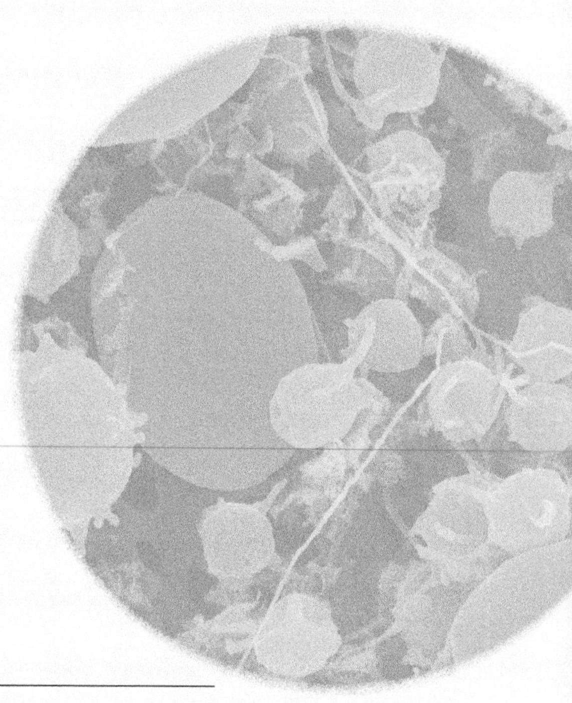

Hoffbrand's Essential Haematology, Ninth Edition. A. Victor Hoffbrand, Pratima Chowdary, Graham P. Collins, and Justin Loke.
© 2024 John Wiley & Sons Ltd. Published 2024 by John Wiley & Sons Ltd.
Companion website: www.wiley.com/go/haematology9e

Lymphoma can be defined as a cancer of mature lymphocytes. Typically it is divided into Hodgkin and non-Hodgkin lymphoma based on the presence or absence of the malignant Reed–Sternberg (RS) cell of Hodgkin lymphoma, embedded within an exuberant inflammatory microenvironment. Two main forms exist: classical Hodgkin lymphoma (cHL) and the less common nodular lymphocyte-predominant Hodgkin lymphoma (NLPHL) which has a distinct pathology and clinical course. cHL has a unique epidemiology with a bimodal age distribution. It is highly curable with current approaches and there is a focus on reducing late, harmful effects of chemotherapy and radiotherapy.

History and pathogenesis

Thomas Hodgkin was curator of the Anatomy Museum at Guy's Hospital in London and described the disease in 1832. Carl von Sternberg in Vienna identified the abnormal cell that defines this subtype of lymphoma in 1898, and in 1902 Dorothy Reed, who was then a pathology trainee at Johns Hopkins, was the first to distinguish the cell from granulomas found in nodal tuberculosis. The characteristic RS cells, and the associated abnormal mononuclear (Hodgkin) cells, are neoplastic, whereas the infiltrating inflammatory cells are reactive.

Immunoglobulin gene rearrangement studies show that the RS cell is of B-lymphoid lineage and that it is often derived from a B cell with a 'crippled' immunoglobulin gene caused by the acquisition of mutations that prevent synthesis of full-length immunoglobulin. Human leukocyte antigen (HLA) class I expression is usually lost on the neoplastic cells and mutation of the β2-microglobulin gene is frequent. The Epstein–Barr virus (EBV) genome has been detected in approximately 50% of cases in Hodgkin tissue, but its exact role in the pathogenesis is unclear.

Clinical features

Classical Hodgkin lymphoma (cHL) can present at any age but has a peak in the 15–35 year age group and as such it is one of the commonest cancers in the teenage and young adult population. There is an almost 2: 1 male predominance. The following symptoms are common:

1 **Most patients present with painless, asymmetrical, firm and discrete enlargement of superficial lymph nodes** (Fig. 19.1). The cervical nodes are involved in 60–70% of patients, axillary nodes in approximately 10–15% and inguinal nodes in 6–12%. In some cases, the size of the nodes decreases and increases spontaneously; they may also become matted. Typically, the disease is localized initially to a single peripheral lymph node region and its subsequent progression is by contiguity within the lymphatic system. Retroperitoneal nodes are also often involved, but usually only diagnosed by computed tomography (CT) or positron emission tomography (PET) scan.

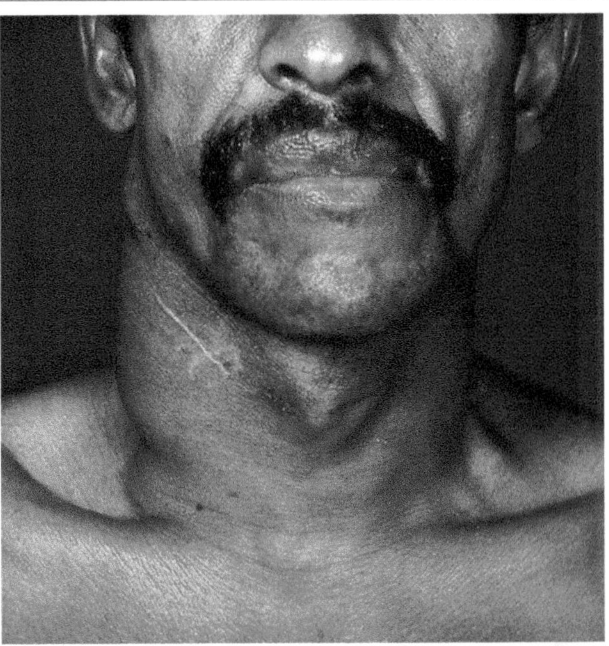

Figure 19.1 Cervical lymphadenopathy in a patient with classical Hodgkin lymphoma.

2 Mediastinal involvement is frequent and may be the dominant site of disease (Fig. 19.2). This may present as a cough or breathlessness, frequently worse on lying flat. An associated pleural effusion or, less commonly, superior vena cava obstruction may be seen.

3 Splenic involvement may occur in more advanced disease but palpable splenomegaly is rare.

4 Other organs may be involved either at presentation or in multiply relapsed disease. Typical sites include the bone, lungs and liver.

5 Constitutional symptoms are prominent in many patients with widespread disease. The following may be seen:
   (a) Fever, which maybe continuous or cyclic
   (b) Pruritus, which is often severe,
   (c) Alcohol-induced pain in the areas where disease is present occurs in some patients;
   (d) Other constitutional symptoms include weight loss, profuse sweating (especially at night), weakness, fatigue, anorexia and cachexia.

Note: so-called B-symptoms are restricted to: fever > 38°C on two or more occasions in the absence of infection, unintentional weight loss of >10% body weight over a period of 6 months or less and drenching night sweats.

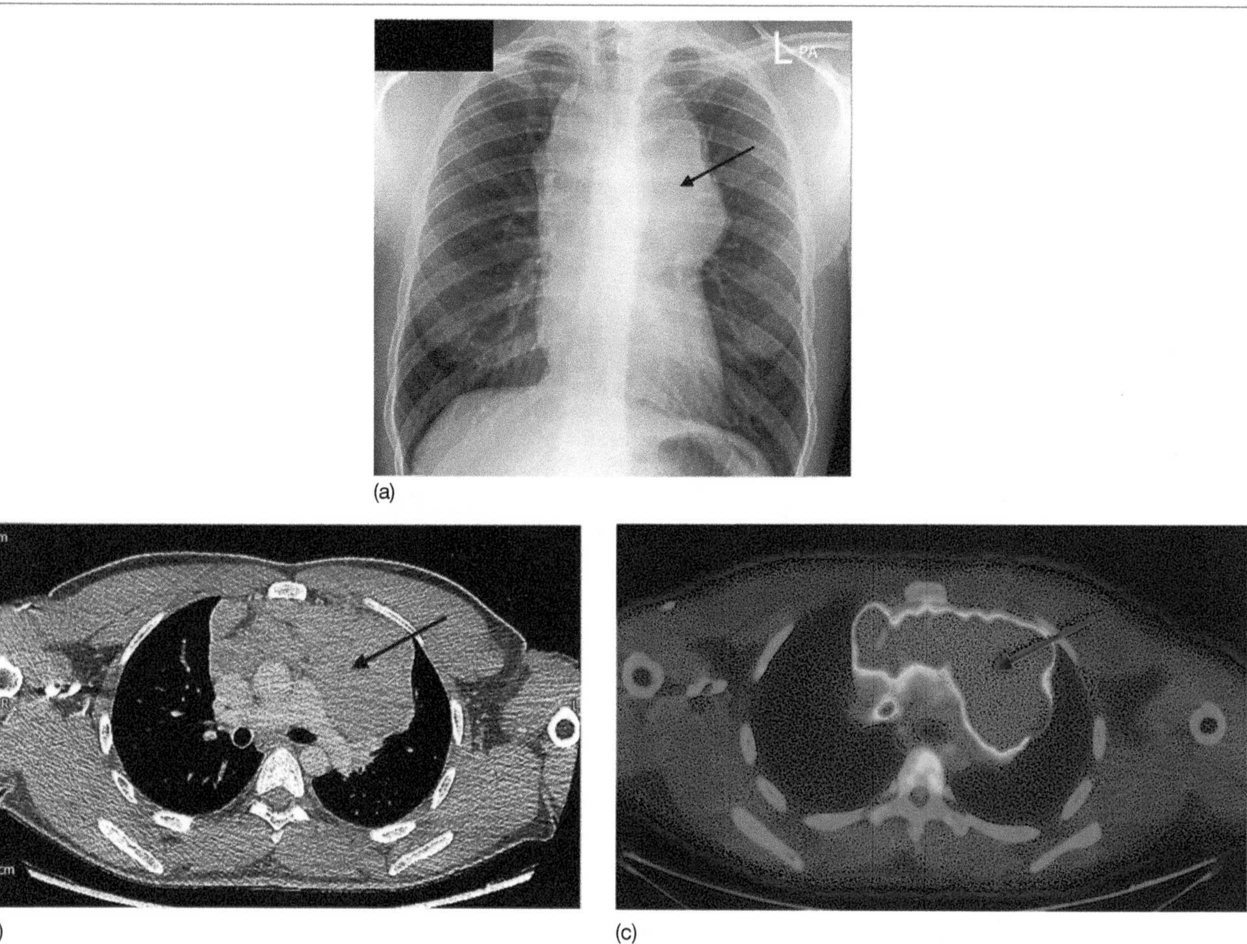

(a)

(b)

(c)

Figure 19.2 Radiological images in classical Hodgkin lymphoma demonstrating a large FDG-avid mediastinal mass (black arrow). **(a)** Chest X-ray **(b)** Axial computer tomography (CT) scan with intravenous contrast in the same patient. **(c)** Axial 18F-Fluorodeoxyglucose (FDG)-PET-CT scan (fused images). Source: Courtesy of the radiology department of Oxford University Hospitals NHS Foundation Trust.

Haematological and biochemical findings

1 Normochromic normocytic anaemia is most common. Bone marrow involvement is unusual in early disease, but if it occurs bone marrow failure may develop with a leuco-erythroblastic anaemia.
2 Neutrophilia and eosinophilia are frequent.
3 Advanced disease is associated with lymphopenia and impairment of cell-mediated immunity.
4 The platelet count is normal or increased during early disease and reduced in later stages.
5 The erythrocyte sedimentation rate (ESR) and C-reactive protein are raised usually in more advanced disease.
6 HIV infection is a risk factor for cHL and HIV status should be determined in all patients.

Diagnosis and histological classification

The diagnosis is made by histological examination of a preferably excised lymph node. The distinctive multinucleate polyploid RS cell embedded within an exuberant inflammatory microenvironment is central to the diagnosis of the four classic types (Figs. 19.3 and 19.4) and mononuclear Hodgkin cells are also part of the malignant clone. These cells always stain strongly with CD30 and frequently (although less strongly) with CD15, but are usually negative for B-cell antigen expression such as CD10, CD19 or CD20. The microenvironment consists of numerous T-cells (often of a regulatory T-cell phenotype), macrophages eosinophils, B-cells and plasma cells. One of the commonest cytogenetic changes in HRS cells is amplification of part of

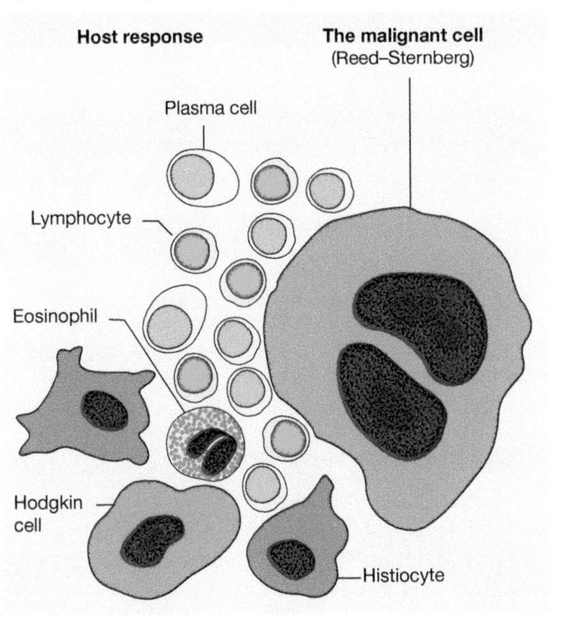

Figure 19.3 Diagrammatic representation of the different cells seen histologically in Hodgkin lymphoma.

chromosome 9 (9p24) which contains the gene for the PD-1 ligand called PDL1. This is often strongly expressed by RS cells which can then interact with PD-1 on immune cells such as T cells and macrophages, protecting them from immune attack.

Classical Hodgkin lymphoma may be further divided into four histological subtypes (Table 19.1). There is no significant difference in the prognosis or management of the different subtypes of classical HL. Nodular sclerosis is the most frequent in Europe and the USA, whereas lymphocyte depletion is more common in developing countries and has a particularly strong association with EBV infection and malnutrition.

Nodular lymphocyte-predominant Hodgkin lymphoma (NLPHL) is distinct from classical Hodgkin lymphoma, does not show RS cells and has many features of non-Hodgkin lymphoma, the tumour cells being polylobated (termed variously 'popcorn' or LP cells) B cells (Fig. 19.4d). Indeed the International Consensus Classification (ICC) system no longer calls this entity Hodgkin lymphoma, preferring the term 'Nodular Lymphocyte Prodominant B-cell Lymphoma'. NLPHL is retained by the WHO (2022) classification system however (Table 19.1).

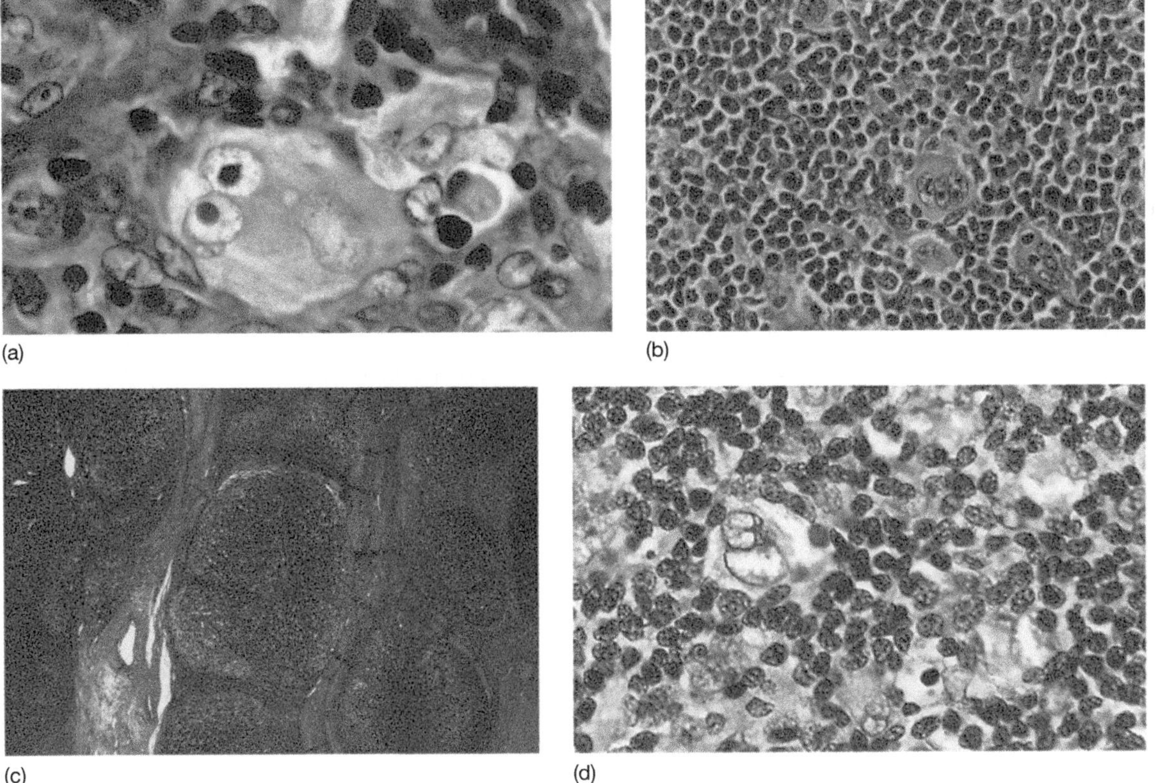

Figure 19.4 Classical Hodgkin lymphoma: **(a)** high-power view of a lymph node biopsy showing two typical multinucleate Reed–Sternberg cells, one with a characteristic owl eye appearance, surrounded by lymphocytes, histiocytes and an eosinophil; **(b)** mixed cellularity; and **(c)** nodular sclerosing Hodgkin lymphoma; **(d)** microscopic appearance of nodular lymphocyte-predominant Hodgkin lymphoma (NLPHL): 'popcorn-like' LP cells surrounded by small lymphocytes. Source: A.V. Hoffbrand *et al.* (2019) *Color Atlas of Clinical Hematology*, 5th edn. Reproduced with permission of John Wiley & Sons.

Table 19.1 World Health Organization (2022) classification of Hodgkin lymphoma.

Classical Hodgkin lymphoma (95% of cases)	
Nodular sclerosis	Collagen bands extend from the node capsule to encircle nodules of abnormal tissue. A characteristic lacunar cell variant of the Reed–Sternberg cell is often found. The cellular infiltrate may be of the lymphocyte-predominant, mixed cellularity or lymphocyte-depleted type; eosinophilia is frequent
Lymphocyte rich	Scanty Reed–Sternberg cells; multiple small lymphocytes with few eosinophils and plasma cells; nodular and diffuse types
Mixed cellularity	The Reed–Sternberg cells are numerous and lymphocyte numbers are intermediate
Lymphocye depleted	There is either a reticular pattern with dominance of Reed–Sternberg cells and sparse numbers of lymphocytes, or a diffuse fibrosis pattern where the lymph node is replaced by disordered connective tissue containing few lymphocytes. Reed–Sternberg cells may also be infrequent in this latter subtype
Nodular lymphocyte-predominant (nodular lymphocyte-predominant B-cell lymphoma)(5% of cases)	
Reed–Sternberg cells are absent. Scattered lymphocyte-predominant (LP) tumour cells with polylobated (popcorn-like) nuclei are present in a background of numerous small lymphocytes which often form nodules (Fig. 19.4d). The malignant cell is called the lymphocyte-predominant (LP) cell and in contrast to RS cells they retain typical B-cell markers. In early stages, the nodules are usually composed of B-cells although a rosette of T-cell often occurs around the LP cells.	

Clinical staging and risk assessment

Selection of appropriate treatment depends on accurate staging of the extent of disease and assessing the disease risk at diagnosis (Table 19.2). Fig. 19.5 shows the Ann-Arbor staging system which is applied to nodal lymphomas. **Staging is performed by clinical examination together with combined positron emission tomography (PET) and CT scans.** CT scan alone (with contrast) can be used if PET is not available (Figs. 19.5 and 19.6). The criteria by which a lymph node is considered normal or abnormal are described in Chapter 9, page xxx. Bone marrow trephine is sometimes carried out although detection of bone involvement is better with a PET-CT scan. **PET-CT scanning is useful in monitoring response to treatment and for detection of small foci of residual disease** (Fig. 19.7). Patients are also classified as A or B according to whether or not the specific constitutional features of fever, drenching night sweats or weight loss are present (Fig. 19.5).

Specific scores can be used to determine the risk of early stage disease which is divided into early favourable or early unfavourable (sometimes called intermediate stage). The main two risk scores used are in Table 19.3. For advanced stage disease the International Prognostic Scoring System (IPSS, sometimes called the Hasenclever index) can be applied (Table 19.4).

Positron emission tomography (PET)

18F-fluorodeoxyglucose positron emission tomography (FDG-PET) is now used widely in the management of lymphoma and other haematological malignancies. It utilizes the fact that in contrast to most normal cells, cancer cells often rely on glycolysis for metabolism, requiring a high uptake of glucose. This phenomenon is known as the Warburg effect. When 18F-fluorodeoxyglucose is taken up by the cells, the radioactive isotope is trapped within the cells enabling detection. Patients have to fast for 6 hours before the injection of FDG and rest for 60–90 minutes prior to scanning. As well as detecting the presence of active disease at the time of diagnosis, PET-CT scans can also be used to assess the response to treatment and to potentially guide the treatment course. Furthermore, research indicates that the volume of active disease at diagnosis (metabolic tumour volume) has prognostic implications and may subsequently help inform treatment strategies.

Table 19.2 Investigations for staging and assessing risk at diagnosis.

Laboratory	Full blood count, ESR, bone marrow aspirate and trephine biopsy (not routine), liver tests, C-reactive protein, albumin, HIV, hepatitis B and C serology also recommended
Radiology	PET-CT including thorax, abdomen, chest and pelvis CT with contrast if PET-CT not available

CT, computed tomography; ESR, erythrocyte sedimentation rate; PET, positron emission tomography.

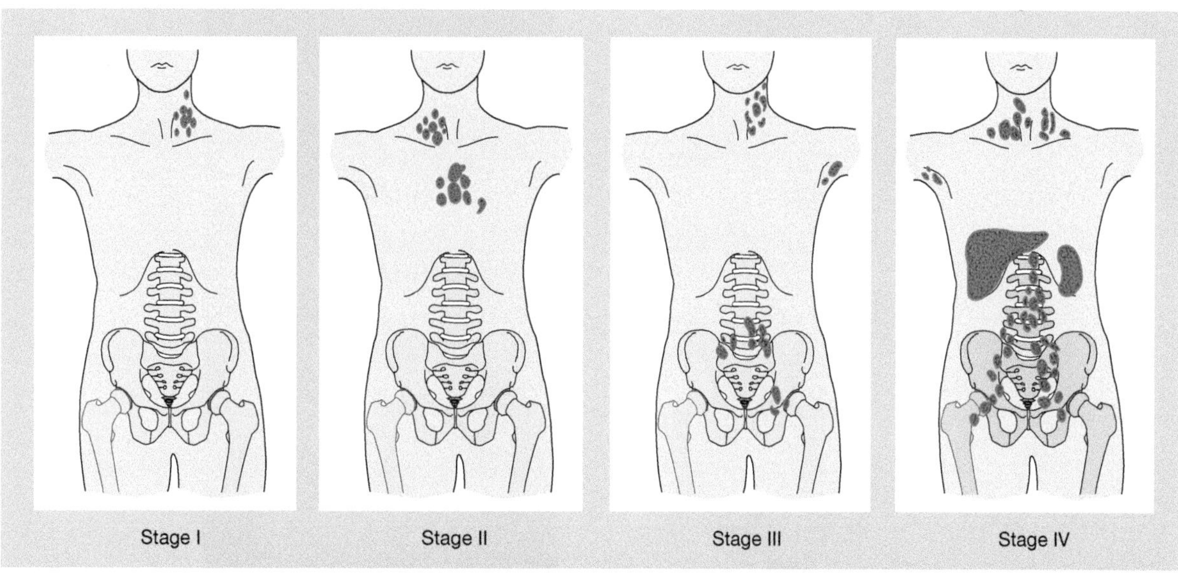

Figure 19.5 Staging of Hodgkin lymphoma. Stage I indicates node involvement in one lymph node area. Stage II indicates disease involving two or more lymph nodal areas confined to one side of the diaphragm. Stage III indicates disease involving lymph nodes above and below the diaphragm. Splenic disease is included in stage III, but this has special significance (see below). Stage IV indicates involvement outside the lymph node areas and refers to diffuse or disseminated disease in the bone marrow, liver and other extranodal sites. N.B. The stage number in all cases is followed by the letter A or B, indicating the absence (A) or presence (B) of one or more of the following: unexplained fever above 38°C; drenching night sweats; or unintentional loss of more than 10% of body weight within 6 months. Localized extranodal extension from a mass of nodes does not advance the stage, but is indicated by the subscript E. Thus, mediastinal disease with contiguous spread to the lung would be classified as IE. As involvement of the spleen is often a prelude to widespread haematogenous spread of the disease, patients with lymph node and splenic involvement are staged as IIIS. Bulky disease (widening of the mediastinum by more than one-third of the transthoracic diameter, or the presence of a nodal mass >10 cm in diameter) may be signalled by the letter X after the stage and may have therapeutic implications.

Deauville score

Interim and end of treatment PET-CT scans are reported according to the Deauville 5-point criteria, which uses the uptake in the mediastinum and liver as an internal control, from which to assess the activity of the tumour. Scores 1, 2 and 3 are generally considered 'negative', whereas 4 and 5 are 'positive'.

- Score 1 no FDG uptake.
- Score 2 nodal uptake present but ≤ mediastinal blood pool.
- Score 3 nodal uptake > mediastinum but ≤ liver.
- Score 4 moderately increased nodal uptake > liver.
- Score 5 markedly increased nodal uptake > liver.

Treatment

Frontline treatment is either with chemotherapy alone or a combination of chemotherapy with radiotherapy. The choice depends primarily on the stage and prognostic factors (Table 19.3). Semen storage for males, if appropriate, should be carried out before therapy is begun. For females of child-bearing age, it is advisable that fertility advice is sought from a specialist. Options for fertility preservation including storage of stimulated eggs and embryos, or cryopreservation of ovarian tissue. If blood transfusion is needed, this must be irradiated to avoid transfusion-associated graft-versus-host disease due to the infusion of live donor lymphocytes, which can engraft due to the impaired cellular immunity of the HL patient.

Early-stage disease

The outcome for early-stage disease is excellent and an important aim is to avoid over-treatment and the risk of late complications. Two broad options are chemotherapy alone or 'combined modality treatment' (CMT) using chemotherapy and radiotherapy (Fig 19.8). CMT achieves better short-term disease control, but in the longer term there is no clear increase in overall survival. Individual treatment decisions will depend on local regimens and patient choice. The most widely used chemotherapy regimen is A (Adriamycin = Doxorubicin), B (Bleomycin), V (Vinblastine), D (Dacarbazine) (ABVD). If radiotherapy is used, the traditional area to irradiate was 'involved field' which also included a fairly high volume of normal tissue. Modern radiotherapy techniques enable smaller field sizes (involved site or even involved node) and

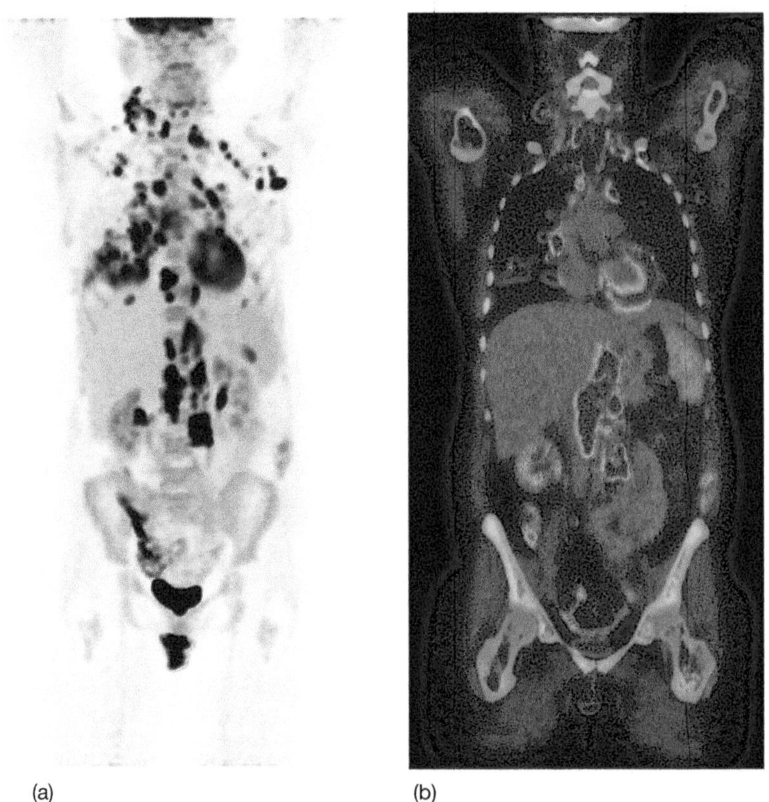

Figure 19.6 Hodgkin lymphoma. Staging positron emission tomography (PET)/computed tomography (CT): 35-year-old female who had disease above and below the diaphragm at presentation. **(a)** Coronal PET image shows multiple foci of uptake above and below the diaphragm. **(b)** Coronal fused PET/CT scan image shows multiple foci of uptake above and below the diaphragm corresponding to nodes, spleen and lung nodules. PET stage IV. Source: Courtesy of Dr Thomas Wagner and the Department of Nuclear Medicine, Royal Free Hospital, London.

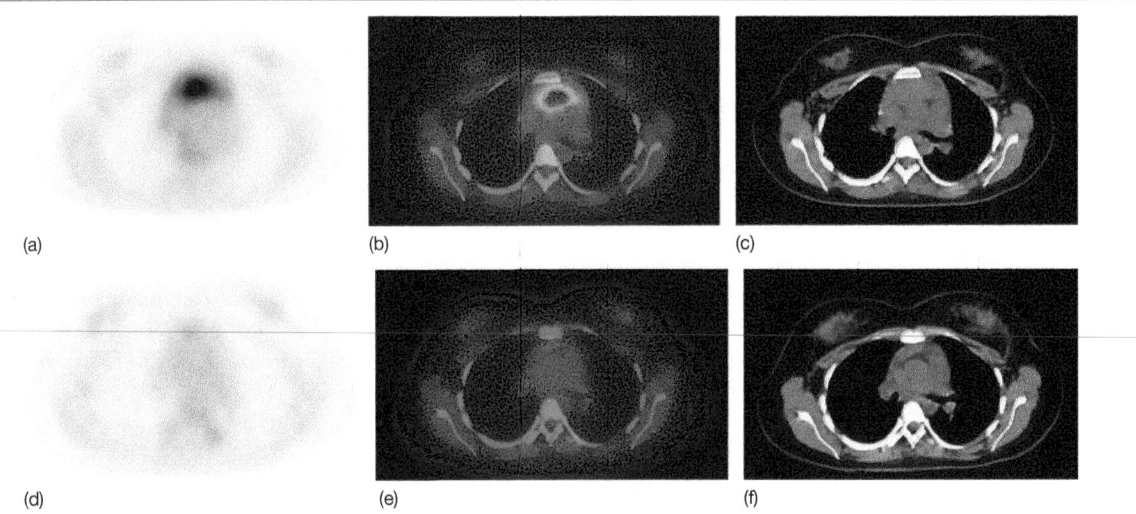

Figure 19.7 Example of the value of imaging in the management of Hodgkin lymphoma. **(a)** Axial positron emission tomography (PET), **(b)** fused PET/computed tomography (CT) and **(c)** CT images at diagnosis demonstrate intense [18]FDG uptake in an anterior mediastinal mass. Following two cycles of ABVD chemotherapy, **(d)** the axial PET, **(e)** fused PET/CT and **(f)** CT images demonstrate no significant [18]FDG uptake in the residual mediastinal mass, in keeping with a complete metabolic response. Source: Courtesy of Dr V.S. Warbey and Professor G.J.R. Cook.

Table 19.3 Different definitions of early stage favourable and unfavourable Hodgkin lymphoma.

EORTC criteria		**GHSG criteria**	
Early stage favourable	*Early stage unfavourable Presence of one or more of the following*	*Early stage favourable*	*Early stage unfavourable Presence of one or more of the following*
No large* mediastinal adenopathy	Large* mediastinal adenopathy	No large mediastinal adenopathy	Large mediastinal adenopathy
ESR <50 without B symptoms	ESR ≥50 without B symptoms	ESR <50 without B symptoms	ESR ≥50 without B symptoms
ESR <30 with B symptoms	ESR ≥30 with B symptoms	ESR <30 with B symptoms	ESR ≥30 with B symptoms
Age ≤50 years	Age <50 years	No extranodal lesions	Extranodal lesions present
1–3 lymph node sites involved	≥4 lymph node sites involved	1–2 lymph node sites involved	≥3 lymph node sites involved

EORTC, European Organisation for the Research and Treatment of Cancer; GHSG, German Hodgkin Study Group.
* Large is defined as mediastinal thoracic ratio >0.35 at the level of T5/6

Table 19.4 The International Prognostic Scoring System (IPSS) for assessment of risk in advanced stage cHL.

IPSS (Hasenclever index): one point for each of the following:
Male Sex
Age ≥ 45 years
Stage IV disease
Haemoglobin < 105 g/dL
White cell counts ≥ 15×10^9/L
Lymphocyte count < 0.6×10^9/L or < 8% of differential
Albumin < 40 g/L

with techniques such as deep inspiration breath hold, further reduction in irradiation of organs such as the heart is achieved.

For early favourable disease (Table 19.3), two cycles of ABVD followed by 20 Gy of radiotherapy leads to very high cure rates (Fig 19.8). For those who are felt to be too high a risk for the late effects of radiotherapy, three cycles of ABVD leading to a negative PET scan after two or three cycles can enable omission of radiotherapy. However, while most are cured, relapse rates are modestly higher with ABVD alone. If the interim PET scan is positive, consideration for two cycles of a more intensive regimen such as escalated BEACOPP (Bleomycin, Etoposide, Adriamycin, Cyclophosphamide, Vincristine = Oncovin, Procarbazine and Prednisolone) should be made, followed by radiotherapy at 30 Gy.

For unfavourable disease (Table 19.3) a number of approaches can be taken (Fig 19.8). Four cycles of ABVD followed by 30Gy of radiotherapy achieves high rates of cure. A strategy of giving the more intensive escalated BEACOPP (or BEAECOPDac where procabarbazine is replaced by dacarbazine) for two cycles followed by ABVD for two cycles means that, if the end of chemotherapy PET scan is negative, radiotherapy can be omitted with no increase in rate of relapse and some of the highest rates of cure described so far. If it is desirable to avoid more intensive chemotherapy, two cycles of ABVD with four cycles of AVD, i.e. ommission of bleomycin if the PET scan after two cycles is negative, also achieves cure for most with a very low requirement for radiotherapy.

Advanced-stage disease

Combination chemotherapy alone is used most often (Fig 19.9). Advanced stage encompasses stage III and IV disease and often stage 2 B disease with a large mediastinal mass or extranodal disease. Three main approaches are used:

- ABVD for two cycles followed by an interim PET scan. If this is negative four more cycles of AVD (no bleomycin) are given. If PET positive (about 15–20% of patients) up to four cycles of escalated BEACOPP are given.
- Escalated BEACOPP for two cycles followed by an interim PET scan. If this is negative, two further cycles of escalated BEACOPP or four cycles of ABVD are given (sometimes without the bleomycin). If PET is positive, four more cycles of escalated BEACOPP are given.
- AVD combined with the anti-CD30 antibody drug conjugate brentuximab vedotin for six cycles. This enables no bleomycin which is desirable due to serious lung toxicity of bleomycin in some patients. A randomized trial compared six cycles of ABVD to the combination of brentuximab vedotin (BV) with doxorubicin, vinblastine and dacarbazine (AVD-BV regimen). Progression-free survival was

improved with AVD-BV and with longer follow-up a small but significant improvement in overall survival was seen. Reported rates of cure, however, were still not as high as those seen with escalated BEACOPP. There was more febrile neutropenia with AVD-BV and a higher rate of peripheral neuropathy. BV is significantly more costly than bleomycin and not funded in a number of countries for routine use.

Trials incorporating a PD-1 inhibitor, e.g. nivolumab, pembrolizumab, in first-line therapy are in progress (Fig. 19.11). Dacarbazine is often used to replace procarbazine in escalated BEACOPP due to reduced gonadotoxicity and bone marow suppression, both seen more frequently with procarbazine.

The outcome for older patients (defined as over 60 years of age) with cHL are relatively poor due partly to distinctive biology of the lymphoma and partly to a worse tolerance of chemotherapy. BEACOPP for example cannot be used safely in this group and age is a significant risk factor for bleomycin-induced pulmonary toxicity. For fitter older patients, AVD or AVD-BV can still be used. For those not fit for anthracycline-based regimens, other regimens such as ChlVPP (chlorambucil, vinblastine, procarbazine, prednisolone) can be tried. Radiotherapy is particularly important in older patients with very little risk of late complications.

Assessment of response to treatment

Clinical examination and imaging (PET/CT scans) are used to assess response to treatment and plan further therapy. Vigilance is needed to recognize complications of therapy such as bleomycin lung toxicity or BV-induced peripheral neuropathy.

PET-CT scanning reveals the areas of residual active disease (Fig. 19.7) and enables evaluation of residual masses which are common following treatments. Only masses which retain metabolic activity (and are therefore positive on a PET scan) are of concern. As described above PET-CT is used to define the management of individual patients. It is widely used after the first two cycles of ABVD or escalated BEACOPP and if

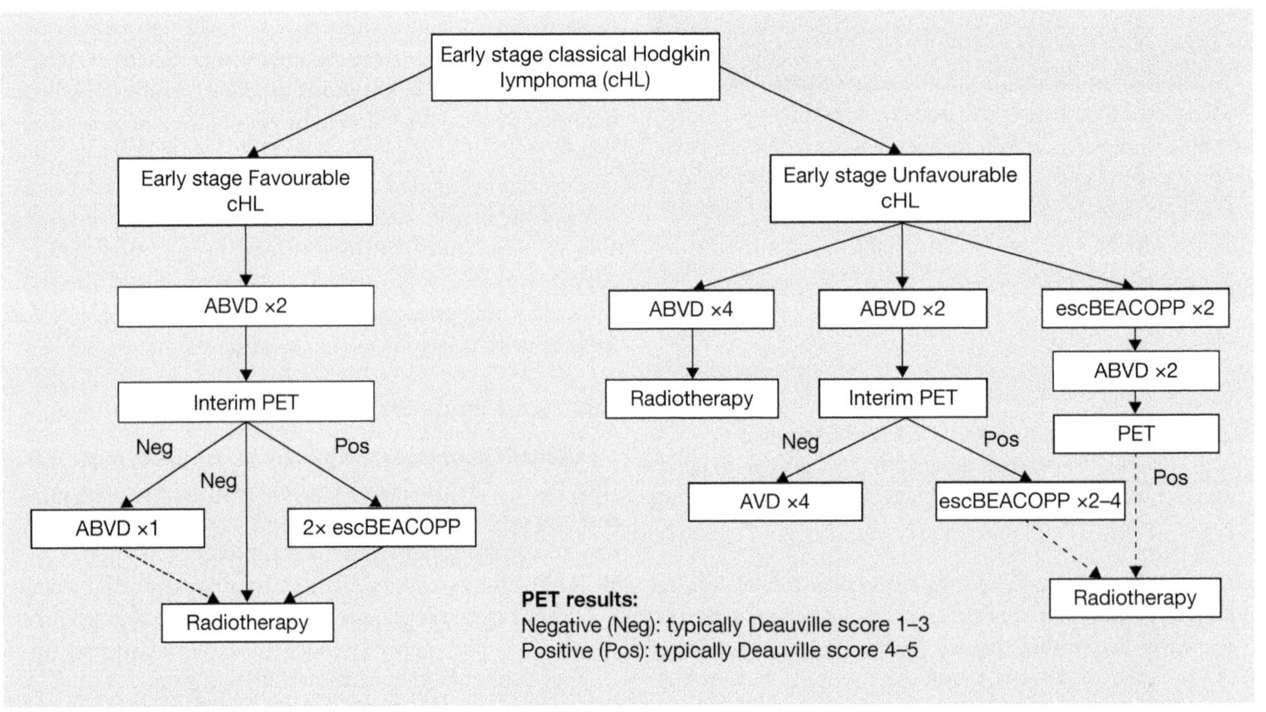

Figure 19.8 Suggested schema for the treatment of early stage classical Hodgkin lymphoma. Favourable or unfavourable maybe based on German Hodgkin Study Group (GHSG) or European Organisation for Research and Treatment of Cancer (EORTC) schemas although for early favourable disease, 2× ABVD followed by 20 Gy of radiothearpy has only been tested in a trial using GHSG criteria (see Table 19.3). For unfavourable disease treated with ABVD and with interim PET positivity, the RATHL trial used four cycles of escBEACOPP with no pre-sepcified radiotherapy (Source: P. Johnson *et al.* (2016) *N. Engl. J. Med.* 374: 2419–29), whereas the H10 trial used two cycles followed by radiotherapy (Source: M.P.E. Andre *et al.* (2017) *J. Clin. Oncol.* 35: 1786–94). The use of radiotherapy for an individual at any stage in their treatment is determined by a number of factors including the PET result and the risk of late effects. Source: Based on G.A. Follows *et al.* (2022) Guideline for the first-line management of Classical Hodgkin Lymphoma – a British Society for Haematology Guideline. *Br. J. Haematol.* 197: 558–72. ABVD: doxorubicin, bleomycin, vinblastine, dacarbazine; escBEACOPP: bleomycin, etoposide, doxorubicin, cyclophosphamide, vincristine, procarbazine and prednisolone. Many centres now replace procarbazine with dacarbazine – escBEACOPDac.

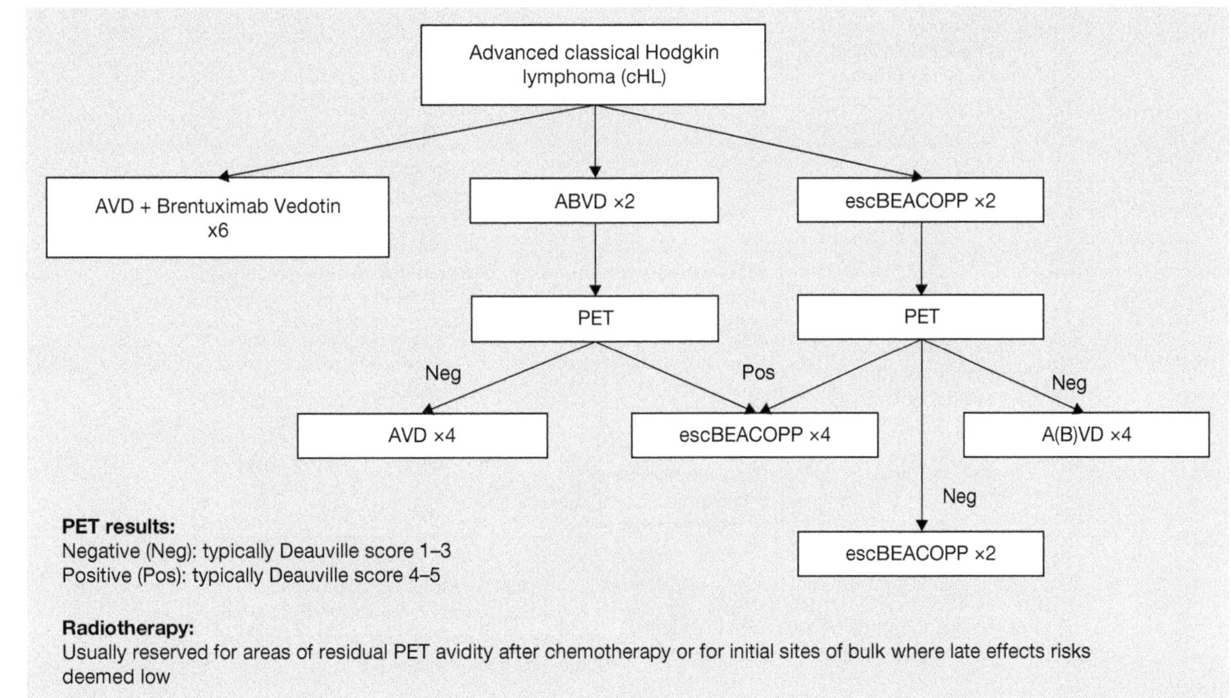

Figure 19.9 Suggested schema for the treatment of advanced stage classical Hodgkin Lymphoma. AVD + Brentuximab Vedotin is not considered a PET-adapted approach as the initial trial had only a few patients who changed treatment on the basis of an interim PET scan. The AHL2011 study continue with four cycles of AVD in those who had achieved a negative PET scan after two cycles of esc BEACOPP (Source: R.O. Casasnovas *et al.* (2022) *J. Clin. Oncol.* 40: 1091–101 although many centres omit the bleomycin, extrapolating results from the RATHL study (referenced in Figure 19.8). Source Based on G.A. Follows *et al.* (2022) Guideline for the first-line management of Classical Hodgkin Lymphoma – a British Society for Haematology Guideline. *Brit. J. Haematol.* 197: 558–72. ABVD: doxorubicin, bleomycin, vinblastine, dacarbazine; escBEACOPP: bleomycin, etoposide, doxorubicin, cyclophosphamide, vincristine, procarbazine and prednisolone. Many centres now replace procarbazine with dacarbazine – escBEACOPDac.

there is residual active disease, treatment might be switched to more intensive or prolonged chemotherapy and if the PET scan is negative, bleomycin can be omitted from subsequent ABVD cycles. There is generally no need to repeat the PET-CT scan at the end of therapy if the interim PET scan was negative. For patients PET-CT positive at the end of therapy, repeat biopsy is preferable although not always possible. In this case, close clinical follow-up and repeat imaging assessments are needed. Inflammatory tissue may cause a false-positive PET scan.

Relapsed disease

Approximately 20% of patients suffer from disease relapse or are refractory to initial therapy. For younger patients, treatment is still with curative intent. Alternative combination chemotherapy (often platinum based) to the initial regimen is often used with the aim to treat responding patients with high-dose chemotherapy with autologous stem cell transplantation (Fig 19.10).

More targeted agents such as BV and monoclonal antibodies e.g. durvalumab which block the inhibitory interaction between PD-1 on T-cells and PDL-1 on RS cells (Fig 19.1) may be used either as single agents or where available, in combination with chemotherapy, including as a bridge to stem cell transplantation. Allogeneic stem cell transplantation may be used in the small minority of patients who are not cured with other approaches. For older patients who are not fit for intensvie approaches, treatment at relapse is aimed at inducing remissions and optimizing quality of life.

New treatments in clinical trials for relapsed cases include CD30-directed chimeric antigen receptor T-cell (CAR-T) therapy and drugs which target other immune checkpoints such as TIM-3 and LAG-3.

Paediatric and adolescent patients

Classical HL is the most common malignancy within the teenage and young adult age group (16–24 years). Regimens have been designed to reduce late effects and preserve fertility. These

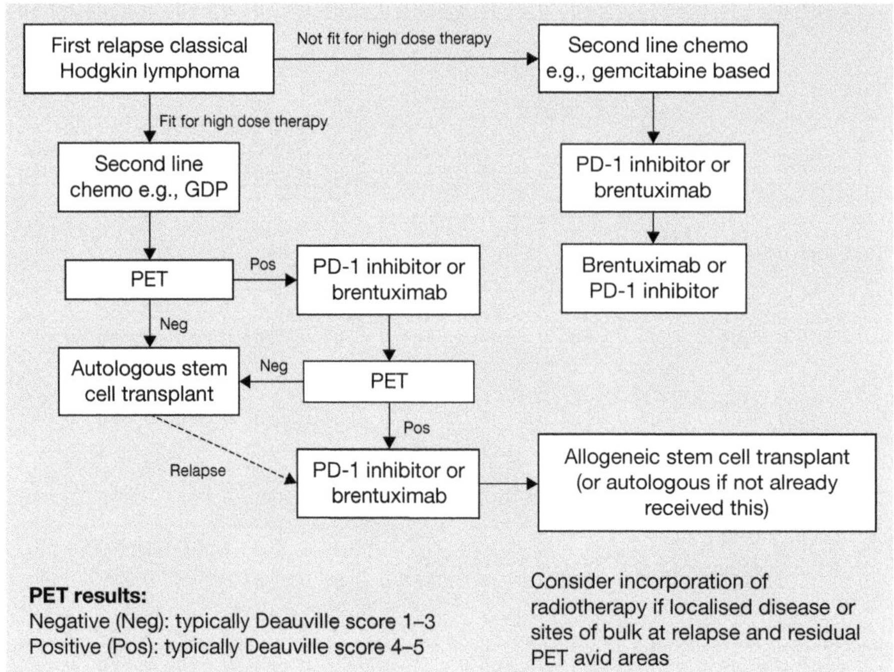

Figure 19.10 Suggested schema for the treatment of relapsed cHL. This is based on use of agents within their licensed indication. GDP: gemcitabine, dexamethasone, cisplatin. The approach each centre adopts often depends on availability of agents such as PD-1 inhibitors or brentuximab vedotin and ability to combine with other treatments. For example, second-line treatment, i.e. treatment at first relapse, may combine a PD-1 inhibitor with chemotherapy if available. Treatment will also depend what the patient has already had and their prior response, e.g. a patient refractory to AVD in combination with brentuximab as first-line treatment is unlikely to respond to further brentuximab vedotin. A large, randomized trial has shown a progression-free survival benefit for brentuximab vedotin as a maintenance treatment following autologous stem cell transplant for high-risk relapse, and this is a licensed indication in many regions. However, lack of reimbursement is an issue in some countries and with more brentuximab use higher up the pathway, its role here is questioned and therefore not included in this schema. Source: Based on Thames Valley Strategic Clinical Network guidelines for relapsed Hodgkin Lymphoma: https://nssg.oxford-haematology.org.uk/lymphoma/, author: Dr Graham Collins.

reduce cumulative doses of anthracyclines, bleomycin, alkylating agents and radiotherapy. These regimens include corticosteroids, a high initial dose but lower cumulative dose, an anthracycline and more vinca alkaloids.

One regimen is two cycles of vincristine, etoposide, prednisolone, doxorubicin (OEPA) followed by cycles of cyclophosphamide, vincristine, prednisolone, dacarbazine (COPDac), the number, dependent on baseline risk. Radiotherapy is given to slow responders on interim PET, with lower doses than used in adults.

Prognosis

Classical HL is a disease which is cured in the majority of patients and prognosis is excellent. In younger patients the chance of cure is approximately 90% whilst this falls significantly over the age of 60 years.

The late effects of Hodgkin lymphoma and its treatment

Long-term follow-up of patients has revealed a considerable burden of late disease following treatment, especially those treated with radiation. Late disease as result of chemotherapy or radiotherapy usually becomes apparent only after 10 years. Cancer of the lung and breast occurs as a consequence of radiotherapy. Radiotherapy involving breast tissue is particularly dangerous in women under the age of 20 years. Annual screening starting 8 years after the radiotherapy or at age 30 years whichever is earlier is recommended as well as avoidance of oestrogen containing medication. Myelodysplastic syndromes or acute myeloid leukaemia, slightly more common after escalated BEACOPP than after ABVD, are more associated with the use of alkylating agents and radiotherapy. Non-Hodgkin lymphoma, gastro-intestinal and other cancers also occur with greater frequency than in controls.

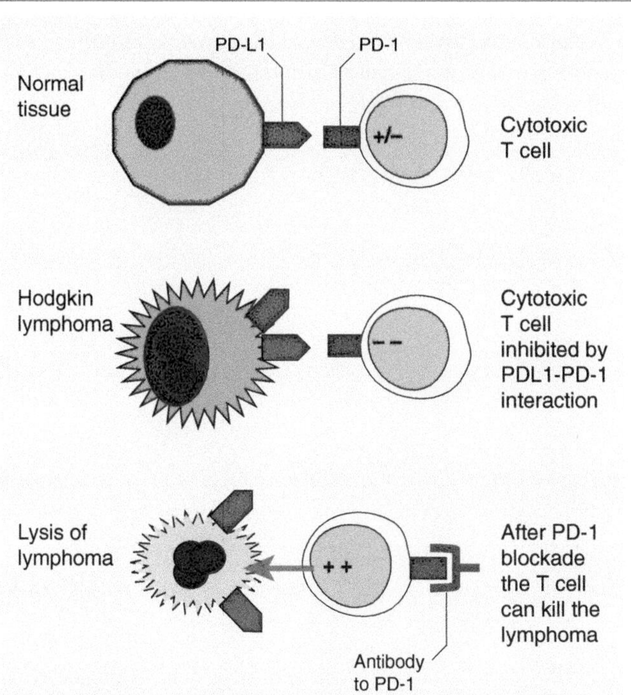

Figure 19.11 Potential mechanism whereby Hodgkin lymphoma is controlled after treatment with antibodies to block PD-1. PD-1 and PD-L1 are natural molecules that limit the attack of normal tissues by cytotoxic T cells. Hodgkin lymphoma overexpresses PD-L1 due to gene amplification or effects of Epstein–Barr virus infection. This delivers a strong negative signal to the T cells around the tumour. If antibody-mediated blockade of PD-1 is used, the T cells can then recognize and kill the tumour.

Non-malignant complications include sterility, more common in men than women after alkylating drug therapy, premature ovarian failure, intestinal complications, osteonecrosis (related to corticosteroid therapy) and pulmonary disease, as a result of mediastinal radiation or bleomycin chemotherapy. Anthracycline use (as well as radiotherapy affecting heart muscle) increaes the risk of heart disease later in life. Substituting procarbazine for dacarbazine to reduce the risk of male infertility is being explored. Vinblastine and brentuximab vedotin may cause a permanent neuropathy. These features are the main reason why less intensive treatment regimens guided by interim PET/CT results are now being explored for this disease.

Nodular lymphocyte-predominant Hodgkin lymphoma

The natural history of NLPHL is similar to low-grade non-Hodgkin lymphoma and the prognosis is generally excellent. Some centres treat NLPHL in a similar way to classical Hodgkin lymphoma. However in recent years there has been a shift to a less intensive approach. For early stage disease surgical excision (for diagnosis) followed by surveillance alone or radiotherapy is usual. For advanced disease, an approach is watch and wait or if symptomatic, chemotherapy with, e.g. R-CVP. For those in stage 3 or 4 with B symptoms, mediastinal or splenic involvement, R-CHOP is appropriate. High-grade transformation to diffuse large B-cell lymphoma occurs in about 10% of cases (a complication which is essentially never seen with cHL).

SUMMARY

- Lymphoma is a cancer of mature lymphocytes frequently leading to accumulation of lymphocytes in lymph nodes (and in other tissues) resulting in lymphadenopathy.
- The major subdivision of lymphoma is into Hodgkin lymphoma and non-Hodgkin lymphoma, based on the presence of Reed–Sternberg cells within an inflammatory background seen in Hodgkin lymphoma.
- Reed–Sternberg cells are neoplastic B cells, but most cells in the lymph node are reactive inflammatory cells.
- The usual clinical presentation is with painless asymmetrical lymphadenopathy – most commonly in the neck although mediastinal involvement is also common.
- Constitutional symptoms of fever, weight loss and night sweats are prominent in patients with widespread disease.
- Blood tests may show anaemia, neutrophilia and raised erythrocyte sedimentation rate (ESR).
- Diagnosis is made by histological examination of an excised lymph node and there are four classical subtypes and a fifth non-classical type called NLPHL.
- Staging of the disease with PET-CT is important for determining treatment and prognosis.
- Treatment is with chemotherapy or a combination of chemotherapy and radiotherapy. The choice depends on a number of disease and patient factors.
- The response to treatment can be monitored by CT and PET scans. The treatment may be modified according to interim PET findings.
- Disease relapse can be treated with alternative chemotherapy, checkpoint inhibitors, targeted antibody–toxin drug conjugates and sometimes with stem cell transplantation, most frequently autologous.

- CAR-T cells and other immunotherapy agents are undergoing clinical trials for relapsed patients.
- The prognosis is excellent and over 85% of patients can expect to be cured.
- Late side effects of treatment including secondary cancers, infertility, cardiac and lung disease are a concern.
- Nodular lymphocyte-predominant disease is treated as for a low-grade B-cell lymphoma and can transform into high grade non-Hodgkin lymphoma.

Now visit **www.wiley.com/go/haematology9e** to test yourself on this chapter.

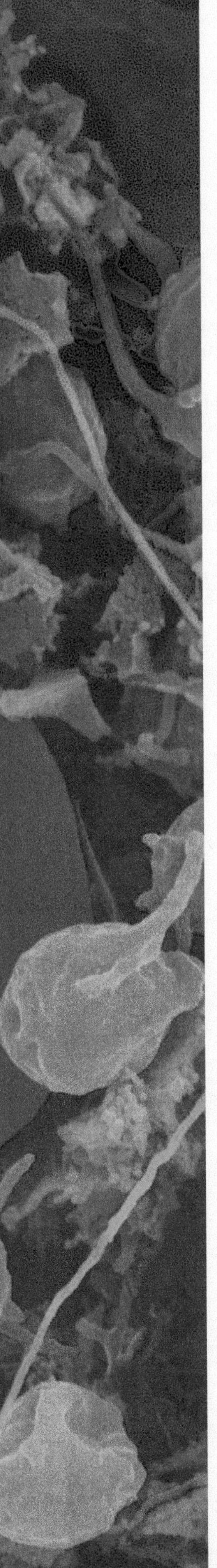

CHAPTER 20

Non-Hodgkin lymphomas 1: General aspects

Key topics

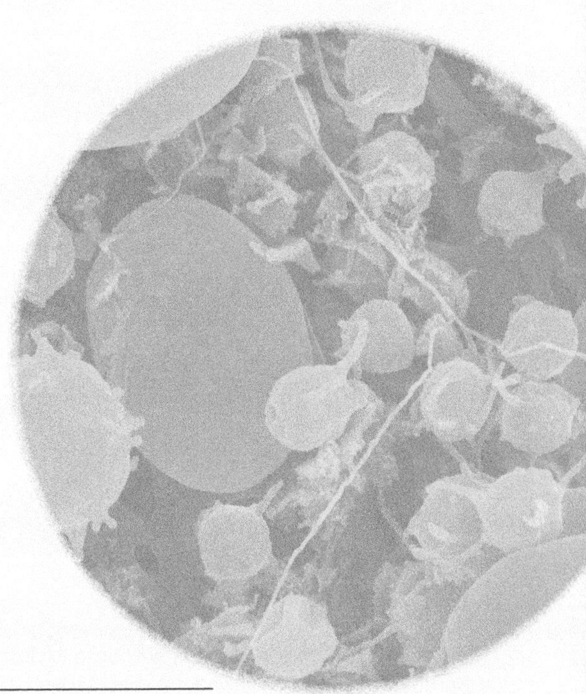

Hoffbrand's Essential Haematology, Ninth Edition. A. Victor Hoffbrand, Pratima Chowdary, Graham P. Collins, and Justin Loke.

© 2024 John Wiley & Sons Ltd. Published 2024 by John Wiley & Sons Ltd.

Companion website: www.wiley.com/go/haematology9e

Definition

Lymphoma is defined as a cancer of mature lymphocytes. The same may be said of chronic lymphocytic leukaemia (CLL) with the key difference being that CLL affects the blood and bone marrow, whereas lymphoma predominantly affects lymph nodes, other lymphoid tissue or, less commonly, extranodal sites. There is overlap, however, in that when CLL does not affect the blood and bone marrow, it is called small lymphocytic lymphoma (SLL).

Due to the complexity of the life cycle of lymphocytes, there are many lymphoma subtypes. Typically the malignant lymphocytes accumulate in lymph nodes and other lymphoid tissue causing the characteristic clinical feature of lymphadenopathy. Less commonly, clonal lymphocytes may spill over into blood ('leukaemic phase') or involve organs outside the lymphoid tissue. Lymphomas may also arise solely within extralymphatic tissue, so-called primary extranodal lymphomas. Some rare lymphoma subtypes arise from lymphoid progenitors, such as T-cell lymphoblastic lymphoma. These are biologically more akin to the acute lymphoid leukaemias which are discussed in Chapter 17.

Classification

In broad terms, lymphomas are initially split into Hodgkin lymphoma (Chapter 19) and non-Hodgkin lymphomas (NHLs). Non-Hodgkin lymphomas are far more common than Hodgkin lymphoma and comprise a heterogeneous group of disorders (Fig. 20.1). They usually arise from a malignant B-cell, with T-cell-derived lymphomas being far less common in Western countries. The relative incidence of T-cell lymphomas is commoner in East Asia, West Africa and the Caribbean.

T-cell non-Hodgkin lymphomas can be divided into cutaneous and peripheral (or systemic) types. B-cell NHL is typically subclassified as high-grade (or aggressive) versus low-grade (or indolent) subtypes. The most common type of high grade NHL is diffuse large B-cell lymphoma, the commonest of all the lymphomas. Follicular lymphoma is the most frequent type of low-grade lymphoma. It is helpful to group low-grade and high-grade forms as separate entities as they share a number of factors in common with each other (Table 20.1).

Table 20.2 lists the main subtypes of B-cell and T-cell lymphoma described in the 5th (2022) edition of the WHO

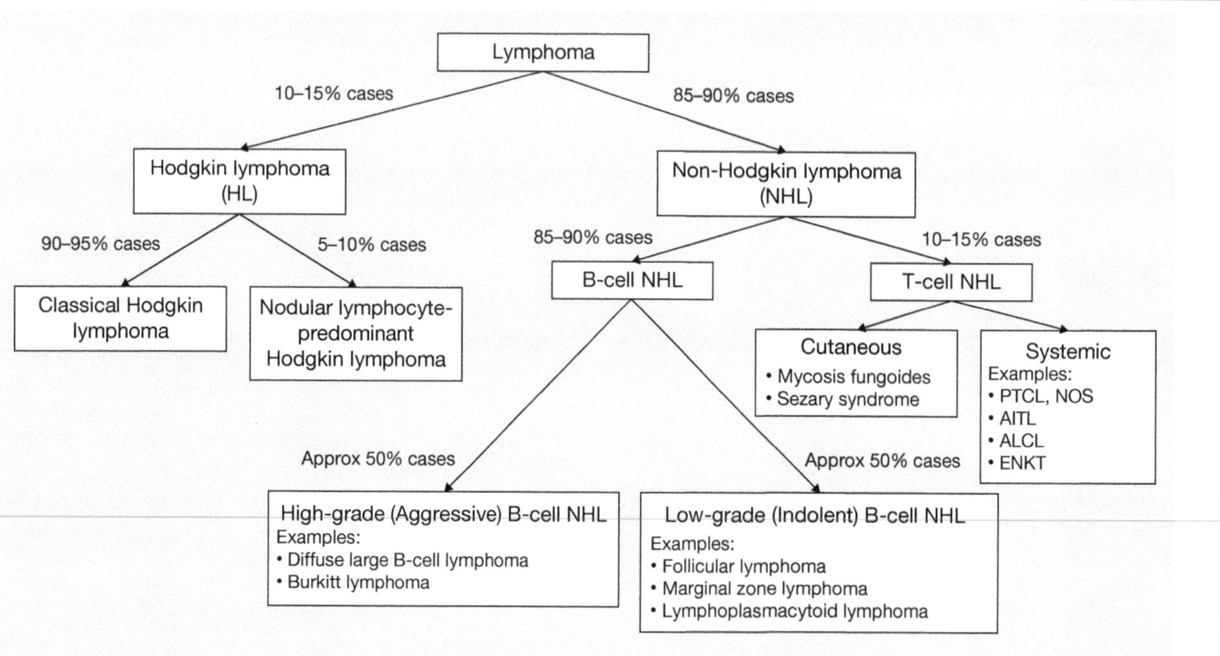

Figure 20.1 A simplified schema illustrating the classification of lymphoma. Percentage incidence are those reported in Western countries. T-cell lymphomas have a relatively higher incidence in East Asia, West African and the Caribbean. Source: K.C. Thandra *et al.* (2021) Epidemiology of non-Hodgkin's Lymphoma. *Med. Sci. (Basel)* 9: 5 and Haematological Malignancy Research Network: https://hmrn.org/. PTCL, NOS: peripheral T-cell lymphoma not otherwise specified; AITL: angioimmunoblastic T-cell lymphoma; ALCL: anaplastic large cell lymphoma; ENKT: extrandoal NK/T-cell lymphoma.

Table 20.1 Characteristics shared by subtypes of high-grade non-Hodgkin lymphoma and low-grade non-Hodgkin lymphoma. BTK, Bruton kinase.

	High-grade B-cell NHL	Low-grade B-cell NHL
Rate of disease progression	Relatively rapid	Slow
Mode of presentation	More likely to present with complications requiring emergency management, e.g. pain, bowel obstruction	Patient usually well at presentation typically presenting with a palpable lump
Age distribution	Commoner in older patients but can present at any age including childhood	Commoner in older patients; extremely rare in children
Aim of first-line treatment	Curative for most patients	Not curative for most patients. Aim is prolong quantity and maintain quality of life
Management options (first-line)	Combination immunochemotherapy +/– radiotherapy (if fit enough to tolerate)	**1** Active surveillance / 'Watch and Wait' **2** Radiotherapy alone **3** Anti-CD20 antibody monotherapy **4** Combination immunochemotherapy **5** Targeted agents, e.g. BTK inhibitors or immunomodulatory agents
Prognosis	Excellent if cured with first line treatment; relatively poor if relapses	Generally good unless early relapse after first-line treatment, or high-grade transformation occurs

Table 20.2 The 2022 World Health Organization (WHO) classification of mature B-cell and T-cell neoplasms (modified), which includes the non-Hodgkin lymphomas. B-cell disorders comprise 85% of cases. T cell and NK cell together comprise 15% of cases. A few rare or provisional subtypes have been omitted (see Appendix).

Mature B-cell neoplasms

- Monoclonal B-cell lymphocytosis
- Chronic lymphocytic leukaemia / small lymphocytic lymphoma
- Hairy cell leukaemia
- Splenic marginal zone lymphoma
- Lymphoplasmacytic lymphoma
- Extranodal marginal zone lymphoma of mucosa-associated lymphoma tissue (MALT)
- Nodal marginal zone lymphoma
- Follicular lymphoma
- Mantle cell lymphoma
- Leukaemic non-nodal mantle cell lymphoma
- Transformations of indolent B-cell lymphomas
- Diffuse large B-cell lymphoma, NOS
- T-cell/histiocyte-rich large B-cell lymphoma
- Diffuse large B-cell lymphoma / high grade B-cell lymphoma with *MYC* and *BCL2* rearrangements
- EBV positive diffuse large B-cell lymphoma
- Primary large B-cell lymphoma of immune-privileged types
- Primary mediastinal large B-cell lymphoma
- Mediastinal grey zone lymphoma
- Burkitt lymphoma

Mature T-cell neoplasms

- T-prolymphocytic leukaemia
- T-large granular lymphocytic leukaemia
- Adult T-cell leukaemia/lymphoma
- Sezary Syndrome
- Mycosis fungoides
- Subcutaneous panniculitis-like T-cell lymphoma
- Enteropathy-associated T-cell lymphoma
- Hepatosplenic T-cell lymphoma
- ALK-positive anaplastic large cell lymphoma
- ALK-negative anaplastic large cell lymphoma
- Breast implant-associated anaplastic large cell lymphoma
- Nodal TFH cell lymphoma, angioimmunoblastic-type
- Nodal TFH lymphoma, follicular-type
- Nodal TFH lymphoma, NOS
- Extranodal NK/T-cell lymphoma

NOS, not otherwise specified; TFH, T follicular helper.

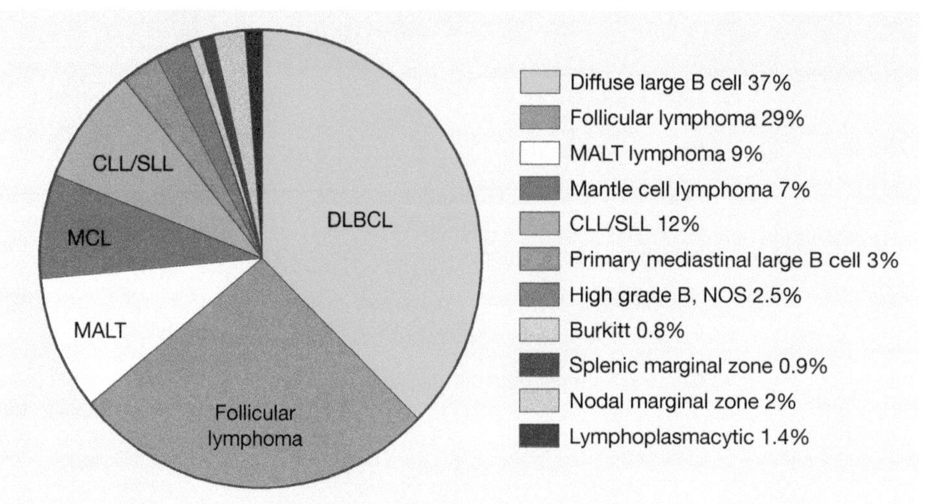

Figure 20.2 The relative frequencies of B-cell non-Hodgkin lymphomas. CLL, chronic lymphocytic lymphoma; DLBCL, diffuse large B-cell lymphoma; MALT, mucosa-associated lymphoid tissue; MCL, mantle cell lymphoma; NOS, not otherwise specified; PMLBCL, primary mediastinal large B-cell lymphoma; SLL, small lymphocytic lymphoma.

classification system. Figure 20.2 illustrates the relative frequency of some of these subtypes.

Pathogenesis

Risk factors

Most cases of lymphoma have no identifiable cause. However a number of risk factors have been identified, some of which can be called causative agents (Table 20.3). In particular, some subtypes of lymphoma more often have an identifiable risk factor than others. Marginal zone lymphomas are an uncommon type of low-grade B-cell NHL which arise in the setting of a chronic inflammatory state. This can be induced by an infectious agent, e.g. *H. Pylori* in gastric marginal zone lymphoma of MALT type or an autoimmune process, e.g. ocular adnexal marginal zone lymphoma of MALT type seen in association with Sjögren syndrome.

A frequently implicated infectious agent in a number of B-cell lymphomas (both Hodgkin and non-Hodgkin) is the Epstein–Barr virus (EBV). This virus infects B cells via its receptor CD21 and causes a latent infection within subsets of memory B cells. A very potent immune response to EBV generally maintains EBV in a latent state although periodic reactivation may occur. Immunosuppressive states (such as occur following a solid organ transplant due to immunosuppressive drugs) may lead to reactivation and malignant transformation of B cells. Furthermore, even in immunocompetent individuals, EBV may be a factor in the development of Hodgkin lymphoma, Burkitt lymphoma and, particularly in older patients, diffuse large B-cell lymphoma. Rarely EBV may infect other cell types such as T cells and is implicated in the pathogenesis of these disorders.

Cell of origin

B-cell lymphomas tend to mimic normal B cells at different stages of development (Fig. 20.3). This is shown by their phenotypic patterns on immune histology or flow cytometry (Tables 20.4, 20.5). They can be divided into those resembling precursor B cells found in the bone marrow, more mature B-cells which have not yet undergone a germinal centre reaction, germinal centre (GC) or post-GC B cells. Finally the terminally differentiated B cell is a plasma cell. Most B-cell lymphomas arise from the germinal centre. This is often due to aberrant somatic hypermutation (the process which introduces single base pair changes into the variable region of immunoglobulin genes to refine the specificity of the molecules). T-cell lymphomas resemble precursor T cells in the bone marrow and thymus, or peripheral mature T cells.

Molecular changes

Cytogenetic abnormalities are frequent, often translocations involving the immunoglobulin genes in the B-cell neoplasms (Table 20.6). Translocations of oncogenes to the immunoglobulin loci on chromosomes 2, 14 or 22 may result in the overexpression of the oncogene under the influence of the highly active promoter elements of an immunoglobulin locus, leading to alteration of the cell cycle, failure of apoptosis or aberrant expression of survival genes (see Chapter 11 and Table 20.6). Specific signalling pathways may be affected and next-generation sequencing has revealed point mutations in genes involved in, for example, chromatin remodelling, the NFκB pathway of B-cell activation and pre-mRNA splicing. As many as 80 somatic mutations may be present in NHL at presentation (Fig. 11.3) and further mutations may appear as the disease progresses.

Table 20.3 Risk factors for the development of lymphoma.

Risk factor	Association
Infectious agent	
Virus	
■ Epstein–Barr virus	Approximately 50% cases of Hodgkin lymphoma have clonal EBV integration Post-solid organ transplant (or other immunosuppressive states) Endemic Burkitt lymphoma (100% case) and approximately 50% of sporadic cases Extra-nodal NK/T-cell lymphoma (100% cases)
■ Human T-cell lymphotropic virus (HTLV)-1	Adult T-cell leukaemia / lymphoma (ATLL) – 100% of cases
■ Human herpesvirus 8 (HHV8)	Primary effusion lymphoma (PEL)
■ Human immunodeficiency virus (HIV)	Lymphoma is more common in individuals with HIV infection who experience more profound and more prolonged immunosuppression. The lymphoma subtypes associated with HIV include HIV-associated Burkitt lymphoma, primary CNS lymphoma, Hodgkin lymphoma, plasmablastic lymphoma.
■ Hepatitis C virus	Splenic marginal zone lymphoma Diffuse large B-cell lymphoma (de novo or transformed) Follicular lymphoma (rarely)
Bacteria	
■ Helicobacter pylori	Gastric marginal zone lymphoma of MALT type
■ Chlamydia psittaci	Ocular adnexal marginal zone lymphoma of MALT type
■ Moraxella Catarrhalis	Nodular lymphocyte-predominant Hodgkin lymphoma (with IgD expression)
Malaria	Endemic Burkitt lymphoma
Autoimmune diseases	
■ Sjögren syndrome	Ocular adnexal marginal zone lymphoma of MALT type
■ Hashimoto thyroiditis	Primary thyroid lymphoma (marginal zone of MALT type of diffuse large B-cell lymphoma)
■ Rheumatoid arthritis	Lymphoma is more common in rheumatoid arthritis with a similar distribution of subtypes
Immunodeficiency states	
Primary	
Many are associated e.g.	
■ Common variable immunodeficiency disorder (CVID)	Approximately 4% prevalence of B-cell lymphoma
■ Ataxia telangiectasia	T-cell and B-cell lymphomas
Secondary	
■ HIV	See above
■ Post-transplant (solid organ or haemopoietic)	These may be EBV positive (often early after transplant in EBV negative organ recipient) or negative (often later after transplant)
Familial predisposition	■ Family history for lymphoma or CLL is a consistent risk factor for non-Hodgkin lymphoma of all subtypes. ■ The relative risk for a first-degree relative is 1.5-2 (although for CLL, the relative risk for developing CLL is approximately 8) ■ Some genetic susceptibility regions are shared between lymphoma subtypes, e.g. HLA regions variants ■ Other regions are subtype specific ■ Genetic testing is usually NOT recommended for relatives of people affected by lymphoma
Other environmental factors	■ Prior radiotherapy (for example, Hodgkin lymphoma treated with radiotherapy increases the risk of non-Hodgkin lymphoma later in life) ■ Prior chemotherapy ■ Exposure to pesticides / herbicides. Large epidemiological studies inconsistently report associations with these chemicals

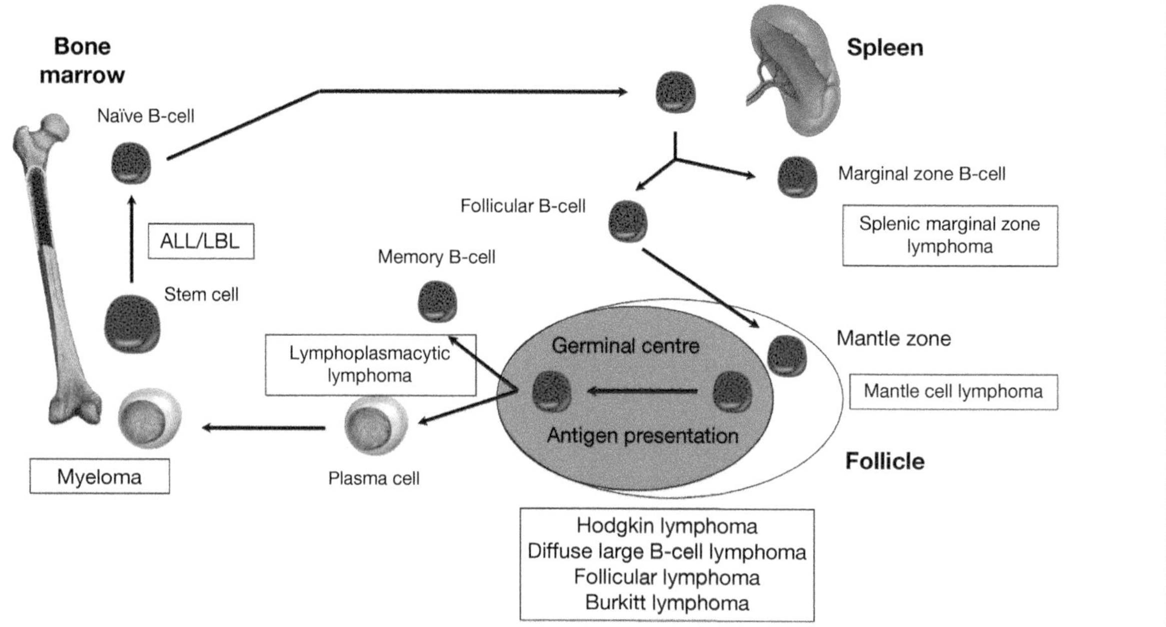

Figure 20.3 A simplified version of the life cycle of a B-lymphocyte. After transitioning through lymphoid progenitor stages in the bone marrow, the naïve B cell transits to the spleen where further maturation occurs. Most B cells become marginal zone B cells (in the spleen, Peyer's patches lining epithelial surfaces and in lymph nodes) or follicular B cell (in lymph nodes or the spleen mainly). After transiting the germinal centre and if it survives the B-cell differentiates into a memory B cell or plasma cell. The various B-cell disorders arise at different stages of this life cycle although some disorders (such as chronic lymphocytic leukaemia) have not had their cell of origin convincingly determined. ALL/LBL, acute lymphoblastic leukaemia/lymphoblastic lymphoma

Diagnosis

Some types of lymphoma may be diagnosed on examination of peripheral blood film (Fig. 20.4) combined with flow cytometry (Table 20.5). However, the diagnosis of lymphoma usually relies on examination of biopsy material by an expert haemato-pathologist. For this, the architecture of the tissue needs to be preserved as this is crucial for both the diagnosis of lymphoma and for accurate subtyping. Two main types of biopsy may be performed:

1 Excision of an involved lymph node. This is the gold standard technique, providing ample tissue for morphology, immunohistochemistry (Table 20.4, Fig. 20.5) and genetic studies. On occasion, different types of lymphoma may exist in the same lymph node, e.g., follicular lymphoma and diffuse large B-cell lymphoma, and provision of a whole lymph node is needed to demonstrate this. However this involves surgical intervention which may present logistical challenges.

2 Core biopsy. This is usually performed under ultrasound or CT guidance. It results in a core of tissue of variable diameter. Whilst sufficient for the diagnosis in many cases, sampling error may give an inadequate picture of the full spectrum of disease within a node and not enough tissue for the range of tests required. Multiple wide-bore cores are preferred. For lymphomas involving deep structures, a core biopsy may be the only possible means of diagnosis.

Fine needle aspirate (FNA) which is used in the diagnosis of some types of cancer is NOT of use in lymphoma diagnosis. This is because it yields disaggregated cells and relies on cytological examination. In some forms of lymphoma (such as many low grade forms), there is little cytological atypia and so a false negative result may result. Even if a high-grade lymphoma is correctly identified, an accurate subtype is needed, which is not possible from an FNA. Once a biopsy is obtained, a number of tests (described in Chapter 11 and Table 20.4) are performed depending on the likely subtype.

Staging

The staging system is the same as that described for Hodgkin lymphoma (Chapter 19), but stage is less clearly related to prognosis than the histological subtype. Staging procedures usually include PET/CT or CT scanning (Fig. 20.6). The criteria by which a lymph node is considered normal or abnormal by CT are described in Chapter 9. PET/CT can also be used to follow treatment response (Fig. 20.6). Bone marrow aspiration and trephine are sometimes performed although may be deferred if the results would not affect management. PET/CT may detect marrow disease when the biopsy is negative especially in high-grade disease. The Deauville criteria by which a lymph node is considered normal or abnormal on PET/CT scanning have been described in Chapter 19.

Table 20.4 Tests performed on a biopsy to aid in the diagnosis and sub-typing of lymphoma. Note, not every technique is required for all cases.

Diagnostic test	Principle involved	Example
Immunohistochemistry	Use of labelled antibodies to determine cell surface or intra-cellular protein expression associated with subtypes of lymphoma. Kappa and lambda light chain staining can confirm clonality (Fig. 20.5)	B-cell lymphomas typically positive for CD19, CD20, CD79a T-cell lymphomas typically positive for CD3, CD5, CD7 See Table 20.5 for the common immunophenotypes for NHL subtypes
Flow cytometry	Performed on cells in suspension which maybe from blood, bone marrow aspirate or from disaggregated nodal tissue. Fluorescent tagged antibodies are used to probe the expression of proteins on the cell surface	Diagnosis of leukaemic forms of NHL such as mantle cell lymphoma (which is positive for CD5, CD19, CD20, FMC7 and CD79b) See Table 20.5 for the common immunophenotypes for NHL subtypes
Fluorescent *in situ* hybridisation (FISH)	Fluorescent DNA probes used to determine whether a chromosomal translocation in present	Probes for *c-MYC* and *BCL2* to determine the presence of 'double hit' lymphoma See Table 20.6 for translocations associated with common lymphoma subtypes
Mutation analysis	DNA sequencing to determine the presence of mutations in specific lymphoma-associated genes	*TP53* mutation as a poor prognostic factor in CLL or mantle cell lymphoma See Table 20.6 for mutations associated with common lymphoma subtypes
Determination of clonality	B-cell clonality can be determined by immunophenotyping demonstrating expression of either κ or λ light chains (Fig. 20.5) There is a specific form of mutation analysis to look for either B-cell receptor, i.e., immunoglobulin, or T-cell receptor clonality	T-cell clonality may help in the determination of a T-cell lymphoma from a reactive T-cell proliferation (NB – T-cell clones can sometimes be seen in reactive phenomena, so interpretation can be difficult)
Gene expression profiling	Determination of which genes are expression by analysis of RNA products	Whilst this was how diffuse large B-cell lymphoma was initially categorized into germinal centre and activated B-cell subtypes, this is not routinely performed in diagnostic laboratories

Clinical features of non-Hodgkin lymphoma

1 **Superficial lymphadenopathy** The majority of patients present with asymmetrical painless enlargement of lymph nodes in one or more peripheral lymph node regions.

2 **Constitutional symptoms** Fever, night sweats and weight loss can occur, but are less frequent than in Hodgkin lymphoma. Their presence is usually associated with more advanced, disseminated disease.

3 **Oropharyngeal involvement** In 5–10% of patients there is disease of the oropharyngeal lymphoid structures

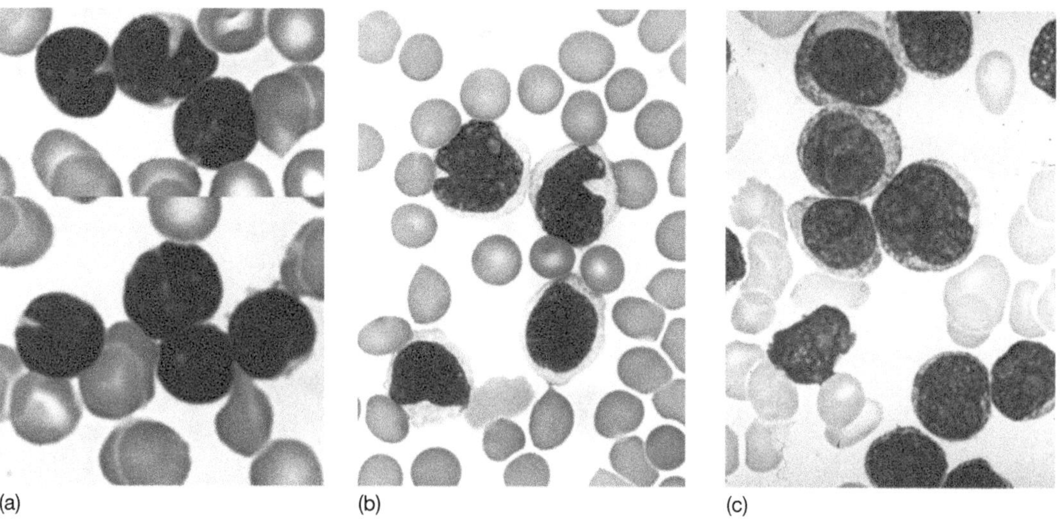

Figure 20.4 Blood involvement by malignant lymphoma: **(a)** small cleaved lymphoid cells in follicular lymphoma; **(b)** mantle cell lymphoma; **(c)** large B-cell lymphoma.

Table 20.5 Characteristic immunophenotype of common B-cell lymphomas. Compare also Table 18.2.

	SIg	CD20	CD5	CD10	CD23	BCL6	MUM1
Small lymphocytic lymphoma/CLL	weak	+	+	–	+	–	–
Hairy cell leukaemia (classical subtype)[1]	+	+	–	–	–	–	–
Lymphoplasmacytic lymphoma	+	+	–	–	–	–	+
MALT lymphoma	+	+	–	–	+/–	–	+/–
Follicular lymphoma	+	+	–	+	+/–	+	–
Mantle cell lymphoma	+	+	+	–	–	–	–
DLBCL, GCB subtype	+/–	+	–	+		+	–
DLBCL, non-GCB subtype	+/–	+	–	–		–	+
Burkitt lymphoma	+	+	–	+	–	+	–

CLL, chronic lymphocytic leukaemia; DLBCL, diffuse large B-cell lymphoma, GCB, germinal centre B-cell type; MALT, mucosa-associated lymphoid tissue; MUM1, a lymphocytic-specific transcription factor; SIg, surface immunoglobulin.

[1] Hairy cell leukaemia is strongly positive for CD11c, CD25, CD103 and annexin A1.

(Waldeyer's ring), which may cause complaints of a 'sore throat' or noisy or obstructed breathing.

4 **Symptoms due to anaemia, infections due to neutropenia or purpura with thrombocytopenia** These may be presenting features in patients with diffuse bone marrow involvement. Cytopenias may also be autoimmune in origin or due to sequestration in an enlarged spleen.

5 **Abdominal disease** The liver and spleen are often enlarged and involvement of retroperitoneal or mesenteric nodes is frequent. The gastrointestinal tract is the most commonly involved extranodal site after the bone marrow, and patients may present with acute or subacute abdominal symptoms.

6 **Other organs** Involvement of the skin, brain, testis or thyroid is not infrequent. The skin is also primarily involved in

Table 20.6 Examples of cytogenetic abnormalities and gene mutations found in cases of mature lymphoid malignancies.

	Cytogenetics	Gene mutations
Chronic lymphocytic leukaemia	Chromosome 13p, 11q or 17p deletions; trisomy 12	*TP53*, *ATM*, *NOTCH1*, *SF3B1*
Hairy cell leukaemia	Non-specific	*BRAF* (>99% in classic subtype)
Lymphoplasmacytic lymphoma	Non-specific	*MYD88* (>90%), *CXCR4* (30%)
MALT lymphoma	t(11;18) *[API2::MALT1]*, t(1;14) *[BCL9::IGH]*	Activation of NFκB pathway
Follicular lymphoma	t(14;18) *[IGH::BCL2]*	Mutations in genes such as *CREBBP*, *EZH2* and *KMT2D* (*MLL2*), which influence chromatin remodelling
Mantle cell lymphoma	t(11;14) *[IGH::CCND1]*	*ATM*, *CCND1*, *TP53* and genes influencing chromatin modification
Diffuse large B-cell lymphoma	t(14;18) *[IGH::BCL2]* and others	*MYD88*, *CD79B*, *NOTCH1/2*, *EZH2*, *BCL2*, *BCL6*, *MYC*
Burkitt lymphoma	t(8;14) *[MYC::IGH]*, t(2;8) *[IGK::MYC]*, t(8;22) *[MYC::IGL]*	Various
Anaplastic large cell lymphoma	t(2;5) *[NPM1::ALK]*	*ALK*

MALT, mucosa-associated lymphoid tissue.

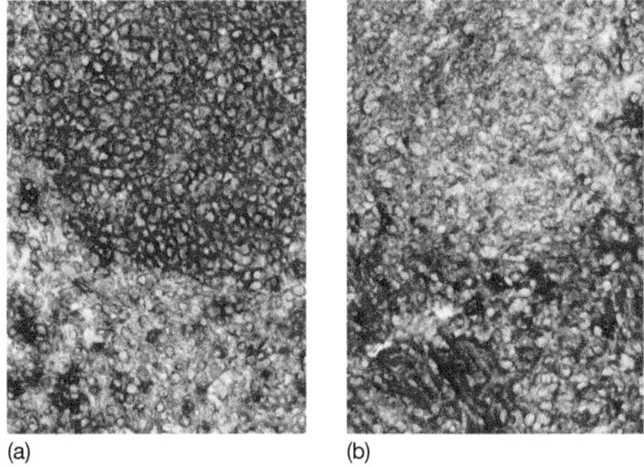

Figure 20.5 Non-Hodgkin lymphoma: lymph node stained by immunoperoxidase shows **(a)** brown ring staining for κ in the malignant lymphoid nodule; and **(b)** no labelling for λ, confirming the monoclonal origin of the lymphoma.

two closely related T-cell lymphomas: mycosis fungoides and Sézary syndrome.

General principles of treatment

The goal of treatment must always be clear when developing a management plan:

1 **Curative.** Patients with high-grade NHL (or very early stage low grade NHL) can often be treated with curative intent. In this case, treatment initiation should be prompt as rates of cure are usually higher with earlier stage, less bulky disease. Maintaining treatment intensity is a priority.

2 **Disease modification.** Whilst many low-grade NHLs cannot be cured, treatment for many is highly effective resulting in long life expectancy for most. Treatment in this situation is generally initiated when symptoms of the disease develop, organ function is impaired by the lymphoma,

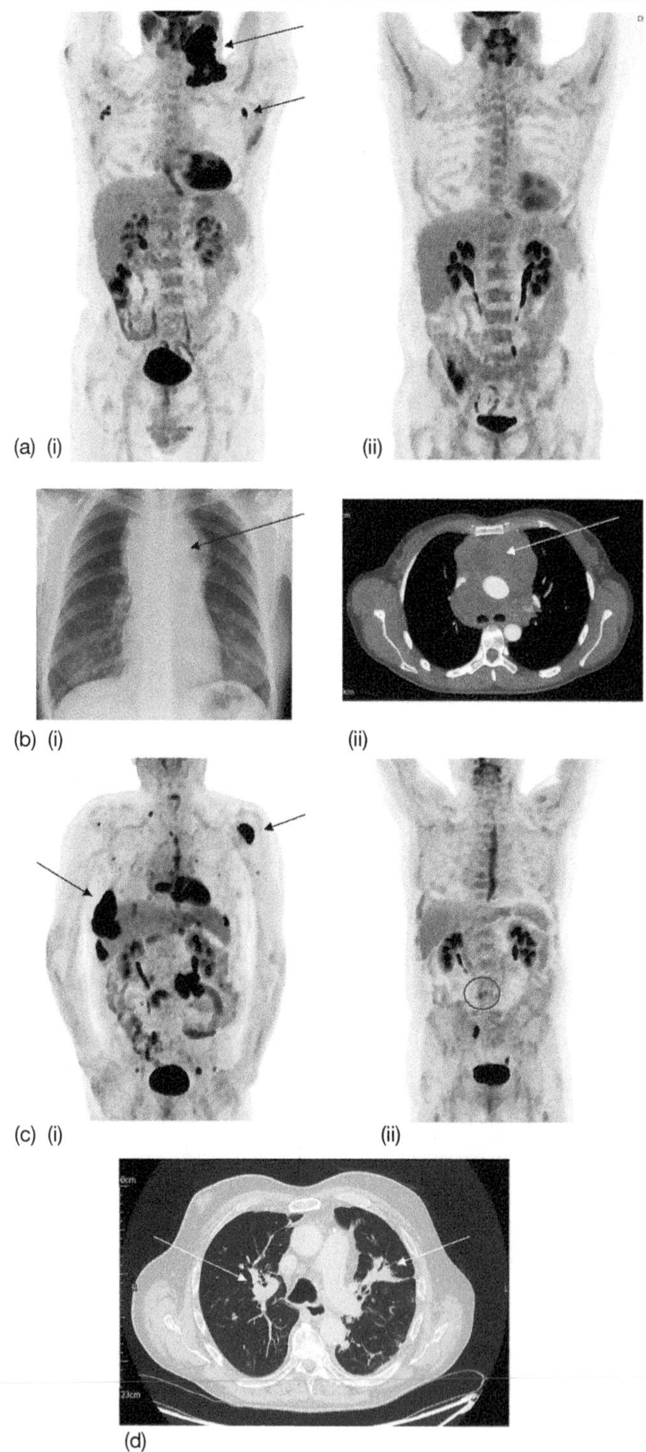

Figure 20.6 **(a)** (i) PET scan of a 64-year-old man who presented with a lump in the left neck and some difficulty swallowing. A bulky FDG-avid mass is seen in the left neck along with bilateral uptake in much smaller axillary lymph nodes. The biopsy confirmed DLBCL and after 2 cycles of R-CHOP, the interim PET scan (ii) was negative (Deauville score 2). **(b)** A 24-year-old woman presented with a cough worse on lying flat and (i) the chest X-ray showed a mediastinal mass; (ii) CT scan confirmed a large mediastinal mass with areas of necrosis. Biopsy confirmed a primary mediastinal B-cell large cell lymphoma. **(c)** A 78-year-old man presented with pain in the right side of his chest followed by the development of a palpable mass. Biopsy showed DLBCL. The PET scan showed an erosive lesion of the right chest wall with other bony sites such as the left humeral head. Interim PET scan after 2 cycles showed a good response with some mild avidity in the mesenteric residuum (circle), Deauville 4. **(d)** a 73 year old man presented with a cough with multiple areas of well-defined nodules and consolidation in both lungs. Biopsy showed a marginal zone lymphoma. Source: Courtesy of Oxford University Hospitals Radiology Department.

Table 20.7 Criteria for treatment initiation in low-grade non-Hodgkin lymphoma management.

GELF criteria	BNLI criteria
High tumour bulk defined by ■ Tumour > 7 cm ■ 3 nodes in 3 distinct areas >3 cm ■ Symptomatic splenic enlargement ■ Organ compression ■ Serous effusion	Rapid disease progression in preceding 3 months
Presence of systemic symptoms	Life-threatening organ involvement
Raised serum LDH or β2-micorglobulin	Presence of systemic symptoms
ECOG performance status 2 or more	Hb < 100 g/l; WBC < 1.5×10^9/l; platelet count < 100×10^9/l
	Bone lesions

BNLI, British National Lymphoma Investigation; GELF, Groupe d'Etude des Lymphomes Folliculaires.

e.g. falling blood counts due to bone marrow involvement, or disease bulk is sufficient to be concerned for continuing observation. Formal criteria for the initiation of treatment have been developed, e.g. GELF or BNLI criteria for follicular lymphoma (Table 20.7). Prior to these criteria being met, a 'watch and wait' or 'active surveillance' strategy is frequently employed.

3 **Palliative.** The goal in this setting is to reduce symptoms burden even if there is no or little expectation of prolonging life expectancy. Treatment may be focused on targeting specific lesions causing symptoms (frequently employing radiotherapy) or systemic treatment if symptoms are due to widespread disease. Treatment toxicity should be carefully weighed against likely benefit.

Specific treatment regimens will be discussed in Chapter 21.

SUMMARY

Non-Hodgkin lymphomas are a large group of clonal lymphoid neoplasms. Approximately 85% are of B-cell origin and 15% derive from T or NK cells.

- Their clinical presentation and natural history are more variable than Hodgkin lymphoma and can range from a very indolent disease to rapidly progressive subtypes that need urgent treatment.
- The NHLs are divided into B- and T-cell subtypes. The B-cell subtypes are divided into low-grade and high-grade disease. Low-grade disorders are typically slowly progressive, respond well to chemotherapy, but are difficult to cure; whereas high-grade lymphomas are aggressive and need urgent treatment, but are more often curable.
- Infections with viruses, e.g. Epstein–Barr, HIV, hepatitis C, HTLV-1; bacteria, e.g. H. pylori and protozoa, e.g. malaria underlie some cases.
- Clinical presentation is most often with an enlarged superficial lymph node or with the effects of an enlarged lymph node mass in the chest or abdomen, systemic symptoms, e.g. fever, weight loss, anorexia, symptoms due to bone marrow, abdominal or other organ involvement.
- Investigation is with lymph node biopsy, blood tests and imaging, usually by PET/CT. Immunohistochemistry of the lymph node is essential and flow cytometry, cytogenetic or gene mutation analysis is helpful in many cases.
- Clinical staging is performed as for Hodgkin lymphoma.

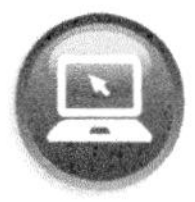

Now visit **www.wiley.com/go/haematology9e** to test yourself on this chapter.

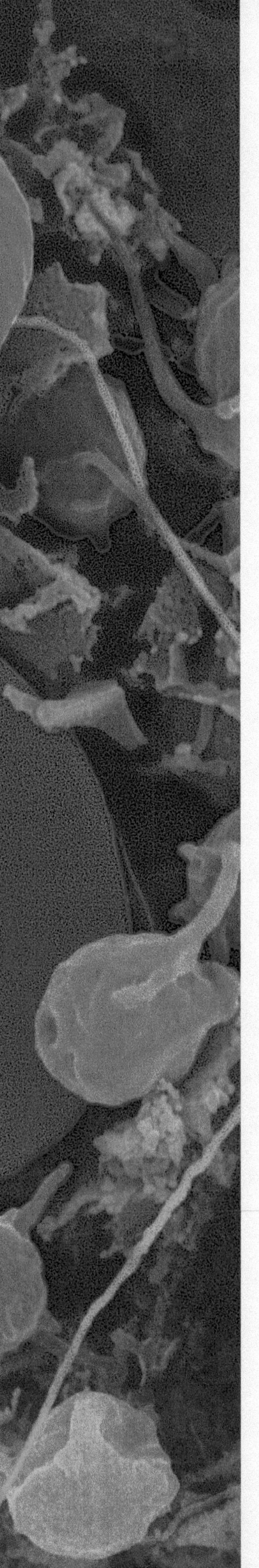

CHAPTER 21

Non-Hodgkin lymphomas 2: Individual diseases

Key topics

Hoffbrand's Essential Haematology, Ninth Edition. A. Victor Hoffbrand, Pratima Chowdary, Graham P. Collins, and Justin Loke.

© 2024 John Wiley & Sons Ltd. Published 2024 by John Wiley & Sons Ltd.

Companion website: www.wiley.com/go/haematology9e

High-grade non-Hodgkin lymphomas

Large B-cell lymphomas

Large B-cell lymphomas are a heterogeneous group of disorders representing the classic 'high-grade' lymphomas. Histologically the biopsy shows large neoplastic cells with prominent nucleoli. A number of subtypes exist such as diffuse large B-cell lymphoma (DLBCL) not otherwise specified (NOS), T-cell/histiocyte-rich large B-cell lymphoma (which in some has transformed from an underlying nodular lymphocyte-predominant Hodgkin lymphoma) and primary mediastinal B-cell lymphoma (PMBCL). DLBCL cases can be subdivided into 'germinal centre B-cell' (GCB) and 'activated B-cell' (ABC) subtypes when using gene expression profiling. As this technique is not routinely available, cases are more often subdivided by immunohistochemistry into GCB (characterized by CD10 and/or BCL6 expression) and non-germinal centre B-cell (non-GCB), which stain with antibodies to MUM1 (Table 20.6; Fig. 21.1).

The clinical presentation is usually with rapidly progressive lymphadenopathy, which may also involve the bone marrow, gastrointestinal tract, brain (Fig. 21.2), spinal cord, kidneys or other organs (Fig. 21.3). Approximately 30–40% of cases may arise within an extranodal site and are termed primary extranodal.

A variety of clinical and laboratory findings are relevant to the outcome of therapy. According to the **International Prognostic Index (IPI)** these include age, performance status, stage, number of extranodal sites and serum LDH (Table 21.1). Two other commonly used prognostic indices are the **Revised IPI** which was initially devised in a more modern era with patients treated with R-CHOP (see below) and the **NCCN-IPI** which also analysed R-CHOP treated patients and divides some of the risk categories into more than two sub-groups (Table 21.1). Bulky disease (major mass >5 cm diameter), prior history of low-grade disease or HIV infection, and ABC compared to GCB subtype are also associated with a poorer prognosis, but are not included in the IPI.

The most common cytogenetic changes involve the *IGH* locus on chromosome 14, the *BCL6* gene at chromosome 3q27, and translocation of the *BCL2* gene occurs in 20%. Somatic mutations are frequent in all types (Table 20.7). So-called **double hit** lymphoma has underlying chromosomal translocations involving the *MYC* and *BCL2* genes. When the partner gene for the *MYC* translocation is an immunoglobulin gene, the disease is associated with a relatively poor prognosis. A **'double expressor'** DLBCL is when the *MYC* and *BCL2* genes are normal but the proteins are aberrantly expressed. They have a somewhat worse outcome, but less poor than for double hit cases. Whilst double expressor lymphomas are more common in the ABC subtype of DLBCL, double hit lymphoma is far more common in the GCB subtype (Fig. 21.4).

Treatment

The mainstay of treatment of advanced stage disease until recently was rituximab in combination with CHOP – cyclophosphamide, doxorubicin (hydroxydaunorubicin), vincristine (oncovin) and prednisolone – given in 3-weekly cycles, typically for six cycles. The Polarix trial demonstrated a progression free (but not overall survival) advantage of 6 cycles of polatuzumab vedotin (an anti-CD79b antibody-drug conjugate) combined with CHP (CHOP with vincristine omitted) compared with 6 cycles of R-CHOP in patients

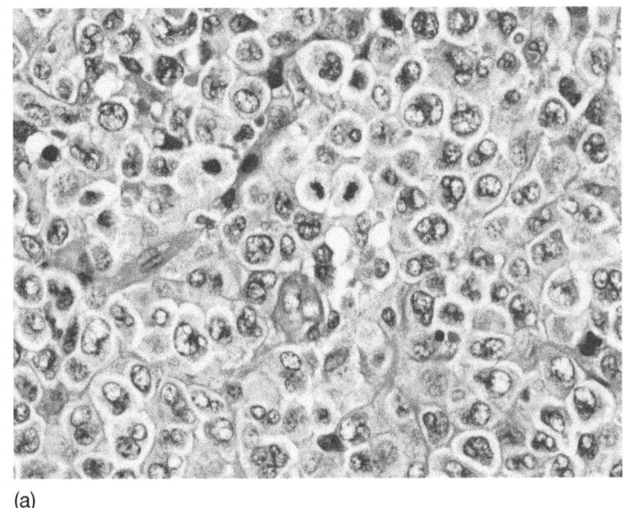

(a)

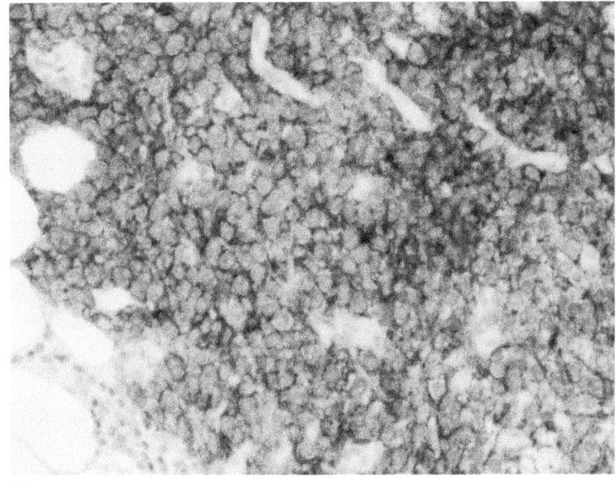

(b)

Figure 21.1 (a) Diffuse large B-cell lymphoma. **(b)** The cells stain positive for CD10. This suggests a germinal centre cell origin in this case. Source: E. Campo, S.A. Pileri. In A.V. Hoffbrand *et al.* (eds) (2016) *Postgraduate Haematology*, 7th edn. Reproduced with permission of John Wiley & Sons.

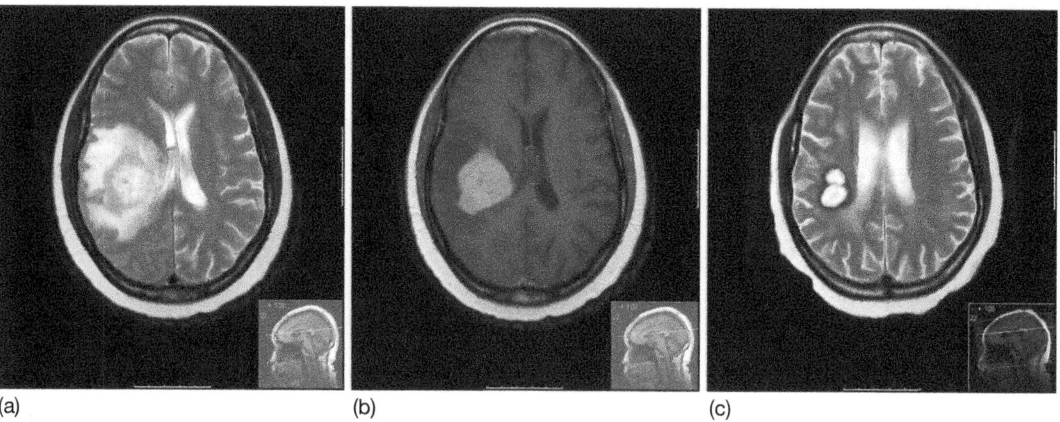

Figure 21.2 Cerebral lymphoma in HIV infection; magnetic resonance imaging (MRI). **(a)** T2-weighted magnetic resonance brain scan showing heterogeneous mass and adjacent oedema in right inferior frontoparietal region. There is compression of the right lateral ventricle and displacement of midline structures. Biopsy showed diffuse large B-cell lymphoma. **(b)** The mass enhances after intravenous gadolinium injection. **(c)** Enhanced image after chemotherapy showing regression of the mass. Source: Courtesy of Department of Radiology, Royal Free Hospital, London.

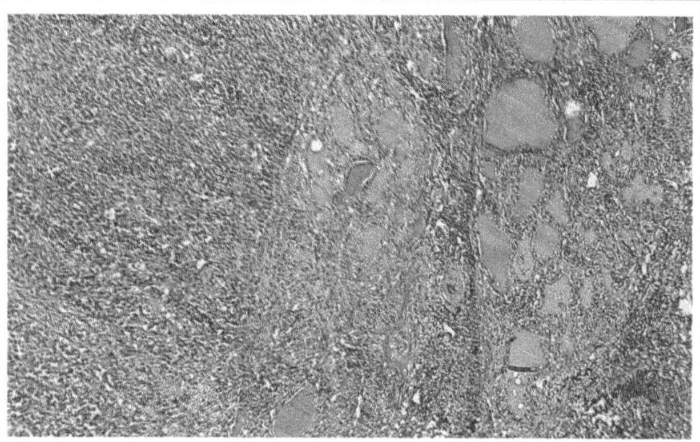

Figure 21.3 Diffuse large B-cell lymphoma of the thyroid. Sheets of neoplastic cells (left) and remaining colloid filled thyroid acini (right). Source: A.V. Hoffbrand *et al.* (2019) *Color Atlas of Clinical Hematology*, 5th edn. Reproduced with permission of John Wiley & Sons.

with an IPI of 2–5. Where available, many centres have adopted this as a standard of care for these patients. Radiotherapy may reduce relapse at sites of initial bulky (e.g. ≥ 7 cm) disease although an alternative approach is to only irradiate residual PET-avid areas. See Fig. 21.5 for treatment algorithm.

For localized disease, combined radiotherapy and immunochemotherapy (e.g. three courses of R-CHOP) may be optimal. Alternative strategies in some patients are 4 or 6 cycles of R-CHOP alone. In some situations such as primary testicular lymphoma, 6 cycles of immunochemotherapy are considered standard even in stage 1 disease. Prophylactic therapy to prevent central nervous system (CNS) disease is controversial. Whilst recent data suggest little benefit in reducing the risk of CNS relapse with intrathecal chemotherapy, e.g. methotrexate and/or cytarabine, or intravenous high dose chemotherapy, e.g. methotrexate, the devastating nature of such an event and the retrospective nature of the data, means than many centres still consider prophylaxis for very high risk patients such as those with testicular involvement, or those with a very high CNS-IPI (score of 5 or 6 with one point for each IPI score and an additional point for renal and / adrenal involvement).

The response to treatment is monitored by repeat CT or PET/CT typical after 2 cycles of chemotherapy and then following completion. The analysis of baseline and post first or second chemotherapy cycle circulating tumour DNA (ctDNA) has also been shown to be a powerful prognostic tool although it is not routinely available.

The optimal treatment for patients with double hit lymphoma is not defined. R-CHOP or Pola-R-CHP are both options although intensification with, for example, DA-EPOCH-R (a regimen containing similar drugs to R-CHOP but with the addition of etoposide, an infusional component, and generally higher doses titrated according to effect on blood counts) may improve outcome.

For patients who relapse, a judgement is made whether the patient is fit for high dose chemotherapy with autologous stem cell transplantation (ASCT) or for chimeric antigen receptor (CAR) T-cell therapy, e.g. with axicabtagene ciloleucel or tisagenlecleucel, (Chapters 9, 12). Where second line CAR T-cell therapy is available, a randomized trial suggests this is the optimal approach compared with ASCT for those who are primary refractory or relapse within 1 year of first line treatment. Where not available, drug regimens such as R-ICE (rituximab, ifosfamide, carboplatin and etoposide) or gemcitabine-based or other platinum-based regimens are used (Fig. 21.6). This is with the aim to proceed to ASCT with curative intent. This approach results in prolonged remissions (and likely cure) in only 20% of patients. For those relapsing after ASCT,

Table 21.1 A comparison of the three commonly used prognostic indices for patients with newly diagnosed diffuse large B-cell lymphoma. The R-IPI and NCCN-IPI were developed using patients treated in the rituximab era although the standard IPI is still commonly used for risk stratification.

International Prognostic Index (IPI) (1 point for each)	Revised IPI (R-IPI) (1 point for each)	National Comprehensive Cancer Network IPI (NCCN-IPI)
Age > 60 years	Age > 60 years	Age: > 75 years: score 3 > 60 years: score 2 > 40 years: score 1 ≤ 40 years: score 0
LDH > upper limit normal	LDH > upper limit normal	LDH > 3× upper limit normal: score 2 > 1× upper limit normal: score 1 ≤ upper limit normal: score 0
ECOG Performance status > 1	ECOG Performance status > 1	ECOG Performance Status > 1: score 1
Number of extranodal sites > 1	Number of extranodal site > 1	Involvement of CNS, GI tract, liver, bone marrow or lung: 1 point if any present
Stage III or IV	Stage III or IV	Stage III or IV: score 1
Score 0/1: low risk **Score 2:** low intermediate risk **Score 3:** high intermediate risk **Score 4/5:** high risk	**Score 0:** very good risk **Score 1/2:** good risk **Score 3/4/5:** poor risk	**Score 0/1:** low risk **Score 2/3:** low intermediate risk **Score 4/5:** high intermediate risk **Score 6/7/8:** high risk

CNS, central nervous system; ECOG, Eastern Cooperative Oncology Group; GI, gastrointestinal tract; LDH, lactate dehydrogenase.

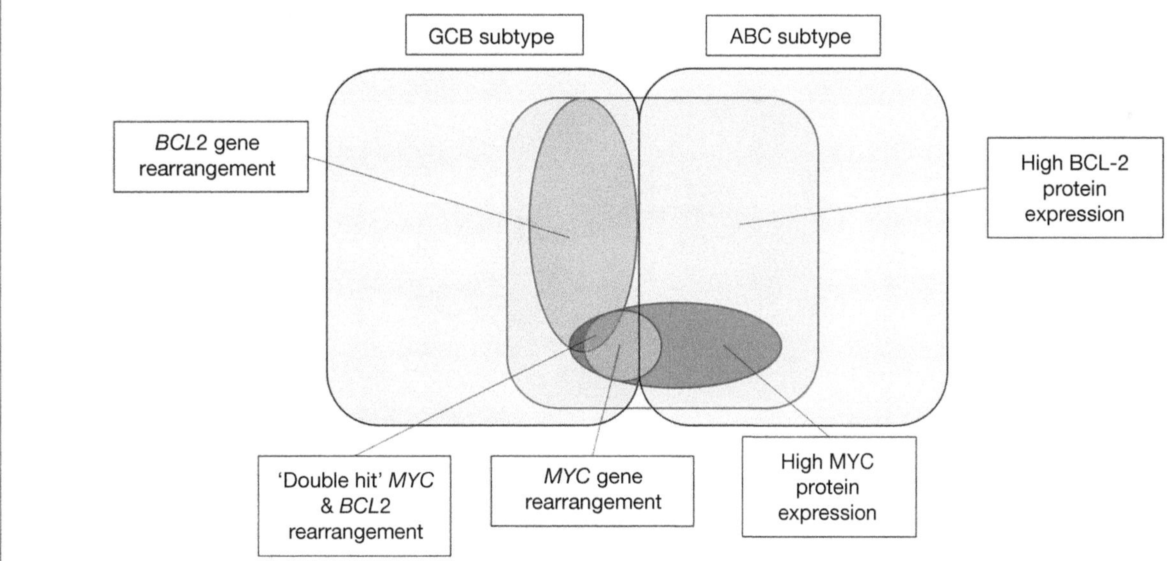

Figure 21.4 Double expressor lymphoma, characterized by high expression levels of BCL-2 and MYC protein, are found in both ABC and GCB subtypes of DLBCL but are more common in ABC. An underlying *MYC* rearrangement is more in the GCB subtype and a *BCL2* rearrangement (and therefore a 'double hit' lymphoma) is almost exclusively found in GBC subtypes.

anti-CD19 directed CAR-T cell therapy is an option and can result in prolonged remissions in about 40% of patients.

The bi-specific antibodies glofitamab and epcoritamab (anti-CD3, anti-CD20) have been shown effective for relapsed DLBCL with cytokine release syndrome and infection the main side effects. Their use, particularly in those relapsing after CAR-T cell therapy, is likely to increase significantly. Other active agents in multiply relapsed DLBCL include the anti-CD19 glyco-engineered antibody tafasitamab combined with lenalidomide, polatuzumab vedotin combined with bendamustine and rituximab

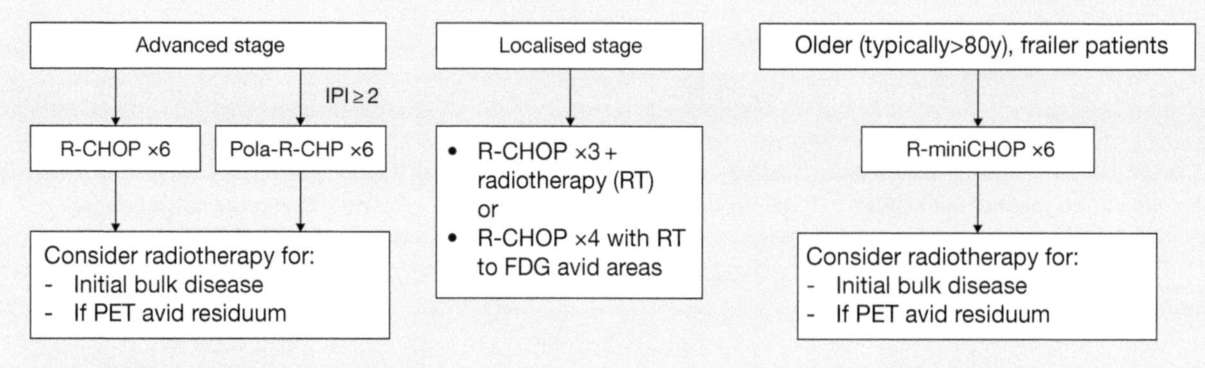

Interim PET scan
Maybe consifered after 2 cycles of chemotherapy in advanced stage disease although there is no evidence to use this to guide treatement

Double hit lymphoma
Consider a more dose intense regimen such as DA-EPOCH-R

CNS prophylaxis
Consider intravenous high dose methotrexate at the end of initial chemotherapy in very high risk disease (e.g. testicular involvement, CNS-IPI 5 or 6)

Figure 21.5 Algorithm for the first line treatment of DLBCL. Advanced stage disease is usually defined as stage III or IV by the Ann-Arbor staging system with localized disease often considered as that which can be safely encompassed in a radiation field. R-CHOP: rituximab, cyclophosphamide, doxorubicin, vincristine, prednisolone; Pola-R-CHP: R-CHOP with polatuzumab vedotin in place of vincristine; R-miniCHOP: same drugs as R-CHOP but with reduced doses of cyclophosphamide, doxorubicin and vincristine; DA-EPOCH-R: dose adjusted (according to effect on blood counts from previous cycle) etoposide, doxorubicin, cyclophosphamide, vincristine, prednisolone and rituximab.

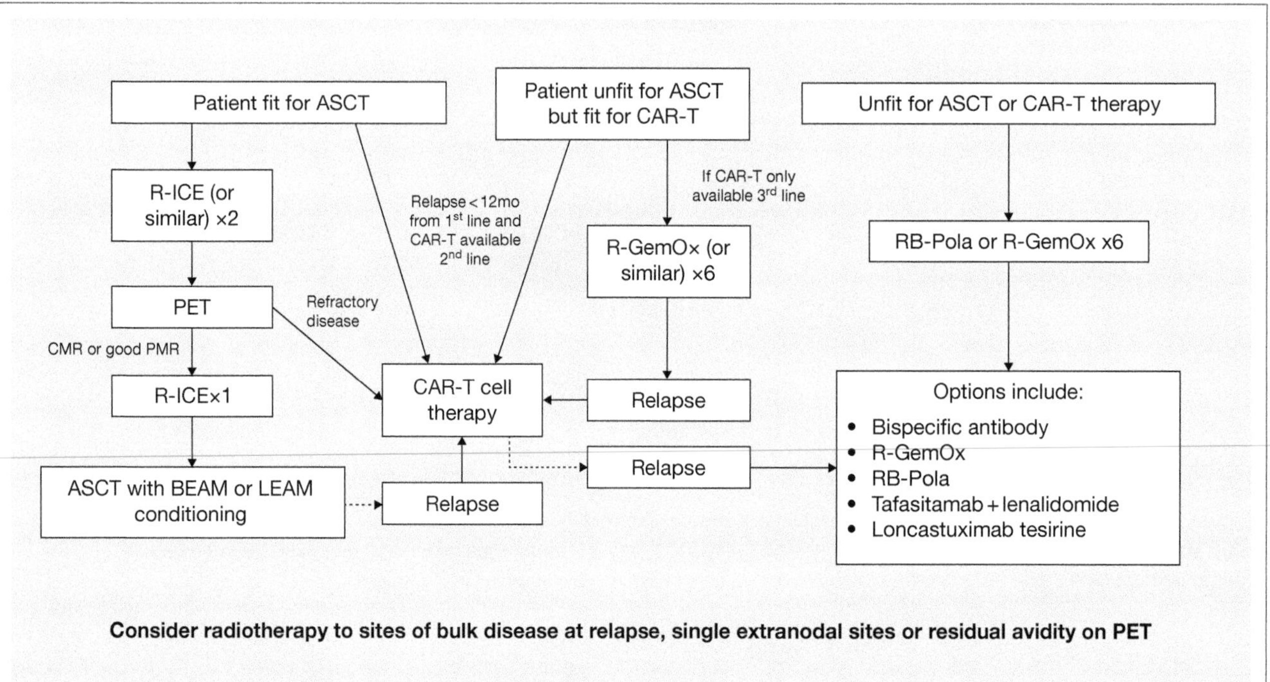

Figure 21.6 Algorithm for the treatment of relapsed DLBCL. ASCT: autologous stem cell transplant; DLBCL: diffuse large B-cell lymphoma; BEAM: BCNU, etoposide, cytarabine, melphalan; LEAM: as for BEAM except for lomustine in place of BCNU; CAR-T: chimeric antigen receptor T-cell; R-GemOx: rituximab, gemcitabine, oxaliplatin; RB-Pola: rituximab, bendamustine, polatuzumab vedotin; CMR: complete metabolic response; PMR: partial metabolic response.

and the anti-CD19 immunoconjugate loncastuzimab tesirine. Conventional chemotherapy with regimens such as R-GemOx (rituximab, gemcitabine, oxaliplatin) is also an option.

Primary central nervous system lymphoma

This is a rare diffuse large B-cell lymphoma, more common in older patients and those with HIV infection. It is generally of the activated B-cell (ABC) subtype with underlying mutations of *MYD88*, *CD79B* and *CDKN2A*. Diagnosis is usually made by stereotactic biopsy; tumour cells are uncommonly found in the cerebrospinal fluid. Contrast-enhanced magnetic resonance imaging (MRI) is recommended for initial imaging and for response assessment. Patients are treated with cycles of high-dose methotrexate with partner cytotoxic agents, e.g. high-dose cytarabine, thiotepa and rituximab (the MATRix regimen). Anti-HIV therapy is added if the patient is HIV positive. Consolidation with high dose chemotherapy (such as with BCNU (carmustine) and thiotepa) and autologous SCT prolongs survival. Whole brain radiotherapy is an alternative and effective consolidation, but subsequent long-term cognitive dysfunction can be a major problem. For relapsed or refractory disease, chemotherapy with drugs such as ifosfamide or thiotepa with or without autologous SCT may be effective in a minority.

Primary mediastinal B-cell lymphoma

This is a rare type of NHL arising in the thymus, presenting mainly in adolescents and young adults and affecting women more commonly than men (Fig. 21.7). The histology may resemble Hodgkin lymphoma, but in contrast to Hodgkin lymphoma, tumour cells are dominant, CD30 expression is often weak and CD15 negative. *PAX5* and *BCL-6* are expressed in most cases, as are B-cell antigens (CD19, CD20, CD22, CD79b). Half of cases have amplification of the *REL* gene on chromosome 2q16, and tumour suppressor *SOCS1* is mutated or deleted in a similar proportion of cases. The tumour invades locally. Treatment is with R-CHOP, preferably at 14-day intervals, or more intensive regimens (such as DA-EPOCH-R) with or without subsequent local radiotherapy. A recent randomized trial has demonstrated that for patients treated with chemotherapy to a complete metabolic remission, there was no benefit for radiotherapy. For relapsed disease in suitable patients and if available, anti-CD19 CAR T-cell therapy is effective and potentially curative. Unusually for a large B-cell lymphoma, PD-1 inhibitors (Chapter 19) are also active.

Burkitt lymphoma

Burkitt lymphoma occurs in endemic or sporadic forms. Endemic (African) Burkitt lymphoma is seen in areas with chronic malaria exposure and is associated with Epstein–Barr virus (EBV) infection. In virtually all cases the *MYC* oncogene is overexpressed because it is translocated to an immunoglobulin gene, usually the heavy-chain locus t(8;14) (Fig. 11.11) and less commonly to one of the light chain loci. As a result, the gene is expressed in parts of the cell cycle during which it should normally be switched off. Typically the patient, usually a child, presents with massive lymphadenopathy, often

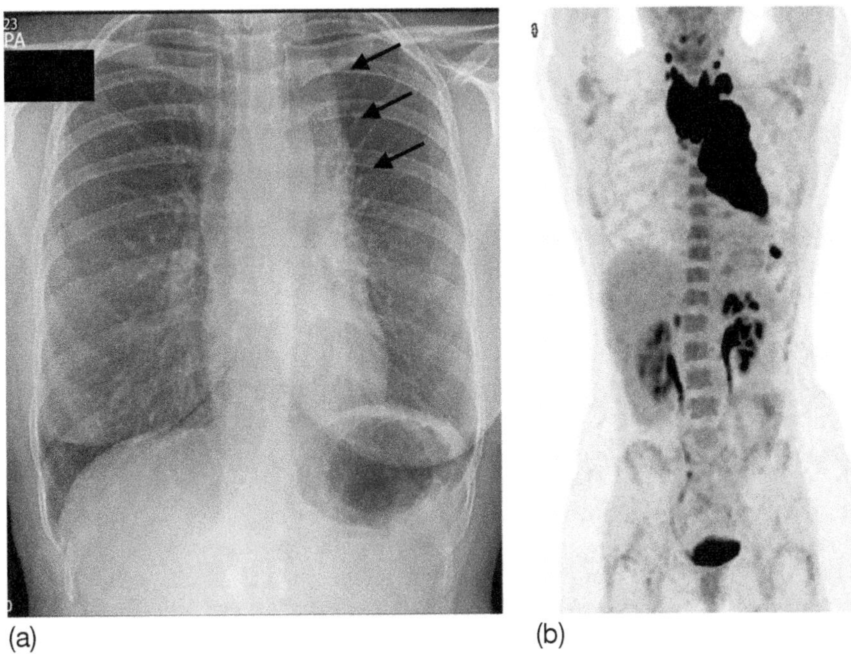

Figure 21.7 (a) Chest X-ray and **(b)** ^{18}FDG-PET scan of a 52 year old woman presenting with cough on lying flat, lump in the base of the neck and intermittent chest pains. The dominant feature is a large anterior mediastinal mass. Biopsy confirmed features in keeping with primary mediastinal B-cell lymphoma (PMBCL). Source: Courtesy of Oxford University Hospitals Dept of Radiology.

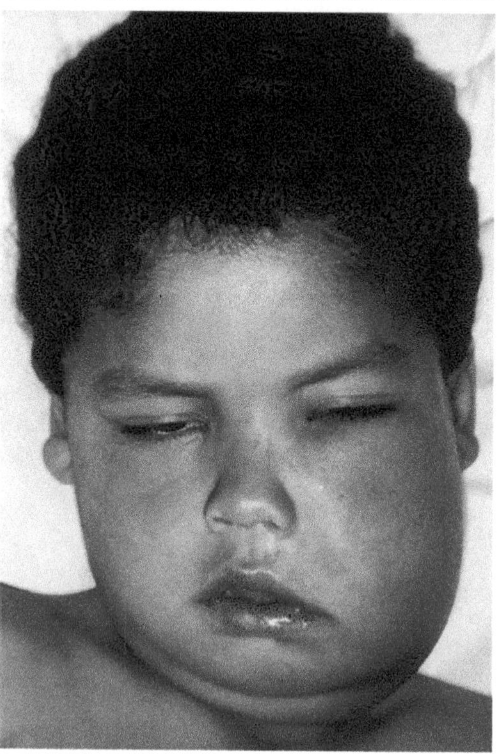

Figure 21.8 Burkitt lymphoma: characteristic facial swelling caused by extensive tumour involvement of the mandible and surrounding soft tissues.

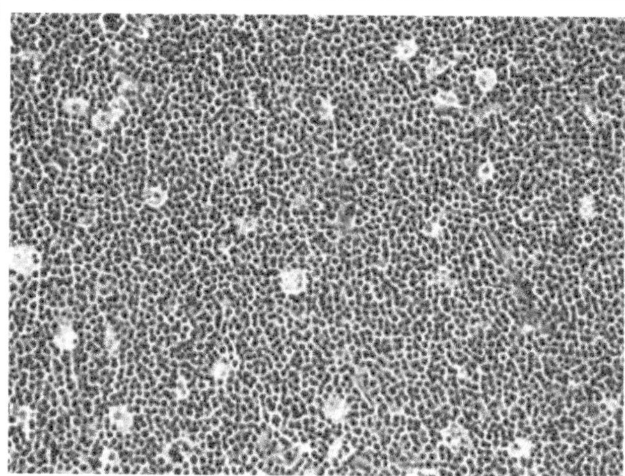

Figure 21.9 Burkitt lymphoma: histological section of lymph node showing sheets of lymphoblasts and 'starry sky' tingible body macrophages.

of the jaw (Fig. 21.8). Whilst initially very responsive to chemotherapy, long-term cure is uncommon due to lack of good supportive care limiting the intensity of therapy given.

Sporadic Burkitt lymphoma may occur anywhere in the world and EBV infection is seen in 20% of cases. There is an increased incidence in HIV infection. The histological picture is distinctive, with a very high proliferative index of over 95% (Fig. 21.9). The prognosis is excellent using chemotherapy regimens which include high doses of methotrexate, cytarabine and cyclophosphamide with rituximab, e.g. R-CODOX-M/R-IVAC (which also includes doxorubicin, ifosfamide and etoposide) or DA-EPOCH-R (which contains an infusional etoposide, doxorubicin and vincristine with adjustment of doses based on the myelosuppression seen in the previous cycle). Intrathecal chemotherapy is also given.

Lymphoblastic lymphoma

Lymphoblastic lymphomas (B or T cell) occur mainly in children and young adults and these conditions merge clinically and morphologically with acute lymphoblastic leukaemia (ALL). The cells, like those in ALL, are terminal deoxynucleotide transferase positive (Chapter 17), whereas this test is negative in all the other B- and T-cell lymphomas. They are treated as ALL using similar protocols.

Low-grade non-Hodgkin lymphomas

Follicular lymphoma

This represents around 25% of NHL, with a median age of onset of 60 years. It is associated with the t(14;18) translocation in the great majority of cases. The translocation leads to constitutive expression of the *BCL2* gene with increased survival of cells because of reduced apoptosis. Additional molecular abnormalities are usually present (Table 20.6). The histology shows complete effacement of lymph nodes by a nodules of B lymphocytes without the normal germinal centre appearances (Fig. 21.10). The cells are typically CD10, CD19, CD20, BCL2 and BCL6 positive (Table 20.5, Fig. 21.11).

Patients are likely to be middle-aged or elderly and their disease is often characterized by an indolent course for many years. The median survival from diagnosis is approximately 20 years. Rarely the disease presents in a benign form in children or as an *in situ* form, e.g. as an incidental finding on duodenal biopsy. Until recently, histological grading (based on the number of centroblasts seen per high powered field) was recommended. However due to a lack of reproducibility of which cells should be classified as centroblasts and which as more differentiated centrocytes and to impact on treatment, the WHO no longer recommends this. The term 'classic follicular lymphoma' encompasses those previously termed grade I-IIIa. Grade 111b (no centrocytes) is now termed 'follicular large B-cell lymphoma' (FLBL) and treated like a large B-cell lymphoma. Bone marrow involvement is frequent.

Presentation is usually with painless lymphadenopathy, often widespread, and the majority of patients will have stage III or IV disease. However, sudden transformation may occur at a rate of about 3% a year to a high grade B-cell lymphoma.

Treatment depends on the stage of the disease and the presence or absence of symptoms. Around 10–20%

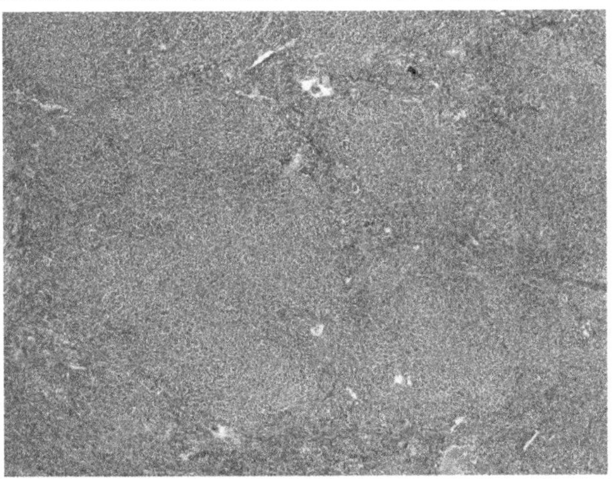

(a)

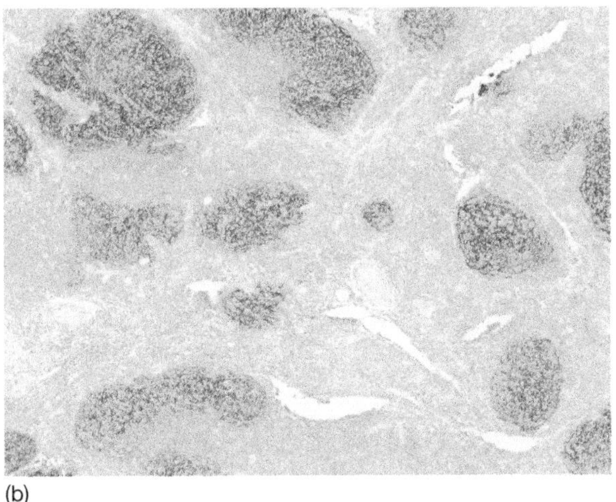

(b)

Figure 21.10 Follicular lymphoma. **(a)** The normal nodal architecture is replaced by lymphocyte proliferation in a nodular pattern. The nodules lack the starry sky pattern of normal germinal centres and the mantle zones are attenuated. **(b)** Staining for CD 21 shows the underlying network of follicular dendritic cells. Source: A.V. Hoffbrand *et al.* (2019) *Color Atlas of Clinical Hematology*, 5th edn. Reproduced with permission of John Wiley & Sons.

of patients have initially localized (stage I or some stage II encompassable in a radiotherapy field) disease and approximately 50% of these may achieve cure with radiotherapy alone (Fig. 21.12). Those with disseminated (stage II–IV) disease are generally not treated in the absence of symptoms ('active surveillance' or 'watch and wait'), but treatment is introduced when either symptoms occur or complications become imminent such as bone marrow failure or other organ compromise (Table 20.8). Single agent rituximab is an alternative to 'watch and wait' and may be preferred for older patients as a way of avoiding subsequent chemotherapy. A number of prognostic scores have been developed. Table 21.2 compares three or them. Whilst the FLIPI-2 was developed in the rituximab era, benefit over FLIPI-1 has not been demonstrated. Whilst helpful prognostically, these scores do not dictate when to initiate treatment or what to use. At the current time, chemotherapy is not a curative option.

First line therapy is with an anti-CD20 monoclonal antibody (such as rituximab or obinutuzumab) either as monotherapy or, more usually, combined with chemotherapy such as bendamustine, CVP or CHOP (Fig. 21.12). Rituximab combined with lenalidomide has been shown to be as effective as an immunochemotherapy approach in this setting. After immunochemotherapy, 2 years of maintenance rituximab or obinutuzumab is frequently used, to prolong remission duration. Maintenance treatment has not, however, been shown to prolong overall survival and is associated with increased infection risk.

Whilst first remission can be durable (often 10 years or more), relapse of advanced stage disease is inevitable. Treatment at relapse depends on what was received first line and the duration of the first remission (Fig. 21.12). Progressive disease within 24 months of first line therapy (so called POD 24) is particularly high risk and second line immunochemotherapy with autologous stem cell transplantation maybe appropriate for some. Otherwise, R-CHOP, R-bendamustine and R-lenalidomide are frequently used. Where available and in

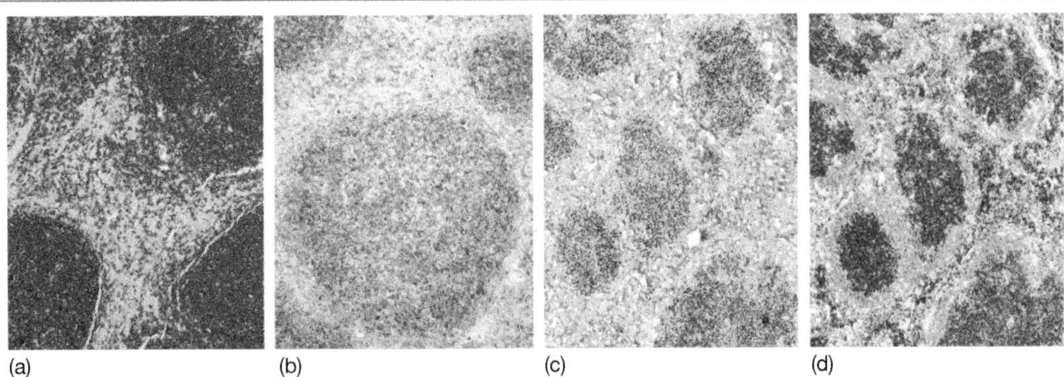

(a) (b) (c) (d)

Figure 21.11 Follicular lymphoma: immunostains. **(a)** The neoplastic cells are diffusely positive for B-cell markers (CD20). **(b)** The neoplastic cells are diffusely positive for CD10, a germinal centre marker, and are located in the follicular and interfollicular areas. **(c)** The neoplastic cells are positive for BCL6, a germinal centre marker. **(d)** The neoplastic cells are positive for BCL2.

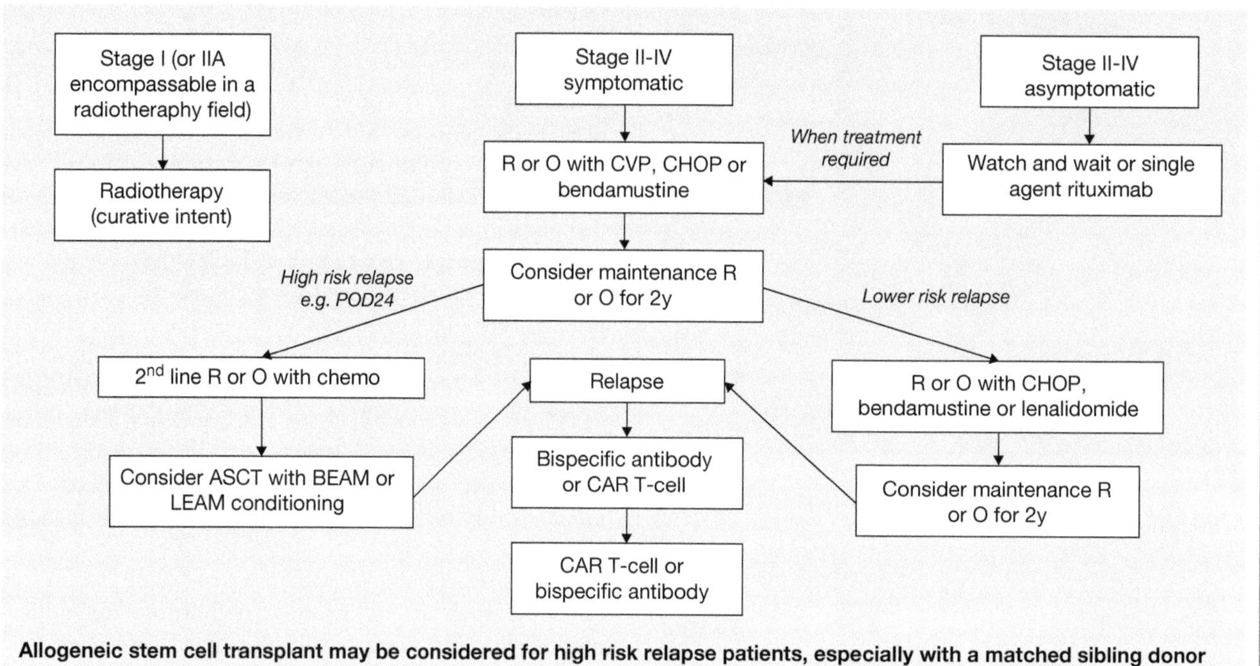

Figure 21.12 Algorithm for the treatment of follicular lymphoma. R: rituximab; O: obinutuzumab; CVP: cyclophosphamide, vincristine, prednisolone; CHOP: cyclophosphamide, doxorubicin, vincristine, prednisolone; POD24: progression of disease within 24 months of first line therapy; CAR T-cell: chimeric antigen receptor T-cell.

Table 21.2 A comparison of three prognostic indices for patients with follicular lymphoma.

Follicular Lymphoma IPI – 1 (1 point for each)	**Follicular Lymphoma IPI – 2 (1 point for each)**	**PRIMA-PI**
Age > 60 years	Age > 60 years	Bone marrow involvement
LDH > upper limit normal	Bone marrow involvement	Serum beta-2-micoglobulin
Haemoglobin < 120 g/L	Haemoglobin < 120 g/L	
Stage III or IV	Greatest diameter of largest involved node > 6 cm	
Number of nodal sites > 4	Serum beta-2-microglobulin > upper limit normal	
Score 0/1: low risk **Score 2:** intermediate risk **Score 3 or more:** high risk	**Score 0:** low risk **Score 1/2:** intermediate risk **Score 3 or more:** high risk	**Low risk:** clear marrow, β2M ≤ 3 mg/L **Intermediate risk:** involved marrow, β2M ≤ 3 mg/L **High risk:** β2M > 3 mg/L

ECOG, Eastern Cooperative Oncology Group; IPI, International prognostic index; LDH, Lactate dehydrogenase; PRIMA PI, Prognostic index developed from analysis of data from the PRIMA study.

suitable patients, subsequent relapses may be treated with anti-CD19 CAR T-cell therapy or with anti-CD20/-CD3 bispecific antibodies. Targeted oral agents may also be active, such as the EZH2 inhibitor tazemetostat.

Mantle cell lymphoma

Mantle cell lymphoma (MCL) is named after the mantle zone of secondary follicles which is composed of pre-germinal centre B-cells. However whilst some cases do appear to derive from naïve B-cells, others are antigen experienced. **WHO 2022**

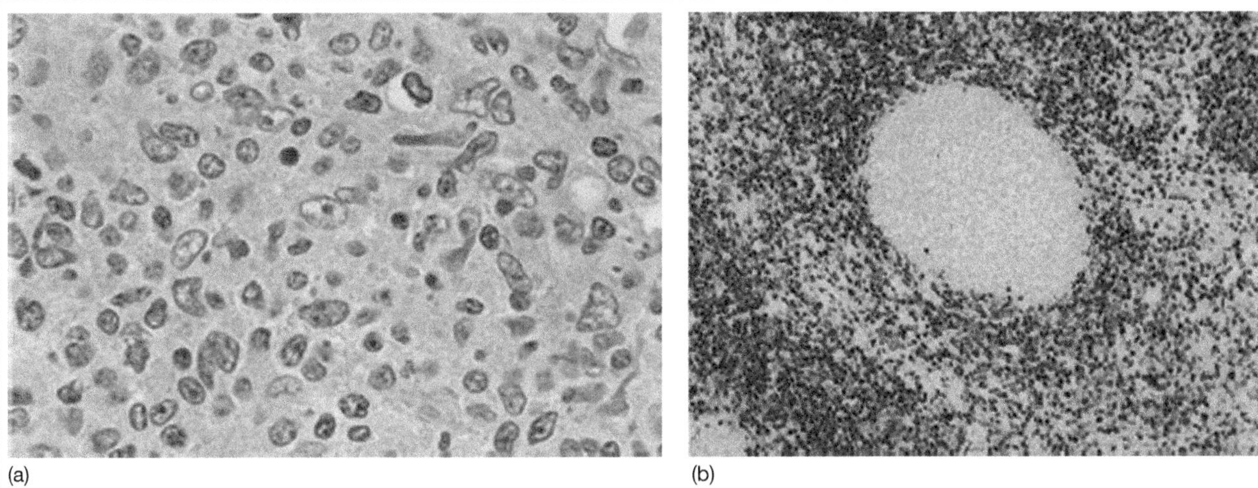

Figure 21.13 (a) Mantle cell lymphoma: showing characteristic deformed pattern of small lymphocytes with angular nuclei ('centrocytes'). **(b)** Mantle cell lymphoma: expression of cyclin D1 shown by immunohistochemistry. Source: A.V. Hoffbrand *et al*. (eds) (2016) *Postgraduate Haematology*, 7th edn. Reproduced with permission of John Wiley & Sons.

recognizes two major subtypes: one classical involving lymph nodes and extranodal sites characterized by expression of SOX11 and the other a leukaemic, non-nodal subtype typically SOX11 negative. The cells usually show angular nuclei in histological sections (Fig. 21.13a) and often circulate in the blood (Fig. 20.4). MCL has a characteristic phenotype of CD19$^+$ and CD5$^+$ (like CLL) but, in contrast to CLL, is CD22$^+$ and CD23$^-$. **A specific t(11;14) translocation juxtaposes the cyclin D1 gene *CCND1* to the immunoglobulin heavy-chain gene and leads to increased expression of cyclin D1 (Fig. 20.13b), which alters cell cycle behaviour.** Presence of this translocation is common but cycle D1 negative cases exist, some of which harbour translocations which involve the gene for cyclin D2. Other mutations are usually present (Table 20.6).

Clinical presentation of the classical type of MCL is with lymphadenopathy and the leukaemic type with blood, bone marrow and splenic disease. A Mantle Cell International Prognostic Index (MIPI), based on age, performance status, serum LDH and leucocyte count exists but generally does not guide treatment. The nodal disease tends to be more aggressive although indolent types are recognised. In addition to the MIPI, a worse prognosis is associated with high expression of Ki67 (marking out cells in the cell cycle) and with acquisition of additional genetic abnormalities such as *TP53* mutations.

For patients with asymptomatic disease, 'watch and wait' is a reasonable initial management (Fig. 21.14). When requiring treatment, fitter patients receive a high dose cytarabine protocol such as R-DHAP (dexamethasone, high dose cytarabine, cisplatin) or the 'Nordic' regimen which alternates R-CHOP with high dose cytarabine. Such patients are normally considered for ASCT in first remission followed by maintenance rituximab. For older patients, rituximab combined with CHOP, bendamustine or bendamustine combined with cytarabine (BAC), with consideration for maintenance rituximab can induce good remissions.

BTK inhibitors (BTKi) are highly active in mantle cell lymphoma and are frequently used at first relapse. Studies using these agents in the frontline setting also show benefit and may enable omission of ASCT if licensed and available in this setting. Subsequent relapses are preferably treated with anti-CD19 CAR T-cell therapy which has demonstrated significant activity even in very high risk disease. Whilst responses are good, relapse still remains a problem and it is unclear whether cure is possible.

Non-covalent BTK inhibitors may circumvent resistance seen with covalent inhibitors and pirtobrutinib is now licensed in the US for multiply relapsed mantle cell lymphoma treated with a covalent BTKi. Other agents under active investigation include venetoclax (a BCL-2 inhibitor), anti-CD3/CD20 bispecific antibodies and anti-ROR1 antibody-drug conjugates. Allogeneic stem cell transplantation is also option but usually reserved for those relapsing after CAR T-cell therapy.

With recent treatment developments, the prognosis for mantle cell lymphoma has been improving with typical life expectancy now of 8–10 years.

Marginal zone lymphomas

Marginal zone lymphomas are low-grade B-cell lymphomas that arise from the marginal zone of lymphoid follicles. It is thought that lymphoid hyperplasia initially occurs in response to antigen or inflammation and then cells acquire secondary genetic damage that leads to lymphoma. Cytogenetic analysis may reveal translocations involving the immunoglobulin loci and molecular tests show point mutations particularly involving the NF-κB pathway.

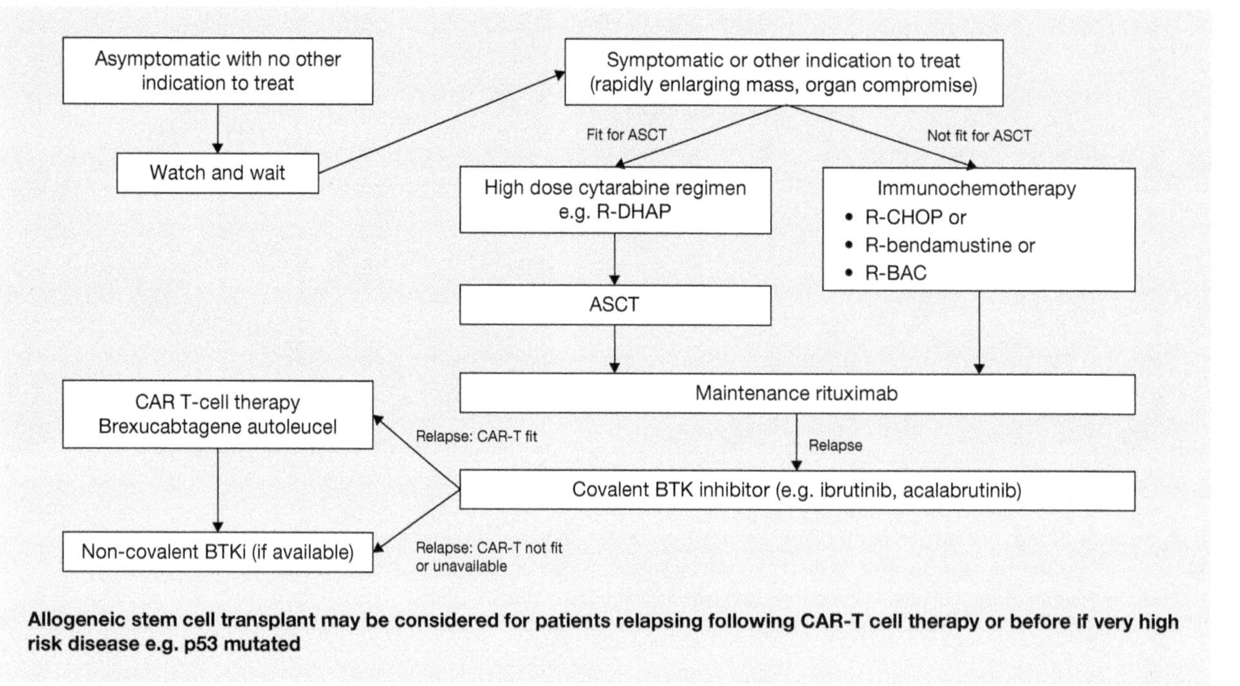

Figure 21.14 Algorithm for the treatment of mantle cell lymphoma. R-CHOP: rituximab, doxorubicin, vincristine, prednisolone; DHAP: dexamethasone, high dose cytarabine, cisplatin; R-BAC: rituximab, bendamustine, cytarabine; ASCT: autologous stem cell transplant; BTKi: Bruton's tyrosine kinase inhibitor; CAR T-cell: chimeric antigen receptor T-cell. Based on British Society for Haematology guideline on the management of mantle cell lymphoma, 2018 (addendum added 2022).

There are three broad types named according to according the anatomical site at which they arise:

- Extranodal marginal zone lymphoma of MALT type (Mucosa Associated Lymphoid Tissue)
- Splenic marginal zone lymphoma
- Nodal marginal zone lymphoma.

MALT lymphomas usually arise in the stomach (Fig. 21.15), respiratory tract, ocular adnexa, salivary glands, thyroid and skin. Gastric MALT lymphoma is the most common form and is preceded by *Helicobacter pylori* infection in many. In the early stages it may respond to antibiotic therapy aimed at eliminating *H. pylori*. Ocular adnexal lymphoma may result from *Chlamydia* infection, while Sjögren syndrome and Hashimoto thyroiditis underlie MALT lymphomas of salivary glands and thyroid. Primary cutaneous marginal zone lymphoma is regarded as a separate entity. Though there are common cytogenetic changes such as trisomy 3 or 18, the cytogenetic and molecular genetic changes generally differ between MALT lymphomas at different sites and from those of nodal MZL.

Splenic marginal zone lymphoma usually presents as splenomegaly and may be associated with circulating 'villous' lymphocytes that may be mistaken for hairy cells. 'Watch and wait' is appropriate if asymptomatic. If systemic therapy is needed, single agent rituximab is frequently used, or regimens used in other low-grade lymphomas such as follicular lymphoma. Splenectomy maybe also useful for symptomatic patients.

Lymphoplasmacytoid lymphoma (Waldenström macroglobulinaemia)

This is an uncommon condition, seen most frequently in men over 50 years of age. A monoclonal immunoglobulin (Ig) M paraprotein is usually present in plasma and the combination of an underlying lymphoplasmacytoid lymphoma (LPL) with an IgM paraprotein is termed Waldenström macroglobulinaemia (WM). The cell of origin is a post-germinal centre B cell with the characteristics of an IgM-bearing memory B cell.

LPL or its precursor, IgM monoclonal gammopathy of undetermined significance (MGUS, Chapter 22.), may be diagnosed by chance in symptomless patients. The disease usually presents clinically with an insidious onset, often with fatigue and weight loss. Hyperviscosity syndrome is a common complication as the IgM paraprotein increases blood viscosity more than equivalent concentrations of IgG or IgA. Symptoms include visual disturbance with associated retinal changes, such as engorged veins, haemorrhages, exudates and a blurred optic disk (Fig. 22.15). If the macroglobulin is a cryoglobulin, features of cryoprecipitation, such as Raynaud phenomenon, may be present.

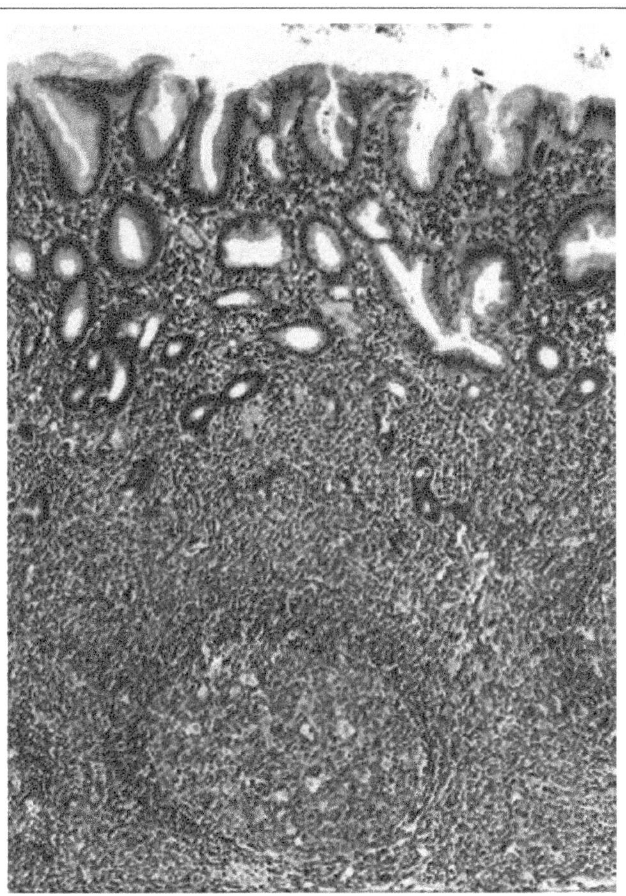

Figure 21.15 Gastric mucosa-associated lymphoid tissue (MALT) lymphoma: the tumour cells surround reactive follicles and infiltrate the mucosa. Lympho-epithelial lesions are characteristic, whereby epithelial structures are distorted by the infiltration of neoplastic B-cells. Source: Courtesy of Professor P. Isaacson.

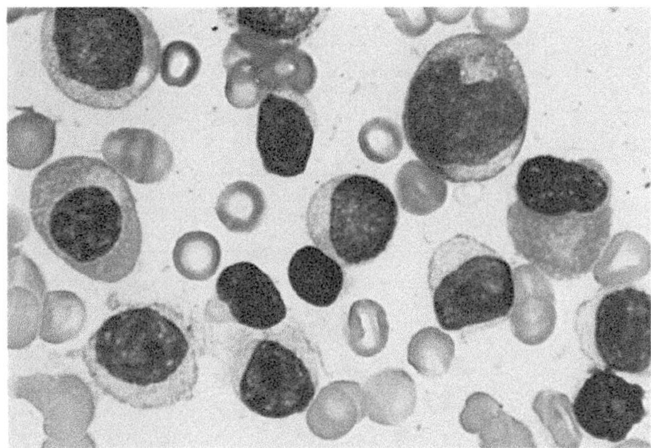

Figure 21.16 Lymphoplasmacytoid lymphoma associated with Waldenström macroglobulinaemia. Bone marrow shows cells with features of lymphocytes and plasma cells.

Anaemia is usually a significant problem and a bleeding tendency may result from interference with coagulation factors and platelet function by the paraprotein. Iron deficiency is often contributory and should be corrected. Neurological symptoms, dyspnoea and heart failure may also be presenting symptoms. Whilst moderate lymphadenopathy and enlargement of the liver and spleen are seen, often the bone marrow is the only involved site. Less common but important complications also include AL amyloidosis and peripheral neuropathy (often in association with anti-MAG (myelin associated glycoprotein) antibodies).

Diagnosis is made by the finding of a monoclonal serum IgM together with bone marrow or lymph node infiltration with lymphoplasmacytoid cells (Fig. 21.16). Sequential measurement of the IgM paraprotein (or total IgM) is helpful as a disease marker and response assessment. **Mutation of *MYD88* is present in nearly all cases and is very helpful diagnostically**. About 30% of patients have *CXCR4* mutations, almost all also with the *MYD88* mutation. These patients tend to have more cytopenias and more extensive disease although routine testing for *CXCR4* mutations is not recommended. Mutation of *TP53* is seen in approximately 10% of patients at diagnosis and is associated with worse outcome. The erythrocyte sedimentation rate is raised and there may be peripheral blood lymphocytosis.

Treatment

No treatment is required for patients without symptoms, but treatment should be started if there are features such as symptomatic organomegaly, symptomatic anaemia, hyperviscosity or other complications such as amyloid or neuropathy (Fig. 21.17. Combination therapy with an anti-CD20 antibody such as rituximab and chemotherapy is generally given. If rituximab is given, the IgM level may transiently rise ('flare'), which can cause hyperviscosity. Omission of rituximab with the first (or more) cycle, or prophylactic plasma exchange may be needed initially. Chemotherapy options include cyclophosphamide, bendamustine, chlorambucil or bortezomib. Chemotherapy choice is dictated partly by patient age and fitness, e.g. DRC – dexamethasone, rituximab and cyclophosphamide – or chlorambucil are suitable for older, frailer patients, and the need for a rapid reduction in paraprotein, e.g. bendamustine or bortezomib combinations are often used for symptomatic hyperviscosity. BTK inhibitors such as ibrutinib and zanubrutinib are effective in cases refractory to other drugs. They are licensed for use in Europe for second and subsequent lines as well as for first line therapy for those not deemed suitable for immunochemotherapy. If BTK inhibitors are available first line, rituximab is usually also used although the benefit of using this in combination with a BTK inhibitor in this setting is unclear. Treatment of relapsed disease is usually with a BTK inhibitor unless used first line. The role of autologous (and indeed allogeneic) stem cell transplantation is

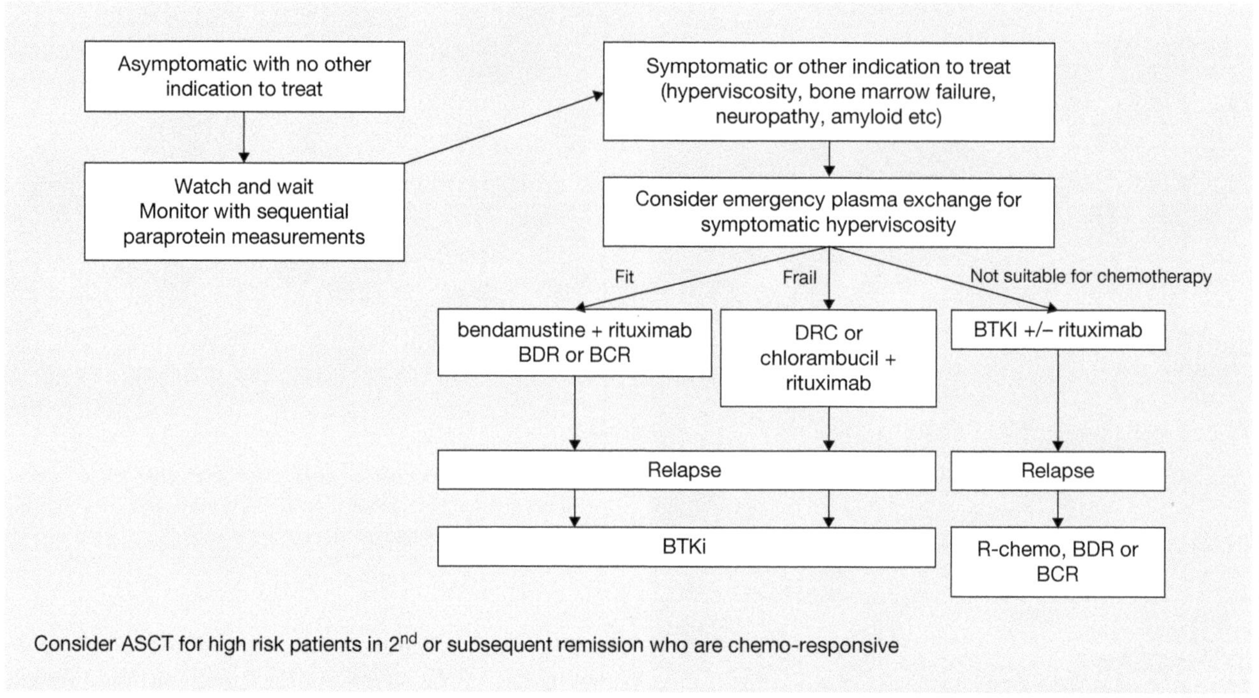

Figure 21.17 Treatment algorithm for the treatment of lymphoplasmacytic lymphoma. Based on the British Society of Haematology Guidelines (2022) *Br. J. Haematol.* 197: 171–87. ASCT, autologous stem cell transplantation; BCR, bortezomib, cyclophosphamide, rituximab; BDR, bortezomib, dexamethasone, rituximab; BTKi, Bruton's tyrosine kinase inhibitor; DRC, dexamethasone, cyclophosphamide, rituximab; R-chemo, rituximab with chemotherapy.

contentious in the era of targeted agents but may be considered in high risk patients. See Fig. 21.17 for treatment algorithm.

Acute hyperviscosity syndrome (p. 300) is treated with repeated plasmapheresis until the underlying disease can be brought under control. As IgM is mainly present in the intravascular space, plasmapheresis is more effective than for IgG or IgA paraproteins, where much of the protein is extravascular and so rapidly replenishes the plasma compartment after plasmapheresis.

Small lymphocytic lymphoma

This term is used for cases with the same morphology and immunophenotype as B-CLL, but with less than 5×10^9/L peripheral blood B cells and no cytopenias due to bone marrow involvement. Lymphadenopathy is typical. Treatment is as for patients with B-CLL (Chapter 18).

T-cell lymphomas

T-cell lymphomas are a heterogeneous group of tumours that present with lymphadenopathy or with extranodal disease. They comprise about 10–15% of NHL in Western countries, but more in Asia, and are usually of CD4$^+$ phenotype. Several variants of T-cell lymphomas exist (Fig. 21.18). Clinically they are best categorized as cutaneous (which includes mycosis fungoides and Sézary syndrome) and peripheral (or systemic).

Cutaneous T-cell lymphomas

Mycosis fungoides

Mycosis fungoides is a chronic cutaneous T-cell lymphoma that presents with severe pruritus and psoriasis-like eczematoid skin lesions that can later become plaques and ulcerated tumours (Fig. 21.19). In contrast to Sézary syndrome, tumour cells do not circulate in the blood. It is relatively indolent at first and early stage disease is associated with a good prognosis. However deeper organs may become affected, particularly lymph nodes, spleen, liver and bone marrow. Treatment is initially often skin directed, e.g. phototherapy or topical creams. More difficult disease may require systemic treatment such as with bexarotene (a retinoid), oral methotrexate, or brentuximab vedotin if CD30 positive. Other agents such as histone deacetylase inhibitors are active but access is limited.

Sézary syndrome

In Sézary syndrome, there is dermatitis and generalized erythroderma, but also lymphadenopathy and circulating T-lymphoma cells. The cells are usually CD4$^+$ and have a folded or cerebriform nuclear chromatin (Fig. 21.20).

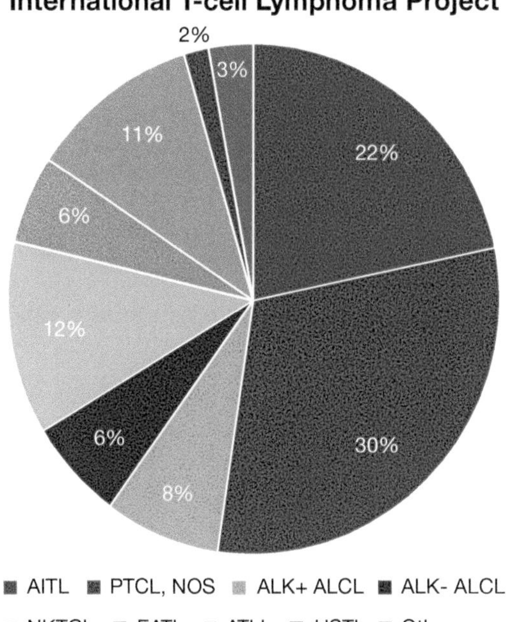

Figure 21.18 The relative frequencies of T-cell non-Hodgkin lymphomas subtypes based on the WHO 2018 classification. AITL, angioimmunoblastic T-cell lymphoma; ALCL, anaplastic large cell lymphoma; ALK+ or ALK−, anaplastic lymphoma tyrosine kinase + or −; ATLL, adult T-cell leukaemia/lymphoma; EATL, enteropathy-associated T-cell lymphoma; HSTL, hepatosplenic T-cell lymphoma; NKTCL, natural killer/T-cell lymphoma; NOS, not otherwise specified; PTCL, peripheral T-cell lymphoma. Source: N. Schmitz *et al.* (2018) *Blood* 132: 246.

Treatment is often with ECP (extracorporeal photopheresis whereby white cells are separated from the blood, exposed to a psoralen and UV light and then returned to the body) often in combination with a systemic therapy such as bexarotene. The anti-CCR4 monoclonal antibody mogamulizumab can also be effective in this condition.

Peripheral T-cell lymphoma (PTCL)

The 2022 version of the WHO classification recognizes that several subtypes of PTCL are derived from the follicular T-helper cell which normally gives help to developing B-cells in the germinal centre. This led to the 'nodal T-follicular helper cell lymphoma' category, the most common subtype of which is angioimmunoblastic lymphoma. The other common subtype is so-called 'peripheral T-cell lymphoma, not otherwise specified'.

Nodal T-follicular helper cell lymphoma

The angioimmunoblastic-subtype is the most frequent diagnosed. It has characteristic features due to cytokine secretion by the malignant cells and effects on surrounding germinal centre structures. Pathologically there is an expansion of the dendritic cell meshwork, proliferation of high endothelial venules, large blastic B cells (immunoblasts) which are frequently positive for EBV and a proliferation of malignant small to medium sized T-cells with a characteristic phenotype (positive for CD10, CXCL13, PDL1, BCL6 and ICOS). These lymphomas frequently harbour mutations in epigenetic modifying genes such as *TET2, DNMT3A* and/or *IDH2.* Clinically patients are typically older and present with small volume lymphadenopathy, rash, joint pains, autoimmune haematological

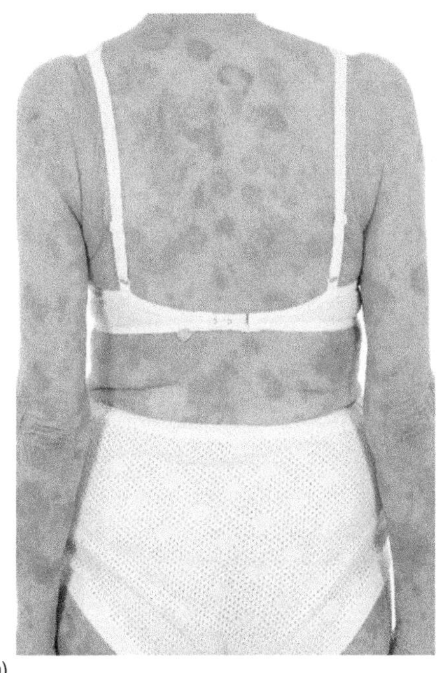
(a)

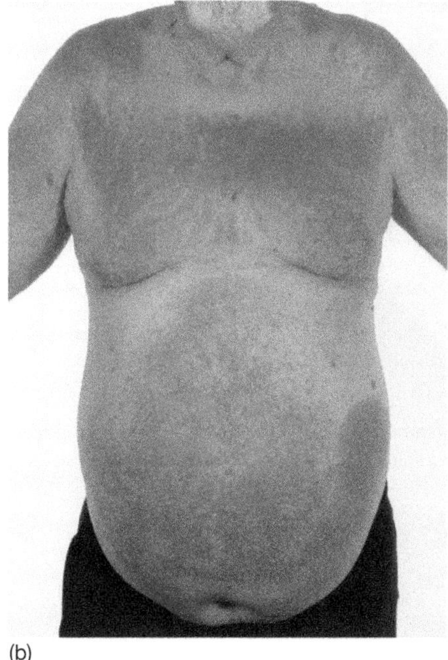
(b)

Figure 21.19 Mycosis fungoides (MF). **(a)** Patch stage MF with annular, scaly, well defined patches and **(b)** erythrodermic MF with morbilliform appearance. Source: Pictures provided by Dr Rubeta Matin, Department of Dermatology, Oxford University Hospitals.

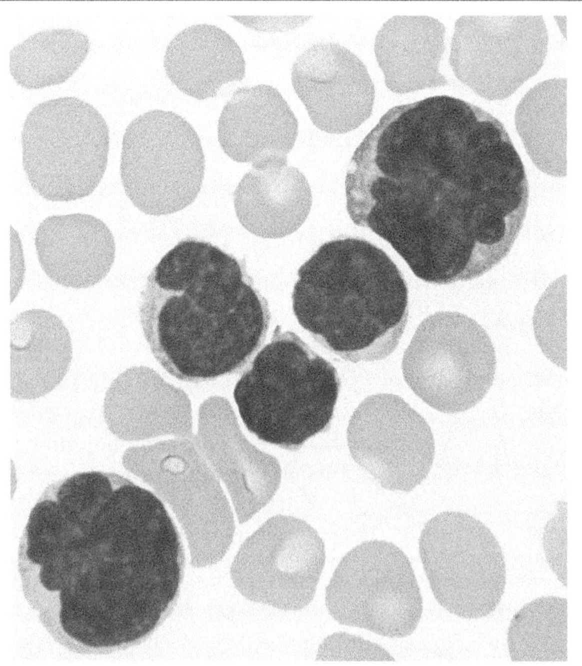

Figure 21.20 Sézary syndrome. Abnormal cells in the peripheral blood have a cerebriform, clefted nucleus, fine chromatin and scanty cytoplasm. Source: A.V. Hoffbrand *et al.* (2019) *Color Atlas of Clinical Hematology*, 5th edn. Reproduced with permission of John Wiley & Sons.

manifestations (haemolytic anaemia or ITP) and hypergammaglobulinaemia. A well recognized but uncommon feature is the development of a synchronous large B-cell lymphoma. Treatment is similar to PTCL-NOS (see below and Fig. 21.21). For relapsed disease, a number of agents show activity but none have yet secured a license in Europe. These include histone deacetylase inhibitors, PI3 kinase inhibitors and demethylating agents such as 5-azacytidine.

Peripheral T-cell non-Hodgkin lymphoma, not otherwise specified

These derive from T cells at various stages of differentiation. Gene expression profiling has identified two subgroups, those associated with high levels of GATA3 expression and those associated with high levels of TBX2 expression and a cytotoxic phenotype. The latter type is associated with a worse prognosis. They are treated with combination chemotherapy (e.g. CHOP; see Fig. 21.21). The addition of etoposide (CHOEP) is controversial. Brentuixmab vedotin combined with CHP is licensed for CD30 expressing non-ALCL subtypes of T-cell lymphoma in the US but not in Europe due to the pivotal study not being powered to show a benefit in these subtypes. The prognosis is poor. Autografting for patients with chemosensitive disease is often performed although the evidence base for this is poor. CAR T-cells are in development for T-cell lymphomas, but

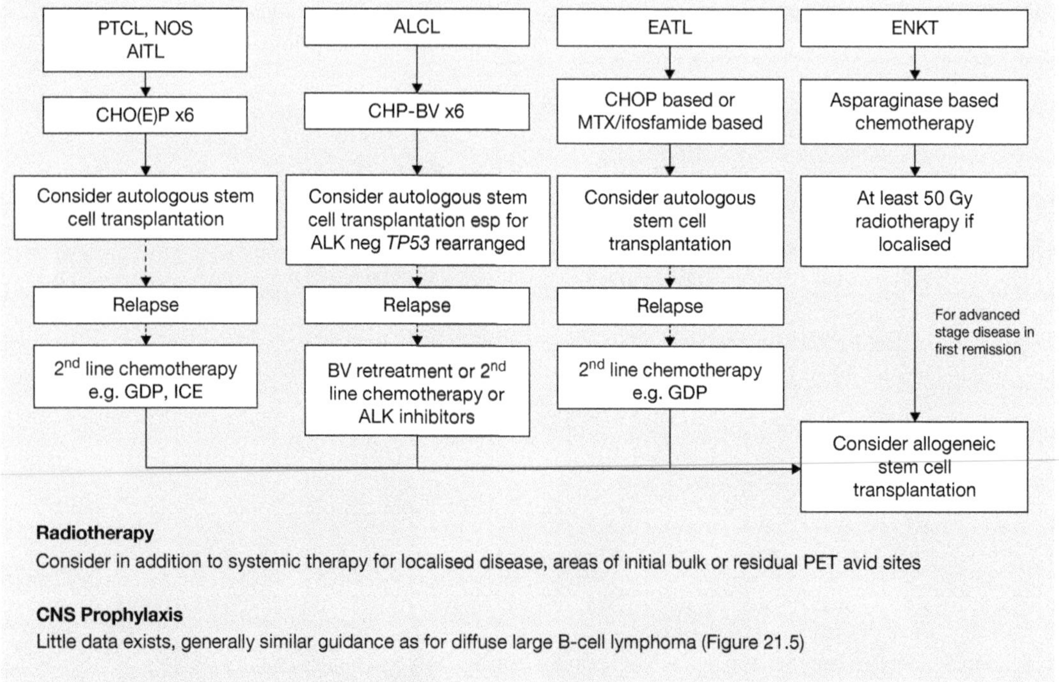

Figure 21.21 Algorithm for the treatment of the more common subtypes of peripheral T-cell Lymphoma (PTCL). ALCL, anaplastic large cell lymphoma; ALK, anaplastic lymphoma kinase; BV, brentuximab vedotin; CHOP, cyclophosphamide, doxorubicin, vincristine, prednisolone; E, etoposide; EATL, enteropathy associated T-cell lymphoma; ENKT, extranodal NK/T-cell lymphoma; GDP, gemcitabine, dexamethasone, cisplatin; ICE, ifosfamide, carboplatin, etoposide; MTX, methotrexate; PTCL, NOS: peripheral T-cell lymphoma, not otherwise specified.

difficulty distinguishing between CAR-T cells, endogenous T cells and neoplastic T cells poses a challenge for this technology.

Anaplastic large cell lymphoma

There are two forms of anaplastic large cell lymphoma: ALK positive (relatively common in children, associated with t(2;5) and generally associated with a good prognosis); and ALK negative (commoner in older people and associated with a worse prognosis). The disease is usually strongly $CD30^{+}$. Genetic studies have shown that ALK negative cases may harbour a disruption of the *TP53* gene associated with a poor prognosis and of the *DUSP22* gene associated with a more favourable prognosis. It has an aggressive course, characterized by systemic symptoms and extranodal involvement. The anti-CD30 antibody drug conjugate brentuximab vedotin (BV) is highly active and a large trial showed overall survival benefit for BV combined with CHP versus CHOP chemotherapy alone. CHP-BV is licensed and used in many countries. For relapsed disease, BV retreatment maybe effective and in ALK positive cases, oral ALK inhibitors are extremely active. A specific subtype of ALCL is breast implant-associated ALCL. This may be seen in patients with textured breast implants and often presents with implant associated effusions, with cytology showing the presence of ALCL cells in the fluid. Treatment is usually removal of the breast implant and associated capsule.

Intestinal T-cell lymphomas

A number of uncommon intestinal T-cell lymphoma are described. Enteropathy-associated T-cell lymphoma (EATL) is associated with gluten-induced enteropathy (coeliac disease). A similar condition in the absence of an underlying enteropathy is termed monomorphic epitheliotropic intestinal T-cell lymphoma (MEITL). Both conditions are difficult to treat, with patients often presenting malnourished and with intestinal perforation. Treatment is outlined in Fig. 21.21. CHOP chemotherapy is frequently used although an alternative regimen based on methotrexate and ifosfamide is also effective.

Extranodal NK/T cell lymphoma

This is a subtype of EBV positive NK/T-cell lymphomas, mainly occurring in Asia and Central and South America. It is associated with EBV infection and usually affects the nose ('nasal-type') (Fig 21.22) The peak age is around 50 years. The disease causes local destruction although it can occur with disseminated disease where it frequently affects extranodal sites such as skin and can be associated with haemophagocytic lymphohistiocytosis (HLH) (Chapter 8) Systemic treatment has improved with the incorporation of asparaginase. For localized disease, high doses of radiotherapy (at least 50 Gy) are essential to maximize the chance of cure. For advanced disease, allogeneic stem cell transplantation in first remission is considered (Fig. 21.21).

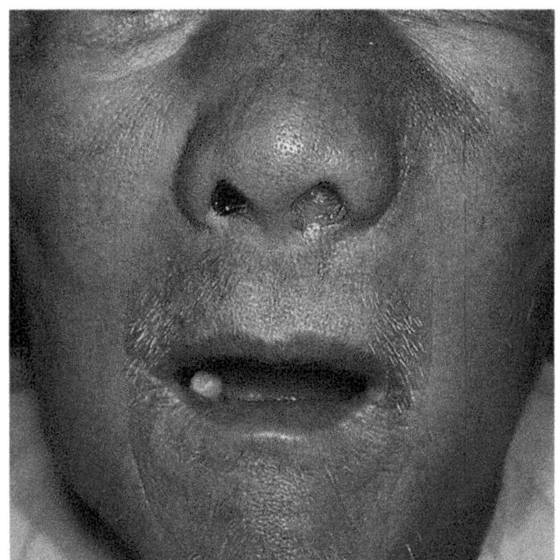

Figure 21.22 T/NK nasal type lymphoma. Mid-line nasal swelling. Source: A.V. Hoffbrand *et al.* (2019) *Color Atlas of Clinical Hematology*, 5th edn. Reproduced with permission of John Wiley & Sons.

Adult T-cell leukaemia/lymphoma

This is associated with human T-cell lymphotrophic virus type 1 (HTLV-1) infection (Chapter 18).

Histiocytic and dendritic cell neoplasms

These rare diseases including dendritic and macrophage-derived sarcomas, which may be localized or disseminated, are discussed in Chapter 8 They usually present as tumours at extranodal sites, especially the intestinal tract, skin and soft tissues. Systemic symptoms are present.

Tumour-like lesions with B-cell predominance

Castleman disease

This is a rare lymphoproliferative disease that occurs in three distinctive sub-types which may progress to a B-cell lymphoma. It occurs in unicentric and idiopathic multicentric (which is usually associated with systemic symptoms) forms, most frequently affecting thoracic or abdominal nodes. In the third sub-type the KSHV/HHV8 associated multicentric form, most common in subjects with HIV infection, the cells contain the human herpesvirus-8 (HHV8). Microscopically the localized form usually shows a hyaline vascular appearance, and the multicentric form usually shows proliferation of plasma cells. Mixed and plasmablastic forms also occur. The localized form may be treated by surgery, the multicentric form by corticosteroids, chemotherapy or immunotherapy with rituximab, siltuximab (an anti-IL6 monoclonal antibody) and other systemic agents such as thalidomide.

SUMMARY

- Non-Hodgkin lymphomas are a large group of clonal lymphoid neoplasms. Approximately 85–90% are of B-cell origin and 10–15% derive from T or NK cells.
- Their clinical presentation and natural history are more variable than Hodgkin lymphoma and can range from a very indolent disease to rapidly progressive subtypes that need urgent treatment.
- The NHLs are divided into high-grade and low-grade disease. Low-grade disorders are typically slowly progressive, respond well to chemotherapy, but are difficult to cure, whereas high-grade lymphomas are aggressive and need urgent treatment, but are more often curable.
- Some of the more common subtypes are:
  - *Diffuse large B-cell lymphoma* is a common subtype and is an aggressive disease which needs urgent treatment. There is a wide variety of subtypes. Over 60-70% of patients are cured with first line rituximab and chemotherapy.
  - *Burkitt lymphoma* is one of the most highly proliferative subtypes of neoplasm. Endemic cases in Africa are associated with EBV infection. Treatment is with aggressive immunochemotherapy regimens.
  - *Follicular lymphoma* represents 25% of all NHL and is associated with the t(14;18) translocation. Treatment usually achieves disease remission, although cure is generally only achieved in early stage disease with radiotherapy or in later stage with allogeneic stem cell transplantation.
  - *Mantle cell lymphoma* is associated with increased expression of the cyclin D1 gene and has clinical features of an 'intermediate grade' lymphoma with nodal and leukaemic subtypes.
  - *Marginal zone lymphomas* arise from marginal zone B cells of lymphoid follicles and can occur as mucosa associated (MALT) lymphoma, most frequent in the stomach.
  - *Lymphoplasmacytic lymphoma* usually produces an IgM paraprotein, when it is also known as Waldenström macroglobulinaemia, and often leads to anaemia and hyperviscosity.
  - *Small lymphocytic lymphoma* is the lymphoma equivalent of chronic lymphocytic leukaemia.
- T-cell lymphomas are less common and include cutaneous forms, e.g. *mycosis fungoides*, and systemic forms, e.g. *angioimmunoblastic T-cell lymphoma* and *anaplastic large cell lymphoma*.
- Treatments for NHL are based on a variety of chemotherapy regimens. Anti-CD20 antibodies are used in most cases of B-cell lymphomas and have markedly improved the prognosis. Antibody-drug conjugates are entering front-line regimens and targeted agents such as BTK inhibitors are used frequently in relapsed disease. CAR T-cells directed against CD19 are being increasingly used for relapsed/refractory patients.

Now visit **www.wiley.com/go/haematology9e** to test yourself on this chapter.

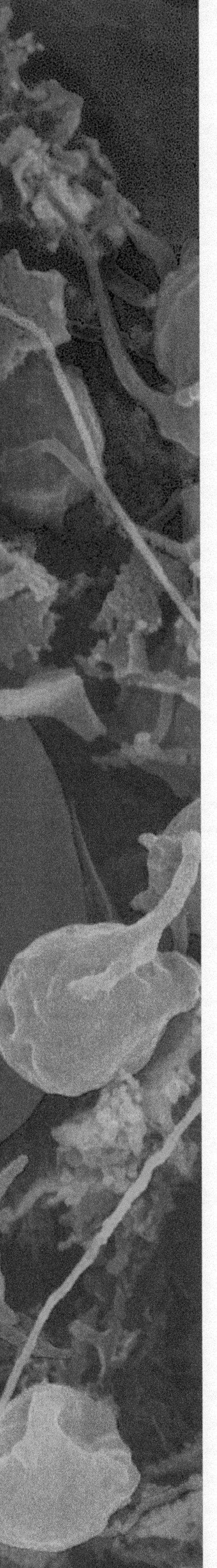

CHAPTER 22

Multiple myeloma and related plasma cell neoplasms

Key topics

Hoffbrand's Essential Haematology, Ninth Edition. A. Victor Hoffbrand, Pratima Chowdary, Graham P. Collins, and Justin Loke.

© 2024 John Wiley & Sons Ltd. Published 2024 by John Wiley & Sons Ltd.

Companion website: www.wiley.com/go/haematology9e

Paraproteinaemia

Normally, serum immunoglobulins are polyclonal, representing the combined output from billions of different plasma cells making antibodies with diverse antigen specificities. **A monoclonal immunoglobulin band (M-protein), or paraprotein, reflects the synthesis of an identical immunoglobulin from a single clone of plasma cells (Fig. 22.1). When a monoclonal immunoglobulin is detected in the blood, it is called paraproteinaemia.** The paraprotein may be the product of a primary (clonal) neoplastic disease of plasma cells, or be secondary to an underlying benign or neoplastic disease affecting other parts of the immune system (Table 22.1).

Usually the monoclonal protein produced by a plasma cell neoplasm is an intact immunoglobulin, but in some cases clonal plasma cells produce only a light chain or heavy chain. A **free light chain** is an immunoglobulin light chain circulating in plasma in an unbound state; it may be excreted in the urine.

Multiple myeloma

Multiple myeloma, also termed myeloma or plasma cell myeloma, is a neoplastic disease characterized by plasma cell accumulation in the bone marrow (Fig. 22.2), the presence of a monoclonal protein in the serum or urine or both and, in symptomatic patients, related tissue damage (Table 22.2, Fig. 22.3). Other plasma cell neoplasms are listed in Table 22.3.

Almost all cases of myeloma occur over the age of 40 years, with a peak incidence between 65 and 70 years. The disease is twice as common in individuals of African compared to those of European or Asian origin.

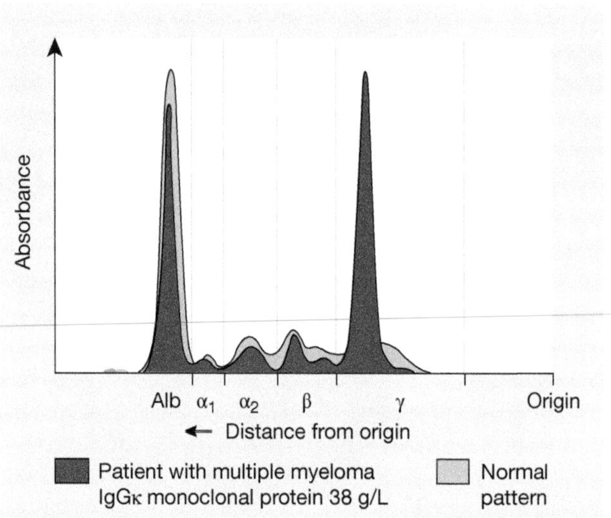

Figure 22.1 Serum protein electrophoresis in multiple myeloma showing an abnormal paraprotein in the γ-globulin region with reduced levels of background β- and γ-globulins.

Table 22.1 Diseases associated with monoclonal immunoglobulins.

Neoplastic
Multiple myeloma
Solitary plasmacytoma
Monoclonal gammopathy of undetermined significance (MGUS)
Osteosclerotic myeloma and POEMS (polyneuropathy, organomegaly, endocrinopathy, monoclonal protein, skin changes) syndrome
Monoclonal gammopathy of renal significance
Waldenström macroglobulinaemia
Non-Hodgkin lymphoma
Chronic lymphocytic leukaemia
Primary (light-chain, AL) amyloidosis
Heavy-chain disease
Cryoglobulinaemia (some forms may have polyclonal immunoglobulins, or a mixture of polyclonal and monoclonal)
Non-neoplastic
Chronic cold haemagglutinin disease
Transient, e.g. with infections
HIV infection
Gaucher disease

Pathogenesis

The myeloma neoplastic cell is a post-germinal centre plasma cell that has undergone immunoglobulin class switching and somatic hypermutation and secretes the paraprotein that is present in serum. Normal plasma cells are located primarily within the haemopoietic bone marrow, and this feature is retained by the neoplastic cell.

Myeloma neoplastic cells contain an average of 35 somatic mutations at the time of diagnosis, more than the median number of mutations for leukaemias (Fig. 11.3). Immunoglobulin heavy and light chain genes are clonally rearranged, with translocations involving the heavy chain on chromosome 14q being the most frequent. Neoplastic cells accumulate complex genetic changes, with chromosomal aneuploidy present in almost all cases. Dysregulated or increased expression of the cyclin D1, D2 or D3 genes, either directly through translocations or indirectly via mutations, is an early unifying genetic event. Later genetic events include secondary translocations, e.g. of *MYC*; point mutations, e.g. of *RAS* or *TP53*; deletions, e.g. of *TP53*; or epigenetic abnormalities.

Analysis of stored serum samples has shown that almost all cases of myeloma develop from a pre-existing monoclonal gammopathy of undetermined significance (MGUS), described further below (Table 22.2; Fig. 22.3). Like myeloma, MGUS is also more common in persons of African descent. Most of the early plasma cell genetic changes characteristic of myeloma are present at the MGUS stage, but the size of the clone is considerably smaller (Fig. 22.3).

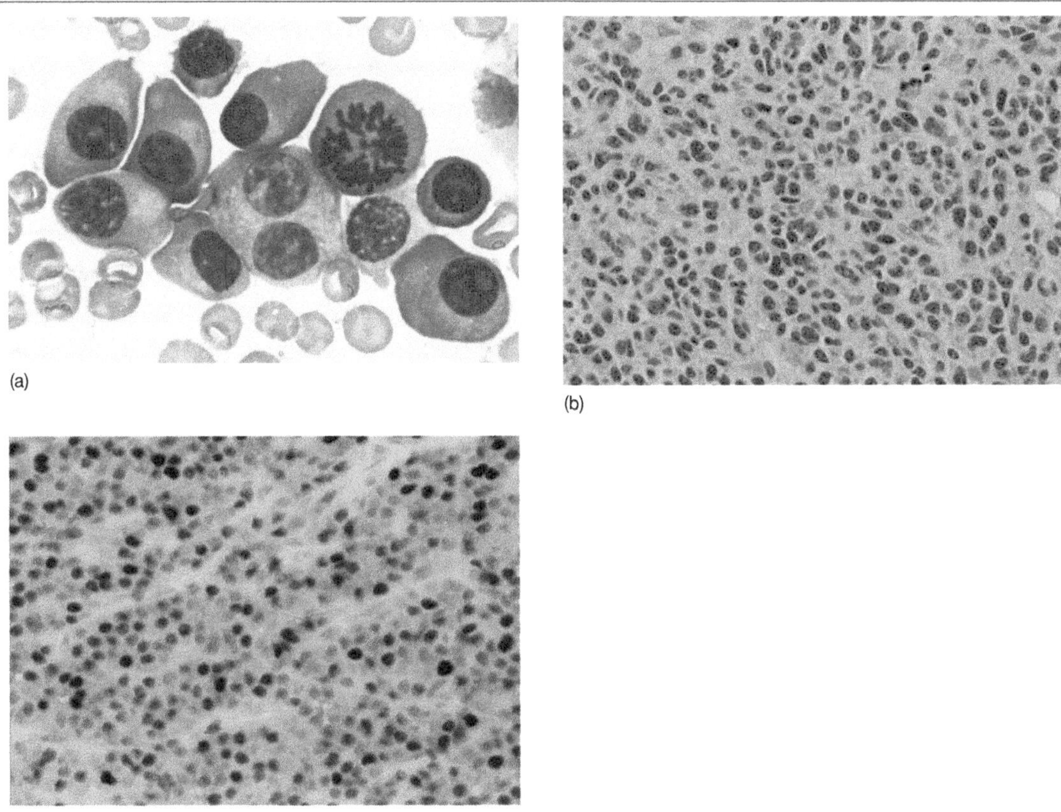

Figure 22.2 **(a)** The bone marrow in multiple myeloma showing large numbers of plasma cells, with many abnormal forms. **(b)** Low-power view showing sheets of plasma cells replacing normal haemopoietic tissue. **(c)** Immunohistochemical staining of the bone marrow in myeloma with antibody to CD138 revealing extensive numbers of plasma cells.

Table 22.2 The clinical and laboratory features of monoclonal gammopathy of uncertain significance (MGUS), smouldering myeloma and symptomatic myeloma.

	MGUS	**Asymptomatic (smouldering) myeloma**	**Symptomatic myeloma**	
Marrow plasma cells	<10%	≥10%	≥10%	
Paraprotein	<30 g/L	≥30 g/L	≥30 g/L	
Normal immunoglobulins	Normal	Reduced	Reduced	
Free light chain ratio	Normal or abnormal	Abnormal	Abnormal	
Clinical features	Usually none (see p. xxx)	None	Hyper**c**alcaemia	C
			Renal failure	R
			Anaemia	A
			Bone lesions	B*
Progression to symptomatic multiple myeloma	1%/year	10%/year	N/A	

* Magnetic resonance imaging (MRI) or positron emission tomography (PET) scan needed to exclude bone lesions, especially of the spine, which may not be detected on plain radiographs. Other clinical features include amyloid, hyperviscosity, recurrent infections, peripheral neuropathy and deep vein thrombosis.

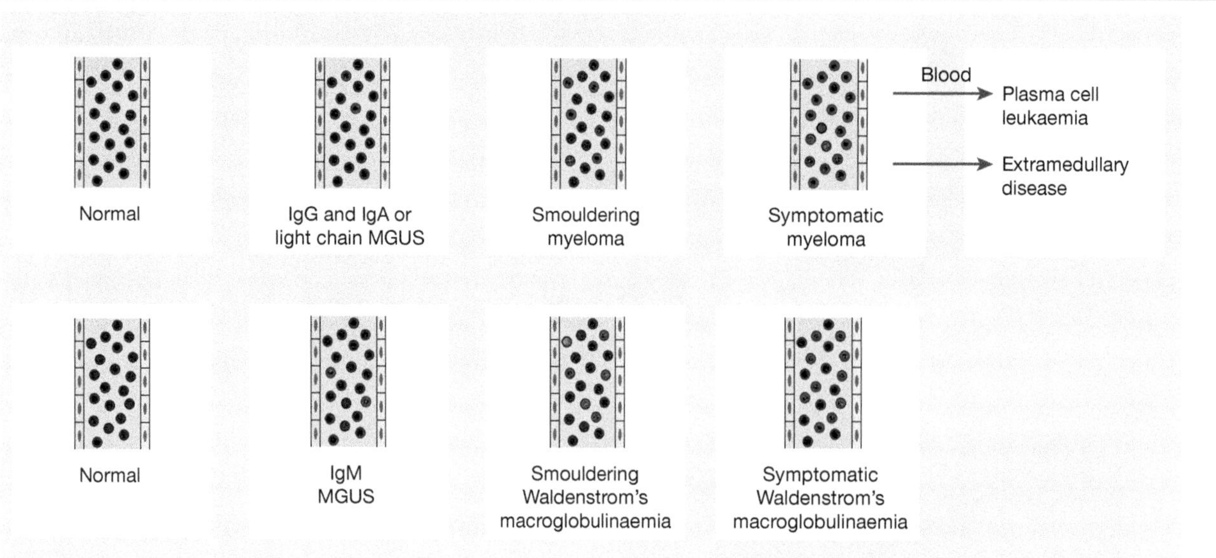

Figure 22.3 The degree of involvement of bone marrow by clonal neoplastic cells in: **(a)** monoclonal gammopathy of undetermined significance (MGUS), asymptomatic and symptomatic myeloma and plasma cell leukaemia associated with a serum immunoglobin (Ig) G or IgA paraprotein; **(b)** MGUS and Waldenström's macroglobulinaemia (lymphoplasmacytic lymphoma) associated with a serum IgM paraprotein.

Table 22.3 Plasma cell neoplasms.

IgM Monoclonal gammopathy of undetermined significance (MGUS) Non-IgM monoclonal gammopathy of undetermined significance (MGUS)
Monoclonal gammopathy of renal significance (MGRS) Plasma cell myeloma *Variants:* Asymptomatic (smouldering) myeloma Non-secretory myeloma Plasma cell leukaemia
Plasmacytoma: Solitary plasmacytoma of bone Extraosseous (extramedullary) plasmacytoma Monoclonal immunoglobulin deposition diseases Heavy chain deposition diseases (μ heavy-chain disease, γ heavy-chain disease, α heavy-chain disease)
Ig, immunoglobin. Source: World Health Organization (2022).

Myeloma cells adhere to bone marrow stromal cells and extracellular matrix through a variety of adhesion molecules. This inhibits their apoptosis and stimulates a cascade of cytokine release. Osteolytic lesions are caused by osteoclast activation resulting from high serum levels of receptor activator of nuclear factor-κB (NF-κB) ligand (RANKL), produced by plasma cells and bone marrow stroma, which binds to activating RANK receptors on the osteoclast surface.

Diagnosis

Symptomatic myeloma is diagnosed if there is:

1 Monoclonal protein in serum, urine or both (Fig. 22.1);
2 Increased clonal plasma cells in the bone marrow (Fig. 22.2); and
3 Disease-related organ or tissue impairment.

A useful acronym for myeloma-associated tissue damage is CRAB (hypercalcaemia, renal impairment, anaemia, bone disease; Table 22.2). Amyloidosis, serum hyperviscosity, recurrent infections, peripheral neuropathy and deep vein thrombosis are other clinical complications of myeloma, which are less frequently presenting features (Fig. 22.4).

Clinical features

1 **Bone pain** (especially backache) resulting from vertebral collapse and pathological fractures (Fig. 22.5).
2 Features of **anaemia**, such as lethargy or dyspnoea.
3 **Recurrent infections** related to deficient antibody production, abnormal cell-mediated immunity and neutropenia.
4 Features of **renal failure** or hypercalcaemia: polydipsia, polyuria, anorexia, vomiting, constipation and mental disturbance.
5 Abnormal **bleeding** tendency: myeloma protein may interfere with platelet function and coagulation factors; thrombocytopenia occurs in advanced disease.
6 **Amyloidosis** (light chain) occurs in 5% with features such as macroglossia, carpal tunnel syndrome, heart failure, periorbital purpura and diarrhoea (Chapter 23).

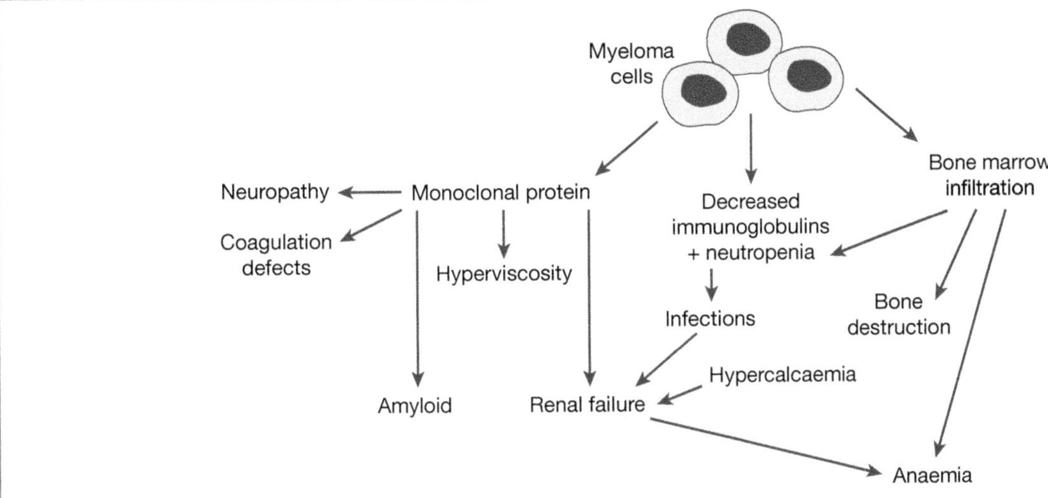

Figure 22.4 The pathogenesis of the clinical features of myeloma.

7 In approximately 2% of cases there is a **hyperviscosity syndrome**, with purpura, haemorrhages, visual changes and central nervous system (CNS) symptoms (see below).

Laboratory diagnosis

1 **Presence of a paraprotein.** Serum and urine protein electrophoresis should be performed. The paraprotein is immunoglobulin (Ig) G in 60% of cases, IgA in 20% and light chain only in almost all the rest. Fewer than 1% have IgD or IgE paraprotein, and a similar number are non-secretory, when neither intact immunoglobulin nor light chain can be found in the serum or urine. Mass spectrometry is a new sensitive method of measuring paraproteins and free light chains.

2 **Elevated serum immunoglobulin free light chains.** Immunoglobulin free light chains (FLC) are κ or λ light chain proteins that have not been paired with heavy chain (Fig. 22.6). They are normally made in small quantities and filtered from the serum into the urine by the kidney, but can be measured in serum. Free light chains are produced by almost all malignant plasma cells and so the **serum free light chain** assay is useful in diagnosis and monitoring of myeloma and other forms of malignant paraproteinaemia. Typically in myeloma there is an increase in either the κ or λ serum free light chain value. The normal κ: λ serum free light chain ratio of 0.6 (range 0.26–1.65) is skewed with an excess of either κ or λ chains. Since free light chains are excreted in the urine, their total levels in plasma increase in the presence of renal insufficiency, but the ratio in the absence of a plasma cell neoplasm will usually remain close to normal.

3 Normal serum immunoglobulin levels (IgG, IgA and IgM) are reduced, a feature known as **immunoparesis**. The urine contains free light chains, **Bence–Jones protein**, in two-thirds of cases. Rare cases of myeloma are non-secretory and therefore not associated with a paraprotein or Bence–Jones proteinuria, although some will still show a disturbed free light chain ratio in the serum.

4 There is usually a normochromic normocytic or macrocytic **anaemia**. Rouleaux formation is marked in many cases (Fig. 22.7). Neutropenia and thrombocytopenia occur in advanced disease. Abnormal plasma cells appear in the blood film in 15% of patients and can be detected by sensitive flow cytometry in over 50%.

5 There is a **high erythrocyte sedimentation rate (ESR)**, due to immunoglobulin coating of erythrocyte surfaces.

6 There are increased plasma cells in the bone marrow (usually more than 20%), often with abnormal forms (Fig. 22.2). **The characteristic immunophenotype of malignant plasma cells is CD38^{high}, CD138^{high} and CD45^{low}. CD19 is negative.** Anti-CD138 is used to measure the number of plasma cells in the marrow biopsy (Fig. 22.2).

7 **Radiological investigation of the skeleton reveals bone lesions such as osteolytic areas without evidence of surrounding osteoblastic reaction or sclerosis in 60% of patients (Fig. 22.8) or generalized osteoporosis in 20% (Fig. 22.5). In addition, pathological fractures or vertebral collapse (Fig. 22.5) are common.** Skeletal survey X-rays do not detect small lesions. **MRI of the spine** is needed in cases considered as asymptomatic (smouldering) myeloma to detect early bone lesions. **Positron emission tomography (PET) scan** is also a sensitive imaging technique to detect bone damage (Fig. 22.5). Cross-sectional imaging by MRI is best for follow-up of bone disease.

8 **Serum calcium elevation** occurs in ~45% of patients. Typically, the serum alkaline phosphatase is normal, except following pathological fractures.

9 **The serum creatinine is raised in >20% of cases.** Proteinaceous deposits from light chain proteinuria, glomerular injury, hypercalcaemia, uric acid, amyloid and pyelonephritis may all contribute to renal failure (Fig. 22.9).

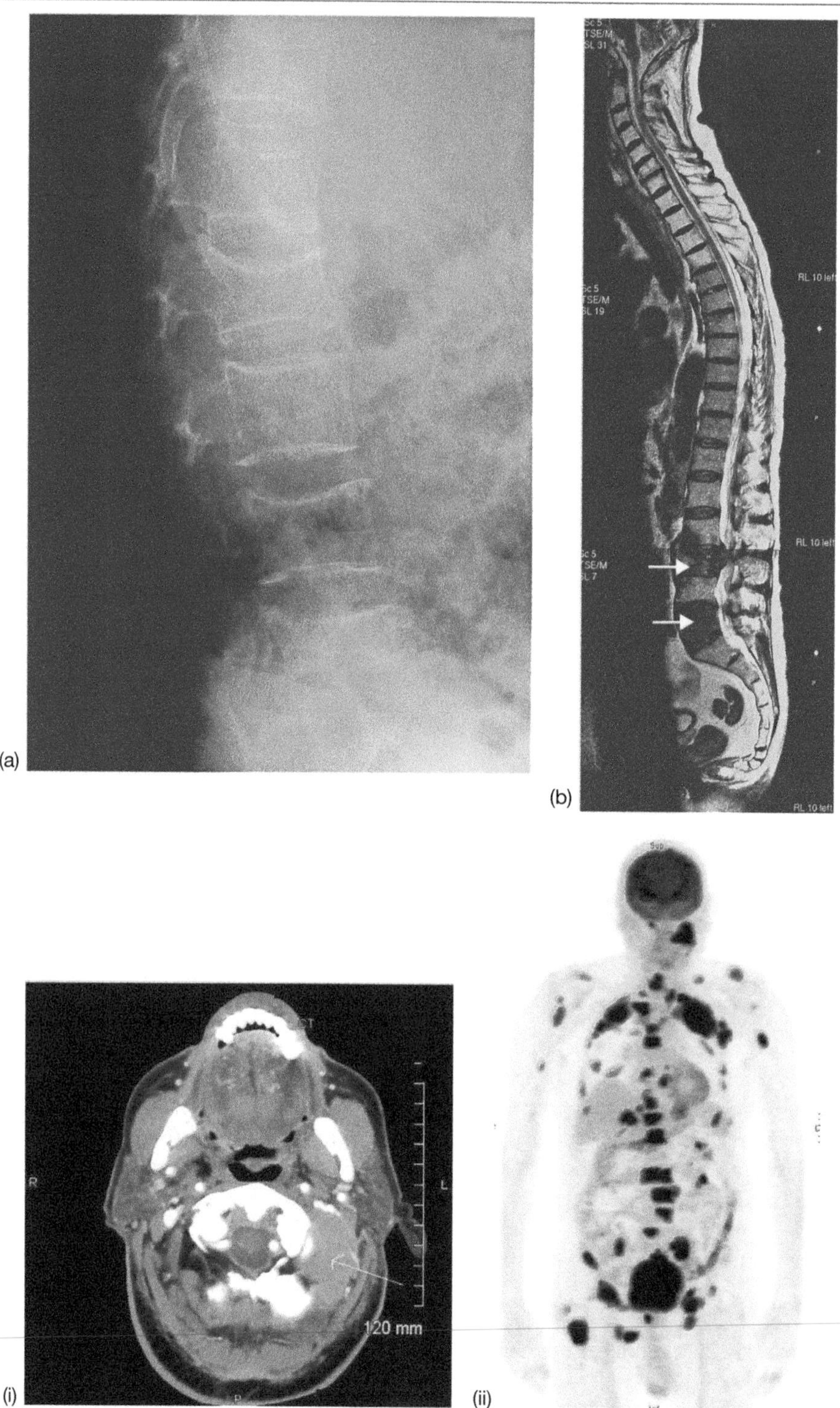

Figure 22.5 **(a)** Multiple myeloma: X-ray of lumbar spine showing severe demineralization with partial collapse of L_3. **(b)** Magnetic resonance imaging (MRI) of spine: T_2-weighted study. There is infiltration and destruction of L_3 and L_5 with bulging of the posterior part of the body of L_3 into the spinal canal compressing the corda equina (arrowed). Radiotherapy has caused a marrow signal change in vertebrae C_2–D_4 because of replacement of normal red marrow by fat (bright white signal). Source: Courtesy of Dr A. Platts. **(c)** (i) Computed tomography (CT) scan of base of skull showing paravertebral soft tissue extramedullary plasmacytoma (white arrow). (ii) Positron emission tomography (PET) scan of the same patient showing extensive medullary and extramedullary involvement. Source: T. Sher *et al*. (2010) *Br. J. Haematol*. 150: 418–27. Reproduced with permission of John Wiley & Sons.

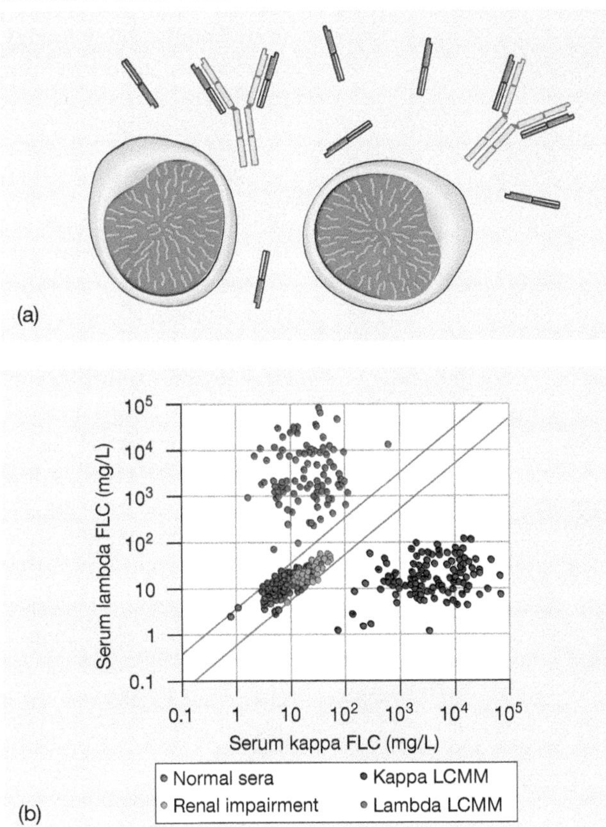

Figure 22.6 The value of serum immunoglobulin free light chain (FLC) measurement in multiple myeloma. **(a)** Serum free light chains are immunoglobulin light chains that are synthesized by plasma cells but not paired with heavy chains before they are released into the blood. Low levels are found in normal individuals and these are increased in patients with myeloma. **(b)** Profile of serum free light chains in healthy controls, patients with renal impairment and those with κ or λ light chain multiple myeloma (LCMM). As light chains are normally filtered by the kidney, their levels rise in patients with renal impairment, although the κ : λ ratio remains normal. Source: Adapted from C. Hutchison (2008) *BMC Nephrology* 9: 11–9. A.R. Bradwell (2003) *Lancet* 361: 489–91.

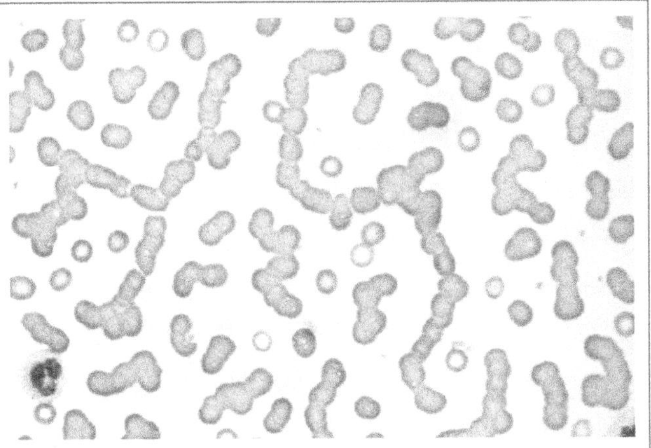

Figure 22.7 The peripheral blood film in multiple myeloma showing Rouleaux formation. Rouleaux differs from agglutination in that the former are more linear, the latter typically clumped.

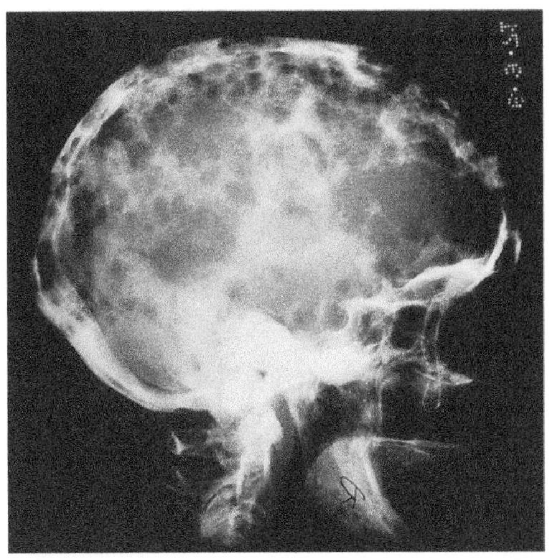

Figure 22.8 Skull X-ray in multiple myeloma showing many 'punched-out' lesions.

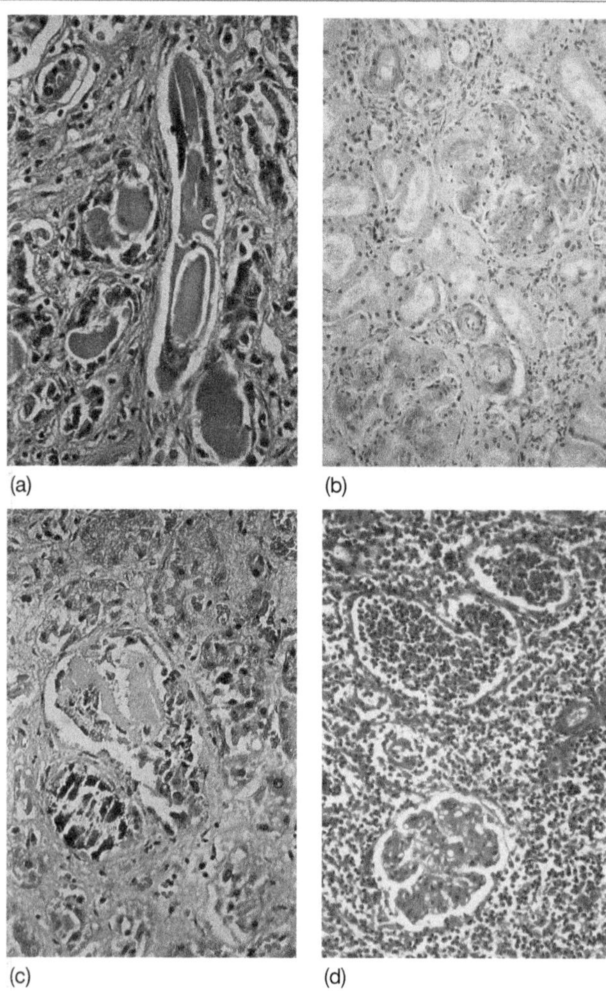

Figure 22.9 The kidney in multiple myeloma. **(a)** Myeloma kidney: the renal tubules are distended with hyaline protein (precipitated light chains or Bence–Jones protein). Giant cells are prominent in the surrounding cellular reaction. **(b)** Amyloid deposition: both glomeruli and several of the small blood vessels contain an amorphous pink-staining deposit characteristic of amyloid (Congo red stain). **(c)** Nephrocalcinosis: calcium deposition (dark 'fractured' material) in the renal parenchyma. **(d)** Pyelonephritis: destruction of renal parenchyma and infiltration by acute inflammatory cells.

10 Serum lactate dehydrogenase (LDH) elevation occurs in advanced disease (Table 22.4).

11 A **low serum albumin** occurs with advanced disease and is a useful indicator of prognosis (Table 22.4).

12 **Serum β2-microglobulin** is often raised and is also a useful indicator of prognosis (Table 22.4), with higher levels correlating with poorer outcomes.

13 **Cytogenetic and molecular genetic abnormalities** (see below).

An International Staging System (ISS) divides patients into three groups, calculated by whether the serum albumin is ≥35 g/L or <35 g/L; and whether the serum β2-microglobulin is <3.5 mg/L, 3.5–5.5 mg/L or >5.5 mg/L. A revised system (R-ISS) also includes chromosome abnormalities and serum LDH (Table 22.4)

Cytogenetics and molecular testing

Interphase fluorescence *in situ* hybridization (FISH) shows that aneuploidy (more or fewer than 46 chromosomes) is almost universal, usually gains or loss involving odd numbered chromosomes. There is also a high incidence of translocations involving the immunoglobulin heavy-chain gene (*IGH*) on chromosome 14 such as t(4;14), t(14;16). These translocations and del(17p) which involves the *TP53* gene (more common in late stage disease), del (1p32) and 1q gains confer a worse prognosis whereas t(11;14) is prognostically neutral. Loss of chromosome 13 is present in 40–50% of newly diagnosed patients and is associated with abnormalities of chromosomes 1,14 and 17. Over-expression of D-cyclin genes occurs in almost all myeloma patients suggesting a unifying event in pathogenesis. Later-stage cases often have more complex cytogenetic findings. The genetic changes may be used (alone or with serum β2-microglobulin, albumin and LDH) to classify the disease into standard, intermediate and high risk (Table 22.4 and annotation to Fig. 22.10).

In later stages of disease deregulation of the oncogene MYC is frequent. Mutations of *KRAS* and *NRAS* (20%), of *TP53, DIS3, FAM46C,* and *BRAF* (all 10%) and other mutations, in about 5% of patients, are also found. The impact of these mutations apart from of *TP53* on survival and response to therapy remains unclear.

Asymptomatic (smouldering) myeloma

The term asymptomatic or smouldering myeloma is used for cases with similar laboratory findings to multiple myeloma, but no organ or tissue damage causing clinical features (Table 22.2). There is about a 10% chance each year of these cases becoming symptomatic and requiring therapy (although the annual risk falls after 5 years). There are different schemes for predicting speed of progression based on the level of paraprotein, degree of free light chain imbalance, proportion of plasma cells in the marrow, degree of immuosuppression and presence or absence of certain unfavourable cytogenetic abnormalities such as t(4;14), t(14;16), gain of 1q21 or hypodiploidy. The risk is greatest if there are more than 60% plasma cells in the marrow, circulating plasma cells, a greatly unbalanced free light chain ratio (see below), unfavourable cytogenetics and more than one focal lesion on spinal magnetic resonance imaging. Treatment as for symptomatic myeloma should be considered in high risk cases as early therapy of this group may improve outcome.

Treatment

This may be divided into specific and supportive (Fig. 22.10; Table 22.5).

Table 22.4 Standard risk factors for multiple myeloma: the Revised International Staging System (R-ISS).

Prognostic Factor	Criteria
ISS stage	
■ I	■ Serum β2-microglobulin <3.5 mg/L, serum albumin ≥35 g/L
■ II	■ Not ISS stage I or III
■ III	■ Serum β2-microglobulin ≥5.5 mg/L
Chromosome abnormalities (CA) by iFISH	
■ High risk	■ Presence of del(17p), del 1p, 1q gains, t(4;14), t(14;16)
■ Standard risk	■ No high-risk chromosome abnormalities
LDH	
■ Normal	■ Serum LDH ≤ the upper limit of normal
■ High	■ Serum LDH > the upper limit of normal
R-ISS stage	
■ I	■ ISS stage I and standard risk CA by iFISH and normal LDH
■ II	■ Not R-ISS stage I or III
■ III	■ ISS stage III and either high-risk CA by iFISH or high LDH

CA, chromosome abnormalities; iFISH, interphase fluorescence *in situ* hybridization; ISS, International Staging System; LDH, lactate dehydrogenase; R-ISS, revised ISS.
Median overall survival of R-ISS I in a series of 3060 patients was not yet reached at >10 years, while that for R-ISS II was 83 months, and for R-ISS III 43 months.
Source: A. Palumbo *et al.* (2015) *J. Clin. Oncol.* 33: 2863–69. Reproduced with permission of American Society of Clinical Oncology.

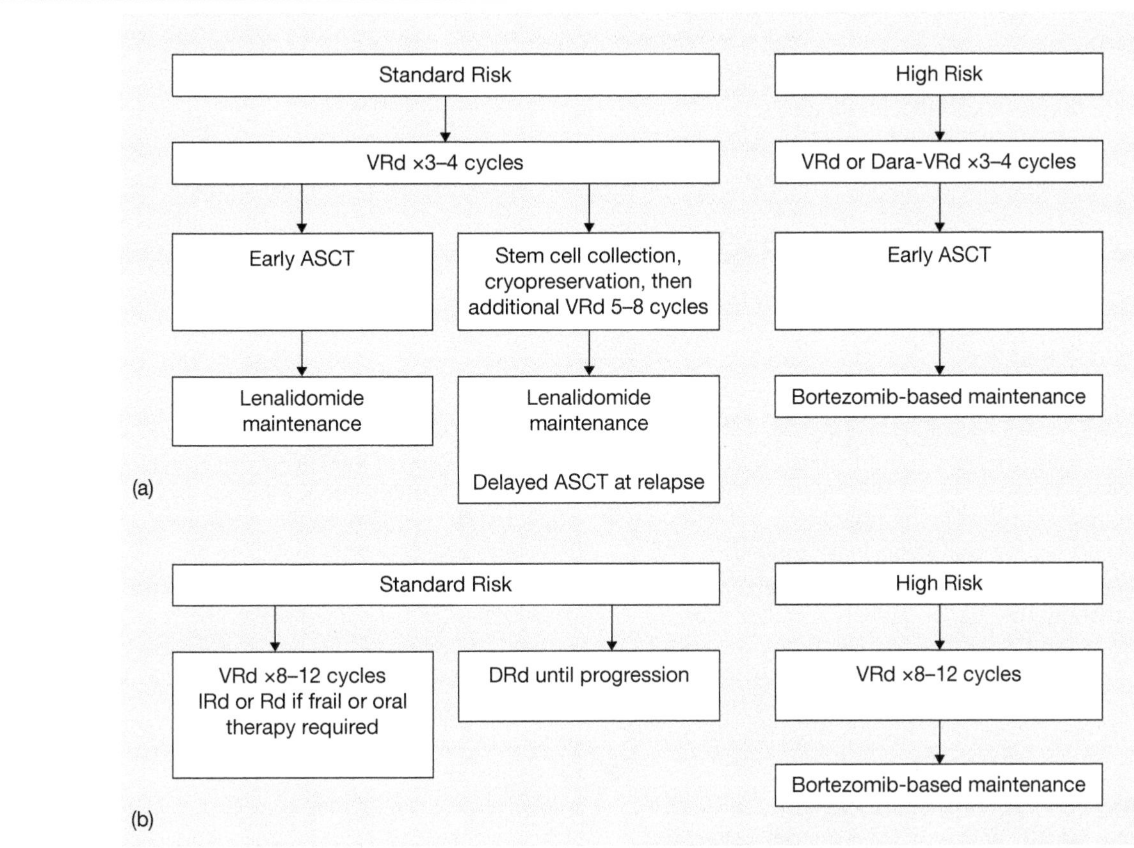

Figure 22.10 Algorithm of potential approaches to the management of multiple myeloma. Treatment approach to the patient with newly diagnosed multiple myeloma who is **(a)** transplant eligible or **(b)** transplant ineligible. Standard risk includes t(11;14), trisomies and t(6;14). High risk includes t(4;14), t(14;16) and del(17p) (Table 22.4). ASCT, autologous stem cell transplantation; VRd, bortezomib, lenalidomide, dexamethasone; Dara-VRd, Daratumumab combined with VRd, DRd, daratumumab, lenalidomide, dexamethasone. Source: Based on S.V. Rajkumar (2020) *Blood Cancer J.* 10: 94.

Table 22.5 Treatment of myeloma.

Modality	Examples or indications
Corticosteroids	Dexamethasone, prednisolone, prednisone
Alkylating agents	Cyclophosphamide, melphalan
Proteasome inhibitors	Bortezomib, carfilzomib, ixazomib (oral)
Immunomodulators (IMID)	Lenalidomide, pomalidomide, thalidomide
Monoclonal antibodies Bi-specific antibodies	Daratumumab, isatuximab (both anti-CD38), elotuzumab (anti-SLAM7); belantamab-mafodotin (anti-BCMA) Teclistamab, elranatamab (both anti-CD3, anti-BCMA); talquetamab (anti-CD3, anti-GPRC5D)
Nuclear export	Selinexor
BCL2 inhibitor	Venetoclax
Cell therapy	Autologous SCT CAR-T cells (ide-cel, ciltacel) anti-BCMA or other myeloma antigens
Radiotherapy	External beam therapy used for painful local lytic lesions or spinal cord/nerve root compression; unstable lesions at risk for fracture, e.g. femoral neck may also require orthopaedic surgery
Plasmapheresis	Used for acute treatment of hyperviscosity, and for monoclonal gammopathies with clinical consequences, e.g. acquired coagulation factor inhibitors, severe neuropathy
Supportive care	Bisphosphonates, e.g. pamidronate, zoledronic acid; denusomab (RANKL inhibitor) Intravenous immunoglobulin for patients with low gamma globulins and recurrent infection. Haemodialysis for severe renal failure

BCMA, B-cell maturation antigen; CAR-T, chimeric antigen receptor T cells; RANKL, receptor activator of nuclear factor κB ligand; SCT, stem cell transplant; SLAM, signalling lymphocytic activation molecule; GPRC5D, G-protein-coupled receptor family C group 5 member D.

Specific

The life expectancy of patients with myeloma has improved markedly with the introduction of proteasome inhibitors, immunomodulatory agents and monoclonal antibodies. The major initial treatment decision is between **intensive combination chemotherapy** (mostly for patients aged less than 70 years, who may be candidates for autologous stem cell transplant, SCT) or **non-intensive therapy** for older or frail patients.

Intensive therapy

Intensive therapy involves four to six cycles to reduce the tumour burden, usually followed by stem cell collection and high-dose chemotherapy with autologous SCT followed sometimes by further consolidation and / or maintenance therapy. The initial chemotherapy is given as repeated intravenous or oral chemotherapy cycles usually combining three or four drugs with distinct mechanisms of action against tumour cells (Table 22.5).

Some commonly used combination therapies for patients who are transplant candidates include:

- VRd (RVd) – bortezomib (Velcade), lenalidomide (Revlimid) and dexamethasone.
- Dara-VRd – daratumumab combined with bortezomib, lenalidomide and dexamethasone, the four drug usually reserved for higher risk disease but becoming preferred care also for standard risk patients. The addition of daratumumab increases minimal residual disease negativity rates and progression free survival.
- KRd – carfilzomib (Kyprolis), lenalidomide and dexamethasone. Less commonly used as a first-line treatment due to higher rate of cardiac, renal and pulmonary side effects compared with bortezomib combinations.

Other drugs including thalidomide and cyclophosphamide are less effective but still used as cheaper options in some countries. Alkylating agents such as melphalan are generally avoided, since their use makes subsequent collection of stem cells difficult.

More intensive therapy may be used in ultrahigh-risk newly diagnosed myeloma and plasma cell leukaemia. Examples include the five-drug combination, daratumumab, cyclophosphamide, bortezomib, lenalidomide, dexamethasone, with intensified consolidation post auto-SCT and the VTD-PACE (bortezomib, thalidomide, dexamethasone, cisplatin, doxorubicin, cyclophosphamide and etoposide) regimen.

Auto-stem cell transplantation (SCT)

After several cycles of treatment, when the number of tumour cells has been reduced, the patient usually undergoes an autologous SCT. Peripheral blood stem cells are collected after mobilization using a combination of chemotherapy and granulocyte colony-stimulating factor (G-CSF). High-dose melphalan is the typical conditioning regimen for SCT.

Minimal residual disease (MRD) monitoring is helpful in deciding on further therapy. It is carried out on peripheral blood or bone marrow by flow cytometry, molecular testing or by mass spectrometry. For patients who become MRD negative on induction and consolidation therapy trials are in place of omitting immediate auto-SCT and instead storing peripheral blood stem cells and starting maintenance therapy. For patients MRD positive before auto-SCT, post SCT further courses of triple or four drug chemotherapy are considered, followed by maintenance therapy.

Maintenance treatment

After autologous SCT maintenance with lenalidomide or bortezomib (or sometimes both agents in high risk disease) is usual. Lenalidomide maintenance after auto SCT shows benefit in progression free and overall survival although it is associated with a 2–3 fold increase in second cancers. For those MRD negative at 6 months it should be continued for at least 3 years in total. For those MRD positive, it should be continued until relapse. There is no cumulative haematological toxicity. Carfilzomib and daratumumab are also in trials as maintenance therapy either alone or in combination with lenalidomide

About 10% of patients who have undergone intensive therapy and autologous SCT appear to be cured. The median life expectancy for myeloma has increased from 2 to 3 years in the 1990s to 5 years or more.

Although **allogeneic stem cell transplantation** may cure the disease, it carries a high procedure-related mortality, so is rarely undertaken. Moreover, patients frequently relapse after the procedure. It is only used in highly selected, multiply relapsed patients.

Non-intensive therapy

Melphalan-based regimens were frequently used in this setting but are no longer recommended due partly to toxicity concerns and also better outcomes with lenalidomide-based regimens. Lenalidomide and dexamethasone (Rd) were shown to be superior to a melphalan-based combination and addition of bortezomib (VRd) led to further benefit although this combination is not reimbursed in all regions. An alternative is daratumumab combined with lenalidomide and dexamethasone (DRd) but treatment until progression is a drawback in this patient group due to infection risk, cost and effect on quality of life. Daratumumab combined with VRd (DVRd) is also an option for some who can tolerate this four drug treatment.

Relapsed/refractory disease

After a variable period of time the disease is likely to progress with rising paraprotein levels and return of symptoms. A wide range of drugs, monoclonal antibodies and cellular therapies is available and various combinations have been used showing a range of responses. Choice of regimen will depend on a number of factors:

- Patient related (such as age and comorbidities)
- Disease related (such as genetic risk)
- Treatment related (such as prior refractoriness or prior toxicities or expense)

If a patient is not resistant to anti-CD38 directed therapy (daratumumab or isatuximab), this generally forms the backbone of treatment. Either a proteasome inhibitor or an immunomodulatory agent is added. Since many patients now are relapsing on lenalidomide maintenance, a proteasome inhibitor or third-generation IMID (such as pomalidomide) is often used.

When patients become refractory to proteasome inhibitors, immunomodulatory agents and CD38 directed antibodies, a number of options have recently become available and/or are in trials. Some are directed against the B-cell maturation antigen (BCMA) such as chimeric-antigen-receptor (CAR-T cells) therapy, e.g. idacebtagene vicleucel; bispecific antibodies, e.g. teclistamab; and antibody-drug conjugates, e.g. belantamab mafadotin. The bispecific antibody talquetamab targets a G-protein-coupled receptor, the monoclonal antibody elotuzumab targets SLAMF7 and selinexor is a small molecule which targets nuclear export.

Notes on some specific drugs used in myeloma

Thalidomide was the first immune-modulator drug to be used in myeloma. It has a number of side effects such as sedation, constipation, embryo toxicity, neuropathy, myelosuppression and venous thrombosis. The addition of dexamethasone increases the response rate, but venous thrombosis becomes a major concern and prophylactic anticoagulation with low-molecular-weight heparin, a direct-acting oral anticoagulants, warfarin or aspirin is needed if this combination is used. **Lenalidomide** is an analogue of thalidomide and is highly active in the management of myeloma. It is used widely both for first-line therapy and for relapsed disease. It is also associated with myelosuppression, but causes increased risk of thrombosis and neuropathy less frequently than thalidomide (Table 22.2). **Pomalidomide** is the most recent addition to this class of drugs and shows a high level of activity against relapsed disease. Like lenalidomide it causes less neuropathy than thalidomide. All three drugs increase ubiquitin-mediated proteasome degradation of Ikaros family zinc finger proteins that are important survival factors for plasma cells.

Bortezomib inhibits cellular proteasome and NF-κB activation. It is highly active in first-line treatment and relapsed disease. Its main side effect is a neuropathy. **Carfilzomib** is a more recently introduced proteasome inhibitor which is less likely to cause a neuropathy although it is associated with certain cardiac, renal and pulmonary complications. **Ixazomib** is an orally active proteasome inhibitor.

Monoclonal antibodies include **daratumumab** (anti-CD38) and **elotuzumab** (anti-SLAMF7). They bind to plasma cell-associated antigens and induce killing of tumour cells. Bi-specific antibodies (anti-BCMA, anti CD3) include teclistamab and elranatamab. BCMA is also the target antigen of the antibody–drug conjugate belantamab-mafodotin and of some CAR-T cells.

Radiotherapy is useful in treating the symptomatic bone disease in myeloma. It is used for areas of bone pain or spinal cord compression.

Supportive care

Renal impairment It is advisable for patients to drink at least 2–3 L of fluid each day throughout the course of their disease in order to limit the accumulation of paraprotein within the kidney. Some patients present with renal failure and treatment should include rehydration and treatment of contributing factors, such as hypercalcaemia or hyperuricaemia (Fig. 22.9). Dialysis is generally well tolerated if required. Assessment of renal function is important in choosing which drugs to use initially and their doses. The outcome of patients presenting with renal impairment has drastically improved with the introduction of newer agents such as proteasome inhibitors.

Bone disease and hypercalcaemia Bisphosphonates, such as pamidronate or zoledronic acid, are effective in reducing the progression of bone disease and may also improve overall survival. Denusomab is an inhibitor of RANKL that may be useful in patients who cannot tolerate bisphosphonates due to renal insufficiency. Acute hypercalcaemia is treated with rehydration using isotonic saline, a diuretic and corticosteroids followed by a bisphosphonate.

Compression paraplegia Surgical decompression laminectomy or irradiation are treatments of choice. Chemotherapy and corticosteroid treatment are usually also given.

Anaemia Transfusion or an erythropoiesis-stimulating agent may be used.

Bleeding Bleeding caused by paraprotein interference with coagulation and hyperviscosity syndrome are treated by repeated plasmapheresis. More durable remission can be obtained with treatment of the underlying disorder.

Infections Rapid treatment of any infection is essential. Prophylactic infusions of immunoglobulin concentrates together with oral broad-spectrum antibiotics and antifungal agents may be needed for recurrent infections in patients with severe hypogammaglobulinaemia.

Prognosis

The outlook for patients with myeloma is improving markedly. The overall median survival is now over 10 years in younger patients (less than 60 years old). High-risk patients (defined Table 22.4) have poorer outcomes so therapy is risk-stratified (Fig. 22.10). **The achievement of negativity for minimal residual disease (<1 tumour plasma cell in 10^6 bone marrow cells by next-generation sequencing) after induction chemotherapy with or without autologous SCT, at the start of maintenance therapy, predicts for excellent progression-free and overall survival.**

Other plasma cell neoplasms

Solitary plasmacytoma

These are isolated plasma cell neoplasms, usually involving bones (where they arise from underlying bone marrow) or soft tissue such as the mucosa of the upper respiratory and gastrointestinal tracts or the skin. An associated paraprotein, if present, disappears following radiotherapy to the primary lesion. Many patients but not all will develop myeloma. Bone plasmacytoma has the highest risk of progression.

Plasma cell leukaemia

This rare disease is characterized by a high number of circulating malignant plasma cells (Fig. 22.3). The clinical features tend to be a combination of those found in acute leukaemia (pancytopenia and organomegaly) with features of myeloma (hypercalcaemia, renal involvement and bone disease). Treatment is with supportive care and systemic chemotherapy, but prognosis is poor.

Osteosclerotic myeloma (POEMS syndrome)

Osteosclerotic myeloma and POEMS (polyneuropathy, organomegaly, endocrinopathy, monoclonal protein, skin changes) syndrome is a rare condition in which a polyneuropathy is associated with a monoclonal plasma cell disorder and osteosclerotic bone lesions. Elevated levels of vascular endothelial growth factor (VEGF) are present and there are often clinical features such as splenomegaly, hepatomegaly or lymphadenopathy, extravascular fluid overload, endocrine abnormalities, skin changes or Castleman disease. Treatment is similar to that described for myeloma.

Monoclonal gammopathy of undetermined significance

Transient or persistent paraproteins can occur in many other conditions as well as in multiple myeloma (Table 22.1). **A persistent serum paraprotein (most frequently IgG, less frequently IgA, IgM or light chain only) may be sometimes be**

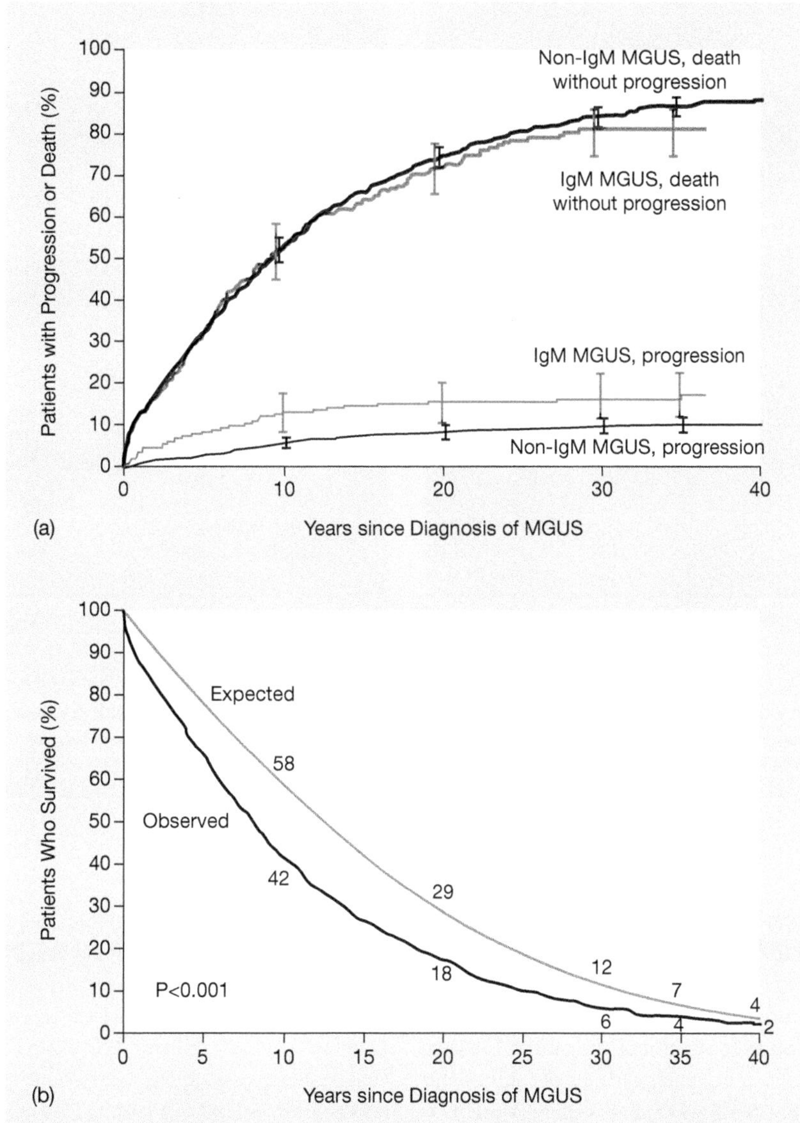

Figure 22.11 (a and b) Survival of patients with monoclonal gammopathy of undetermined significance (MGUS) ($n = 1384$) is reduced compared to the control population; median 8.1 vs 12.4 years, respectively ($p < 0.001$). Among the subset of patients with immunoglobin (Ig) M MGUS, adverse risk factors for progression included an abnormal serum free light-chain ratio and higher serum M protein level (≥1.5 g/dL). Both risk factors were associated with a risk of progression at 20 years of 55%, compared to 41% among patients with one risk factor and 19% among patients with neither risk factor. Source: R.A. Kyle *et al.* (2018) *N. Engl. J. Med.* 378: 241–9. Reproduced with permission of Massachusetts Medical Society.

detected without any evidence of myeloma or other underlying disease and is termed monoclonal gammopathy of undetermined significance (MGUS). It is increasingly common with age, being present in 3–4% of persons older than 50 years and more than 10% by age 80 years.

MGUS was formerly called 'benign monoclonal gammopathy', but the recognition of a disease progression risk as well as of an increased incidence of venous and arterial thrombosis, infections, osteoporosis, kidney and skin diseases, and of bone fractures compared to controls led to adoption of the MGUS term. Rarely, paraneoplastic changes including acquired haemophilia or neuropathy will result from monoclonal proteins with specific antigen binding properties.

The proportion of plasma cells in the marrow in MGUS is normal (less than 4%) or slightly raised (less than 10%; Table 22.2; Fig. 22.3). The concentration of monoclonal immunoglobulin in serum is less than 30 g/L and other serum immunoglobulins are not depressed. The κ or λ light chain is

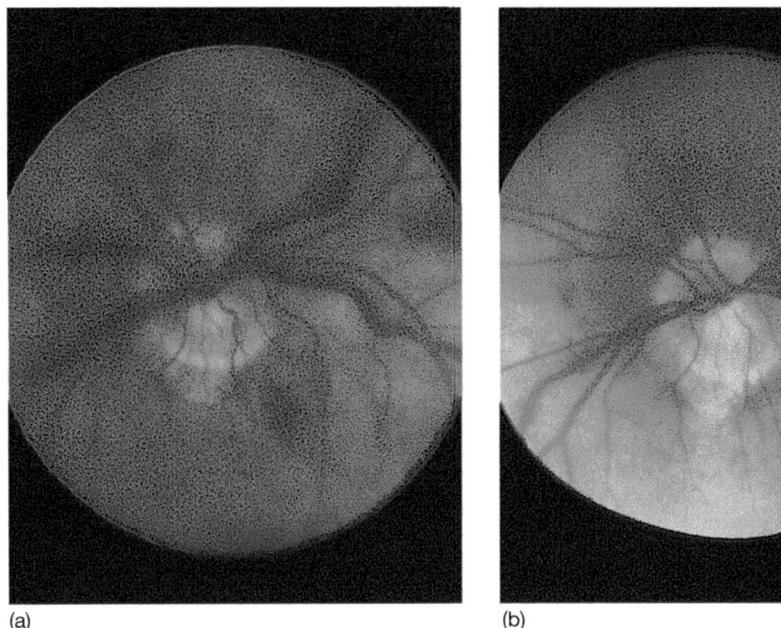

Figure 22.12 Hyperviscosity syndrome in Waldenström's macroglobulinaemia. **(a)** The retina before plasmapheresis shows distension of retinal vessels, particularly the veins, which show bulging and constriction (the 'linked sausage' effect) and areas of haemorrhage. **(b)** Following plasmapheresis the vessels have returned to normal and the areas of haemorrhage have cleared.

increased in serum in one-third of patients; the greater the imbalance, the more the risk of transformation.

No treatment is needed for most patients unless a complication such as neuropathy or nephropathy occurs. Patients with IgG or IgA MGUS develop overt myeloma at a rate of 1% each year and so are usually followed up regularly in the outpatient clinic. Patients with IgM MGUS are classified separately, as their risk is for development of lymphoplasmacytic lymphoma rather than myeloma, and their risk of progression is higher (Fig. 22.11a). The survival of patients with MGUS is modestly reduced compared with control populations and this effect increases with duration of follow-up and age (Fig. 22.11b).

Hyperviscosity syndrome

Hyperviscosity may occur in patients with myeloma or Waldenström macroglobulinaemia or in polycythaemia. A related condition, hyperleucocytosis, can affect patients with chronic myeloid or acute leukaemias associated with very high white cell counts. The clinical features of the hyperviscosity syndrome include visual disturbances, lethargy, confusion, muscle weakness, nervous system symptoms and signs, and congestive heart failure. The retina may show a variety of changes: engorged veins sometimes with sausage-like changes, haemorrhages, exudates and a blurred disc (Fig. 22.12).

Emergency treatment varies with the cause:

1. Correct dehydration in all patients, but do not transfuse unless absolutely necessary.
2. Venesection or isovolaemic exchange with a plasma substitute for red cells in a polycythaemic patient.
3. Plasmapheresis in myeloma, Waldenström disease or hyperfibrinogenaemia.
4. Leucopheresis or chemotherapy in myeloid leukaemias associated with high white cell counts.

The long-term treatment depends on control of the primary disease with specific therapy.

SUMMARY

- The term *paraproteinaemia* refers to the presence of a monoclonal immunoglobulin band in serum, and reflects the synthesis of immunoglobulin or portion of an immunoglobulin from a single clone of plasma cells.
- Multiple myeloma is a neoplasm of plasma cells that accumulate usually to >20% of cells in the bone marrow. In >98% of cases there is a paraprotein and/or an excess kappa or lambda immunoglobulin light chain in plasma which can cause tissue damage. The disease has a peak incidence in the seventh decade.
- Almost all cases of myeloma develop from a preexisting monoclonal gammopathy of undetermined significance (MGUS) in which there is low-level paraprotein and no evidence of tissue damage. Approximately 1% of cases progress to myeloma each year.
- A useful reminder for the spectrum of tissue damage in symptomatic myeloma is *CRAB* – hyper**c**alcaemia, **r**enal impairment, **a**naemia, **b**one disease (lytic lesions or osteoporosis).
- Magnetic resonance imaging (MRI) or positron emission tomography (PET) scan is needed to exclude bone lesions, especially of the spine, which may not be detected on plain radiographs. Other clinical features include amyloid, hyperviscosity, recurrent infections, peripheral neuropathy and deep vein thrombosis.
- Asymptomatic (smouldering) myeloma describes patients with bone marrow and protein findings of myeloma but without CRAB or other clinical symptoms or findings.
- The serum albumin and β2-microglobulin concentrations as well as the cytogenetic findings are important for determining prognosis.
- In patients younger than 70 years, symptomatic myeloma is usually treated by intensive chemotherapy with a three-or four- drug combination followed by an autologous stem cell transplant, using stem cells harvested from the patient.
- Maintenance therapy with lenalidomide alone or with other drugs or combinations improves survival.
- Minimal residual disease monitoring helps to plan treatment and maintenance protocols.
- In older (>70 years) and frail patients, less intensive chemotherapy is usually given. Autologous SCT is not used.
- Support care is vital and includes prevention and treatment of bone and renal disease, infections and bleeding and thrombotic complications.
- Radiotherapy may be needed to treat bone lesions
- Immunomodulatory drugs (lenalidomide, thalidomide, pomalidomide) and proteasome inhibitory drugs (bortezomib, ixazomib, carfilzomib), usually used in combination with dexamethasone, with or without the monoclonal antibody daratumumab (anti-CD38) are improving the outlook for patients and median survival is now >10 years. Other monoclonal antibodies including elotuzumab (anti-SLAM7) and belantamab-mafodotin (anti-BCMA) and bi-specific antibodies are also effective.
- CAR-T cells against BCMA or other plasma cell-associated antigens are highly active and are in clinical trials.
- A *plasmacytoma* is a localized mass of malignant plasma cells and is usually treated with radiotherapy. Many cases progress to myeloma.
- Osteosclerotic myeloma and POEMS syndrome is a rare variant form of multiple myeloma
- *Hyperviscosity syndrome* may occur in paraproteinaemia or in patients with a very high red or myeloid white cell count. Clinical features include visual disturbances, confusion and heart failure. Venesection, plasma exchange or chemotherapy may be required.

Now visit **www.wileyessential.com/haematology9e** to test yourself on this chapter.

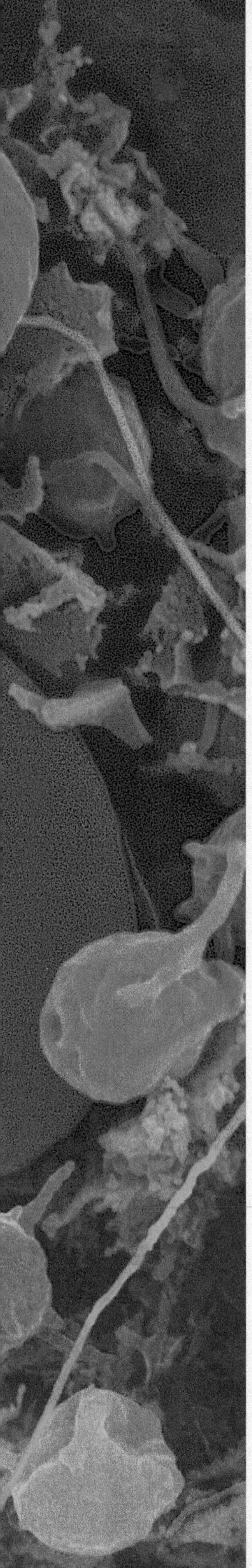

CHAPTER 23

Amyloid

(Written with Professor Ashutosh Wechelaker)

Key topics

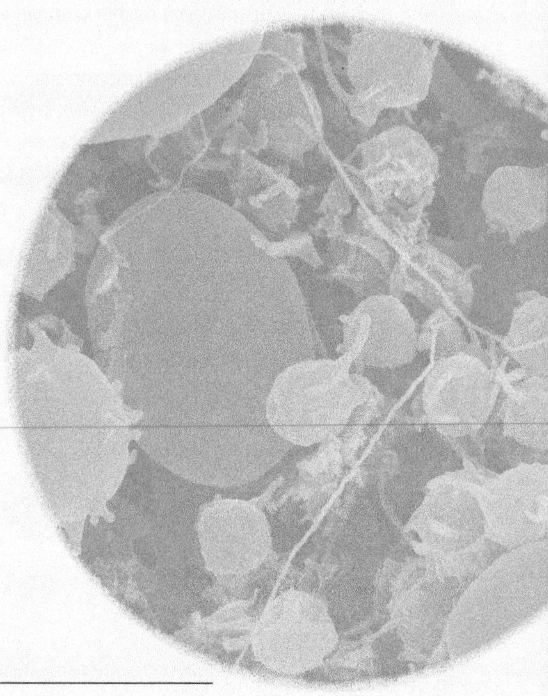

Hoffbrand's Essential Haematology, Ninth Edition. A. Victor Hoffbrand, Pratima Chowdary, Graham P. Collins, and Justin Loke.

© 2024 John Wiley & Sons Ltd. Published 2024 by John Wiley & Sons Ltd.

Companion website: www.wiley.com/go/haematology9e

Introduction

The amyloidoses are a heterogeneous group of disorders characterized by the extracellular deposition of normally soluble proteins in an abnormal fibrillar form. These deposits interfere with the normal function of the host tissue both by their physical presence and by direct toxicity. Amyloidosis may be hereditary or acquired, and deposits may be localized or systemic in distribution (Table 23.1).

Amyloid may be formed by over 30 proteins. The pattern of organ distribution varies with the different fibril types and even within the same type. In systemic amyloidosis, the dominant organs involved are the liver, spleen, kidneys, bone marrow, heart and tongue (Fig. 23.1) autonomic and peripheral nerves, skin and eyes. Cardiac amyloid is most frequently the dominant cause of morbidity and death. Except for intracerebral amyloid plaques, all amyloid deposits contain a non-fibrillary glycoprotein amyloid P,

Table 23.1 Classification of amyloidosis (in order of clinical frequency).

Type	Chemical nature	Organs involved
Systemic (primary) AL amyloidosis Associated with an occult plasma cell proliferation	Immunoglobulin light chains (AL)	Kidney, heart, nerves, liver, soft tissues
Associated with myeloma, MGUS, Waldenström's macroglobulinaemia, other lymphomas		
May also occur in localized form with local 'immunocyte' proliferation		
Wild type transthyretin amyloidosis (wATTR) (previously known as senile systemic amyloidosis)	Normal transthyretin	Heart, connective tissues (carpal tunnel syndrome)
Systemic amyloidosis with predominant renal involvement	Leucoyte chemotactic Factor II (LEC2)	Kidney, liver
Systemic amyloidosis associated with chronic inflammation		
Rheumatoid arthritis, tuberculosis, bronchiectasis, chronic osteomyelitis, inflammatory bowel disease, Hodgkin lymphoma, carcinomas; also familial genetic causes including familial Mediterranean fever *Systemic amyloidosis associated with chronic dialysis*	*Protein A (AA)* *β2 microglobulin*	Kidney, liver Joints, muscular- skeletal
Familial(genetic) amyloidoses	Genetic variants of transthyretin, apoprotein-A1and -A2, lysozyme, fibrinogen and other proteins	Nerves, heart, kidney, liver
Localized amyloidosis		
Central nervous system	β-Amyloid protein	Alzheimer's disease
Endocrine Type 2 diabetes	Peptide hormones	Endocrine Pancreatic islets
Senile	Various	Heart, brain, joints, prostate, etc.

Source: A. Mead *et al.* (eds) *Hoffbrand's Postgraduate Haematology*, 8th edn (2025, in press).

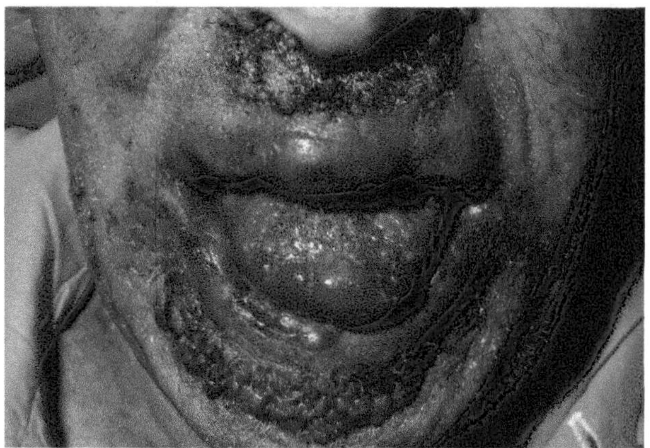

Figure 23.1 Multiple myeloma: the tongue and lips are enlarged because of nodular and waxy deposits of amyloid.

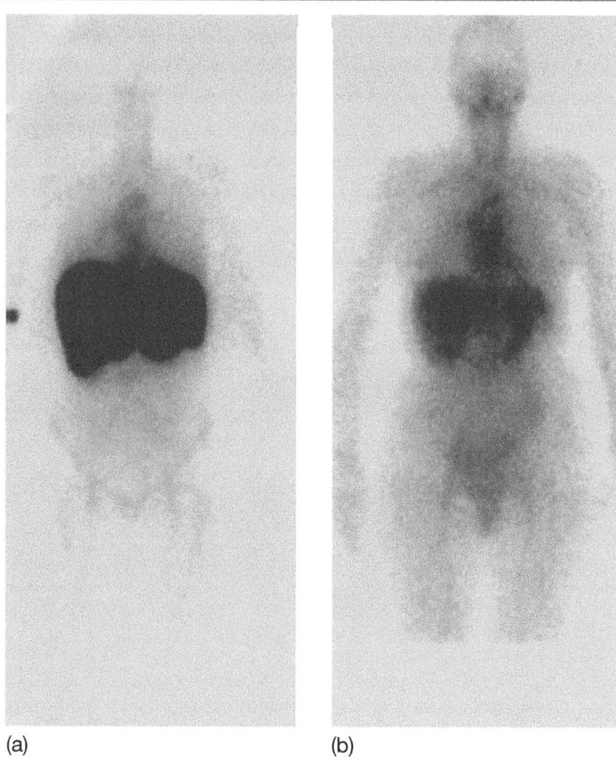

Figure 23.2 Serial anterior whole body ^{123}I-labelled serum amyloid P component (SAP) scans of a 52-year-old woman who presented with renal failure resulting from systemic AL amyloidosis. **(a)** The initial scan demonstrates a large amyloid load with hepatic, splenic, renal and bone marrow deposits. The underlying plasma cell dyscrasia responded to high-dose melphalan followed by autologous stem cell rescue. **(b)** Follow-up SAP scintigraphy 3 years after chemotherapy showed greatly reduced uptake of tracer, indicating substantial regression of her amyloid deposits. Source: Courtesy of Professor P.N. Hawkins, National Amyloidosis Centre, Royal Free Hospital, London.

which is derived from a normal serum precursor structurally related to C-reactive protein (CRP). Normal serum amyloid P component can be radiolabeled and used to determine the sites of amyloid deposition (Fig. 23.2). Glycosaminoglycans may stabilize amyloid deposits. **The classic diagnostic histological test is apple green birefringence after staining with Congo red and viewing under polarized light (Figs. 22.9 and 23.3).**

Systemic amyloidosis has three groups of underlying causes:

1 Sustained high concentration of a normal protein such as serum amyloid A protein (SAA) in chronic inflammation or β2-microglobulin in renal failure
2 Normal concentration over a prolonged period of a normal (wild type) protein with an amyloid tendency. The most frequent example is of transthyretin (named as the carrier protein of thyroid hormone and retinol), deposited in wild type transthyretin (wATTR) amyloidosis with predominant cardiac involvement.
3 An acquired or inherited abnormal protein such as a monoclonal light chain in AL amyloidosis, or inherited variants of transthyretin, lysozyme, apolipoprotein A-1 and of other proteins.

There are no histological signs of tissues reacting to amyloid deposits. These can be cleared by complement mediated macrophage ingestion. If new deposition can be prevented, amyloid may be slowly cleared with improvement in organ function.

Systemic (primary) amyloid light chain (AL) amyloidosis

Systemic AL amyloidosis, one of the most frequent systemic amyloidosis in Western countries, is caused by deposition of monoclonal light chains produced from a clonal plasma cell proliferation, most often monoclonal gammopathy of uncertain significance (MGUS) but can also be due to other plasma cell neoplasms including myeloma, Waldenström's macroglogulinaemia and other B-cell lymphomas. The disease is about 5 times less frequent than myeloma. The mutational landscape of the clonal plasma cells is similar to that of myeloma (Chapter 22) with the translocation t(11,14) present in 45% of cases and in contrast to myeloma, associated with an unfavourable prognosis. The level of paraprotein may be very low and is not always detectable in serum or urine, but the serum free light chain ratio is usually abnormal (Fig. 22.6). The organs most involved are the kidneys, heart (in 70% of cases), liver and peripheral nerves.

Clinical features

These are caused by involvement of the heart (in more than 70% of patients, usually with a restrictive cardiomyopathy), kidneys (Fig. 22.9), tongue (Fig. 23.1), gastrointestinal tract, peripheral nerves and autonomic nervous system. The joints,

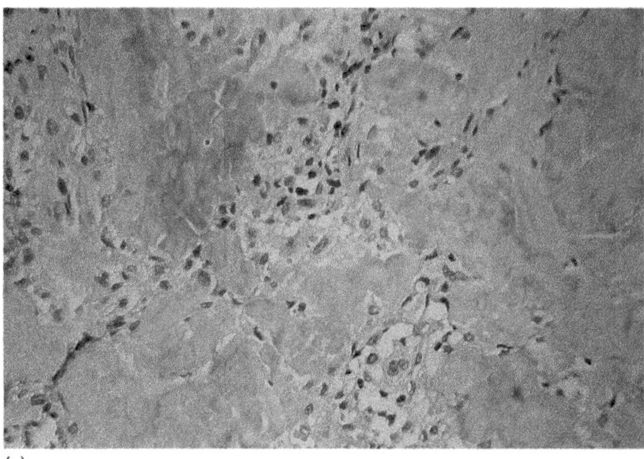

(a)

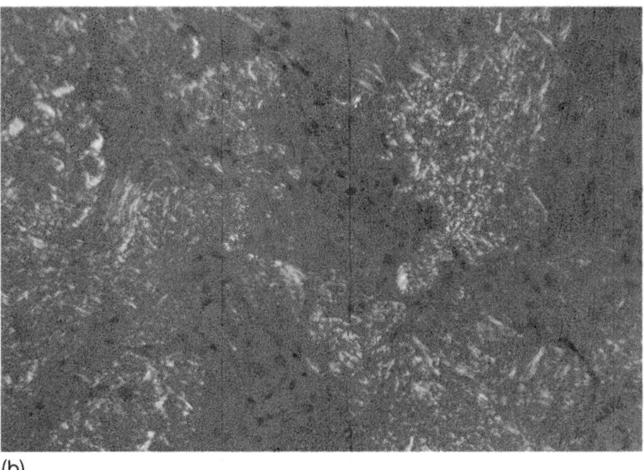

(b)

Figure 23.3 Amyloidosis. Abdominal fat biopsy: **(a)** Congo red staining of extracellular pink amorphous material **(b)** blue–green birefringence under polarized light.

tendons and other soft tissues, skin and lymph nodes may also be affected. The patient may present with non-specific symptoms such as fatigue, anorexia or weight loss, or with heart failure, renal failure including the nephrotic syndrome, macroglossia, peripheral neuropathy or carpal tunnel syndrome. Bleeding may be due to a low coagulation factor X.

Assessment of organ involvement

Cardiac and renal involvement are frequent and will affect choice of treatment.

Heart. Electrocardiogram and more sensitively Doppler with longitudinal strain on echocardiography and cardiac MRI are used to detect and monitor cardiac amyloid, often showing symmetric left ventricular hypertrophy. A mean wall thickness >12 mm with loss of longitudinal function with no other cause suggests amyloidosis. A more recently introduced sensitive technique for detecting cardiac amyloid is a radioactive technetium (^{99}Tc) DPD scan which helps to differentiate AL from wATTR amyloidosis (a negative DPD scan does not rule out cardiac amyloidosis). Cardiac markers troponin and N-terminal pro-brain natriuretic peptide (NT-pro-BNP) are useful to determine the severity of cardiac damage and predict prognosis (see below).

The serum amyloid P (SAP) scan available in specialized centres can be used to determine the extent and severity of disease in other organs (Fig. 23.2).

Kidney. Renal function is measured by serum and 24 hour urine creatinine. Albuminuria >0.5 g in 24 hours is present in almost all cases with renal involvement.

Diagnosis

1 **Histological diagnosis is usually by abdominal fat and/or bone marrow biopsy.** Rarely biopsy of an affected organ is needed. The deposits are in interstitial tissue and the blood vessels and appear as amorphous pink material on conventional staining but show up as birefringent under polarized light on Congo Red staining (Fig. 23.3).
2 **Serum amyloid P scanning** is used in major centres to determine organ involvement and to monitor treatment.
3 PET scan using special tracers may also be used. FDG-PET, MRI or CT is needed to exclude the bone lesions of myeloma.
4 The bone marrow usually shows between 5% and 9% of clonal plasma cells.
5 Serum and urine are tested for monoclonal protein with electrophoresis and immunofixation. Light chain concentrations are measured.
6 Fibril typing and DNA analysis to diagnose hereditary types is carried out in special centres. It is important to establish by fibril analysis in the elderly whether or not a mononoclonal gammopathy (more frequent in the elderly) is the cause of the systemic amyloidosis or is incidental to transthyretin amyloidosis; also to determine whether transthyretin amyloidosis is hereditary or acquired.

Prognosis

Four Mayo prognostic stages are based on the levels in serum of N-terminal prohormone of brain natriuretic peptide (NT-proBNP), cardiac troponin and the difference between the involved and the uninvolved free light chains. In Stage 0, none of these is abnormal (as defined for the staging), though the exact level of NT-pro BNP still has prognostic value. In Stage 4, with the poorest prognosis, all three are abnormal. Survivals have improved to a median over 5 years with the introduction of proteasome inhibitors, lenalidomide and daratumumab and other new drugs into therapeutic protocols,

Treatment

Chemotherapy

Treatment of AL amyloid is with combination chemotherapy similar to that used in myeloma (Fig. 23.4). Daratumumab-cyclophosphamide/bortezomib/dexamethasone (Dara-CyBorD)

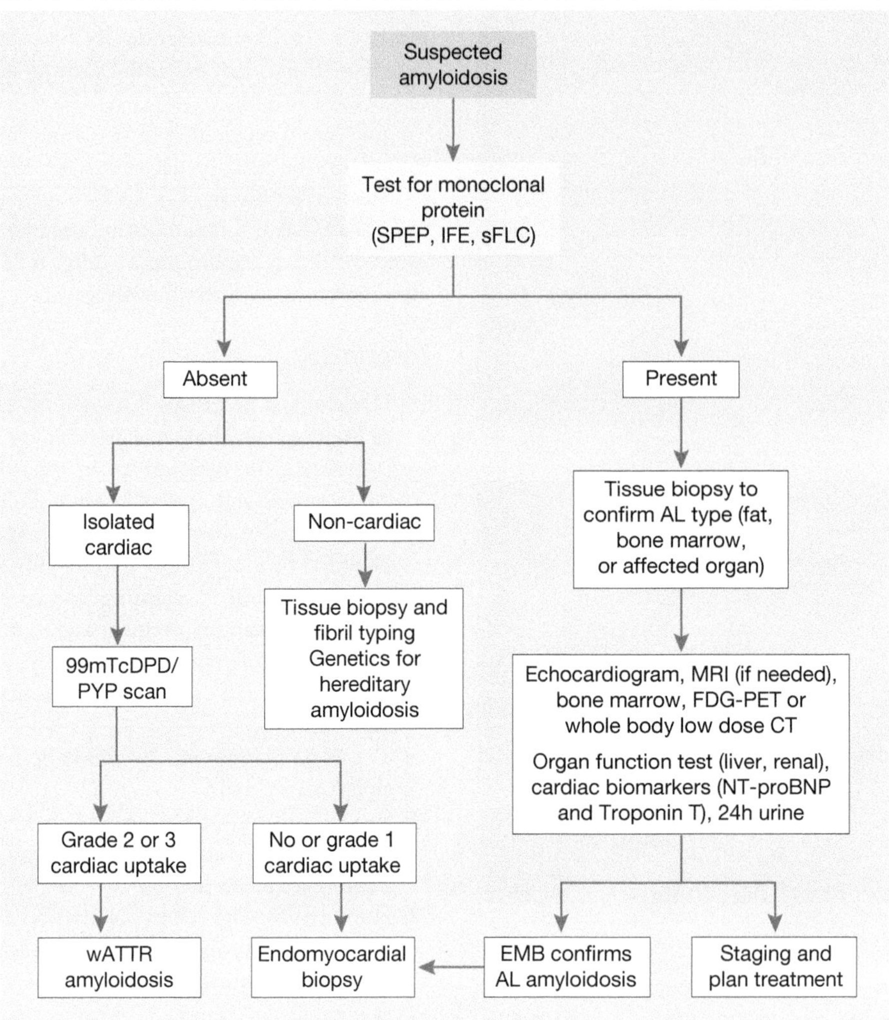

Figure 23.4 Suggested approach to the investigation of suspected amyloidosis. EMB, endomyocardial biopsy; IFE, immunofixation electrophoresis; NT-proBNP, N-terminal pro-brain natriuretic peptide; sFLC, serum free light chains; SPEP, serum protein electrophoresis. Other abbreviations see text. Source: A. Mead *et al.* (eds) (2025) *Hoffbrand's Postgraduate Haematology*, 8th edn (2025, in press). Reproduced with permission of John Wiley and Sons.

is the preferred induction regimen. This has the highest reports response rates. CyBorD (when daratumumab is not accessable) is an acceptable alternative. The triple combination of ixazomib, lenalidomide and dexamethasone, all oral drugs, is an alternative protocol (Fig. 23.5).

In those with a peripheral neuropathy, bortezomib is omitted and treatment with daratumumab and/or lenalidomide and dexamethasone substituted. In younger fit patients with little end-organ damage (or who achieve this with initial therapy), high-dose melphelan and autologous stem cell transplantation (ASCT) improve survival. Patients may be selected for ASCT as having: 1. >10% plasma cell infiltration of the marrow at presentation, and 2. failing to go into complete remission on first line chemotherapy but there are no firm guidelines. Patients with amyloidosis are often at more risk of serious side effects than those with myeloma, especially if there is significant cardiac, autonomic nervous system or renal involvement. Lenalidomide and pomalinomide are used in relapsed disease, if not used in induction. Venetoclax may also be tried, especially in those with the t(11; 14) translocation.

Birtamimab is a humanized monoclonal antibody that neutralizes and disaggregates circulating soluble toxic light chain aggregates. Early clinical trials show it improves survival in stage IV disease and is well tolerated. CAEL101 is another anti-fibril antibody shown to improve organ function in phase I studies.

Cardiac and renal transplantation may be performed in younger subjects who enter remission and have otherwise good organ function so are able to survive these procedures.

Supportive treatment is essential such as diuretics for cardiac failure, amiodarone or pacemakers for dysrhythmias, dialysis for renal failure, diet advice and protein/calorie supplements

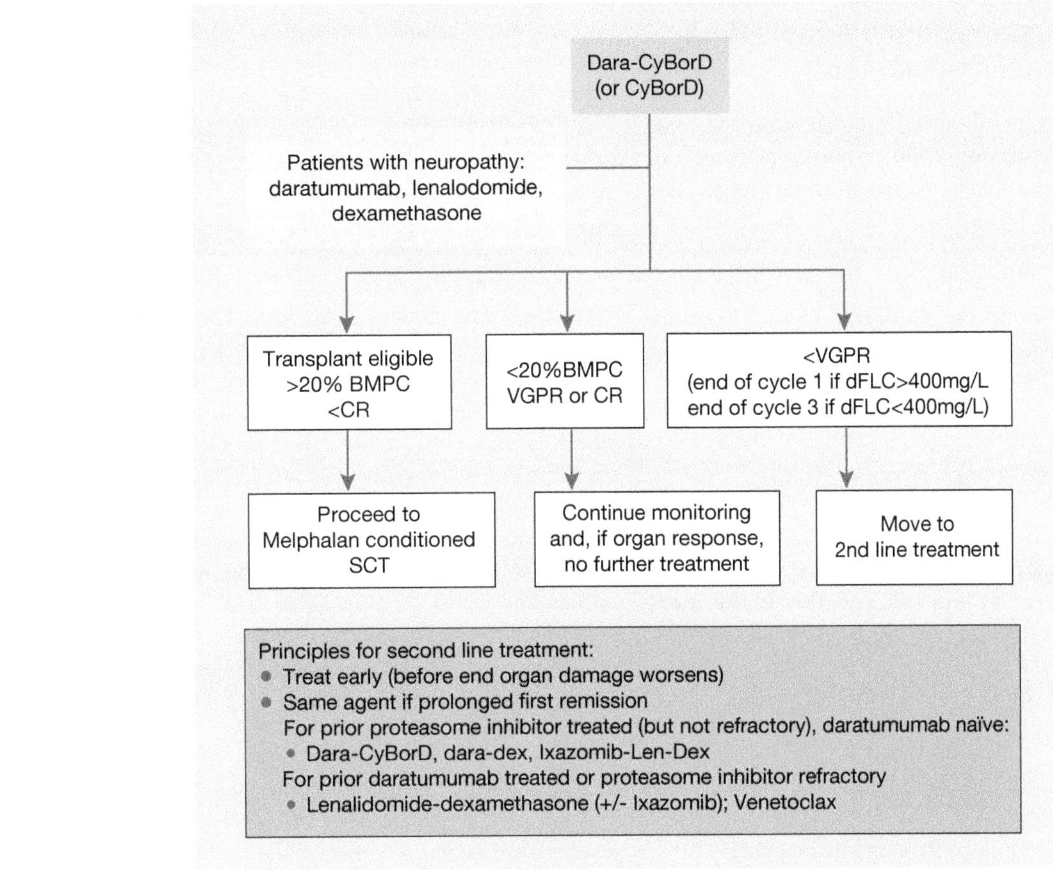

Figure 23.5 A proposed treatment algorithm for AL amyloidosis (BMPC, bone marrow plasma cells; CR, complete remission; CyBorD, cyclophosphamide-bortezomib-dexamethasone; dara, daratumumab; dFLC, difference between the involved and uninvolved free light chains; Len, lenalidomide; SCT, stem cell transplantation; VGPR, very good partial remission). Source: A. Mead *et al.* (eds) (2025) *Hoffbrand's Postgraduate Haematology*, 8th edn (2025, in press). Reproduced with permission of John Wiley and Sons.

for those with malnutrition due to anorexia, chemotherapy, gut or tongue involvement. Some may need direct acting oral anticoagulation, others tranexamic acid for a bleeding tendency.

Localized AL amyloid

Localized deposits of AL amyloid may occur almost anywhere in the body, with the most usual sites the skin, airways, conjunctivae and urogenital tract. They are associated with a focal infiltrate of clonal plasma cell producing amyloidogenic light chains. Progression of localized AL amyloid into a systemic disease is exceedingly rare, and conservative management is usually appropriate. Direct or laser excision or local radiotherapy may be appropriate.

Other forms of localized amyloidosis include that of the brain in Alzheimer's disease, of endocrine glands due to hormone peptide deposits and senile amyloid with deposits in the heart, brain and other organs.

Systemic A protein (AA) amyloid

This is an increasingly rare disease in Western countries due to a lower incidence of chronic inflammatory diseases such as tuberculosis and to improved management of them. Serum amyloid A is an acute-phase reactant which deposits as amyloid in a few per cent of patients with chronic inflammation after a latency of up to 20 years. Rheumatoid arthritis, juvenile arthritis and inflammatory bowel disease are the most frequent causes in developed countries but chronic infections are the dominant causes elsewhere. Familial Mediterranean fever is a potent cause.

Renal dysfunction with proteinuria, liver and gastrointestinal abnormalities cause clinical presentation but heart and nerve involvement are rare. Treatment is of the underlying inflammatory disease aimed at bringing the serum AA protein, which can be raised to over 1000 mg/L, to normal (<10 mg/L). This prevents further amyloid deposition and allows slow clearance of amyloid deposits.

Leucocyte chemotactic factor II (ALEC2) amyloidosis (systemic amyloidosis with predominant renal involvement)

This disease was the third most frequent after AL and systemic AA amyloid among 4000 Mayo Clinic amyloid patients. It occurs in the elderly in certain ethnic groups. The LECT 2 protein made by the liver has, like transthyretin, a tendency to form insoluble fibres. This tendency is greater in certain genetic types. The nephrotic syndrome or gradually progressive renal failure is the dominant clinical features. Diagnosis is by histology with histochemistry to identify the LECT2 fibrils. Treatment is supportive with renal transplantation for end-stage renal disease.

Wild type transthyretin amyloidosis (wATTR)

Transthyretin is a transport protein for thyroxine and retinols. It may deposit as amyloid and this is the most frequent cause of systemic amyloidosis in older adults (especially men). It is increasingly recognized and may become the commonest type of amyloidosis globally. It presents clinically as heart failure with preserved left ventricular ejection fraction, carpal tunnel syndrome, spinal canal stenosis or rupture of the biceps tendon. There are probably many more individuals with the same disease but without clinical symptoms. The drug tafamidis stabilizes the TTR molecule and improves prognosis.

Hereditary systemic amyloidosis

Many different mutations in the TTR gene are the most common cause of hereditary amyloidosis. The disease is labelled as a 'familial amyloidotic neuropathy' as it presents as a progressive peripheral and autonomic neuropathy. There may be cardiac and eye (vitreous) involvement. It occurs in many different ethnic groups. Treatment is with a small interfering RNA (patisiran) or an anti-sense oligonucleotide (inotersan).

Mutations of other proteins listed in Table 23.1, all inherited in a dominant fashion with variable penetrance, cause systemic amyloidosis usually presenting in adult life. Renal, cardiac and nerve damage occur with different frequencies depending on which abnormal protein is responsible. DNA analysis is needed to diagnose these diseases if AL or AA fibril type amyloidosis cannot be diagnosed for certain.

SUMMARY

- The amyloidoses are caused by the extracellular deposition of normally soluble protein in an abnormal fibrillar form. This may damage the tissues and organs where the deposits occur.
- The disease may be localized or widespread (systemic), hereditary or acquired.
- In systemic amyloid the organs involved include the liver, spleen, kidneys, bone marrow, heart and tongue, nerves, skin and eyes.
- Histological diagnosis is usually by abdominal fat and/or bone marrow biopsy. The deposits appear as amorphous pink material on conventional staining but as birefringent under polarized light on Congo Red staining.
- Serum amyloid P protein scanning is used in major centres to determine organ involvement and to monitor treatment.
- Systemic AL amyloid disease is caused by monoclonal light chains produced from a clonal plasma cell proliferation in the bone marrow, with heart failure the dominant cause of death. Treatment is similar to that for myeloma.
- Localized AL amyloid occurs predominantly in the skin, conjunctivae, airways or urogenital tract. It does not progress to systemic amyloidosis. Other forms of localized amyloid include those in the brain in Alzheimer's disease, in endocrine glands and in the elderly 'senile' amyloid deposits.
- Serum amyloid A is an acute-phase reactant which deposits as amyloid in a few per cent of patients with chronic inflammation.
- Leucocyte chemotactic factor II (LEC2) is a protein made by the liver which may in the elderly deposit as amyloid causing renal failure or the nephrotic syndrome.
- Wild type transthyretin (wATTR), the transport protein for thyroxine and retinols may deposit as amyloid in the elderly causing heart failure and tendon damage including carpal tunnel syndrome.
- Hereditary amyloidosis is caused by a variety of genetic abnormalities, most frequently of transthyretin.

Now visit **www.wiley.com/go/haematology9e** to test yourself on this chapter.

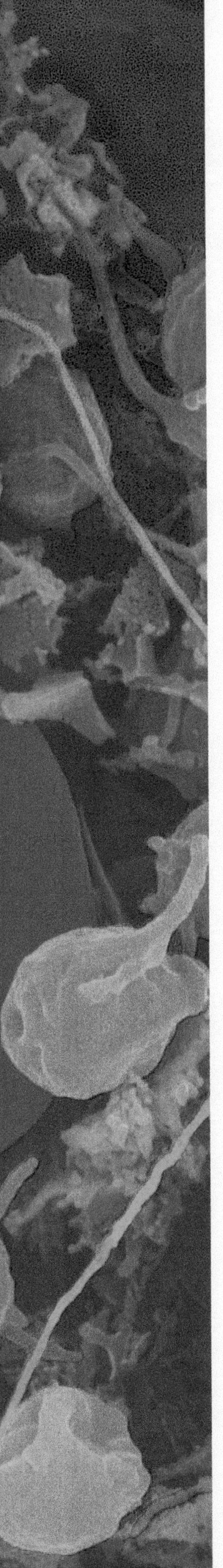

CHAPTER 24

Aplastic anaemia and bone marrow failure syndromes

Key topics

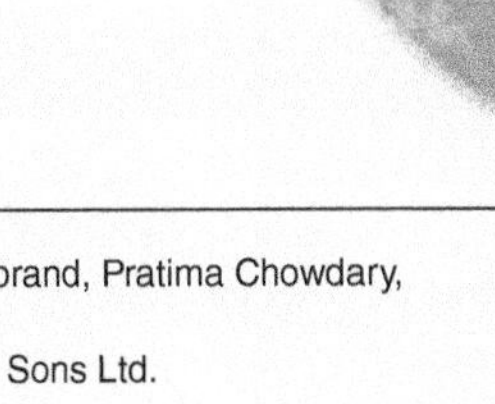

Hoffbrand's Essential Haematology, Ninth Edition. A. Victor Hoffbrand, Pratima Chowdary, Graham P. Collins, and Justin Loke.

© 2024 John Wiley & Sons Ltd. Published 2024 by John Wiley & Sons Ltd.

Companion website: www.wiley.com/go/haematology9e

Pancytopenia

Pancytopenia is a reduction in the blood count of all three major cell lines – red cells, white cells and platelets. Pancytopenia has several causes (Table 24.1), which can be broadly divided into decreased bone marrow production or increased peripheral destruction of blood cells. One cell line may be affected to a greater degree than the others.

Table 24.1 Causes of pancytopenia.

Decreased bone marrow function (but marrow still cellular), e.g. during an acute infection
Aplastic anaemia/paroxysmal nocturnal haemoglobinuria
Acute leukaemia, myelodysplasia (MDS)
Infiltration with lymphoma, myeloma, metastatic solid tumours, tuberculosis
Megaloblastic anaemia
Myelofibrosis, both primary (myeloproliferative neoplasm) and reactive
Haemophagocytic lymphohistiocytosis
Increased peripheral destruction, e.g. due to a microangiopathic process
Splenomegaly

Aplastic anaemia

Aplastic (hypoplastic) anaemia is defined as pancytopenia resulting from hypoplasia of the bone marrow (Fig. 24.2). It can be classified into primary (congenital or acquired) or secondary types (Tables 24.2 and 24.3).

Pathogenesis

The underlying defect in all cases is a substantial reduction in the number of haemopoietic pluripotential stem cells, and a fault in the remaining stem cells or an immune reaction against them, which makes them unable to divide and differentiate sufficiently to populate the bone marrow and blood.

Congenital bone marrow failure syndromes

These are characterized by a range of accompanying systemic clinical features in addition to bone marrow failure (Fig. 24.1).

Fanconi anaemia

Fanconi anaemia (FA) is one of the congenital bone marrow failure syndromes which affect either a single lineage or cause pancytopenia (Table 24.2). It has a recessive pattern of inheritance. The pancytopenia (Fig. 24.3) is often associated with growth retardation and congenital defects of the skeleton alongside other malformations (Fig. 24.1, Fig. 24.4). Sometimes there is hydrocephalus and/or learning disability, but most often intelligence is normal. With increasing age there is a risk of cancers such as gynaecological, head and neck squamous cell and other cancers.

The syndrome is genetically heterogeneous with at least 19 different genes involved: *FANCA–Q*. *FANCD1* is identical to *BRCA2*, the breast cancer susceptibility gene. The proteins coded for by these genes cooperate in a common cellular pathway which results in ubiquitination of the FAN-CD2:FANCI dimer, which is important for normal DNA repair and protects cells against genetic damage. **Cells from FA patients show an abnormally high frequency of spontaneous chromosomal breaks**, and the diagnostic test is elevated breakage after incubation of peripheral blood lymphocytes with a DNA cross-linking agent such as diepoxybutane (DEB test) or mitomycin C. *In vivo* reactive aldehydes resulting from cell metabolism damage DNA by forming cross-links which Fanconi cells are unable to repair.

Table 24.2 The inherited bone marrow failure syndromes.

Pancytopenia
Fanconi anaemia
Dyskeratosis congenita
Shwachman–Diamond syndrome
Pearson syndrome
Familial aplastic anaemia (autosomal and X-linked forms) Myelodysplasia Non-haematological syndromes (Down, Dubowitz syndromes)
Single cytopenia (usually)
Anaemia Diamond–Blackfan anaemia Congenital dyserythropoietic anaemia
Neutropenia Severe congenital neutropenia (Chapter 8)
Thrombocytopenia Congenital amegakaryocytic thrombocytopenia (Chapter 27) Amegakaryocytic thrombocytopenia with absent radii (Chapter 27)

Source: A. Mead *et al.* (eds) (2025) *Hoffbrand's Postgraduate Haematology*, 8th edn (2025, in press). Reproduced with permission of John Wiley and Sons.

Table 24.3 Causes of aplastic anaemia.

Primary	Secondary
Congenital (Fanconi anaemia), other inborn marrow failure syndromes	*Ionizing radiation*: accidental exposure (radiotherapy, radioactive isotopes)
Idiopathic acquired, usually with an autoimmune pathophysiology	*Chemicals*: benzene, organophosphates and other organic solvents, DDT and other pesticides, recreational drugs (ecstasy)
	Drugs: Those that regularly cause marrow depression, e.g. busulphan, melphalan, cyclophosphamide, anthracyclines, nitrosoureas. Those that occasionally or rarely cause marrow depression, e.g. chloramphenicol, sulphonamides, gold, anti-inflammatory, anti-thyroid, psychotrophic, anticonvulsant/anti-depressant drugs
	Viruses: viral hepatitis (non-A, non-B, non-C, and non-G in most cases), EBV, other undefined viruses
	Autoimmune diseases: systemic lupus erythematosus
	Transfusion associated GVHD (Chapter 25)
	Thymoma (more usually associated with red cell aplasia)

DDT, dichlorodiphenyltrichloroethane; EBV, Epstein–Barr virus; GVHD, graft-versus-host disease.

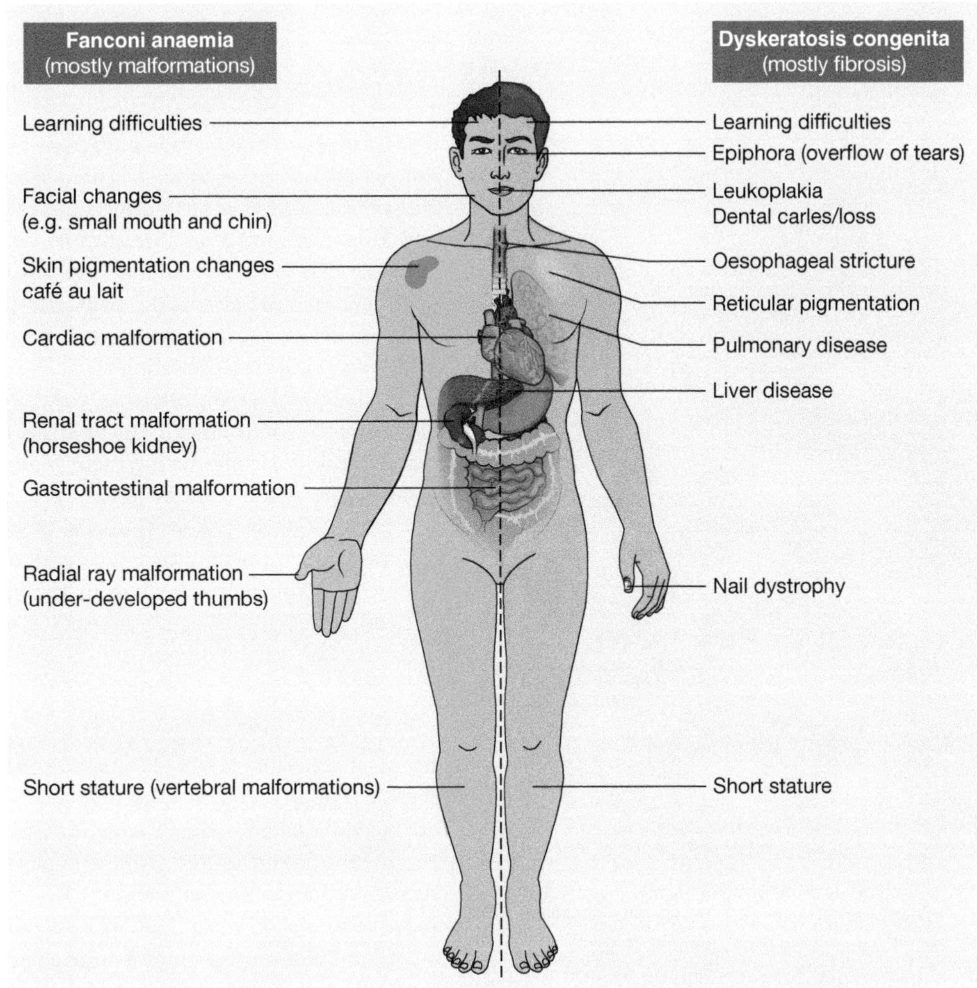

Figure 24.1 Summary of systemic manifestations of Fanconi anaemia (left) and dyskeratosis congenita (right).

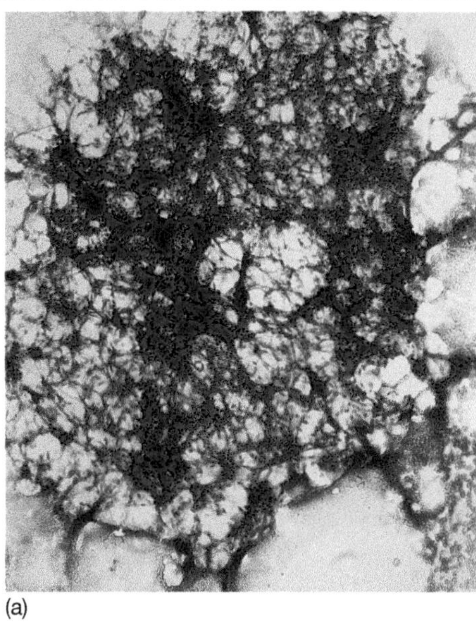
(a)

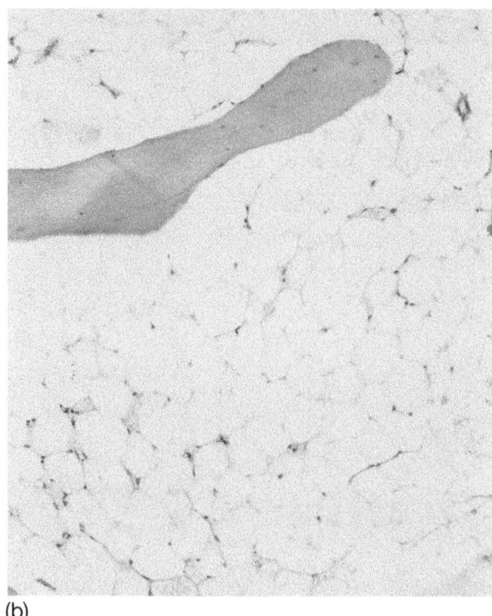
(b)

Figure 24.2 Aplastic anaemia: low power views of bone marrow show severe reduction of haemopoietic cells with an increase in fat spaces. **(a)** Aspirated fragment showing primarily stromal elements with absent haemopoietic cells. **(b)** Trephine biopsy.

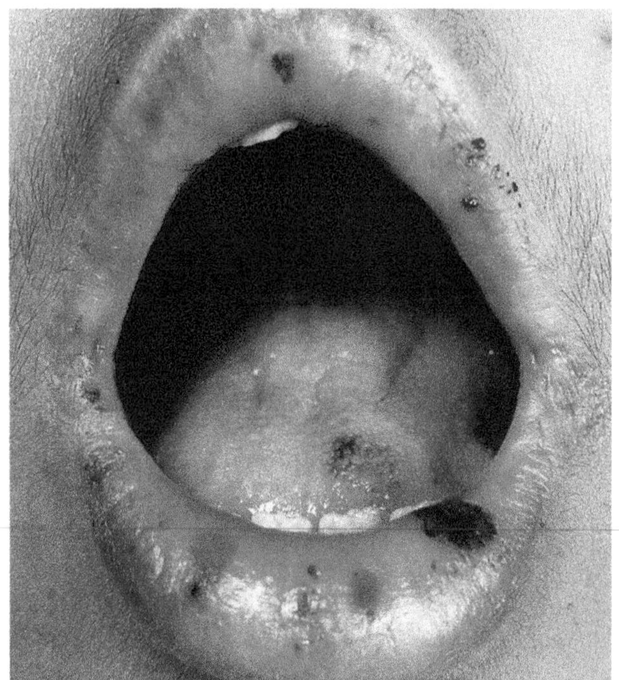

Figure 24.3 Aplastic anaemia: spontaneous mucosal haemorrhages in a 10-year-old boy with severe Fanconi anaemia. Platelet count <5 × 10^9/L. Source: A.V. Hoffbrand *et al.* (2019) *Color Atlas of Clinical Hematology*, 5th edn. Reproduced with permission of John Wiley & Sons.

The usual age of presentation of FA is 3–14 years, but 10% of patients present in adulthood. These 'adult' cases usually lack the typical features of birth defects and early onset of bone marrow failure and many are identified by testing the siblings of more severely affected children. Approximately 10% of patients develop myelodysplastic neoplasias (MDS) or acute myeloid leukaemia (AML). Treatment is usually with androgens or by stem cell transplantation (SCT).

The blood count usually improves with androgens, but side effects, especially in children, can be distressing, including virilization and liver abnormalities; remission with androgens rarely lasts more than 2 years. SCT may cure the patient of the marrow failure, but the risk for epithelial cancers continues to be increased and growth retardation and other congenital defects are not influenced. Because of the sensitivity of the patient's cells to DNA damage, conditioning regimes for SCT in FA patients are mild and irradiation is avoided.

Dyskeratosis congenita

Dyskeratosis congenita (DKC) is a rare disorder characterized by a classic triad of nail dystrophy, lacy reticular pigmentation of the upper chest and neck, and oral leukoplakia (Fig. 24.1). Other systemic manifestations are illustrated in Fig. 24.1.

Autosomal dominant and recessive DC are heterogeneous diseases due to mutations in *TERT, TERC* (telomerase reverse transcriptase RNA template) or other genes encoding components of telomerase, an enzyme complex which is involved in the maintenance of telomere length.

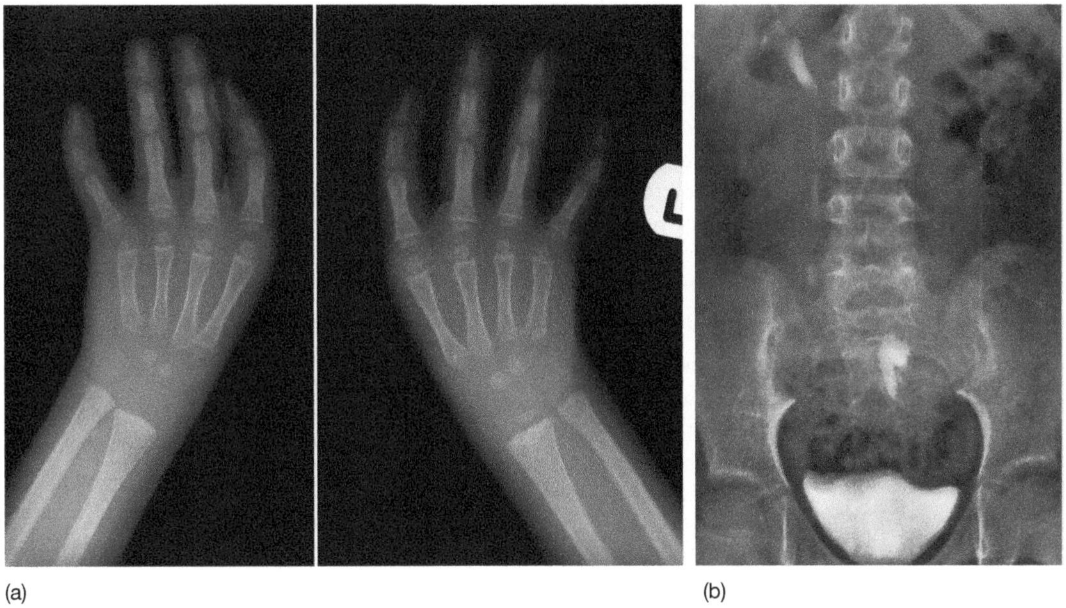

(a) (b)

Figure 24.4 **(a)** X-rays showing absent thumbs in a patient with Fanconi anaemia (FA). **(b)** Intravenous pyelogram in a patient with FA showing a normal right kidney but a left kidney abnormally placed in the pelvis.

X-linked DC is associated with mutations in the *DKC1* (dyskerin) gene. A severe form, the Hoyeraal-Hreidarsson (HH) syndrome is a multisystem disorder starting as an intrauterine growth failure.

Diagnosis is by measuring length of lymphocyte telomeres (granulocyte telomeres can also shorten in acquired marrow failure syndromes) and by genetic testing for mutations in telomere complex genes. Androgens can be helpful in improving blood counts and may lengthen telomeres. SCT can cure the marrow failure, but transplanted patients are still at risk for epithelial cancer, cirrhosis or pulmonary fibrosis.

Shwachman–Diamond syndrome

Shwachman–Diamond syndrome (SDS) is a rare, usually autosomal recessive syndrome characterized by varying degrees of cytopenia, especially neutropenia with a propensity to transform to MDS or AML. Exocrine pancreatic dysfunction is a common feature, while skeletal abnormalities, hepatic impairment and short stature are frequent. The disorder in over 90% of cases results from inherited mutations in the gene *SBDS*, located on chromosome 7q involved in ribosome assembly (Fig. 24.7).

Other congenital marrow failure syndromes

(Table 24.2)

Pearson syndrome is due to a fault in mitochondrial DNA with bone marrow failure and pancreatic defects with diabetes and malabsorption. Ring sideroblasts are characteristic (p. xxx). Germline mutations of the *GATA2* transcription factor can cause pancytopenia, a hypoplastic marrow and predisposition to MDS or AML. This syndrome's presentation is highly variable. *GATA2* mutations are also associated with defects in cellular immunity. Other inherited bone marrow failure syndromes affecting dominantly one lineage include Diamond–Blackfan anaemia (DBA; p.317), severe congenital neutropenia (p.109), amegakaryocytic thrombocytopenia (p. xxx) and thrombocytopenia with absent radii (p.364) (Table 24.2). In DBA as in SDS there are genetic defects in ribosomal biosynthesis and function (Fig. 24.7).

Idiopathic acquired (immune) aplastic anaemia

This is the dominant type of sporadic aplastic anaemia, accounting for at least two-thirds of acquired cases. In most patients, haemopoietic tissue is the target of an autoimmune process with oligoclonal expression of cytotoxic $CD8^+$ T cells, possibly initiated by an infection or an acquired mutation in the STAT3 signalling pathway. T-regulatory cells (Tregs) are decreased. It is associated in a minority of cases with other immune diseases including seronegative hepatitis, eosinophilic fasciitis and thymoma. Clonal haemopoiesis occurs in 50% of cases with somatic mutations of genes including *PIGA*, *BCOR*, *BCORL1*, *ASXLI*, *RUNX1* or *DNMT3A*. Also there are frequent mutations with loss of expression of the human leukocyte antigen (HLA) genes.

This clonal haemopoiesis presumably arises by selection for survival of pre-existing clones in a failed marrow.

The disease may be difficult to distinguish from a late onset of a congenital form of aplastic anaemia and from hypoplastic MDS. Mutations of the telomere repair complex and short telomeres may be present, apparently as acquired abnormalities. The favourable responses to anti-lymphocyte globulin (ALG)/ anti-thymocyte globulin (ATG) and ciclosporin support the concept of an autoimmune disorder.

Secondary causes

Aplastic anaemia may be caused iatrogenically by direct damage to the haemopoietic marrow by radiation or cytotoxic drugs. The antimetabolite drugs, e.g. methotrexate and mitotic inhibitors, e.g. daunorubicin cause only temporary aplasia, but the alkylating agents, particularly busulphan, may cause a more prolonged aplasia closely resembling idiopathic aplastic anaemia. **Some individuals develop aplastic anaemia as a rare idiosyncratic side effect of drugs such as chloramphenicol or gold (Table 24.3)**.

Patients may also develop the disease during or within a few months of **viral hepatitis** (most frequently negative for all known hepatitis viruses). Because the incidence of marrow toxicity is particularly high for chloramphenicol, this drug should be reserved for treatment of infections that are life-threatening and for which it is the optimum antibiotic, e.g. typhoid. Chemicals such as benzene may be implicated; industrial exposure to benzene was a frequent cause but is now negligible except in China with its rapid industrialization. Rarely, aplastic anaemia may be a presenting feature of acute lymphoblastic or myeloid leukaemia, especially in childhood. MDS (Chapter 16) may also present with a hypoplastic marrow, and distinction of hypoplastic MDS from aplastic anaemia may be difficult, especially given the presence of clonal mutations in many patients with aplastic anaemia and occasional responses to immunosuppressive therapy in MDS.

Clinical features

The onset of the idiopathic disease is at any age, with bimodal peak incidences around 10–25 and over 60 years. It is more frequent in Asia, e.g. China or Vietnam, than in Europe or the Americas. **It can be insidious or acute, with symptoms and signs resulting from anaemia, neutropenia or thrombocytopenia**. Bruising, bleeding gums, epistaxes and menorrhagia are the most frequent haemorrhagic manifestations and the usual presenting features (Fig. 24.3), often with symptoms of anaemia. Retinal haemorrhage may impair vision. Infections, particularly of the mouth and throat, are common and generalized infections are frequently life threatening. The lymph nodes, liver and spleen are not enlarged. A careful history and examination (including chest CT scan, abdominal ultrasound) for heart, lung, kidney bone deformities are needed at all ages to exclude inherited forms.

Laboratory findings

1. **In aplastic anaemia, there must be at least two of the following:**
   - **Anaemia (haemoglobin <100 g/L)**. This is normochromic, normocytic or macrocytic, with MCV often 95–110 fL. The reticulocyte count is usually extremely low in relation to the degree of anaemia.
   - **Neutrophil count <1.5 × 10^9/L.**
   - **Platelet count <50 × 10^9/L.**

   Severity of AA is defined by the modified Camitta criteria and helps guide management strategies. Severe cases are defined by marrow cellularity <25% and at least two of neutrophils <0.5 × 10^9/L, platelets <20 × 10^9/L, reticulocytes <20 × 10^9/L; very severe cases as for severe AA but also show neutrophils <0.2 × 10^9/L. Non-severe cases are those which do not meet either severe or very severe criteria.
2. **There are no abnormal cells in the peripheral blood that would indicate leukaemia.**
3. **The bone marrow shows hypoplasia, with loss of haemopoietic tissue and replacement by fat which comprises over 75% of the marrow**. Trephine biopsy is critical; this should be of adequate length, and care taken to ensure a non-subcortical sample is taken. Trephine biopsy may show patchy cellular areas in a hypocellular background. The main cells present are lymphocytes and plasma cells; megakaryocytes in particular are severely reduced or absent.
4. Cytogenetic and, more recently, molecular analysis is performed to exclude inherited forms (especially Fanconi anaemia or dyskeratosis congenita), or MDS. Aplastic anaemia cases may occasionally exhibit numerical chromosomal abnormalities such as monosomy 7 or trisomy 8, but usually the karyotype is normal. Conventional karyotyping may fail as a result of low cell numbers, in which case FISH may be of use. *PIGA*, *BCOR* and *BCORL1* mutations predict for a better prognosis and higher likelihood of response to immunosuppressive therapy, while mutations of *ASXL1*, *RUNX1* and splicing factor genes and short leucocyte telomeres predict lower response rates and higher likelihood of progression to MDS/AML. Telomeres are presumably shortened due to increased mitotic turnover of a reduced number of stem cells.
5. Paroxysmal nocturnal haemoglobinuria (PNH), discussed further below, must be excluded by flow cytometry testing for CD55 and CD59 on red cells and CD14,16 and 24 on white cells.

Diagnosis

The disease must be distinguished from other causes of pancytopenia (Table 24.1). This may require further radiological imaging for example. In older adults especially, care should be undertaken to differentiate with hypocellular/hypoplastic MDS (Chapter 16, Table 24.4).

Table 24.4 Comparison of varying features in AA and hypoplastic MDS.

	Age	Cytogenetics	PNH clone	Blasts	Morphology	Macrocytosis	Other mutations
Aplastic Anaemia	Bimodal distribution (young and old)	Normal	Maybe present	No excess	Dyserythropoiesis	In context of PNH	Maybe present, but at low allelic frequency
Hypoplastic MDS	Older adults	Abnormal in half of patients	Usually absent/ smaller clone	Maybe increased	Multilineage dysplasia	Common	Common, classic MDS associated mutations including spliceosome mutations

Source: Adapted from J. Durrani, J.P. Maciejewski (2019) *Hematol. Am. Soc. Hematol. Educ. Program* 2019: 97–104.

Treatment

This is best carried out in a specialized centre.

General

If a primary cause such as a drug has been identified, this is removed. Initial management consists largely of supportive care with blood transfusions, platelet concentrates and treatment and prevention of infection. All blood products should be leucodepleted, to reduce the risk of alloimmunization, and irradiated, to prevent grafting of live donor lymphocytes. An antifibrinolytic agent, e.g. tranexamic acid, may be used to reduce haemorrhage in patients with severe prolonged thrombocytopenia. If a patient is a transplant candidate, transfusions prior to transplant should be minimized. CMV serology should be taken prior to transfusions to enable donor selection. Granulocyte transfusions are rarely used, but may be given to patients with severe bacterial or fungal infections not responding to antibiotics. Oral antibacterial and antifungal drugs are used to reduce infections. To reduce iron overload from blood transfusions, iron chelation may be needed. Alternatively, venesections may be required after successful stem cell transplantation.

Specific

This must be tailored to the severity of the illness as well as the age of the patient and availability of stem cell donors. Severe cases have a high mortality in the first 6–12 months unless they respond to specific therapy. Less severe cases may have an acute transient course or a chronic course with ultimate recovery, although the platelet count often remains subnormal for many years. Relapses, sometimes severe and occasionally fatal, may also occur and rarely the disease transforms into MDS, AML or PNH (see below).

The two main lines of treatment are immunosuppression with either a combination of the three drugs, anti-thymocyte (lymphocyte) globulin, ciclosporin and eltrombopag or stem cell transplantation.

1 ***Anti-thymocyte globulin*** (ATG), also called anti-lymphocyte globulin (ALG) is prepared by immunizing animals (usually horse or rabbit in the West, pig in China) with human thymocytes. Alone it is of benefit in approximately 50–60% of acquired cases. Given with ciclosporin there is a 75% haematological response rate. Eltrombopag may improve the rate of response still further so now this three-drug combination is preferred first-line treatment for less severe cases and older severe cases or those without a suitable donor. Corticosteroids are given short term to reduce the immediate allergic effects and the incidence and severity of serum sickness (fever, rash and joint pains), which may occur approximately 7 days after ATG administration. The platelet count should be maintained $>10\times10^9$/L. If there is no response after 3–4 months a second course of triple therapy may be tried, with ATG prepared from the same or another species. A randomized trial showed superiority of horse ATG to rabbit ATG, maybe because rabbit ATG depletes CD4 and Tregs more severely. Responses are not usually complete and relapses occur. As discussed above certain clonal mutations predict for a favourable response whereas other mutations predict for a less favourable response.

2 ***Ciclosporin*** This is an effective agent which is particularly valuable in combination with ATG. In older subjects it is sometimes used alone as ATG is poorly tolerated. Some centres substitute tacrolimus, which may have fewer adverse events.

3 ***Eltrombopag*** This is a TPO-receptor agonist (Chapter 26) which stimulates platelet production but may result in a durable tri-lineage improvement in blood cell counts in aplastic anaemia. It is given in combination with ATG and ciclosporin.

4 ***Stem cell transplantation*** (SCT) Allogeneic SCT offers the chance of permanent cure in selected patients. In general, SCT is favoured in patients less than 35 years old with severe aplastic anaemia and an HLA matching sibling donor. SCT is an important option for others, e.g. older patients, for whom IST immunosuppression has failed. It is the only cure for constitutional bone marrow failure syndromes. Conditioning in idiopathic aplastic anaemia is typically with

cyclophosphamide without irradiation, and prolonged course of ciclosporin is used to reduce the risks of graft failure and graft-versus-host disease (GVHD). GVHD can be maximally avoided as there is no benefit from a graft vs host phenomenon (in contrast to management of leukaemias, where a graft vs leukaemia effect is desired). ATG is included in the conditioning regimen. Cure rates of more than 90% in young children and more than 80% in adolescents are obtained, but with a survival rate of about 50% in those older than 50 years. Marrow rather than peripheral blood is the preferred source of stem cells, since the risk of GVHD is lower with marrow grafts.

Non-myeloablative transplants (Chapter 25) are used in congenital aplastic anaemia and for selected patients with acquired idiopathic aplastic anaemia over the age of 40 years. SCT using umbilical cord blood, unrelated volunteer donors and haplo-identical family members is used in carefully selected patients. *In vivo* T-cell depletion and high-dose cyclophosphamide a few days after the stem cell infusion reduce the risk of severe GVHD (see Chapter 25).

5 ***Alemtuzumab*** (anti-CD52 antibody) This has proved effective in about 50% of patients in small studies but is toxic and so is only used if at all, after ATG and other therapies have failed.
6 ***Androgens, e.g. danazol*** These are beneficial in improving blood counts in some patients, but do not improve survival. Side effects from chronic use are marked, including virilization, salt retention and liver damage with cholestatic jaundice or rarely hepatocellular carcinoma. If there is no response in 4–6 months, androgens should be stopped. If there is a response, the drug should be withdrawn gradually.
7 ***Haemopoietic growth factors*** Granulocyte colony-stimulating factor (G-CSF) may produce minor responses but does not lead to sustained improvement. Other growth factors besides eltrombopag have not proved helpful.
8 ***Iron chelation therapy*** This may be needed in patients who require regular red cell transfusion.

Paroxysmal nocturnal haemoglobinuria

Paroxysmal nocturnal haemoglobinuria (PNH) is a rare, acquired, clonal disorder of marrow stem cells in which there is deficient synthesis of the glycosylphosphatidylinositol (GPI) anchor, a structure that attaches several surface proteins to the cell membrane. This deficiency results in the clinical triad of chronic intravascular haemolysis, venous thrombosis and bone marrow failure. PNH results from acquired mutations in the X chromosome gene coding for phosphatidylinositol glycan protein class A (*PIGA*), which is essential for the formation of the GPI anchor (Fig. 24.5). The net result is that GPI-linked proteins (such as CD55 and CD59) are absent from the cell surface of all the cells derived from the abnormal stem cell including white cells and platelets (Fig. 24.5). **The lack of the surface molecules decay-activating factor (DAF, CD55) and membrane inhibitor of reactive lysis (MIRL, CD59) renders red cells sensitive to lysis by complement, which is normally cleared from the surface of cells by these factors, and the result is chronic intravascular haemolysis.**

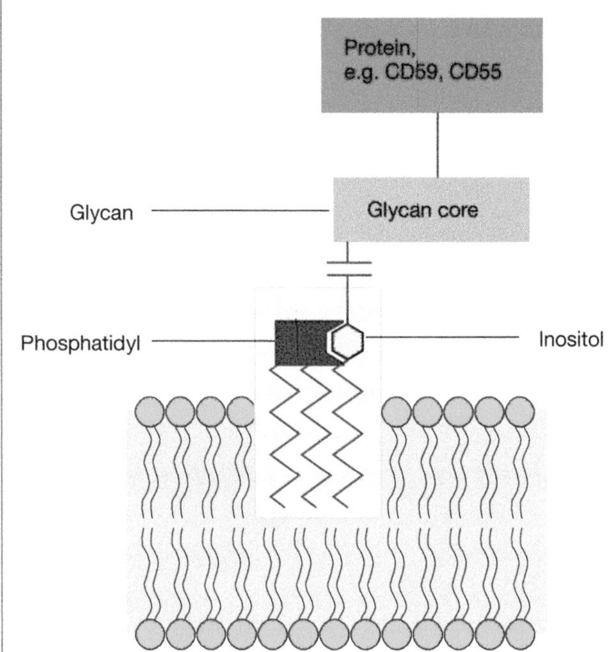

Figure 24.5 Schematic representation of the phosphatidylinositol glycan which anchors many different proteins to the cell membrane, e.g. CD59 (MIRL, membrane inhibitor of reactive lysis).

Haemosiderinuria is a constant feature of PNH and can give rise to iron deficiency, which may exacerbate the anaemia. The haemolysis is typically continuous and rarely paroxysmal or limited to the nocturnal period, despite the name of the condition. Haptoglobins are absent; free haemoglobin may damage the kidney and it removes nitric oxide from smooth muscle, causing oesophageal spasm and dysphagia, erectile dysfunction and pulmonary hypertension. The serum LDH is raised and the level can be used to monitor progress of the disease.

The other main clinical problem in PNH is of venous thrombosis. Patients may develop recurrent thromboses in any venous distribution including large vessels, such as the portal, hepatic and mesenteric veins and dural sinuses. Arterial thrombosis, such as strokes or myocardial infarction, can also occur. Intermittent abdominal pain due to mesenteric vein thrombosis is a common feature.

PNH is almost invariably associated with some form of bone marrow hypoplasia and there may even be complete aplastic anaemia. The PNH clone may expand as a result of a selective pressure, possibly immunologically mediated, against cells that have normal GPI-linked membrane proteins.

PNH is diagnosed by flow cytometry, which shows loss of expression of the GPI-linked proteins CD55 and CD59 or by the fluorescent aerolysin (FLAER), this dye binding to normal but not to PNH cells.

Eculizumab and ravulizumab are humanized antibodies against complement C5 which inhibit the activation of terminal components of complement and reduce haemolysis, transfusion requirements and the incidence of thrombosis. Ravulizumab is longer-acting and is given only once in eight weeks, whereas eculizumab, with which there is much longer experience, is given every fortnight. **Pegcetacoplan is a more recently introduced pegylated peptide that targets the proximal complement protein C3.** Trials have shown it to be superior to eculizumab in controlling extravascular and intravascular haemolysis, improving haemoglobin and clinical and haematological outcomes. **Iptacopan**, an oral drug that inhibits complement factor B, is also approved for preventing haemolysis in PNH.

Iron therapy is used for iron deficiency and long-term anticoagulation may be needed. Immunosuppression can be useful and allogeneic SCT is a definitive treatment. The disease occasionally remits spontaneously. The median survival is over 10 years. As for aplastic anaemia, transformation to MDS or AML may occur.

Red cell aplasia

This is a rare group of syndromes characterized by anaemia with normal leucocytes and platelets and grossly reduced or absent erythroblasts in the marrow (Fig. 24.6).

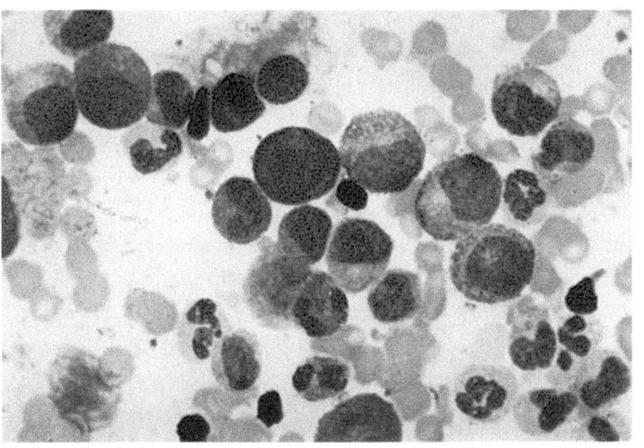

Figure 24.6 The bone marrow in red cell aplasia. There is selective loss of erythropoiesis.

Chronic forms

Diamond–Blackfan anaemia

This congenital disease is inherited as a recessive condition. It is associated in 50% of cases with a varying number of somatic abnormalities, e.g. of the face, skeleton, urogenital tract or heart and is typically diagnosed in the first two years of life. The anaemia is macrocytic or normocytic and sometimes accompanied by mild neutropenia or thrombocytopenia. Raised red cell foetal haemoglobin and deaminase levels are frequent. Mutation of one of several genes that encode ribosomal proteins underlies most cases (Fig. 24.7). Both the Shwachman–Diamond syndrome and the acquired myelodysplasia 5q- syndrome (Chapter 16) also affect ribosome synthesis (Fig. 24.7). DBA must be differentiated from viral or immune-mediated red cell aplasia and rare congenital immune diseases accompanied by red cell aplasia. Corticosteroids are the first line of treatment with an 80% initial response rate. Long-term doses must be tapered and if possible stopped to avoid serious side effects such as impaired growth, endocrine dysfunction, osteoporosis and infections. Spontaneous remission of the disease may occur.

Stem cell transplantation from an HLA matching sibling or unrelated donor may be curative but has many possible immediate and long-term side effects. It is considered in corticosteroid refractory cases, those with serious side effects from steroids and those needing regular chronic blood transfusions.

Severe iron organ overload from blood transfusions, including of the heart, occurs relatively early compared with thalassaemia major. The absence of erythropoiesis in DBA is thought to lead to high levels of non-transferrin bound iron. Iron chelation is needed but deferiprone is avoided if possible as the incidence of agranulocytosis caused by the drug is particularly high in DBA.

Acquired chronic red cell aplasia

Acquired chronic red cell aplasia can occur without any obvious associated disease or precipitating factor (idiopathic), or may be seen with autoimmune diseases (especially systemic lupus erythematosus), with thymoma, lymphoma or chronic lymphocytic leukaemia (Table 24.5). Monoclonal antibodies, such as rituximab (anti-CD20), are being used increasingly in treatment of refractory acquired red cell aplasia and other autoimmune cytopenias. In some cases, other immunosuppressive drugs can be helpful.

Table 24.5 Classification of red cell aplasia.

Acute, transient	Chronic congenital	Chronic acquired
Parvovirus infection Infancy and childhood Drugs, e.g. azathioprine, co-trimoxazole	Diamond–Blackfan anaemia	Idiopathic Associated with thymoma, systemic lupus erythematosus, rheumatoid arthritis, lymphoma, chronic lymphocytic leukaemia, T-cell large granular lymphocytic leukaemia, myelodysplasia, viral infection, drugs

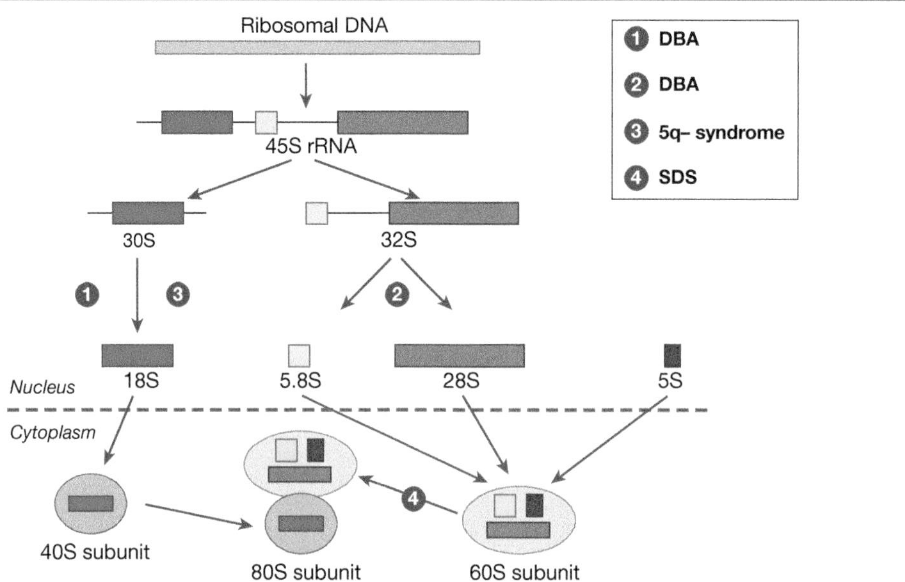

Figure 24.7 Ribosomal RNA processing and the sites of disruption in bone marrow failure syndromes. The different RNA species have roles in cell stress response, proliferation and apoptosis. Source: Courtesy of Professor I. Dokal. DBA, Diamond–Blackfan anaemia; SDS, Shwachman–Diamond syndrome.

If regular blood transfusions are needed, iron chelation therapy will also be necessary. SCT has been carried out in some severe cases.

Transient form

Parvovirus B19 infects red cell precursors via the P antigen and causes a transient (5–10 days) red cell aplasia. This can result in rapid onset of severe anaemia in patients with pre-existing shortened red cell survival, such as those with sickle cell disease or hereditary spherocytosis (Fig. 24.8). Transient red cell aplasia with anaemia may also occur in association with drug therapy (Table 24.3) and in normal infants or children, often with a history of a viral infection in the preceding three months.

Congenital dyserythropoietic anaemias

Congenital dyserythropoietic anaemias (CDAs) are a group of hereditary refractory anaemias characterized by ineffective erythropoiesis and often erythroblast multinuclearity. The patient may be jaundiced with splenomegaly. Skeletal and other non-haematological abnormalities may be present. The white cell and platelet counts are normal. The reticulocyte count is low for the degree of anaemia, despite increased marrow cellularity. The anaemia is of variable severity and is usually first noted in infancy or childhood. Iron overload may develop.

The CDAs are classified into several types based on the degree to which megaloblastic changes, giant erythroblasts and dyserythropoietic changes are present. CDA Type 1 is due to mutation of the gene *CDAN1* (codanin), active during the S phase of the cell cycle. Somatic abnormalities are common. CDA Type 2 is known as HEMPAS (hereditary erythroblast multinuclearity with a positive acidified serum lysis test). The test is positive with some sera, but not with the patient's serum. The basic lesion is a defect in the gene *SEC23B* coding for a protein involved in synthesis of endoplasmic reticulum-derived vesicles destined for the Golgi component.

Osteopetrosis

This is a rare heterogeneous group of disorders due to failure of bone resorption by osteoclasts. Inheritance may be recessive or dominant. The bones are dense but brittle and fractures are common. The marrow space is reduced and a leucoerythroblastic anaemia occurs. The liver and spleen are enlarged. Early death from the consequences of bone marrow failure is usual. SCT offers a chance of cure.

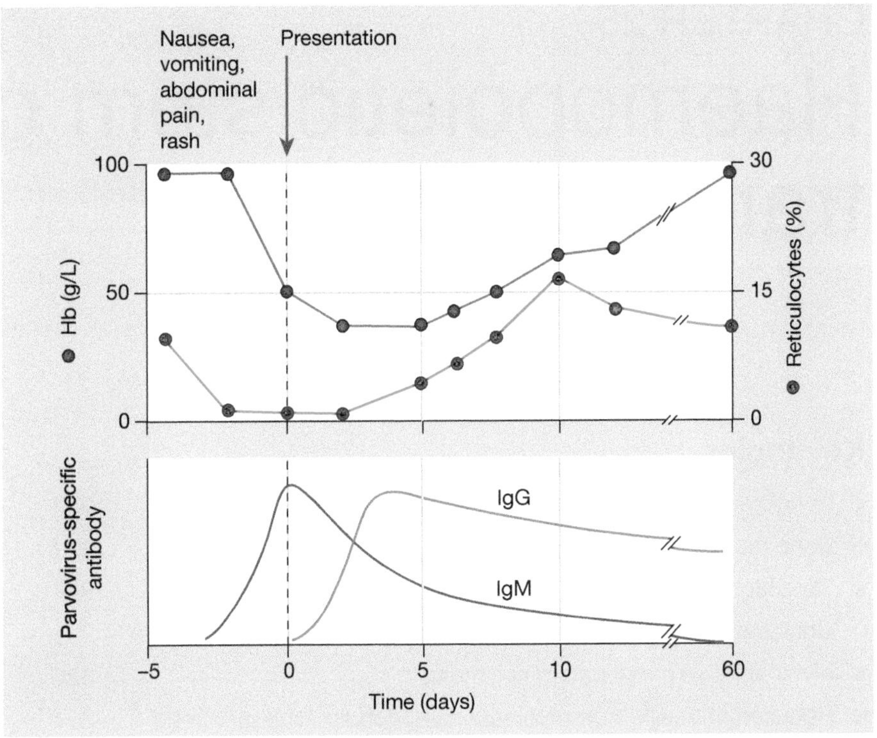

Figure 24.8 Parvovirus infection: flow chart showing transient fall in haemoglobin and reticulocytes in a patient with hereditary spherocytosis.

SUMMARY

- Aplastic anaemia presents as pancytopenia (subnormal haemoglobin, neutrophils and platelets) associated with a hypoplastic bone marrow.
- Marrow failure syndromes may be congenital, e.g. Fanconi anaemia, dyskeratosis congenita, Shwachman–Diamond syndrome or acquired-idiopathic or due to drugs, viral infection or toxins.
- Fanconi anaemia is usually autosomal recessive, associated with congenital skeletal, skin and renal abnormalities. It is caused by inherited mutations of genes involved in DNA repair.
- Dyskeratosis congenita is due to short telomeres resulting from inherited mutations of genes encoding proteins of the telomerase complex. It is associated with nail dysplasia, oral leukoplakia and skin abnormalities.
- Acquired aplastic anaemia if severe is treated with anti-thymocyte globulin, ciclosporin and eltrombopag or by stem cell transplantation.
- Paroxysmal nocturnal haemoglobinuria is an acquired clonal haemolytic anaemia associated with pancytopenia arising in a hypoplastic marrow. There is defective synthesis of the glycosylphosphatidylinositol anchor for many membrane proteins. It is treated with complement inhibitors and often anticoagulation.
- Other rare congenital syndromes are associated with pancytopenia or with selective anaemia, neutropenia or thrombocytopenia.
- Red cell aplasia causes anaemia with normal white cell and platelet counts. It may be transient, usually caused by parvovirus infection, or chronic. Chronic forms may be congenital (Diamond–Blackfan anaemia) or acquired, e.g. associated with systemic lupus erythematosus, lymphoma or chronic lymphocytic leukaemia.
- Congenital dyserythropoietic anaemias are a group of rare inherited disorders of erythropoiesis.

Now visit **www.wiley.com/go/haematology9e** to test yourself on this chapter.

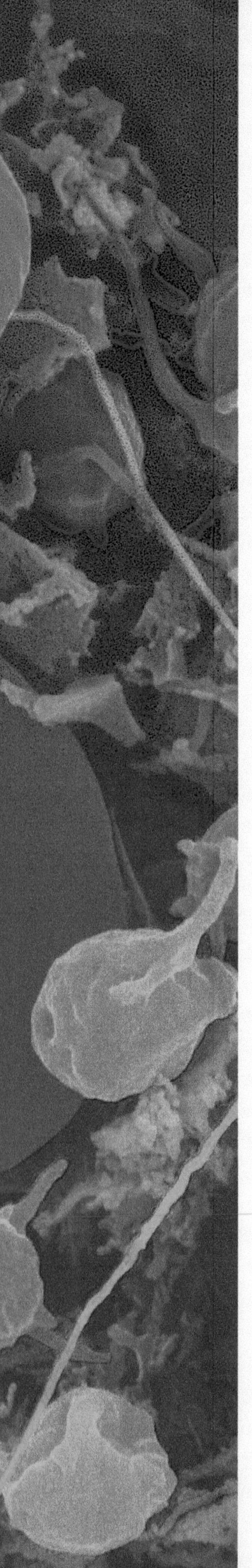

CHAPTER 25

Haemopoietic stem cell transplantation

Key topics

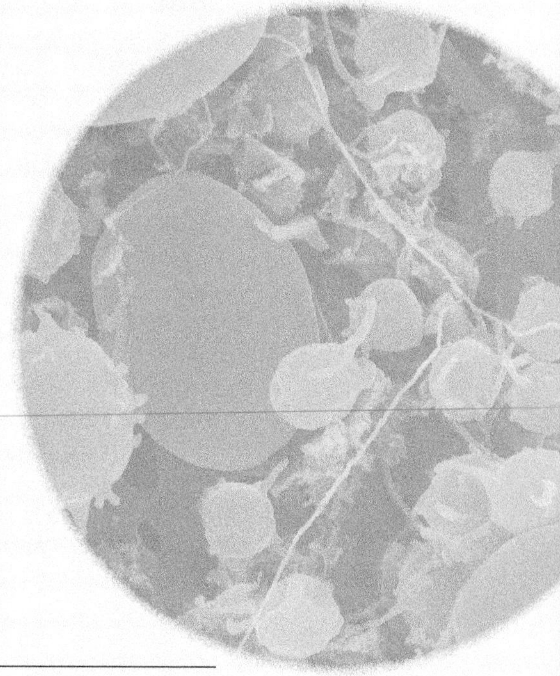

Hoffbrand's Essential Haematology, Ninth Edition. A. Victor Hoffbrand, Pratima Chowdary, Graham P. Collins, and Justin Loke.
© 2024 John Wiley & Sons Ltd. Published 2024 by John Wiley & Sons Ltd.
Companion website: www.wiley.com/go/haematology9e

Principles of stem cell transplantation

Haemopoietic stem cell transplantation (SCT) involves replacing the patient's haemopoietic and immune systems with stem cells either from another individual or with a previously harvested portion of the patient's own haemopoietic stem cells (Fig. 25.1). Depending on the source of the stem cells, the term includes *bone marrow transplantation* (BMT), *peripheral blood stem cell* (PBSC) transplantation and *umbilical cord blood* transplantation. Depending on the type of donor and source of stem cells, SCT may be *syngeneic* (identical twin), *allogeneic* (family member or unrelated person) or *autologous* (self) (Table 25.1).

The principal diseases for which allogeneic and autologous SCT are performed are shown in Fig. 25.2. However, the exact role of SCT in the management of each disease is complex and depends on factors such as disease severity and subtype, remission status, patient age and co-morbid conditions, and, for allogeneic transplantation, availability of a donor. The advent of CAR-T cell therapy and improvements in first- and second-line treatments for acute lymphoblastic leukaemia, lymphomas and myeloma are also changing the indications for autologous and allogeneic transplants in these disorders.

Collection of stem cells

Stem cells can be collected from the peripheral blood, bone marrow or umbilical cord blood. Regardless of source, the collection typically includes harvest of not just true pluripotential stem cells, but other more differentiated progenitor cells that may be important in facilitating early post-transplant engraftment and haemopoietic recovery.

Peripheral blood normally contains too few haemopoietic stem cells to allow collection of sufficient numbers for transplantation, so stem cells must be 'mobilized' into the blood in greater numbers to facilitate collection (Fig. 25.3). Growth factors can increase the number of circulating stem cells by around 10–100 times. Granulocyte colony-stimulating factor (G-CSF) is given to patients (for autologous transplantation) or donors (for syngeneic or allogeneic transplant) as a course of injections until the white cell count starts to rise. Plerixafor, an inhibitor of CXCR4, a stem cell adhesion molecule, helps to mobilize bone marrow stem cells and is also given to increase the yield. For autologous transplant, cytotoxic chemotherapy, e.g. salvage therapy for relapsed lymphoma, may also given both to reduce malignant cells and to mobilize stem cells, since during recovery after this chemotherapy the circulating stem cell numbers transiently increase. A large dose cyclophosphamide may also be given to patients (but not to healthy donors) since this may enhance subsequent stem cell mobilization and harvesting.

Using G-CSF-based mobilization strategies, **the minimum target cell dose of 2×10^6 CD34$^+$ cells/kg to be harvested,** is achieved in more than 80% of patients. The adequacy of the collection is assessed by CD34$^+$ cell count, as CD34 is a marker of stem and progenitor cells (Chapter 1). In patients who fail to mobilize the target number of CD34$^+$ cells, as described above, the CXCR4 antagonist plerixafor can be combined with G-CSF. This permits mobilization of the required numbers of PBSC in more than 95% of autograft candidates.

After mobilization, PBSC collections are harvested by apheresis. Depending on the typical outpatient protocol is G-CSF on days 1–4 and plerixafor on days 5, 6 and 7 with efficiency of stem cell mobilization, repeated collections may be needed for up to 4 days with harvests on days 5, 6, 7 and 8 (Fig. 25.3).

Bone marrow collection

The donor is given a general anaesthetic and 500–1200 mL of marrow are harvested from the pelvis. The marrow is anticoagulated and a mononuclear cell count is taken periodically while marrow is being obtained, in order to assess the yield. This should be approximately $2–4 \times 10^8$ nucleated cells/kg body weight of the recipient. Compared to PBSCs, bone marrow reduces the risk of graft failure, but increases the risk of chronic graft-versus-host disease (GVHD). The risk of relapse of the primary disease and risk of acute GVHD is similar between stem cell sources.

Cord blood collection

Foetal blood is a rich source of haemopoietic stem cells, which may be collected from cord blood at the time of delivery. Because of the relatively small numbers of stem cells collected from a single cord, these collections are most useful for children who do not have a fully matching sibling or unrelated donor. Two cord donations may be needed to obtain sufficient stem cells for adult recipients. Less stringent HLA matching is needed due to the immunological naïveté of the stem cells, resulting in less GVHD. On the other hand, immune reconstitution is slower after cord blood transplantation.

Choice of donor

The most frequently used donor for allogeneic transplant is a fully human leucocyte antigen (HLA)-matching sibling donor. The HLA system is described further below. Multiparous female donors are more likely than male donors to result in GVHD in the recipient due to previous alloimmunization to paternal antigens of the female donor during prior pregnancies with a male foetus. An identical twin can also be used as donor, but there is no graft versus leukaemia/lymphoma effect from a syngeneic donor, so relapse of the original disease is more likely.

An HLA-matching unrelated donor may be sought from international volunteer donor panels. Mismatched and one-half HLA-matching 'haplo-identical' donors – i.e. father, mother, child or sibling donors can also be used. For haploidentical transplants, a large dose of cyclophosphamide is given alone or with other immunosuppressive drugs 3 or 4 days after the stem cell infusion. This protocol reduces the risk of donor T cells proliferating

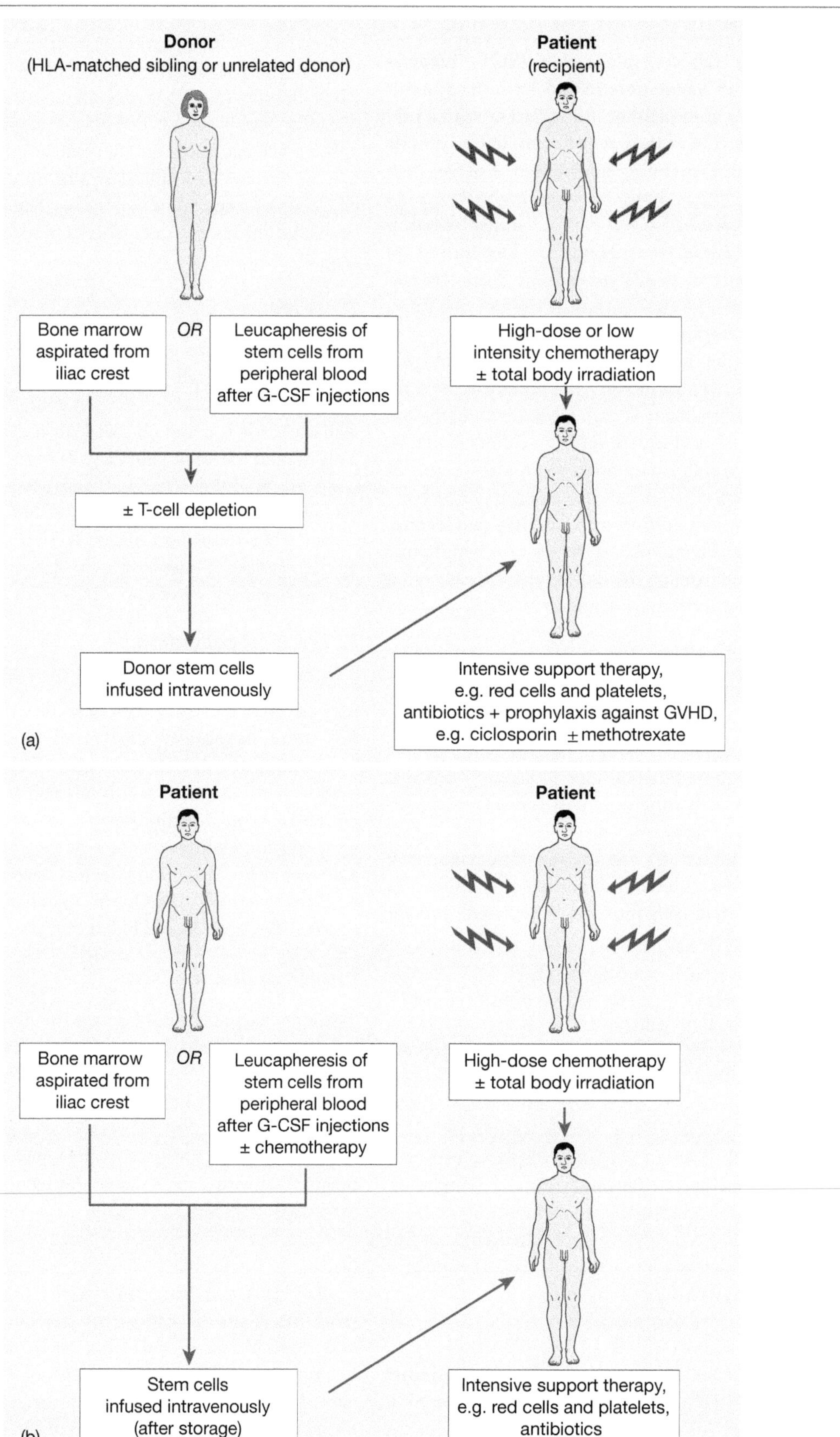

Figure 25.1 Procedures for **(a)** allogeneic and **(b)** autologous stem cell transplantation. G-CSF, granulocyte colony-stimulating factor; GVHD, graft-versus-host disease.

Table 25.1 Haemopoietic stem cell transplantation: potential donors.

Donor	Type of transplant
HLA-matching sibling Unrelated fully HLA-matching or nearly fully HLA-matching volunteer Haploidentical (half HLA-matching) family member Umbilical cord blood	Allogeneic
Identical twin	Syngeneic
Self	Autologous

HLA, human leucocyte antigen.

and causing severe acute GVHD. It is now employed in mismatched transplants and is also being used in identical sibling and fully matched transplants. Haploidentical transplants are more successful for younger donors and recipients and with certain types of HLA matching. For some indications a young haplo-matched or matched unrelated donor may be preferable to an older matched sibling donor. Subjects with clonal haemopoiesis of undetermined prognosis (CHIP) are not excluded as donors.

Stem cell processing

CD34⁺ stem cells may be selected from both types of harvest. After collection, the stem cell harvest is processed with removal of red cells and concentration of the mononuclear cells. In some protocols, antibodies to remove T lymphocytes are used *in vitro*. This reduces the risk of GVHD, but increases the risk of non-engraftment, viral infections and, if the transplant is being done for malignant disease, relapse. *In vivo* T-cell depletion is generally preferred (see below).

Conditioning

Prior to infusion of haemopoietic stem cells, patients receive chemotherapy, sometimes in combination with total body irradiation (TBI; Fig. 25.1) in a procedure called conditioning. The primary goal is to induce a state of immunosuppression so that the recipient's body does not immediately reject the donor cells. In the case of malignant disease, the conditioning regimen may also reduce or even eliminate any remaining neoplastic cells.

Myeloablative conditioning regimens

These regimens aim at irreversibly destroying the haemopoietic function of the bone marrow with high doses of chemotherapy, with or without TBI. The conditioning is also aimed at destroying the patient's immune system and any malignant cells in the bone marrow. TBI is usually used in patients with malignant disease and is most frequently

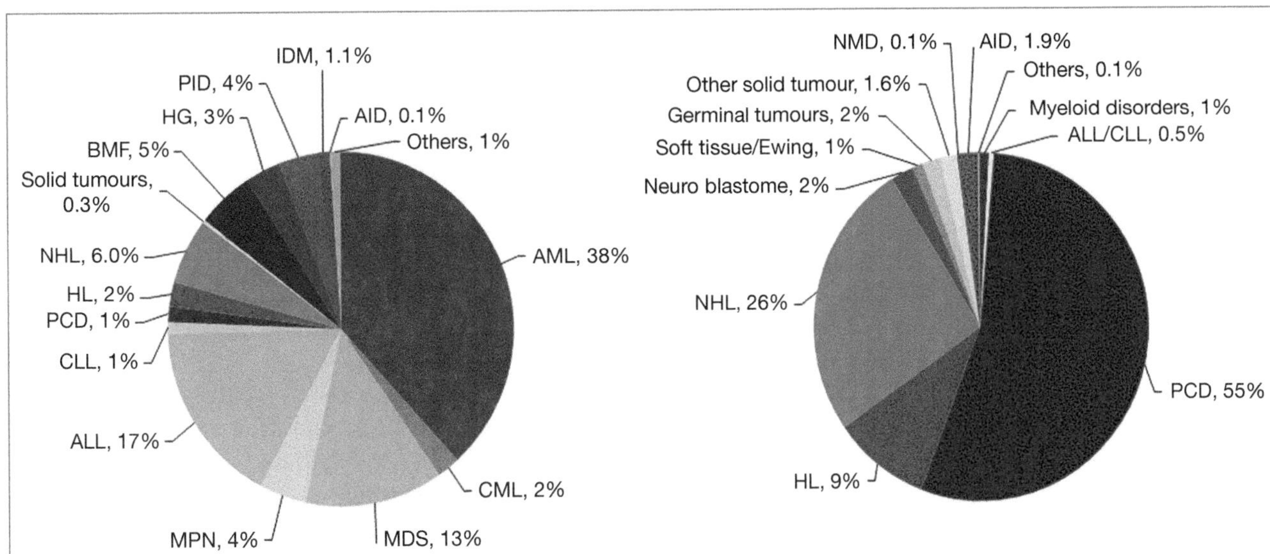

Figure 25.2 Relative proportion of disease indications for SCT in Europe 2021. Green shades: myeloid malignancies, blue: lymphoid malignancies, brown: solid tumours and red: non-malignant disorders. Left figure allogeneic HCT(SCT). Right figure autologous HCT(SCT). Source: J.R. Passweg *et al.* (2023) *Bone Marrow Transpl.* 58: 647–58/Springer Nature/CC BY 4.0. AID, autoimmune diseases; ALL, acute lymphoblastic leukaemia; AML, acute myeloid leukaemia; BMF, bone marrow failure; CLL, chronic lymphocytic leukaemia; CML, chronic myeloid leukaemia; HG, haemoglobinopathies (thalassemia and sickle cell disease); HL, Hodgkin lymphoma; IDM, inherited diseases of metabolism; MDS, myelodysplasia; MPN, myeloproliferative neoplasia; NHL, non-Hodgkin lymphoma; NMD, non-malignant disorders; PCD, plasma cell disorders; PID, primary immune deficiencies.

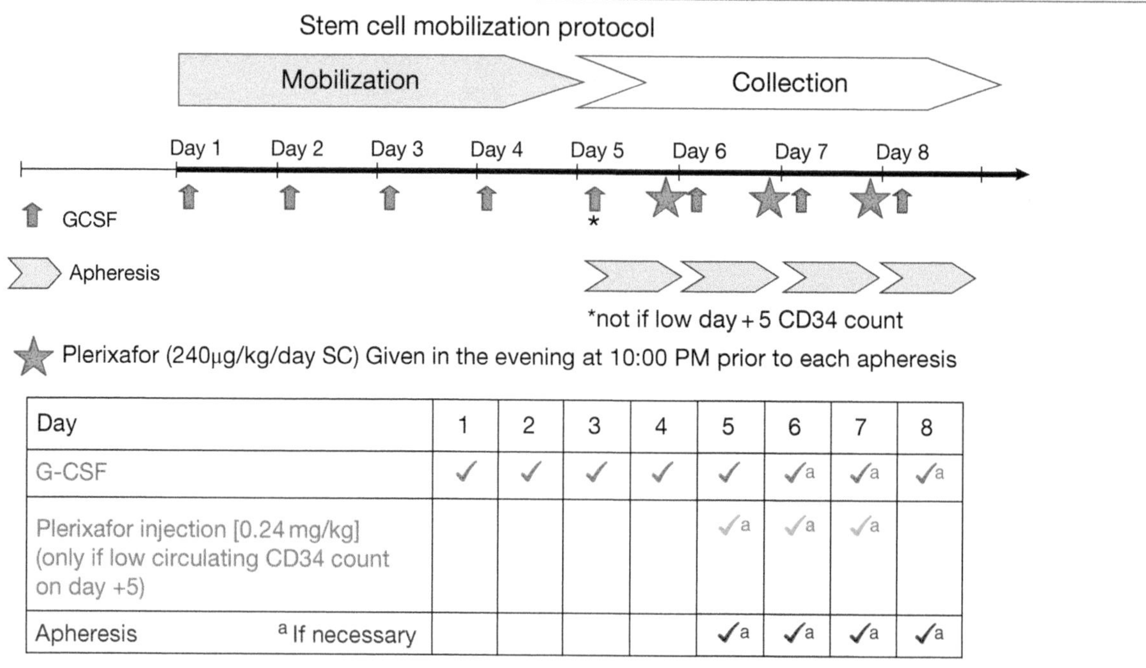

Day	1	2	3	4	5	6	7	8
G-CSF	✓	✓	✓	✓	✓	✓[a]	✓[a]	✓[a]
Plerixafor injection [0.24 mg/kg] (only if low circulating CD34 count on day +5)					✓[a]	✓[a]	✓[a]	
Apheresis [a] If necessary					✓[a]	✓[a]	✓[a]	✓[a]

Figure 25.3 'Pre-emptive' mobilization schedule. Source: C. Craddock, R. Chakraverty. In A. Mead *et al.* (eds) (2025) *Hoffbrand's Postgraduate Haematology*, 8th edn (2025, in press). Reproduced with permission of John Wiley & Sons.

administered over several days (**fractionated**). High-dose cyclophosphamide with TBI (CY/TBI) or with busulphan (Bu/CY) are standard regimens. Fludarabine (F) with busulphan (Bu) is a another commonly used myeloablative regimen, especially used for myeloid disease indications.

At least 36 hours are typically allowed for the elimination of these drugs from the circulation following the last dose of conditioning chemotherapy before donor stem cells are infused. Conditioning is often complicated by mucositis, and patients must be scrupulous about oral hygiene and sometimes need parenteral nutrition.

Myeloablative regimens cause greater degree of post-transplant complications and transplant-related mortality but result in fewer relapses of the original disease, compared with reduced intensity (RIC) transplants. They are generally preferred in fit patients under the age of 50 and especially in those with resistant disease such as AML in first remission but with positive minimal residual disease (MRD).

For patients over the age of 50, RIC transplants, discussed next, are preferred because of the excess toxicity of myeloablative regimens. There is also some evidence that RIC regimens give better outcomes in younger patients with lymphoid disease such as ALL or Hodgkin lymphoma.

Reduced-intensity (non-myeloablative) conditioning regimens

Reduced-intensity (RIC) regimens are used to reduce the morbidity and mortality of allogeneic transplantation. These regimens in contrast with myeloablative conditioning do not completely destroy the host bone marrow. Instead, the aim in reduced-intensity transplants is to use enough immunosuppression to allow donor stem cells to engraft without completely eradicating host marrow stem cells.

Such regimens extend the age range of feasibility for transplant to above 70 years and increase the treatment indications for allogeneic transplantation. RIC regimens divide into those based on fludarabine and those based on low-dose irradiation. The fludarabine regimens include also busulphan (lower dose than that used for myeloablative regimens), treosulfan, melphalan and/or cyclophosphamide. The TBI regimens also usually incorporate fludarabine. Engraftment and full donor chimerism (over time) are achieved with these RIC regimens but chronic GVHD and disease relapse are major complications. *In vivo* T-cell depletion with ATG or alemtuzumab (see below) is used as GVHD prophylaxis.

Donor leucocyte infusions (DLIs) are commonly used at a later stage after RIC allografting in order to encourage complete donor engraftment or to enhance a graft-versus-leukaemia (GVL) or -lymphoma effect (see below). They can also be used in the event of loss/persisting mixed chimerism or relapse of malignant disease post-allografting, including after myeloablative transplant.

Conditioning regimens for non-malignant diseases

For aplastic anaemia, cyclophosphamide alone suffices. For thalassaemia, sickle cell anaemia and other benign diseases with a cellular bone marrow, busulphan, fludarabine and *in vivo* ATG or alemtuzumab are added to cyclophosphamide.

Prevention of graft-versus-host disease

Immunosuppressive drugs, usually tacrolimus or ciclosporin (both calcineurin inhibitors) with a short course of methotrexate, mycophenolate mofetil (MMF) or sirolimus (a MTOR inhibitor), are given post-transplantation to reduce the risk of GVHD. Ciclosporin and tacrolimus levels are monitored; the intensity and duration are reduced if the risk of relapse is particularly high. The duration of immunosuppression following transplantation for aplastic anaemia is longer than that for haematological malignancies.

As mentioned above a high dose of cyclophosphamide 3 or 4 days after the stem cell infusion reduces the risk of acute (but not of chronic) GVHD without causing graft rejection or loss of the GVL effect. These high-dose post-transplant cyclophosphamide (PT-CY)-based regimes are standard of care for haploidentical and mismatched transplants.

T-cell depletion (TCD) effectively reduces the risk of acute and chronic GVHD. TCD can be achieved both by *in vitro* and *in vivo* manipulations. *In vitro* T-cell depletion of harvested stem cells reduces the risk of GVHD, but results in increased graft failure, graft rejection and relapse of malignant disease, viral infections and of post-transplant lymphoproliferative disease. *In vivo* T-cell depletion of the donor stem cells with anti-thymocyte immunoglobulin (ATG) or alemtuzumab (anti-CD52) carries increased risk of these complications but less so. ATG is now commonly used *in vivo*, especially in matched unrelated transplants. T-cell depletion is not undertaken in all centres internationally, with some centres using a T-replete donor protocol. Post-transplant immunosuppression to some extent is tailored to the patient's risk of relapse of malignant disease.

Post-transplant engraftment and immunity

After a period of typically 1–3 weeks of severe pancytopenia, the first signs of successful engraftment are the appearance of monocytes and neutrophils in the blood, with a subsequent increase in platelet count (Fig. 25.4). G-CSF may be used to reduce the period of severe neutropenia. Engraftment is usually a few days faster following PBSC transplantation compared with BMT.

The marrow cellularity gradually returns towards normal, but the marrow reserve remains impaired for 1–2 years and in some cases is impaired permanently. There is profound T-cell immunodeficiency for 3–12 months with a low level of CD4 helper cells. The patient's blood group changes to that of the donor, and antigen-specific immunity becomes that of the donor (including predisposition to allergic reactions) after approximately 60 days. Revaccination against common childhood viruses is usually carried out beginning at 9–12 months post-transplant. Immune recovery is quicker after autologous and syngeneic SCT than following allogeneic SCT.

Autologous stem cell transplantation

Stem cells are harvested from the patient and stored before high-intensity chemotherapy is given and are then reinfused to rescue the patient from the myeloablative effects of the chemotherapy (Fig. 25.1). The re-infused stem cells allow the delivery of a high dose of myelotoxic chemotherapy, with or without radiotherapy, which otherwise would result in prolonged bone marrow aplasia and severe infection risk.

High-dose melphalan is given for myeloma and a combination regimen, e.g. 'BEAM' (carmustine (BCNU), etoposide, cytarabine and melphalan) for lymphoma. Thiotepa is added in some protocols e.g. for relapsed CNS lymphoma.

A limitation of the autologous procedure is that, in the setting of neoplastic disease, malignant cells contaminating the stem cell harvest may be reintroduced into the patient. Nevertheless, autografting has a major role in the treatment of haematological diseases such as lymphoma and myeloma. Autografting is also used in gene therapy for inherited bone marrow diseases (Chapter 7).

The major problem associated with autografting is recurrence of the original disease, especially if the indication for transplant was a neoplasm (Fig. 25.5). GVHD is not an issue. Other complications depend on the conditioning regimen and may include intestinal, lung, mucous membrane, renal, liver (including veno-occlusive disease), cardiac damage and late development of myelodysplasia or AML. Procedure-related mortality is generally well below 2%.

The human leucocyte antigen system

One of the major reasons for failure of allogeneic transplantation is the immunological incompatibility between donor and patient despite matching of the HLAs. This mismatch may manifest as immunodeficiency, GVHD or graft failure (Fig. 25.5). There is also a beneficial GVL or graft-versus-lymphoma effect in which donor immune cells identify remaining neoplastic cells in the recipient and destroy them. This underlies much of the success of the procedure.

Allografting would be impossible without the ability to perform HLA typing. **The short arm of chromosome 6 contains a cluster of genes known as the major histocompatibility complex (MHC) or the HLA region (Fig. 25.6a).** Genes in this region encode the HLA antigens and many other molecules, including complement components, tumour necrosis factor (TNF) and proteins associated with antigen processing.

HLA molecules are of two types: class I and II (Table 25.2). Their role is to bind intracellular peptides and 'present' these to T lymphocytes for antigen recognition (Chapter 9). Class I HLA molecules (HLA-A, -B and -C) present antigens such as virus peptide fragments to CD8$^+$ T cells, resulting in destruction of the infected cell. Class II molecules (HLA-DR, -DQ and -DP) present antigens to

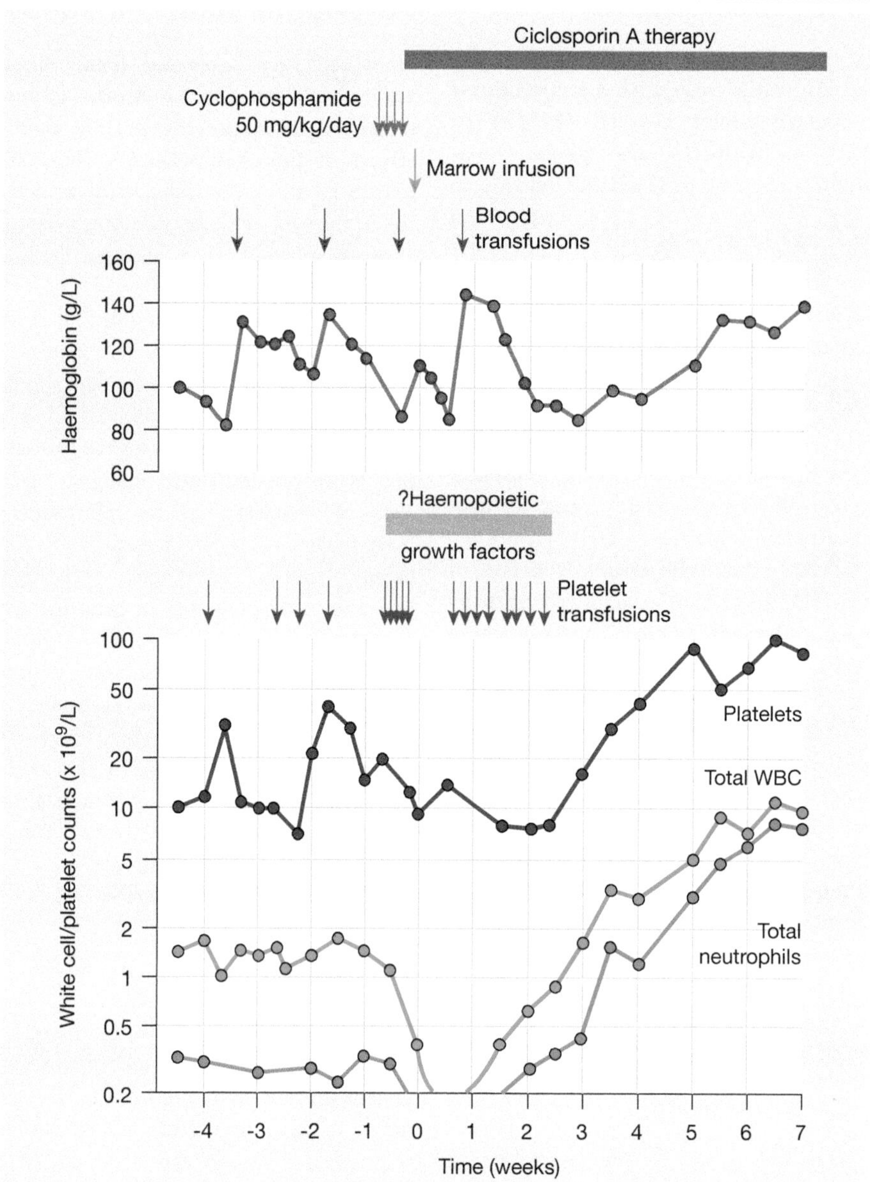

Figure 25.4 Typical haematological chart of a patient undergoing allogeneic bone marrow transplantation for aplastic anaemia. WBC, white blood cells.

CD4+ T cells, which results in proliferation of these T cells and of B cells which make antibodies to the relevant antigen (Fig. 25.6b). Natural killer cells also possess receptors for HLA molecules.

As there are 12 antigen-presenting HLA molecules, each highly polymorphic, the chances of two unrelated individuals matching at all 12 loci, even in the same ethnic group (since specific HLA markers generally cluster within ethnic groups), is very unlikely. Allelic diversity among HLA markers arose as a result of climate, geography, infectious pathogen differences and is greater in some ethnic groups, such as those of African or South Asian descent, than others such as Northern Europeans. Overall there are more than 18 000 HLA alleles, of which more than 13 000 are class I and more than 5000 class II (Fig. 25.6a).

Class I HLA molecules are present on most nucleated cells and on the cell surface they are associated with β2-microglobulin. The α chain is encoded on chromosome 6, whereas β2-microglobulin is encoded on chromosome 15. **Class II HLA molecules have a more restricted tissue distribution.** These comprise α and β chains, both encoded by genes on chromosome 6 in the HLA region (Fig. 25.6a).

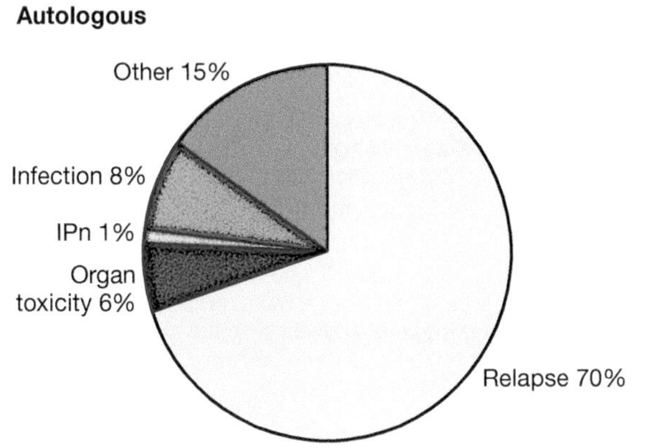

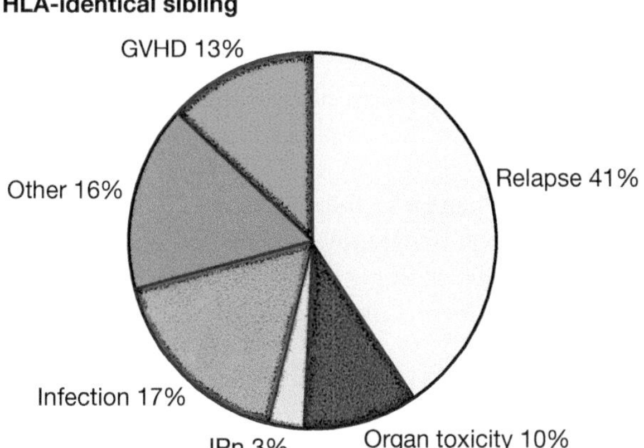

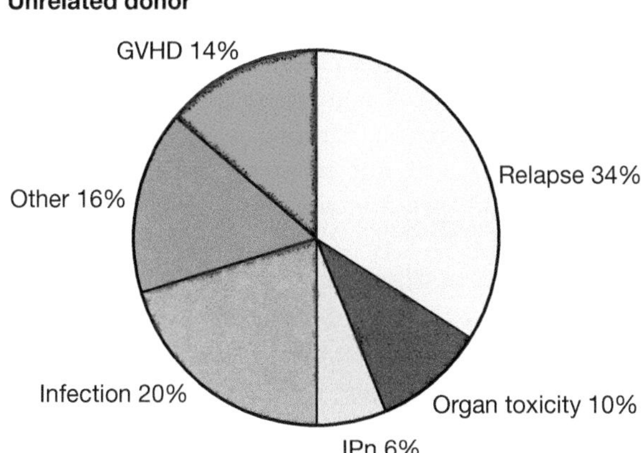

Figure 25.5 The causes of death following autologous, HLA-matched sibling and unrelated allogeneic transplantation IPn, interstitial pneumonitis. Source: C. Craddock, R. Chakraverty (2016) *Postgraduate Haematology*, 7th edn. Reproduced with permission of John Wiley & Sons.

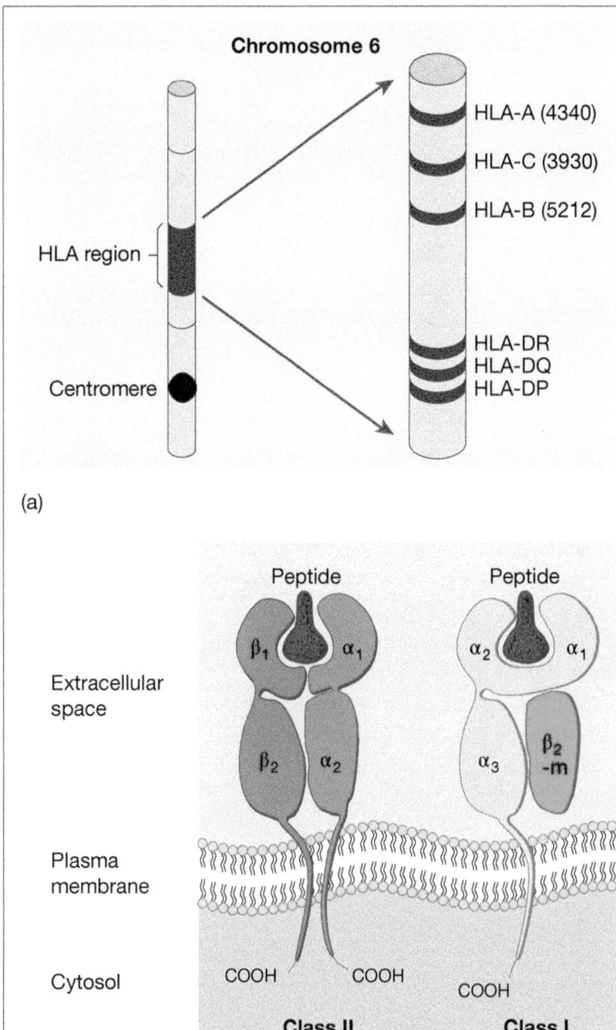

Figure 25.6 **(a)** The human leucocyte antigen (HLA) complex. The number of allele variants at each locus identified to date is shown. **(b)** HLA class I and II molecules showing protein domains and bound peptide. Class I alpha chains are encoded by genes *HLA-A, HLA-B* or *HLA-C*. Class II alpha DR chains are encoded by gene *HLA-DRA*, and beta chains by genes *HLA-DRB1, -DRB3, -DRB4* or *-DRB5*. *DRB2* is a non-protein-coding pseudogene. Class II DP alpha chains are encoded by gene *HLA-DPA*, while beta chains are encoded by *HLA-DPB*. Class II DQ alpha chains are encoded by gene *HLA-DQA*, while beta chains are encoded by *HLA-DQB*.

The inheritance of the HLA loci is closely linked: one set of loci is inherited from each parent, so that there is approximately a one in four chance of two full siblings having identical HLA antigens (Fig. 25.7a). Crossing-over of genes during meiosis and non-paternity accounts for occasional unexpected disparities. The inheritance of HLA molecules is independent of sex or blood group.

Human leucocyte antigen and transplantation

The natural role of HLA molecules is in directing T-lymphocyte responses and the greater the HLA mismatch, the more severe is the immune response between transplanted cells and host tissues. HLA typing is critical in donor selection for allogeneic SCT.

Minor histocompatibility antigens, e.g. HA-1, HA-2 and Hy, are peptides that are presented by HLA molecules and are able to act as antigens in SCT, either because they are polymorphic in the population or because they are encoded on the Y

Table 25.2 The human leucocyte antigens (HLA).

	Class I	Class II
Antigens	HLA-A, B, C	HLA-DR, -DP, -DQ
Distribution	All nucleated cells, platelets	B lymphocytes Monocytes Macrophages Activated T cells
Structure	Large polypeptide chain and a β2-microglobulin	Two polypeptide chains (α and β)
Interacts with	CD8 lymphocytes	CD4 lymphocytes

chromosome and therefore represent novel antigens to a female immune system that has engrafted in a male. The woman may have already been primed against these antigens by a pregnancy with a male baby. They are likely to be important antigens in GVHD and the GVL reaction despite complete matching at the major HLA loci (see below).

HLA typing may be carried out by serological or molecular techniques, most recently high-throughput, low-cost, automatic next-generation technologies. The nomenclature for *HLA* alleles is standardized. A single antigenic specificity defined by serological typing, e.g. HLA-A2 can be divided into different alleles by DNA sequencing. Each allele is given in numerical designation. The gene name is followed by an asterisk. The first field of digits indicates the allele group. The second field of digits lists subtypes, which differ in the protein sequence. The third field is used for alleles that differ by synonymous nucleotide substitutions (also called silent or non-coding). The fourth field indicates minor differences in non-coding regions. As an example, alleles at the *HLA-A* loci are written as *HLA-A*01:01* to *HLA-A*80:01*. The nomenclature for the class II genes is similar, but complicated by the fact that there may be more than one *HLA-DRB* gene on each chromosome (Fig. 25.7b).

When searching for an unrelated donor, the aim is to match HLA-A, -B –C and **-DRB1 and –DQB1 between recipient and donor, and this is then called a 10/10 match.** A 9/10 match may also be acceptable in the absence of a full 10/10 match. An exception is when a donor with only a single HLA haplotype match, usually a parent or sibling, is used in a **haploidentical SCT**. There are over 30 million volunteer donors registered on international registries, and the chance of identifying a matched unrelated donor for a patient lacking an HLA identical sibling is greater than 70% in populations of European descent but much lower in other ethnic groups.

Chimerism analysis

Following allogeneic SCT, the recipient's blood shows the presence of both donor and recipient cells (chimerism). This admixture can be detected by fluorescence *in situ* hybridization (FISH) analysis (Chapter 11) of the proportion of Y chromosome-containing cells if there is a sex mismatch, or by DNA analysis techniques regardless of donor and recipient sex, e.g., using microsatellite amplification by PCR. Persisting mixed chimerism is frequently seen following RIC transplants and may be converted to full donor chimerism with DLI. Following successful engraftment, loss of donor chimerism may be a harbinger of impending graft failure or relapse of a malignant disease.

Complications of stem cell transplantation

Complications of stem cell transplantation are outlined in Table 25.3, with the leading causes of death shown in Fig. 25.5. The overall rate from the procedure itself is lowest (< 2%) for autologous SCT and highest in unrelated and haploidentical SCT. Estimates for risk of non-relapse mortality following an allogeneic stem transplant maybe undertaken using a Hematopoietic Cell Transplantation-specific Comorbidity Index Score (http://www.hctci.org).

Graft-versus-host disease

GVHD is caused by donor-derived immune cells, particularly T lymphocytes, reacting against recipient tissues. Its incidence increases with increasing age of donor and recipient and the degree of HLA mismatch between them. Donor alloimmunization, e.g. a female who has had multiple pregnancies, and, in the recipient, viral infection, e.g. cytomegalovirus, CMV, liver, inflammatory bowel or rheumatological disease and use of PBSC also increase the risk of acute GVHD. GVHD prophylaxis has been described above.

In acute GVHD, occurring in the first 100 days but often persisting beyond that time frame, the skin, gastrointestinal tract and liver are affected (Table 25.4). Its severity is graded giving a guide to prognosis and to treatment needed. An overall clinical grade can be calculated (Table 25.5). The skin rash typically affects the face, palms, soles and ears, but may, in severe cases, affect the whole body (Fig. 25.8). The gut

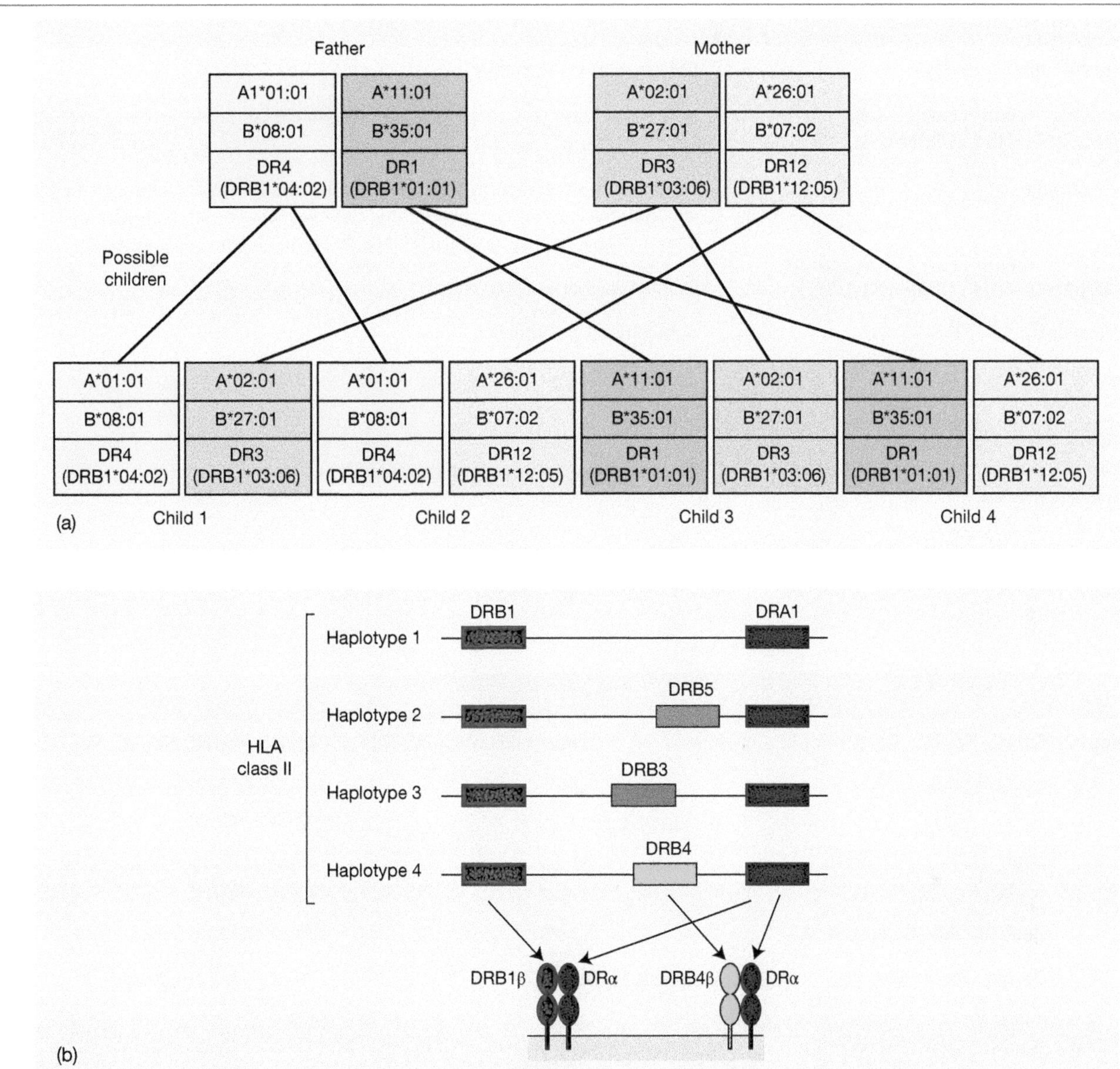

Figure 25.7 **(a)** An example of the possible pattern of inheritance of the A, B and DR (*DRB1*) series alleles of the human leucocyte antigen (HLA) complex. **(b)** Molecular genetics of the HLA class II gene complex. There are four major haplotypes of MHC class II genes in the population and each individual may have up to two (one on each chromosome). The *DRA1* gene codes for the DRα protein and the *DRB1*, *DRB3*, *DRB4* and *DRB5* genes encode DRβ chains. Expression from the *DRB1* gene is higher than from the other genes. The number of alleles at each gene is shown in Fig. 23.6a. Alleles at each locus have a standard nomenclature, e.g., the alleles at the *DRB1* gene are termed *DRB1*0101* to *DRB1*1608*.

microbiome is altered and diarrhoea may lead to fluid and electrolyte depletion. Typically, bilirubin and alkaline phosphatase are raised, but the other hepatic enzymes are relatively normal. Acute GVHD is usually treated by high doses of corticosteroids, intravenous, oral or topical depending on the severity. They are effective in the majority of cases. Second-line therapy is with ruxolitinib, a JAK2 inhibitor. Trials of other agents including sirolimus, other JAK1, e.g., itacitinib or JAK2 inhibitors, various monoclonal antibodies and faecal microbiota transplants are in progress. Intensive support is needed with fluids, nutrition, pain control and prevention of infection.

In chronic pattern GVHD, which usually occurs after 100 days and may evolve from acute GVHD, these tissues are involved, but also the joints and other serosal surfaces, the oral mucosa and lacrimal glands. Fibrosis is a main feature resulting from repair of damaged tissues by myofibroblasts that deposit excess collagen. Features of an autoimmune disease with scleroderma, Sjögren's syndrome, myositis, lichen planus and

Table 25.3 Complications of stem cell transplantation.

Early (usually <100 days)	Late (usually >100 days)
Infections, especially bacterial, fungal, herpes simplex virus, CMV, BK polyoma virus	Infections, especially varicella-zoster, capsulate bacteria
Haemorrhage	Chronic-pattern GVHD (arthritis, malabsorption, hepatitis, scleroderma, sicca syndrome, lichen planus, pulmonary disease including bronchiolitis obliterans, serous effusions); acute GVHD may also persist beyond 100 days
Acute-pattern GVHD (skin, liver, gut)	Chronic pulmonary disease
Graft failure	Autoimmune disorders
Haemorrhagic cystitis	Cataract
Interstitial pneumonitis	Infertility
Others: veno-occlusive disease, cardiac failure	Second malignancies, lymphoproliferative diseases

CMV, cytomegalovirus; GVHD, graft-versus-host disease.

Table 25.4 Acute pattern graft-versus-host disease: clinical staging (Glucksberg score).

Stage	Skin	Liver (bilirubin, μmol/L)	Gut (diarrhoea, L/day)
0	No GVHD rash	<34	No nausea or vomiting, stool <0.5 or <3 episodes/day
I	Rash <25% body surface	34–51	Persistent nausea or 0.5–1.0 or 3-4 episodes/day
II	Rash 25–50% body surface	52–101	1.0–1.5 or5-7 episodes/day
III	Generalized erythroderma >50% body surface	102–255	>1.5 or>7 episodes/day
IV	Bullae, desquamation + erythrodermia >50% body surface	>255	Severe pain, ileus, bloody diarrhoea

Table 25.5 Overall clinical grade (based upon most severe target organ involvement).

Grade 0: No stage 1–4 of any organ
Grade I: Stage 1–2 skin without liver, upper GI or lower GI involvement
Grade II: Stage 3 rash and/or stage 1 liver and/or stage 1 upper GI and/or stage 1 lower GI
Grade III: Stage 2–3 liver and/or stage 2–3 lower GI, with stage 0–3 skin and/or stage 0–1 upper GI
Grade IV: Stage 4 skin, liver or lower GI involvement, with stage 0–1 upper GI

cytopenias may develop. The immune system is also impaired (including hyposplenism) with increased risk of infection. Malabsorption and pulmonary abnormalities, e.g. bronchiolitis obliterans, are frequent. Treatment is with corticosteroids. Second-line drugs, include ibrutinib (most recently approved), JAK1/2 inhibitors, ciclosporin, rituximab, sirolimus, mycophenolate mofetil. Extracorporeal photopheresis is also used in resistant cases. The response to all these measures may be poor.

Infections

Prophylaxis

In the early post-transplant period, bacterial or fungal infections are frequent (Fig. 25.9). These may be reduced by reverse barrier nursing with laminar or positive-pressure air

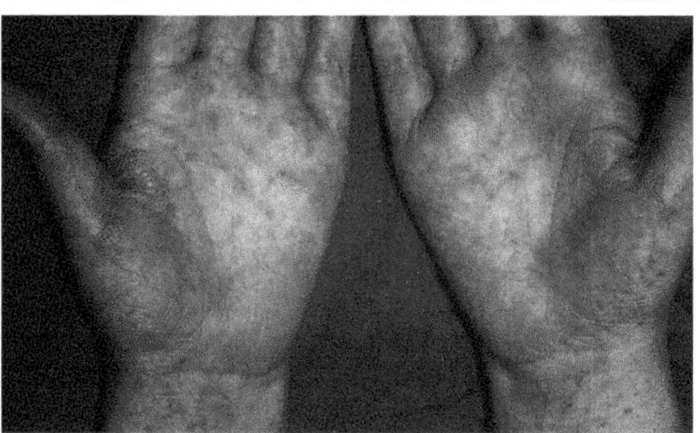

Figure 25.8 Widespread erythematous skin rash in acute graft-versus-host disease following allogeneic stem cell transplantation.

flow and the use of skin and mouth antiseptics. Prophylactic therapy with aciclovir (continued for one year) and an antifungal agent, e.g. fluconazole, are given. Some units also give a prophylactic quinolone oral antibiotic, e.g. ciprofloxacin but this depends on local microbiological advice. Cotrimoxazole prophylaxis (or dapsone or atovaquone if allergic to cotrimoxazole) against *Pneumocystis jirovecii* is given from the time of neutrophil engraftment. This also protects against toxoplasmosis. Lifelong protection against encapsulated bacteria with penicillin V or erythromycin is needed in all allogeneic transplant recipients. Letermovir is now first choice for prophylaxis against CMV infection (see below).

Treatment

If a fever or other evidence of an infection occurs, broad-spectrum intravenous antibiotics are commenced immediately after blood cultures and other appropriate microbiological specimens have been taken. Failure of response to antibacterial agents is usually an indication to commence systemic antifungal therapy with liposomal amphotericin, caspofungin, micafungin, voriconazole, posaconazole or isavucanozium. Fungal infections, especially *Candida* and *Aspergillus* species (Chapter 12), are a particular problem because of prolonged neutropenia or the use of corticosteroids to treat GVHD. Further details of their prevention, diagnosis and treatment are given in Chapter 12.

Viral infections, particularly with the herpes group of viruses, are frequent with herpes simplex, CMV and varicella zoster virus (VZV) occurring at different peak intervals

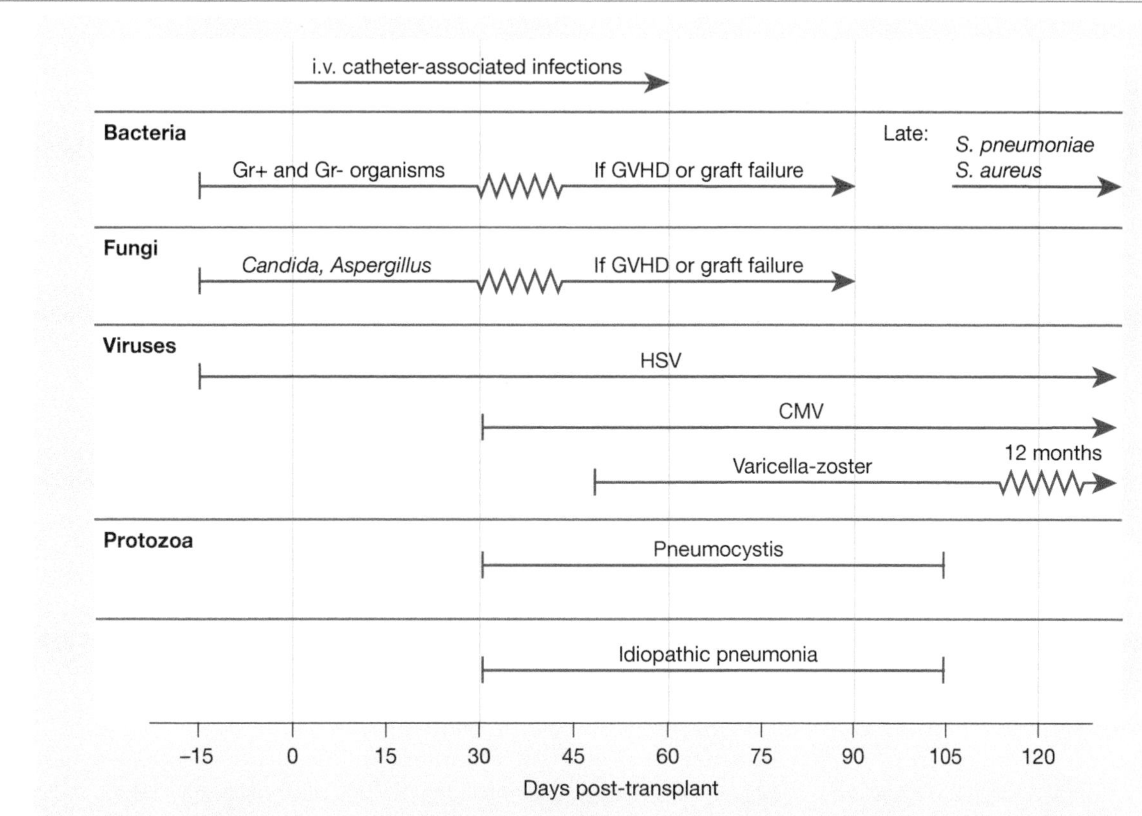

Figure 25.9 Time sequence for development of different types of infection following allogeneic stem cell transplantation. CMV, cytomegalovirus; Gr+, Gr–, Gram-positive or -negative; GVHD, graft-versus-host disease; HSV, herpes simplex virus.

(Fig. 25.9). CMV presents a particular threat and is associated with a potentially fatal interstitial pneumonitis (Fig. 25.10), as well as with hepatitis and falling blood counts. The infection may be caused by reactivation of CMV in the recipient or a new infection transmitted by the donor. Letermovir, a CMV terminal complex inhibitor, is given from the time of engraftment to 100 days post-transplant. It substantially reduces the risk of CMV infection. Patients are screened regularly (usually weekly in the first few months after transplant) for evidence of CMV reactivation following allogeneic transplantation. If these tests become positive, valganciclovir may suppress the virus before clinical complications occur. Ganciclovir, foscarnet, cidofovir and CMV immunoglobulin may be tried for established CMV infection, e.g. pneumonitis. Risk of CMV reactivation also increases subsequently if immunosuppression is required again, e.g. for treatment of GVHD.

VZV infection with painful shingles, headache or abdominal pain is also frequent post-SCT but occurs later, with a median onset at 4–5 months. Rarely, disseminated VZV infection occurs. Intravenous aciclovir is indicated for this complication. Antivirals are also helpful in Epstein–Barr virus (EBV) infections and EBV-associated lymphoproliferative disease (Fig. 25.12). In refractory viral infections, T cells with specificity for these organisms can be selectively harvested from donors and administered to patients. HHV-6 causing an encephalitis is another viral complication, particularly after T-cell depleted or cord blood transplants.

Pneumocystis jirovecii (Fig. 25.10) is a cause of pneumonitis that should, as mentioned above, be prevented by prophylactic cotrimoxazole (or dapsone or atovaquone).

Interstitial pneumonitis

CMV is a frequent cause but other herpes viruses and *P. jirovecii* account for other cases (Fig 25.10). In most cases, however, no specific cause other than the previous radiation and chemotherapy can be implicated. Diffuse alveolar haemorrhage may also occur. Trans-bronchoscopic biopsy or open lung biopsy may be needed to establish the diagnosis. High-dose corticosteroids are usually administered if no infection is detected.

Blood product support

Blood transfusions and platelets given in the post-transplant period must be irradiated prior to administration in order to kill any passenger live lymphocytes that might cause transfusion-associated graft-versus-host disease. ABO blood

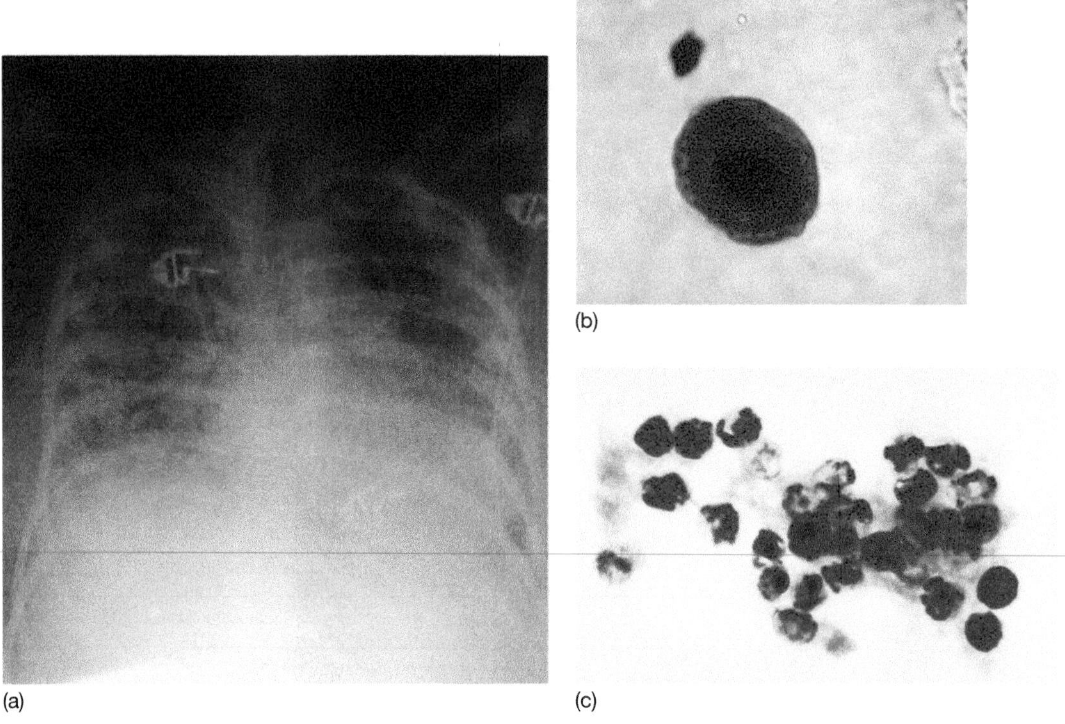

Figure 25.10 (a) Chest radiograph showing interstitial pneumonitis following bone marrow transplantation. Widespread diffuse mottling can be seen. The patient had received total body irradiation and had grade III graft-versus-host disease. No infective cause of the pneumonitis was identified. Possible causes include pneumocystis, cytomegalovirus, herpes zoster, fungal infection or a combination of these. **(b)** Sputum cytology: intranuclear cytomegalovirus inclusion body in a pulmonary cell. Papanicolaou stain. **(c)** *Pneumocystis jirovecii* in bronchial washings, Gram–Weigert stain.

group matching can present problems during the weeks when the recipient's blood group is changing to that of the donor (Chapter 12). Platelet concentrates are given to maintain a count of 10×10^9/L or more.

Other complications of allogeneic transplantation

Graft failure

This is indicated by failure of neutrophil recovery 4 weeks post-transplantation. The risk of graft failure is increased if the patient has aplastic anaemia, a low dose of donor CD34+ cells, increasing HLA disparity between donor and recipient and if T-cell depletion (especially *in vitro*) is used as GVHD prophylaxis. This is because donor T cells are needed to overcome host resistance to engraftment of stem cells. Occasionally, even after myeloablative regimens, the patient's own marrow will eventually recover after several months. It is over 50% fatal. If there is no donor engraftment a second transplant from an alternative donor can be tried. If there is poor donor engraftment, then booster donor stem cells can be given.

Secondary graft failure may occur after haploidentical and unrelated transplants. It has various causes including viral infection, drugs, ABO incompatibility or late graft rejection. Autoimmune cytopenias may also occur. The cause of the secondary failure should be sought and treated.

Haemorrhagic cystitis

This can be caused by the cyclophosphamide metabolite acrolein. Mesna, a cytoprotectant, is given in an attempt to prevent this. Certain viruses, e.g. adenovirus or the BK polyomavirus, may also cause this complication. Therapy is typically supportive care, since specific antivirals are not available. Impaired renal function from ciclopsorin, amphotericin, other drugs and fluid imbalance is frequent.

Other complications

Oral mucositis following radiotherapy or chemotherapy may be severe. Palifermin, a recombinant form of keratinocyte growth factor, may help to prevent or treat this.

Veno-occlusive disease (VOD) of the liver, also called sinusoidal obstruction syndrome (SOS), manifests as jaundice, painful hepatomegaly and ascites with weight gain. In severe cases there is hepatic venous occlusion with portal hypertension, widespread organ failure and death. Patients who have received busulphan and high-dose TBI are at increased risk, as are those who have received calicheamicin-containing antibody–drug conjugates such as gemtuzumab or inotuzumab prior to transplant. Defibrotide, a mixture of single-stranded oligonucleotides derived from pig mucosa, is approved for treatment of VOD/SOS. Ciclosporin which can cause a similar clinical picture should be temporarily stopped.

Cardiac failure may develop as a result of the conditioning regime (especially high doses of cyclophosphamide) and previous chemotherapy. *Haemolysis* because of ABO incompatibility between donor and recipient may cause problems in the first weeks. *Microangiopathic haemolytic anaemia* (Chapter 6) may also occur due to ciclosporin or to endothelial injury from the conditioning regimen. It responds poorly to plasma exchange.

Late complications

For patients undergoing transplant for neoplastic disorders, relapse of the original disease, e.g., myelodysplasia or acute or chronic leukaemia, is the leading cause of post-transplant death (Fig. 25.5). Bacterial infections remain frequent even after neutrophil recovery, especially with encapsulated organisms affecting the respiratory tract. Prevention of bacterial and other infections has been discussed above.

Delayed pulmonary complications include restrictive pneumonitis and bronchiolitis obliterans. *Endocrine complications* include hypothyroidism, growth failure in children, impaired sexual development and infertility. The endocrine problems are more marked if TBI has been used. Clinically apparent *autoimmune disorders* are infrequent and include myasthenia, rheumatoid arthritis, anaemia, thrombocytopenia or neutropenia. Autoantibodies are frequently detected in the absence of symptoms. *Second malignancies* (especially non-Hodgkin lymphoma) occur with a six- or sevenfold incidence compared with controls. *Central nervous system complications* include neuropathies and eye problems caused by chronic GVHD (sicca syndrome) or cataracts.

Iron overload may be present due to repeated red cell transfusions before and after transplantation. This can be treated by iron chelation or, when there is adequate red cell recovery, venesections. It is not necessary to 'de-iron' before the transplant procedure. There is usually not time for adequate chelation and it has not been proven to be of benefit.

Graft-versus-leukaemia effect and donor leucocyte infusions

After allogeneic transplantation, the donor immune system helps to eradicate the patient's leukaemia, a phenomenon known as the graft-versus-leukaemia, GVL) effect. Graft-versus-lymphoma and -myeloma effects also exist, though these terms are rarely used. Evidence for GVL includes the decreased relapse rate in patients who have GVHD (the GVHD provides evidence of immunocompetence of the graft), the increased relapse rate after T-cell depletion of donor stem cells and in identical twins. The most convincing evidence is the ability of donor lymphocyte infusion (DLI) to cure relapsed leukaemia after allogeneic SCT in some patients. The protocol of DLI is that peripheral blood mononuclear cells including T cells are collected from the original allograft donor and directly infused into the patient. A lower dose is used to correct mixed donor chimerism, as compared to that used at the time of leukaemia relapse, detected by molecular, cytogenetic techniques or morphologically (Fig. 25.11).

There is a large difference in the outcome of different diseases treated by DLI. Chronic myeloid leukaemia (CML) is most sensitive with >80% success rate in producing a durable

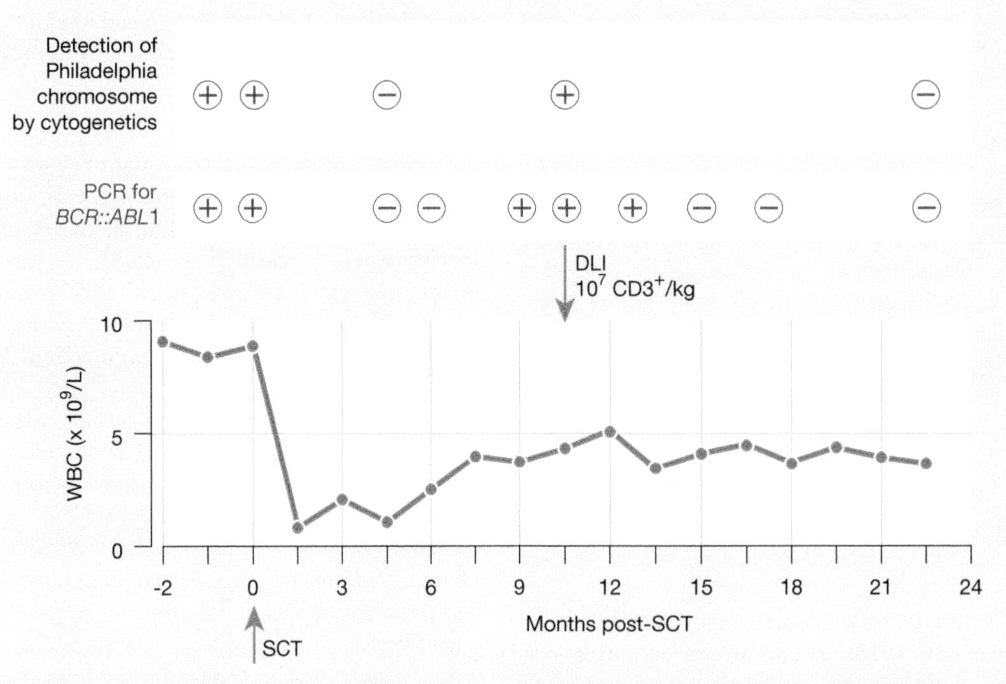

Figure 25.11 Donor leucocyte infusions. Example of donor leucocyte infusion (DLI) in the treatment of chronic myeloid leukaemia (CML) which relapsed following allogeneic stem cell transplantation (SCT). Polymerase chain reaction (PCR) analysis of the blood for the *BCR::ABL1* transcript shows that there was transient loss of the transcript, but molecular and cytogenetic relapse occurred at 10 months. One infusion of donor leucocytes led to re-establishment of a durable complete remission.

molecular remission, although transplant is now rarely necessary for chronic-phase CML given the availability of multiple highly effective tyrosine kinase inhibitors (Chapter 14). Success rates are lower in Hodgkin lymphoma and indolent NHL lymphomas while acute lymphoblastic leukaemia rarely responds. Polymerase chain reaction can be used to monitor serial blood samples for evidence of recurrence of the *BCR::ABL1* transcript or other known molecular abnormality of the original disease before karyotypic or clinical relapse occurs (Fig. 25.11). DLI risks causing GVHD. This risk is reduced by giving DLIs late, e.g. >12 months after the transplantation and by giving escalating doses rather than a single infusion.

Positron emission tomography (PET) scans can be used to detect residual disease in cases of lymphoma and to guide the requirement for DLI and determining the disease response (Fig. 25.12).

Post-transplant lymphoproliferative disease (PTLD)

These are a range of polyclonal or monoclonal, usually B-cell lymphoid proliferations that occur in recipients of stem cell or more frequently solid organ allografts, as a result of the intensive immunosuppression. The polyclonal lymphocytosis or lymphoma is EBV driven. PTLD in solid organ recipients occurs in those who were EBV seronegative before the transplant and develop primary infection from the donor subsequently while still on immunosuppressive therapy. This explains why PTLD is more common in children than adults. After SCT PTLD is due to failure of T-cell control of proliferation of EBV infected B cells. This depends mainly on the degree of HLA matching and the use of T-cell depletion protocols. The highest incidence is in haploidentical transplants, but this may diminish with the increased use of high-dose cyclophosphamide after SCT, instead of T-cell depletion to prevent GVHD.

The incidence of non-Hodgkin lymphoma in solid-organ transplant recipients is about 10 times normal and of Hodgkin lymphoma about 4 times depending mainly on which organ is being transplanted. For recipients of allogeneic haemopoietic stem cell transplants, the overall incidence of lymphoma is about 3%. It usually occurs in the first year post-transplantation.

There is often extranodal involvement of bowel, lung, brain or bone marrow (Fig. 25.13). EBV negative cases resemble closely diffuse large B cell non-Hodgkin lymphoma (DLBCL), with many of the same genomic aberrations, whereas EBV positive cases have fewer genomic abnormalities. Treatment is by withdrawing immunosuppression (if feasible), anti-CD20 antibodies such as rituximab, and chemotherapy, local radiotherapy or surgery for selected cases. Newer strategies involve therapy with Bruton kinase and proteasome inhibitors.

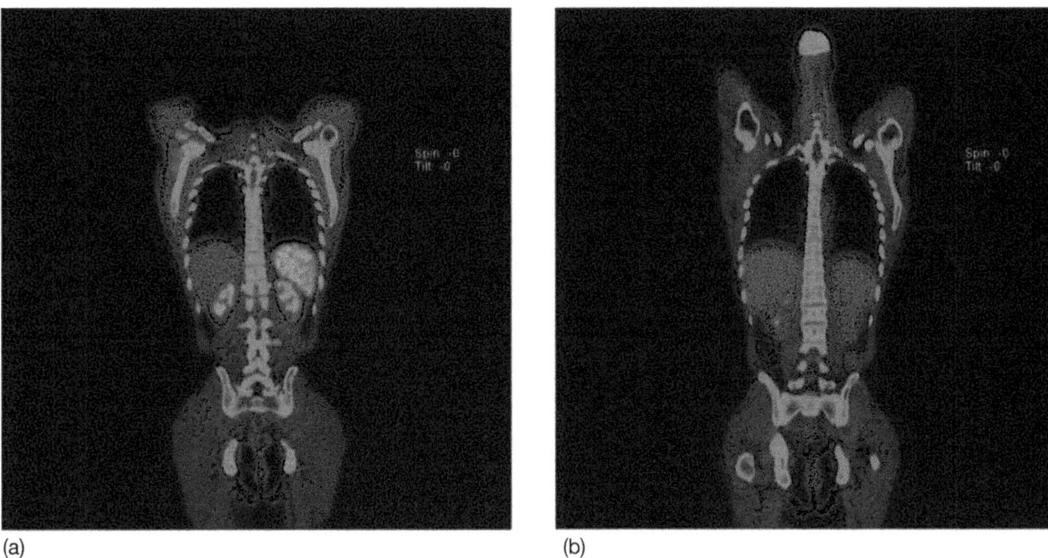

Figure 25.12 Example of disease control following administration of a donor leucocyte infusion (DLI) after stem cell transplantation. **(a)** A positron emission tomography (PET) scan revealed residual disease activity in a patient at 6 months following allogeneic transplantation for non-Hodgkin lymphoma. The bright signals reflect the metabolic activity of malignant cells in the spleen and axillary lymph nodes. Donor leucocyte infusion was then given and after 3 months a repeat PET scan **(b)** revealed no evidence of residual disease. Source: Courtesy of Professor Nigel Russell.

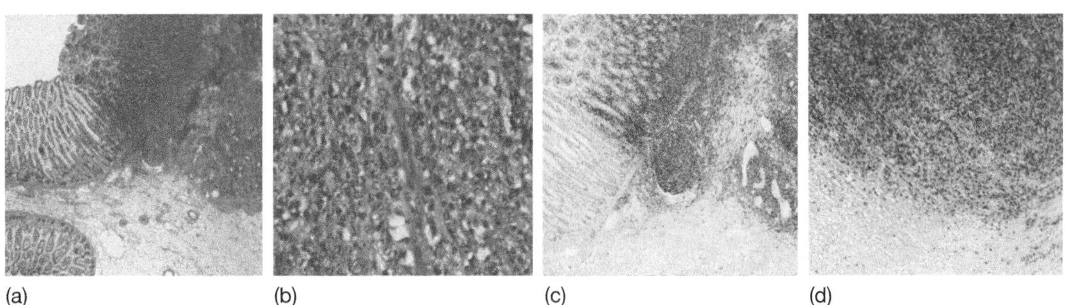

Figure 25.13 Post-transplantation lymphoproliferative diseases: 17-year-old male 5 months after renal transplantation had small bowel perforation caused by diffuse large B-cell lymphoma. **(a)** Low-power view of lymphoid mass invading small bowel. **(b)** High-power view of lymphoid mass. **(c)** Immunostaining for CD20. **(d)** EBV-ISH (*in situ* hybridization) stain showing the tumour cells are positive for Epstein–Barr virus. Source: Courtesy of Professor P. Amrolia and Dr N. Sebire.

SUMMARY

- Haemopoietic stem cell transplantation (SCT) involves replacing the patient's haemopoietic and immune systems by stem cells from either the same subject (autologous) or another individual (allogeneic). The donor stem cells can be harvested from bone marrow, peripheral or umbilical cord blood.
- Autologous SCT is most frequently performed for lymphomas or myeloma. It is also used in gene therapy protocols for inherited bone marrow diseases.
- For allogeneic SCT the recipient's own haemopoietic and immune systems are either eliminated by myeloablative conditioning by chemotherapy, radiotherapy and monoclonal antibody 'conditioning,' or partly eliminated by reduced-intensity (non-myeloablative) conditioning.
- Allogeneic SCT requires a tissue (HLA) matching sibling, a matching unrelated or an haploidentical family member donor.
- The human leucocyte antigens (HLAs, class I or II) are coded for by genes on chromosome 6. They are extremely polymorphic and are involved in presentation of antigens to T lymphocytes.
- Allogeneic SCT is indicated in selected cases of acute leukaemia, other malignant bone marrow diseases, and severe acquired or genetic marrow diseases, e.g. aplastic anaemia, thalassaemia major.
- Reduced-intensity conditioning SCT is preferred in older subjects.
- Early (first 100 days) complications of allogeneic SCT include acute graft-versus-host disease, infections, graft failure and veno-occlusive disease. Long-term complications include relapse of the original disease, chronic GVHD, damage to many different organs, e.g., skin, heart, lungs and liver, and post-transplant lymphoproliferative disease.
- Infections (bacterial, fungal, viral and other) are major causes of morbidity and death after SCT.
- Donor leucocyte infusions may be given to treat relapse of leukaemia post-allogeneic SCT, by a 'graft-versus-leukaemia' effect.

Now visit **www.wiley.com/go/haematology9e** to test yourself on this chapter.

CHAPTER 26

Platelets, coagulation and normal haemostasis

Key topics

Hoffbrand's Essential Haematology, Ninth Edition. A. Victor Hoffbrand, Pratima Chowdary, Graham P. Collins, and Justin Loke.

© 2024 John Wiley & Sons Ltd. Published 2024 by John Wiley & Sons Ltd.

Companion website: www.wiley.com/go/haematology9e

Haemostatic response

The normal haemostatic response is an efficient and rapid mechanism to stop bleeding from sites of blood vessel injury and essential for survival. This results in the formation of a blood clot when vessel walls are damaged (Fig. 26.1). The subsequent restoration of vessel wall integrity through tissue regeneration is associated with clot removal. Such a response must be tightly controlled to ensure clot formation is localized to the site of injury.

The haemostatic response requires a coordinated interaction between endothelium, blood vessel wall, platelets and coagulation factors (Fig. 26.2). Four stages are distinguishable within the response:

1. **Vasoconstriction of the vessel wall**
2. **Primary haemostasis (platelet activation and platelet plug formation)**
3. **Secondary haemostasis (thrombin generation and clot formation)**
4. **Fibrinolysis (clot breakdown and tissue repair)**

Understanding the normal haemostatic response is essential as disorders of haemostasis are secondary to dysfunction or hyperfunction of the individual components.

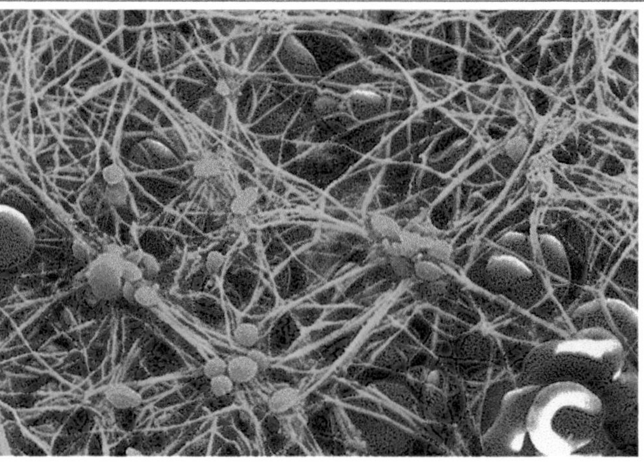

Figure 26.1 Colourized scanning electron micrograph of a blood clot formed *in vitro*. Fibrin (green); adherent platelets (purple); red blood cells (red). Source: Image by Yuri Veklich and John W. Weisel, University of Pennsylvania, with permission.

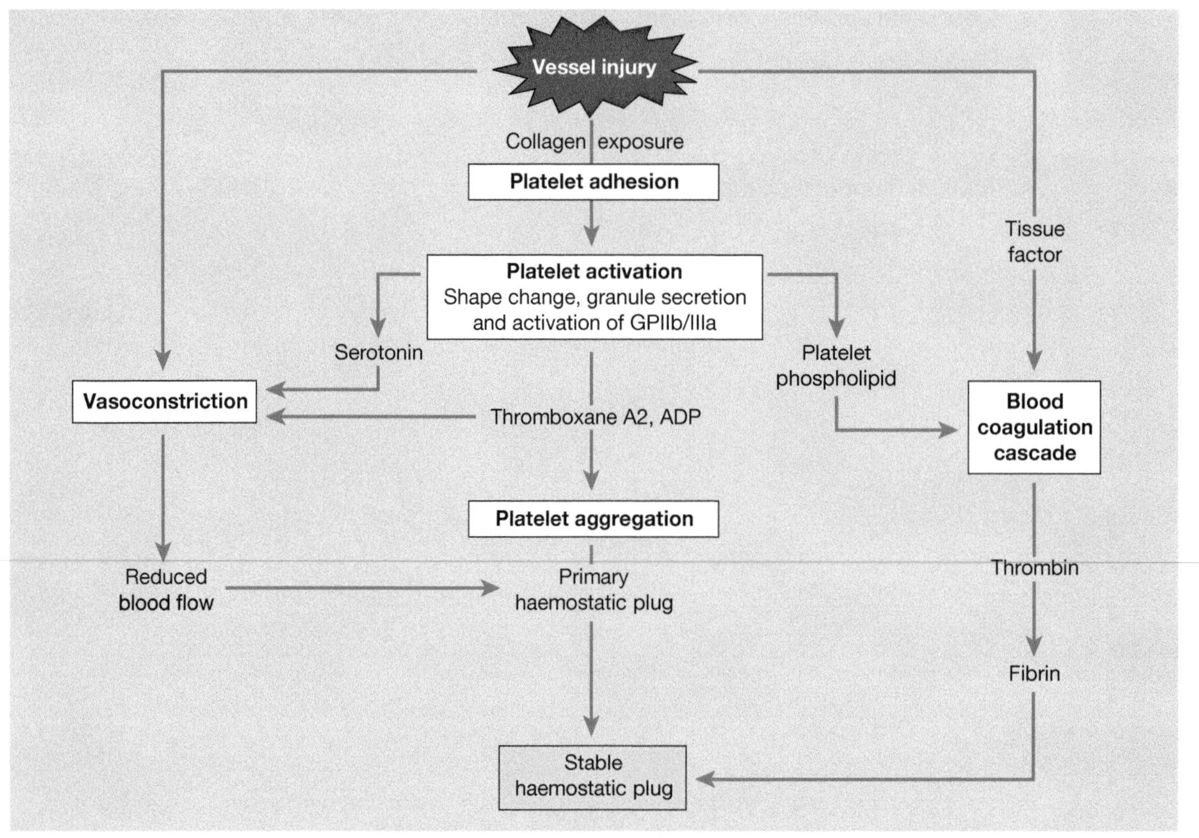

Figure 26.2 Interplay of blood vessels, platelets and blood coagulation in normal haemostasis. ADP, adenosine diphosphate.

Vasoconstriction

Immediate vasoconstriction of the injured vessel and reflex constriction of adjacent small arteries and arterioles following injury reduces blood flow to the affected area. When there is a severe injury, this vascular reaction prevents exsanguination. The reduced blood flow facilitates contact of platelets and coagulation factors with subendothelial collagen and tissue factor. Vasoactive amines and thromboxane A2 liberated from platelets also have vasoconstrictive activity (Fig. 26.2) and aid the process.

Platelets

Platelets are anucleate fragments of megakaryocyte cytoplasm. The smallest of the blood cells, platelets mediate primary haemostasis that results in platelet plug formation. Mature platelets are discoid in shape with an average diameter of 3.0 µm, thickness of 0.5 µm and volume of 7 fL (Fig. 26.4d).

The normal platelet count ranges from 150 to 400 × 10^9/L, with an average lifespan of around 10 days (range 8–12) (Table 2.1). Two-thirds of the total platelet pool normally circulates in blood vessels, with a third trapped in the spleen (Fig. 27.4). On average, 10–12% of circulating platelets are removed each day by the mononuclear phagocyte system, primarily macrophages in the spleen and liver.

Megakaryopoiesis and platelet formation

Megakaryocytes and platelets develop in specialized bone marrow microenvironments (niches) that influence proliferation and maturation.

Platelet formation is characterised by two phases. The first is megakaryopoiesis, which includes the commitment of haemopoietic stem cells (HSCs) to the megakaryocyte lineage and proliferation of the progenitors (Figs. 1.2, 26.4a). The second phase includes megakaryocyte differentiation, maturation, platelet formation and release (Figs. 26.3, 26.4). The time interval from the differentiation of the human stem cell to the production of platelets averages 7–10 days.

Following proliferation, the differentiation and maturation of megakaryocytes include nuclear duplication without cell division (endomitosis), resulting in polyploidy (typically 16–32 N). This creates some of the largest cells in the marrow; 100–150 µm in diameter. Cytoplasmic content markedly increases with the synthesis of various granules and organelles (Fig. 26.3b). During this period, a characteristic demarcation membrane system (DMS) appears composed of an extensive network of cisternae and tubules, which are continuous with the plasma membrane (Fig. 26.3c). The DMS acts as a membrane reservoir for the development of platelets. A cytoskeletal machinery of microtubules, actin filaments, spectrin and other proteins develop to support proplatelet and platelet formation.

The assembly of platelets from megakaryocytes converts the cytoplasm into 100–500 µm long-branched proplatelets over 4–10 hours, with each megakaryocyte releasing approximately 1000–5000 platelets (Figs. 26.3d, 26.4c). Proplatelet formation is driven by cytoskeletal proteins and proximity to vascular sinusoids with transendothelial proplatelet migration.

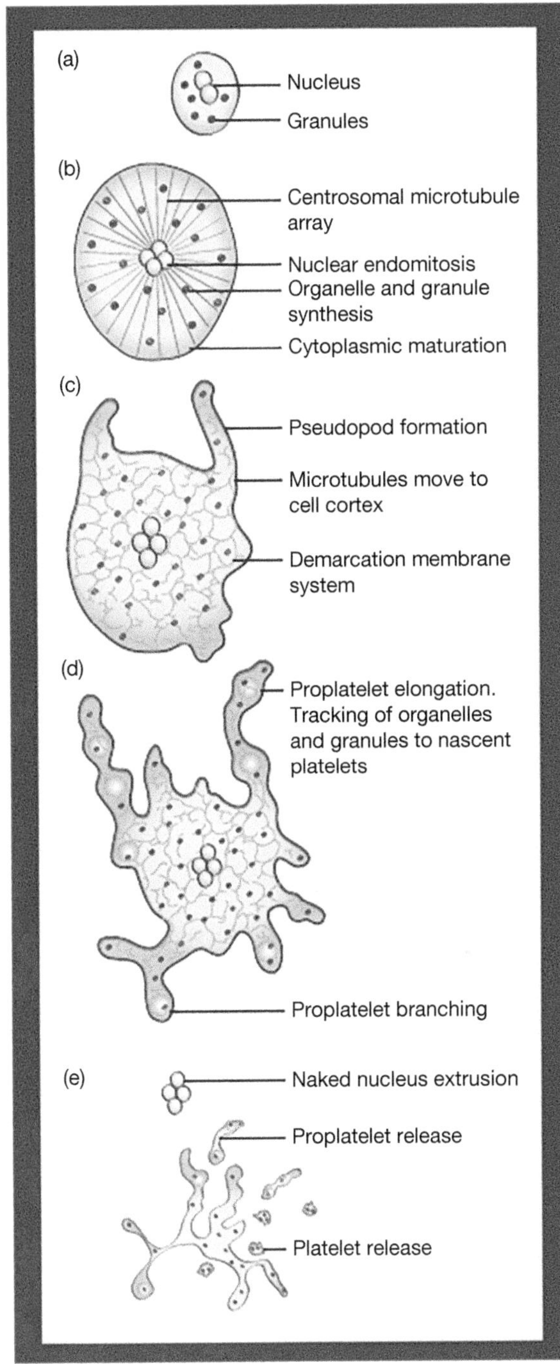

Figure 26.3 Overview of megakaryocyte development and platelet release. **(a)** Immature megakaryoblast. **(b)** Nuclear and cytoplasmic maturation; nuclear endomitosis. **(c)** Proplatelet formation, early phase. **(d)** Expansion of proplatelets with branching. **(e)** Proplatelet and platelet release.

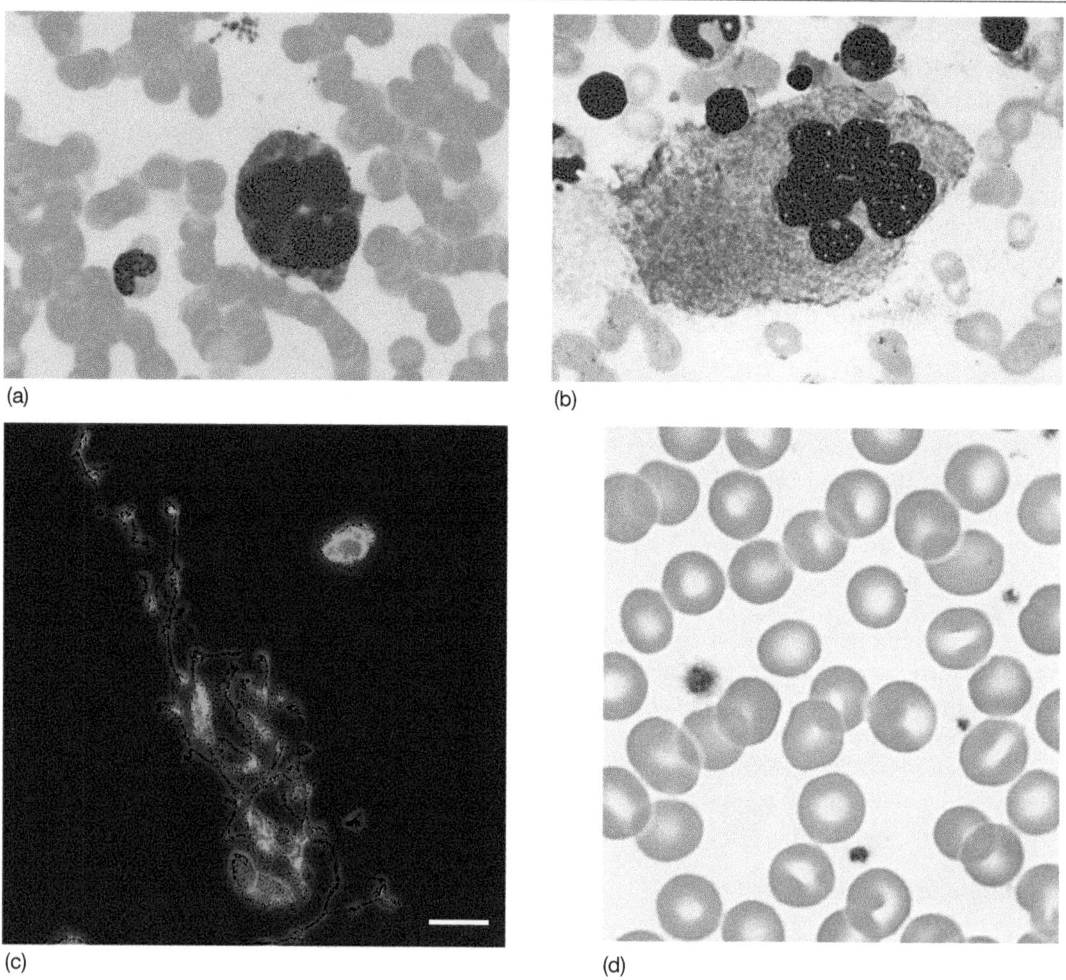

Figure 26.4 Megakaryocytes and platelets. **(a)** Immature megakaryocyte with basophilic cytoplasm. **(b)** Mature megakaryocyte with multi-lobed nuclei and pronounced granulation of the cytoplasm. **(c)** Megakaryocyte in culture, stained for α-tubulin (green), demonstrating branching proplatelets. **(d)** Normal red cells, 8 μm in diameter, with minor variations in size and shape. The majority show a central pale area of diminished staining. Platelets, 1–3 μm across, are also evident. Source: (a)–(c) A. Pecci et al. (2009) *Thromb. Haemost.* 109: 90–6. (d) A.V. Hoffbrand *et al.* (2019) *Color Atlas of Clinical Hematology*, 5th edn. Reproduced with permission of John Wiley & Sons.

Fragmentation into platelets and proplatelet fragments is facilitated by the shear forces generated by circulating blood.

Thrombopoietin

The cytokine thrombopoietin (TPO) is the principal regulator of megakaryocyte and platelet production, signalling via its receptor TPO-R. TPO-R is encoded by the human *MPL* (myeloproliferative leukaemia protein) gene and expressed on the surface of HSCs, megakaryoblasts, megakaryocytes and platelets. TPO increases the proliferation and differentiation of HSCs through to increased megakaryocyte number and size.

TPO is a glycoprotein constitutively expressed by the liver (contributes 95%), kidneys and marrow. Binding to TPO receptors on platelets is an important route of its elimination, and plasma levels of TPO are inversely proportional to platelet and megakaryocyte mass. Plasma levels are high if this mass is low, as in aplastic anaemia, and low if this mass is high, seen in patients with raised platelet counts.

Hepatic expression of TPO mRNA is increased when desialylated, senile platelets bind to the hepatic asialoglycoprotein receptor (ASGPR, also known as Ashwell–Morell receptor), triggering the production of new platelets (Fig. 26.5). Interleukin-6 (IL-6), which mediates the acute phase response, can induce hepatic TPO expression with thrombocytosis.

Although TPO is the primary regulator, transcription factors (e.g. GATA-1, RUNX1) and other cytokines (IL-3, IL-6) work in conjunction to regulate megakaryocyte development. Mutation in these genes is associated with severe thrombocytopenia.

Platelet antigens

Platelet surface proteins called human platelet antigens (HPA) are important in platelet-specific autoimmunity. Platelets also

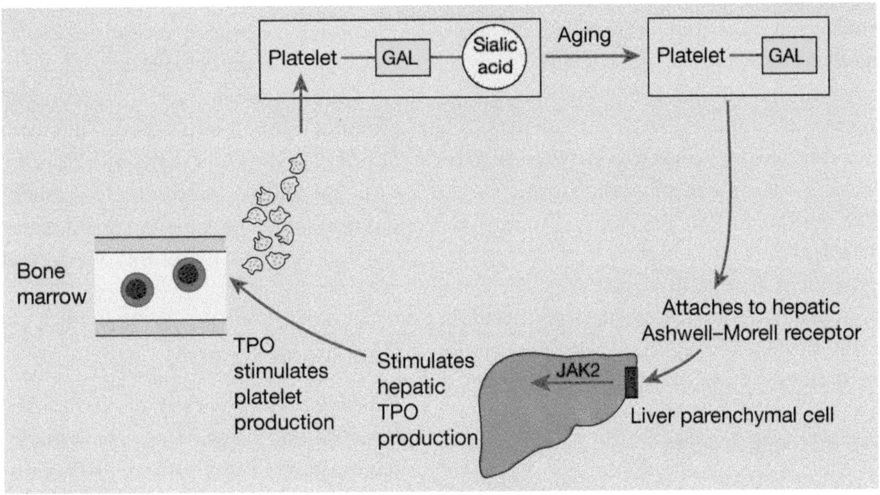

Figure 26.5 Regulation of platelet production is facilitated through hepatic clearance of desialylated platelets, which attach to the Ashwell–Morell hepatic receptor. This initiates a signal via JAK2 for further TPO production and subsequent platelet production. GAL, galactose.

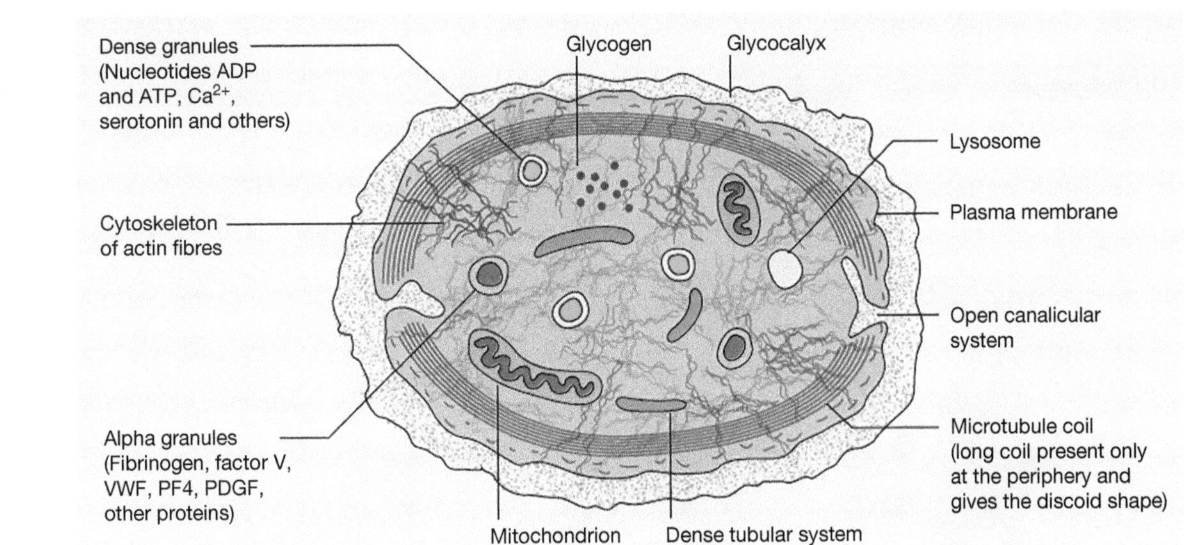

Figure 26.6 Ultrastructure of platelets with the various organelles. The plasma membrane and open canalicular system are a source of phospholipids, supporting the membrane-bound complexes of the coagulation cascade. ADP, adenosine diphosphate; ATP, adenosine triphosphate; Ca^{2+}, calcium ion; PDGF, platelet-derived growth factor; PF4, platelet factor 4; VWF, von Willebrand factor.

express ABO and human leucocyte antigen (HLA) class I but not class II (Table 25.2).

Platelet ultrastructure

The ultrastructure of platelets at rest can be described in three zones (Fig. 26.6). The peripheral zone includes a fuzzy glycocalyx coat with adsorbed proteins, platelet membrane and platelet receptors. The adjacent sol-gel zone has the microtubule coil, open canalicular and dense tubular systems. The inner organelle zone contains various granules, mitochondria and actin filaments.

Platelet cytoskeleton and membrane systems

The platelet cytoskeleton has three components and supports the discoid shape at rest, and shape change following activation. A **marginal microtubule coil at the widest diameter is responsible for the discoid shape. A spectrin-based skeletal framework underneath the plasma membrane and a rigid network of actin filaments also provide support.** Actin filaments enable shape change and are the most abundant platelet proteins that traverse the cytoplasm.

The resting platelet has two distinct membrane systems: a surface-connected open canicular system (OCS) and a closed dense tubular system (DTS). The OCS is an invaginated tubular extension of the plasma membrane forming a complex, anastomosing network of varying diameters. The OCS is necessary for transporting substances between platelets and plasma, facilitating the uptake of plasma proteins and diffusion of granule contents upon release. It also acts as a reservoir of plasma membrane and membrane receptors for a rapid, activation-dependent increase in surface area. The closed DTS network represents the residual endoplasmic reticulum. It appears as long, thin tubules and regulates platelet activation through the release or sequestration of calcium.

Platelet granules and organelles

Platelets contain three storage granules: alpha granules (α), dense granules (δ), lysosomes and other organelles, including peroxisomes and mitochondria (Fig. 26.6). Alpha granules are the most common, with 50–80/platelet, accounting for around 10% of the platelet volume. They contain a variety of proteins, including clotting factors, e.g. factor V, von Willebrand factor, fibrinogen, angiogenic factors, vascular endothelial growth factor, anti-angiogenic factors, PF4, membrane-associated receptors, e.g. GPIIb/IIIa, growth factors, proteases and cytokines.

Dense granules are the second most abundant platelet granules, with 5–8/platelet. They contain nucleotides (ADP and ATP), bioactive amines (serotonin, histamine) and cations, particularly calcium. The name is attributed to their electron-dense appearance on electron microscopy due to high calcium content. Lysosomes (1–3/platelet) contain hydrolytic enzymes.

Platelet receptors

Platelets have a variety of surface receptors and associated intracellular signalling pathways essential for their haemostatic functions of adhesion (platelet–vessel wall interaction) and aggregation (platelet–platelet interaction). Glycoprotein (GP) and other classes of receptors also perform non-haemostatic roles in innate immunity, inflammation and tumour growth, which requires interactions with leucocytes, endothelial cells and coagulation factors (Chapter 29). The receptors essential for normal haemostasis include the following (Fig. 26.7):

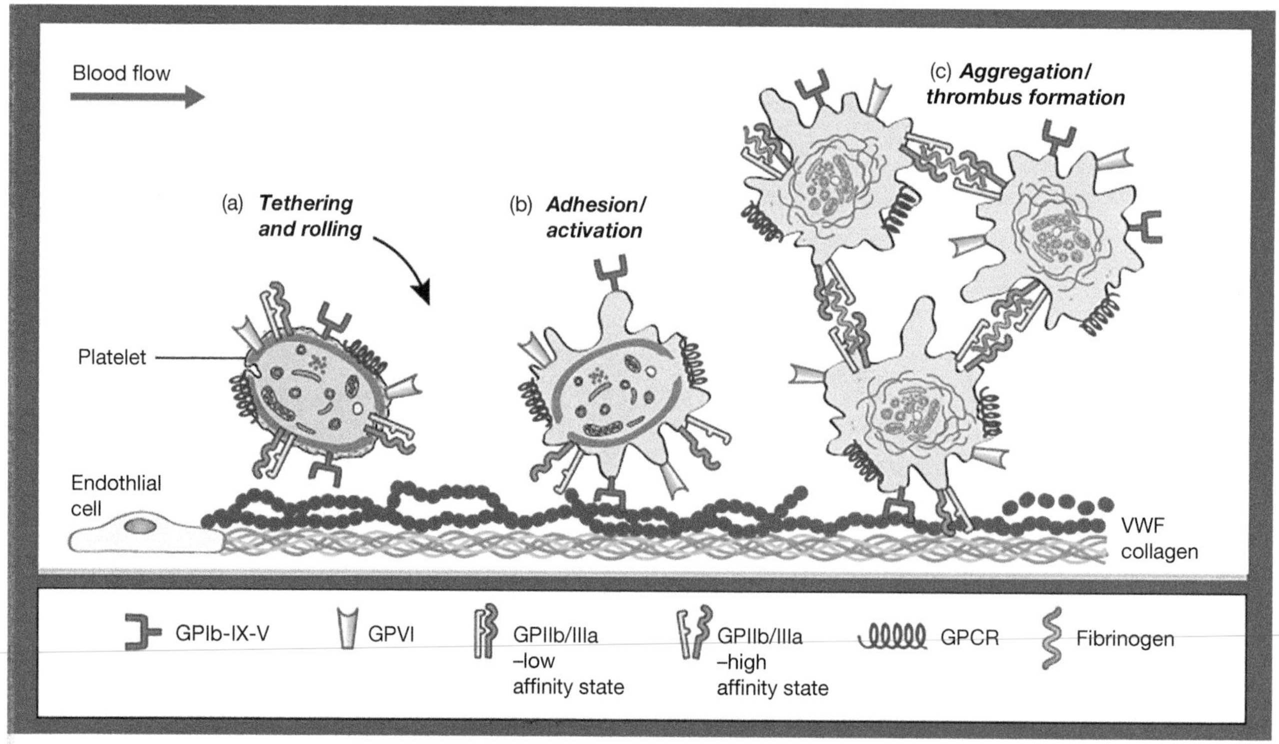

Figure 26.7 Overview of platelet receptors, platelet adhesion and aggregation. Platelets under normal flow conditions are marginalized, placing them adjacent to the endothelium. Injury results in multiple adhesive receptor-ligand interactions. **(a)** Exposure of platelets to sub-endothelial collagen results in rapid interactions between collagen-bound von Willebrand factor (VWF) and glycoprotein (GP) Ib-IX-V (tethering). Tethering enables collagen to bind directly to GPVI. **(b)** The initial adhesion leads to the activation of platelet integrins (GPIIb/IIIa and GPIa/IIa) to a high-affinity state, enabling binding with their ligands. **(c)** Interactions between GPIIb/IIIa with subendothelial VWF or fibrinogen and GPIa/IIa (not shown) and collagen lead to irreversible platelet activation with shape change and granule release. Platelet aggregation requires the bridging of GPIIa/IIIb receptors on adjacent platelets by fibrinogen. The platelet clot is stabilized by cross-linked fibrin generated in secondary haemostasis. GPCR, G protein-coupled receptor.

Platelet receptors for adhesion and aggregation

- **GPIb-IX-V complex:** This transmembrane complex is a platelet mechano-sensor with three subunits, GPIbα, GPIbβ and GPIX. GPIbα is the largest subunit linked covalently to GPIbβ subunits and non-covalently to GPIX-GPV. GPV is weakly associated with the complex and appears to regulate the activity of the complex. GPIbα mediates binding to various ligands, principally von Willebrand factor (VWF) (Fig. 26.7).
- **Glycoprotein IIb/IIIa (integrin αIIbβ3):** The dominant platelet integrin receptor, a transmembrane receptor, mediates interactions with other platelets and extracellular matrix. Resting platelets express integrin receptors in a **low-affinity state** to avoid interactions with their ligands. Following activation, these receptors undergo a conformational change to a **high-affinity state** that enables binding to their ligands, including fibrinogen and VWF. The switch to a high-affinity state is triggered by intra-platelet signalling, initiated by adhesion or activation **(inside-out signalling)**. It enables fibrinogen to bridge GPIIb/IIIa receptors on adjacent platelets **(platelet aggregation)** (Fig. 26.7). Fibrinogen binding activates intracellular pathways with irreversible changes **(outside-in signalling)**, including platelet spreading and receptor clustering.
- **GPIa/IIa (integrin α2β1):** This receptor mediates stable adhesion to exposed collagen on the vessel wall when activated.

Platelet activation and signalling receptors

- **G protein-coupled receptors (GPCRs):** This cell surface receptor family mediates platelet activation and recruitment to growing platelet thrombi. Important agonists and corresponding receptors are thrombin and protease-activated receptors (PAR1 and PAR4), ADP, purinergic receptors (P2Y1 and P2Y12), TXA2 and thromboxane receptor (TP). Platelet activation via GPCRs involves three major G-protein–mediated signalling pathways initiated by activation of the G proteins. The GPCRs are a popular target for antithrombotic drug development.
- **GPVI:** This belongs to the immunoglobulin (Ig) superfamily of receptors and is necessary for stable adhesion to collagen. It exists in a high-affinity complex with the FcRγ chain.
- **FcγRIIa**: A second Ig superfamily receptor which can activate platelets when bound to immune complexes, causing pathological thrombosis.

von Willebrand factor

von Willebrand factor (VWF) is a multidomain adhesive plasma glycoprotein necessary for primary haemostasis (Fig. 26.7). VWF is synthesized as a large 600 kDa protein and undergoes extensive post-translational modifications, including glycosylation, sufation, dimerization and multimerization. It has binding sites for factor VIII, heparin, collagen and platelets (Fig. 28.10). VWF circulates in plasma as a heterogeneous mixture of disulphide-linked multimers that range in size from dimers to multimers containing up to 50 dimeric units (Fig. 28.10). High molecular weight VWF multimers are haemostatically more active than low molecular weight VWF multimers.

VWF is synthesized in megakaryocytes and endothelial cells. In megakaryocytes and platelets, it is stored in the alpha granules (Fig. 26.6). Endothelial VWF is the source of all circulating VWF. VWF typically exists as a globular protein, but under shear stress, it unfolds with exposure of the platelet binding sites (Fig. 28.10), allowing the capture of platelets. **VWF has two key roles in haemostasis; it supports platelet adhesion at sites of injury (Fig. 26.7) and protects circulating FVIII from premature proteolytic degradation.**

Primary haemostasis

Primary haemostasis is initiated when circulating platelets make contact with the subendothelial extracellular matrix (ECM) following damage to the integrity of the vessel wall. This immobilization of platelets at the site of injury requires adhesion, activation and aggregation of platelets (Fig. 26.7). The ECM of the vessel walls is rich in collagens and other proteins that play essential roles in thrombus formation by supporting platelet adhesion and activation.

Platelet adhesion

The shear rates in the flowing blood influence specific platelet receptor and ECM interactions. Under high shear e.g. in arterioles, adhesion depends on the rapid reversible association between the VWF A1 domain and GPIb-IX-V, i.e. tethering (Fig. 26.7). VWF binds to collagen through various domains; once immobilized, the unfolded molecule provides multiple A1 domains for platelet binding. Tethering also facilitates the binding of GPVI with sub-endothelial collagen. The engagement of GPIb-IX-V and GPVI initiates intracellular signalling, activating platelet integrins (GPIIb/IIIa, GPIa/IIa) and other receptor-ligand interactions. At static or low shear rates e.g. in veins, the interaction of platelet GPVI with subendothelial collagen is likely more important for the initiation of platelet adhesion. The binding of ligands to their respective integrin receptors results in platelet activation.

Platelet activation

Platelet activation can either be triggered by adhesion or soluble agonists. Initial activation is potentially reversible. Receptor-ligand interactions mediate intra-platelet signalling through various pathways that include second messengers and signal integrators 26.8. The net effect of activation is:

- **Integrin activation** results in a change in the ligand affinity state. GPIIb/IIIa and GPIa/IIa switch from low to high-affinity state. Activated GPIIb/IIIa and GPIa/IIa bind VWF and subendothelial collagen, respectively, triggering platelet activation with shape change and granule release.
- **Reorganization of the cytoskeleton with platelet shape change.** A transition from a discoid to a spherical shape is

facilitated by the disassembly of the microtubule ring. Actin polymerization facilitates filopodia formation (Fig. 26.7).

- **Alpha and dense granule secretion** results in the release of ADP, calcium, serotonin, VWF, FV, FVIII and fibrinogen. These act in an autocrine and paracrine fashion, augmenting platelet activation and recruiting additional platelets.
- **Exposure of negatively charged phosphatidylserine (PS)** on the platelet membrane for assembly of coagulation complexes.
- **De novo synthesis of thromboxane A2 (TXA2)** from arachidonic acid released by phospholipase A2 from membrane phospholipids following platelet activation. Sequential action of cyclooxygenase-1 and thromboxane synthase in platelets results in generation of thromboxane A2 (TxA2). TXA2 potentiates platelet aggregation by amplifying platelet activation through autocrine and paracrine mechanisms by binding to thromboxane receptor. TXA2 also has potent vasoconstrictive activity. In the vascular endothelial cells sequential action of cyclooxygenase-1 and prostacyclin synthase results in generation of prostacyclin I2 (PGI2) that results in vasodilation and platelet inhibition. (Fig. 26.8). TxA2 and PGI2 mediate their vascular effects via specific G-protein coupled receptors called thromboxane receptor and prostacyclin receptor.

Platelet aggregation

Cross-linking of platelets through fibrinogen, VWF and fibronectin, bridging activated GPIIb/IIIa receptors on adjacent platelets promotes platelet aggregation (Fig. 26.7).

Coagulation proteins

Blood clot formation requires stabilization of the platelet plug by the fibrin meshwork. The generation of fibrin from soluble fibrinogen is catalysed by thrombin, the final enzyme in the coagulation cascade of haemostasis.

The procoagulants include serine proteases, cofactors and glycoproteins (Table 26.1). Most coagulation factors circulate as inactive precursor zymogens (inactive precursors of enzymes). Predominantly belonging to the serine-protease enzyme family, the activation of each zymogen is depicted by suffixing the letter 'a' to the Roman numeral identifying that clotting factor. Notably, factors VIII and V are glycoprotein cofactors and not protease enzymes. These circulate in a precursor form and require limited cleavage by thrombin for the expression of full cofactor activity. The activity of some procoagulants and anticoagulants is dependent on vitamin K (Table 26.1, Fig. 31.4).

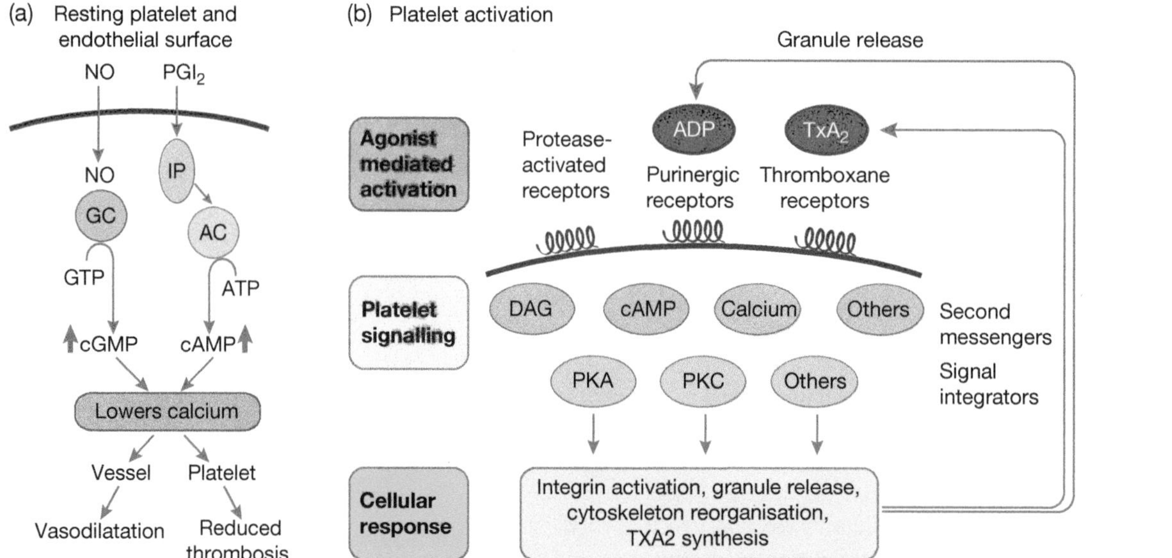

Figure 26.8a Platelets in the circulation are kept in a quiescent state by nitric oxide (NO) and prostacyclin (PGI2), both generated by the vascular endothelium. Nitric oxide diffuses into endothelial cells and platelets, where it activates guanylyl cyclase (GC), which converts GTP to cGMP. Prostacyclin activates its cell surface receptors (IP) and adenylate cyclase (AC), leading to the conversion of ATP to cAMP. The increased levels of cGMP and cAMP reduce calcium levels, promote vasodilation, and inhibit platelet activation. **26.8b** Platelets can be activated by multiple agonist receptor interactions. Platelet signalling includes the generation of second messengers (e.g., calcium, DAG, cAMP, cGMP) through the action of various enzymes (e.g., PLC, PI3K, AC, GC) that then integrate via effector pathways, which include protein kinases and other small proteins. NO, nitric oxide; PGI2, prostacyclin; GC, guanylyl cyclase; GTP, guanosine triphosphate; cGMP, cyclic guanosine monophosphate; AC, adenylate cyclase ATP, adenosine triphosphate; cAMP, cyclic adenosine monophosphate; TP, thromboxane receptor; IP, prostacyclin receptor; DAG, diacylglycerol; PLC, phospholipases; PI3K, phosphoinositide 3-kinase; PKA, protein Kinase A; PKB, protein kinase B.

Table 26.1 Key proteins in coagulation and haemostasis.

Common name	Abbreviation	Mean plasma concentration (μg/mL)	Mean plasma half-life (hrs)	Function
Procoagulants				
Fibrinogen	FGN	3000	90	Glycoprotein, which forms fibrin meshwork.
Prothrombin	FII	90	65	Serine protease, VKD*
Tissue factor	TF	NA	NA	Receptor/cofactor
Factor V	FV	10	15	Cofactor
Factor VII	FVII	0.5	5	Serine protease, VKD
Factor VIII (antihaemophilic factor)	FVIII	0.1	10	Cofactor
Factor IX (Christmas factor)	FIX	5	25	Serine protease, VKD
Factor X	FX	8	40	Serine protease, VKD
Factor XI	FXI	5	45	Serine protease
Von Willebrand factor	VWF	10	12	Glycoprotein multimer
Factor XIII	FXIII	30	200	Transglutaminase
Contact pathway				
Factor XII (Hageman (contact) factor	FXII	30	50	Serine protease
Prekallikrein (Fletcher factor)	PK	50	35	Serine protease
High molecular weight kininogen (Fitzgerald factor)	HMWK	70	144	Cofactor, activation is not required.
Anticoagulants				
Antithrombin	AT	58	140	Serpin (serine protease inhibitor)
Protein C	PC	4	6	Serine protease, VKD
Protein S	PS	10	42	Glycoprotein, VKD
Tissue factor pathway inhibitor	TFPI	0.08	1	Serpin (serine protease inhibitor)
Thrombomodulin	TM	NA	NA	Endothelial cell surface thrombin receptor
Endothelial cell protein C receptor	EPCR	NA	NA	Transmembrane receptor
Fibrinolysis				
Plasminogen	PLG	200	50	Serine protease
Alpha2 antiplasmin	α2-AP	70	72	Serpin (serine protease inhibitor)
Tissue plasminogen activator	tPA	0.005	0.03	Serine protease
Urokinase plasminogen activator	uPA	NA	NA	Serine protease
Plasminogen activator inhibitor 1	PAI-1	10	0.1	Serpin (serine protease inhibitor)
Thrombin activatable fibrinolysis inhibitor	TAFI	5	0.2	Carboxypeptidase

* VKD – Vitamin K-dependent proteins.
Source: A.V. Hoffbrand *et al.* (2016) *Postgraduate Haematology*, 7th edn. Reproduced with permission of John Wiley & Sons.

Cell-based model of thrombin generation

The cell-based model of thrombin generation explains the localization of the haemostatic response to the procoagulant surfaces at sites of injury. Following injury, in addition to subendothelial collagen, tissue factor (TF) is exposed, triggering coagulation.

In vivo, thrombin generation is a complex network of amplification and negative feedback loops. This ensures the response is localised and proportionate to the tissue injury. Three enzyme macromolecular complexes are responsible for thrombin generation (Fig. 26.9), namely extrinsic tenase, intrinsic tenase and prothrombinase. Each complex has an enzyme and cofactor that activate a precursor protease on a phospholipid surface (from injured cell or platelet) in the presence of calcium. Generation of thrombin is a two step process with FXa generated by tenase complexes and thrombin by prothrombinase (Fig. 26.9).

Three overlapping phases of thrombin generation are recognized, which generate thrombin in two waves of very different magnitudes. During the initiation and amplification phases, small amounts of thrombin are generated by activated FXa. This thrombin leads to a second larger burst (a million times higher) of thrombin in the propagation phase (Fig. 26.9).

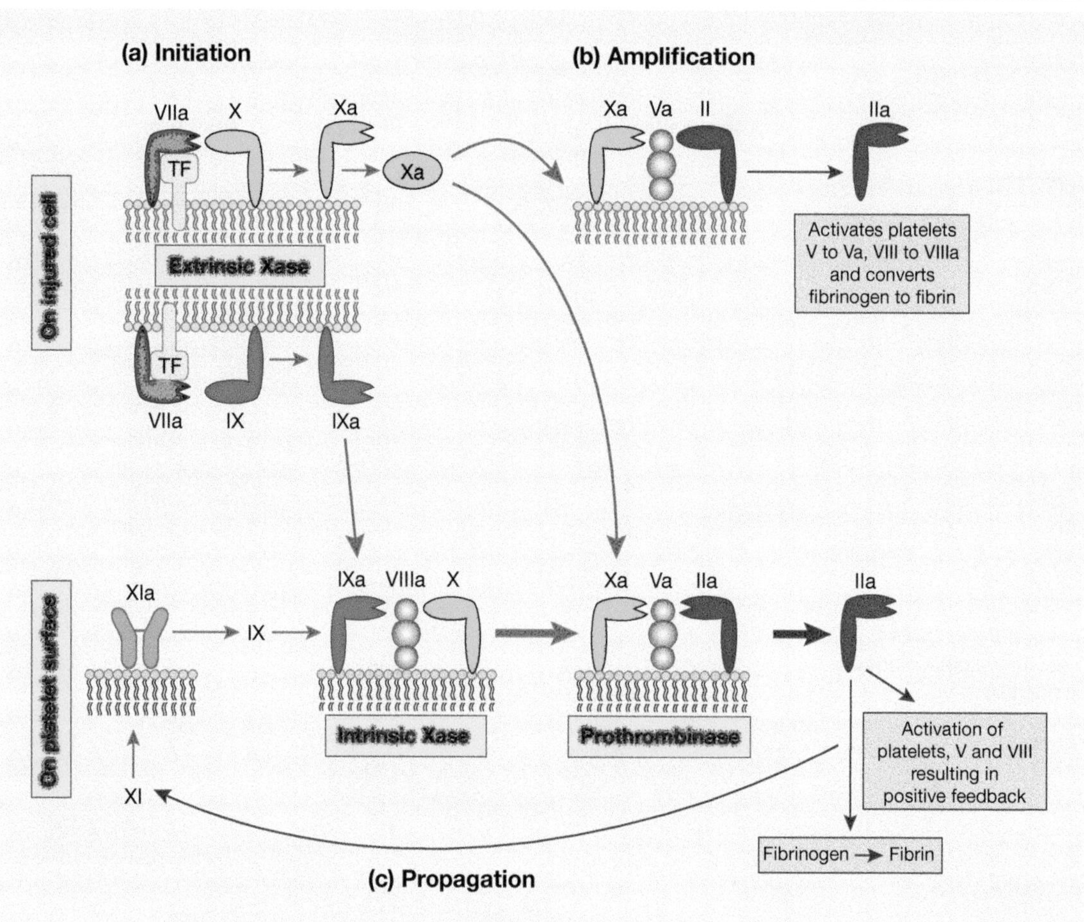

Figure 26.9 Cell-based model of coagulation (see text for detailed explanation) (a) During the initiation phase, small amounts of FXa and FIXa are generated by the extrinsic tenase complex. (b) In the amplification phase, small amounts of thrombin are generated on the injured cell by the FXa, which is necessary to establish the foundation for the propagation phase. (c) Propagation phase is characterised by thrombin burst which results in clot formation. Contact factor XIIa can also activate FXI, a feature used in laboratory. Assays but of doubtful clinical relevance. (green – PL from injured cell; purple – PF from platelet).

Initiation

TF is a transmembrane receptor that acts as a cofactor for circulating FVIIa, which represents 1–2% of the total circulating FVII. Under physiological conditions, TF is constitutively expressed by specific cells surrounding the vessel wall, including vascular smooth muscle cells and fibroblasts. **Exposure of TF following injury initiates coagulation. The extrinsic Xase complex is formed of TF-FVIIa on a phospholipid surface provided by the injured cells. This generates small quantities of FXa and FIXa from FX and FIX, respectively, FX being the more efficient substrate (Fig 26.9). The initiation complex is regulated by tissue factor pathway inhibitor (TFPI), which binds free and bound FXa.**

Amplification phase

FXa that bypasses TFPI inhibition activates small amounts of prothrombin to thrombin. Only picomolar amounts of thrombin are generated during the early or initiation phase. The thrombin activates platelets by cleaving protease-activated receptors, cofactors V and VIII, and FXI (Figs. 26.9, 26.10).

The cell surface hosting the macromolecular complexes distinguishes the amplification and propagation phases. The amplification phase continues on the injured cell, and the propagation phase is based on activated platelet surface.

The initiation and amplification phases are also called the extrinsic pathway, as the TF that initiates the pathway is extrinsic or outside of blood.

Propagation phase (thrombin burst)

The bulk of thrombin (≈95%) is formed during the propagation phase and is based on the platelet surface. FXa here is generated by the intrinsic Xase complex (FIXa, FVIIIa, PL, Ca2+) (Fig. 26.9). This complex is the primary activator of FX; it is 50-fold more efficient than FVIIa-TF in catalysing FX

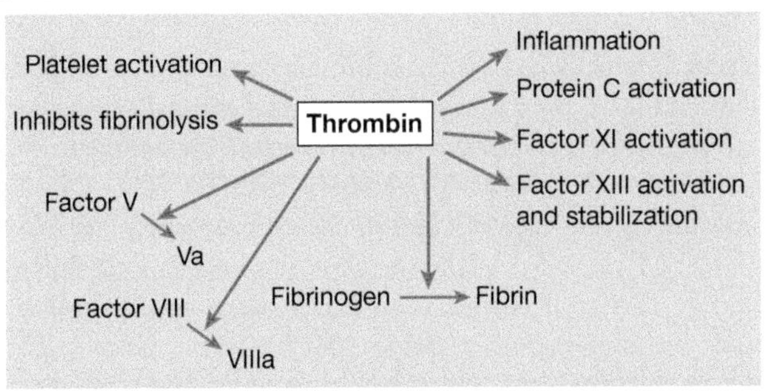

Figure 26.10 The heterogeneous actions of thrombin in haemostasis and inflammation.

activation. FIXa in the intrinsic Xase complex can originate following activation by the TF-FVIIa complex or by FXIa.

FXa and FVa form the **prothrombinase complex**, cleaving prothrombin to thrombin on platelet membranes (Fig. 26.9c). The generated thrombin mediates platelet activation and fibrin deposition, enabling blood clot formation. Under normal conditions, the concentration of FXa is the rate-limiting component of the prothrombinase complex.

The propagation phase is also called the intrinsic pathway, as all the constituents are within the blood. Under normal physiological conditions, FXI activation is catalysed by thrombin (Fig. 26.10). FXI can also be activated by FXIIa, seen *in vitro*, where autoactivation of FXII is facilitated by glass or silica to form FXIIa (Fig. 26.15). Indeed, FXII deficiency is not associated with a bleeding disorder.

FIXa and FXa in the enzyme complexes are protected from inhibition by antithrombin (AT) and other plasma protease inhibitors. Thrombin, in addition to its procoagulant effect, has anticoagulant effects and myriad other roles in haemostasis and immune response (Fig. 26.10).

Fibrinogen and fibrin formation

Fibrinogen (FGN) is a 340 kDa, multi-chain soluble glycoprotein. After activation by thrombin, it forms an insoluble clot providing a mechanical scaffold (fibrin network) for the blood clot. It is essential for haemostasis, wound healing, inflammation, angiogenesis and other biological functions.

Fibrinogen molecule is a homodimer with each unit made of three different polypeptide chains (Aα, Bβ and γ). The molecule is organized into a trinodular structure with a central globular region (E domain) and two peripheral symmetric units (D domains) with an elongated coiled-coil region in between (Fig 26.11). The central E domain contains the amino-terminal ends of the six polypeptide chains, and globular carboxyl-terminal domains of Bβ and γ form the terminal D domain. The terminology of the polypeptide chains arises from the cleavage of peptides (fibrinopeptide A and B) by thrombin at the N-terminal ends of the Aα and Bβ chains, necessary for polymerisation.

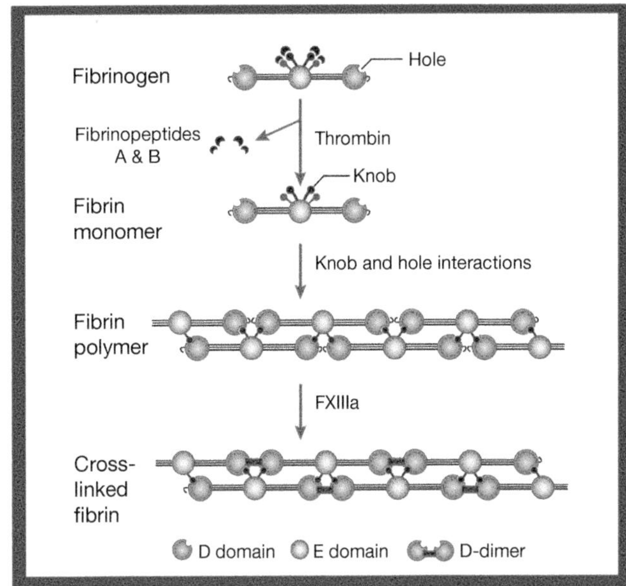

Figure 26.11 The formation and stabilization of fibrin meshwork. The fibrinogen molecule has a trinodular structure with a central E domain and two peripheral D domains. Thrombin activation results in the generation of monomers, where 'knobs' are generated by cleavage of the fibrinopeptides A and B at the N-terminal ends of the Aα and Bβ chains respectively in the central E domain. Fibrin polymer is generated by the interactions of the exposed 'knobs' in the E domain with the existing 'holes' in the D domains of adjacent molecules (violet lines). FXIIIa creates cross-linked fibrin (red horizontal lines) by covalently linking adjacent D domains, creating D-dimers.

Fibrin formation

Cleavage of fibrinopeptides A and B by thrombin results in fibrin monomers, initiating fibrin polymerization. (Fig. 26.11). The fibrin monomers continue to aggregate longitudinally to form oligomers and laterally to form protofibrils, creating the fibrin polymer (Fig. 26.11).

Cross-linking of fibrin

Cross-linking of fibrin by FXIIIa increases the resistance of fibrin clots to fibrinolysis. FXIIIa is a transglutaminase that cross-links fibrin γ- and α-chains into γ-chain dimers and α-chain polymers, respectively (Fig. 26.11). The 'γ-dimers' are the D-dimers measured for diagnosing venous thrombosis, exemplifying clot formation and lysis. Polymerized fibrin enhances the activation of FXIII ~100-fold.

Physiologic anticoagulants and coagulation regulation

The haemostatic response is localized temporally and spatially, crucial for limiting blood loss without compromising blood flow through excessive clot formation. **Thrombin generation**

is tightly regulated in the circulation and on the endothelial surface. This is achieved through the inactivation of active enzymes by serine protease inhibitors (serpins), tissue factor pathway inhibitor (TFPI) and antithrombin (AT) (Table 26.1), and inactivation of cofactors FVa and FVIIIa by activated protein C (APC) (Fig. 26.12).

Tissue factor pathway inhibitor

Tissue factor pathway inhibitor is the primary physiologic inhibitor of the initiation pathway/extrinsic Xase complex (Fig. 26.12). TFPI, mediates FXa-dependent inhibition of FVIIa. TFPI has two major isoforms, with more than 95% of TFPI bound to endothelial cells (TFPIβ) in the microcirculation.

TFPIα is the primary circulating form.

Antithrombin

Antithrombin is the principal circulating serpin. AT binds to its target and irreversibly inhibits the protease with the complex removed by the reticuloendothelial system. AT inhibits active serine proteases thrombin (FIIa), FIXa, FXa, FXIa and FXIIa, with thrombin and FXa being the primary targets. The inhibitory activity of AT is increased 1000-fold when bound to exogenous heparin or endogenous glycosaminoglycans present in the endothelial glycocalyx (Chapter 31).

Alpha2-macroglobulin, α2-antiplasmin, C1 esterase inhibitor and α1-antitrypsin also exert inhibitory effects on circulating serine proteases. AT also inhibits tissue plasminogen activator, urokinase, trypsin and plasmin.

Proteins C and S

Protein C is activated by thrombin associated with thrombomodulin (TM), the endothelial cell surface thrombin receptor. Activation is more efficient when protein C is bound to the endothelial cell protein C receptor (EPCR) (Fig. 26.12). Activated protein C (APC) and its cofactor protein S inactivate cofactors FVa and FVIIIa through proteolysis and downregulate thrombin generation. APC has a profibrinolytic effect through the inactivation of PA1-1 (see below). The microvasculature has the highest concentration of both glycosaminoglycans and EPCR. As for other serine proteases, activated protein C is subject to inactivation by serpins.

Fibrinolysis

Fibrinolysis is the tightly regulated process of clot dissolution, which coincides with wound repair. The central enzyme is plasmin, and the plasmin–antiplasmin system consists of two main protein families: serine proteases including plasminogen (PLG), tissue plasminogen activator (tPA) and urokinase plasminogen activator (uPA), and their inhibitor serpins that include α2-antiplasmin and plasminogen activator inhibitor 1 and 2 (PAI-1 and PAI-2) (Fig. 26.13).

Plasmin

Plasmin is generated from plasminogen following activation by tPA and uPA via different mechanisms (Fig. 26.13). Activation by tPA requires colocalization on cross-linked fibrin with plasminogen. In contrast, uPA activates plasminogen when both are associated with their cellular receptors. This mechanism is

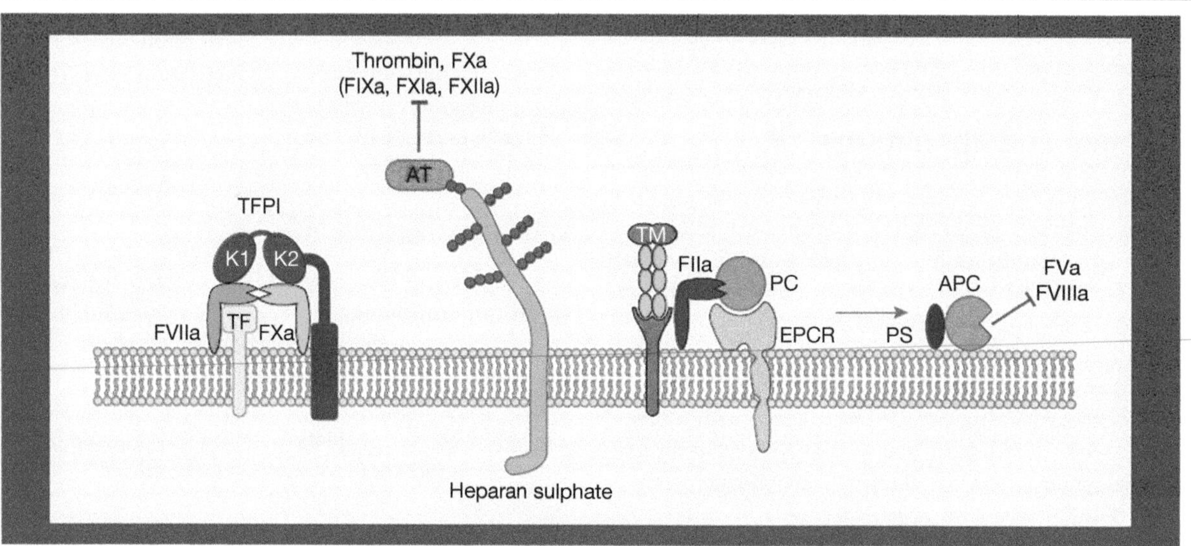

Figure 26.12 Physiologic anticoagulants and regulation of coagulation. The three principal physiologic anticoagulants that downregulate thrombin generation are tissue factor pathway inhibitor (TFPI), antithrombin (AT) and protein C (PC). TF, tissue factor; TFPI, tissue factor pathway inhibitor; K1 and K2, Kunitz domains of TFPI; AT, antithrombin; PC, protein C; APC, activated protein C; EPCR, endothelial cell protein C receptor; PS, protein S; TM, thrombomodulin.

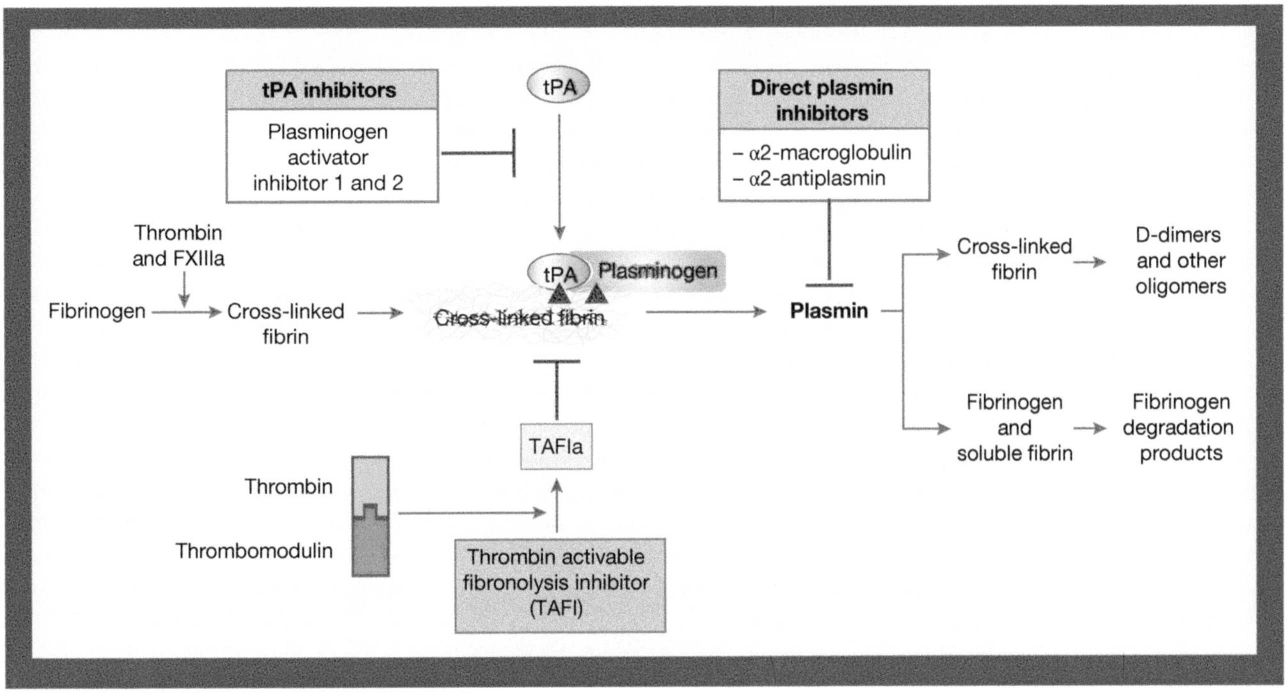

tPA inhibitors
Plasminogen activator inhibitor 1 and 2
tPA
Direct plasmin inhibitors
– α2-macroglobulin
– α2-antiplasmin
Thrombin and FXIIIa
Fibrinogen → Cross-linked fibrin →
tPA Plasminogen
Cross-linked fibrin → Plasmin
Cross-linked fibrin → D-dimers and other oligomers
Fibrinogen and soluble fibrin → Fibrinogen degradation products
TAFIa
Thrombin
Thrombomodulin
Thrombin activable fibronolysis inhibitor (TAFI)

Figure 26.13 Plasmin–antiplasmin system. Plasmin is generated from plasminogen when cleaved by tissue plasminogen activator (tPA). This activation requires colocalization of cross-linked fibrin, tPA and plasminogen, i.e. a ternary complex. The colocalization is facilitated by exposed lysine residues (red triangles) on fibrin monomers binding tPA and plasminogen through their lysine binding sites, producing an open confirmation of plasminogen susceptible to tPA. Plasmin, as shown, can act on both cross-linked fibrin and fibrinogen, giving rise to different fibrin degradation products. Plasminogen activation is inhibited by plasminogen activator inhibitor -1 (PAI-2, not shown) through inhibition of tPA. Plasmin is directly inhibited by α2-antiplasmin and α2-macroglobulin. Activated thrombin-activated fibrinolysis inhibitor (TAFIa) cleaves lysine residues from partially degraded fibrin and thus prevents the colocalization of plasminogen and tPA and reduces plasminogen activation.

important in the extracellular matrix, where plasmin has an essential role in tissue turnover.

Excess plasmin in addition to cross-linked fibrin, can also digest fibrinogen, non-cross linked fibrin, FV, FVIII and other proteins (Fig. 26.13). Cleavage of cross-linked fibrin as part of clot resolution results in D-dimers, which are measurable in plasma.

Regulation of fibrinolysis

Regulation of fibrinolysis is achieved by controlling the generation of plasmin or through inhibition of its activity (Fig. 26.13). PAI-1 and 2 inhibit tPA and uPA, preventing the activation of plasminogen. Plasmin is directly inhibited by α2-antiplasmin, a fast-acting inhibitor present at high concentration in plasma and by α2-macroglobulin, a broad-spectrum protease inhibitor. Finally, thrombin activated fibrinolysis inhibitor (TAFIa) is a carboxypeptidase that downregulates the binding of tPA and plasminogen and reduces plasmin generation. TAFIa is generated from TAFI by the action of thrombin/thrombomodulin complex.

Endothelial cells

Endothelial cells have an active role in the maintenance of vascular integrity and permeability. They exhibit both antithrombotic and prothrombotic properties (Fig. 26.14). Endothelial cells provide the basement membrane that separates collagen, elastin and fibronectin of the subendothelial connective tissue from the circulating blood.

The luminal surface of endothelium is covered by the glycocalyx/endothelial surface layer. The glycocalyx is secreted by the endothelial cells. It consists of membrane-binding proteoglycans with glycosaminoglycan side chains, e.g. heparan sulphate, which increase the catalytic efficiency of antithrombin at the cell surface. The glycocalyx also contains TFPI and thrombomodulin, which have anticoagulant activity. The endothelium actively synthesizes substances with antithrombotic properties (Fig. 26.14).

Any loss or injury to endothelium activates haemostasis. Sepsis can disrupt the glycocalyx, promoting the expression of various ligands, facilitating leucocyte and platelet adhesion, and microthrombi development in the microcirculation.

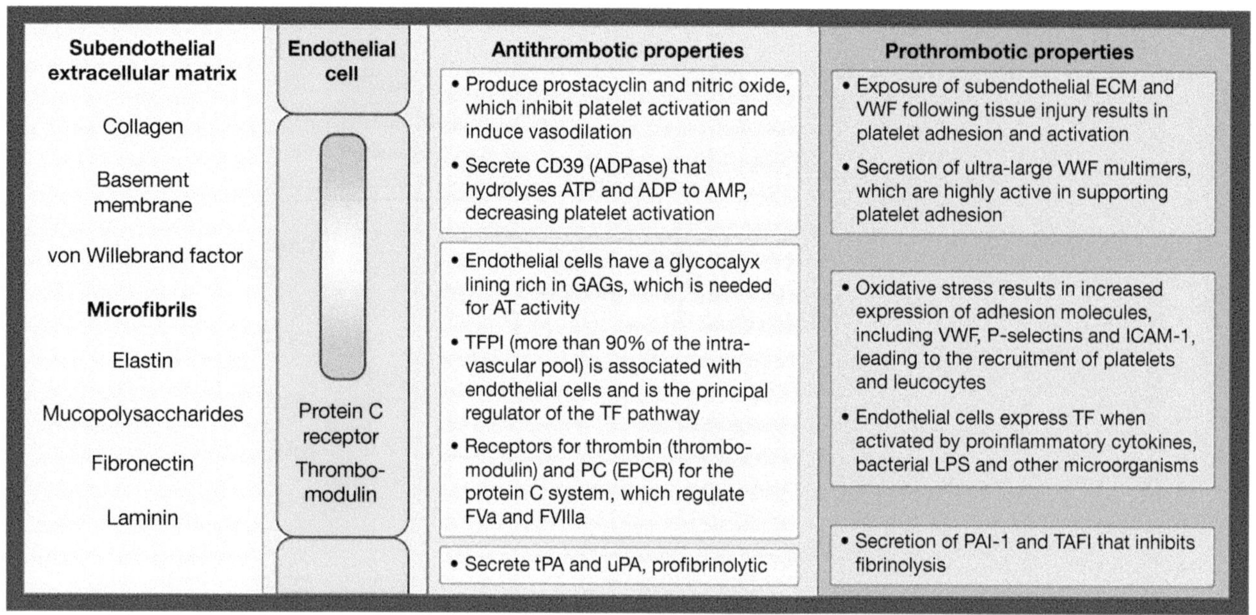

Figure 26.14 The endothelial cell forms a barrier between platelets and plasma clotting factors and the subendothelial connective tissues. Endothelial cells exhibit antithrombotic properties by generating substances that inhibit platelets and coagulation, reduce their activation and promote fibrinolysis. Following tissue injury or activation, exposure of blood to the subendothelial extracellular matrix enables normal haemostasis. In addition, it can also express molecules during inflammation and infection that can promote thrombosis even in the absence of tissue injury. CD39 – ectonucleotidase; ATP, adenosine triphosphate; ADP, adenosine diphosphate; AT, antithrombin; TFPI, tissue factor pathway inhibitor; EPCR, endothelial cell protein C receptor; tPA, tissue plasminogen activator; uPA, urokinase plasminogen activator; ECM, extracellular matrix; VWF, von Willebrand factor; ICAM-1, intercellular adhesion molecule 1; TF, tissue factor; LPS, lipopolysaccharide; PAI-1, plasminogen activator inhibitor-1; TAFI, thrombin activatable fibrinolysis inhibitor.

Tests of haemostatic function

Investigations for bleeding tendency aim to identify the cause suggested by the clinical history. Defective haemostasis with abnormal bleeding may result from:

1 A vascular disorder
2 Disorder of platelet number or function
3 Defective thrombin generation
4 Abnormalities of clot stability

Broadly, the investigations can be categorized as screening or specific assays. Specific assays can be antigen or activity assays. Activity assays can be global, i.e. measuring multiple components, or specific, measuring only one component.

In order to analyse the cellular and haemostatic components of peripheral blood, *in vitro* coagulation must be prevented. Sodium citrate solution is the anticoagulant of choice when investigating platelets and coagulation. Sodium citrate chelates calcium, preventing coagulation and is easily reversed with additional calcium. Ethylenediaminetetraacetic acid (EDTA) is the anticoagulant of choice for analysing cellular components as it preserves the cells and does not interfere with the staining. EDTA is also a potent chelator of calcium, and the anticoagulant effect is not reversible with the addition of calcium. Therefore, it is not appropriate for coagulation assays.

Blood count and blood film examination

The first steps in investigating a bleeding tendency are a full blood count (FBC) and a coagulation screen with a fibrinogen assay.

An FBC will detect thrombocytopenia, and any other blood cell abnormalities that hint at bone marrow pathology. Further investigations of thrombocytopenia are detailed in Chapter 27.

Modern counters measure platelet volume, and immature platelets (which contain RNA) that correlates with increased platelet production,. Both may not be available routinely.

Tests of blood coagulation

Most coagulation assays are functional bioassays; they provide a quantitative/semiquantitative assessment of the potency of the coagulation factors in the plasma by measuring their ability to form a fibrin clot. The result, often presented in seconds or minutes, reflects the time to initial clot detection and is compared to the normal range. The result can also be compared to a standard with a known activity level and expressed in units per millilitre or decilitre.

Coagulation assays - extrinsic and intrinsic pathways

Thrombin generation is not measured routinely in clinical practice. A deficiency of thrombin generation is inferred by measuring low factor levels. Prothrombin time (PT) and activated partial thromboplastin time (APTT) are *in vitro* approximations of the initiation, amplification and propagation phases of thrombin generation and are affected by low factor levels. They are functional assays as the endpoint is clot formation, and this is detected by a change in light transmittance. **The PT assay based on the *in vitro* extrinsic and common pathways reflects the initiation and amplification phase of thrombin generation (Fig. 26.15a). The APTT based on the *in vitro* intrinsic and common pathways reflects the propagation phase of thrombin generation (26.15b).**

Prothrombin time and international normalized ratio (INR)

TF and phospholipid together are referred to as thromboplastin reagent (Fig. 26.15a). The tissue thromboplastin used may be synthetic or derived from animal brain and other tissues. The normal time for clotting is 9–12 s with minor interlaboratory variation. It may be expressed as the international normalized ratio (INR). The INR allows interlaboratory comparison that corrects for the sensitivities of the various thromboplastin reagents.

Activated partial thromboplastin time

Coagulation is triggered by activating contact factors (Fig. 26.15b). The contact factors have no role in normal coagulation but help isolate the intrinsic pathway for laboratory evaluation. The normal time for clotting is approximately 30–40 s.

Mixing studies and thrombin time

Prolonged clotting times in PT and APTT caused by factor deficiency can be corrected by the addition of normal plasma to the test plasma (50:50 mix). If there is no correction or incomplete correction with normal plasma, the presence of a coagulation inhibitor is suspected.

The thrombin (clotting) time (TT) is sensitive to fibrinogen deficiency or thrombin inhibition. Diluted bovine thrombin is added to citrated plasma, and concentration is adjusted to give a clotting time of 14–16 s in normal subjects.

PT and APTT - clinical use

While easy to use and sensitive, PT and APTT tend to be abnormal in sick, hospitalized patients in intensive care due

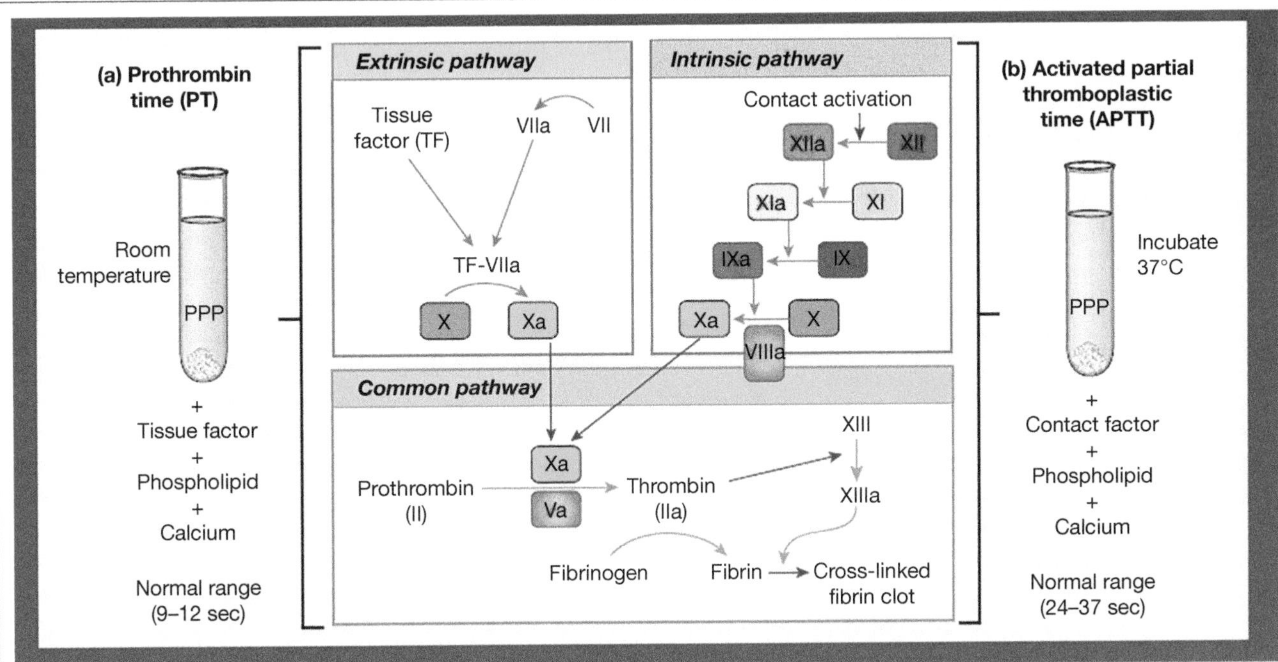

Figure 26.15 Prothrombin time (PT) and activated partial thromboplastin time (APTT) are the standard screening coagulation assays. **(a)** PT is performed by adding tissue factor and phospholipid to platelet poor plasma (PPP) at room temperature in the presence of calcium. Here, supraphysiological concentrations of TF drive the generation of FXa and FIIa via extrinsic and common pathways, resulting in the rapid formation of a fibrin clot. **(b)** APTT measures the plasma clotting time following the activation of the contact factor FXII. Autoactivation of FXII to FXIIa is facilitated by the addition of contact activators kaolin, silica or ellagic acid to PPP, followed by incubation. FXIIa activates FXI and generates FXa and FIIa through intrinsic and common pathways and fibrin clot formation. Under normal physiological conditions, FXI activation is catalysed by thrombin rather than FXIIa. Deficiencies in any of the factors along the pathway result in the prolongation of PT and APTT.

Table 26.2 Screening tests used in the diagnosis of coagulation disorders.

Screening tests	Abnormalities indicated by prolongation	Most common cause of coagulation disorder
Prothrombin time (PT)	Deficiency or inhibition of factors in extrinsic (VII) or common pathway (X, V, II, fibrinogen)	Liver disease, warfarin therapy, DIC*
Activated partial thromboplastin time (APTT)	Deficiency or inhibition of factors in intrinsic (FXII, FXI, FIX, FVIII) or common pathway (X, V, II, fibrinogen) or lupus anticoagulant	Haemophilia A (FVIII), haemophilia B (FIX), warfarin therapy, DIC
Thrombin time (TT)	Deficiency or abnormality of fibrinogen or inhibition of thrombin by heparin or FDPs*	DIC, heparin therapy
Fibrinogen quantitative	Fibrinogen deficiency	DIC, haemodilution, inherited disorders and liver disease

* DIC, disseminated intravascular coagulation; Lupus anticoagulant is an antibody against phospholipid that interferes with APTT assays but is not associated with bleeding (Chapter 30); FDPs, fibrinogen degradation products.

to low-grade consumption of multiple factors and, therefore, not always reflective of isolated factor deficiency. Despite this, there is an association between PT/INR, APTT and factor levels, and they continue to be used in routine clinical practice to identify patients for further investigations (Table 26.2).

Fibrinogen assay

The Clauss fibrinogen assay is a quantitative, clot-based, functional assay. It measures the conversion of fibrinogen to fibrin clot after exposure to a high amount of thrombin. Another method sometimes used is derived fibrinogen. The latter is based on the change in light transmittance in the PT test beyond the initial clot formation. Although popular as there are no additional costs, it is not sensitive to low levels and can give inaccurate results in anticoagulated patients.

Specific assays

Most coagulation assays are functional biological assays that use clot formation as the endpoint. Several chemical, chromogenic and immunological methods are available for quantifying proteins such as fibrinogen, VWF, FXa and FVIII.

Tests of platelet function

There are no simple, reliable screening assays for detecting platelet function abnormalities. One assay in practice across centres is the platelet function analyser -100/200 (PFA-100/PFA-200), but the gold standard for platelet function testing continues to be light transmission aggregometry (LTA) (Fig. 26.16).

The standard panel of agonists includes different concentrations of ADP, adrenaline, collagen, ristocetin and arachidonic acid. Response to agonist is read at 3–5 min. LTA requires fresh blood and a minimum platelet count of 80×10^9/L.

Variations of the assay and equipment allow the aggregometry to be performed on whole blood, with simultaneous measurement of ATP released from platelet granules, a measure of platelet activation and granule release. The response pattern enables a diagnosis in most platelet function disorders (Chapter 27). Flow cytometry is increasingly used to identify platelet glycoprotein defects in routine practice. Dense granule content and release (nucleotide) often require specialist assays.

In the PFA-200 test, citrated blood is aspirated through a capillary tube onto a thick membrane with apertures coated with collagen/ADP or collagen/adrenaline. Under shear, platelets adhere and aggregate, primarily via VWF interactions with GPIb and GPIIb/IIIa, resulting in occlusion of the aperture. The PFA-200 is prolonged in VWD and other defects of platelet function but is not always sensitive to mild platelet function abnormalities. It is not a reliable tool for screening mild platelet function defects.

Tests of fibrinolysis

Testing for hyperfibrinolysis by traditional methods, such as euglobulin clot lysis times, are rarely performed. A clinically significant hyperfibrinolytic state, e.g. during liver transplantation, can be detected by visco-elastic measurement of clot stability described below.

The detection of D-dimers suggests lysis of cross-linked fibrin and thus indicates sequential action of thrombin and plasmin on fibrinogen. There are many causes of elevated D-dimers, including infection, cancer, pregnancy and venous thromboembolism. Plasma levels are very high

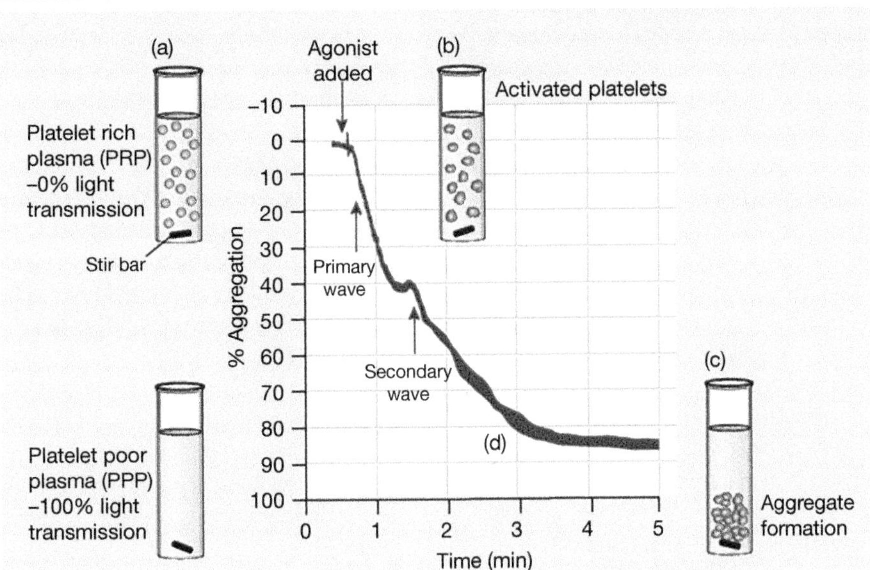

Figure 26.16 Light transmission aggregometry (LTA) for evaluation of platelet function. LTA measures the change in light transmittance in platelet-rich plasma as platelets aggregate. **(a)** Light transmission through platelet-rich plasma (PRP) and platelet-poor plasma (PPP) are set at 0% and 100%, respectively. A stir bar at the bottom of the tubes keeps the platelets suspended in plasma. **(b)** The addition of agonists to PRP results in the activation of platelets. **(c)** Activation is followed by shape change, granule release and aggregate formation. Platelet aggregates sink to the bottom of the tube, increasing light transmission. **(d)** Most agonists increase light transmittance to 70–90% of PPP at 3–5 min. Typically, a single curve demonstrating increasing light transmission over time is seen. A biphasic response can be seen at critical concentrations of weak agonists like ADP. The primary wave reflects the response to an exogenous agonist and is reversible. The secondary wave reflects the irreversible activation and release of an endogenous pool of agonists.

in disseminated intravascular coagulation and following thrombolysis.

Thrombin generation assays

These assays measure the amount of thrombin that can be generated over time. Coagulation is initiated by adding TF at physiological concentrations. The assay is performed in plasma or platelet-rich plasma and is sensitive to procoagulants and anticoagulants. The amount of thrombin generated is detected through the cleavage of a chromogenic or fluorogenic substrate. Thrombin production correlates with factor deficiencies or the use of anticoagulants. Their role in routine clinical practice is yet to be determined.

Viscoelastic tests (VET)

These tests assess whole blood clot formation *ex vivo* by monitoring changes in the physical properties (viscoelastic) of blood by shear or resonance. The main instruments are TEG® (thromboelastography), ROTEM® (thromboelastometry) and Sonoclot®. They have proprietary triggers to activate different parts of the coagulation pathway. They also use different technologies for monitoring the change in the viscoelastic properties of an evolving clot. All instruments display results graphically. These changes represent the interaction between platelets, coagulation factors and other cellular components, and resulting changes, including fibrin polymerization and platelet fibrin interactions.

They are typically available as point-of-care tests on whole blood with or without an anticoagulant, and results are available quite rapidly. They have a role in clinical situations with gross rapidly changing haemostatic abnormalities, e.g. traumatic or obstetric haemorrhage, liver transplantation and cardiopulmonary bypass. In these situations, they can guide the use of various blood products through algorithm-based haemostatic interventions. They are not sensitive to moderate to mild deficiencies of coagulation factors, platelet dysfunction or anticoagulants and antiplatelet agents. They are good for diagnosing hyperfibrinolysis.

SUMMARY

- Normal haemostasis requires a coordinated response to tissue injury that involves vasoconstriction, platelet plug formation and a fibrin meshwork. It culminates in the formation of a blood clot to arrest bleeding.
- Intact endothelial cells separate blood from collagen and other subendothelial connective tissues that potentially initiate platelet adhesion. The endothelial cells actively maintain an antithrombotic surface by secreting several substances, including prostacyclin, nitric oxide and endothelial glycocalyx, which inhibit platelet aggregation and coagulation.
- Platelets are produced from megakaryocytes in the bone marrow, a process regulated by thrombopoietin. Platelets mediate primary haemostasis, which includes adhesion, activation and aggregation to form the platelet plug.
- Platelet adhesion is mediated by GP1b-IX-V receptor tethering to subendothelial VWF. This results in intracellular signalling and platelet activation, reinforced by granule release and additional activation. The intracellular signalling also activates GPIIb/IIIa receptors, enabling binding to fibrinogen and cross-linking of platelets, resulting in aggregation.
- Blood coagulation *in vivo* in response to vascular injury commences with tissue factor binding to clotting factor VIIa. Thrombin generation occurs in two waves of different magnitudes, the initiation and amplification phase generating less than 5%, and the propagation phase generating most of the thrombin. The key steps are the generation of FXa by extrinsic Xase and intrinsic Xase complexes respectively and the generation of thrombin by prothrombinase.
- Thrombin generation is tightly regulated. The three principal physiologic anticoagulants are tissue factor pathway inhibitor, the principal regulator of the initiation complex, antithrombin that irreversibly inhibits thrombin and FXa, and protein C and protein S inhibiting cofactors FVa and FVIIIa.
- Dissolution of fibrin clots (fibrinolysis) occurs following the activation of plasminogen to plasmin, facilitated by colocalization of plasminogen with its activators on cross-linked fibrin. Regulation of fibrinolysis includes reducing the amount of plasmin generated and its activity.
- Platelet function tests include the light transmission aggregometry and other point-of-care assays.
- Coagulation tests include screening assays prothrombin time (PT), activated partial thromboplastin time (APTT) and specific assays for individual clotting factors.
- Global point-of-care viscoelastic assays visually chart the formation and dissolution of clots and play a role in targeted resuscitation during haemorrhage.

Now visit **www.wiley.com/go/haematology9e** to test yourself on this chapter.

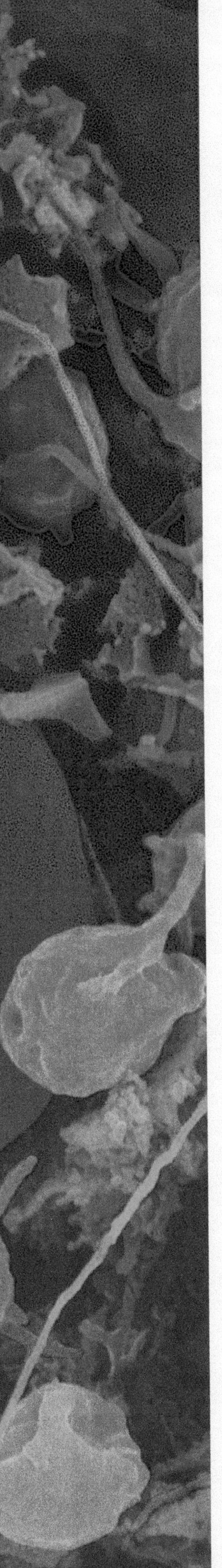

CHAPTER 27

Bleeding disorders caused by platelet and vascular abnormalities

Key topics

Hoffbrand's Essential Haematology, Ninth Edition. A. Victor Hoffbrand, Pratima Chowdary, Graham P. Collins, and Justin Loke.

© 2024 John Wiley & Sons Ltd. Published 2024 by John Wiley & Sons Ltd.

Companion website: www.wiley.com/go/haematology9e

Severe bleeding disorders, inherited or acquired, are potentially life-threatening. Mild and moderate bleeding disorders are often associated with increased morbidity secondary to excessive bleeding post-trauma or surgery. Post-surgical bleeding contributes to impaired wound healing and infections. A high degree of suspicion is key to the diagnosis of mild to moderate bleeding disorders.

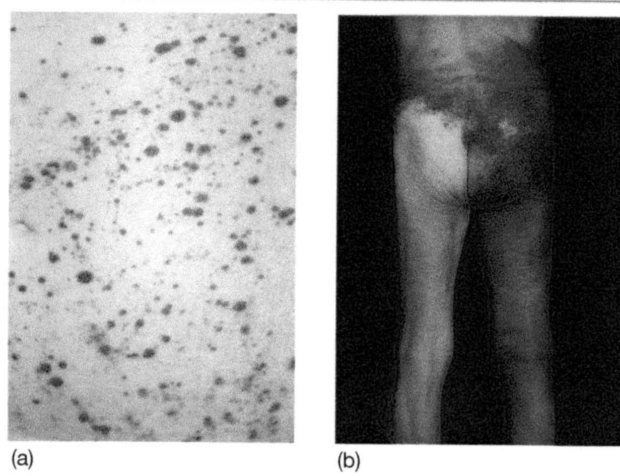

Figure 27.1 (a) Typical purpura. (b) Massive subcutaneous haemorrhage in a patient with immune thrombocytopenia (drug-induced).

Abnormal bleeding

This may result from the following:

- **Low platelet count (thrombocytopenia)**
- **Defective platelet function**
- **Vascular (connective tissue) defects**
- **Defective coagulation**
- **Abnormalities of fibrinolysis**

The bleeding pattern can hint at the underlying defect in patients with severe bleeding tendency but is of less help in patients with a mild bleeding tendency. Bleeding due to inherited or acquired thrombocytopenia, abnormal platelet function and vascular abnormalities is dealt with in this chapter. Chapters 28 and 29 cover inherited and acquired abnormalities of coagulation and fibrinolysis. In a small minority of patients, the cause of excessive bleeding cannot be identified.

Bleeding history

Bleeding is a common symptom; whilst bleeding caused by severe disorders is easily identifiable as abnormal, distinguishing normal from abnormal bleeding can be challenging in mild bleeding disorders.

History and evaluation of bleeding symptoms

The age of onset and family history help identify heritable disorders, particularly severe disorders where bleeding is typically spontaneous. Bleeding can present in the neonatal period or the first few years of life. Neonatal bleeding includes umbilical stump bleeding, cephalhaematoma, cheek haematoma caused by sucking during breast/bottle feeding, conjunctival haemorrhage or excessive bleeding following circumcision or venepuncture.

The bleeding pattern may provide clues to the underlying disorder. Mucosal bleeding (nose bleeding, gum bleeding, haematuria, heavy menstrual bleeding, haematemesis and melaena) can be seen in any bleeding disorder. Cutaneous and mucosal petechiae and purpura are typical of thrombocytopenia (Figs. 24.3, 27.1a), whereas ecchymoses and subcutaneous haematomas are seen with any bleeding disorder (Fig. 27.1b). Petechiae, caused by the extravasation of red cells from dermal capillaries, relate to the role of platelets in maintaining vascular integrity. Spontaneous joint and muscle bleeds are typical of patients with severe coagulation factor deficiencies. Bleeding into vital organs and nervous system can be seen with any severe bleeding disorder.

A bleeding history should evaluate the clinical significance of bleeding symptoms (Table 27.1) and cover the following areas:

1. Sites of bleeding – cutaneous, mucosal (nose, gum and oral cavity bleeding, haematuria, heavy menstrual bleeding), internal organs (gastrointestinal, pulmonary or central nervous system bleeding) or musculoskeletal system.
2. Spontaneous or precipitated by activities of daily living, surgery or trauma.
3. Age of onset – neonatal period or lifelong history with onset in childhood or new onset bleeding tendency.
4. Duration of bleeding – superficial or minor injuries bleeding for more than 5 to 10 minutes, nose bleeds longer than half hour, bleeding requiring intervention, anaemia due to recurrent blood loss.
5. Severity of bleeding – exacerbation of normal blood loss through gastrointestinal tract or menstrual bleeding, or more than expected following a haemostatic challenge.
6. Frequency of bleeding – the number of events over days, months and years. The clinical presentation of the various bleeding symptoms and minimal criteria that determine potential significance are presented in Table 27.1.

Bleeding assessment tools

Several bleeding assessment tools (BATs) have been developed to standardize the assessment of bleeding severity. Scores based on these tools are used to assess the pretest probability of identifying a bleeding disorder. The World Health Organization

Table 27.1 Bleeding symptoms and assessment of clinical significance.

Site of bleeding	Description and criteria for clinical significance
Mucosal	
Epistaxis	Nosebleeds are common and can be seasonal. They are considered significant if there is no identifiable cause, > 10 minutes or > 5 episodes per year, require hospitalisation and treatment, or have other symptoms
Oral cavity bleeding	Gum bleeding with frank blood in sputum or bleeding after bites to lips, cheek and tongue > 10 minutes on more than one occasion. Some patients may present with blisters
Tooth extraction	Prolonged bleeding after a procedure or requiring a review after leaving the dental unit
Haematuria	Macroscopic haematuria without identifiable disease
Cutaneous and mucosal	
Petechiae and purpura	Petechiae – pinpoint haemorrhages <3 mm; Purpura – haemorrhagic spots 3–10 mm. Ten or more in palm-sized areas distributed across the body
Ecchymoses	Haemorrhages >1 cm in size. Five or more in exposed body areas, spontaneous or disproportionate to trauma
Haematoma	Large palpable bruise, both in number and size. If more than two to three in different areas, along with other symptoms
Uterine	
Heavy menstrual bleeding (menorrhagia)	Change of pads more frequently than every 2 hours; bleeding lasting seven or more days; history of flooding with clots >1 cm
Postpartum haemorrhage (PPH)	Primary (within 24 hours) – when blood loss from the genital tract is >500 mL or requires intervention (additional uterotonics, tranexamic acid, blood or blood products, mechanical or surgical haemostatic measures). Secondary PPH (after 24 hours and up to 12 weeks) – excessive vaginal bleeding that requires changing pads or tampons more frequently than every 2 hours or is considered abnormal by the clinician responsible for routine care
Organ	
Gastrointestinal	Haematemesis, melena, and haematochezia NOT explained by the presence of a specific disease
Central nervous system	Any subdural or intracerebral haemorrhage requiring diagnostic or therapeutic intervention with no apparent cause
Musculoskeletal	
Muscle haematomas or haemarthrosis	Any spontaneous joint/muscle bleed (unrelated to traumatic injuries) or minimal trauma
Haemostatic challenge	
Surgical bleeding	Any bleeding judged by the surgeon as abnormally prolonged or requiring supportive treatment
Minor cutaneous Wound	Any prolonged (> 10 minutes) bleeding episode caused by surperficial cuts (e.g., by shaving razor, knife) on more than occasion

Source: Modified from the International Society of Haemostasis and Thrombosis scientific subcommittee bleeding assessment tool (F. Rodeghiero *et al.* (2010) *J. Thromb. Haemost.* 8: 2063–65), International Working Group Standardization of bleeding assessment for ITP (F. Rodeghiero *et al.* (2013) *Blood* 121: 2596–606) and European Haematology Association consensus report on mild and moderate bleeding disorders (F. Rodeghiero *et al.* (2019) *Hemasphere* 3: e286).

Bleeding Scale, designed for chemotherapy, is the most commonly applied criterion in thrombocytopenia and is given in Table 27.2.

The International Society of Haemostasis and Thrombosis (ISTH) published a version of BAT (ISTH-BAT) in 2011 for the evaluation of mild to moderate inherited coagulation and platelet disorders. The international working group for immune thrombocytopenic purpura (ITP) and other groups have published assessment tools for assessing bleeding severity in ITP.

Table 27.2 World Health Organization bleeding grades.

Grade 0	None
Grade 1	Petechiae, ecchymoses, occult blood loss, mild spotting
Grade 2	Gross bleeding, i.e. epistaxis, haematuria, haematemesis not requiring transfusion
Grade 3	Haemorrhage requiring transfusion
Grade 4	Haemorrhage with haemodynamic compromise, retinal haemorrhage with visual impairment, central nervous system haemorrhage, fatal at any location

Thrombocytopenia

Thrombocytopenia, acquired or inherited, is an important cause of bleeding. The severity of thrombocytopenia determines the bleeding risk, extent of investigations and management. Mild thrombocytopenia may be defined as counts between 100 and 139 × 10⁹/L, moderate 50 and 99 × 10⁹/L, severe < 50 × 10⁹/L, and very severe < 20 × 10⁹/L.

Causes of thrombocytopenia

Two principal mechanisms contribute to thrombocytopenia: decreased production and increased consumption. The causes based on the primary mechanism are listed in Table 27.3. Although classified by primary mechanism of action, some of the listed disorders may operate via both mechanisms.

Occasionally, artefactual thrombocytopenia may be due to EDTA-mediated platelet clumping, an *in vitro* phenomenon. This is mediated by non-pathogenic antibodies against new epitopes exposed on platelet receptors by strong calcium chelation. This can be resolved by performing a platelet count on a citrated sample.

Investigation of thrombocytopenia

The normal platelet count is 140–400 × 10⁹/L, with some normal individuals having counts below normal. Increased destruction, most frequently immune mediated, is the most common mechanism of isolated thrombocytopenia in patients referred from the community.

Clinical

History and physical examination can point to systemic causes of thrombocytopenia.

- Life-long history of bleeding or asymptomatic platelet abnormalities suggests heritable platelet disorders.
- Features of systemic sepsis or inflammation suggest a secondary cause.
- Palpable purpura suggests vascular inflammation.
- Drug history and timing of thrombocytopenia in relation to drug initiation

Table 27.3 Thrombocytopenia: causes listed by the primary mechanism.

Thrombocytopenia due to increased consumption

- Autoimmune thrombocytopenia
  - Idiopathic
  - Secondary — associated with other autoimmune disorders, e.g. systemic lupus erythematosus, antiphospholipid syndrome
  - Secondary to chronic lymphocytic leukaemia or lymphoma
  - Drug-induced
- Alloimmune
  - Post-transfusional purpura
  - Feto-maternal alloimmune thrombocytopenia
- Infections
  - *Helicobacter pylori*
  - HIV
  - Other viruses
  - *Plasmodium* parasites (malaria)
  - COVID-19
- Consumptive coagulopathies
  - Thrombotic microangiopathies (TMA), e.g. thrombocytopenic Purpura (TTP) or haemolytic uraemic syndrome (HUS)
  - Heparin-induced thrombocytopenia
  - Disseminated intravascular coagulation
  - Haemangiomas
- Gestational thrombocytopenia
- Pregnancy specific TMA
  - Pre-eclampsia
  - Hemolysis, elevated liver enzymes, low platelets (HELLP) Syndrome
  - Acute fatty liver of pregnancy
- Abnormal distribution of platelets
  - Splenomegaly, e.g. liver disease
- Multiple mechanisms
  - Liver disease
  - Massive transfusion of stored blood

Thrombocytopenia due to impaired production

- Inherited platelet disorders
- Selective megakaryocyte depression
- Bone marrow failure syndromes
  - Secondary to primary haematological malignancy, e.g. leukaemia
  - Myelodysplastic syndromes
  - Marrow infiltration, e.g. carcinoma, lymphoma, Gaucher's disease
  - Aplastic anaemia
- Nutritional deficiencies
  - Folate and B12 deficiency
- Acute alcohol intoxication
- Viral infections, including HIV
- Drugs and chemicals
  - Chemotherapy
  - Radiotherapy
  - Other toxic substances

Laboratory

1 Full blood count and morphology – the critical first step to confirm isolated thrombocytopenia.
- Presence of other cytopenias or abnormal cells suggests other primary haematological disorders.
- Presence of red cell fragments and anaemia suggests thrombotic microangiopathic haemolytic anaemia (Chapter 29).

2 Low fibrinogen and elevated D-dimers with or without thrombosis suggest consumptive coagulopathy

3 Tests for infections
- Hepatitis C and B
- HIV
- *Helicobacter pylori*
- Polymerase chain reaction for Epstein–Barr virus, parvovirus and cytomegalovirus in selected populations.

4 Autoantibody screen
- Antinuclear antibodies and antiphospholipid antibodies
- Thyroid function tests and anti-thyroid antibodies
- Direct antiglobulin test

5 Immunoglobulin levels
- To exclude immunodeficiency syndromes, particularly in children.

6 Bone marrow biopsy
- Confirm marrow failure as the cause of thrombocytopenia, selective or multilineage.
- Diagnoses of infiltration or other haematological neoplasias.

7 Thrombopoietin (TPO) levels and antiplatelet antibodies
- Are not used routinely and do not help with the differential diagnosis.

Immune (idiopathic) thrombocytopenia purpura

Definitions

This is a relatively common disorder and the most common cause of isolated thrombocytopenia. Asymptomatic presentation is frequent; symptoms, if present, range from mild mucocutaneous bleeding to life-threatening bleeds. Approximately a fifth of patients require hospital admission within five years of diagnosis.

Immune thrombocytopenia (ITP) is a heterogeneous disorder with a complex pathophysiology. To address this, in 2009, an International Working Group proposed standardized terminology, definitions and outcome assessment for use in clinical trials and routine care.

Pathogenesis

The pathogenesis of ITP is complex; a range of alterations in humoral and cellular immunity have been observed. (Fig. 27.2). Platelet survival is decreased to a few hours or days. Megakaryocytes in the marrow are normal or mildly increased in number, showing that platelet production is inappropriately low. In the majority, TPO levels are normal or moderately elevated.

In most, autoantibodies responsible for the immune destruction of platelets are directed against the GPIIb/IIIa receptors, with antibodies against other receptors in a minority of patients. Antibodies may be present against multiple antigens. Rarely antibodies cannot be detected. Various abnormalities of cell-mediated immunity have been documented, including an increase in autoreactive T cells, a reduction in regulatory T-cell activity and an increase in cytotoxic T cells (Fig. 27.2).

Clinical features: children

ITP is of acute onset in children, often presenting with a purpuric rash of less than a week's duration. Approximately three-quarters of episodes follow vaccinations or infections like chickenpox or infectious mononucleosis. Most cases are caused by non-specific immune complex deposition on platelets. The diagnosis is one of exclusion.

Spontaneous remissions are usual, but in 5–10% of cases, the disease becomes chronic (Table 27.4). Morbidity and mortality in paediatric ITP are very low. The main risk is cerebral haemorrhage, fortunately rare. Most children do not bleed even with platelet counts $<10 \times 10^9$/L, but they must avoid trauma such as contact sports.

Although there is a correlation between platelet count and bleeding risk, there is active debate about a threshold platelet count that is sensitive and specific for severe bleeding. Clinical studies have suggested that no treatment is indicated if the counts are $>30 \times 10^9$/L, and the bleeding risk increases when platelets are $<20 \times 10^9$/L. However, as bleeding is unusual, many clinicians adopt a wait-and-watch approach even with platelet counts $<10 \times 10^9$/L in the absence of bleeding. A clinical decision to treat a child with ITP is based on the severity of their clinical symptoms and impending haemostatic challenges, not solely on the platelet count. In addition, a risk–benefit analysis should include time for regular tests and reviews, access to urgent care and parenteral anxiety before embarking on a wait-and-watch option.

Clinical features: adults

In adults, the highest incidence is in women aged 15–50 years. Asymptomatic presentation through a routine FBC is seen in about a third of new patients. In symptomatic patients, the onset is often insidious with petechial haemorrhage, easy bruising and, in women, menorrhagia when platelet counts drop below 50×10^9/L. Mucosal bleeding occurs in severe cases. Intracerebral bleeding is a rare cause of death. Fatigue is a commonly reported symptom in patients with a low platelet count.

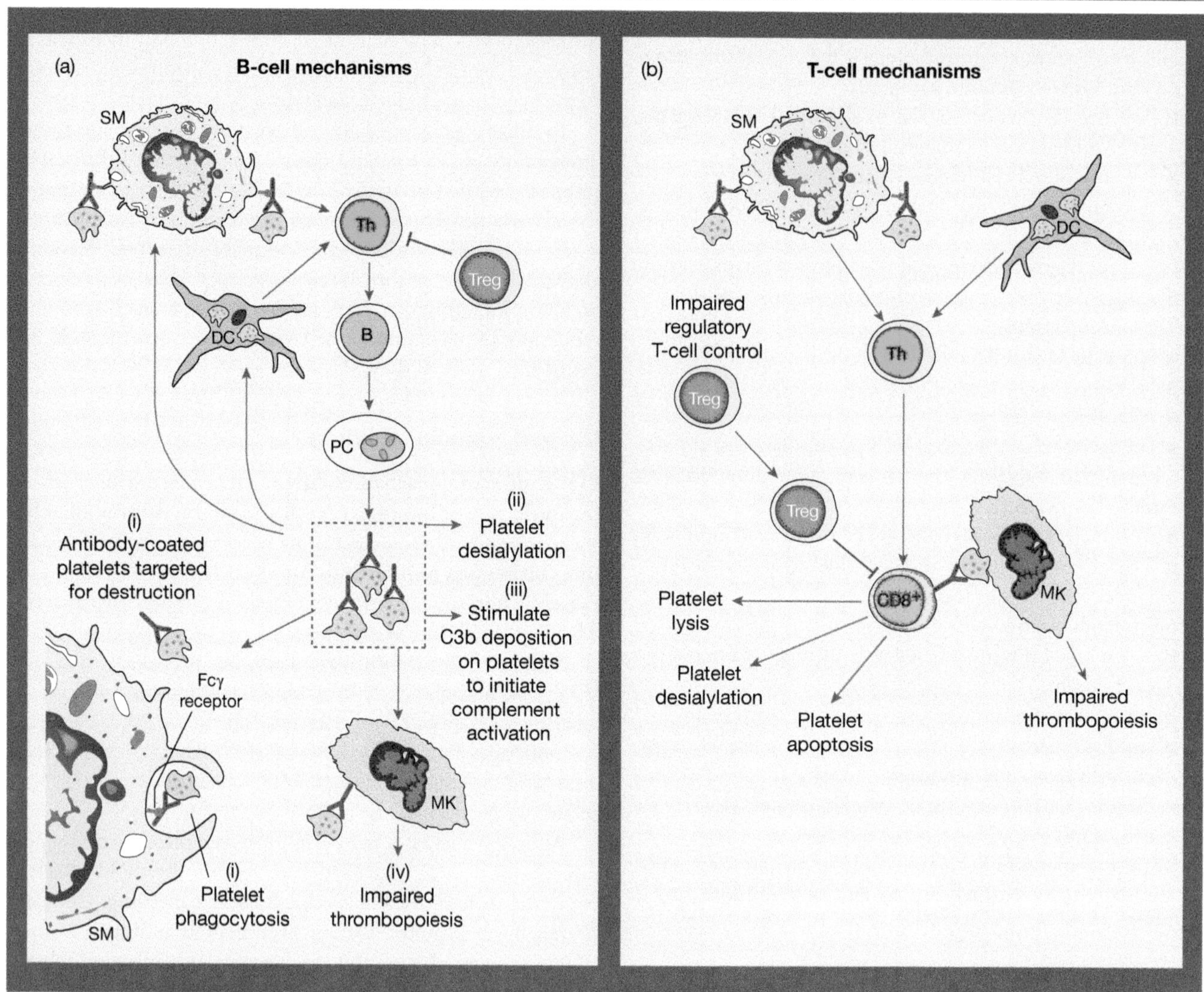

Figure 27.2 Pathogenesis of immune thrombocytopenic purpura (ITP) involving B- and T-cell mechanisms. (a and b) Splenic macrophage and dendritic cells phagocytose platelet fragments with antigens presented to T-helper (Th) cells. Th cells enable the development of B and plasma cells that secrete platelet autoantibodies or stimulate cytotoxic T-cell effector mechanisms. **(a)** Autoantibodies against platelet components contribute to thrombocytopenia by four potential mechanisms: (i) removal by reticuloendothelial system via Fcγ-receptor-mediated phagocytosis, primarily in the spleen and, to a lesser extent, in the liver and bone marrow, (ii) contribute to desialylation and (iii) stimulate complement deposition leading to activation and platelet lysis, (iv) against platelet receptors can interfere with maturation and proplatelet formation. **(b)** Cytotoxic (CD8+) T cells inhibit megakaryopoiesis by targeting megakaryocyte cells and responsible for shortened platelet life span through increased platelet apoptosis, desialylation, and direct lysis. SM, splenic macrophage; DC, dendritic cell; Th, T CD4+ helper cell; Treg, regulatory T cell; B, B lymphocyte; PC, plasma cell; MK, megakaryocyte. Source: Adapted from M. Swinkels *et al.* (2018) *Front. Immunol.* 9: 880.

The severity of bleeding in ITP is usually less than that seen in patients with comparable degrees of thrombocytopenia from bone marrow failure. This is attributed to the circulation of predominantly young, larger and functionally superior platelets. Chronic ITP tends to relapse and remit spontaneously. The spleen is not palpable unless there is an associated disease-causing splenomegaly.

Diagnosis of ITP

1. Diagnosis of ITP is one of exclusion. The blood film shows reduced numbers of platelets, often large, with no other morphological abnormalities.
2. History confirms a new onset bleeding history; if there is a long-standing history or family history, then inherited thrombocytopenias must be excluded.

Table 27.4 Immune thrombocytopenia purpura (ITP) definitions.

Aetiology	
Primary ITP (Idiopathic)	An autoimmune disorder characterized by isolated thrombocytopenia (<100 × 10^9/L) that is transient or persistent, affecting both adults and children without any identifiable pathology
Secondary ITP	Immune thrombocytopenia associated with other diseases such as viral infections (hepatitis C, HIV), autoimmune disorders (e.g. SLE), lymphoproliferative disorders (e.g. CLL) or drug-induced (excludes alloimmune thrombocytopenias)
Duration of illness	
New diagnosis ITP	Within 3 months of diagnosis
Persistent ITP	Between 3 and 12 months after diagnosis, have not achieved stable remission (spontaneous or on treatment)
Chronic ITP	More than 12 months
Severity	
Severe ITP	Present with bleeding symptoms that mandate treatment or when new symptoms develop that require additional therapeutic intervention

Source: Adapted from the International Working Group report on standardisation of terminology, definitions and outcome criteria in immune thrombocytopenic purpura of adults and children, Rodeghiero *et al.* (2009) *Blood* 113: 2386–93.

3 Routine investigations should exclude secondary causes of immune thrombocytopenia.
4 A bone marrow examination is not essential. It is reserved for patients with atypical presentations or those not responding to ITP treatment. It shows normal or increased numbers of megakaryocytes without dysplasia.

Treatment of ITP

Many therapeutic agents are available to treat ITP, manage acute bleeding, prevent bleeding and achieve long-term remission.

1 **Corticosteroids** are usually first-line therapy, with 60–80% of patients responding. Steroids suppress B- and T-cell-mediated autoantibody production and impair destruction by macrophages. A response is seen in 4–14 days, with a third achieving a sustained response. Prednisolone 1 mg/kg/day in adults (in children up to 2 mg/kg), continued for 1–2 weeks, followed by a slow taper over 4–6 weeks, is a usual regime. The dosage is reduced more slowly in poor responders. A proton pump inhibitor and glucose monitoring are required. An alternative is high-dose dexamethasone 40 mg daily for 4 days for 1–4 cycles, given at 7–21-day intervals.
2 **Intravenous immunoglobulins (IVIg) or anti-D immunoglobulin (anti-D)** rapidly increase platelet count by blocking macrophage Fc receptors. A 2 grams/kg regimen over 2–5 days raises the platelet count within 14 days in 80% of patients, but the effect lasts only 1–2 weeks. IVIg is used to rapidly increase counts in patients with acute bleeding, life-threatening haemorrhage and steroid-refractory ITP during pregnancy or before surgery.
3 **Thrombopoietin receptor (TPO-R) agonists (mimetics)** bind TPO-R to stimulate platelet production with three approved agents available. Romiplostim is an Fc fusion recombinant protein given subcutaneously which binds TPO-R at the same sites as native TPO. Eltrombopag and avatrombopag are orally active non-peptide agonists that bind to the transmembrane part of the receptor. Response is achieved in 40–60% of patients, with around half maintaining remission on discontinuation. The time to response varies between the three drugs. These agents have been associated with a slightly higher risk of thromboembolism with no other significant side effects.
4 **Rituximab, an anti-CD20 monoclonal antibody,** targets CD20+ B cells and lowers the production of antiplatelet antibodies. It produces a sustained response in 60% of patients at six months and 30% at two years. Treatment can be repeated. Some use it with corticosteroids as first-line therapy.
5 **Fostamatinib, a spleen tyrosine kinase inhibitor,** is approved for patients with chronic ITP in whom one previous steroid-sparing therapy has failed. It impairs the FcR signalling pathway involved in the phagocytosis of autoantibody-coated platelets (Chapter 9).
6 **Splenectomy** induces a durable response in 60–80% when used as second-line therapy. There are no clinical or laboratory markers that predict response. Splenectomy is now limited to patients who cannot receive immunosuppression or are intolerant or refractory to standard medical therapies. Bone marrow examination and genomic testing should be considered to exclude alternative diagnoses before splenectomy. Splenunculi must be removed; otherwise, subsequent relapse of ITP can occur.
7 **Non-specific immunosuppressive agents are** often given as third-line therapies. The most commonly used are mycophenolate mofetil and azathioprine. Less commonly used are danazol, dapsone, ciclosporin, cyclophosphamide and vincristine.
8 **Other treatments** aim to treat any underlying cause. *Helicobacter pylori* infection should be treated as it is reported to improve platelet counts, particularly in countries where the infection is common.
9 **Platelet transfusions** are used only in life-threatening emergencies, e.g. cerebral bleeding. Transfused platelets have a much shorter life span than normal, so concurrent transfusions of IVIg are required.

The aim is to achieve and maintain a platelet count above the level at which spontaneous bruising or bleeding occurs. Generally, a platelet count >30 × 10^9/L without symptoms or with minor mucocutaneous bleeding does not require treatment. Treatment should be considered in patients requiring an invasive procedure, positive history of significant or recurrent bleeding, comorbidities that increase the risk of bleeding and concurrent use of antiplatelets or anticoagulants. Female sex, exposure to nonsteroidal anti-inflammatory drugs, a platelet count <20 × 10^9/L and exposure to anticoagulant drugs are risk factors for bleeding at diagnosis.

In the long run, both bleeding and infection secondary to treatment contribute equally to mortality. Due to the chronic nature of ITP, treatment decisions need to be personalized, considering the risk of bleeding in the context of lifestyle and activities, comorbidities, duration of illness, other symptom severity, patient preferences and side effects.

Increased platelet destruction: other causes

Drug-induced thrombocytopenia

An immunological mechanism is the cause of many drug-induced thrombocytopenias with increased clearance (Fig. 27.3). Quinine (including that in tonic water), quinidine and heparin are particularly common causes (Table 27.5). The platelet count is often <10 × 10^9/L, and the bone marrow shows normal or increased megakaryocyte numbers. Drug-dependent antibodies against platelets may be demonstrated in the sera of some patients. The immediate treatment is to stop all suspected drugs. Platelet concentrates should be given to patients with severe bleeding, and IVIg may also be considered.

Other mechanisms including marrow suppression related to the use of chemotherapy; platelet-activating antibodies, as in heparin-induced thrombocytopenia (Chapter 29), can result in platelet activation, consumption and thrombocytopenia.

Post-transfusion purpura

This presents as thrombocytopenia approximately 10 days after a blood transfusion (Chapter 33). Treatment with high-dose IVIg and transfusion of HPA-1a-negative platelets may be necessary.

Gestational thrombocytopenia

A low platelet count during pregnancy is not uncommon. It explains 70–80% of all cases of thrombocytopenia in pregnancy (Chapter 34). Hypertensive disorders account for approximately 20%, and ITP for about 3–4%.

Splenomegaly

The major factor responsible for thrombocytopenia in splenomegaly is platelet 'pooling' by the spleen. In splenomegaly, up to 90% of platelets may be sequestered in the spleen with a normal platelet lifespan, compared with the normal 30% (Fig. 27.4). In the absence of additional haemostatic defects, the thrombocytopenia of splenomegaly is not usually associated with bleeding.

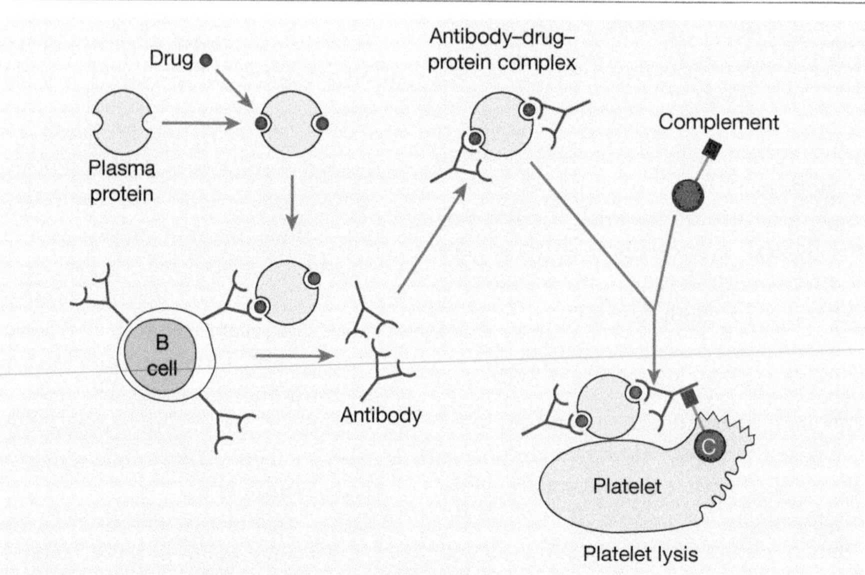

Figure 27.3 Usual type of platelet damage caused by drugs in which antibody, drug and protein complexes are deposited on the platelet surface. If the complement is attached, and the sequence goes to completion, the platelet may be lysed directly. Otherwise, it is removed by reticuloendothelial cells through opsonization with immunoglobulin and/or the C3 component of complement.

Table 27.5 Drugs associated with thrombocytopenia.

Drug-induced immune thrombocytopenia (DITP) – definite or probable
- Anti-inflammatory drugs
  - Gold salts
  - Ibuprofen
- Antimicrobials
  - Penicillins
  - Rifamycin
  - Trimethoprim/sulfamethoxazole
  - Vancomycin
  - Ceftriaxone
- Quinine, quinidine
- Glycoprotein IIb/IIIa (GPIIb/IIa) inhibitors
  - Abciximab
  - Tirofiban
  - Eptifibatide
- Sedatives, anticonvulsants
  - Diazepam, sodium valproate, carbamazepine
- Diuretics
  - Acetazolamide, chlorathiazides, furosemide
- Antidiabetics
  - Chlorpropamide, tolbutamide
- Others
  - Digitoxin, methyldopa, mirtazapine, oxaliplatin and suramin

Platelet-activating antibodies
- Heparin-induced thrombocytopenia
- Vaccine-induced thrombocytopenia

Bone marrow suppression
- Predictable (dose-related)
  - Ionizing radiation
  - Cytotoxic drugs
  - Ethanol
- Occasional
  - Chloramphenicol, idoxuridine, penicillamine, organic arsenicals, benzene etc.

Massive transfusion

Platelets are unstable in blood stored at 4°C, and the platelet count rapidly falls in blood stored for more than 24 hours. Patients transfused with massive amounts of stored blood such as those treated for trauma frequently show abnormal clotting and thrombocytopenia (p. 392).

Infections

Thrombocytopenia associated with many viral and protozoal infections is mainly immune-mediated. In HIV infection, reduced platelet production is also involved (Chapter 32).

Thrombocytopenic microangiopathic haemolytic anaemias (TMA) and disseminated intravascular coagulation (DIC)

Thrombocytopenia secondary to consumption due to TMA or DIC is common and covered in Chapter 29.

Thrombocytopenia due to impaired platelet production

Failure of platelet production may be isolated or part of a generalized bone marrow failure (Table 27.3, Chapter 24). Selective impairment of platelet production may present as isolated heritable macrothrombocytopenia. Bone marrow failure usually results in pancytopenia or bicytopenia. Selective megakaryocyte depression may result from drug toxicity or viral infection. Alcohol may induce thrombocytopenia and is a common cause of low platelet count in acute settings. Bone marrow examination is crucial for the diagnosis of impaired platelet production.

The use of platelet transfusions in treating and preventing bleeding due to thrombocytopenia is discussed below and in Chapter 33.

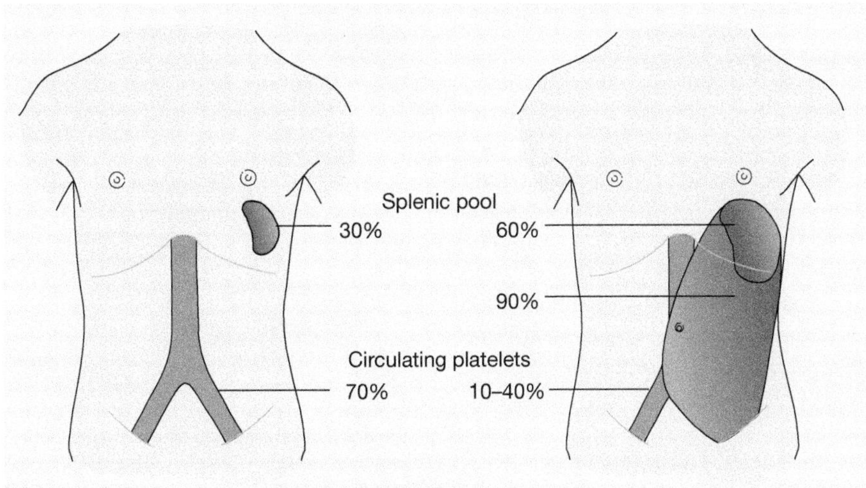

Figure 27.4 Platelet distribution between the circulation and spleen in normal individuals (left) and patients with moderate or massive splenomegaly (right).

Inherited platelet disorders

Inherited platelet disorders (IPDs) due to abnormalities of megakaryopoiesis and platelet formation are uncommon causes of a bleeding tendency. They are heterogeneous in clinical presentation, ranging from asymptomatic laboratory abnormalities to life-threatening bleeds. They can be isolated findings or be part of clinical syndromes.

IPDs present with thrombocytopenia (platelet size can be normal, small or large), impaired function, or both. They are often misdiagnosed as ITP and may receive inappropriate treatment. A diagnosis helps identify other syndromic features or organ abnormalities which may need long-term monitoring and intervention.

Representative IPDs due to defects in specific pathways such as thrombopoietin signalling, transcriptional regulation, granule formation and secretion, proplatelet formation and transmembrane glycoprotein signalling are described below.

Disorders of early megakaryopoiesis and maturation

Pathogenic mechanisms include abnormalities in megakaryocyte differentiation, e.g. thrombocytopenia absent radius syndrome. Disorders of maturation are often secondary to mutations in genes associated with cellular signalling and transcription factors, e.g. GATA1-related diseases. Variants of specific transcription factors, such as RUNX1 or ETV6, are associated with an increased risk of haematological malignancies.

Disorders of proplatelet formation and granule formation

Megakaryocyte maturation, proplatelet formation and release are affected by mutations in genes encoding cytoskeletal and microtubule components (e.g. macrothrombocytopenias, see below) and those involved in granule biogenesis.

Inherited macrothrombocytopenias

Inherited thrombocytopenias most frequently are macrothrombocytopenias. Several classification systems are in place and a clinically relevant classification identifies three patient groups: (1) abnormalities limited to platelets; (2) platelet abnormalities with other congenital defects (syndromic with skeletal deformities e.g absent radii, malformations of the central nervous or cardiovascular system, or immunodeficiencies); (3) patients at risk of acquiring other diseases during their lifetime (e.g. haematological malignancies, bone marrow aplasia, or increased risk for end-stage renal disease seen with MYH9 disorders).

Other inherited thrombocytopenias with normal or small platelets

Wiskott–Aldrich syndrome (WAS) is an X-linked recessive disorder characterized by microcthrombocytopenia, eczema and immune dysregulation. It is caused by mutations in the *WAS* gene, and the gene product is a cytoplasmic protein expressed exclusively in hematopoietic cells.

α-Storage pool disease or Grey (Gray) platelet syndrome (GPS)

An infrequent disorder characterized by thrombocytopenia, with a characteristic grey appearance of platelets by light microscopy, due to the absence or reduction of α-granules and their constituents (Fig. 27.5). The qualitative and quantitative deficiency results in mild to moderate bleeding tendency. GPS is an autosomally recessive inherited disease due to mutation in the *NBEAL2* gene, the product of which is involved in granule trafficking. Patients demonstrate abnormalities in other haemopoietic cells with low white cell counts, impaired neutrophil function, immune dysregulation and autoimmune defects. Myelofibrosis and splenomegaly may develop with disease progression.

δ-Storage pool disease (δ-SPD)

A deficiency of dense granules in megakaryocytes and platelets characterizes this congenital abnormality. It can be part of syndromic disorders, including Hermansky-Pudlack and Chediak-Higashi (Chapter 8), or associated with albinism and other immune deficiencies. Bleeding is typically mild to moderate. Platelet aggregometry shows impaired responses to ADP and other agonists. However, aggregometry may be normal when assays of nucleotide content are required for diagnosis.

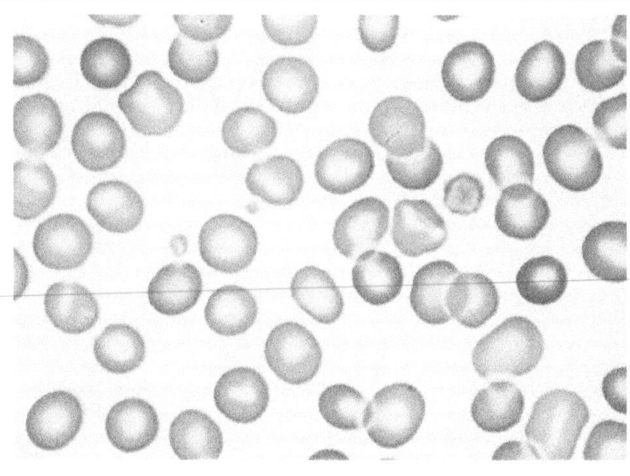

Figure 27.5 Blood film of Grey (gray) platelet syndrome showing large and colourless platelets due to lack of α-granules. Source: A.V. Hoffbrand *et al.* (2018) *Color Atas of Clinical Hematology*, 5th edn. Reproduced with permission of John Wiley & Sons.

Disorders of membrane glycoproteins

Glanzmann thrombasthenia

Glanzmann thrombasthenia (GT) is the most common severe inherited disorder of platelet dysfunction. It is due to qualitative or quantitative abnormalities of platelet GPIIb (integrin αIIb) and GPIIIa (integrin β3) receptors; it is autosomal recessive in inheritance. Platelet counts and morphology are normal, with a bleeding tendency that is moderate to severe. Platelet aggregation is absent with multiple agonists, except ristocetin, which promotes agglutination through GPIb receptors. Flow cytometry can determine the quantitative absence or reduction of GPIIb (CD41) or GPIIIa (CD61) receptors but will not detect qualitative defects. Based on the degree of deficiency or dysfunction of the receptors, type 1 GT with receptors less than 5% (most common) and type II with receptor density between 5 and 20% are recognized.

Bernard–Soulier syndrome

Bernard–Soulier syndrome (BSS) is an inherited recessive disorder secondary to mutations in genes encoding for GPIbα (*GPIBA*), GPIBβ and GPIX, three of the four subunits that make the GPIb-IX-V complex. The disorder is characterized by thrombocytopenia, giant platelets (Fig. 27.6) and a failure of platelets to bind various GPIb ligands, including VWF and thrombin. The genotype/phenotype correlation is weak. Platelet aggregometry shows a normal pattern with multiple agonists and absent response to ristocetin.

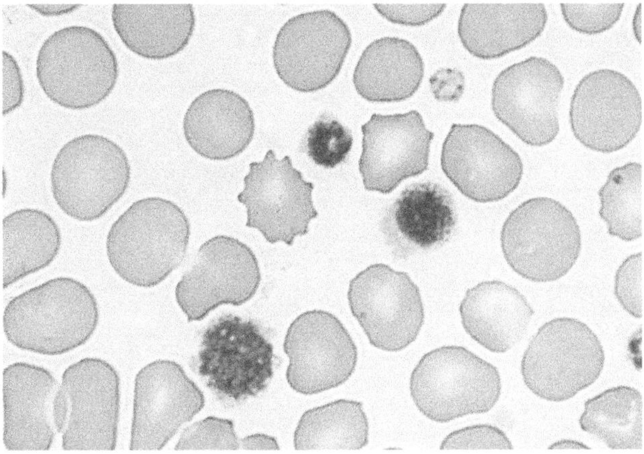

Figure 27.6 Bernard–Soulier syndrome. Blood film showing abnormally large platelets. Source: A.V. Hoffbrand *et al.* (2018) *Color Atas of Clinical Hematology*, 5th edn. Reproduced with permission of John Wiley & Sons.

Platelet-type von Willebrand disease

A rare autosomal dominant disorder characterized by a mutation in *GP1BA* that increases the affinity of GPIbα for VWF multimers. The net result is an increase in spontaneous binding of high molecular weight VWF multimers to platelets, resulting in platelet clumping and increased clearance with intermittent thrombocytopenia.

Investigation of inherited platelet disorders

Diagnosis of IPDs can be challenging as they often present as asymptomatic thrombocytopenia or with a history of mild to moderate bleeding tendency that can also be due to factor deficiencies. A detailed history of the bleeding tendency, including standardised scores, is invaluable in determining its severity and the extent of investigations needed. Physical examination for any syndromic features also provides clues to diagnosis. The following laboratory investigations are usually needed.

1 Full blood count and blood film. See Laboratory on page 359.
2 Exclusion of other mild to moderate coagulation factor deficiencies
3 Platelet function testing by light transmission aggregometry (LTA) using various agonists.
4 Flow cytometry for platelet glycoprotein abnormalities confirms a diagnosis of GTS and BSS. Platelet nucleotide content and secretion assays are required to evaluate the function of dense granules.
5 Genotyping by conventional and novel techniques. The increasing availability of DNA sequencing has transformed the diagnosis of inherited platelet disorders. Gene panels have been established, including the most commonly affected genes. This helps identify disorders where additional interventions have a long-term impact (e.g. MYH9 disorders and renal function), but also identifies abnormalities with potentially severe consequences later in life e.g. mutations predisposing to haematological malignancy.

Acquired platelet dysfunction

The most common cause is antiplatelet drugs (Chapter 30). Other acquired causes present as new onset bleeding tendency in the context of another disorder. Table 27.6 details common causes of platelet dysfunction and their underlying mechanisms.

Table 27.6 Acquired platelet dysfunction – causes and mechanisms.

Cause or disorder	Mechanism of platelet dysfunction
Drugs	
Antiplatelet drugs ■ Anti-receptor drugs ■ Drugs affecting intra-platelet signalling (Fig. 31.8)	Antiplatelet drugs have been developed to inhibit platelet function. They tend to affect platelet receptor function or intra-platelet cell signalling pathways, thus interfering with adhesion and or aggregation.
Other drugs ■ Antibiotics ■ Anticoagulants and fibrinolytic agents ■ Cardiovascular drugs (nitrates and calcium antagonists [at high doses]) ■ Volume expanders ■ Psychotropic agents ■ Oncologic drugs	As with antiplatelet drugs, inhibition is not severe
Haematologic disorders	
Paraproteinaemia ■ Monoclonal gammopathy of unknown significance (MGUS) ■ Chronic lymphocytic leukaemia (CLL) ■ Multiple myeloma ■ Waldenström's	Low levels in the context of MGUS and CLL can result in acquired von Willebrand disease. High levels of paraprotein potentially seen in multiple myeloma or Waldenström's disease may cause interference with platelet adherence, release and aggregation
Myeloproliferative	High platelet counts may be associated with acquired von Willebrand disease. In some instances, platelet function abnormalities are present
Myelodysplastic syndromes	Acquired storage pool defect is not uncommon in this disorder, exacerbated by thrombocytopenia
Systemic disorders associated with abnormal platelet function	
Uraemia	Abnormalities of platelet activation and acquired storage pool disorder have been demonstrated. The severity is related to the degree of uraemia
Cardiopulmonary bypass	Bleeding tendency is multifactorial, in addition to platelet dysfunction due to drugs and degranulation.
Autoimmune disorders	During an acute flare, patients sometimes demonstrate symptoms suggestive of mild to moderate immune thrombocytopenia with normal counts, suggesting auto-antibodies against various receptors

Treatment of inherited platelet disorders and acquired platelet dysfunction or thrombocytopenia due to failure of production

Supportive treatment

If the acquired dysfunction is due to drugs, immediate cessation is essential. As the life span of platelets is 7 to 10 days, the effect is not immediate.

Treatment of the underlying cause

A stem cell transplant may be considered in patients with severe inherited platelet disorders, e.g. GTS and BSS, when recurrent life-threatening bleeding in childhood is progressively unresponsive to treatment. TPO-R agonists have been used in some inherited thrombocytopenias with benefits.

Tranexamic acid and desmopressin

A combination of tranexamic acid and desmopressin may be adequate for managing mild bleeds in most patients with mild to moderate bleeding tendencies. Tranexamic acid and aminocaproic acid are anti-fibrinolytic drugs that reduce bleeding by stabilizing the clot (Chapter 28). They are relatively contraindicated in the presence of haematuria from the upper renal tract.

Desmopressin improves primary haemostasis by releasing high molecular weight VWF multimers from Weibel–Palade bodies of the endothelium (Chapter 28). It also seems to improve platelet function. Desmopressin can be administrated intranasally or subcutaneously. Once administered, there should be a strict fluid restriction of less than one litre a day. Plasma sodium must be measured if treatment for more than 1–2 days is required.

Platelet transfusions

In patients with severe IPD or severe bleeding due to acquired platelet dysfunction or thrombocytopenia, including life-threatening bleeds and before major surgery, the mainstay of treatment is platelet transfusions. If patients have had a previous haemostatic challenge, interventions that achieved post-procedural haemostasis help guide management. In patients with IPD, platelet transfusion should be avoided as long as possible to prevent the development of alloantibodies. Where possible, HLA-matched platelets should be used.

Recombinant activated VIIa.

Recombinant activated factor VII alone can be used for mild to moderate bleeding patients with GTS and, potentially, in BSS. In most of these patients, monitoring the individual response to treatment is essential.

Vascular bleeding disorders

Vascular disorders are a heterogeneous group of inherited and acquired disorders characterized by easy bruising and spontaneous bleeding from the small vessels. The underlying abnormality is either in the vessels or the perivascular connective tissues. Most cases of bleeding caused by vascular defects alone are not severe. Frequently, the bleeding is mainly in the skin, causing petechiae, ecchymoses or both. In some disorders, there is also bleeding from mucous membranes. Investigations for platelet and coagulation abnormalities are normal. Well-characterized inherited vascular disorders include hereditary haemorrhagic telangiectasia and connective tissue disorders.

Hereditary haemorrhagic telangiectasia

Hereditary haemorrhagic telangiectasia (HHT) is an autosomally dominant inherited vascular dysplasia. Various genetic defects underlie the disease, including mutations of endothelial

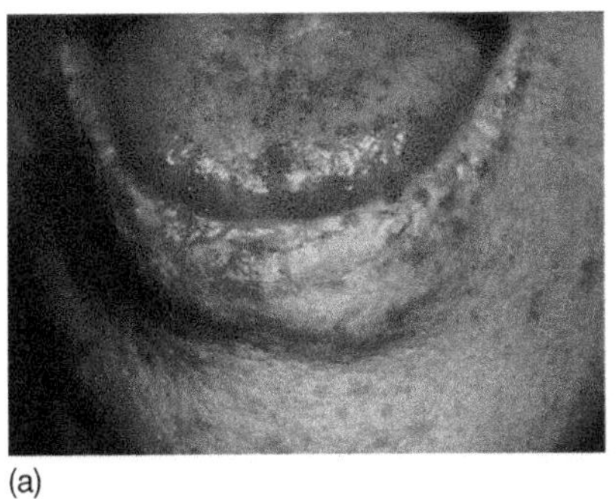

(a)

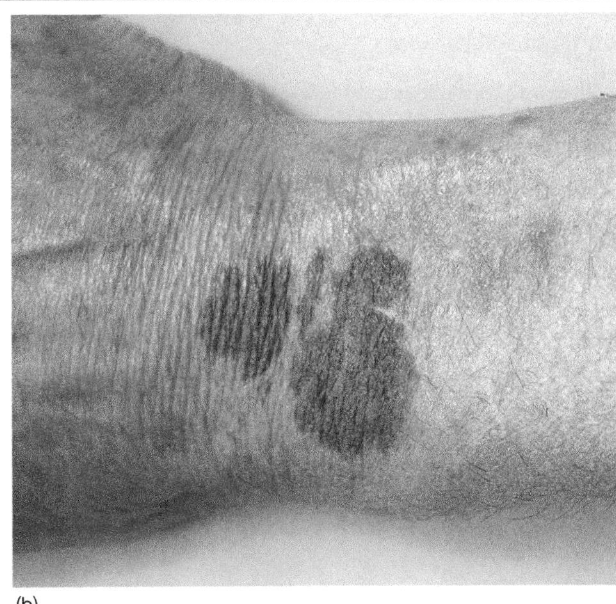

(b)

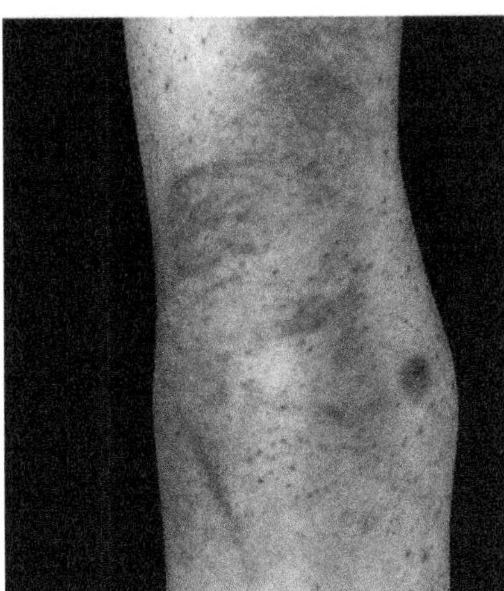

(c)

Figure 27.7 (a) Hereditary haemorrhagic telangiectasia: characteristic small vascular lesions are obvious on the lips and tongue. **(b)** Senile purpura. **(c)** Characteristic perifollicular petechiae in vitamin C deficiency (scurvy).

protein endoglin that affect blood vessels throughout the body. Clinical symptoms are heterogeneous, and spontaneous and recurrent nosebleeds starting in the second decade of life is the most common presentation. Defects in the endothelial cell junctions, endothelial cell degeneration and weakness of the perivascular connective tissue are thought to cause dilation of capillaries and postcapillary venules, manifesting as telangiectasias.

Telangiectasias (small arterio-vascular malformations, AVMs) are characteristically found on the lips, tongue, buccal and gastrointestinal (GI) mucosa, face, and fingers (Fig. 27.7a). Large arteriovenous (AV) shunts may occur in the pulmonary, hepatic, splenic and cerebral circulation, where they can cause bleeding or obstruction. All patients need to be screened for pulmonary AV shunts. Recurrent epistaxes can be challenging to treat, and recurrent GI tract haemorrhage may cause chronic iron deficiency anaemia. A diagnosis requires three of four criteria: nose bleeds, telangiectasia, AV malformations and a first-degree relative with HHT. Genomic testing of a limited panel of causative genes may confirm the diagnosis.

Treatment involves embolization, laser therapy, oestrogens, tranexamic acid, and iron supplementation. Thalidomide, lenalidomide, danazol, epsilon-aminocaproic acid and bevacizumab (anti-vascular endothelial growth factor) have been used to reduce GI bleeding and bleeding at other sites in severe cases.

Connective tissue disorders

Hereditary collagen abnormalities in Ehlers–Danlos syndromes present with purpura resulting from defective platelet adhesion, hyperextensibility of joints and hyperelastic friable skin. Pseudoxanthoma elasticum is associated with arterial haemorrhage and thrombosis. Patients may present with superficial bruising and purpura following minor trauma or after the application of a tourniquet. Bleeding and poor wound healing after surgery may be a problem. Platelet aggregometry most often does not show abnormalities.

Acquired vascular defects

Simple easy bruising is a common benign disorder which occurs in otherwise healthy women, especially those of childbearing age.

Senile purpura is caused by atrophy of the supporting tissues of cutaneous blood vessels. Seen mainly on the dorsal aspects of the forearms and hands (Fig. 27.7b).

Purpura associated with infections is secondary to vascular damage by infections (e.g. measles, dengue fever or meningococcal septicaemia), disseminated intravascular coagulation or immune complexes.

Scurvy due to vitamin C deficiency results in the formation of defective collagen, which may cause perifollicular petechiae, bruising and mucosal haemorrhage (Fig. 27.7c).

Steroid purpura, associated with long-term steroid therapy or Cushing's syndrome, is caused by defective vascular support tissue.

Henoch–Schönlein syndrome is an IgA-mediated vasculitis usually seen in children and often follows an acute upper respiratory tract infection. It presents with a characteristic purpuric rash accompanied by localized oedema and itching. The rash is most prominent on the buttocks and extensor surfaces of the lower legs and elbows (Fig. 27.8). Painful joint swelling, haematuria and abdominal pain may also occur. It is usually a self-limiting condition, but occasionally patients develop renal failure. Corticosteroids are indicated in these cases.

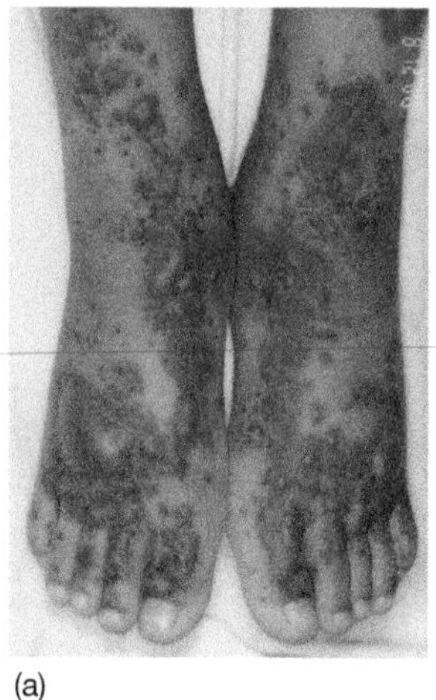

(a)

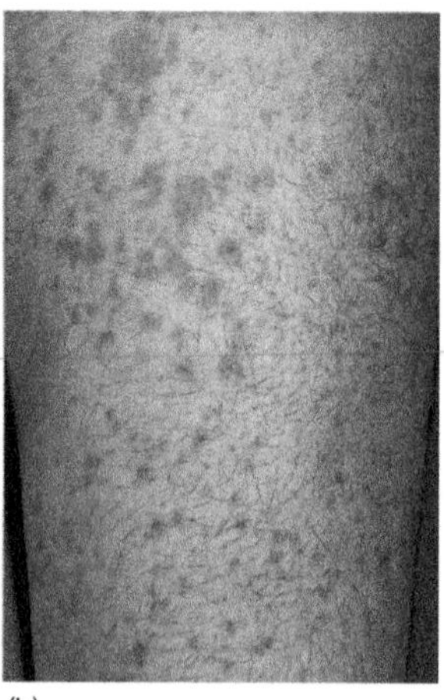

(b)

Figure 27.8 Henoch–Schönlein purpura: **(a)** unusually severe purpura on legs with bulla formation in a 6-year-old child; **(b)** early urticarial lesions.

SUMMARY

- Abnormal bleeding can be due to vessel wall abnormalities, impaired primary haemostasis or coagulation or excessive fibrinolysis.
- A thorough bleeding history focussing on the duration of symptoms is critical to distinguishing acquired and inherited disorders of platelets.
- Thrombocytopenia can be caused by many conditions, and mechanims include increased consumption seen with immune thrombocytopenias and consumptive coagulopathies; and impaired production due to inherited or acquired abnormalities of megakaroypoiesis.
- Immune(idiopathic) thrombocytopenia (ITP) is a chronic disorder. Treatment strategies include corticosteroids, rituximab, high-dose immunoglobulin, thrombomimetics, splenectomy or immunosuppressive drugs alone or in various combinations.
- Hereditary thrombocytopenias often present as asymptomatic abnormalities or are referred for evaluation of a long-standing mild to moderate bleeding tendency.
- Disorders of platelet function may rarely be hereditary, as in Glanzmann's thrombasthenia and Bernard–Soulier syndrome.
- Acquired disorders of platelet function are far more common. Causes include antiplatelet drugs (e.g. aspirin, clopidogrel and dipyridamole), nonsteroidal anti-inflammatory drugs and a wide range of medical disorders.
- Tranexamic acid is useful for patients with mild recurrent bleeding
- Platelet transfusions with concurrent tranexamic acid to ensure stable clot formation are required for severe bleeding in patients with thrombocytopenia or platelet dysfunction.
- Desmopressin and activated factor VII can also be used in select indications.
- Vascular bleeding disorders such as hereditary haemorrhagic telangiectasia and scurvy may cause bleeding.
- Purpura may also be due to vascular abnormalities such as senile purpura, viral infections and Henoch–Schönlein purpura.

Now visit **www.wiley.com/go/haematology9e** to test yourself on this chapter.

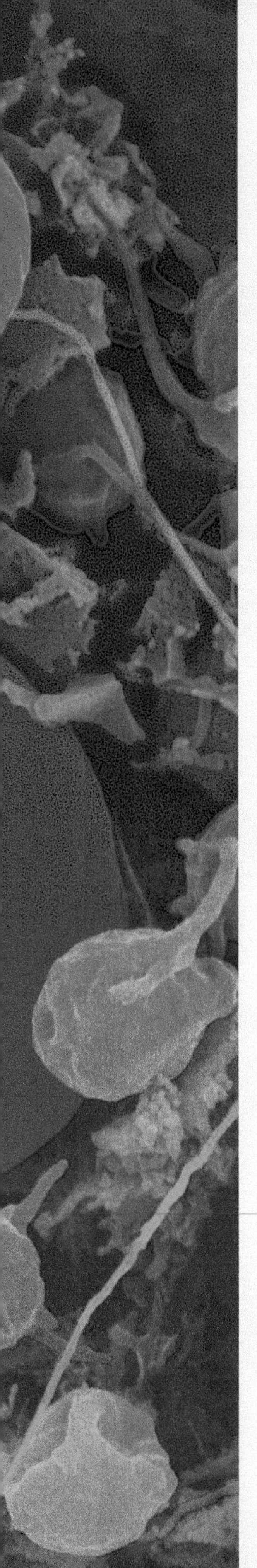

CHAPTER 28

Hereditary coagulation disorders

Key topics

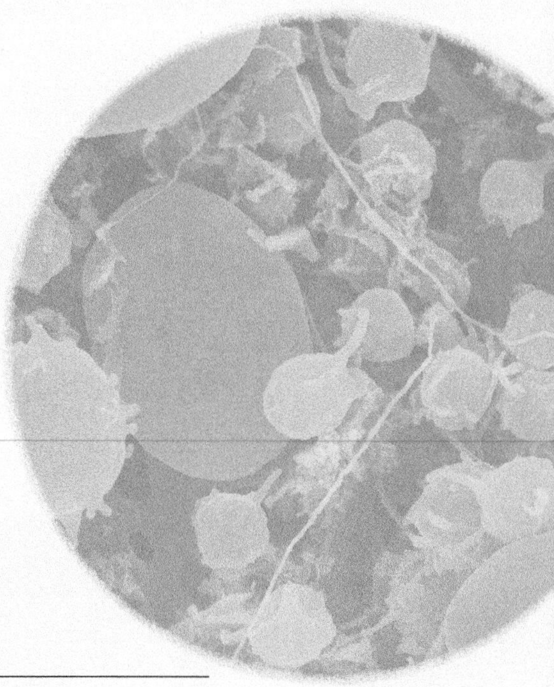

Hoffbrand's Essential Haematology, Ninth Edition. A. Victor Hoffbrand, Pratima Chowdary, Graham P. Collins, and Justin Loke.
© 2024 John Wiley & Sons Ltd. Published 2024 by John Wiley & Sons Ltd.
Companion website: www.wiley.com/go/haematology9e

Deficiency of procoagulant clotting factors results in a reduction in the amount of thrombin generated, leading to impaired clot formation and increased bleeding tendency. Inherited deficiencies of each coagulation factor have been described. Although von Willebrand disease is the most common inherited bleeding disorder (IBD), factor VIII deficiency (FVIII), in its severe form, is the most common severe IBD. Disorders of fibrinolysis result in poor wound healing and excess bleeding tendency.

Haemophilia A (FVIII deficiency)

Haemophilia A (HA) is due to deficiency or complete absence of FVIII. It is caused by mutations in *F8* gene, located on the long arm of the X chromosome. For all severities of haemophilia, the estimated incidence is 1 in 5000 live male births. Inheritance is X-linked, with a third of patients having no family history (Fig. 28.1).

FVIII is a large 330 kDa glycoprotein synthesized in endothelial cells. It is organized into six domains denoted as A1-A2-B-A3-C1-C2. FVIII circulates as a heterodimer, made of a heavy chain (A1-A2 domains, plus parts of the B domain) and a light chain (A1-C1-C2 domains) linked non-covalently via divalent metal cations; 95–97% circulates in complex with von Willebrand factor (VWF), which protects against its proteolytic degradation and clearance. Without VWF, the half-life is about 1–2 hours.

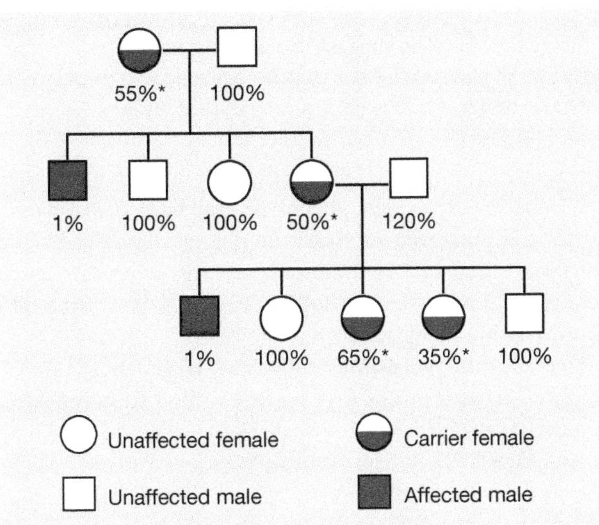

Figure 28.1 A typical family tree in a family with haemophilia. Note the variable levels of FVIII activity in carriers (*) because of random X chromosome inactivation (Lyonization). FVIII activity is shown as a percentage of normal levels.

Haemophilia B (FIX deficiency, Christmas disease)

Haemophilia B (HB) is caused by deficiency or complete absence of factor IX (FIX). FIX is a serine protease that forms the intrinsic Xase complex with cofactor FVIIIa and activates FX to FXa, necessary for adequate thrombin generation. The incidence of haemophilia B is one-fifth that of haemophilia A.

FIX is synthesized in the liver, and the mature protein consists of four distinct domains: the N-terminal Gla-domain, the epidermal growth factor like domain, the activating peptide domain and the C-terminal serine protease domain. An important post-translational modification is the vitamin K dependent carboxylation of glutamic acid residues to form γ-glutamic acid (Gla) in the Gla domain.

The *F9* gene is located close to *F8*, near the tip of the long arm of the X chromosome. The inheritance and clinical features of FIX deficiency are identical to FVIII deficiency and only distinguishable by specific factor assays.

Clinical features and investigations

The clinical presentation of haemophilia A and B is related to the severity of the disease. The International Society of Thrombosis and Haemostasis (ISTH) has proposed a classification for disease severity based on coagulation activity, which correlates strongly with the clinical picture (Table 28.1).

Table 28.1 Haemophilia disease severity by factor levels.

Severity of disorder	Coagulation factor activity	Clinical manifestations
Severe haemophilia	<1%	■ Frequent spontaneous bleeding into joints, muscles, and internal organs from early life ■ Joint deformity that is crippling, if not adequately prevented or treated ■ Bleeding after minor and major trauma and surgery
Moderate haemophilia	1–5%	■ Occasional spontaneous episodes ■ Bleeding after minor and major trauma and surgery
Mild haemophilia	>5%	■ Bleeding only after significant trauma, surgery

Source: Adapted from G.C. White *et al.* (2001) On behalf of the Factor VIII and Factor IX Subcommittee of ISTH. Definitions in hemophilia. *Thromb. Haemost.* 85: 560.

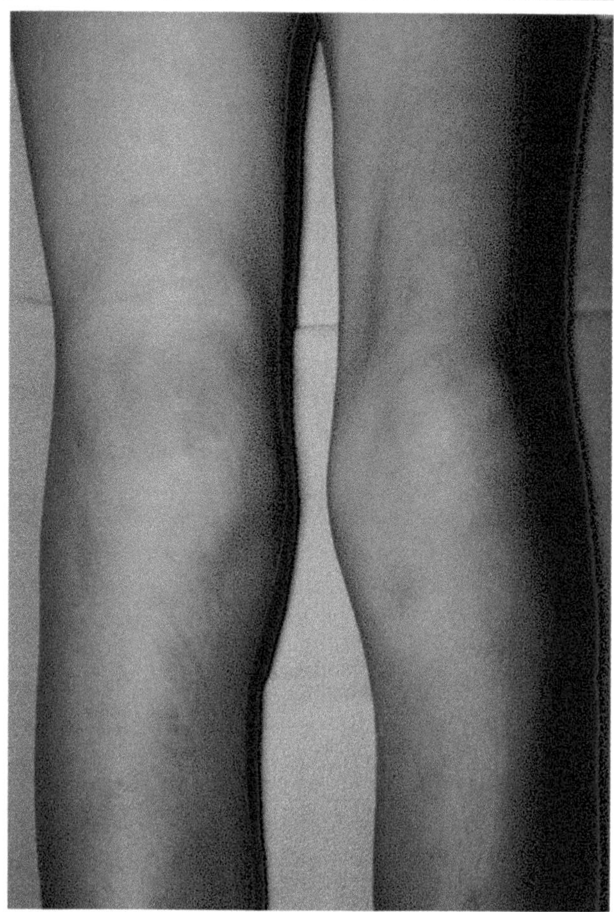

Figure 28.2 Haemophilia A: acute haemarthrosis of the right knee joint with swelling of the suprapatellar region. There is wasting of the quadriceps muscles, particularly on the left.

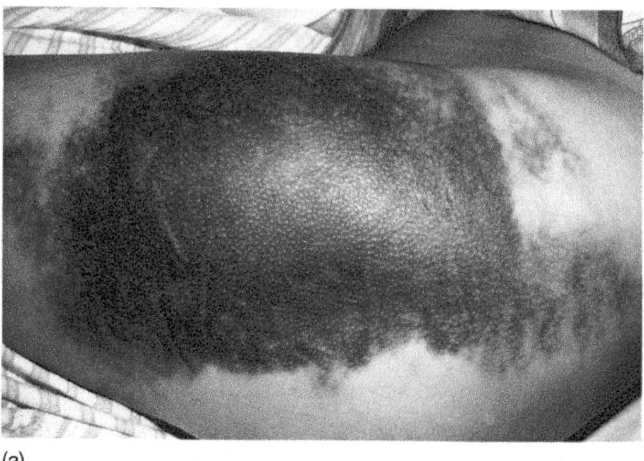

(a)

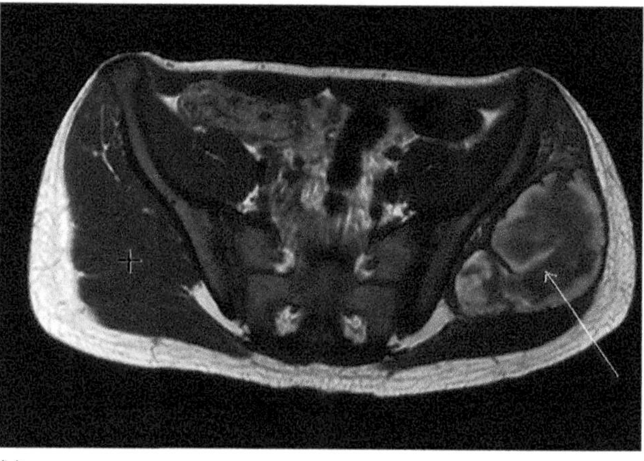

(b)

Figure 28.3 (a) Haemophilia A: massive haemorrhage in the right buttock area. **(b)** 15-year-old boy with sudden left hip pain and haemophilia A. Magnetic resonance imaging (MRI) axial image, T2-weighted, revealing large left spontaneous haematoma (yellow arrow) in left gluteus maximus muscle compared with the normal right side (red cross). Source: Courtesy of Dr P. Wylie.

Patients with severe deficiency present in the first few years of life with excessive bruising, prolonged bleeding from minor trauma, such as cut lips or tongue, prolonged bleeding post-circumcision or decreased movement due to joint or muscle bleeds (Figs. 28.2). The defining feature is spontaneous bleeding, i.e. bleeds with no apparent trauma (Fig. 28.3). Patients also present with bleeds that are disproportionate to the tissue injury. Fatal bleeding is not uncommon due to intracerebral haemorrhage or bleeding into other internal organs. Before the advent of modern treatment, the average life span was around 11 years.

Following the introduction of replacement therapy, the clinical picture is dominated by recurrent spontaneous joint and muscle bleeds that limit mobility and result in arthropathy. The severity of arthropathy is related to access to treatment, age at initiation of a treatment regimen for prevention of joint bleeds, and appropriate management of joint bleeds. Inadequate treatment can result in joint destruction, with fixed flexion deformities or joint replacement, as early as young adulthood (Fig. 28.4, Fig. 28.5).

A patient with a severe phenotype may have 20–40 bleeding episodes a year without treatment that prevents bleeds. The annualized bleed rate is commonly used in clinical trials to assess the efficacy of a drug and, increasingly, in routine care to ensure adequacy of treatment.

Haemophilic pseudotumours are large encapsulated haematomas with progressive cystic swelling from repeated haemorrhage. They are best visualized by magnetic resonance imaging (MRI). They may occur in large muscle groups, long bones and any fascial plane. They arise from large haematomas that have been poorly treated. Other complications of bleeding are related to the entrapment of nerves and compartment syndromes due to increased tissue pressure.

Patients with moderate haemophilia tend to have fewer spontaneous bleeds but may bleed with minimal trauma and excessively following dental extractions or other surgical

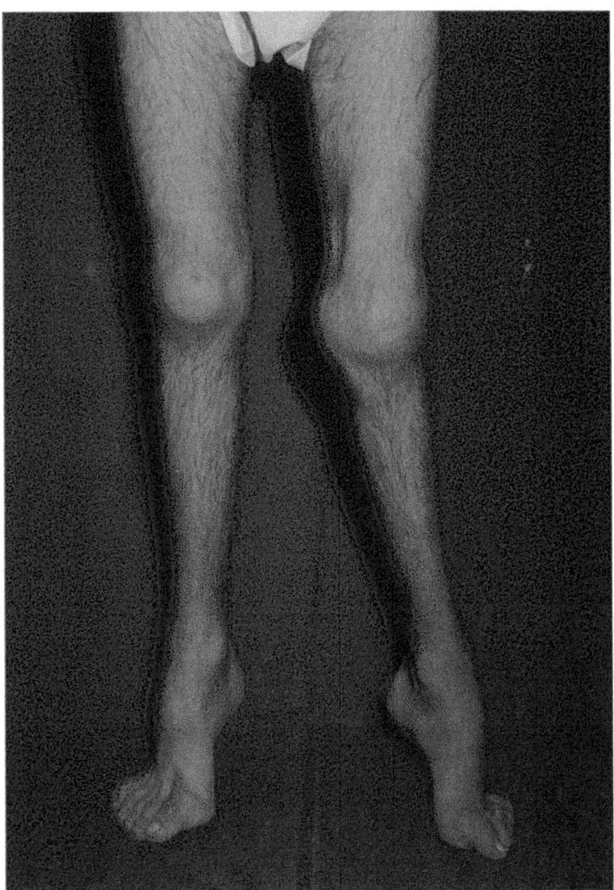

Figure 28.4 Haemophilia A showing severe disability. The left knee is swollen with posterior subluxation of the tibia on the femur. The ankles and feet show residual deformities of talipes equinus, with some cavus and associated toe clawing. There is generalized muscle wasting. The scar on the medial side of the left lower thigh is the site of a previously excised pseudotumour (encapsulated haematomas).

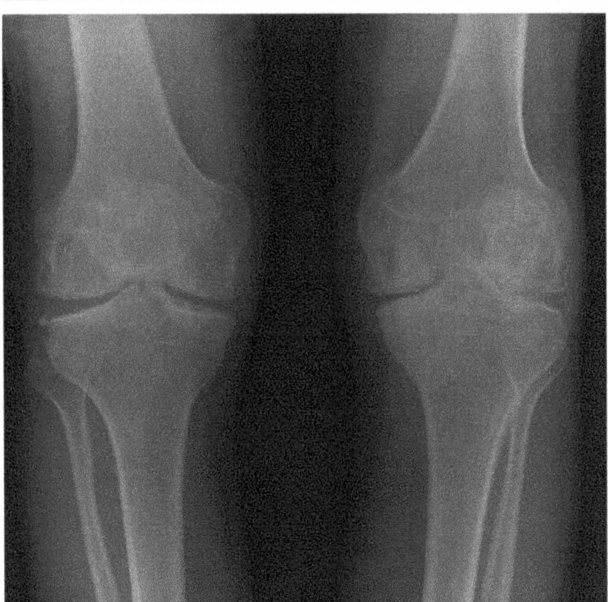

Figure 28.5 Haemophilia A: X-ray of the knee joints shows destruction and narrowing of the left joint space.

interventions. Patients with mild deficiency typically present with bleeding after surgery. Diagnosis in this group may be delayed to the second or third decade of life. In the context of family history a diagnosis often precedes clinical bleeding episodes.

Laboratory findings

Suspicion is key to diagnosis; investigations show:

1 Prolonged activated partial thromboplastin time (APTT)
2 Normal PT and normal platelet function
3 FVIII or FIX clotting assay confirms the diagnosis.
4 In patients with mild FVIII deficiency, evaluation should include an analysis of VWF parameters to exclude VWD.
5 A genetic diagnosis can be undertaken through mutation analysis. This provides information on the phenotype and risk of inhibitor development and helps screen carriers.

Mutation analysis

Mutations reported in the *F8* gene are heterogeneous and include nonsense, missense, splice site, frameshift mutations or large insertions/deletions. A characteristic intron 22 inversion (Inv22) of the *F8* gene accounts for around half of severe HA cases. This involves recombination between homologous sequences located in intron 22 and upstream of the *F8* gene, resulting in a characteristic 'flip-tip' inversion and disruption of the *F8* gene. A single nucleotide change causes variants responsible for mild or moderate haemophilia A. In haemophilia B, 75% of variants are single nucleotide changes. No genetic variant is identifiable in about 5% of familial haemophilia cases.

Most variants are detectable by direct sequencing. This is increasingly performed in developed healthcare systems through next-generation (massively parallel) sequencing. Inv22 can be detected using specific, tailored polymerase chain reaction (PCR) assays. Genetic diagnosis of severe haemophilia A incorporates these PCR techniques alongside direct sequencing.

Carrier detection and antenatal diagnosis

Following identification of the causative variant in an index case (usually an affected male), any potential female carriers in the pedigree may be detected using the same techniques. Antenatal diagnosis can be confirmed on chorionic biopsies at 8–10 weeks gestation, providing sufficient foetal DNA is available for analysis. Free foetal DNA isolated from maternal peripheral blood can be used to identify the causative mutations.

Therapeutic options and comprehensive care

The mainstay of treatment is the correction of factor deficiency and, therefore, bleeding tendency. There are two main therapeutic aims:

1. **Management of bleeds (spontaneous or trauma) and haemostatic insults, for example trauma and surgery**
2. **Prophylaxis aimed at prevention of spontaneous bleeds and excessive bleeding with trauma, thus altering the clinical phenotype of the disorder.**

Therapeutic options in use can be categorized as replacement therapies, non-replacement therapies, gene therapies or adjunctive treatments. Some, like replacement therapy, can treat and prevent bleeds. Therapeutic categories and drugs, including those in clinical trials, are listed in Table 28.2.

Comprehensive care

Two innovations improved outcomes even before the advent of definitive treatment regimens. The first was home treatment; the second was comprehensive care. The availability of factor concentrates stored in domestic refrigerators dramatically altered haemophilia management. At the earliest indication of bleeding, a patient can be treated at home reducing the need for hospitlization. Most patients in developed countries attend specialized haemophilia centres with a multidisciplinary team. The team includes specialist nurses providing advisory services and teaching self-infusion, specialist physiotherapists for joint assessment and rehabilitation and a psychologist to help with the many challenges they might face. Comprehensive care is now offered to almost all patients with inherited bleeding disorders.

With modern treatment, the lifestyle of a haemophilic child is almost normal, but certain activities, such as extreme contact sports, should be avoided or undertaken with extra prophylaxis.

Replacement therapies

Until 2020, the standard of care was replacement therapy with FVIII or FIX. Replacement therapy is feasible in haemophilia and other coagulation disorders as proteins are in the extracellular milieu. Intravenous injection allows the protein to disperse in the intravascular and extravascular spaces based on size and other characteristics.

Replacement therapy in the form of plasma or cryoprecipitate was used as early as the mid-19th century. Plasma contains both FVIII and FIX, while cryoprecipitate is rich in FVIII and VWF, but large volumes are required and are no longer used in routine clinical practice. The early 1980s saw the introduction of plasma-derived clotting factor concentrates (CFCs). A decade later, recombinant FVIII and FIX CFCs with normal or standard half-life (SHL) were introduced into clinical practice (Table 28.2). Currently extended half-life (EHL) CFCs are in routine clinical use, allowing less frequent infusions. EHL FVIII confers a 1.5- to 2-fold increase in half-life compared to SHL FVIII, and a 3- to 4-fold increase is seen with EHL FIX.

Coagulation factor half-life extension has been achieved by employing different protein modification strategies. The first involves fusion with a protein with known long half-life, such as albumin (albumin fusion) or immunoglobulin (Fc fusion) (Chapter 9). The second involves post-translational modification with polyethene glycol (PEG) or biodegradable protein polymer. PEGylation increases the hydrodynamic volume of the molecule, with reduced renal clearance and decreased receptor-mediated clearance, contributing to prolonged half-life.

An ultra-long half-life (UHL) FVIII has also been licensed. Two strategies were employed to achieve a 4-fold increase in half-life compared to SHL factor VIII. The first uncoupled FVIII from VWF by blocking its VWF binding site with a recombinant VWF fragment. The second involved the fusion of FVIII with protein polymer called XTEN, increasing the circulating half-life. XTEN works similarly to PEGylation.

Table 28.2 Therapeutic options in haemophilia (A and B).

Factor replacement therapies	Non-replacement therapies	Gene therapies	Adjunctive therapies

■ Plasma-derived CFC
■ Recombinant, standard half-life CFC
■ Recombinant, extended half-life CFC
■ Recombinant, ultra long half-life CFC
 	
CFC = clotting factor concentrates
	■ FVIIIa mimetics
	  ■ Emicizumab
	  ■ Denecimig
	■ Monoclonal antibodies against TFPI
	  ■ Concizumab
	  ■ Marstacimab
	■ Antithrombin knockdown
	  ■ Fitusiran
	■ Bypass agents
	  ■ Recombinant activated factor VII
	  ■ Activated prothrombin complex concentrates
		■ Haemophilia B – adeno-associated viral vector
		  ■ Etranocogene dezaparvovec
		■ Haemophilia A – adeno-associated viral vector
		  ■ Valoctocogene roxaparvovec
		■ Clinical trials
		  ■ Lentiviral vectors
		  ■ Gene editing
			■ Desmopressin
			■ Tranexamic acid
			■ Fibrin glue

Prophylaxis with replacement therapy

Prophylaxis describes the institution of regular treatment with replacement or non-replacement therapies to prevent spontaneous bleeding (Table 28.2). Regular prophylaxis is superior to on-demand treatment (treatment of bleeds and surgery) and represents the current standard of care for patients with severe haemophilia. Prophylaxis with FVIII or FIX is initiated after the first spontaneous bleed or in the second year of life. The frequency of infusion depends on the product used. EHL FVIII can be infused twice a week, and EHL FIX can be infused once a week, compared to SHL FVIII (3/week) and SHL FIX (2/week).

Early prophylaxis aimed to keep trough levels (lowest level between infusions) around 1%, based on the observation that moderate haemophilia patients have substantially less severe joint damage. Recent guidance has recommended trough levels of 3–5% to reduce joint damage further.

Typically, on a well-planned prophylactic regimen, patients can expect to have 0-2 spontaneous bleeds in a year. Severely affected patients are now reaching adult life with little or no arthropathy.

Venous access can be issue for regular intravenous infusions, especially in the very young and older patient groups. Various strategies are used to manage this, including venous access devices, e.g. portacath or permanent arterio-venous fistulae.

Complications of FVIII and FIX treatment

Inhibitors

One of the most serious complications of haemophilia is the development of alloantibodies or inhibitors to FVIII and FIX. Inhibitors decrease and abrogate response to CFCs. In severe HA, inhibitors are detected in 25–35% of patients, usually within the first 50 exposures. Immunosuppression and immune tolerance (daily exposure to high doses of FVIII) regimens have been used in an attempt to eradicate the antibody. This is achieved in about two-thirds of cases but at significant expense. Inhibitors are seen in 1–5% of patients with severe HB.

HIV and HCV infections due to contaminated blood products

Contamination of plasma-derived factors with blood-borne viruses in the late 70s and early 80s resulted in large numbers of patients being infected with human immunodeficiency virus (HIV) and hepatitis C (HCV) and excess mortality

The recognition that blood and blood products could transmit blood-borne viruses resulted in rigorous screening of blood donors alongside the development and introduction of viral inactivation procedures. All plasma and recombinant factor treatments are now dual virally inactivated to prevent transmission of viral infections, a significant milestone in making blood products safe for patient use.

Management of bleeds and surgery

Replacement therapy

Treatment with replacement therapy is typically required prior to minor and major surgery to increase factor levels to prevent bleeding in the peri-operative period. Levels within the mild to normal range are required to achieve this. Response to treatment is determined by measuring factor levels pre-infusion (trough) and immediately after infusion (peak). Treatment response and type of procedure determine the treatment regimen (dose and frequency) for control of bleeding and prevention of rebleeding. National and international guidelines have described desired peak and trough levels and duration of treatment for best outcomes.

a Joint and muscle bleeds are best managed with peak plasma levels of 50–80%. Joint bleeds require treatment for 1–2 days, and muscle bleeds for 2–3 days.
b Peak levels of 100% or higher are required for major surgery, major trauma, or haemorrhage at a dangerous site. The required trough levels determine the frequency of infusion. Trough levels are maintained at > 50–80% for the first 3 days and slowly reduced to prevent rebleeding from the wound. Treatment is continued until complete wound healing or resolution of haematoma.
c Local supportive measures used in treating haemarthroses and haematomas include resting the affected part and applying ice.

Desmopressin (1-Diamino-8-D-arginine vasopressin, DDAVP)

Desmopressin is a selective agonist for the vasopressin 2 receptor (V2R), expressed on the kidney collecting duct and endothelial cells. It mimics the antidiuretic effects of vasopressin and promotes exocytosis of VWF from Weibel–Palade bodies (WPB) in the endothelial cells. Desmopressin also has vasodilator properties, with a slight increase in the heart rate, a decrease in systolic and diastolic blood pressure, and facial flushing. **Following intravenous administration, a 2- to 6-fold rise in FVIII levels is seen after 60 minutes. This correlates with the release of FVIII and VWF, stored in endothelial cells, into circulation.**

Desmopressin may also be given subcutaneously or intranasally; this has been used as immediate treatment for mild haemophilia after accidental trauma or haemorrhage. The antidiuretic effect of desmopressin lasts longer than the haemostatic effect. It should be avoided in older adults with multiple comorbidities. Fluid restriction to less than one litre over 24 hours is essential. Repeated administration can be associated with tachyphylaxis, i.e. loss of response with time, but also accumulation of fluid with hyponatremia and subsequent convulsions.

Bypass therapies

Bypassing agents are used to treat and prevent bleeding when patients develop inhibitors, when FVIII and FIX are ineffective. Two bypass agents are available to achieve haemostasis with different mechanisms of action. Recombinant activated factor VIIa (rFVIIa) promotes coagulation through tissue factor-dependent and independent pathways. The second is activated prothrombin complex concentrate (aPCC), which contains non-activated FII, FIX, FX, and mainly activated FVII.

Antifibrinolytics

Tranexamic acid is an essential intervention for managing bleeding disorders of any severity. It decreases plasminogen activation by occupying lysine binding sites and preventing co-localization with tissue plasminogen activator on cross-linked fibrin (Fig. 26.13, Fig. 28.6).

Non-replacement therapies

The natural history of haemophilia has demonstrated that higher factor levels are required for managing bleeds, but bleed prevention can be achieved at lower levels. This understanding, combined with biotechnological advances, has enabled the development of novel molecules that restore thrombin generation adequate for bleed prevention. Bleed management requires additional treatment as they do not restore thrombin generation into the normal range.

Non-replacement therapies or thrombin incrementing therapies can be broadly categorized into bypass agents (see above), FVIIIa mimetics, e.g. emicizumab, and rebalancing therapies based on their mechanisms of action (Table 28.2).

Emicizumab

Emicizumab is a bispecific monoclonal antibody that acts as an FVIIIa mimetic and binds FIXa and FX, with activation of FX to FXa (Fig. 28.7). Emicizumab represents a new approach with excellent success at decreasing the frequency of major bleeds in HA patients with and without inhibitors. It has a half-life of 4 weeks, similar to immunoglobulins, and can be dosed every 1–4 weeks. Similar to prophylaxis with FVIII, it significantly decreases spontaneous and mild trauma-associated bleeds. **Emicizumab has the greatest impact in haemophilia A patients with inhibitors offering a prophylactic strategy for the first time.**

Emicizumab: bleed management

The thrombin generation with emicizumab is inadequate for managing major or minor bleeds that have not improved over a day. In patients without inhibitors, bleeds are managed with FVIII as the binding affinity of FIXa to FVIIIa is much higher than that of emicizumab. In patients with inhibitors, bleeds are managed with bypassing agents. rFVIIa is used preferentially over aPCC due to drug interaction with the latter.

Emicizumab: thrombosis risk

A drug-drug interaction has been reported with aPCC, with patients developing thrombotic microangiopathy and thrombosis with repeated doses. This is because emicizumab is 'always on', and the magnitude of thrombin generation is related to the amount of FIXa in circulation, that increases with repeated administration of aPCC. No such interaction has been reported with rFVIIa.

Rebalancing therapies

The advent of emicizumab established the principle that restoration of thrombin generation is adequate to prevent spontaneous bleeding and bleeding in relation to minor

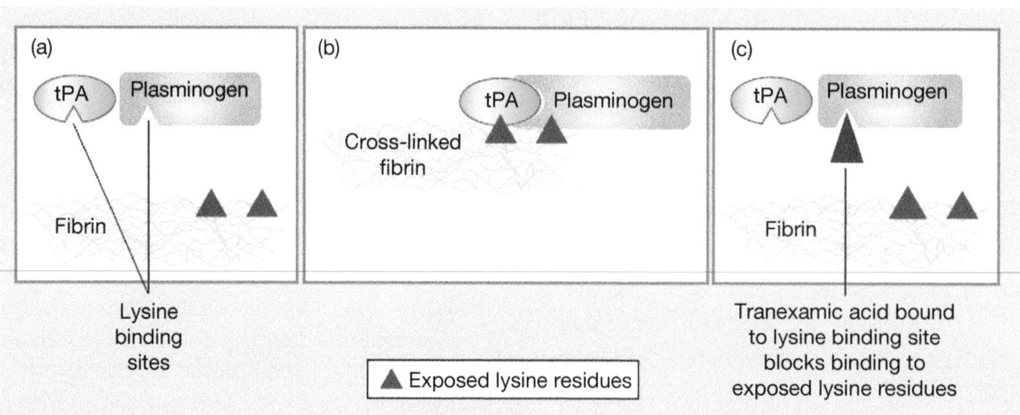

Figure 28.6 Tranexamic acid mechanism of action. **(a)** Plasminogen is the zymogen for plasmin and has lysine binding sites, as does tissue plasminogen activator (tPA) to facilitate molecular interactions with substrates. **(b)** Formation of fibrin exposes lysine residues, enabling attachment of plasminogen and tissue plasminogen activator (tPA) through their lysine binding sites. This colocalization changes plasminogen conformation and increases its activation to plasmin by tPA. **(c)** Tranexamic acid (TXA) binds with lysine binding sites on plasminogen only and decreases its activation.

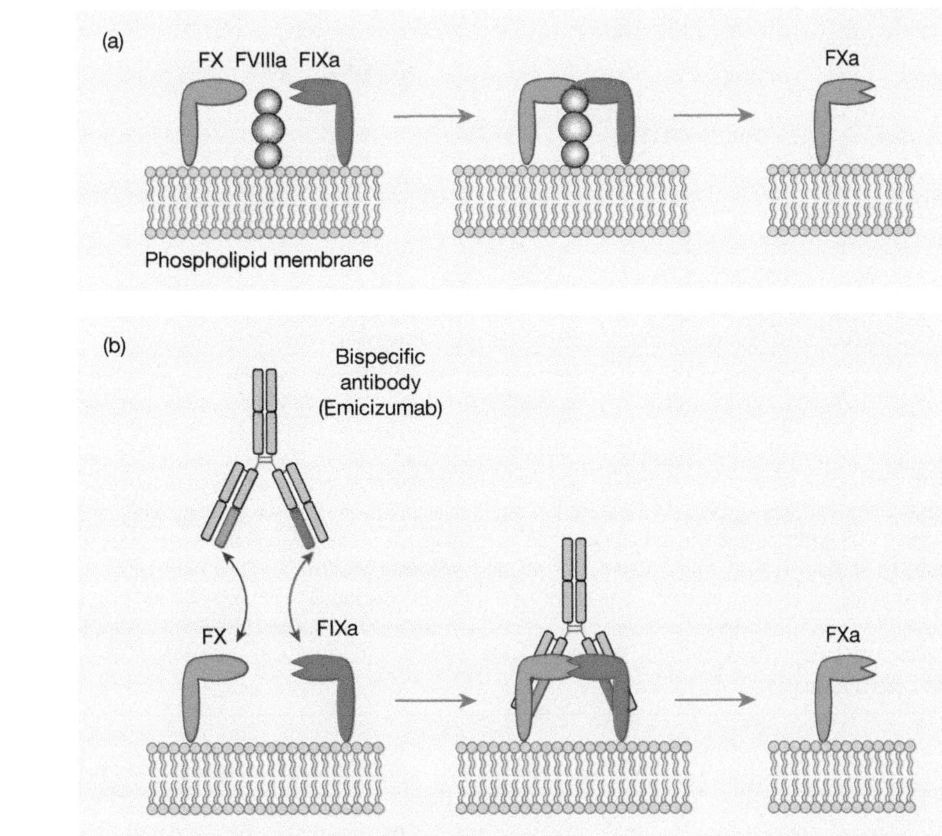

Figure 28.7 Intrinsic Xase and mechanism of action of emicizumab. **(a)** The intrinsic Xase complex on the phospholipid membrane has FVIIIa as a cofactor that supports the interaction between FIXa and FX by binding to both factors and increasing the activation of FX to FXa. **(b)** Emicizumab is a bispecific antibody with one arm binding FIXa and another FX, which are spatially positioned to enable activation of FX by FIXa.

trauma. **Rebalancing therapies include molecules that target physiologic anticoagulants (inhibit the inhibitors), including antithrombin (AT), tissue factor pathway inhibitor (TFPI) and activated protein C (APC) (Fig. 28.8). Reduction or inhibition of these anticoagulants increases thrombin generation and clot formation. Human clinical trials in HA and HB patients with and without inhibitors have demonstrated a reduction in bleeding tendency. The overall effectiveness needs to be determined.**

Like emicizumab, thrombin generation is adequate for preventing spontaneous bleeds and resolving minor bleeds. It is inadequate to manage major or significant bleeds, and additional treatment is required. In patients without inhibitors, bleeds are managed with FVIII; in patients with inhibitors, bypass agents are used with rFVIIa used preferentially over aPCC.

Rebalancing therapies: bleed management

Thrombin generation with rebalancing therapies is adequate for preventing spontaneous bleeds and managing minor bleeds. Major bleeds or bleeds that have not resolved over 24 hours require treatment. Current recommendations suggest using the lowest possible dose of FVIII or FIX. Similarly, lower doses of bypass agents have been recommended.

Rebalancing therapies: thrombosis

Replacement with standard doses of FVIII or FIX results in thrombin generation that is potentially supraphysiological. Thrombotic events have been reported with extended duration of treatment with CFCs or bypass agents.

Gene therapy

Gene therapy for HA and HB was licensed for clinical practice in 2022. Both use liver-directed adeno-associated viral vectors, the most commonly used vectors for gene therapy in haemophilia (Fig. 28.9). AAV is a small, non-enveloped DNA parvovirus that is replication incompetent. Therefore, AAV requires co-infection with adenovirus or other helper viruses

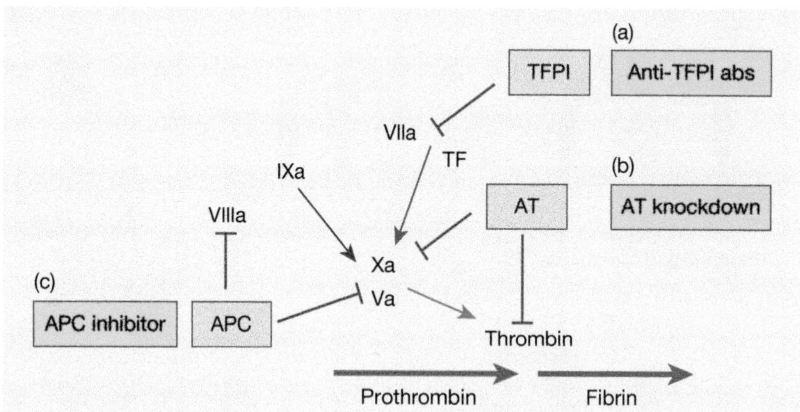

Figure 28.8 Rebalancing therapies in haemophilia A and B. They inhibit the inhibitors and restore thrombin generation into the mild to normal range. **(a)** Tissue factor pathway inhibitor (TFPI) is inhibited by monoclonal antibodies, e.g. concizumab and marstacimab. **(b)** Inhibition by antithrombin (AT) is diminished when the plasma concentration is reduced through the degradation of hepatic AT messenger RNA mediated by fitusiran, a nucleic acid therapy based on RNA interference (RNAi). Small interfering RNAs (siRNA) are double-stranded RNAs that enable post-transcriptional gene silencing through the degradation of target mRNA **(c)** Serpin PC is an engineered serine protease inhibitor modified from α1-antitrypsin with three substitution mutations and targets activated protein C (APC) specifically, the key inhibitor of cofactors FVa and FVIIIa. All three classes are in various phases of clinical development and are to be licensed for use in routine clinical practice.

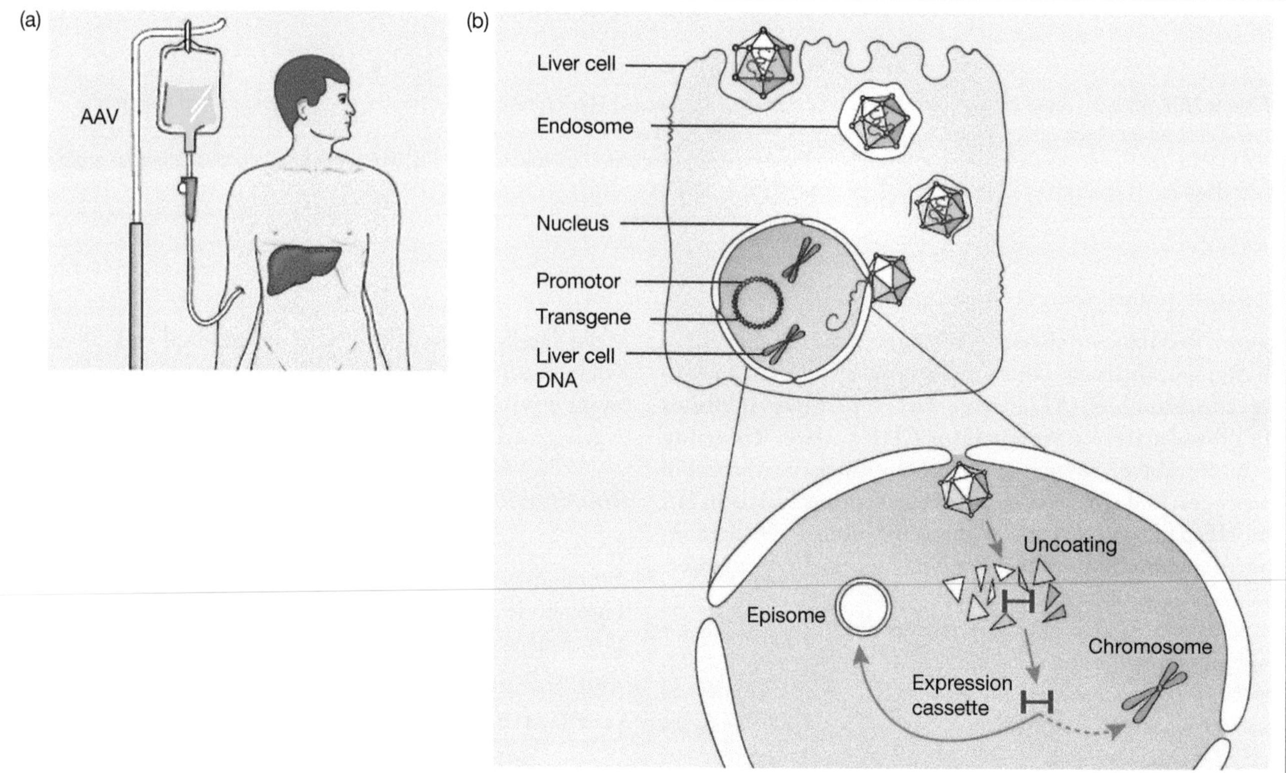

Figure 28.9 AAV gene therapy. **(a)** Recombinant AAV-based gene therapy is administered as a peripheral intravenous infusion. **(b)** Specific cell surface viral receptors mediate the cellular entry of AAV viral vectors. The virus particle is uncoated in the nucleus, and the expression cassette is deposited episomally (intranuclear, extrachromosomal). The DNA is transcribed, and the mRNA transcript diffuses into the cytoplasm, where it is translated into a protein product (not shown).

to replicate. AAV is non-pathogenic, i.e. it is not associated with any known disease.

AAV vectors are made of the virus protein shell, the capsid packaging the expression cassette that has replaced the viral DNA. The expression cassette includes a modified *F8* or *F9* gene (the transgene) and a liver-specific promotor. Major gene modifications include B domain deletion in *F8* and gain of function mutation in *F9* gene (FIX Padua). Following uptake by the hepatocyte, the transgene is placed episomally, i.e. intranuclear, but extrachromosomal (Fig. 28.9). Factor level expression varies between none to levels within the normal range.

Elevation of liver enzymes (transaminitis) after the vector infusion can herald an immune response to the vector. The immune response contributes to loss of expression, impacting the predictability and durability of factor expression. It can be controlled by steroid therapy. FIX Padua (8 times more potent than wild-type FIX) results in higher FIX activity levels for lower protein expression. Whilst long-term stable expression of FIX has been observed with HB gene therapy, loss of expression with time is notable in HA gene therapy. Moreover, inter-individual variability is an issue in both HA and HB.

Despite the challenges, it is a great leap forward for managing patients with severe HA and HB.

von Willebrand disease

von Willebrand disease (VWD), due to reduced von Willebrand factor (VWF) function, either quantitative or qualitative, is the most common inherited bleeding disorder. The estimated prevalence varies from 1:100 to 1:10,000 depending on the assessment criteria. Symptomatic presentation requiring assessment and care is observed in about 1 in 1,000 individuals. The gene is located on the short arm of human chromosome 12, and inheritance depends on the type of VWD.

Pathogenesis of VWD

von Willebrand factor (VWF) is a large, multidomain, adhesive plasma glycoprotein with binding sites for FVIII, heparin, collagen and platelets (GPIb, GPIIb–IIIa) (Fig. 28.10a). Abnormalities of function may be restricted to a single aspect, e.g. binding FVIII or more extensive when multimerization is interrupted.

VWF is synthesized as a pre-pro-VWF molecule with a signal peptide, a propeptide and mature VWF. In the endoplasmic reticulum, signal peptide removal is followed by the formation of disulphide bonds, protein folding and dimerization. In the Golgi, VWF molecules undergo glycosylation, sulfation and multimerization (Fig. 28.10b). Further, furin cleaves the VWF propeptide (VWFpp) from the mature VWF. The endothelium is the source of circulating VWF, with secretion occurring via three main routes. Low molecular weight VWF multimers (LMWM) are secreted constitutively into the subendothelial matrix. High molecular weight VWF multimers (HMWM) are condensed and packaged into Weibel–Palade bodies (WPBs).

WPBs are endothelial granules that store VWF necessary for haemostasis and P-selectin essential for inflammation. Basal secretion from WPBs occurs continuously, releasing a full range of VWF multimers into circulation. WPB exocytosis can be triggered by a wide range of physiological stimuli like adrenaline (epinephrine), thrombin, histamine, exercise, desmopressin, and pathological signals (inflammation and infection). This regulated secretion can release a full range of multimers, including ultra-large VWF multimers that bind platelets via the GPIb subunit under high shear conditions (Fig. 26.7).

Patients with blood group O have a slightly shorter VWF half-life related to alternations in post-translational glycosylation. VWF levels can change with age, as does the bleeding phenotype. Stress affects plasma levels, and VWF is also an acute phase protein. The average half-life of VWF is around 15 hours.

Clinical features

Patients experience excessive mucocutaneous bleeding, including easy bruising, oral bleeding, epistaxis, gastrointestinal bleeding, prolonged bleeding from minor trauma and heavy menstrual bleeding (Table 27.2). Excessive bleeding can also be seen after childbirth. The severity of bleeding is highly variable, depending on the absolute level of VWF activity, FVIII level and mutation type. Haemarthroses and muscle haematomas are rare, except in Type 3, where VWF is absent. Women are more severely affected than men at a given VWF level due to heavy menstrual bleeding.

VWD is a heterogeneous disorder with multiple variants consolidated into three groups per the current ISTH classification (Table 28.3).

Laboratory investigations

The complex structure of VWF supports platelet adhesion and protects circulating FVIII from premature degradation. Investigations measure these two functions and aim to diagnose and classify subtypes. The assays used are listed below.

1 **VWF: Ag** (antigen) levels are measured by ELISA assay, a measure of protein concentration.
2 **VWF: Rco (ristocetin cofactor activity)** assay is a functional assay and uses fixed platelets and ristocetin. Ristocetin alters VWF conformation, facilitating the interaction between the VWF A1 domain and platelet GP1b receptors; shear mediates this *in vivo*. HMWMs are more active as they contain more binding sites than smaller multimers. This defines the platelet-dependent function of VWF.
3 **VWF: Activity assays** also measure the interaction between the VWF A1 domain and platelet GPIbα receptor and have superseded VWF: Rco in many centres. GP1bR uses

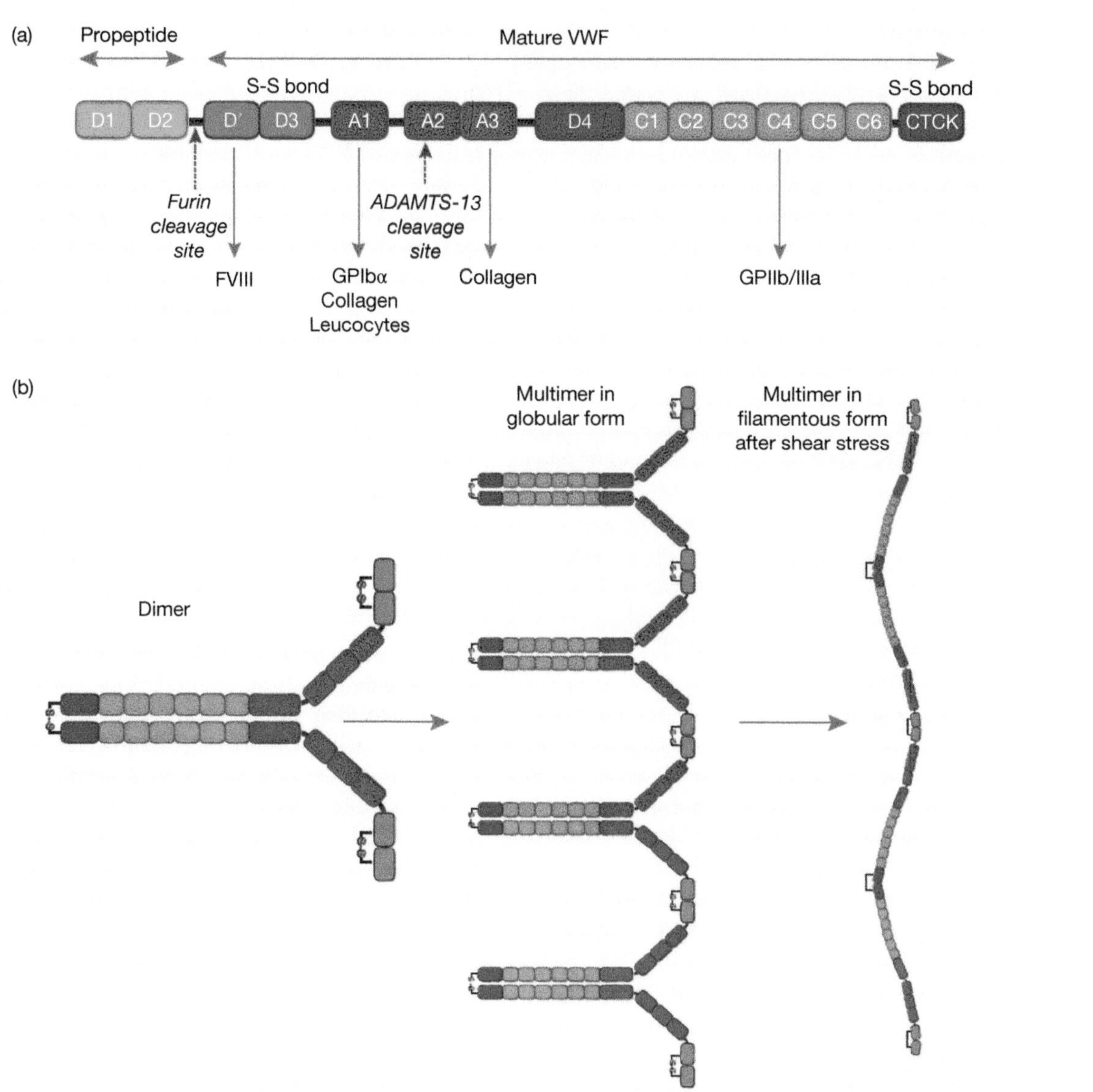

Figure 28.10 Structure and function of von Willebrand factor (VWF) relevant to VWD. **(a)** von Willebrand factor (VWF) monomer domains and multiple binding sites for ligands. A1 domain has a binding site for platelet GP1bα (GP1b-IX-V), A1 and A3 for collagen facilitating adhesion, C4 for platelet GPIIb/IIIa, and D'D3 for FVIII. Cleavage in the A2 domain by ADAMTS13 ensures the appropriate size of VWF multimers. The C domains facilitate VWF flexibility. Gene mutations can affect interaction with any ligand and provide a genetic basis for type 2 VWD. **(b)** VWF is present in a range of multimers, from dimers to high-molecular weight multimers. Interruption of VWF post-translational modification or multimerization can result in the loss of active multimer function with a relatively preserved antigen. VWF monomers are dimerized in the C-terminal cysteine knot (CTCK) through disulphide bonds. Other disulphide bonds bind VWF dimers in D domains to form multimers. Multimers have a higher number of platelet binding sites and help in bringing platelets together. ADAMTS13 (a disintegrin and metalloproteinase with a thrombospondin type 1 motif 13)

recombinant GPIb instead of fixed platelets, and VWF: GPIbM uses recombinant GPIbα with a gain of function mutation, dispensing the need for ristocetin.

4 **VWF: CB** is measured by ELISA assay and measures VWF collagen-binding (CB) activity.

5 **VWF multimers** are evaluated by electrophoresis. Loss of HMWMs impacts VWF: RCo and other VWF activity assays.

6 **Ristocetin-induced platelet aggregation (RIPA)** uses low-dose ristocetin to induce platelet agglutination when a

Table 28.3 Classification of von Willebrand disease.

Types	
Quantitative	
Type 1	Partial quantitative deficiency of VWF
Type 3	Complete deficiency of VWF
Qualitative	
Type 2	Qualitative abnormalities of the VWF molecule
Type 2A	Decreased VWF-dependent platelet function (adhesion) and a selective deficiency of HMW VWF multimers
Type 2B	Decreased VWF-dependent platelet function (adhesion) AND increased affinity of VWF for platelet GPIbα
Type 2M	Decreased VWF-dependent platelet function (adhesion) without a selective deficiency of HMW VWF multimers
Type 2N	Markedly decreased binding affinity for FVIII

HMW, High molecular weight multimers.
Source: Adapted from J.E. Sadler *et al.* (2006) *J. Thromb. Haemost.* 4: 2103–14. E.J. Favaloro (2020) *Res. Pract. Thromb. Haemost.* 4: 952–7.

gain of function mutation in VWF increases affinity to platelets.

7 **FVIII binding** measures the ability of VWF to bind FVIII.

VWD subtypes

Type 1 VWD

Partial quantitative deficiency manifests as concordant reductions of VWF antigen and activity (Table 28.4). It is autosomal dominant in inheritance, with incomplete penetrance. Diverse mechanisms underlie the disease, including reduced synthesis, abnormalities of retention, secretion, and survival. Some variants cause a dominant negative effect, i.e. an abnormal VWF molecule interferes with the function of a normal molecule.

Patients with VWF activity levels of < 30 IU/dL, immaterial of bleeding history, should be diagnosed as Type 1. This group is very likely to have abnormalities in the VWF gene. Patients with levels between 30 and 50 IU/dL and bleeding history can also be labelled as having Type 1; genetic abnormalities are less common.

Type 3 VWD

Autosomal recessive in inheritance, patients have a complete or near complete deficiency, with VWF: Ag <2 IU/dL and FVIII: C of < 10 IU/dL.

Type 2A, 2B, 2M and 2N

Subtypes 2A, 2B and 2M are all associated with the loss of VWF activity disproportionate to the antigen levels, presenting with activity/antigen ratios < 0.7 (range of 0.5–0.7). The mechanism of activity loss is different in each subtype; this is reflected in the RCo/CB ratios (see laboratory tests above).

- In 2A, the loss of VWF activity is due to the selective loss of HMWM. The variants affect the intracellular processing of VWF, resulting in intracellular retention or degradation, defective multimerization, loss of regulated storage and increased proteolysis by ADAMTS13 (Chapter 29).
- In 2B, a gain of function mutation in the A1 domain results in increased binding to platelet GPIbα receptors, forming platelet–VWF complexes that are cleared rapidly. This results in thrombocytopenia and loss of HMWM. RIPA with low dose ristocetin shows an exaggerated response, and mutation analysis is diagnostic.
- In 2M, the mechanisms are poorly understood; multimerization and collagen binding are unaffected with preserved HMWM. Other subtle multimer abnormalities may be identifiable.
- In 2N, a mutation results in reduced binding to FVIII, with increased clearance of FVIII and low levels. The differential diagnosis is mild haemophilia A.

Treatment

Therapeutic strategies

a Local measures and antifibrinolytic agents can be used for mild bleeding and as adjunctive measures.

b Desmopressin injection increases VWF levels by releasing endothelial stores 30 minutes after intravenous infusion. This is effective in VWD Type 1 and some Type 2M and 2A cases. A therapeutic trial is indicated before using it for a planned procedure or in an emergency. Precautions have been detailed (page 375)

c VWF concentrates are indicated in patients with low levels and major surgery. The concentrates include plasma-derived, intermediate purity factor VIII/VWF concentrates and high-purity VWF-only concentrates.

d Recombinant VWF concentrate is available for the management of bleeds and surgery.

e When using VWF-only containing concentrates, a low FVIII at baseline necessitates additional FVIII replacement for management of a bleed. Otherwise, treatment should be started 8–12 hours pre-surgery to allow FVIII levels to rise to normal range.

Major surgery

Haemostatic levels of FVIII and VWF should be maintained for at least three days, aiming for trough levels of >50 IU/dL for both rather than just FVIII. Extended duration may be appropriate for patients with low levels until wound healing is complete. Concomitant tranexamic can be used unless contraindicated.

Table 28.4 – VWD subtypes - Laboratory abnormalities and usual treatment.

Type	FVIII: C	VWF: Ag	VWF: RCo or VWF: GP1b assays	VWF: CB	RCo/ag ratio	RCo/CB ratio	VWF multimer structure/ comments	Treatment
1	N, ↓	↓	↓	↓	>0.7	>0.7	Normal	Desmopressin, TXA and VWF only concentrates or Factor VIII/VWF concentrates
3	very low	not detected	not detected	not detected	N/A	N/A	Absent	VWF only concentrates or Factor VIII/VWF concentrates; desmopressin has no effect
2A	N, ↓	N, ↓	↓↓	↓↓	<0.7	<0.7	High and medium MWM absent	VWF only concentrates or Factor VIII/VWF concentrates; subset can use desmopressin
2B	N, ↓	N, ↓	↓	↓	<0.7	<0.7	HMWM absent, with agglutination to low dose ristocetin	VWF only concentrates or Factor VIII/VWF concentrates; desmopressin should be avoided
2M	N, ↓	N, ↓	↓↓	↓	<0.7	>0.7	Normal	VWF only concentrates or Factor VIII/VWF concentrates; subset can use desmopressin
2N	↓↓	N, ↓	N, ↓	N, ↓	>0.7	NA or > 0.7	Normal and FVIII< VWF	VWF only concentrates or Factor VIII/VWF concentrates

Ag, antigen; CB, collagen binding; FVIII: C, factor VIII activity; GP1b, glycoprotein 1b assays; N, normal; ↑ increased; ↓ reduced; Rco, ristocetin cofactor; RIPA, ristocetin induced platelet agglutination; TXA, tranexamic acid; VWF, von Willebrand factor.

Minor surgery

The bleeding risk assessment needs to be individualized to the patient, procedure and baseline levels. For minor surgery or invasive procedures, achieving a VWF activity level of > 50IU/dL with desmopressin or factor concentrates and tranexamic acid is appropriate. In patients with levels between 30 and 50 IU/dL, tranexamic acid may be adequate.

Heavy menstrual bleeding

The first line of treatment is hormonal therapy in the form of combined hormonal contraception or levonorgestrel-releasing intrauterine system. Tranexamic acid can be added to this regimen. In patients who wish to conceive, tranexamic acid is the first-line treatment, followed by desmopressin. In some patients, targeted concentrate prophylaxis is not unreasonable.

Rare coagulation disorders

Rare bleeding disorders include inherited deficiencies of coagulation factors: fibrinogen, prothrombin, FV, combined FV and FVIII, FVII, FX, FXI, FXIII and combined deficiencies of vitamin-K-dependent factors. Incidence is 1 in 500,000 to 1 in 2 million and increases with consanguinity.

Bleeding tends to be prominently mucocutaneous; central nervous system bleeding is not unusual. Data analysis by the European Network on Rare Bleeding Disorders shows a good correlation between bleeding tendency and factor levels in patients with fibrinogen, combined FV and VIII, FX and FXIII deficiencies. The association is weak with FV and FVII deficiencies and minimal with FXI deficiency. Further, the minimum level where symptoms are absent varies across all the disorders. In addition to factor assays, mutation analysis confirms the diagnosis.

Treatment involves a combination of tranexamic acid with strategies to increase factor levels. Fresh frozen plasma (FFP) contains all factors, with virally inactivated FFP preferred in patients with inherited conditions. Plasma-derived single-factor concentrates are available for certain factors (fibrinogen, FXI, FVII, FX, FXIII), with a few recombinant options (rFVIIa, rFXIII). Prothrombin complex concentrates rich in factors II, VII, X and IX; proteins C and S can also be used.

Congenital fibrinogen disorders (CFDs)

CFDs are a group of heterogeneous disorders arising from a wide spectrum of mutations in the fibrinogen genes. Quantitative disorders include afibrinogenemia (complete absence of fibrinogen) and hypofibrinogenemia (proportional decrease of functional and antigenic fibrinogen levels). Qualitative disorders include dysfibrinogenemia (decreased functional and normal antigenic fibrinogen levels) and hypodysfibrinogenemia (discrepant decrease of functional and antigenic fibrinogen levels). The severity is categorized based on the level of functional fibrinogen as: complete absence, severe (<0.5 g/L), moderate (0.5–1.0 g/L), and mild (>1.0 g/L and less than 1.5 g/L, lower limit of normal). The severity of the deficiency correlates with the bleeding risk.

Patients with afibrinogenemia are homozygotes or compound heterozygotes, while individuals with hypofibrinogenemia are usually heterozygotes. Dysfibrinogenemia is usually associated with autosomal dominant inheritance.

Most patients with afibrinogenemia suffer from major bleeding, with recurrent foetal loss uniquely described in this group. Some patients are asymptomatic; paradoxically, patients can develop thrombosis with and without fibrinogen replacement. In dysfibrinogenemia, the bleeding phenotype is usually mild, with some variants strongly associated with a high risk of thrombosis (up to 20%).

Patients are treated as needed to prevent or manage bleeds with plasma-derived fibrinogen concentrates. Prophylaxis may be indicated in patients with CNS bleeds.

Factor VII deficiency

FVII deficiency is the most common autosomal recessive coagulation disorder (1 in 500,000). Several polymorphisms modulate plasma levels with a wide normal range. Bleeding symptoms range from mild to fatal and do not always correlate with levels. Even with levels <1 IU/dL, patients may not show a severe bleeding tendency. The clinical phenotype determines the need for treatment. The age at diagnosis and previous bleeding history in relation to haemostatic challenges help with management decisions. Some case series reported a high incidence of CNS bleeding; trauma during birth was a significant risk factor. Thrombosis has also been reported. Treatment with tranexamic acid may be adequate. Single FVII plasma-derived concentrate or recombinant FVIIa (which can be used at very low doses) are preferred. FFP and PCCs can also be used.

Factor X deficiency

Severely affected patients (levels < 1 IU/dL) present early in life with umbilical stump, CNS or GI bleeding. Patients with severe deficiencies also commonly experience haemarthroses and haematomas. Treatment is with tranexamic acid for minor bleeding for patients with levels > 5 IU/dL. Patients with FX deficiency can be treated with factor X concentrate and prothrombin complex concentrates for acute bleeding and surgical interventions.

Factor XI deficiency

Factor XI deficiency is inherited usually in an autosomal recessive manner with a worldwide prevalence of 1 in 100,000 people, being more common in Askenazi Jews. Bleeding tendency is variable and the relationship between FXI levels in plasma and bleeding tendency is less certain, with some patients with significant deficiency (FXI: C ≤15 IU/dL) not demonstrating any bleeding and vice versa. However, when a site of injury with high local fibrinolytic activity is involved, e.g. urogenital tract, oral cavity after dental extraction or tonsillectomy, the risk of bleeding is increased (49–67%) in comparison to sites with less local fibrinolytic activity (1.5–40%). Treatment is with tranexamic acid, FFP or factor XI concentrate.

Factor XIII deficiency

FXIII deficiency, an autosomal recessive disorder, is a rare but potentially life-threatening cause of a haemorrhagic diathesis. Patients with severe deficiency are often diagnosed early because of bleeding in the first few years of life. This ranges from umbilical stump bleeding to CNS bleeding. Treatment is by replacement with plasma-derived or recombinant XIII concentrate every 4 weeks to prevent bleeding.

Prothrombin (FII) deficiency

Prothrombin deficiency is one of the rarest inherited coagulation disorders, with a 1 in 2 million prevalence. Severe deficiency of FII (plasma levels <5 IU/dL.) in homozygous or double heterozygous patients is always characterized by severe bleeding. Treatment is with prothrombin complex concentrates.

Other disorders

In factor V deficiency, the bleeding does not correlate with factor levels. Treatment is with plasma infusions; platelets are indicated if there is a poor response to plasma. Combined mild FV and FVIII deficiency is caused by mutations in the *LMAN1* gene, which codes for a cargo receptor transporting FV, FVIII and other glycoproteins from the endoplasmic reticulum (ER) to the ER-Golgi intermediate compartment. Inherited abnormalities of gamma-glutamyl carboxylase and vitamin K epoxide reductase, involved in the recycling of vitamin K (Chapter 31), result in the reduction of vitamin-K-dependent coagulation factors.

Disorders of primary fibrinolysis

These rare disorders are of interest as they help elucidate physiological pathways and redundancies. Patients present with mild bleeding, notably post-surgical bleeding. Bleeding may be delayed with impaired wound healing, and there are instances of catastrophic bleeds.

Bleeding in this group is because of accelerated fibrinolysis. The causes include:

1. Decreased inhibition of fibrinolysis as a result of an inherited deficiency of the main inhibitors, plasminogen activator inhibitor-1 (PAI-1) or α2-Antiplasmin (α2-AP).
2. Increased fibrinolysis due to excess tissue plasminogen activator (tPA) or urokinase-type plasminogen activator (uPA), such as Quebec platelet disorder.

Treatment is with antifibrinolytic agents to help control the bleeding.

SUMMARY

- Severe haemophilia A, with FVIII activity < 1 IU/dL, is the most common inherited severe bleeding disorder. Haemophilia B (FIX deficiency), five times less frequent, has identical clinical features.
- Patients with severe deficiency present with spontaneous bleeding, particularly joint and muscle bleeds. Patients with deficiencies of all severities have excess bleeding with trauma and surgery.
- Treatment advances in haemophilia A and B have resulted in a near-normal life span. Prevention of bleeding is the current standard of care for patients with severe deficiency or severe phenotype, thus decreasing long-term joint morbidity.
- Therapies for haemophilia A and B include replacement therapies, non-replacement therapies that restore thrombin generation, and gene therapy that restores endogenous expression of the deficient factor.
- VWD is the most common inherited bleeding disorder, with an estimated prevalence of symptomatic disease of 1 in 1000. Mild quantitative deficiency is the most common subtype, with multiple qualitative subtypes and severe deficiency recognized. Mucocutaneous haemorrhages are common presenting symptoms, and symptomatic presentation is more common in women.
- Desmopressin is a valuable treatment for mild VWD and mild haemophilia A by releasing endothelial stores of VWF and FVIII.
- VWF-containing plasma-derived and recombinant concentrates are appropriate for managing patients with severe VWD and qualitative defects.
- It is crucial to diagnose rare coagulation disorders as they are associated with increased mortality and morbidity.
- Most rare coagulation disorders can be treated with recombinant or plasma-derived concentrates. A few continue to require treatment with plasma.

Now visit **www.wiley.com/go/haematology9e** to test yourself on this chapter.

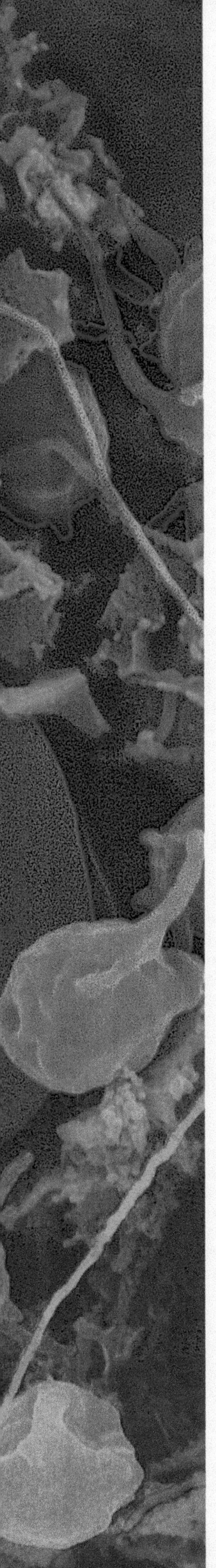

CHAPTER 29

Acquired coagulation disorders and thrombotic microangiopathies

Key topics

Hoffbrand's Essential Haematology, Ninth Edition. A. Victor Hoffbrand, Pratima Chowdary, Graham P. Collins, and Justin Loke.

© 2024 John Wiley & Sons Ltd. Published 2024 by John Wiley & Sons Ltd.

Companion website: www.wiley.com/go/haematology9e

Introduction

Acquired coagulation disorders and thrombotic microangiopathies are a diverse group of disorders. The clinical presentation varies from asymptomatic laboratory abnormalities to rapidly progressive fatal conditions.

Acquired coagulation disorders

Acquired coagulation disorders are more common than inherited disorders and the most common frequent indication for haemostatic interventions in hospitalized patients. The disorders are characterized by abnormal coagulation assays, such as prolonged prothrombin time (PT), prolonged activated partial thromboplastin time (APTT), and thrombin clotting time (Table 26.2). Abnormal PT and APTT can be associated with abnormalities of fibrinogen and raised plasma D-dimers.

The haemostatic abnormalities may be part of the clinical presentation of established disorders. The absence of an obvious explanation should prompt investigations to identify an underlying disease. The abnormalities may be asymptomatic or associated with a bleeding or thrombotic tendency.

Three main groups of acquired coagulation disorders are identifiable:

1 **Acquired isolated factor deficiencies**
2 **Acquired coagulopathy secondary to systemic disorders**
3 **Drug-induced acquired coagulopathy**

Systemic disorders are the most common cause of acquired coagulopathy and are seen primarily in hospitalized patients. Antithrombotic medications, including anticoagulants and thrombolytics, can cause abnormalities in routine screening assays and contribute to a bleeding tendency.

Acquired isolated factor deficiencies

These have a clearly defined mechanism; notable examples are summarized in Table 29.1. Patients typically present with new onset bleeding tendency of variable duration, and other haemostatic components are not affected. An important differential diagnosis for this group are the acquired disorders of platelet function (Table 27.7).

Acquired haemophilia A

Acquired haemophilia A (AHA) is a rare disorder characterized by the development of neutralizing autoantibodies against FVIII. The incidence is 1.4–6 cases/million per year. It affects both men and women, with 70 years being the average age at diagnosis. It is usually idiopathic, but in 30–50% of patients, it is associated with malignancy, other autoimmune disorders or pregnancy, usually in the postpartum period.

Table 29.1 Acquired coagulation disorders due to isolated factor deficiencies

Disorder	Mechanism of action
Acquired haemophilia A (FVIII deficiency)	Autoantibody against FVIII resulting in decreased or no activity
Acquired von Willebrand syndrome	Multiple mechanisms for impaired VWF levels and function: increased proteolysis, increased clearance and impaired multimerization
FX deficiency due to amyloidosis	Adsorption of FX by the amyloid fibrils
Acquired FXIII deficiency	Autoantibody against FXIII

Clinical features

Typically, patients present with a new onset bleeding tendency or are found to have an isolated prolonged APTT during routine investigations. The bleeding tendency does not always correlate with FVIII level. Unlike inherited HA, cutaneous and muscle (including iliopsoas) bleeds dominate the clinical picture, while joint bleeds are uncommon.

Diagnosis

1 FVIII activity is <1% in approximately half of the patients, with others demonstrating detectable FVIII.
2 Neutralizing antibody and titre are detected by the Bethesda assay, which measures the ability of the inhibitor in patient plasma to inhibit FVIII activity of normal plasma.
3 Patients should be investigated for underlying malignancy and autoimmune disorders.

Treatment

The management of acquired HA includes bleed management and inhibitor eradication.

1 **Bleed management:** Clinically significant bleeding is treated using bypassing agents or recombinant porcine factor VIII (rpFVIII). Bypassing agents include recombinant activated factor VII (rFVIIa) or activated prothrombin complex concentrate (aPCC) (Chapter 28). Tranexamic acid can be used as an adjunct agent, particularly for mucocutaneous bleeds, or as a single agent for minor bleeds. While recombinant porcine FVIII is effective, there is a high risk of developing antibodies that reduce efficacy. Human FVIII is typically ineffective, except in rare cases with low inhibitor levels. Emicizumab is used in some patients to prevent bleeding but is ineffective in managing bleeds.
2 **Inhibitor eradication:** Immunosuppression is the mainstay for inhibitor eradication. Regimens include corticosteroids, rituximab and/or cyclophosphamide. Caution should be

exercised in the elderly where infection and bleeding equally contribute to death. The time to response is related to the presenting FVIII level and inhibitor titre. Patients with underlying malignancy rarely respond to treatment. Recurrences are uncommon except in those with underlying autoimmune disorders.

Acquired von Willebrand syndrome (AVWS)

AVWS includes disorders that result in acquired quantitative, structural or functional VWF abnormalities associated with an increased risk of bleeding. Three main mechanisms contribute to AVWS, and each is associated with specific disorders:

1 **Antibody-mediated clearance** with or without functional interference:
   (a) Monoclonal gammopathy of unknown significance (MGUS)
   (b) Lymphoproliferative disorders
   (c) Autoimmune disorders
2 **Adsorption to surfaces** of transformed cells or platelets:
   (a) Myeloproliferative neoplasms and thrombocytosis
   (b) Wilms tumour in children
3 **Increased proteolysis** due to shear-induced unfolding of VWF:
   (a) Cardiovascular disorders with increased shear stress, including aortic valve stenosis, ventricular assist devices and extracorporeal membrane oxygenation
   (b) Hypothyroidism

Clinical features

A diagnosis of VWD, of any subtype, in a patient with a new onset bleeding tendency and negative family history suggests AVWS. Clinical presentation is indistinguishable from acquired platelet dysfunction or isolated coagulation factor deficiency.

Diagnosis

1 Investigations show low VWF levels in one of the assays (Chapter 28).
2 A therapeutic trial with VWF concentrate or intravenous immunoglobulins (IVIg) may help to establish the diagnosis. Measurement of VWF levels after infusion of VWF concentrate demonstrates shortened half-life. IVIg infusion can improve VWF levels in antibody-mediated clearance.
3 Once AVWD is diagnosed, investigations for underlying causes must be completed.

Treatment

1 Treatment of the underlying condition, particularly cardiac disorders, solid tumours, and hypothyroidism, results in complete remission.
2 Control of platelet count reverses AVWD in myeloproliferative neoplasms.
3 Intravenous IVIg can induce temporary remission in patients with a low paraprotein level. Antibody (especially IgM) removal may also be achieved by plasmapheresis. Remission is rare with low-grade lymphoproliferative neoplasms or MGUS.
4 Because of its heterogeneous nature, more than one therapeutic approach is often required to treat acute bleeds and prevent recurrence.
5 Bleed management options include desmopressin, VWF concentrates, IVIg, plasmapheresis or recombinant FVIIa.

Acquired coagulation disorders due to systemic disorders

Systemic disorders are the most common cause of acquired coagulation abnormalities/coagulation disorders. Multiple clotting factor deficiencies are common and may be associated with abnormalities of platelets and fibrinolysis (Chapter 32). The disorders maybe asymptomatic or associated with bleeding or thrombotic tendency and listed in Table 29.2.

Bleeding tendency mechanisms

Bleeding in these situations is often multifactorial, as described below and requires a multipronged intervention.

Impaired platelet function

- Thrombocytopenia – reduced production, increased consumption/destruction
- Platelet dysfunction – medications, including antiplatelet agents, or degranulation due to extracorporeal circuits or other medications.

Impaired coagulation

- Low levels of factors – reduced synthesis, increased catabolism, increased loss into extravascular spaces secondary to increased vascular permeability, increased consumption and dilution.
- Low FXIII is typically due to reduced hepatic synthesis.
- Low fibrinogen and FVIII are due to increased consumption.
- Inhibition of coagulation factors by anticoagulants
- Fibrin polymerization defects

Increased fibrinolysis

- Activation of plasminogen
- Other proteolytic enzymes

Vitamin K deficiency

Several vitamin K-dependent proteins are involved in coagulation, bone metabolism and other physiologic processes. Vitamin K-dependent (VKD) proteins undergo a specific post-translational modification called gamma-carboxylation necessary for serine protease activity (Chapter 31). Vitamin K includes a group of fat-soluble compounds. There are two naturally occurring forms: vitamin K1 (phylloquinone), found in green

Table 29.2 Acquired coagulation disorders secondary to systemic disorders.

Disorder	Dominant mechanism for coagulopathy
Vitamin K deficiency	Reduction in the production of vitamin K-dependent proteins
Liver disease	Acute liver failure or chronic liver disease due to reduced synthesis of coagulation factors (procoagulants and anticoagulants) and complex dysregulation
Disseminated intravascular coagulation (DIC)	Activation of coagulation, which is disseminated, results in consumption with low factors, low platelets, low fibrinogen and low FXIII. Some disorders demonstrate evidence of hyperfibrinolysis.
Consumptive coagulopathy (chronic DIC)	Consumption due to local vascular malformation or device or extracorporeal circuit with low factors, low platelets, low fibrinogen and low FXIII
Massive transfusion, including trauma-induced coagulopathy	Consumption secondary to unstable clots, increased clot formation due to excessive activation of coagulation and increased breakdown of key clotting factors. These mechanisms can lead to severe coagulopathy, especially when combined with significant fluid resuscitation.
Coagulopathy of critical illness	Often seen in patients in intensive care units due to increased consumption and impaired synthesis
Dilutional coagulopathy	Seen perioperatively when a combination of excess fluid replacement and blood loss can result in coagulopathy
Post-cardiac surgery bleeding	Combination of platelet dysfunction, low factors and heparin secondary to the use of extracorporeal circuit extracorporeal circulation
Non-specific inhibitors	Diseases with paraprotein can non-specifically interfere with coagulation. Similarly, non-specific inhibitors may be seen in autoimmune disorders
Venom-induced coagulopathies	Activate specific coagulation factors with secondary DIC
L-asparaginase	Reduced synthesis of clotting factors from the liver
Factitious disorder	Munchausen syndrome

leafy vegetables, fruits, and oils; and vitamin K2 (menaquinone), produced through fermentation of dairy products or produced by the gut microbiota. Vitamin K3, also known as menadione, is a synthetic preparation. Deficiency is caused by an inadequate diet, malabsorption or inhibition of vitamin K by vitamin K antagonist drugs such as warfarin (Chapter 31). Deficiency may occur in newborns (haemorrhagic disease of the newborn) or later in life.

Haemorrhagic disease of the newborn

At birth, newborns have low to undetectable levels of vitamin K because of inefficient placental transfer, a sterile gut, and an immature liver. This is exacerbated by prematurity and low levels in breast milk. **Vitamin K deficiency may cause haemorrhagic disease of the newborn (HDN), also referred to as vitamin K deficiency bleeding. It presents as cutaneous, gastrointestinal or intracranial bleeding. It was a common cause of infant mortality before routine vitamin K supplementation.**

There are three recognizable categories of HDN based on the timing of the presentation.

1 Early - presents within 24 hours of birth
2 Classic - presents between days 1 and 7
3 Late - presents between 1 and 12 weeks

Vitamin K is administered after birth as a preventive measure against HDN. However, the early forms of HDN cannot be prevented. Without vitamin K supplementation, the incidence of classic HDN is estimated to be 0.25-1.7%.

Diagnosis

- PT and APTT are abnormal due to reduced factors II, VII, X and IX.
- Platelet count and fibrinogen are normal
- No evidence of disseminated intravascular coagulation (DIC)

Treatment

1 Prophylaxis can be administered as a single 1 mg vitamin K intramuscular injection or as a series of oral doses. Oral preparations are not available in all countries.
2 In bleeding infants, vitamin K 1 mg intramuscularly is given every 6 hours, supplemented with prothrombin complex concentrate if the bleeding is severe.

Vitamin K deficiency in children or adults

In children and adults, deficiency is due to inadequate absorption, as in liver disease, biliary obstruction, and pancreatic or small bowel disease (tropical sprue, gluten-induced enteropathy). Rarely, prolonged antibiotic use can result in deficiency due to impaired gut bacterial synthesis, mainly seen in patients with suboptimal reserves.

The abnormalities are similar to HDN, and mild PT may be the only abnormality. Patients are treated with oral vitamin K daily. Intravenous vitamin K can be used for three or more days to correct the deficiency in hospitalized patients before a planned procedure. Prothrombin complex concentrates may be necessary in the context of bleeding or for an urgent procedure.

Liver disease

Multiple haemostatic abnormalities may contribute to a bleeding tendency and exacerbate haemorrhage from oesophageal varices.

1 Biliary obstruction results in impaired vitamin K absorption and decreased synthesis of factors II, VII, IX and X by liver parenchymal cells.
2 With severe hepatocellular disease, there are often reduced factors, particularly FV and fibrinogen, as most are synthesized in the liver. VWF and FVIII levels which are not synthesized in the liver are elevated.
3 Functional abnormality of fibrinogen (dysfibrinogenaemia).
4 Hypersplenism associated with portal hypertension frequently results in thrombocytopenia. Decreased thrombopoietin production from the liver contributes to thrombocytopenia.
5 Disseminated intravascular coagulation (DIC; see below) may be related to the release of thromboplastins from damaged liver cells and reduced concentrations of antithrombin, protein C and α_2-antiplasmin. In addition, there is impaired removal of activated clotting factors and increased fibrinolytic activity.
6 **Haemostasis in liver disease is dysregulated with some rebalancing of haemostasis. The management should be based on the clinical picture, including the risk of procedure-related bleeding, the presence of active bleeding and concurrent haemostatic abnormalities.**

Disseminated intravascular coagulation (DIC)

Disseminated intravascular coagulation (DIC) is a complication of an underlying disorder which can independently predict mortality. It is characterized by the systemic activation of coagulation with vascular endothelial damage. The subcommittee on DIC of the International Society on Thrombosis and Haemostasis (ISTH) in 2001 has described it as an acquired syndrome secondary to intravascular activation of coagulation with loss of localization resulting in damage to the microvasculature, potentially resulting in organ dysfunction. Acute DIC generally develops over hours and chronic DIC over days to weeks (Table 29.3). Some cases of chronic DIC do not consistently demonstrate evidence of loss of localization.

Table 29.3 Causes of disseminated intravascular coagulation.

Acute DIC	Disorders
Sepsis/ severe infection from any organism	Gram-negative and meningococcal septicaemia; severe falciparum malaria; viral infections (varicella, HIV, hepatitis, cytomegalovirus)
Obstetric complications	Abruption, amniotic fluid embolism, eclampsia, HELLP (haemolysis, elevated liver enzymes and low platelet count) syndrome, acute fatty liver
Malignancy	Acute promyelocytic leukaemia
Trauma	Serious tissue injury, head injury, freshwater drowning, heat stroke, burns
Organ destruction	Pancreatitis, fulminant hepatic failure
Severe toxic or immunological reactions	Snake bite, recreational drug use, severe transfusion reaction, transplant rejection
Other	Homozygous protein C and S deficiency (infants)
Subacute DIC	
Malignancy	Mucinous adenocarcinoma (Trousseau syndrome)
Obstetric	Retained dead foetus
Vascular abnormalities	Haemangioma, leaking or ruptured aortic or other aneurysms, haemangioendothelioma and other vascular malformations

Pathogenesis

Three factors contribute to DIC (Fig. 29.1):

1 Coagulation activation
2 Platelet aggregation
3 Endothelial damage

The central abnormality is coagulation activation with thrombin generation driven by tissue factor (TF). The source of TF is related to the underlying disease. It can be released into circulation from damaged tissues or tumour cells (Table 29.3). Upregulation of TF on circulating monocytes or endothelial cells in response to pro-inflammatory cytokines, e.g. interleukin-1, tumour necrosis factor, endotoxin, may also contribute to TF-mediated coagulation activation (Fig. 29.1). The damaged cell membranes are also a source of phosphatidylserine supporting thrombin generation, that is inadequately neutralized due to impaired regulation by physiologic anticoagulants. The impaired regulation is caused by low circulating AT levels or loss of antithrombotic properties of the endothelial surface (Fig. 26.13).

Endothelial damage impairs the antithrombotic milieu of the vascular lumen. Platelet activation and aggregation are stimulated by thrombin and other inflammatory mediators. Platelet activation and endothelial damage can be secondary to excess thrombin generation or be part of the initial disorder. Platelets release von Willebrand factor and platelet factor 4 (PF4), neutralizing glycosaminoglycans on the endothelial surface. The endothelium becomes prothrombotic with the expression of adhesion molecules facilitating interactions with neutrophils and increasing vascular permeability.

Sepsis is the classic example where DIC is initiated by widespread endothelial damage and activation of monocytes, neutrophils and platelets, e.g. Gram-negative and meningococcal septicaemia, septic abortion. Activated neutrophils release damage-associated molecular patterns after cell death and expel extracellular traps (NETs) that facilitate inflammation (see Chapter 8 and Immunothrombosis below).

Intravascular thrombin formation produces large amounts of circulating fibrin monomers, which can interfere with fibrin polymerization. In most patients, this is accompanied by an increase in plasminogen activator inhibitor-1 (PAI-1) (Fig. 26.12) that slows clot removal with organ dysfunction.

In some patients, there is excess fibrinolysis with the consumption of clotting factors and bleeding from the start. This can be due to the release of proteolytic substances into the circulation or systemic activation of plasminogen, as seen in acute promyelocytic leukaemia (Chapter 13).

Progressive clot formation and lysis result in depletion of fibrinogen, low platelet count, decreased coagulation factor levels and bleeding tendency, i.e. a consumptive coagulopathy.

Clinical features

1 The clinical presentation reflects the balance between coagulation activation (microthrombi formation) and fibrinolysis (Fig. 29.2).
2 The most common presentation is with asymptomatic laboratory abnormalities.

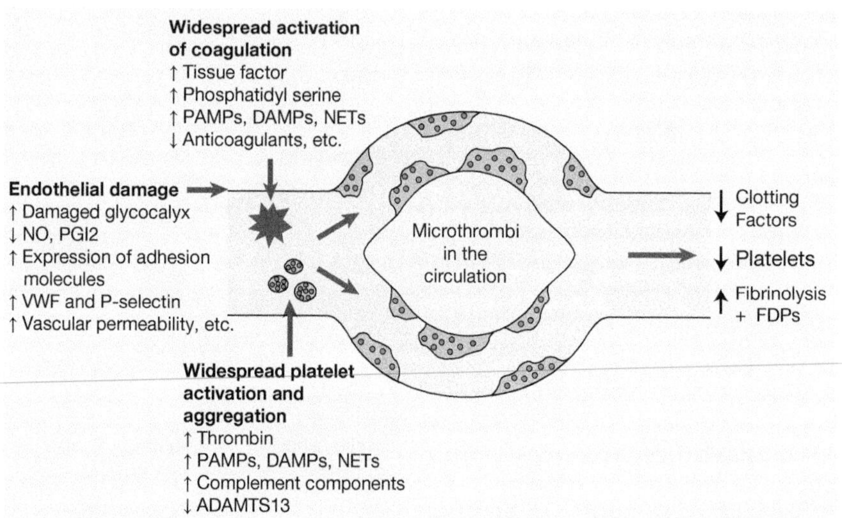

Figure 29.1 Pathogenesis of disseminated intravascular coagulation (DIC) and haemostatic changes over time. Coagulation activation, platelet aggregation and endothelial damage that is widespread contribute to DIC. PAMPs, pathogen-associated molecular patterns; NETs, neutrophil extracellular traps; DAMPs, damage-associated molecular patterns; ADAMTS13, a disintegrin and metalloproteinase with a thrombospondin type 1 motif, member 13; NO, nitric oxide; PGI2, prostaglandin I_2; VWF, von Willebrand factor; FDPs, fibrin degradation products.

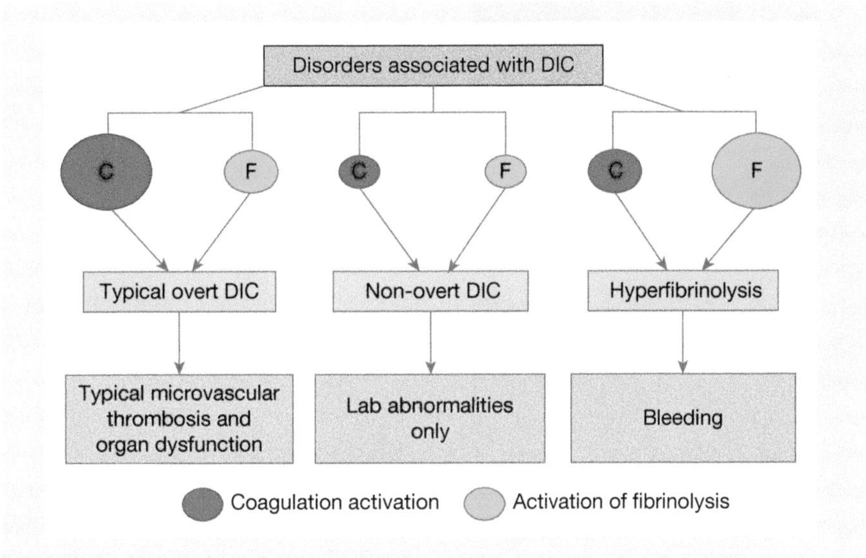

Figure 29.2 Disseminated intravascular coagulation – clinical and laboratory phenotypes. The clinical or laboratory phenotype is related to the magnitude of endothelial damage, platelet and coagulation activation **and the balance between coagulation activation and thrombus formation and fibrinolysis.** Source: Adapted from J. Thachil (2019) The elusive diagnosis of disseminated intravascular coagulation: does a diagnosis of DIC exist anymore? *Semin. Thromb. Hemost.* 45: 100–7.

3 Microthrombi present as organ dysfunction e.g. elevated liver enzymes, renal impairment, myocardial ischemia, neurological dysfunction, decreased gas exchange and other organ abnormalities.
4 Less frequently, microthrombi may cause skin lesions, renal failure and gangrene of the fingers or toes (Fig. 29.3b).
5 A microangiopathic haemolytic anaemia (see below) may also complicate the clinical picture.
6 Bleeding is seen when DIC is advanced with the consumption of clotting factors or if the fibrinolytic phenotype predominates (Fig. 29.2). There may be generalized bleeding, especially in the gastrointestinal, respiratory and urogenital tracts and skin (Fig. 29.3a). In obstetric cases, vaginal bleeding may be particularly severe.
7 Some patients may develop subacute or chronic DIC, especially with mucin-secreting adenocarcinoma.

Laboratory findings

The International Society for Thrombosis and Haemostasis (ISTH) DIC score was developed to distinguish overt from non-overt DIC, identify patients who might benefit from intervention and guide prognosis. It includes four laboratory tests that help establish the score: (1) severity of thrombocytopenia, (2) elevation of fibrin-related marker including D-dimers and fibrin degradations products, (3) prolonged PT, (4) fibrinogen level. Due to a lack of sensitivity, APTT is not included in the DIC score. The timing of onset is used to categorize the DIC as acute, subacute/chronic DIC (Table 29.3).

Treatment

Treatment of the underlying cause is key to management. The management of bleeding patients differs from that of patients with thrombotic problems.

Actively bleeding

If PT/INR is high (>1.7), treatment is with fresh frozen plasma (FFP) and/or prothrombin complex concentrates (PCCs). Fibrinogen concentrate or cryoprecipitate is appropriate if the fibrinogen is low (<1-1.5 mg/L), and platelet concentrates if the platelets are low ($<50 \times 10^9$/L). Antifibrinolytic therapy can also be used judiciously.

Thrombosis

Heparin or antiplatelet drugs are used in those with thrombotic problems such as skin ischemia. There have been numerous trials of anticoagulants that have not demonstrated unequivocal benefits. Anti-fibrinolytics should not be used because of failure to lyse thrombi in organs such as the kidney.

Other systemic causes of acquired coagulopathy

Coagulopathy of critical illness

Patients admitted to intensive care commonly have abnormal coagulation. The earliest abnormality is elevated fibrinogen due to increased hepatic synthesis as part of interleukin-6

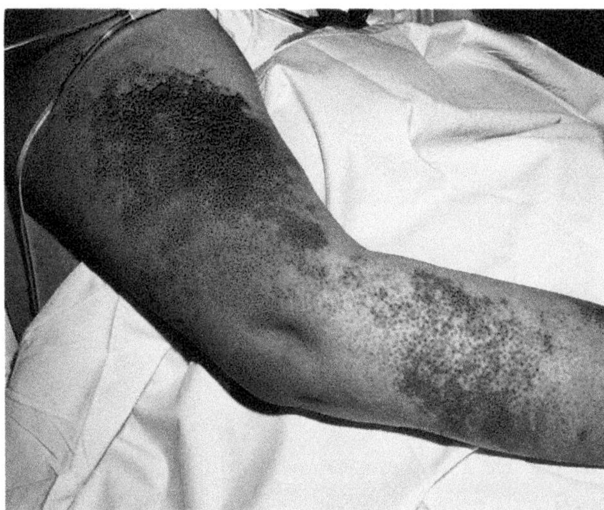

(a)

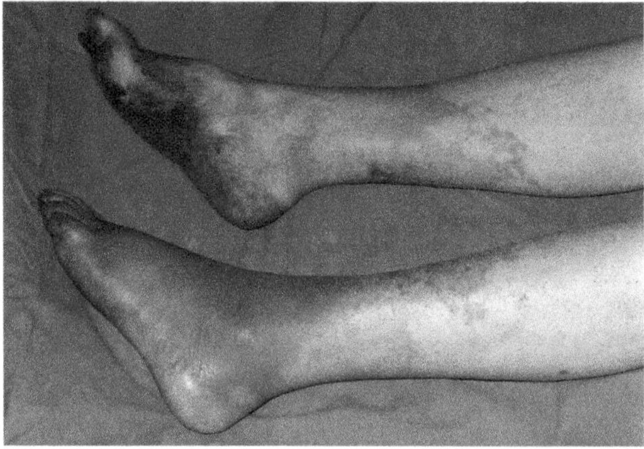

(b)

Figure 29.3 Clinical features of disseminated intravascular coagulation. **(a)** Indurated and confluent purpura of the arm. **(b)** Peripheral gangrene with swelling and discolouration of the skin of the feet in fulminant disease.

driven acute phase response. This is commonly followed by a prolongation of APTT due to the activation of FXII through multiple mechanisms. Prolonged APTT is more common than prolonged PT. The aetiology of coagulopathy of critical illness and DIC are almost similar; the distinction is the severity of the abnormalities. The prolonged APTT does not require treatment. It does influence the APTT ratio used for monitoring heparin infusions.

Massive transfusion syndrome (see also Chapter 33)

Many factors may contribute to the bleeding tendency following a massive transfusion. Blood loss results in reduced levels of platelets, coagulation factors and inhibitors. Further dilution of these factors occurs during replacement with red cells. Management is discussed next under trauma -induced coagulopathy.

Trauma-induced coagulopathy

Trauma-induced coagulopathy describes the abnormal coagulation seen with massive trauma and is a subset of DIC. **The trinity of hypothermia, acidosis and coagulopathy, the lethal triad of trauma, predicts high mortality**. The severity of the injury and resuscitation interventions contribute to the outcome.

Both tissue injury and shock with hypoperfusion contribute to this evolving coagulopathy. The widespread activation of endothelium, platelets and immune system impairs thrombin generation and platelet function. The impaired clot formation is further compromised by fibrinolysis. The coagulopathy in the early resuscitation phase is secondary to hypocoagulability, resulting in bleeding. This progresses to hypercoagulability, associated with thrombosis and multiorgan failure.

Treatment aims to stop blood loss and reverse the shock. Interventions include damage control surgery, haemostatic resuscitation and permissive hypotension (maintaining low blood pressure to decrease blood loss), all of which have improved outcomes. Various blood products can be used for restoring circulating blood volume, but there is no international consensus on the optimal transfusion components. Tranexamic acid has been used in pre-hospital settings.

1. **Red cells are given to replenish the lost blood.** For women under 50 years of unknown blood group, type O Rh− blood is given until the blood group is known. For males, O Rh+ is given initially. Red cell salvage is practised in some obstetric, trauma, cardiac and vascular centres.
2. **Platelet concentrates are given to maintain a platelet count above 50–75 × 10^9/L or 100 × 10^9/L in cerebral injury or after massive trauma.**
3. **The PT and APTT should be kept to less than 1.5 times normal, with FFP given initially at 15 mL/kg. It is usually necessary to give 4–6 units of FFP for every 6 units of red cells transfused. FFP is started early with red cell transfusion. Some protocols include a 1:1:1 ratio for red cells: platelet packs: FFP.**
4. **Cryoprecipitate or fibrinogen concentrate is given to keep fibrinogen above 1.5 g/L.** Trials of fibrinogen concentrates have been performed in obstetric emergencies and perioperative bleeding during cardiac surgery with good results.
5. **Intravenous tranexamic acid** can be given for bleeding.
6. Monitoring by platelet count, PT and fibrinogen level is essential to find the appropriate balance of different products. Near-patient and viscoelastic testing can also be used (p. 353). Viscoelastic testing is often used in conjunction with transfusion algorithms to help avoid over-transfusion.

Immunothrombosis

The relationship between inflammation and the development of thrombosis has gained prominence during the COVID-19 pandemic. Inflammation and thrombosis are interlinked processes that contribute to innate defence for containing pathogens. Immunothrombosis is recognized as an important thrombotic mechanism in some systemic disorders and infections. The key players are platelets and neutrophils, with secondary activation of complement and coagulation. Extensive activation of coagulation and complement results in thrombo-inflammation, manifesting as microvascular and macrovascular thrombosis.

Platelets have numerous immune receptors that recognize pathogen-associated molecular patterns on bacteria and other pathogens. This results in activation, degranulation and aggregation, trapping the pathogen. **Activated platelets release several substances that promote inflammation, coagulation and recruitment of neutrophils.** Interactions between platelets and neutrophils are orchestrated by their surface and secreted molecules. This includes surface molecule interactions between P-selectin on platelets and P-selectin glycoprotein ligand-1 on neutrophils, thus allowing for physical interactions between the cells.

Inflammation is also associated with endothelial dysfunction. This leads to the release of VWF and the expression of various adhesion molecules that recruit platelets, neutrophils and monocytes, resulting in platelet activation and aggregation. The glycocalyx is also perturbed, impairing the antithrombotic environment. **Tissue factor expressed on monocytes and macrophages stimulated by inflammatory cytokines may trigger coagulation and fibrin formation. Fibrinogen levels are also increased in inflammation.** Free protein S (a natural anticoagulant) levels are reduced due to the binding of protein S by complement C4b-binding protein, the levels of which rise during inflammation.

NETosis is an important pathogenic mechanism in many inflammatory disorders, infections, cancer, atherosclerosis and other diseases (Chapter 8). Targeting inflammation using the anti-interleukin-1β monoclonal antibody canakinumab has been shown to reduce recurrent cardiovascular events in those with a previous myocardial infarction and raised CRP. This further demonstrates the link between atherothrombosis and inflammation.

Heparin-induced thrombocytopenia

Heparin-induced thrombocytopenia (HIT) is a significant, unpredictable, adverse reaction to heparin that is immune-mediated. Thrombocytopenia can be accompanied by thrombosis (venous and arterial).

HIT is caused by pathological antibodies against platelet factor 4 (PF4) and heparin complexes. The mechanism of thrombocytopenia is shown in Fig. 29.4.

Clinical presentation

1 HIT is a disease of hospitalized patients who often have other causes for thrombocytopenia. It is is a clinicopathologic syndrome that needs to fulfil both laboratory and clinical criteria for diagnosis.
2 Clinical criteria include venous or arterial thrombosis and skin or acute systemic reactions after intravenous heparin.
3 The laboratory findings are:
   (a) Thrombocytopenia that occurs between 4 and 14 days after the start of heparin, the timing consistent with immune sensitization. It is typically moderate, with median counts of $60–70 \times 10^9/L$, but may be severe ($<20 \times 10^9/L$).
   (b) The detection of HIT antibodies confirms the diagnosis. These are detected by platelet activation or ELISA assays. Although less specific, ELISA is readily available. The concentration of HIT antibodies and clinical features confirm the diagnosis.
4 Pre-test probability assessment is undertaken before testing improves diagnostic accuracy. Criteria include the severity of thrombocytopenia, timing of thrombocytopenia in relation to heparin exposure, presence of thrombosis and other explanations for thrombocytopenia. Patients with low pre-test probability are not tested, while those with intermediate or high pre-test probability are tested for HIT antibodies.
5 The antibody tests are also helpful in ruling out a diagnosis when the clinical probability is low. Some patients develop antibodies but have no clinical features or thrombocytopenia.
6 Patients develop thrombosis concurrently, following thrombocytopenia, or, more rarely, before thrombocytopenia.
7 Risk factors for HIT include the use of unfractionated heparin rather than low-molecular-weight heparin; surgical patients; age > 40 years; female sex; and previous history of HIT.

Treatment

The risk of thrombosis in HIT is very high, with around half the patients developing thrombosis. Current guidelines recommend anticoagulation even in the absence of thrombosis.

The management of suspected HIT includes:

1 Immediate withdrawal of heparin anticoagulant
2 Clinical assessment for thrombosis
3 Imaging of the lower limb deep veins
4 Anticoagulation with intravenous (danaparoid, fondaparinux) or oral (rivaroxaban, apixaban) FXa inhibitors or with direct thrombin inhibitors (argatroban, bivalirudin, dabigatran). Patients must be anticoagulated with warfarin or other direct-acting oral anticoagulants for at least three months following parenteral intravenous anticoagulants.
5 High-dose intravenous immunoglobulin (IVIg) has been used to rapidly inhibit platelet activation, improving the platelet count and decreasing the thrombotic risk.

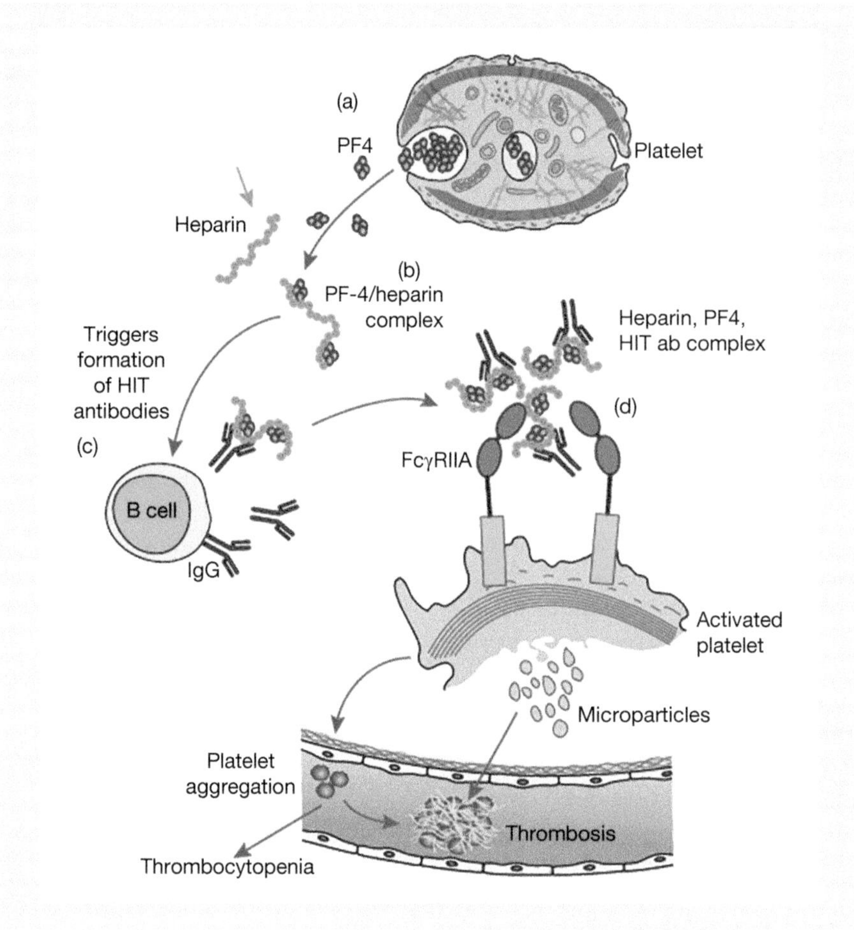

Figure 29.4 Heparin-induced thrombocytopenia (HIT). HIT is underpinned by the formation of antibodies against platelet factor 4 (PF4)–heparin complex. **(a)** PF4 is present in the alpha granules of platelets, released on activation. **(b)** PF4, a positively charged molecule, binds the negatively charged heparin. **(c)** The HIT antigen forms when heparin brings together two PF4 tetramers, uncovering new epitopes that stimulate HIT antibody development. **(d)** HIT antibody–heparin–PF4 complexes bind FcγRIIA receptors on platelets. This binding results in receptor clustering with platelet activation, thrombocytopenia and thrombosis.

Vaccine-induced immune thrombotic thrombocytopenia (VITT)

Vaccine-induced immune thrombotic thrombocytopenia (VITT) is a rare and severe complication of adenovirus-based COVID-19 vaccine. VITT diagnosis requires the following criteria:

1 A COVID-19 vaccine 4-42 days before symptom onset
2 Venous or arterial thrombosis, which can occur at uncommon sites such as cerebral and splanchnic vessels
3 Thrombocytopenia
4 Positive ELISA for PF4/heparin antibodies (certain assays only)
5 Elevated D-dimer levels

VITT resembles HIT, with some differences. VITT antibodies can form immune complexes with PF4 without heparin, and the complexes activate platelets through FcγRIIA receptors. In addition, these antibodies contribute to neutrophil activation and NETosis.

Patients are usually treated with immunoglobulin infusions to disrupt activation and anticoagulants to prevent or treat thrombosis. There is no indication for long-term anticoagulation.

COVID-19 (SARS-CoV-2) infection

The clinical and laboratory haematological findings in SARS-CoV-2 infection are described in Chapter 32. The infection is associated with a significantly increased risk of venous and, less commonly, arterial thrombosis. The pathophysiology is driven by endothelial injury, hypercoagulability and inflammation. Pulmonary thrombi in COVID-19 represent *de novo* thrombus formation, secondary to local inflammation and infection of endothelial cells. Autopsy studies have demonstrated that fibrin thrombi in alveolar capillaries are nine times more frequent in COVID-19 patients than in influenza patients, in whom post-capillary venule thrombosis is more common.

In addition, in COVID-19 infection, there is a high prevalence of deep vein thrombosis and pulmonary embolism. Multiple mechanisms contribute to hypercoagulability, including elevated VWF, FVIII and fibrinogen levels. Reduced thrombomodulin and ADAMTS13, with an altered VWF: ADAMTS13 ratio, also occur in severe disease. All abnormalities are more prominent in patients requiring ventilatory support. Meta-analysis shows a higher prevalence of venous thrombo- embolism (VTE), ischemic stroke and myocardial infarction in intensive care patients compared to ward patients.

Anticoagulation

Prophylactic anticoagulation is recommended in all hospitalized patients with acute COVID-19. Therapeutic anticoagulation with LMWH is recommended only for patients requiring oxygen and not on mechanical ventilation. Prophylactic anticoagulation is not needed in outpatients with COVID-19, except for patients with previous VTE.

Thrombotic microangiopathies (TMA)

Thrombotic microangiopathies (TMAs) are a heterogeneous group of syndromes with similar phenotype; the clinical triad of:

1. **Microangiopathic haemolytic anaemia (MAHA) (Chapter 6)**
2. **Thrombocytopenia**
3. **Ischemic organ damage due to microthrombi**

The disorders can be life-threatening due to varying degrees of end-organ ischemia/infarction. As the presenting symptoms are extremely varied, a high degree of suspicion is necessary to ensure relevant investigations that lead to the diagnosis.

Thrombotic thrombocytopenic purpura (TTP) and haemolytic uraemic syndrome (HUS) are the two most common TMAs. The disorders may be inherited or acquired and primary or secondary to other systemic disorders (Table 29.4).

Thrombotic thrombocytopenic purpura (TTP)

TTP is a rare thrombotic microangiopathic disorder characterized by inherited or acquired deficiency of ADAMTS13 (a disintegrin and metalloproteinase with a thrombospondin type 1 motif, member 13). ADAMTS13 is a VWF-cleaving protease that targets specific regions in the VWF A2 domain, decreasing the size of the ultra-large multimers secreted by the endothelium. Inherited or acquired deficiency results in the development of platelet thrombi in the microcirculation, rich in VWF with barely detectable fibrin (Fig. 29.5). Thrombi in large arterial and venous blood vessels

Table 29.4 Differential diagnosis of TMAs.

Primary thrombotic microangiopathies
Thrombotic thrombocytopenic purpura (TTP)
■ Congenital
■ Acquired
Haemolytic uraemic syndrome (HUS)
■ STEC- HUS (Shiga toxin-producing *Escherichia coli*)
■ Atypical
Secondary thrombotic microangiopathies
■ Malignant hypertension
■ Pregnancy-associated thrombotic microangiopathy, preeclampsia/ eclampsia and HELLP (haemolysis, elevated liver enzymes, low platelet count) syndrome
■ Drugs – immune (quinine, ticlopidine) and toxic (cyclosporine, tacrolimus)
■ Autoimmune disease, e.g. systemic lupus erythematosus, scleroderma-associated renal crisis, antiphospholipid syndrome
■ Transplantation, e.g. solid organ, haematopoietic stem cell
■ Infections, e.g. influenza, HIV, Epstein–Barr virus, parvovirus
■ Cancer

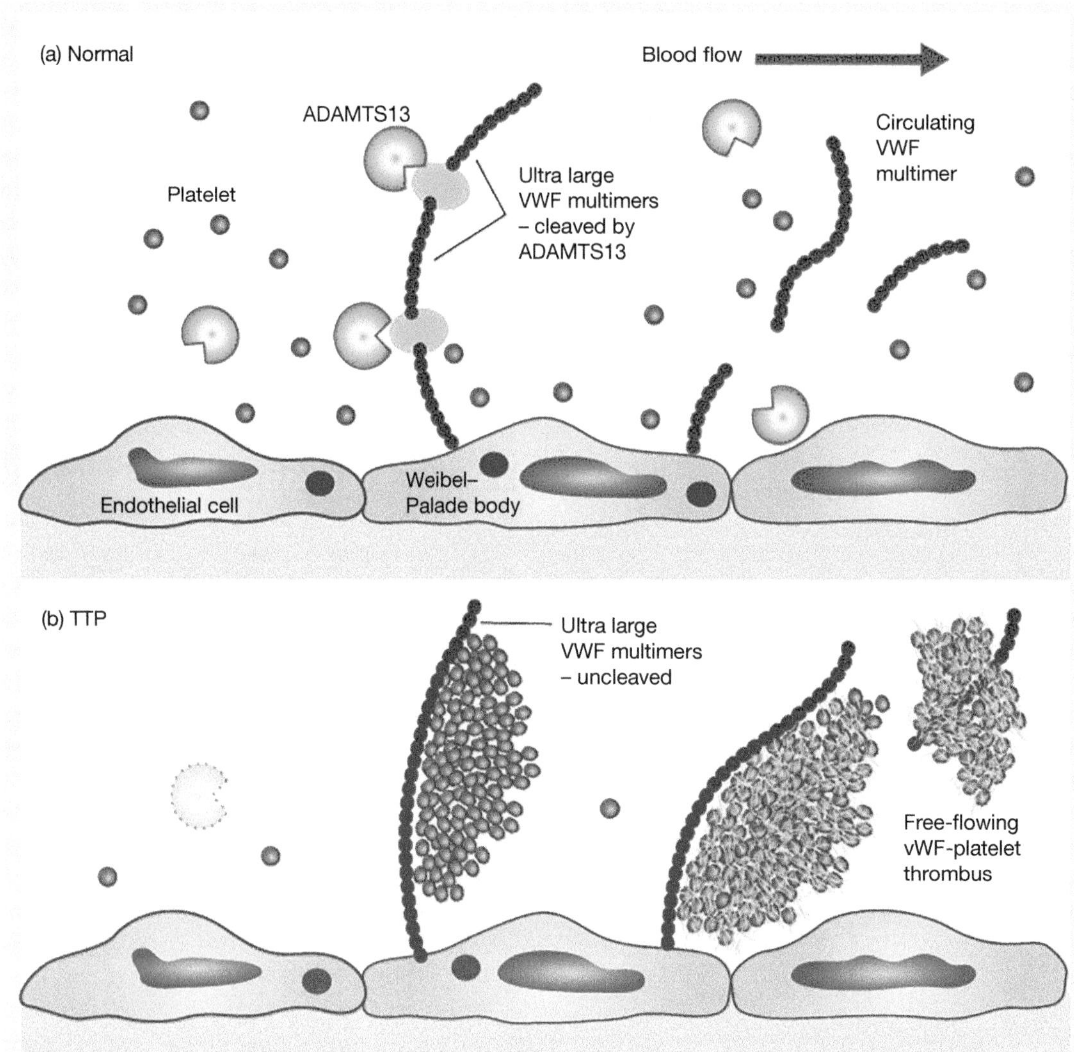

Figure 29.5 Pathogenesis of thrombotic thrombocytopenic purpura (TTP). **(a)** Ultra-large von Willebrand factor (VWF) multimers released from the Weibel–Palade bodies of the endothelial cells under normal flow are cleaved by ADAMTS13, a plasma VWF cleaving protease. **(b)** In TTP, deficiency of ADAMTS13 results in the generation of ultra-large VWF multimers that recruit platelets and result in the development of platelet-rich microthrombi. These microthrombi are responsible for organ ischemia and dysfunction.

are unusual. Microvascular thrombosis increases shear with consumptive thrombocytopenia, microangiopathic haemolytic anaemia (MAHA), ischemic organ damage and multiorgan failure (Fig. 29.6).

Congenital TTP

This is caused by homozygous or, more frequently, double heterozygous mutations in the *ADAMTS13* gene. It can present in infancy or adulthood during infections or pregnancy. Acute episodes are triggered by increased secretion of ultra-large VWF multimers. Clinical presentation is variable with respect to the severity of presentation, number of relapses and need for long-term prophylactic replacement therapy.

Acquired TTP (immune-mediated TTP)

Acquired TTP is secondary to autoantibodies that inactivate ADAMTS13. It can be idiopathic or, rarely, associated with infections, autoimmune disorders, drugs and organ transplantation. There is a higher prevalence in pregnancy and postpartum. Mortality of both TTP types was very high (80–90%) until plasma exchange was introduced. The disease continues to have high mortality, partly related to delay in diagnosis.

Clinical features

1 In severe cases, microvascular thrombi and organ dysfunction present with:
   (a) Fluctuating neurological symptoms (confusion, headache, paresis, seizures, aphasia, dysarthria and visual problems)

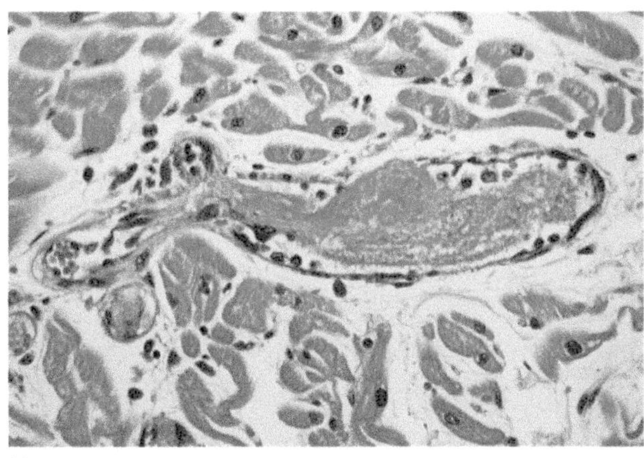

(a)

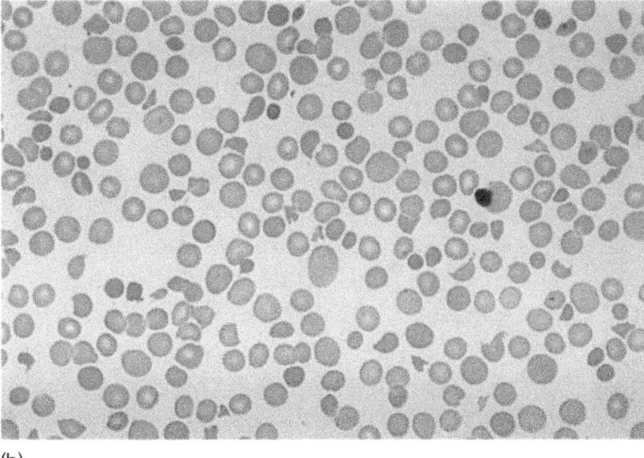

(b)

Figure 29.6 Thrombotic thrombocytopenic purpura. **(a)** Platelet thrombus in a small cardiac vessel with minor endothelial and inflammatory reaction. Source: Courtesy of Dr J.E. McLaughlin. **(b)** Peripheral blood film showing red cell fragmentation

  (b) Cardiac symptoms (chest pain, hypotension)
  (c) GI symptoms (abdominal pain, nausea)
2 Jaundice is frequent due to haemolysis and liver dysfunction
3 Renal failure is also a feature of severe disease, with multiple factors contributing.
4 Non-specific clinical features such as fatigue, nausea and fever.

Investigations

The presence of thrombocytopenia and MAHA is essential for the diagnosis of both congenital and acquired TTP. Platelet counts are low in the acute phase. Despite the pathogenesis, ultra-large VWF multimers are not consistently detected in patient plasma, probably due to trapping in the microvasculature.

1 Anaemia, with fragmented red cells (schistocytes) on blood film (Fig. 29.6)
2 Evidence of haemolysis - low haptoglobins, elevated LDH
3 Renal impairment
4 D-dimers are moderately elevated, with a normal coagulation screen.
5 ADAMTS13 activity is <10%
6 Demonstration of antibody against ADAMTS13
7 Typical HUS is distinguishable from TTP because of its diarrhoeal prodromes and more frequent and severe renal impairment (see below).

Treatment of acute episodes

1 **Replenish ADAMTS13 activity with therapeutic plasma exchange (TPE) using fresh frozen plasma (FFP), starting as soon as possible.** TPE should be continued until the platelet count is in the normal range for at least 3–4 days and the serum LDH is also normal.
2 **Inhibit the formation of platelet and VWF thrombi with caplacizumab,** a humanized anti-von Willebrand factor (VWF) antibody that binds the A1 domain of VWF (Chapter 26). VWF-platelet microthrombi formation is prevented through inhibition of the interaction between ultra-large VWF multimers and the platelet glycoprotein Ib-IX-V. It shortens the duration for restoring the platelet count to normal range, reducing the duration of TPE and potentially reducing mortality.
3 **Eradicate the inhibitor,** e.g. with prednisolone, rituximab (anti-CD20) and other immunosuppressive agents.
4 In at least one-third of cases, the disease recurs at varying intervals from the acute episode. Recurrences are more frequent during the first year and, in patients with persistently low levels of ADAMTS13, after the first remission.
5 Congenital TTP is managed by replacement therapy. FFP, specific intermediate-purity plasma-derived FVIII-VWF concentrates and recombinant preparations can be used.

Infection-associated haemolytic uraemic syndrome

Shiga-toxin-secreting *Escherichia coli* (STEC) causing HUS is the most common infection associated with TMA. It is mainly seen in children infected with Shiga toxin-secreting *Escherichia coli* O157:H7, although other infections have also been associated.

Clinical manifestations range from uncomplicated diarrhoea to haemorrhagic colitis and post-diarrheal HUS. The clinical picture is one of MAHA, thrombocytopenia and acute kidney injury, with neurological and cardiac involvement seen in severe forms. The disease is mediated by increased complement activation and membrane attack complex formation (Chapter 9), increased pro-inflammatory cytokines, endothelial injury and increased platelet and platelet-leucocyte aggregates, all of which support the development of microthrombi. Treatment is supportive and symptomatic.

Complement-mediated HUS

CM-HUS is a rare complement-mediated thrombotic microangiopathy characterized by MAHA, thrombocytopenia and acute kidney injury. It presents for the first time in children or adults. Unusual presentations include hypertension, isolated renal impairment and extrarenal complications. The primary differential diagnoses are TTP and infection associated HUS. Complement mediated HUS patients have ADAMTS 13 activity greater than 5% and are negative for Shiga toxin-producing infection. In this disorder, mutations in complement activators or regulators result in dysregulated activation of the alternative complement pathway with endothelial injury (Chapter 9). Triggering events, such as infection or pregnancy, can result in uninhibited, continuous activation of this pathway, resulting in a membrane attack complex responsible for endothelial injury and microthrombi, a presentation very apparent in renal glomeruli. Treatment is supportive, involving inhibition of complement with an anti-C5 monoclonal antibody (eculizumab or ravulizumab).

SUMMARY

- Acquired coagulation disorders are more common than inherited disorders. They can be due to isolated factor deficiencies, antithrombotic drugs, or secondary to systemic disorders.
- Acquired coagulation disorders are characterized by abnormal coagulation assays such as prolonged PT, APTT and thrombin clotting time.
- Acquired coagulation disorders can present with asymptomatic laboratory abnormalities or bleeding complicating procedures or spontaneous bleeding. Typically the bleeding tendency is of new onset and slowly progressive. More often, the bleeding tendency and laboratory abnormalities may complicate the clinical course of hospitalized patients.
- The most common isolated factor deficiency is acquired haemophilia A, followed by acquired von Willebrand syndrome.
- Disseminated intravascular coagulation (DIC) is a complication of many acute life-threatening disorders. It is characterized by the systemic activation of coagulation and platelets with widespread vascular endothelial damage, all contributing to organ dysfunction. The bleeding tendency in DIC is related to consumption and/or hyperfibrinolysis.
- Inflammation and thrombosis are interconnected processes that have a role in host defence. The interaction between neutrophils and platelets is increasingly recognized for its pathogenicity in inflammatory disorders and other thrombotic conditions, i.e. immunothrombosis.
- Heparin-induced thrombocytopenia (HIT) and thrombosis is an adverse immune reaction to heparin. Heparin binding to platelet factor 4 results in the exposure of neoantigens that trigger antibody formation (HITabs). The resulting immune complexes contribute to platelet activation and activation of other cells with thrombocytopenia and thrombosis.
- Vaccine-induced immune thrombotic thrombocytopenia (VITT) is a rare and severe complication of adenovirus-based COVID-19 vaccines, which resembles HIT. VITT antibodies can form immune complexes with PF4 without heparin. The complexes activate platelets with thrombosis.
- COVID-19 is associated with excess pulmonary intravascular thrombi, DVT and PE. The pathophysiology is a combination of endothelial injury, hypercoagulability and inflammation.
- Thrombotic microangiopathies (TMAs) are a heterogeneous group of syndromes with a similar phenotype: the clinical triad of microangiopathic haemolytic anaemia (MAHA), thrombocytopenia and ischemic organ damage due to microthrombi.
- Thrombotic thrombocytopenic purpura is a rare TMA characterized by inherited or acquired deficiency of a VWF-cleaving protease, ADAMTS13, which regulates the size of ultra-large VWF multimers secreted by the endothelium.
- Fresh frozen plasma is used to treat acquired coagulation disorders with multiple coagulation defects or specific defects if the appropriate concentrate is not available and for plasma exchange in the management of TTP.

Now visit **www.wiley.com/go/haematology9e** to test yourself on this chapter.

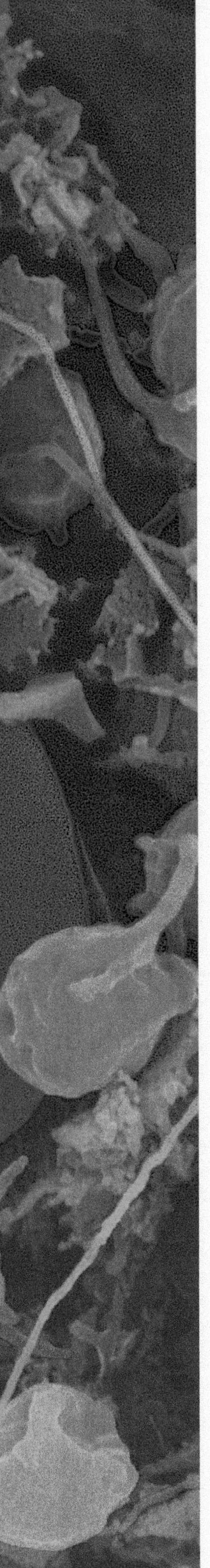

CHAPTER 30

Thrombosis 1: Pathogenesis and diagnosis

Key topics

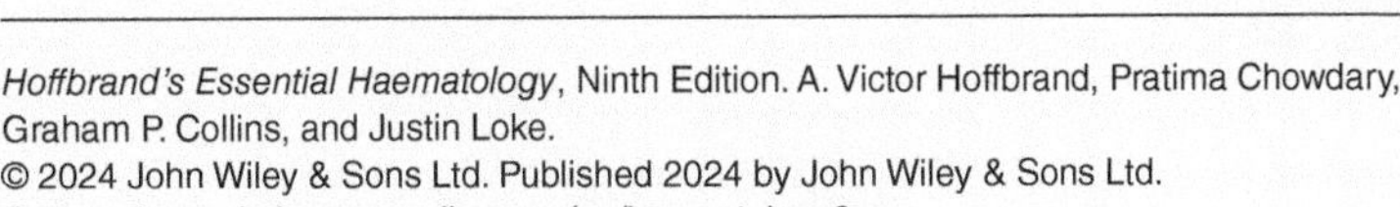

Hoffbrand's Essential Haematology, Ninth Edition. A. Victor Hoffbrand, Pratima Chowdary, Graham P. Collins, and Justin Loke.

© 2024 John Wiley & Sons Ltd. Published 2024 by John Wiley & Sons Ltd.

Companion website: www.wiley.com/go/haematology9e

Introduction

Thrombosis is the clotting of blood within the vasculature in the absence of injury, i.e. pathological. Thrombosis can affect the vascular tree at any level, including major arteries, arterioles, capillaries, large veins and venules. Pathological thrombi can cause occlusion of the blood supply, resulting in end-organ damage through ischemia or symptoms secondary to proximal congestion. The thrombus can embolize to a distal organ, leading to vascular occlusion. Thrombosis and thrombotic emboli are leading causes of disability and death.

Pathological thrombosis is categorized by location as venous (often in the legs and called deep venous thrombosis, DVT), arterial, intracardiac or microcirculation. When venous thrombi break and migrate to the lungs, they obstruct the pulmonary arterial tree, i.e. pulmonary embolism (PE). Arterial thrombosis includes myocardial infarction and cerebrovascular thrombosis. Intracardiac blood clots in the atria and ventricles can lead to systemic embolism, potentially causing strokes and other ischemic events.

Pathological thrombosis requires the interaction of cellular and molecular components (biochemical), as well as contributions from blood flow (biophysical).

Venous and arterial thrombi differ in composition. Arterial thrombi, also known as white thrombi, are composed mainly of platelets. Venous thrombi are rich in red cells and fibrin and are called red thrombi (Fig. 26.1). Thrombosis of small blood vessels and microcirculation is primarily observed in the context of inflammation.

Blood flow not only brings together the necessary components for clot formation but also helps remove excess factors, thereby localizing the clot formation. Physiological flow is laminar, with maximal velocity in the centre of the vessel lumen with minimal to no movement adjacent to the vessel wall. Under conditions of normal haematocrit, the red cells tend to converge in the centre, and platelets marginate towards the vessel wall. This creates a plasma layer adjacent to endothelial cells, rich in platelets, facilitating their binding to adhesive ligands at the sites of vascular damage.

Blood flow varies throughout the vascular tree due to its pulsatile nature and complex vessel geometry. Blood flow also exerts forces on the vessel wall and blood cells, which affect the dynamics, structure and stability of blood clots. Under normal physiological conditions, the wall shear rates in the large arteries range from 300–800 s^{-1}, 15–200 s^{-1} in veins and 450–1,600 s^{-1} in microarterioles.

Pathophysiological mechanisms of thrombosis

The pathophysiological mechanisms underlying arterial and venous thrombosis can be categorised into three groups; the Virchow's triad, described by Rudolf Virchow in the 19th Century. These are altered blood flow, increased coagulation (hypercoagulability) and vessel wall damage.

Altered blood flow/stasis

Obstruction to flow due to vessel wall narrowing or diseased heart valves disrupts the laminar flow and causes turbulence. Turbulence increases contact between cellular components and the vessel wall, triggering platelet adhesion and activation. Increased shear forces on the vessel wall can activate endothelium and release von Willebrand factor (VWF) and FVIII from the endothelium. Stasis leads to the accumulation of factors and platelets, creating a nidus for clot formation.

Indeed, DVT in leg veins starts in the valve sinus behind the valve leaflets. Stiffness of the valve, abnormal flow through the vessel, hypoxia and shear stress can result in dysfunctional endothelium or accumulation of the procoagulants, platelets and leucocytes in the sinus, facilitating the initial development of deep vein thrombosis.

Hypercoagulability

This refers to alterations in cellular and molecular components of blood that increase the tendency of blood clot formation (prothrombotic state) in the absence of injury or other provoking factors. Thrombophilia is a term used to describe a group of inherited or acquired hypercoagulable disorders that persist over time and increase the risk of developing thrombosis. Temporary hypercoagulability is common and related to transient risk factors, e.g. during hospitalization and pregnancy.

Vessel wall damage/endothelial injury

Intact endothelium acts as a physical barrier between the blood and the subendothelial matrix. Normally, the endothelium displays antithrombotic properties (Fig. 26.14); however, this can be impaired by physical disruption, inflammation, or infection.

Increased coagulability of the blood and changes in blood flow (e.g. stasis in the legs due to immobility) are the main factors that contribute to venous thrombosis, while vessel wall damage or dysfunction is more pertinent in arterial thrombosis. However, vessel wall damage may be significant in patients with sepsis, in-dwelling catheters and scarring from previous thrombosis.

Venous thrombosis

Epidemiology

Venous thromboembolism (VTE) which includes DVT and PE is a major worldwide cause of morbidity and mortality with an annual incidence of 1-2 events per 1000 person-years. Globally, VTE is the third most common cardiovascular cause of death after coronary heart disease and ischemic stroke. It is more common in men than women, and the incidence increases with age, particularly after 55 years. Deep vein thrombosis commonly occurs in the lower extremities, with around half of the patients affected by pulmonary embolism, which may or may not be symptomatic. Pulmonary embolism is fatal in approximately 10% of acute cases; most deaths occur within the first few hours of symptom onset.

Risk factors

VTE is a multifactorial disease. Risk factors for VTE can be categorized by the nature of the risk (Table 30.1) as genetic or related to patient characteristics and comorbidities and by strength of risk factor (Table 30.2). **VTE is considered provoked in the presence of transient risk factors and unprovoked when there are no apparent transient risk factors.**

Table 30.1 Risk factors for venous thromboembolism categorized by nature of risk.

Patient characteristics and life style
- Older age
- Male sex
- Pregnancy and post partum
- Obesity
- Strenuous work (arm thrombosis)
- Sedentary life style

Genetic risk factors
- Coagulation
  - Factor V Leiden
  - Prothrombin G20210A variant
  - Antithrombin deficiency
  - Protein C deficiency
  - Protein S deficiency
  - Dysfibrinogenaemia
  - Non-O blood group
- Platelet
- Endothelial
- Family history of thrombosis
- Others

Medications
- Combined oral contraceptive pill
- Oral hormone replacement therapy
- *In vitro* fertilisation
- Chemotherapeutic agents (thalidomide, pegylated asparaginase)
- Steroids
- Heparin induced thrombocytopenia
- Vaccine induced thrombocytopenia
- Erythropoiesis stimulating agents

Environmental
- Hospitalisation
- Intravascular catheters
- Prolonged seated immobility (work related or computer related)
- Prolonged immobility – bed rest >3 days
- Long haul travel 6 hours or longer (sedation, alcohol)

Medical
- Cancer
- Myeloproliferative disorders
- Paroxysmal nocturnal haemoglobinuria
- Autoimmune disorders – acute flare
- Antiphospholipid syndrome
- Heart failure and respiratory failure
- Paralytic stroke
- Chronic renal impairment
- Nephrotic syndrome
- Cushing syndrome
- Infection (intraabdominal, oral, systemic, pneumonia)
- COVID-19
- Immobility (bedrest, neurologic, plaster cast)

Surgical
- Major surgery
- Trauma/injury, especially of legs/spine
- Lower limb orthopaedic surgery (hip joint replacement > knee joint replacement)
- Plaster cast of legs
- Neurosurgery
- Indwelling catheter
- Prostatectomy
- Varicose veins
- Following major haemorrhage
- Structural abnormalities of the venous system

Source: Adapted from J.A. Heit (2015) *Nature Rev. Cardiol.* 2: 464–74. P.L. Lutsey, N.A. Zakai (2023) *Nature Rev. Cardiol.* 20: 248–62. F.A. Anderson Jr, F.A. Spencer (2003) *Circulation* 107: 1–9. S.V. Konstantinides *et al.* (2020) Task force of European Society of Cardiology and European Respiratory Society. *Eur. Heart J.* 41: 543–603. UK National Institute of Clinical Excellence guidelines on VTE (NG 158, 2020; NG 89, 2018).

The aim of identifying risk factors is to facilitate subsequent risk reduction through pharmacological, e.g. anticoagulants, and non-pharmacological means, e.g. mechanical calf compression and lifestyle changes. In determining whether risk reduction is indicated, either lifelong or during and after periods of increased risk, it is important to consider the strength of individual risk factors and the cumulative effect of all risk factors. In rare instances of severe hypercoagulability, VTE can present early in life.

Table 30.2 Venous thrombosis risk factors categorized by the magnitude of risk.

Strong risk factor (odds ratio >10)
- Fracture of lower limb
- Spinal cord injury
- Major trauma
- Major surgery (especially abdomino-pelvic cancer surgery, hip and knee replacement)
- Hospitalization for heart failure or atrial fibrillation (within previous 3 months)
- Myocardial infarction (within previous 3 months)
- Paroxysmal nocturnal haemoglobinuria
- Antiphospholipid syndrome
- Heparin-induced thrombocytopenia
- Previous VTE

Moderate risk factor (odds ratio 2-9)
- Arthroscopic knee surgery
- Autoimmune diseases
- Inflammatory bowel disease
- Postpartum period
- Systemic oestrogen therapy (oral contraceptive and hormone replacement therapy)
- Paralytic stroke
- Myeloproliferative neoplasms
- Congestive heart and respiratory failure
- Intravascular catheters (central venous lines, peripherally inserted venous catheters)
- Hospitalization (for the next 90 days)
- Nephrotic syndrome
- COVID- 19
- Chemotherapy
- Blood transfusions
- Erythropoiesis stimulating agents
- Malignancy (highest with metastatic disease)
- Previous superficial vein thrombosis
- Hereditary thrombophilia
- Non-O ABO blood group
- Deep vein thrombosis in a first-degree relative (especially if unprovoked)
- Infections (specifically intraabdominal, oral, systemic, lower respiratory tract and HIV)

Weak risk factors (odds ratio < 2)
- Prolonged immobility (bed rest > 3 days)
- Long haul travel (6 hours or longer)
- Laparoscopic surgery
- Varicose veins
- Age
- Obesity
- Chronic inflammation
- Cigarette smoking
- Diabetes and hypertension
- Pregnancy

Variable
- Extravascular compression of pelvic veins, e.g. by large fibroids or other masses
- Hyperviscosity
- Secondary polycythaemia
- Dehydration
- Raised plasma levels of factor VIII
- Raised plasma levels of fibrinogen
- Raised plasma levels of homocysteine (uncertain)

Source: F.A. Anderson Jr, F.A. Spencer (2003) *Circulation* 107: 1–9. S.V. Konstantinides *et al.* (2020) *Eur. Heart J.* 41: 543–603. UK National Institute of Clinical Excellence guidelines on VTE (NG 158, 2020; NG 89, 2018).

Genetic variants associated with venous thrombosis

The prevalence of inherited disorders associated with an increased risk of thrombosis (heritable thrombophilia) is higher than that of hereditary bleeding disorders. Approximately a third of VTE patients have an identifiable heritable thrombophilia. This may include deficiency of antithrombin, protein C or protein S, or the common variants affecting factor (F)V or prothrombin (Table 30.1). The prevalence of thrombophilia among patients with VTE is related to age and ethnicity, with approximately half the patients younger than 20 demonstrating thrombophilia. This decreases to a fifth in patients older than 70 years. Caucasians also have a higher prevalence of heritable thrombophilia.

VTE frequently results from gene-environment interaction. Most patients with heritable thrombophilia do not develop VTE. In those who develop VTE, frequently there are other acquired risk factors. Therefore, the presence of heritable thrombophilia per se is not an indication for therapeutic anticoagulation. However, it should prompt the physician to minimize additional acquired risk factors. Appropriate pharmacologic thromboprophylaxis should be considered for these patients during high-risk periods such as pregnancy, hospitalization, surgery and long-distance travel.

Factor V Leiden mutation

The most commonly inherited thrombophilia is a point mutation of the *F5* gene eliminating one of three cleavage sites in FV and FVa proteins (Fig. 30.1). The pattern of inheritance is autosomal dominant, with incomplete penetrance. Prevalence is approximately 3–7% of the white population, lower in Asian, African and Hispanic populations. Diagnosis is by molecular techniques or coagulation assays (which can result in false positive results).

Heterozygosity for factor V Leiden is associated with a four to five-fold increased risk of VTE, and 5–10% develop thrombosis during their lifetime. Homozygous individuals have an

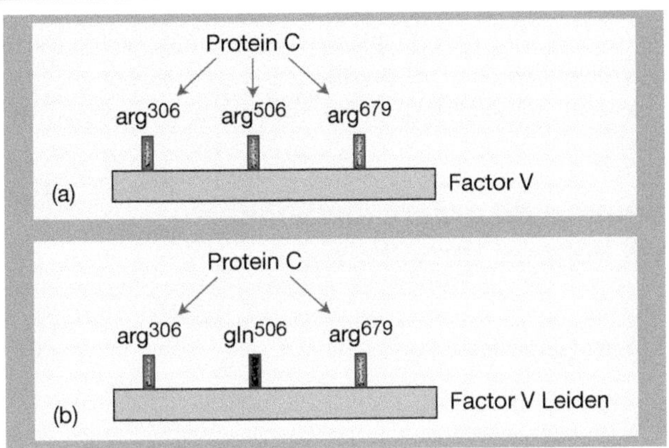

Figure 30.1 Genetic basis of factor V Leiden (FV Arg506Gln). **(a)** Activated protein C (APC) inactivates FVa by proteolytic cleavage at three arginine sites in the FVa heavy chain. **(b)** FV Leiden, a single-point mutation in the FV gene (guanine to adenine at nucleotide 1691), leads to a single amino acid change (replacement of arginine with glutamine at amino acid 506). This abolishes the Arg506 cleavage site for activated protein C in FV and FVa. This slows the rate of FVa inactivation by activated protein C (APC), prompting a state of 'activated protein C resistance'

11–80-fold increased risk, with lower estimates reported in more recent studies.

Prothrombin allele G20210A

Prothrombin gene mutation in the 3′ untranslated region results in a G to A change at nucleotide 20210. The change results in a 30% increase in prothrombin levels in heterozygous individuals, with most having prothrombin levels >115%, i.e. in the highest quartile. Prevalence is 1–3% of the white population and less common in African and Asian population. Heterozygosity is associated with a 3- to 4-fold increased risk of VTE, higher in the homozygous state. Molecular techniques are used for diagnosis.

Compound heterozygosity for FV Leiden and prothrombin G20210A is associated with a 20-fold increased risk.

Antithrombin deficiency

Antithrombin (AT) is a serine protease inhibitor (SERPIN) synthesized by the liver that irreversibly inactivates all active serine proteases (Chapter 26).

Congenital deficiency is autosomal dominant in inheritance with variable penetrance; the homozygous state is incompatible with life. AT deficiency may be type 1 (quantitative, reduced antigen and activity) or type II (qualitative, reduced activity and normal antigen), with mutations affecting the thrombin-binding or heparin-binding sites (less risk of thrombosis). Population prevalence is 0.02-0.6% and associated with an 8- to 16-fold increased risk of VTE. The risk appears to associated with the type of mutation and some mutations result in thrombosis in all affected individuals.

Diagnosis is by molecular techniques, activity and antigen assays. Low AT may result in heparin resistance, but most patients are managed with standard anticoagulation. Antithrombin concentrates are restricted to high-risk patients during surgery or childbirth when anticoagulation needs to be interrupted. It is also used if heparin monitoring assays identify evidence of heparin resistance.

Acquired AT deficiency is due to decreased synthesis (liver disease, pegylated asparaginase), increased renal excretion (nephrotic syndrome) or increased consumption (disseminated intravascular coagulation (DIC), heparin).

Protein C deficiency

Protein C inactivates cofactors FVa and FVIIIa and is one of the physiologic anticoagulants (Chapter 26).

Protein C is a vitamin K-dependent serine protease synthesized by the liver. Congenital deficiency is autosomal dominant in inheritance with variable penetrance. Population prevalence is 0.2–0.5%, with a 4- to 7-fold increase in the risk of VTE. Deficiency can be type I (quantitative) or II (qualitative). Diagnosis is by molecular techniques, activity and antigen assays.

Children born with severe deficiency due to homozygous mutations present with neonatal purpura fulminans. It presents as a purpuric rash due to small vessel thrombosis, progressing to a haemorrhagic rash due to necrosis and DIC. Treatment is with protein C concentrate, and lifelong prophylaxis is indicated. Heterozygous patients may develop skin necrosis due to dermal vessel occlusion caused by rapid reduction in protein C when started on warfarin alone. A similar complication has been noted even in the absence of inherited deficiency when treated with warfarin without concurrent heparin (page 424).

Acquired protein C deficiency can be due to decreased synthesis (liver disease, vitamin K deficiency and warfarin) or increased consumption (sepsis, DIC.)

Protein S deficiency

Protein S acts as a cofactor for APC and contributes to the inactivation of FVa and FVIIIa (Chapter 26). It also directly inhibits prothrombinase and tenase independent of its APC cofactor function.

Protein S is a vitamin K-dependent anticoagulant glycoprotein synthesized in the liver, endothelial cells and megakaryocytes. It exists in bound and free states in plasma, with 60-70% bound to C4b-binding protein (C4bBP). The remaining PS circulates as free-form (free PS), the biologically active form functioning as cofactor to APC.

Congenital deficiency is autosomal dominant in inheritance with variable penetrance. The population prevalence is difficult to estimate as variants do not always contribute to deficiency. It is associated with a 5- to 7-fold increase in the risk of VTE. Three types of assays are used for assessing PS levels: free PS activity (functional assay), free PS antigen (ELISA) and total PS (ELISA). Diagnosis of deficiency and classification is influenced by the measurement of different fractions of protein S. PS deficiency can be type I (quantitative), type II (qualitative), or type III (reduced free protein S but normal total protein S). The clinical features of protein S deficiency are similar to those of protein C deficiency. These include a tendency to skin necrosis with warfarin and neonatal purpura fulminans in those with homozygous mutations and severe deficiency.

Acquired protein S deficiency is seen with pregnancy and contraception (mechanisms incompletely understood), decreased synthesis (liver disease, vitamin K deficiency, warfarin) and increased consumption (DIC). Low levels have been seen with HIV and other inflammatory conditions due to increased C4bBP levels.

Defects of fibrinogen

Thrombosis is often seen in patients with congenital dysfibrinogenaemias, occasionally with congenital afibrinogenemia, and unusual in hypofibrinogenemias. The pathophysiology is likely due to resistance of certain dysfibrinogenaemias to cleavage by plasmin. Rarely, it may be caused by enhanced thrombin generation and platelet aggregation. Routine testing for dysfibrinogenaemia is not indicated in patients with venous or arterial thrombosis.

ABO blood group

Non-O blood group individuals have a higher risk of VTE than those of group O. This is related to elevated VWF and FVIII plasma levels (25–30% higher), although other mechanisms may contribute. Blood group demonstrates an additive effect to FV Leiden and prothrombin G20210 variant in the general population.

Family history of thrombosis

History of unprovoked DVT in a first-degree relative increases individual risk of DVT, even if no known genetic predisposition can be identified.

Hyperhomocysteinaemia

Homocysteine is derived from dietary methionine. It is removed through methylation, to methionine (Fig. 5.3) or through conversion to cysteine via a trans-sulfuration pathway. Classic homocystinuria is a rare autosomal recessive disorder caused by cystathionine beta-synthase (CBS) deficiency, the enzyme responsible for trans-sulfuration. Vascular disease and thrombosis are significant features of CBS deficiency. These are accompanied by other manifestations, including cognitive abnormalities.

Methylenetetrahydrofolate reductase (MTHFR) is involved in the methylation of tetrahydrofolate (THF) to methyl-THF, the methyl donor for the synthesis of methionine from homocysteine (Fig. 5.3). A common thermolabile MTHFR variant is present in up to 25% of the global population, but is not associated with venous thrombosis.

Acquired risk factors for hyperhomocysteinaemia include deficiency of vitamin B6, folate, drugs (e.g. ciclosporin), chronic renal disease and smoking. Risk levels also increase with age and are higher in men and post-menopausal females. Mild hyperhomocysteinaemia is not associated with VTE. Two meta-analyses indicate that the risk of VTE is increased two to three-fold **only** in patients with homocysteine levels greater than two standard deviations above the mean. The role of elevated homocysteine in arterial events is discussed on page 415.

Acquired disorders associated with venous thrombosis

These are more common than inherited disorders, with many being strong risk factors.

Age

Several physiological changes contribute to hypercoagulability in older age, such as an increase in coagulation factors (e.g. VWF, FVIII, FIX, fibrinogen), enhanced platelet activity and reduced fibrinolytic activity. These changes are accompanied by elevated IL-6 and CRP levels, indicating an inflammatory state and underlying endothelial dysfunction.

Hereditary or acquired disorders of haemostasis

High plasma FVIII or fibrinogen levels are also associated with venous thrombosis, although the association is weak. This might be an age-related reactive phenomenon. No genetic mechanisms for increased FVIII or fibrinogen levels have been identified.

Pregnancy and oestrogen therapy

Pregnancy and puerperium are major risk factors for VTE. VTE is one of the top ten causes of death in pregnancy worldwide. A pregnant woman is four times more likely to experience VTE than a non-pregnant woman. The raised oestrogen levels are associated with increased levels of fibrinogen, factors II, VII, VIII and X, VWF and a decline in protein S. Fibrinolysis is inhibited by elevated levels of PAI-1 and PAI-2 produced by placenta and α2-macroglobulin (Chapter 26). These changes enable brisk generation of thrombin and blood clot that is resistant to fibrinolysis, ensuring stable haemostasis after placental separation.

Pregnancy is also associated with venous dilatation and compression of the intra-abdominal veins by the gravid uterus, resulting in venous stasis. The risk is equally raised in all three trimesters and increased further in the puerperium. High-risk women are offered antepartum prophylaxis. This includes patients with heritable thrombophilia, medical comorbidities or previous thrombosis.

Oestrogen based combined oral contraceptive pill and oral hormone replacement therapy (HRT) are also associated with an increased risk of VTE in women. The risk is significantly lower with progestogen-only contraception or topical or transdermal HRT. Women considered at high risk of VTE due to other risk factors or with a strong family history of VTE are advised to use non-oestrogen based contraception. In the case of HRT, topical or transdermal preparations have not been associated with any excess risk of thrombosis. Routine testing for hereditary thrombophilia before commencing either treatment is not advised.

Postoperative venous thrombosis

Surgery is another major risk factor for VTE (Table 30.2). The risk is greatest in the first 6 weeks after surgery but remains elevated up to 12 weeks. The risk is highest with orthopaedic lower limb surgery (especially total joint replacements), abdomino-pelvic and cancer surgery. Elasticated stockings, mechanical compression and pharmacological prophylaxis are used to reduce the risk of DVT. With joint replacements, patients are routinely discharged on thromboprophylaxis for one to four weeks (Chapter 31).

Hospital-acquired thrombosis

Hospital-acquired thrombosis (HAT) is responsible for up to 50% of cases of VTE and is a significant cause of preventable morbidity and mortality. HAT is now regularly defined as VTE occurring within 90 days of hospitalization, and multiple risk factors are common. In most institutions, patients are reviewed at admission for VTE risk factors, and those at high risk are given pharmacological thromboprophylaxis, usually with low-molecular-weight heparin unless contraindicated. Multiple risk assessment algorithms are available that help determine the thrombosis and bleeding risk; an example is given in Fig. 30.2.

Risk assessment for venous thromboembolism - to be completed for all patients at admission.
Patients to be reassessed within 24hrs and whenever the clinical condition changes

Assess all patients admitted to hospital for level of mobility

☐ Surgical patient ☐ Medical patient expected to have ongoing reduced mobility relatve to normal state ☐ Medical patient NOT expected to have significantly reduced mobility relative to normal state

Assess for thrombosis and bleeding risk
Any tick for THROMBOSIS RISK should prompt thromboprophylaxis
Any tick for BLEEDING RISK should prompt clinical staff to consider if bleeding risk is sufficient to preclude pharmacological intervention

Thrombosis risk:

Patient related
- ☐ Active cancer or cancer treatment
- ☐ Age > 60
- ☐ Dehydration
- ☐ Known thrombophilias
- ☐ Obesity (BMI >30 kg/m²)
- ☐ One or more significant medical comorbidities (e.g. heart disease; metabolic, endocrine or respiratory pathologies; acute infectious diseases: inflammatory conditions)
- ☐ Personal history or first-degree relative with a history of VTE
- ☐ Use of hormone replacement therapy
- ☐ Use of oestrogen-containing contraceptive therapy
- ☐ Varicose veins with phlebitis
- ☐ Pregnancy or < 6 weeks post partum (see NICE guidance for specific risk factors)

Admission related
- ☐ Significantly reduced mobility for 3 days or more
- ☐ Hip or knee replacement
- ☐ Hip fracture
- ☐ Total anaesthetic + surgical time > 90 minutes
- ☐ Surgery involving pelvis or lower limb with a total anaesthetic + surgical time > 60 minutes
- ☐ Acute surgical admission with inflammatory or intra-abdominal condition
- ☐ Critical care admission
- ☐ Surgery with significant reduction in mobility

Bleeding risk:

Patient related
- ☐ Active bleeding
- ☐ Acquired bleeding disorders, e.g. acute liver failure
- ☐ Concurrent use of anticoagulants known to increase the risk of bleeding, e.g. Warfarin with INR >2
- ☐ Acute stroke
- ☐ Thrombocytopaenia (platelets< 75x10^{9}/l)
- ☐ Uncontrolled systolic hypertension (230/120 mmHg or higher)
- ☐ Untreated inherited bleeding disorders, e.g. haemophilia and von Willebrand disease

Admission related
- ☐ Neurosurgery, spinal surgery or eye surgery
- ☐ Other procedure with high bleeding risk
- ☐ Lumbar puncture/epidural/spinal anaesthesia within the previous 4 hours
- ☐ Lumbar puncture/epidural/spinal anaesthesia expected within the next 12 hours

Assessment at admission Date:
Doctor sign:

Assessment post 24 hours Date:
Doctor sign:

Figure 30.2 Risk assessment tool for venous thromboembolism to evaluate the risk-benefit for the use of pharmacological (anticoagulants) thromboprophylaxis. The above algorithm was adapted from the UK National Institute for Health and Care Excellence guideline, NG89 (2018).

Cancer-associated thrombosis (CAT)

CAT accounts for 20–30% of all reported VTE. Occasionally, venous thrombosis may be the first manifestation of an underlying cancer. CAT is multifactorial, with both cancer and interventions contributing to the pathogenesis. The risk of CAT is heterogeneous and influenced by the following:

a Patient-related characteristics (including demographics and underlying comorbidities)
b Disease-specific (including type and stage of cancer)
c Treatment-related factors (including cancer surgery, radiotherapy, central venous access devices, hormonal treatments or specific chemotherapy agents).

The highest thrombotic risk has been observed with cancers of the pancreas, stomach and primary brain tumours. Similarly, the risk is higher with regional and disseminated disease than with local disease. CAT can contribute to mortality, representing an adverse prognostic marker unrelated to the type, stage of cancer and risk of VTE.

Abnormalities seen in patients with CAT include thrombocytosis and elevated fibrinogen secondary to increased IL-6; platelet activation; elevated VWF levels; and increased tissue factor (TF) expression by monocytes, all of which increase thrombin generation and clot formation. Leucocytosis with neutrophilia generates neutrophil extracellular traps (Chapter 8) and proteases, which contribute to endothelial glycocalyx degradation. Cancer cells also directly express TF, released into circulation, with increased FXII activators and PAI-1 levels.

Chemotherapy drugs can also contribute to thrombosis, with many mediating thrombogenicity by more than one mechanism. Drugs can decrease anticoagulants (L-asparaginase), increase procoagulants (oestrogen receptor modulators), activate platelets (immunomodulatory agents and checkpoint inhibitors), activate endothelium: (anthracylines and platinum-based agents) and contribute to endothelial dysfunction (anti-VEGF molecules).

Ambulatory outpatients with active cancer can be assessed for risk of VTE using several risk stratification scores. For example, the Khorana score (**www.mdcalc.com**) can be used for assessing thrombosis risk and the need for prophylactic anticoagulation. It is essential to exclude risk factors for bleeding.

Blood disorders

a **Myeloproliferative neoplasms (MPN) demonstrate, in many cases an activating somatic point mutation of the *JAK2* gene (*JAK2-V617F*) (Chapter 15). The mutation is associated with an increased risk of thrombosis not seen with *CALR* mutations that can also cause MPN.** The risk appears to be related to neutrophil activation. Testing for the *JAK2 V617F* mutation should be considered in patients with unexplained significant venous and arterial thrombosis, with or without a suggestive blood count. **All patients with splanchnic vein thrombosis should be screened for this mutation.**
b **Haemolytic anaemias,** especially with intravascular haemolysis, are also associated with an increased risk of VTE due to increased exposure of anionic phospholipids, such as phosphatidylserine and free haemoglobin, which promotes coagulation. Importantly, free haemoglobin can also elicit an inflammatory reaction.
c **Sickle cell disease** contributes to an increased risk of venous thrombosis due to microvascular occlusions, endothelial injury, exposure to phosphatidylserine and pro-inflammatory milieu.
d **Paroxysmal nocturnal haemoglobinuria** is also associated with an increased risk of VTE (Chapter 24). Intravascular haemolysis causes the release of free haemoglobin, procoagulant microparticles and increased complement. This, with the associated pro-inflammatory state, deficiency of GPI-anchored anticoagulants and impaired fibrinolysis, leads to venous thrombosis or, less commonly, arterial thrombosis. PNH should be considered where there are unexplained cytopenias, evidence of biochemical haemolysis and thrombosis, particularly at atypical locations such as cerebral or splanchnic vascular beds.
e **Hyperproteinaemic states such as myeloma and Waldenström macroglobulinaemia** can lead to hyperviscosity when paraprotein levels are high and contribute to thrombosis. Thalidomide and, less so, lenalidomide are associated with thrombosis.
f **Splenectomy**, especially if the elevated platelet count persists, is also associated with an increased risk of venous thrombosis.

Renal disease and nephrotic syndrome

The risk of VTE is increased across the spectrum of renal disorders, including patients with mild renal impairment, nephrotic syndrome, renal transplant and dialysis. Pathophysiologic mechanisms include endothelial and monocyte activation, impaired endothelial thrombomodulin and protein C activity, and increased plasma fibrinogen, FVII, VWF and FVIII levels. There is an impairment of platelet function, but the overall balance leans towards thrombosis. Nephrotic syndrome is peculiarly associated with renal vein thrombosis, partly related to loss of AT and hypoalbuminaemia is an important predictor.

Superficial venous thrombosis

The most common cause is intravenous cannula related thrombophlebitis, followed by varicose vein thrombophlebitis and non-varicose superficial vein thrombosis. Patients with superficial vein thrombosis are at increased risk of DVT in the adjacent deep vein if:

1 The thrombus is long (greater than or equal to 5 cm)
2 Close to the junction with a deep vein (within 3 cm)
3 The patient has other risk factors for VTE.

Superficial vein thrombosis is also a risk factor for future VTE.

Heparin-induced thrombocytopenia

This hypercoagulable state is discussed in Chapter 29.

Antiphospholipid syndrome (APS)

APS is an autoimmune disease characterized by recurrent thrombosis and/or obstetrical morbidity and systemic symptoms induced by the persistent presence of antiphospholipid antibodies (aPL). These include lupus anticoagulant (LA), anti-β2-GP1 (anti-beta 2 glycoprotein 1(anti-β2-GP1)) and/or anticardiolipin antibodies (aCL). The diagnosis requires at least one clinical and one laboratory criterion (Table 30.3).

The pathophysiology of the APS is complex. Studies demonstrate that antiphospholipid antibodies are heterogeneous and bind phospholipid (PL), PL-binding proteins and their complexes. β2-GP1 is the main protein antigen, but protein C and prothrombin can also be targets. PL targets include cardiolipin, phosphatidylserine and others. β2-GP1 is a plasma glycoprotein synthesized in the liver with an affinity for anionic phospholipids. It is ubiquitous, acts as a scavenger protein, and has several other roles. aPL exert their clinical effect by activating various cells (endothelial cells, monocytes, platelets, endometrial and decidual cells), leading to the expression of adhesion molecules, pro-inflammatory cytokines and tissue factor. This results in a pro-inflammatory and procoagulant state.

Histological studies of the placenta in pregnancy loss demonstrate placental infarction, impaired vascularization, inflammation of decidua and complement deposition. This suggests a combination of thrombotic, antiangiogenic and inflammatory factors in the pathological process.

a Laboratory investigations

1 Lupus anticoagulant (LAC) is an antibody that interferes with phospholipid-dependent coagulation assays *in vitro*. LAC prolongs APTT *in vitro*, which does not correct with the addition of plasma but completely corrects with the addition of phospholipid (Chapter 26). This phenomenon must be demonstrated in two different assays, commonly the dilute Russell viper venom test clotting time in which the snake venom directly activates FX and an APTT with low phospholipid content, e.g. silica clotting time.

2 Cardiolipin and β2-GP1 antibodies are measured by ELISA.

Persistence is an essential feature as transient antiphospholipid antibodies in the general population are not uncommon after viral infections or other acute illnesses. APS can be primary idiopathic or secondary, most commonly associated with systemic lupus erythematosus but also with other autoimmune disorders, with certain infections (viral most often), drugs (such as phenytoin and hydralazine) and malignancy (including lymphomas, myeloproliferative disorders and solid organ tumours).

In long-term studies, DVT was the most common presentation, followed by stroke, PE, foetal loss and myocardial infarction. Common non-criterion symptoms include thrombocytopenia, livedo reticularis, skin ulcers and renal issues. Livedo reticularis and renal complications can be seen due to microthrombi. Rare cardiac and neurologic manifestations not attributable to thrombosis have also been noted.

Patients with APS who express all three antibodies are at higher risk of thrombosis and are identified as 'triple positive APS'. Rarely, patients may develop a life-threatening form of APS called catastrophic APS. This is characterized by rapid onset multi-organ thrombosis, ischemia or microvascular occlusions leading to organ damage over days to weeks.

In patients with thrombosis, which appears unprovoked or with poor obstetric history, screening for aPL is indicated.

Table 30.3 Clinical and laboratory criteria for diagnosis of antiphospholipid syndrome.

Clinical criteria	
Thrombosis	**Pregnancy complications**
■ Venous ■ Arterial ■ Small vessel thrombosis with no evidence of inflammation on histopathology	■ Foetal death after the 10th week of gestation ■ Premature birth before the 34th week of gestation because of preeclampsia or placental insufficiency ■ Three early miscarriages before the 10th week of gestation
Laboratory criteria	
■ One antiphospholipid antibody tested positive on at least two occasions 12 weeks apart. The antibody tests include; 1 Lupus anticoagulant 2 Anticardiolipin antibodies (aCL) of IgG and/or IgM isotype (medium/high titer, i.e. >40 GPL or MPL*, or > the 99th percentile of the general population) 3 Anti-β2glycoprotein-1 (β2-GP1) of IgG and/or IgM isotype (in titer > the 99th percentile of the general population)	

** MPL refers to IgM phospholipid units. One MPL unit is 1 microgram of IgM antibody. GPL refers to IgG phospholipid units.*

Additional requirements - Not more than five years between clinical event and aPL testing.

Which patients should be tested for thrombophilia?

There is no consensus on who should be offered testing for thrombophilia, although it is universally agreed that there is overtesting. Patients with provoked VTE and those with arterial thrombosis should not be routinely tested for thrombophilia. The following situations should prompt clinicians to consider thrombophilia testing. However, each patient should have an individualized assessment to evaluate if the results could influence long-term management.

1 Patients under 45 years with unprovoked VTE, particularly with a family history of unprovoked VTE in a first-degree relative at a young age.
2 Patients with a family history of a definable hereditary thrombophilia, where results would change the management, may be tested for the particular thrombophilia.
3 Patients with warfarin-induced skin necrosis should undergo testing for protein C and protein S deficiencies.
4 Patients with unprovoked VTE or minimally provoked VTE should be screened for aPL.
5 Patients with venous thrombosis at unusual sites and abnormal haematological parameters should be offered testing for PNH and screening for myeloproliferative disorders (MPNs) and the *JAK2* mutation.
6 Patients with splanchnic vein thrombosis or cortical vein sinus thrombosis, even without clear provoking factors and a normal FBC, should be tested for the *JAK2* mutation.
7 Women with recurrent (3 or more consecutive) miscarriages or late-pregnancy vascular complications such as placental abruption should only be tested for APS.
8 Genetic testing to predict a first episode of venous thrombosis is not recommended.

Laboratory investigation of thrombophilia

If a full thrombophilia screen is indicated, the following tests should be requested:

1 Full blood count
Increased counts (MPN) or cytopenias (PNH)
2 Blood film examination
For evidence of haemolytic anaemia, MPN; leuco-erthroblastic features may indicate malignant disease. Rouleaux may be seen in hyperviscosity related to myeloma or other paraproteins.
3 PT and APTT – a shortened APPT is often seen in thrombotic states and may indicate the presence of activated clotting factors. A prolonged APTT test, not corrected by the addition of normal plasma, suggests a lupus anticoagulant or an acquired inhibitor to a coagulation factor.
4 Antiphospholipid antibodies:
Lupus anticoagulant by two techniques – usually dilute Russell viper venom test and silica clotting time.
Anti-cardiolipin IgG and IgM (ELISA test)
Anti-beta-2-glycoprotein 1 IgG and IgM (ELISA test)
5 Fibrinogen assay
6 FV Leiden and FII *G20210A* genotype by DNA analysis
7 Antithrombin, protein C and S antigen and activity levels
8 Screening for MPN mutations, particularly in patients with thrombosis of unusual sites and/or if there are myeloproliferative features on the blood film
9 PNH screen (flow cytometry for loss of CD55 and CD59 expression)
10 Appropriate cancer screening by focused history, examination and symptom-directed imaging and laboratory tests (CT chest abdomen pelvis is not routinely indicated in patients with unprovoked PE; screening should be targeted).

Deep vein thrombosis of the lower limbs

DVT usually starts in the calf veins, where most resolve spontaneously. The thrombus in the calf veins can progress and extend into the distal and proximal veins, from where it can break free and embolize to cause PE. Thrombosis at each site may be silent or symptomatic and is related to clot burden, the extent of thrombosis, temporal progression, the establishment of collateral circulation, vascular congestion or compromise.

Lower limb DVT can be distal, i.e. beyond the popliteal vein, or proximal, which includes popliteal DVT and above (Fig. 30.3). The location of DVT is important as it determines the risk of pulmonary embolism and duration of treatment. Proximal DVT is more likely to result in symptomatic PE when compared to distal DVT. Superficial thrombosis rarely extends into the deep veins to cause significant DVT and PE.

Most surgery-related DVTs start during the intra-operative period, but serial studies have demonstrated that they can develop any time after surgery. In orthopaedic surgery, DVT on the operated leg is most common. The timing of postoperative thrombosis may vary with the type of surgery. The risk of symptomatic VTE is highest within 2 weeks of surgery but remains elevated for 2 to 3 months.

A DVT is suspected in patients presenting with a painful, swollen, warm or erythematous limb. Findings on examination may include asymmetry with unilateral oedema, erythema/warmth, tenderness and dilated superficial veins. An objective diagnosis requires diagnostic imaging as only 5–20% of patients with clinically suspected DVT have confirmed DVT. Homan's sign (pain in the calf on flexing the ankle) lacks sensitivity and specificity and is no longer performed.

Unusual sites of thrombosis

1 **Cerebral venous and sinus thrombosis (CVST)**
Obstruction of cerebral veins causes cerebral oedema and venous infarction, while occlusion of venous sinuses causes intracranial hypertension. CVST should be considered in the differential diagnosis of new-onset neurological symptoms, particularly in young people with unusual headaches

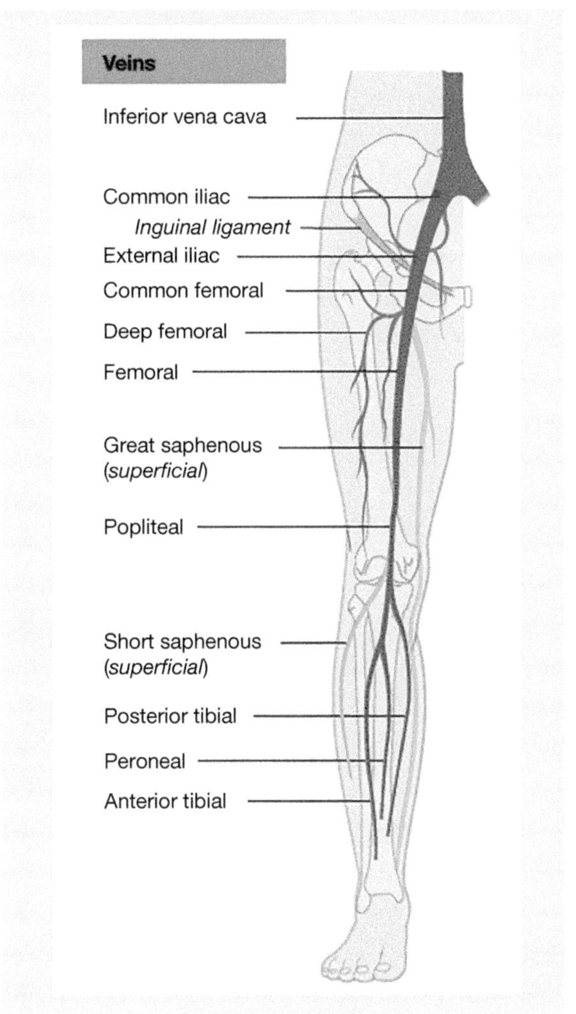

Figure 30.3 Lower limb venous system showing superficial (light blue) and deep veins (dark blue). The femoral vein is also referred to as the superficial femoral vein to distinguish it from the deep femoral vein. It is most commonly involved in proximal deep vein thrombosis.

or stroke-like symptoms. The most sensitive diagnostic test is magnetic resonance venography. Infection and inflammatory causes dominate, in addition to the combined contraceptive pill.

2 **Central retinal vein occlusion**
The typical presentation is an acute, painless visual loss in one eye, and diagnosis is by clinical examination. It is mainly seen in the older group, although younger patients with autoimmune disorders are also affected. Open-angle glaucoma and raised intraocular pressure are local risk factors. There is no strong association with hereditary thrombophilia.

3 **Axillary, subclavian and brachial vein thrombosis – upper extremity DVT**
This can be idiopathic but often related to upper limb effort or thoracic outlet syndrome. The compression of the neurovascular bundle in this syndrome may be due to bony structures, such as the first rib and clavicle, or muscle bulk. Patients typically present with unilateral swelling or effort-related pain and swelling; PE is rare. The most common secondary cause is indwelling central venous catheters.

4 **Superior vena cava obstruction**
This large vein is often obstructed by compression from surrounding malignancy. Patients present with facial puffiness that does not improve with rest and breathlessness.

5 **Inferior vena cava (IVC) thrombosis**
The clinical presentation is similar to that of DVT. In addition to compression from malignancy, the other common causes are congenital anomalies that result in turbulent blood flow and thrombosis. Most cases of IVC thrombosis present with signs and symptoms of a lower limb DVT (unilateral or bilateral) or PE. Patients presenting with bilateral lower limb DVTs should have the IVC imaged.

6 **Abdominal vein thrombosis**
Abdominal vein thrombosis includes hepatic venous outflow obstruction or thrombosis of the splanchnic veins. Hepatic venous outflow obstruction (Budd–Chiari syndrome) presents with abdominal pain, ascites and hepatomegaly. Portal vein or mesenteric vein thrombosis or a combination present with acute abdominal pain, fever and nausea or chronically with symptoms of portal hypertension (variceal bleeding, ascites, hypersplenism). Visceral ischemia leading to abdominal pain is often due to insufficient collateral circulation. Doppler ultrasound or MRI confirms the presence of a thrombus.

7 **Renal vein thrombosis**
This is an uncommon condition with a variable clinical presentation. It is peculiarly associated with nephrotic syndrome and in neonates with dehydration.

Diagnosis of venous thrombosis

Clinical prediction rules

Clinical prediction rules aim to estimate the probability of clinical condition or future outcome by considering a small number of valid markers that are based on history, examination and investigations. The purpose of the rules is to support clinical decision making.

Patients presenting with symptoms suggestive of DVT to emergency is common. Several clinical prediction rules have been developed and validated to increase the likelihood of identifying patients with DVT and PE (the pretest probability) for imaging to limit unnecessary investigations, treatment and radiation exposure.

Currently, an algorithmic approach that includes clinical pretest probability, D-dimer testing and ultrasound of the leg veins allows for safe and effective evaluation of suspected lower limb DVT. The modified Wells score is the most used clinical

Table 30.4 Clinical prediction rule for deep vein thrombosis - the modified Wells score.

Two-level Wells Score for DVT	
Clinical features	**Points**
Active cancer (treatment ongoing, within 6 months, or palliative)	1
Paralysis, paresis or recent plaster immobilization of the lower limb	1
Recently bedridden for 3 days or more or major surgery within the previous 12 weeks requiring general or regional anaesthesia	1
Localized tenderness along the distribution of the deep venous system	1
Entire leg swelling	1
Calf swelling at least 3 cm larger than that of the asymptomatic leg (measured 10 cm below the tibial tuberosity)	1
Pitting oedema confined to the symptomatic leg	1
Collateral superficial veins (non-varicose veins)	1
Previously documented DVT	1
Alternative diagnosis at least as likely as DVT	−2
Interpretation of clinical pretest probability score	
Low probability of DVT	1 or less
Intermediate/high probability of DVT	2 or more

Source: Adapted from P.S. Wells *et al.* (2003) *N. Engl. J. Med.* 349: 1227–35. Scores can be calculated at the MDCalc online tool: https://www.mdcalc.com.

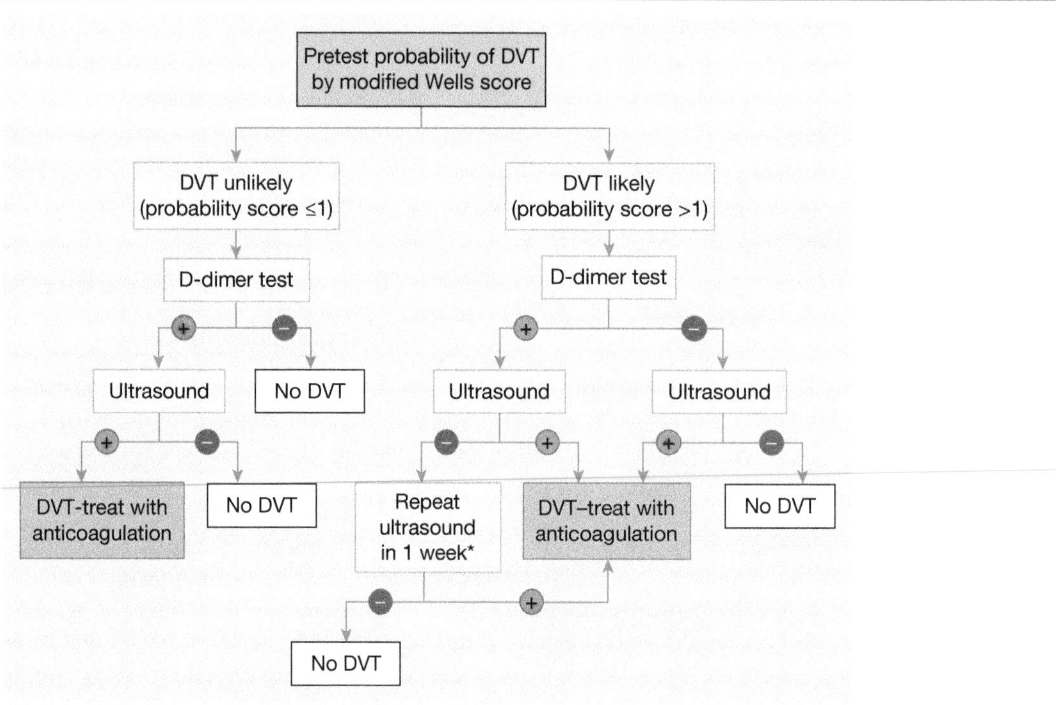

Figure 30.4 Diagnostic algorithms for deep vein thrombosis (DVT) based on clinical pretest probability by modified Wells score (Table 30.4) and D-dimer testing. The cut-off values for the significant D-dimer results can be set as per the manufacturer or the upper limit of normal. As imaging is often available the next working day, the assessment also helps determine the need for immediate bridging treatment until a definitive diagnosis. *Repeat scanning is required if compression ultrasound is used. A scan of proximal and distal veins by colour-coded Doppler does not require a repeat ultrasound.

prediction rule for assessing the pretest probability of DVT (Table 30.4). The addition of D-dimer increases the sensitivity and specificity of the clinical prediction rules.

Investigations

Plasma D-dimers are generated when cross-linked fibrin is degraded by plasmin, and levels increase when there is clot turnover, as in acute thrombosis. The test is of value in patients with low to intermediate pretest probability of DVT, where a negative test rules out DVT. D-dimers can be raised in infection, inflammation, post-surgery, trauma, pregnancy, malignancy and therefore are not specific for thrombosis. A positive test is followed by a confirmatory ultrasound. In patients with a high pretest probability of DVT, imaging is indicated. An algorithm is provided in Fig. 30.4.

Duplex ultrasound combines two-dimensional (2-D) imaging with compression, colour and/or spectral Doppler (Fig. 30.5a). The lack of compressibility of a venous segment under the ultrasound probe is diagnostic for DVT. This is a reliable and practical method for patients presenting for the first time with a suspicion of DVT in the legs, particularly proximal leg DVT; the sensitivity for distal DVT is poor. Colour-coded Doppler ultrasound has additional value by visualizing flow colour-coded for velocity and direction. This increases diagnostic sensitivity, particularly for distal DVT (Fig. 30.5a). It also allows for the quantification of residual thrombus. The distinction between old and fresh thrombus is not always easy. Scanning for residual thrombus is not routine practice, although residual thrombus is a risk factor for recurrence.

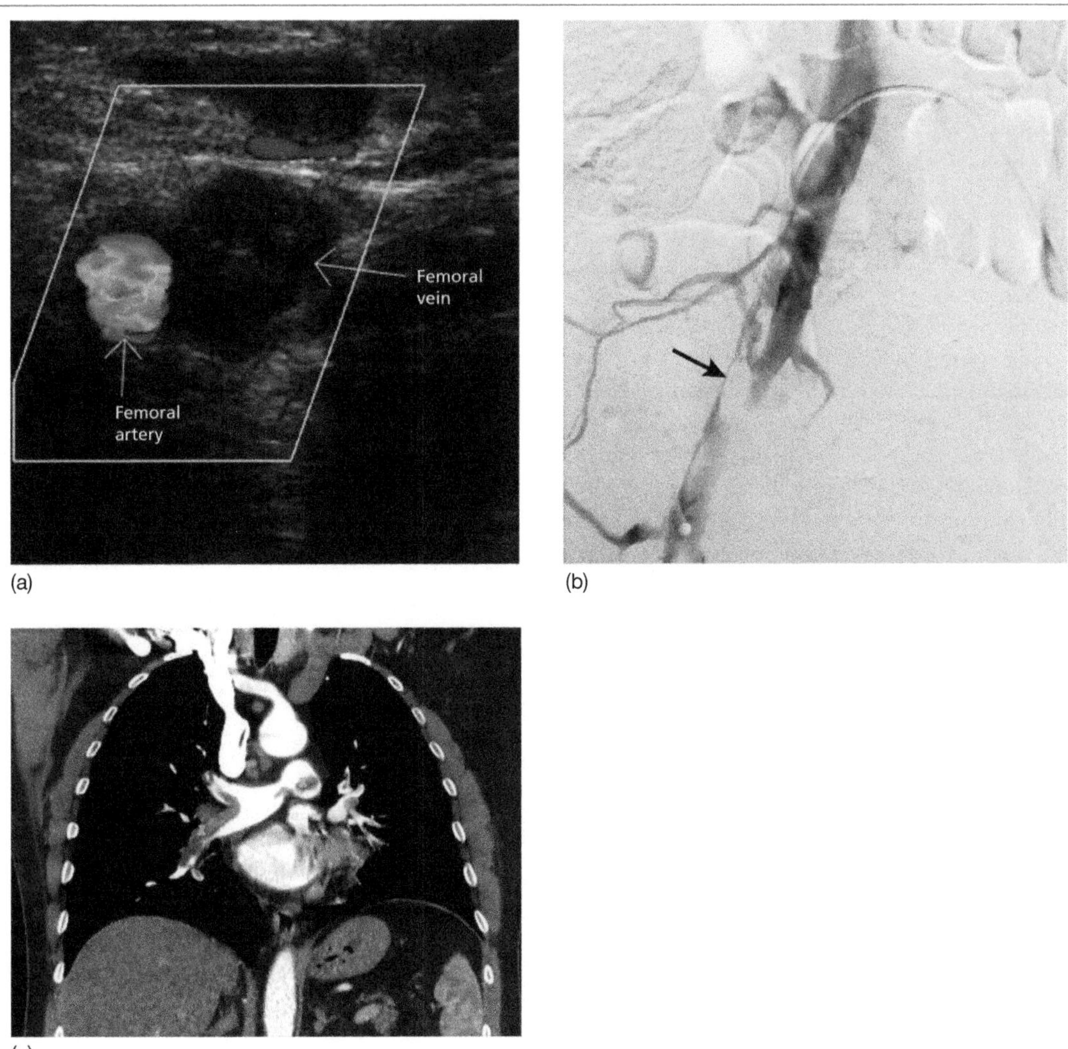

Figure 30.5 Diagnostic imaging of deep vein thrombosis (DVT) and pulmonary embolus (PE). **(a)** Colour power Doppler ultrasound of the right femoral vessels with compression shows normal flow in the femoral artery but absent flow in the vein because of thrombus. A normal vein would collapse with compression of the probe. Source: Courtesy of Dr Tony Young. **(b)** Femoral venogram demonstrating extensive thrombus within the right external iliac vein. Source: Courtesy of Dr I.S. Francis and Dr A.F. Watkinson. **(c)** Computed tomography (CT) pulmonary angiography: a coronal image shows bilateral filling defects (green crosses) in the central pulmonary arteries, indicating pulmonary emboli. Source: Courtesy of Dr Tony Young.

Contrast venography has been the gold standard for diagnosis in many clinical trials but is now rarely performed. Iodinated contrast medium is injected into a vein distal to the suspected DVT. This permits visualization of the site, size and extent of the thrombus by X-ray (Fig. 30.5b). However, it is an invasive technique, with a risk of contrast reaction and procedure-induced DVT.

Computed tomography (CT) with venous phase contrast is particularly indicated for detecting thrombosis at atypical sites, e.g. cerebral venous sinuses, hepatic veins, splanchnic veins, renal veins, gonadal vein, inferior vena cava and the proximal common iliac veins.

Magnetic resonance imaging (MRI) is rarely used due to cost and slow turnaround time. It is indicated when ultrasound might be inaccurate or difficult, e.g. because of obesity or visualizing pelvic and ileal veins.

Pulmonary embolism

Pulmonary embolism (PE) occurs when a thrombus originating from venous circulation obstructs the blood flow in the pulmonary artery or its branches, with or without interference with gas exchange. Clinical symptoms are related to the size and location of the clots and the extent of the vascular bed affected. Larger emboli tend to obstruct the main pulmonary artery, with smaller emboli blocking the segmental and subsegmental branches in the lung. Pulmonary infarction occurs in about 10% of patients.

The obstruction induces vasoconstriction, mediated by the release of thromboxane A2 and serotonin, contributing to the initial increase in pulmonary vascular resistance. The impaired gas exchange is due to physical obstruction of the vessels and vasospasm of the unaffected vessels secondary to the mediators. This results in ventilation-perfusion mismatch with normal ventilation despite impaired flow.

Pulmonary artery pressure increases if more than 30 to 50 % of the total cross-sectional area of the pulmonary arterial bed is occluded. Right ventricular failure due to acute pressure overload is the primary cause of death in severe PE. Saddle PE is a rare presentation that can lead to sudden hemodynamic collapse and death. The definition of saddle PE is a visible thrombus located at the bifurcation of the main pulmonary artery. Recurrent PE may lead to chronic thromboembolic pulmonary hypertension.

Clinical presentation

The clinical signs and symptoms of acute PE are non-specific. It may be asymptomatic or present with cardiovascular collapse. Symptoms include breathlessness, chest pain, cough, haemoptysis, palpitations or syncope. A massive PE may cause cardiogenic shock or cardiac arrest. Chest pain can present as pleuritic chest pain due to distal emboli and pulmonary infarction. Central angina-like symptoms may occur with right ventricle ischemia. Concomitant symptoms of DVT may be present. In some patients, the diagnosis of PE may be an incidental finding, particularly in patients with cancer undergoing staging and surveillance scans.

Clinical signs include sinus tachycardia, atrial tachyarrhythmias, signs of haemodynamic instability or features of consolidation in the case of pulmonary infarction, or a pleural rub in the case of secondary pleuritis. PE should be suspected in patients with signs or previous history of DVT, recently hospitalized or immobilized, or having risk factors for venous thrombosis. Some patients present with significant or sudden changes in exercise capacity in the absence of obvious risk factors.

PE is a diagnosis that should not be missed as the fatality of untreated PE is high. Several clinical prediction rules have been developed to identify patients who should be scanned to limit unnecessary radiation. Some in clinical use are pulmonary embolism rule-out criteria rule; Wells score; revised Geneva score (Table 30.5); and Years criteria. They have similar negative predictive values of around 95% but slightly different sensitivities.

Investigations

Chest X-ray is often normal but may show evidence of pulmonary infarction or pleural effusion.

Electrocardiogram is performed to determine the presence of right heart 'strain', seen in severe cases. Findings may include

Table 30.5 Clinical prediction rule for pulmonary embolism – the revised Geneva score.

Variable		Points
Age > 65 years		+1
Previous venous thromboembolism		+3
Surgery requiring anaesthesia or fracture of the lower limb in the past month		+2
Active malignancy		+2
Unilateral leg pain		+3
Haemoptysis		+2
Unilateral leg oedema		+4
Heart rate 75-94 bpm		+3
Heart rate > 95 bpm		+5
Probability of PE	***Score***	***Prevalence of PE***
Low	≤ 3	8%
Intermediate	4 – 10	29%
High	> 11	74%

Source: Adapted from G. Le Gal *et al.* (2006) *Ann. Intern. Med.* 144: 165–71. Scores can be calculated at the MDCalc online tool: https://www.mdcalc.com.

sinus tachycardia (most common finding), right axis deviation, right bundle branch block and S1Q3T3 (large S wave in lead I, Q wave in lead III and an inverted T wave in lead III).

Plasma D-dimer measurement has a similar negative predictive value in patients with PE as with DVT. PE can be reliably excluded in a patient with a low or intermediate pretest probability score and a normal D-dimer test.

Ventilation perfusion (VQ) scintigraphy is a well-established nuclear medicine technique useful when the chest X-ray is normal. Perfusion scans are combined with ventilation scans with tracers to increase specificity. In acute PE, ventilation is expected to be normal in hypoperfused segments (mismatched).

Multidetector CT pulmonary angiography (CTPA) is used for imaging the pulmonary vasculature in patients with suspected PE. It allows adequate visualization of the pulmonary arteries down to the sub-segmental level (Fig. 30.5c). CTPA is now the gold standard for the diagnosis of PE. In patients with low and intermediate clinical probability, the CTPA has a high negative predictive value, but this decreases in patients with high pretest probability. Further testing is indicated in patients with discordance between clinical judgement and CTPA results.

Magnetic resonance pulmonary angiography that is gadolinium-enhanced is a relatively new and expensive but accurate technique. It is rarely used.

Pulmonary angiography was the traditional reference method but is invasive with complications, such as arrhythmia or contrast reaction.

Echocardiography is done in unstable patients to look for surrogate signs of a massive PE, such as severe right ventricular strain. In the chronic phase, it can also evaluate secondary pulmonary hypertension.

Clinical risk stratification

Risk stratification predicts the risk of fatal outcomes and enables appropriate interventions. There are several scores based on clinical criteria and investigations. A patient is considered to have acute high-risk PE when the following features are present:

- Cardiac arrest requiring resuscitation
- Obstructive shock – with systolic BP < 90 mmHg, or vasopressors required to achieve a BP ≥ 90 mmHg despite adequate filling status along with evidence of end-organ hypoperfusion (altered mental status; cold, clammy skin; oliguria/anuria; increased serum lactate).
- Persistent hypotension with systolic BP < 90 mmHg, or systolic BP drop ≥ 40 mmHg, lasting longer than 15 minutes, that is not caused by new-onset arrhythmia, hypovolaemia, or sepsis.

Patients with no evidence of high-risk PE can be further stratified based on investigations that include echocardiogram, troponin and vitals (heart rate, BP, oxygen saturation, respiratory rate). The patient is considered to have intermediate-risk PE if there is evidence of right ventricle strain on echocardiogram, elevated troponin and increased heart rate. These features suggest a high clot burden and the need for multiple therapeutic approaches.

Pulmonary embolism severity index

The pulmonary embolism severity index (PESI) or the simplified pulmonary embolism severity index (sPESI) can also aid decision-making, mainly in deciding between ambulatory care or hospitalization (Table 30.6). PESI was developed to predict

Table 30.6 Pulmonary embolism severity index (PESI) and simplified (s)PESI.

Parameter	Original PESI	sPESI
Age		1 point (if age >80 years)
Sex, Male	+10	-
History of cancer	+30	1 point
History of heart failure	+10	1 point
History of chronic lung disease	+10	
Heart rate ≥ 110/min	+20	1 point
Systolic BP < 100 mmHg	+30	1 point
Respiratory rate ≥ 30/min	+20	
Temperature < 36°C/ 96.8°F	+20	
Altered mental status (disorientation, lethargy, stupor, or coma)	+60	
O2 saturation < 90%	+20	1 point
Score interpretation	**Total score**	**Total score**
Very low *	≤ 65	
Low risk *	66-85	
Intermediate**	86-105	
High risk**	106-125	
Very high **	>125	
Low risk		0
High risk		≥1

*This group can be managed in an outpatient setting.
** This group has a high risk of mortality and severe morbidity and should be admitted. The mortality increases from 1% in the very low-risk group to 25% in the very high-risk group.
Source: PESI adapted from D. Aujesky *et al.* (2005) *Am. J. Crit. Care. Med.* 172: 1041–6. sPESI adapted from D. Jiménez *et al.* (2010) *Arch. Intern. Med.* 170: 1383–89. Scores can be calculated at the MDCalc online tool: https://www.mdcalc.com.

30-day mortality; the highest score is associated with a 10–25% mortality rate. A PESI, coupled with a holistic assessment of the patient's circumstances, including adherence to treatment and the ability to present promptly to the hospital should they deteriorate, can help decide which patients can be safely managed on an outpatient basis.

Long-term sequelae of venous thromboembolism

Post-thrombotic syndrome

Post-thrombotic syndrome (PTS) symptoms are seen in up to 50% of patients after DVT in the legs, but these are only severe in 5–10%. Destruction of valves with impaired venous return results in venous hypertension and fluid accumulation in the extravascular space.

Symptoms include pain, cramps, heaviness, itching and paraesthsesiae. These are worse at the end of the day and after standing for long periods. The lower leg shows redness, induration, patchy hyperpigmentation, venous ectasia and venous ulceration in severe cases (Fig. 30.6). The early use of compression stockings for up to 2 years after thrombosis has been shown to reduce the risk of PTS in some studies, but not others.

Risk factors for PTS include patient-related factors (older age, obesity, pre-existing varicose veins), DVT-related factors (recurrent DVT, proximal DVT, failure to recanalize at 6 months) and treatment-related factors (delayed or inadequate anticoagulation). Catheter-directed thrombolysis, with or without mechanical thrombolysis, reduces the risk of severe PTS in patients with acute ilio-femoral DVT but has no survival benefit.

Management includes physical exercise, weight loss, compression bandaging, and skin care. Venous surgery can be considered in selected severe cases where feasible. There is no evidence that prolonged anticoagulation reduces the risk of PTS.

Chronic thromboembolic pulmonary hypertension

This subtype of pulmonary hypertension occurs in 1 to 5% of patients with previous pulmonary embolism.. Risk factors include inadequate or delayed treatment of PE, large volume thrombi, unprovoked PE and recurrent PE. Sometimes, the diagnosis is made without a previous documented history of VTE. The diagnosis requires high degree of clinical suspicion, particularly in patients with new or persistent dyspnoea after three months of therapeutic anticoagulation. Diagnosis requires a combination of imaging (V/Q scan, CTPA, digital subtraction angiography) to demonstrate thromboembolic disease and the demonstration of raised pulmonary arterial pressure (which requires a right heart catheterization). Management options include medical therapy (anticoagulation, pulmonary vasodilators), pulmonary thromboendarterectomy or endovascular interventions. Refractory cases may be considered for a double heart and lung transplant.

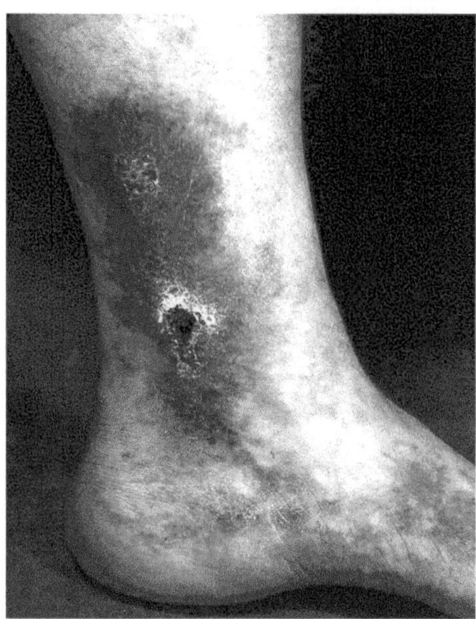

Figure 30.6 Post-thrombotic syndrome: healing venous ulcer with surrounding pigmentation. Source: Courtesy of Professor G. Hamilton; A.V. Hoffbrand *et al.* (2019) *Color Atlas of Clinical Hematology*, 5th edn. Reproduced with permission of John Wiley & Sons.

Arterial thrombosis

Atherosclerosis is a disease of the vascular intima and the leading cause of mortality worldwide. It includes myocardial infarction and stroke. Atherosclerosis is the gradual accumulation of fibro-fatty plaque in the sub-intimal region of an artery, leading to luminal stenosis and ischemia. The plaque has a central core of fatty material covered by a fibrous cap. Arterial thrombi form due to ulceration and rupture at the shoulder of the plaque, which exposes sub-endothelial collagen and tissue factor. This initiates the formation of a platelet-rich thrombus, leading to occlusion of the blood vessel lumen and acute ischemia. Emboli of platelets and fibrin may also break away from the primary thrombus to occlude distal arteries, as seen in carotid artery thrombi, leading to cerebral ischemia. Atherosclerotic plaques may also ulcerate at the cap under conditions of high shear or may develop intra-plaque haemorrhage, both of which lead to luminal occlusion. Pathogenic mechanisms underpinning the development of atherosclerosis are beyond the scope of this chapter.

Arterial thrombosis: clinical risk factors

Thrombosis secondary to atherosclerosis

The risk factors for arterial thrombosis are related to the development of atherosclerosis or a mechanism for thromboembolism (Table 30.7). The identification of patients at risk is primarily based on clinical assessment. Risk factors for atherosclerosis can be classified as non-modifiable, such as age, sex, family history and ethnicity (although the latter may be confounded by over representation of other risk factors) and modifiable risk factors, such as dyslipidaemia, cigarette smoking, hypertension and diabetes mellitus.

Several epidemiological studies have resulted in the development of cardiovascular disease risk algorithms - such as the Atherosclerotic Cardiovascular Disease Risk algorithm and the Joint British Societies recommendations on the prevention of cardiovascular disease. These risk assessment tools predict the 10-year risk of heart attack and stroke. They are valuable in counselling a lifestyle change or recommending medical therapy for at-risk individuals as primary prevention.

Non-atherosclerosis risk factors

There are other risk factors for arterial thrombosis that do not act through atherosclerosis. Atrial fibrillation, endocarditis, intracardiac tumours, left ventricular myocardial scar and abdominal aortic aneurysms can lead to arterial thromboembolism. Trauma can lead to intimal injury, triggering thrombosis. Vasculitis and cancer are systemic disorders associated with an increased risk of arterial thrombosis. There appears to be a relationship between high homocysteine levels and arterial damage. However, high doses of pyridoxine and folic acid, which lower homocysteine, have not been found to decrease the risk for recurrent arterial events such as myocardial infarction. A reduction in incidence of stroke in subjects with hypertension has been found, however, in Chinese trials (Chapter 5). Routine testing for hyperhomocysteinaemia in patients with arterial and/or venous thrombosis is not advised. Clonal haemopoiesis of indeterminate prognosis (CHIP) is a more recently recognized predisposing factor for arterial thrombosis (Chapter 16).

Atrial fibrillation

Atrial fibrillation (AF) is the most common serious cardiac arrhythmia. It is associated with significant morbidity and mortality, including an increased risk of embolic stroke. While long-term use of oral anticoagulants, warfarin or direct-acting oral anticoagulants (DOACS) decrease the risk of thromboembolic events, they carry a risk of serious bleeding. There is considerable interest in using algorithms to predict thromboembolic risk and bleeding in patients to assess who might and who might not benefit from treatment (Chapter 31).

Table 30.7 Risk factors for arterial thrombosis.

Risk factors for atherosclerosis
Non-modifiable
Age
Positive family history (especially first-degree relative with premature atherosclerotic disease (<55 years in males or <65 years in females)
Male sex
Ethnicity (South Asian, African, Polynesian)
Modifiable
Dyslipidaemia (elevated LDL cholesterol and triglycerides)
Hypertension
Diabetes mellitus
Visceral adiposity
Insulin resistance
Cigarette smoking
Chronic kidney disease
High glycaemic index, low-fibre diets
Lack of physical inactivity
Obesity and overweight
Chronic inflammation (CRP, interleukin-6)
HIV
Mediastinal radiation
Risk factors for non-atheromatous arterial disease
Atrial fibrillation
Left ventricular mural thrombus
Endocarditis
Intracardiac tumours (e.g. atrial myxoma)
Abdominal aortic aneurysm
Cancer
Vasculitis
Arterial trauma (e.g. neck trauma leading to vertebral dissection, thoracic trauma leading to thoracic aortic dissection)

LDL, low-density lipoprotein; CRP, C-reactive protein.

SUMMARY

- Pathological thrombi are clinically symptomatic when they compromise blood flow to a organ or through proximal congestion secondary to impaired drainage.
- Thromboembolic conditions are the leading cause of mortality worldwide.
- The pathophysiology of thrombosis has three components (Virchow's triad): hypercoagulability, altered blood flow and vascular/endothelial injury.
- Venous 'red' thrombi are rich in red cells and fibrin, whereas arterial 'white' thrombi are dominated by platelets.
- Venous thromboembolism (VTE) is a multi-causal disease. Symptomatic disease involves the interaction of environmental and genetic risk factors. A combination of hypercoagulability and stasis are the leading causes of VTE.
- Heritable thrombophilias are common and increase the risk but require a second event to trigger VTE development.
- The management of VTE is primarily dictated by site, severity and whether spontaneous or provoked rather than by the presence or absence of an underlying thrombophilia.
- Myeloproliferative neoplasms, antiphospholipid syndrome and paroxysmal nocturnal haemoglobinuria predispose to arterial and venous thrombosis. They should be considered in unprovoked thrombosis at unusual sites.
- Diagnosis of deep vein thrombosis is aided by an algorithmic approach that utilizes clinical prediction rules, which include symptoms and risk factors and D-dimer assay. Confirmation is by imaging with Doppler ultrasound and, less frequently, with CT or MRI venograms.
- Diagnosis of pulmonary embolism requires suspicion and is aided by clinical prediction rules that consider symptoms and risk factors. Multidetector CT pulmonary angiography (CTPA) is the current standard for diagnosis. Mortality is related to clot burden in the pulmonary artery.
- Arterial thrombosis is mainly related to atherosclerosis of the vessel wall or embolic phenomena. Risk factors for atherosclerosis include age, diabetes mellitus, smoking, hypertension and dyslipidaemia.
- Atrial fibrillation is the most common cause of embolic stroke. Oral anticoagulation reduces morbidity and mortality.

Now visit **www.wiley.com/go/haematology9e** to test yourself on this chapter.

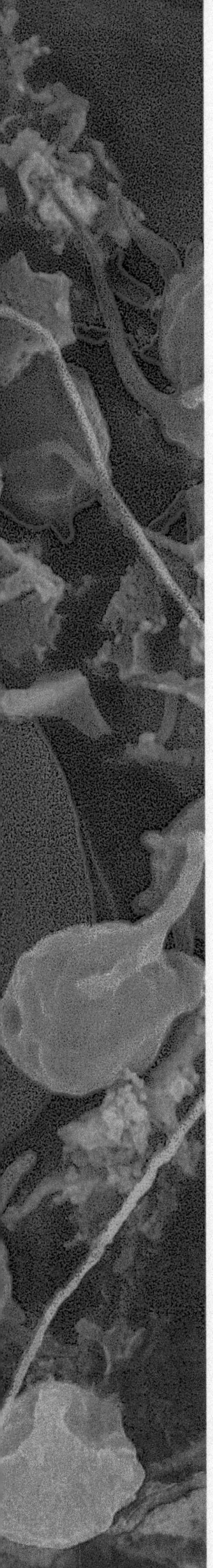

CHAPTER 31

Thrombosis 2: Treatment

Key topics

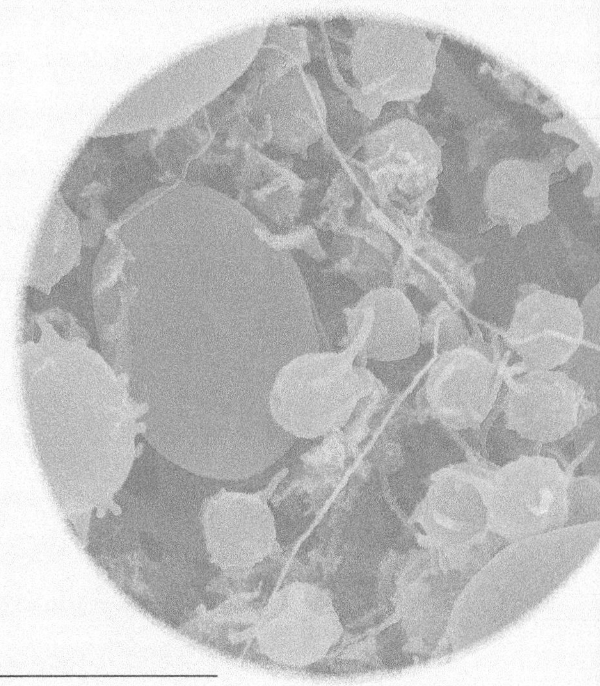

Hoffbrand's Essential Haematology, Ninth Edition. A. Victor Hoffbrand, Pratima Chowdary, Graham P. Collins, and Justin Loke.

© 2024 John Wiley & Sons Ltd. Published 2024 by John Wiley & Sons Ltd.

Companion website: www.wiley.com/go/haematology9e

Introduction

Antithrombotics are used for the prevention and treatment of thrombosis. They can impair clot formation through interference with thrombin generation (anticoagulants) or platelet activity (antiplatelets) or promote clot lysis (fibrinolytics). Anticoagulants and antiplatelets prevent the formation of a thrombus or impair the growth of newly formed clots. Fibrinolytics and interventional techniques such as angioplasty and stenting ensure rapid recanalization. The choice of agents depends on the purpose of the treatment and the pathophysiological mechanisms underpinning clot formation.

Anticoagulation is the mainstay of treatment of venous thromboembolism (VTE). Management of arterial thrombosis is complex and necessitates the use of all three classes of medications based on clinical presentation. The therapeutic armamentarium has expanded in the last two decades with the introduction of direct-acting oral anticoagulants (DOACs) and more potent antiplatelet agents.

Anticoagulants: indications

Anticoagulation aims to prevent the growth of preexisting clots and stop the development of new thrombi. **Anticoagulation does not break down clots (which requires endogenous fibrinolysis) or prevent embolism.** It can reduce the impact of the embolism. Anticoagulants reduce thrombin generation by inhibiting different components of the coagulation cascade (Fig. 31.1).

Prophylactic anticoagulation aims to decrease the risk of thrombus formation, as in atrial fibrillation or hospital-acquired thrombosis. The doses can be lower or similar to those used in therapeutic anticoagulation. The balance of thrombotic risk against bleeding risk determines the dose and duration of anticoagulation.

Therapeutic anticoagulation aims to stop the extension of preexisting thrombosis at the site of formation or the propagation of thrombi at the sites of embolization.

Indications for anticoagulation include:

1 Treatment of deep vein thrombosis (DVT) and pulmonary embolism (PE)
2 Prevention of DVT and PE
3 Prevention of intracardiac thrombi and secondary arterial embolism in patients with cardiac abnormalities, including atrial fibrillation, artificial heart valves and regional wall motion abnormalities
4 Acute coronary syndromes
5 Selected cases of arterial thrombosis
6 Prevention of clot formation in extracorporeal circuits, e.g. haemodialysis, haemofiltration, extracorporeal membrane oxygenation and others.
7 During intravascular procedures to prevent thrombus formation around catheters, e.g. cardiac catheterization

Anticoagulants: classification

Anticoagulants can be categorized by their mechanism of action and route of administration (Table 31.1). **Direct anticoagulants** reduce thrombin generation through direct inhibition of activated serine proteases or cofactors without any intermediate steps. **Indirect anticoagulants** utilize intermediate pathways, usually by activating physiologic anticoagulants

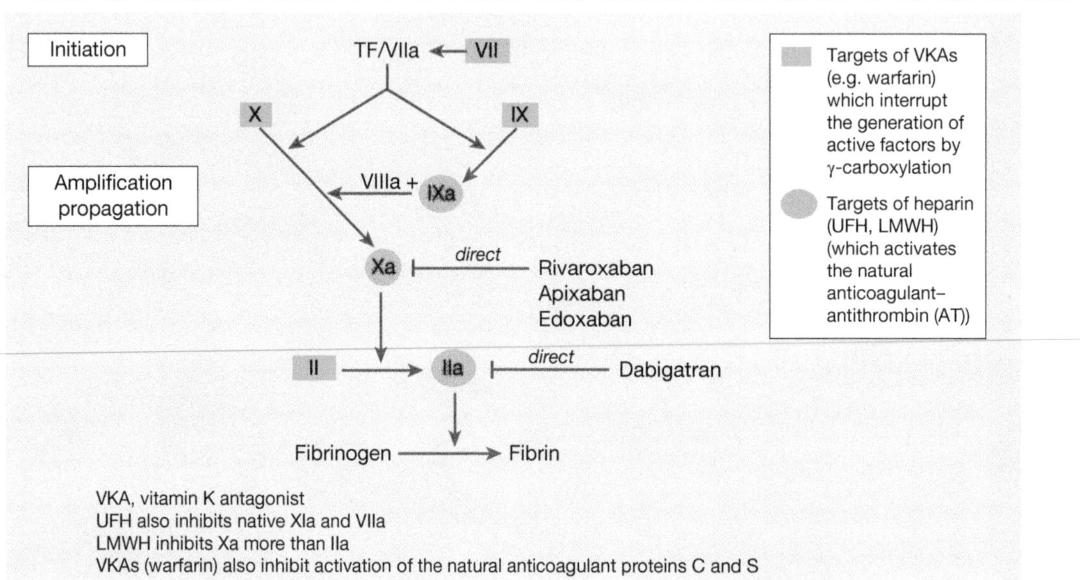

Figure 31.1 Sites of action of the more frequently used anticoagulants. UFH, unfractionated heparin; LMWH, low-molecular-weight heparin; TF, tissue factor. Source: Adapted from R. De Caterina *et al.* (2013) *Thromb. Haemost.* 109: 569–79.

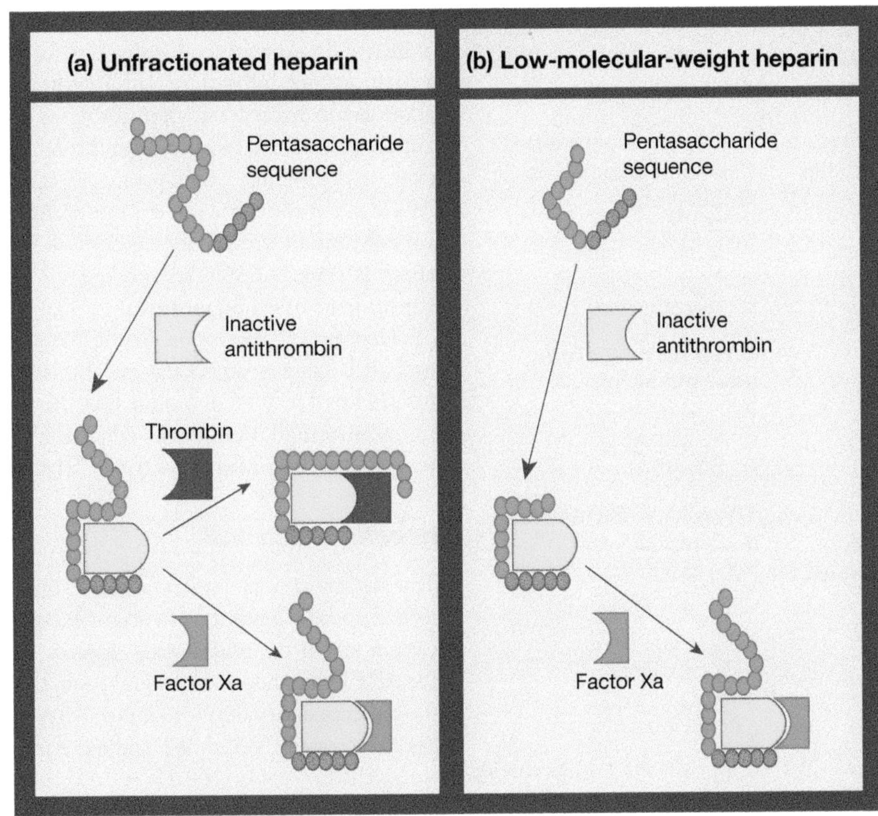

Figure 31.2 Heparin mechanism of action. Heparin mediates its anticoagulant activity indirectly through antithrombin (AT). Binding to AT is mediated by a unique pentasaccharide sequence in heparin that alters AT conformation (allosteric activation) and increases activity. **(a)** Unfractionated heparin (UFH) binds to antithrombin and thrombin (FIIa), inhibiting both FIIa and FXa. Inhibition of thrombin requires the heparin molecule to have at least 18 saccharide units to bind both AT and thrombin, thus ensuring the necessary steric configuration. **(b)** Low-molecular-weight heparins (LMWHs) bind to antithrombin but not to FIIa and predominantly inhibit FXa. The only requirement for FXa inhibition is the activation of AT.

or reducing the substrate, thus reducing thrombin generation. The drugs can be administered orally or parenterally.

Heparins and heparinoids

Heparins are the oldest anticoagulant in clinical use, dating back to the 1930s. They continue to be the most commonly used parenteral anticoagulants (Table 31.1). Heparin is a naturally occurring polysaccharide belonging to the family of glycosaminoglycans (GAG). GAGs are composed of repeating disaccharide units that are negatively charged and ubiquitously expressed; they are abundant on cell surfaces and in the extracellular matrix. GAGs are classified based on their core disaccharide units and include four primary groups: heparin/heparan sulfate; chondroitin sulfate/dermatan sulfate; keratan sulfate; and hyaluronic acid. The core disaccharide unit in heparin and heparan sulfate contains *N*-acetylglucosamine and hexuronic acid (glucuronic and iduronic acid) residues. **Unfractionated heparin and low-molecular-weight heparins consist of heparin and heparan sulfate units. Heparinoids are a mixture of heparan sulfate, dermatan sulfate and chondroitin sulfate.**

Mechanism of action

Heparins and heparinoids share a similar mechanism of action (Fig. 31.2). They exert their anticoagulant activity indirectly by binding antithrombin (AT). AT is the irreversible inhibitor of active serine proteases, which inactivates all activated serine proteases (Chapter 26). Binding to AT is mediated by a unique pentasaccharide sequence that alters AT conformation (allosteric activation), increasing its inhibitory activity 2,000 to 10,000-fold, primarily against thrombin (FIIa) and FXa. The relative inhibition of FIIa vs. FXa is also related to the size of the heparin molecule (Fig. 31.2). AT also inactivates FVIIa, FIXa and FXIa.

Unfractionated heparin and low-molecular-weight heparins

Unfractionated heparin (UFH) is the least processed GAG usually obtained from porcine intestinal mucosa. It is highly sulfated and one of the most negatively charged biological molecules. Preparations are heterogeneous in their molecular size, anticoagulant activity and pharmacokinetic properties. The

Table 31.1 Anticoagulant drug categorization based on route of administration and mode of action.

Parenteral anticoagulants	Oral anticoagulants
Indirect anticoagulants	***Indirect anticoagulants***
Heparins and heparinoids	**Vitamin K antagonists**
■ Unfractionated heparin (UFH)	■ Coumarins
■ Low-molecular-weight heparins (LMWH)	■ Warfarin
■ Enoxaparin	■ Acenocoumarol
■ Dalteparin	■ Phenindione
■ Tinzaparin	■ Nicoumalone
■ Oligosaccharides	***Direct anticoagulants***
■ Fondaparinux	**FXa inhibitors**
■ Indraparinux	■ Rivaroxaban
■ Heparinoid	■ Apixaban
■ Danaparoid	■ Edoxaban
Direct anticoagulants	**Thrombin (FIIa) inhibitor**
Thrombin (FIIa) inhibitors	■ Dabigatran
■ Lepirudin	
■ Bivalirudin	
■ Argatroban	

average molecular weight is 15 kDa, approximately 45 saccharide units in length.

Low-molecular-weight heparins (LMWHs) are derived from UFH through chemical or enzymatic depolymerization. There are several LMWHs in clinical practice, with unique manufacturing processes resulting in specific molecular and structural differences. They have an average molecular weight of 4-5 kDa.

UFH inhibits both FIIa and FXa equally, and LMWHs inhibit FXa more than FIIa (Fig. 31.2). The ratio of anti-FXa to FIIa varies among different LMWHs due to the differences in molecular weights (Table 31.2). Fondaparinux, the synthetic pentasaccharide molecule, inhibits FXa only. The potency (strength) assignment of international units (IU) is based on the WHO standard; this evaluates the ability of UFH and LMWHs to inhibit thrombin and FXa. Key properties of UFH, LMWH and fondaparinux are provided in Table 31.2.

Unfractionated heparin

UFH has a short half-life of approximately 30 to 60 minutes. It is administered intravenously when rapid action is needed. Subcutaneous (sc) administration is chosen for long-term use or thromboprophylaxis. Clearance is by non-specific binding to plasma proteins and endothelial surface, uptake by the reticuloendothelial system,with small amounts excreted unchanged in the urine.

Dosing and monitoring

Standard doses include a loading dose of 80 IU/Kg followed by a maintenance infusion of 18IU/kg/hr. A wide dose response relationship necessitates monitoring to avoid under and over anticoagulation. UFH prolongs the APTT due to the inhibition of thrombin; a therapeutic effect is achieved when the APTT is 2-3 times the upper limit of the normal (ULN) value. Initially, monitoring is done every 6–8 hours until the desired effect is observed. Several nomograms are available for dose adjustments based on measured APTT.

Heparin concentration in the blood can be measured in units/mL using an anti-Xa assay. The assay measures the ability of UFH or LMWH to inhibit FXa. An anti-Xa assay is useful for monitoring UFH in cases where the baseline APTT is prolonged. The target levels are 0.3-0.7 IU/mL.

Heparin resistance

True resistance occurs when no detectable heparin is present due to non-specific binding with acute phase proteins and increased clearance. On the other hand, apparent resistance occurs when the APTT does not show prolongation, but anti-Xa assays reveal the presence of heparin. This is due to hypercoagulability secondary to increased FVIII, VWF and other substances.

UFH advantages

Although LMWHs have mostly replaced UFH, it has specific advantages.

1. It is not renally cleared, therefore, can be safely used in advanced renal failure without dose adjustment.
2. Its rapid onset and offset mean it can be used in patients with imminent surgery or at a very high risk of bleeding, where anticoagulation may need to be stopped and heparin neutralized by protamine sulfate at short notice.

Low-molecular-weight heparins (LMWHs)

LMWHs are administered by subcutaneous injection every 12 or 24 hours. The dose is specific to each type of LMWH. Each LMWH has a specific manufacturing process, and key features of commonly used LWMHs are presented in Table 31.3.

Other LMWHs approved in different countries include ardeparin, bemiparin, certoparin, nadroparin, parnoparin, reviparin

Advantages of LMWH over UFH

The advantages of LMWH over UFH listed below improve efficacy and safety.

1. Ease of subcutaneous administration
2. Higher bioavailability – 90% (LMWH) vs. 30% (UFH)

Table 31.2 UFH, LMWH and fondaparinux: differences in properties, indications and side effects.

	Unfractionated heparin	Low-molecular-weight heparin	Fondaparinux
Mean molecular weight in kDa (range)	15 (4–30)	4.5 (2–10)	1.5
Indications	■ Arterial and venous thromboembolism ■ Extracorporeal circuits ■ Maintenance of in-dwelling arterial and venous catheters and lines ■ Renal failure	■ Arterial and venous thromboembolism ■ VTE in pregnancy* ■ VTE prophylaxis for hospitalized patients and post-joint arthroplasty	■ Arterial and venous thromboembolism ■ HIT*
Anti-Xa: anti-IIa	1:1	2:1 to 4:1	Anti-Xa only
Half-life			
Intravenous	1 hour	2 hours	Not applicable
Subcutaneous (SC)	2 hours	4 hours	17–20 hours
Bioavailability after SC injection	20–30%	90%	100%
Elimination	Reticuloendothelial system, minor renal	Renal	Renal
Monitoring	APTT ratios, anti-Xa if baseline APTT prolonged	Anti-Xa assay (usually not needed)	Anti-Xa assay (usually not needed)
Neutralization by protamine sulfate	Yes	Partial	No
Frequency of HIT	High	Low	Can be used to treat HIT*
Osteoporosis	Yes	Less frequent/unclear	

*HIT (heparin induced thrombocytopenia) is an adverse reaction to heparin that results in thrombocytopenia and thrombosis (Chapter 29).

Table 31.3 Commonly used LMWHs in clinical practice.

LMWH	Anti Xa/IIa ratio	Mean molecular weight (kDa)	Dosage for DVT	Target range (anti-Xa units/mL)*
Enoxaparin sodium (Clexane®, Lovenox®)	3.9	4.5	1.5 mg/kg OD; 1 mg/kg BD	>1.0 for OD; 0.6-1.0 on BD
Tinzaparin (Innohep®)	1.9	6.5	175 units/kg OD; 100 units/kg BD	0.85 for OD
Dalteparin (Fragmin®)	2.7	6	200 units/kg OD; 100 units/kg BD	1.05 for OD

BD, twice daily; OD, once daily.
*Peak levels taken ~4 hours post-administration of LMWH.
Source: Adapted from J. Fareed *et al.* (2008) *Clin. Appl. Thromb. Hemost.* 14: 385–92.

3 Longer plasma half-life enabling once or twice a day dosing
   a 4–6 hours vs. 0.5–1 hour
   b Slower renal clearance
4 Predictable dose response
   a Routine laboratory monitoring is generally not indicated
5 Weight-based dosing
6 Lower incidence of heparin-induced thrombocytopenia (HIT)
7 Lower incidence of osteopenia and osteoporosis

Monitoring of LMWH is by an anti-Xa assay. Peak levels are measured 4 hours after the last dose. Routine monitoring is not necessary, but monitoring is desirable in patients with extreme body weights (<40 kg or >120 kg), renal failure, therapeutic failures and complex situations such as pregnant women with mechanical valves. Dose adjustment is required at creatinine clearance <20-30 mL/min, depending on the LMWH, particularly with enoxaparin.

LMWH is commonly used for the treatment of VTE, as well as acute coronary syndrome, atrial fibrillation, anticoagulation for metallic valves, in the acute phase of VTE and as a bridge until oral anticoagulants can be used.

UFH and LMWH: Side effects and reversal

1 The most common side effect is bleeding. Protamine is used to reverse the anticoagulant effect of heparin. It is a highly basic protein that forms a stable 1:1 neutral charge complex with the strongly acidic heparin. This complex has no anticoagulant activity and is cleared by the reticuloendothelial system. The half-life is shorter than heparin (~7 minutes), and repeat doses may be required. As the neutralization is charge-dependent, the inactivation of LMWHs is partial (65–85%).
2 Heparins are biological products, and allergic reactions are not uncommon.
3 Long-term use is associated with osteopenia and osteoporosis due to stimulation of osteoclasts, which is significantly less with LMWH.
4 A significant side effect is heparin-induced thrombocytopenia and thrombosis, an immune adverse reaction that can be fatal (Chapter 29).

Fondaparinux

Fondaparinux is a synthetic pentasaccharide that activates AT and inhibits FXa only. It is cleared by the kidneys, and its use is avoided if the creatinine clearance is <30 mL/min. It is given for acute coronary syndromes and can be used instead of LMWHs. Clinical experience is limited when compared to LWMHs.

Danaparoid

Danaparoid is a mixture of glycosaminoglycans with a low molecular weight. It inhibits FXa; the anti-FIIa effect is weak. It is administered as a continuous intravenous infusion (mainly for HIT) or subcutaneously. It is only available in a few countries.

Direct thrombin inhibitors

Bivalirudin

Bivalirudin is a synthetic peptide that acts as an irreversible direct thrombin inhibitor. It is administered as a continuous intravenous infusion. Dose adjustment is required with reduced creatinine clearance. It is primarily used in HIT and primary coronary intervention.

Argatroban

Argatroban is a small molecule that acts as a direct reversible thrombin inhibitor. It is administered as a continuous intravenous infusion. It is metabolized in the liver with no renal excretion. Dose adjustment is required in cases of severe synthetic hepatic dysfunction. Like bivalirudin, it is primarily used in HIT and primary coronary intervention.

Oral anticoagulants

Oral anticoagulants are the mainstay of long-term anticoagulation in patients with atrial fibrillation, venous thromboembolism (both in treatment and prevention) and mechanical heart valves. They are also used in selected patients with arterial thromboses. They include warfarin and direct-acting oral anticoagulants (DOACs), which include FIIa inhibitor (dabigatran) and FXa inhibitors (apixaban, edoxaban and rivaroxaban) (Fig. 31.1). Their use in VTE is compared with warfarin in Fig. 31.3.

DOACs have become the new standard of care. The use of warfarin has declined and is now reserved for patients with mechanical valves, antiphospholipid syndrome and a few other select indications.

Warfarin and other vitamin K antagonists

Warfarin and other vitamin K antagonists were the mainstay of oral anticoagulation until a decade ago. Although effective, warfarin has a narrow therapeutic index requiring close monitoring and personalized dosing for clinical effectiveness and reduced bleeding risk by avoiding under- and over-anticoagulation.

Mechanism of action

Warfarin inhibits the generation of active forms of vitamin K-dependent (VKD) proteins, factors II, VII, IX, X and proteins C and S. VKDs undergo a post-translational modification whereby specific glutamate residues (Glu) are converted into gamma-carboxyglutamate residues (Gla). Gla residues are necessary for calcium-dependent conformational changes, which enable binding to cofactors on phospholipids. Vitamin K is efficiently recycled, and warfarin interferes with the recycling by inhibiting vitamin K epoxide reductase (VKOR) with the generation of inactive factors; proteins induced by vitamin K antagonism or absence (PIVKAs) (Fig. 31.4).

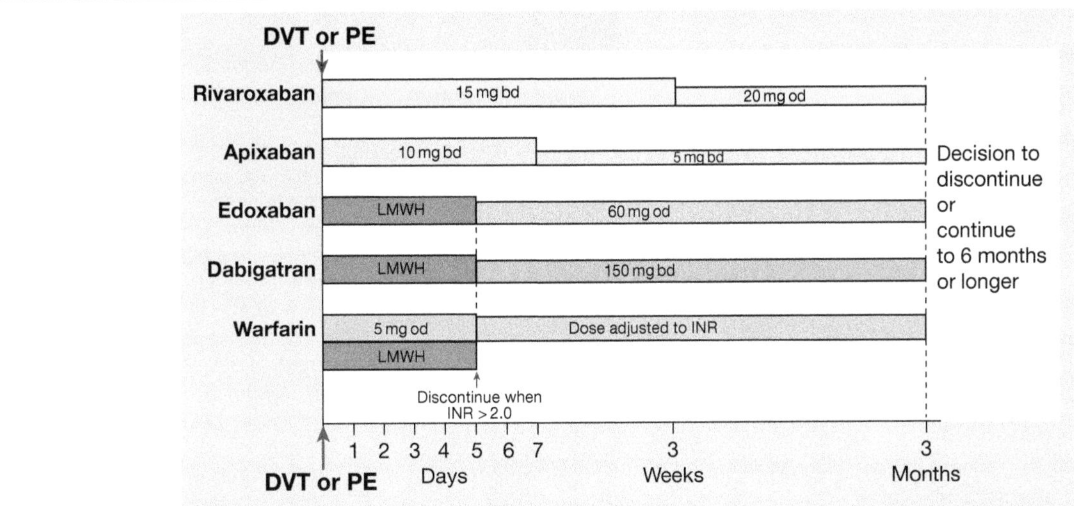

Figure 31.3 Drug regimens and doses for outpatient anticoagulant treatment of deep vein thrombosis (DVT) and pulmonary embolism (PE) of standard risk. Renal impairment, obesity, childhood or old age and other factors affect doses. **Recommended doses and protocols in National Formularies and Guidelines should be consulted for treating individual patients**. OD, once daily; BD, twice daily; LMWH, low-molecular-weight heparin; INR, international normalized ratio.

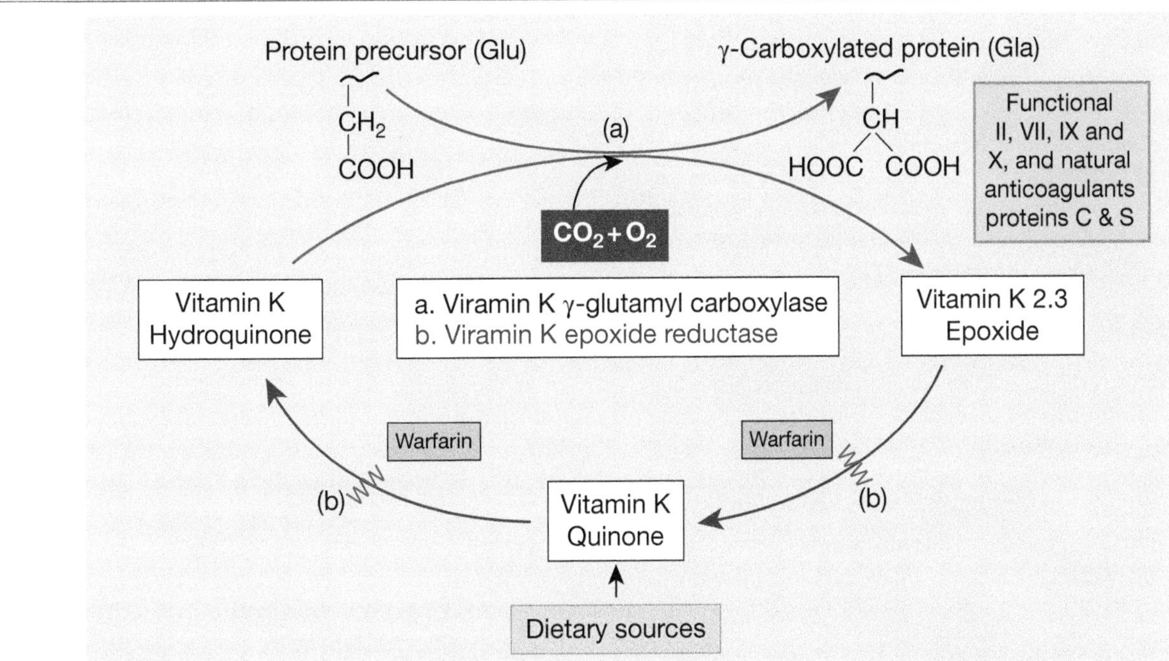

Figure 31.4 Recycling of vitamin K and the effect of warfarin. **(a)** Vitamin K hydroquinone functions as a cofactor for γ-glutamyl carboxylase, the enzyme catalysing γ-carboxylation of specific glutamate residues (Glu) into gamma-carboxyglutamate residues (Gla). During this process, the hydroquinone form is oxidized to the epoxide form. **(b)** Vitamin K epoxide reductase (VKOR) catalyses the reduction of epoxide to quinone before further reduction, generating a hydroquinone. Warfarin competitively inhibits VKOR, thus inhibiting vitamin K recycling. Glu, glutamate; Gla, γ-carboxyglutamate.

Monitoring

The effect of VKAs is monitored by the prothrombin time (PT)/ international normalized ratio (INR). Prolongation of PT occurs as early as 24–36 hours due to a reduction in FVII level. The antithrombotic effect is delayed until FX and FII levels are reduced. This reduction takes approximately four days due to their longer half-life. For the initial treatment of a thrombotic event, warfarin is therefore combined with heparin or another anticoagulant for at least 4-5 days until the desired prolongation of INR is achieved for two consecutive days (Fig. 31.3). This ensures the patient is adequately anticoagulated until the antithrombotic effect of warfarin takes effect. It also addresses the temporary increase in prothrombotic risk due to decreased protein C levels.

The international normalized ratio (INR) allows for the standardization and normalization of PT measurement for VKA therapy, addressing the impact of thromboplastin reagent variation between laboratories.

Table 31.4 Target international normalized ratio (INR) by clinical indication.

Target INR (range)	Clinical state
2.5 (2.0–3.0)	■ Deep vein thrombosis Pulmonary embolism ■ Atrial fibrillation ■ Left ventricular mural thrombus ■ Before direct current (DC) cardioversion for atrial fibrillation and flutter ■ Bioprosthetic (tissue) valves – usually only first 3 to 6 months unless concurrent indication ■ Uncomplicated antiphospholipid syndrome ■ Standard risk mechanical aortic valves (bileaflet) without additional risk factors*
3.5 (3.0–4.0)	■ Recurrent deep vein thrombosis while on warfarin ■ High-risk antiphospholipid syndrome (or antiphospholipid syndrome with breakthrough thrombosis on INR 2.0-3.0) ■ Mechanical mitral or aortic valves (valves of medium to high thrombogenicity or presence of patient-related risk factors)

* Patient-related risk factors for thrombosis: mitral, tricuspid or pulmonary position; previous arterial thromboembolism; atrial fibrillation; left atrium diameter > 50 mm; mitral stenosis of any degree; left ventricular ejection fraction < 35%; and left atrial dense spontaneous ECHO contrast.
Source: Adapted from D. Keeling *et al.* (2011) British Society for Haematology Warfarin Guideline – fourth edition. *Br. J. Haematol.* 154: 311–24.

Warfarin use: principles

Warfarin is predominantly bound to albumin; the free fraction responsible for the anticoagulant effect is less than 1-2%. Warfarin is metabolized via the cytochrome P450 system with a mean half-life of 40 hours. Treatment response is highly variable and related to changes in protein binding, polymorphisms and variants of VKOR and cytochrome P450 enzyme systems, and vitamin K stores.

A standard initial loading regimen for warfarin is 5 mg for 3 days, after which an INR check is performed to determine the appropriate dosage. Higher loading doses, such as 10 mg, are not recommended as they increase the risk of excessive anticoagulation without significantly reducing the time to achieve the desired range. Monitoring is done frequently initially, then at longer intervals once a stable INR has been reached. A stable patient can have their INR monitored every 8–12 weeks. Dose adjustments (up or down) should be done in 5-20% increments depending on how far the INR is from the target level (Table 31.4).

Drug interactions

Interference with the hepatic metabolism and protein binding are the most common mechanisms for drug-drug interaction in patients receiving warfarin. The variation in warfarin dose from person to person can be attributed to modifiable factors (diet, alcohol and other drugs) and non-modifiable factors (age, liver function, genetic variants of key enzymes) or combination (Table 31.5).

Side effects

Haemorrhage, as with any other anticoagulant, is a significant side effect influencing mortality and morbidity. The risk factors for bleeding include: age >75 years, variability in INR, high target INR (intensity of anticoagulation), concurrent use of antiplatelet agents, non-steroidal anti-inflammatory drugs (NSAIDS) and serotonin uptake inhibitors, frailty and predisposition to falls.

Warfarin-induced skin necrosis is a unique side effect related to the reduction of proteins C and S when warfarin is introduced to manage thrombosis without concurrent direct anticoagulant treatment.

Foetal warfarin syndrome, related to the teratogenicity of warfarin, develops when a foetus is exposed between the 6th and 12th week. Women in the reproductive age group are advised on the need to switch to LMWHs by the fifth week of gestation and potentially for the remainder of the pregnancy. Warfarin can be used cautiously from second trimester onwards.

Systemic atheroemboli and cholesterol microemboli may result due to the release of plaque emboli after the initiation of warfarin.

Management of supratherapeutic INR with or without bleeding on warfarin

Generally, patients with severe or life-threatening bleeding require rapid and complete reversal of any warfarin effect. Minor bleeding requires withholding warfarin only, especially if the underlying thrombotic risk is high.

Clinical decision-making is helped by understanding the time taken for each reversal strategy to be effective. Reversal strategies are based on the presence and severity of bleeding and measured INR (Table 31.6).

Table 31.5 Clinical characteristics influencing response to warfarin.

Characteristics	Mechanism of potentiation or inhibition
Age	Older patients require a smaller dose, partially related to low vitamin K stores.
Displacement from albumin	97–98% bound to albumin; minor displacement can disproportionately influence INR with increased effect, e.g. sulfonamides.
Hepatic cytochrome P450 enzyme system	Drug interactions involving the P450 isoforms are due to enzyme induction or inhibition with multiple drugs affecting its metabolism. A review of the product literature for drug interactions helps identify drugs that require close monitoring. The INR should be tested more frequently for few weeks after the introduction of new drugs. e.g. phenytoin and amiodarone inhibit metabolism, whilst barbiturates and rifampicin increase the metabolism.
Genetic variants	Genes for the key enzymes are *CYP2C9* (Cytochrome P450 family 2 subfamily C member 9) and *VKORC1* (vitamin K epoxide reductase) and variants increase sensitivity to warfarin.
Vitamin K absorption and stores	A diet restricted in fruit and vegetables tends to be low in vitamin K with increased sensitivity to warfarin, often seen in malnourished patients.
Food and supplements	Cranberry juice increases the effect, as do some herbal supplements. Some supplements (St. John's wort) increase warfarin metabolism. Multivitamin supplements with vitamin K require an increased warfarin dose.
Liver disease and heart failure	The excretion is slowed with an increased effect.
Antibiotics	A minor component may be related to the inhibition of vitamin K synthesis in the intestine. The major contribution is the inhibition of hepatic degradation of warfarin. Some antibiotics are highly associated with increased INR, e.g. trimethoprim/sulfamethoxazole, ciprofloxacin, levofloxacin, metronidazole, fluconazole, azithromycin and clarithromycin, An INR check 2 to 3 days after completing a week of antibiotics is ideal.
Alcohol	Acutely, drinking more alcohol will inhibit the metabolism of warfarin.

Table 31.6 Recommendations for the management of a supratherapeutic INR with and without bleeding.

Bleeding	INR	Warfarin	Vitamin K	Prothrombin Complex Concentrate (PCC)	Other actions
Major Bleed	≥ 4.0 < 4.0	Stop	5 mg Slow IV bolus	20–35 IU/Kg based on the INR	Resuscitate Give vitamin K <u>and</u> PCC Repeat INR 15 min and 6 hours post-infusion to assess the need for additional PCC.
Minor Bleed	> 4.5	Stop	1 mg IV or 2 mg PO*	Not indicated	Repeat INR in 24 hours Investigate for underlying cause of bleeding e.g. gastrointestinal pathology.
	2.0–4.5	Stop	1 mg PO high-risk patients only**	Not indicated	
No Bleeding	>8.0	Stop	2 mg PO for all patients	Not indicated	Repeat INR in 24 hours
	>4.5	Stop	1 mg PO high-risk patients only**	Not indicated	

IV, intravenous; PO, by mouth.

*Vitamin K consistently reverses the effect of warfarin and can be administered intravenously or orally. The need for rapid action dictates the route of administration. The earliest effect is seen after 6 hours with IV administration.

**Patients at high risk of bleeding include the elderly (>70 years), patients with cancer, and those with a recent history of bleeding or surgery. Patients with uncontrolled hypertension, diabetes, renal or liver failure and patients on antiplatelet medication are also at high risk.

Vitamin K has a slow onset of action when given orally (16-24 hours). Intravenous preparations have an onset of action within 2-4 hours, with a peak effect at approximately 12 hours. Immediate reversal is achieved with prothrombin complex concentrates (PCCs); plasma-derived clotting factor concentrates of vitamin K-dependent factors. Plasma and activated FVIIa can also be used; however, they are less effective than PCCs. A shortcoming of plasma is the volume and time taken for infusion. Vitamin K must always be given to maintain reversal.

Management of surgery for patients receiving warfarin: bridging anticoagulation

Minor surgery, e.g. dental extraction, cataracts, skin biopsies, can be done with an INR at the lower end of the 2-3 range. This is easily achieved by missing one to two doses. Topical tranexamic acid can be used for haemostatic support.

For more invasive procedures, major surgery and high-risk patients, warfarin must be stopped at least five days before surgery.The decision to bridge the patient with LMWH in the perioperative setting depends on the indication for anticoagulation, the nature of the surgery and the consequences of any minor bleeding. Patients with low or standard risk atrial fibrillation (AF) or previous history of VTE do not require bridging. In general, the following groups are considered high-risk and should receive bridging:

1. Atrial fibrillation (AF): patients with stroke or transient ischemic attack (TIA) in the last 3 months, or very high CHADSVASc score (7-9) (Chapter 30), or stroke/TIA/systemic embolism during previous warfarin interruption.
2. Recent VTE within three months (except calf DVT) or VTE on long-term anticoagulation
3. Mechanical heart valves: all mechanical valves except new-generation aortic valves without additional risk factors.
4. Antiphospholipid syndrome

During bridging anticoagulation, LMWH is administered when the INR becomes sub-therapeutic. It is restarted at prophylactic doses postoperatively, increasing to therapeutic doses once haemostasis is secured (usually 48 hours postoperatively, 24 hours for high-risk valves).

Direct-acting oral anticoagulants

DOACs are FXa or FIIa (thrombin) inhibitors and are now the first-line treatment for AF and VTE. Current products in routine clinical use are listed in Table 31.1.

For both conditions, DOACs are as effective as VKAs in most situations and have an improved safety profile, especially with a decreased risk of intracranial haemorrhage in patients with AF. The advantages and disadvantages of DOACs and VKAs are compared in Table 31.7.

DOACs: key pharmacokinetic properties

DOACs are small molecules that reversibly inhibit free and clot-bound activated factors. The advantages are related to

Table 31.7 DOACs vs warfarin: advantages and disadvantages.

Direct-acting oral anticoagulants	Warfarin
Advantages	
■ Rapid onset of action ■ Fixed dosing ■ Immediate acting, and no need for bridging therapy ■ No monitoring, reduction in the number of hospital visits ■ No food interactions ■ Few drug interactions ■ Less major bleeding	■ Long clinical experience ■ INR is validated for monitoring ■ Therapeutic effect is less impacted by missed and delayed doses ■ Monitoring encourages compliance ■ Suited for extremes of body weight ■ Multiple options for reversal ■ Safe in renal failure ■ Less gastrointestinal bleeding
Disadvantages	
■ Dose adjustments required for renal impairment ■ Avoid in liver dysfunction ■ Fixed dosing at extremes of body weight can result in overdosing or underdosing ■ Compliance is more important due to short half-life ■ Not recommended in pregnancy ■ Not recommended for antiphospholipid syndrome and mechanical heart valves ■ Bleeding risk	■ Narrow therapeutic range ■ Regular visits for monitoring and personalized dosing ■ Slow onset (need for heparin at initiation and bridging) ■ Food and drug interactions ■ Not recommended in pregnancy ■ Bleeding risk

Table 31.8 DOACs in clinical practice: pharmacokinetic properties.

Variable	Dabigatran	Rivaroxaban	Apixaban	Edoxaban
Target	FIIa	FXa	FXa	FXa
Pro-drug	Yes	No	No	No
Bioavailability (%)	3–7	90 (with food)	50	62
Site of absorption	Lower stomach and duodenum	Proximal small intestine, some gastric absorption	Proximal small intestine, some gastric absorption	Proximal small intestine
Peak level (h)	1–3	2–4	2–4	1–2
Plasma protein binding (%)	35	93	93	55
Half-life (h)	12–17	5–13 (age dependent)	9–14	10–14
Volume of distribution (litres)	60–70	50	21	107
Unchanged drug renal excretion (%)	~80	~33	~27	~50
Hepatic metabolism (%)	~4	~67	~25	<10
Unchanged drug faecal excretion (%)	~6	Minimal	~50	~40

Source: Adapted from R. Padrini (2019) *Eur. J. Drug. Metab. Pharmacokinet.* 44: 1–12.

their pharmacokinetic (PK) properties (Table 31.8). They show varying bioavailability, protein binding, metabolism and renal elimination, which influence their use in select populations.

Dabigatran is not absorbable orally and is administered as a pro-drug (dabigatran etexilate) that is converted to its active form in the liver. The three FXa inhibitors are absorbed in the active form. Despite being different chemical compounds, the plasma half-life (t½) is approximately 10–12 hours for most of the DOACs.

DOACs show considerable differences in bioavailability and plasma protein binding. Dabigatran has the lowest bioavailability at 3-7%. Food increases the absorption of rivaroxaban, and patients are advised to take it with a meal.

The volume of distribution of DOACs shows a five-fold variation. This influences their plasma levels when drugs are stopped in the event of bleeding or surgery. Rivaroxaban and apixaban are highly protein-bound compared to others. As such, any changes in plasma proteins due to hepatic dysfunction, hypercatabolism and massive bleeding will likely influence their levels.

DOACs can be eliminated in their active form or after metabolism; the proportion eliminated by renal and non-renal routes varies. Most dabigatran is excreted by the kidneys unchanged or in the form of active glucuronides, whilst edoxaban is eliminated unchanged in bile and rivaroxaban is highly metabolized.

Indications

The initial doses of apixaban or rivaroxaban used for the treatment of DVT or PE are higher at the beginning of treatment, as these DOACs are used without a parenteral agent lead-in (Fig. 31.4). Dabigatran and edoxaban require five to ten days of lead-in with a parenteral agent, either LMWH or UFH, before switching to the DOAC alone (Fig. 31.3).

The indications, dosages and dose adjustments are detailed in Table 31.9. Low-intensity anticoagulation with DOACs has been trialled for long term management to diminish the bleeding risk, alone or in conjunction with antiplatelet therapies. Dose adjustments are recommended to prevent supratherapeutic levels in the context of advanced age, low body weight, renal dysfunction and/or drug interactions.

Special populations

1 **Children:** Clinical trials have led to the license of dabigatran and rivaroxaban.

2 **Cancer-associated thrombosis (CAT):** Apixaban and rivaroxaban have demonstrated non-inferiority to LMWH in the management of CAT.
3 **Antiphospholipid syndrome (APS)**: DOACs are contraindicated in patients with triple-positive APS and are not recommended for patients with single-positive APS (Chapter 30).
4 **Mechanical heart valves**: DOACs are contraindicated as a randomized study with dabigatran was terminated due to valve thrombosis.
5 **Cerebral vein thrombosis:** Trials have demonstrated efficacy similar to warfarin.
6 **Pregnancy:** Limited data are available. Patients must be counselled and switched to LMWHs as soon as possible. If the pregnant woman has a mechanical heart valve, LMWH is used for the first trimester. British Society of Haematology guidelines recommend switching to warfarin during second and third trimesters over high doses of LWMH to decrease the risk of thrombosis.
7 **Obesity:** DOACs are not recommended for patients with BMI > 40 kg/m^2 or weight > 120 kg with potential for low levels and therapeutic failure. However, rivaroxaban and apixaban can be used with caution and monitoring actively considered.
8 **Splanchnic vein thrombosis:** Case series suggest DOACs might be as effective as warfarin.
9 **Cardiovascular and peripheral vascular disease interventions:** Used concomitantly with antiplatelet drugs. In these situations, they are used for the shortest time possible and at the lowest recommended dose.
10 **Renal impairment:** DOACs are variably excreted through the kidneys, and numerous dose adjustments exist based on indication and patient characteristics (Table 31.9). None of the drugs are recommended for use when creatinine clearance is < 15 mL/min or on haemodialysis, except for apixaban in patients on haemodialysis.
11 **Liver disease:** Most have an element of hepatic metabolism and should be avoided in severe liver disease.
12 **Drug interactions:** Similarly, caution must be exercised with concurrent use of inhibitors (e.g. some anti-HIV and anti-fungal drugs) or inducers (e.g. St. John's Wort) of cytochrome 3A4 and P- glycoprotein systems, with DOACs avoided with strong inducers or inhibitors.

Monitoring

The thrombin time is very sensitive to the presence of dabigatran, and a normal thrombin time excludes dabigatran, while a dilute thrombin time, or a dabigatran level, can be used for therapeutic drug monitoring. PT is often raised in the presence of therapeutic levels of rivaroxaban and edoxaban, though there is no specific reference range. APTT is not raised unless the levels are supratherapeutic. PT and APTT are both normal in the presence of therapeutic doses of apixaban.

Monitoring of levels is not routinely needed; commercial assays are now available to measure drug levels. The reference ranges are specific to the indication and vary between loading and ongoing treatment or prophylactic phase. They are helpful in patients with specific characteristics that might affect DOAC concentration, such as renal impairment, extremes of body weight, children and patients at high risk of drug interactions. The assays can also be of benefit to assess levels before an invasive procedure and to assess compliance. In most hospitals, there is limited availability out of hours, and their utility in the management of patients with bleeding on DOACs is limited.

Side effects

1 DOACs increase the risk of bleeding or contribute to the volume of blood loss secondary to other pathological bleeding. Clinical decision regarding use of specific reversal agents is made based on the severity of bleeding and local availability of reversal agent (Table 31.9). The monoclonal antibody idarucizumab is a specific reversal agent for dabigatran. Andexanet alfa is a non-specific reversal agent for FXa inhibitors. It is a recombinant FX molecule that lacks catalytic activity and acts as a decoy. It binds and sequesters all the oral FXa inhibitors and is also effective for reversing LMWH and fondaparinux. It has restricted approval for use in certain life-threatening bleeding situations. Prothrombin complex concentrates are frequently used to counter the effect of FXa inhibitors in major and life-threatening haemorrhages.
2 Approximately 10% of patients on dabigatran and rivaroxaban suffer dyspepsia or gastroesophageal reflux disease, which usually responds to a proton pump inhibitor (PPI). If there is no improvement with a PPI, a change is appropriate.

Peri-procedure management of DOACs

The short onset of action and short half-lives of DOACs make temporary interruption of anticoagulation for procedures less cumbersome than VKAs. For major procedures with a high risk of bleeding, the last dose can be given 48 hours before the procedure; although a longer interval, such as 72 hours, may be required for patients with renal impairment. For minor procedures or procedures with low bleeding risk, procedures can be done 18–24 hours after the last dose. Resumption of anticoagulation post-procedure can begin when haemostasis is achieved, although prophylactic doses of DOAC or LMWH may be required while hospitalized with uncertain haemostatic status. Once the risk of bleeding has been minimized, full-intensity anticoagulation can be restarted.

Bridging with LMWH is not required for the majority of patients on DOACs. Exceptions include interruptions in the

Table 31.9 DOACs: indications, doses, dose adjustments and reversal.

Indication	Dabigatran	Rivaroxaban	Apixaban	Edoxaban
Acute management of DVT and PE	150 mg BD, following parenteral anticoagulant for at least 5 days	15 mg BD for the first 3 weeks, then 20 mg OD	10 mg BD for the first 7 days, then 5 mg BD	60 mg OD following parenteral anticoagulant for at least 5 days
VTE prevention post-surgery	Start dose of 110 mg, then 220 mg OD for 10 days post knee surgery, 4-5 weeks post hip surgery	10 mg OD for 2 weeks post-knee surgery 5 weeks post hip surgery; first dose 6–10 hours after surgery	2.5 mg BD for 2 weeks post knee surgery, 5 weeks post hip surgery; first dose 12–24 hours after surgery	
Prevention of arterial thromboembolism in non-valvular AF	150 mg BD	20 mg OD	5 mg BD	60 mg OD
Reduced dose	110 mg BD	15 mg OD	2.5 mg BD	30 mg OD
Clinical criteria for reduced dose	≥ 1 of: ■ Age ≥ 80 years ■ On verapamil ■ Consider for ■ Reflux/gastritis ■ Age 75-80 years ■ CrCl 30-50 mL/min ■ Bleed risk		≥ 2 of: ■ Age ≥ 80 years ■ weight ≤ 60 kg ■ Cr ≥ 133 μmol/L	≥ 1 of: ■ weight ≤ 60 kg ■ CrCl 15-50 mL/min ■ On ciclosporin, dronedarone, erythromycin, ketoconazole
Renal				
CrCl 30-50 mL/min	Consider if at risk of bleeding	15 mg OD	5 mg BD	30 mg OD
CrCl 15-29 mL/min	Contraindicated	15 mg OD	2.5 mg BD	30 mg OD
CrCl < 15 mL/min	Contraindicated	Contraindicated	Contraindicated	Contraindicated
Monitoring	Dabigatran level or thrombin time	Rivaroxaban level or anti-Xa level	Apixaban level or anti-Xa level	Edoxaban level or anti-Xa level
Reversal	Idarucizumab	PCC or andexanet alfa	PCC or andexanet alfa	PCC or andexanet alfa

OD, once daily; BD, twice daily; CrCl, creatinine clearance; PCC, prothrombin complex concentrate.

first 6 weeks after VTE; those with active malignancy; and those with previous recurrences of stroke/TIA during brief DOAC interruptions.

Venous thromboembolism: management

Several issues should be considered upon diagnosis of acute VTE to facilitate the initial treatment and subsequent management. Some of the key issues are listed below.

1 What is the extent and severity of the thrombosis?
2 Does the patient require admission?
3 Is the thrombosis provoked or unprovoked?
4 What is the anticoagulant of choice?
5 What is the duration of anticoagulation?
6 Are other treatments required?
7 Does the patient require an assessment for underlying thrombophilia?

Initial treatment

Venous thrombosis at any site requires treatment with anticoagulation. Several patient and thrombosis related factors determine the need for hospitalization. Uncomplicated DVT and PE can be managed in the ambulatory setting with appropriate safety netting, i.e. the patient understands the symptoms that require representation to the hospital. If patients have conditions that interfere with self-care, multiple comorbidities, require pain control or live far away from the hospital consideration should be given to admitting the patient. Thrombosis assessment includes location, burden and evidence of tissue compromise to determine the need for admission.

What is the anticoagulant of choice?

For most uncomplicated DVT and PE patients, DOACs represent the standard of care with treatment initiated as described (Fig. 31.3, Tables 31.3 and 31.9). This group has been expanded to include cancer-associated thrombosis. The type of DOAC determines the need for initial anticoagulation with LMWHs. There are no head-to-head studies comparing the efficacy of different DOACs. The selection depends on local availability, liver and renal function, potential drug-drug interactions and preference for once-daily dosing (rivaroxaban and edoxaban) versus twice-daily dosing (apixaban and dabigatran).

LMWH is often used in clinically unstable patients, those awaiting invasive procedures, those with GI disturbances that affect drug absorption or who are nil by mouth, and those who require frequent interruptions of anticoagulation due to other reasons such as chemotherapy-induced thrombocytopenia. Patients are switched to a DOAC or warfarin at discharge.

Warfarin is the preferred treatment for the following groups:

1 Antiphospholipid syndrome, particularly high-risk group (triple positive and arterial APS)
2 Mechanical heart valves
3 Advanced renal failure (CKD stage 5 with or without renal replacement therapy)
4 Concurrent use of strong CYP450 enzyme inducers, e.g. phenytoin or rifampicin
5 Breakthrough thrombosis on therapeutic doses of DOACs (these patients are offered warfarin with a higher INR range, 2.5–3.5, or 3–4).
6 Extremes of body weight (<50 kg or > 120 kg).
7 Thrombosis at atypical sites (splanchnic, portal, cerebral); there is increasing evidence for the use of DOACs in these patients, particularly cerebral vein thrombosis.
8 Heparin-induced thrombocytopenia, with increasing evidence of the use of DOACs in these patients

Are other treatments required?

Thrombolysis for PE (systemic and catheter-directed): Anticoagulation alone is efficacious for low-risk PE but is associated with a 3–10% mortality in intermediate- and high-risk PE patients. This risk is related to right ventricular (RV) failure.

Systemic thrombolysis with tissue plasminogen activator (tPA), followed by anticoagulation, improves RV function with reduced mortality but is associated with a high risk of intracranial bleeding. It is indicated in patients with cardiogenic shock. There is increasing interest in using catheter-directed thrombolysis (CDT), wherein clot burden in the obstructed pulmonary artery is reduced by direct administration of thrombolytic therapy at doses lower than with systemic approaches. There are multiple variations of CDT in clinical practice, with local protocols determining the eligibility for treatment. Typically, it is considered in high to intermediate-risk patients with evidence of right heart strain but not yet in cardiogenic shock.

Catheter-directed thrombolysis for deep vein thrombosis: CDT is an endovascular technique that delivers the thrombolytic agent into the clot with or without high-frequency, low-energy ultrasound waves. It enables early recanalization, which is anticipated to reduce the incidence of post-thrombotic syndrome. It is restricted to patients with symptomatic ilio-femoral DVT who have been symptomatic for less than 14 days, with good functional status and a low risk of bleeding. Thrombolysis is followed by anticoagulation, and the placement of a stent is decided on an individual basis. The major complication is stent occlusion.

Transjugular intrahepatic porto-systemic shunt (TIPS): This is often required in patients with hepatic vein obstruction (Budd–Chiari syndrome) or complete portal vein thrombosis to restore blood flow. This may be preceded by CDT, with case series showing favourable outcomes in improving portal vein patency and increasing recanalization. The procedure should be considered if the facilities and expertise are available.

Graduated compression stockings: Graduated compression stockings can be used following the development of lower extremity DVT to improve lower extremity symptoms such as oedema. The data on the long-term effectiveness of the stockings worn for two years in primary prevention of post-thrombotic syndrome have been conflicting. An individualized assessment and duration of therapy based on post-thrombotic symptoms/signs is increasingly being used. The stockings should be replaced regularly and only worn on the affected leg.

Inferior vena cava (IVC) filters: Temporary IVC filters are reserved for patients with PE and ilio-femoral DVT who have an absolute contraindication to systemic anticoagulation such as major haemorrhage, cerebral haemorrhagic metastases or major surgery. Organizing a removal date as soon as an IVC filter is inserted is essential to maximize the chances of successful retrieval. An IVC filter is not an alternative to anticoagulation, and systemic anticoagulation should be commenced post-IVC filter insertion as soon as it is considered safe.

Length of anticoagulation

Is the thrombosis provoked or unprovoked?

This is important as it dictates the duration of anticoagulation. Transient risk factors that help distinguish between provoked and unprovoked DVT are given in Chapter 30.

What is the duration of anticoagulation?

The duration of anticoagulation is determined by the location of DVT, i.e. proximal or distal, and the presence of provoking

Table 31.10 Risk of VTE recurrence.

Type of VTE	Recurrence rate at 1 year after stopping anticoagulation	Recurrence rate at 5 years after stopping anticoagulation
First VTE provoked by major surgery or major trauma	1%	3%
First VTE provoked by transient risk factor (non-surgical)	5%	15%
Provoked VTE with persistent risk factors, e.g. active cancer	15%	45%
First unprovoked distal DVT	5%	15%
First unprovoked proximal DVT or PE	10%	30%
Second episode of unprovoked VTE	15%	45%

Source: Adapted from guidelines from the Thrombosis and Haemostasis Society of Australia and New Zealand for the diagnosis and management of venous thromboembolism by H.A. Tran *et al.* (2019) *Med. J. Aust.* 210: 227–35.

factors. The risk of recurrence based on these criteria is provided in Table 31.10.

Proximal DVT and PE

- Provoked proximal DVT and PE secondary to major trauma or surgery or transient other risk factors should be anticoagulated for three months if the provoking factor has resolved. This is extended to 6 months for active cancer.
- Patients with a persistent provoking factor should continue on anticoagulation until it is resolved. This can be reduced to prophylactic anticoagulation with low-dose rivaroxaban or apixaban after 6 months.
- Unprovoked proximal DVT and PE should be treated with oral anticoagulation for 3–6 months. Extended anticoagulation for secondary prevention should be considered, and a discussion with the patients should include the risk of recurrence (high lifetime risk), risk of bleeding (related to comorbidities, concurrent medications, age) and treatment options (standard vs. low dose).
- If proximal DVT is recurrent, anticoagulation indefinitely with full doses is indicated. Treatment options should be discussed if the recurrence is due to a transient risk factor, including low-dose DOACs.
- Predictive models could be employed if a patient strongly prefers cessation of anticoagulation, such as the DASH score (older age > 50 and male sex are at higher risk for recurrence, while hormonal VTE is a lower risk once the trigger is removed). An elevated D-dimer level, one month after cessation of anticoagulation, is also associated with a higher risk of recurrence.
- If patients at extremes of body weight (<50 kg and >120 kg) are prescribed DOACs, therapeutic monitoring is indicated to ensure the adequacy and safety of treatment.
- The presence of inherited thrombophilia should not impact the duration of anticoagulation if the thrombosis is truly provoked.
- Patients with antiphospholipid syndrome require indefinite anticoagulation with warfarin.

Distal DVT

- Distal DVT caused by a major provoking factor no longer present should be treated for 6 weeks.
- Distal DVT that is unprovoked or with persistence of risk factor is treated for 3 months.
- Expectant management has been suggested if patients are minimally symptomatic and the thrombus involves a short segment in a single calf vein with no risk factors for propagation. This requires close monitoring and a follow-up scan at 7–10 days.

Superficial vein thrombosis

- Superficial vein thromboses do not all require anticoagulation once an ultrasound has ruled out concomitant DVT.
- Patients with isolated low-risk superficial vein thromboses who are minimally or mildly symptomatic can be managed expectantly.
- Superficial vein thrombosis within 3 cm of the junction with deep veins (sapheno-femoral or sapheno-popliteal junctions) is treated like distal DVTs.
- Anticoagulation with prophylactic doses for 6 weeks is recommended in patients with longer thrombi (>5 cm), those within 3-5 cm of the junction of a deep vein, and those who have risk factors for propagation such as older age, previous VTE, reduced mobility, malignancy, or hormonal causes.
- Anticoagulation reduces the risk of propagation and hastens clot resolution in this setting.

Cancer-associated DVT and PE

Cancer-related VTE is treated for a minimum of six months. However, anticoagulation is often continued until the patient is cancer-free and has completed chemotherapy and individualized risk benefit analysis is helpful. Patients with cerebral cancers who develop VTE also require anticoagulation, but the risk-benefit ratio needs to be considered. Patients with metastatic disease, multiple lesions and a history of intratumoral haemorrhage are at particularly high risk of CNS haemorrhage with anticoagulation.

Antiphospholipid syndrome

- Treatment of APS involves anticoagulation with warfarin. Maintaining an INR between 2.0 and 3.0 with warfarin is usual. In patients with arterial thrombosis, low-dose aspirin may be added. Patients who have recurrence require a higher target INR.
- DOACs have been associated with a higher risk of recurrent thrombotic events and are not preferred, particularly in patients with arterial APS.
- Obstetrics APS is treated with preconception low-dose aspirin and LMWH at prophylactic doses from the moment of the positive pregnancy test. Usually, both are continued through pregnancy and 6 weeks postpartum.
- Pregnant women with previous thrombosis are managed with therapeutic dose LMWH plus low dose aspirin during pregnancy and warfarin after delivery in the long-term.
- There is increasing interest in using biologics and immuno-modulatory agents to decrease inflammation and antibody titres.

Venous thromboembolism (VTE) prophylaxis

Chemical thromboprophylaxis

Patients admitted to hospitals are risk-assessed for VTE and bleeding and prescribed pharmacological thromboprophylaxis. Typical doses include enoxaparin, 40 mg once daily; tinzaparin, 4500 units once daily; fondaparinux, 2.5 mg once daily; and dalteparin, 5000 IU once daily. FXa inhibitors are used at reduced doses: apixaban, 2.5 mg twice daily; and rivaroxaban, 10 mg once daily. Dabigatran is only dose-reduced on the first day. Thromboprophylaxis is continued for the hospital stay. Extended prophylaxis at discharge is provided in the context of lower limb joint replacement surgery and cancer surgery.

Mechanical methods of DVT and PE prevention

Graduated compression stockings

These are often used postoperatively, postpartum and during long-haul flights to reduce the risk of DVT. Thromboembolic (TED) stockings are class 1 (light compression) and exert an ankle pressure of 14–17 mmHg.

Intermittent compression devices

Intermittent pneumatic compression and mechanical foot pumps are used in high-risk patients in whom bleeding due to LMWH is likely. They reduce the risk of thrombosis in medical and surgical patients. They are often used intra-operatively on anaesthetized patients and patients who cannot receive chemical thromboprophylaxis due to a high risk of bleeding.

Antiplatelet drugs

Arterial thrombi are platelet-rich thrombi. Inhibition of platelets is key for the prevention and treatment of arterial thrombosis. Antiplatelet agents decrease platelet activation and aggregation by inhibiting various pathways.

Multiple agonists mediate platelet activation. The three key agonists that independently mediate platelet activation are thromboxane A2 (TXA2), adenosine diphosphate and thrombin. They represent non-redundant inhibition targets reflected in the additive effects of combined antiplatelet therapy. Common antiplatelet agents in use inhibit TXA2 generation (aspirin), act as ADP antagonists/ P2Y12 receptor blockers (clopidogrel, prasugrel, ticagrelor and cangrelor), GP IIb/IIIa receptor inhibitors (abciximab and tirofiban) and thrombin receptor antagonists (vorapaxar) (Fig. 31.5).

Platelet cyclo-oxygenase-1 (COX-1) inhibitor: aspirin

TXA2 is an agonist released by activated platelets. TXA2 supports both autocrine (self) and paracrine (adjacent) platelet activation through the thromboxane receptor. TXA2 is synthesized from arachidonic acid (AA) via cyclo-oxygenase (COX) and thromboxane synthase (Fig. 26.8). Arachidonic acid is released during platelet activation. Thromboxane receptor is a G protein coupled receptor that contributes to shape change and granule release.

Aspirin (aminosalicylic acid) irreversibly inactivates COX-1 and suppresses TXA2 generation with impaired aggregation to various agonists(Figs. 31.5 and 31.6). The inhibition lasts for the lifespan of the platelet (7–10 days). Complete inhibition of platelet COX1 results in modest inhibition of platelet function *in vivo*.

The loading dose is 300 mg, and a daily dose of 75–150 mg is often used for its antiplatelet effect. The main adverse effect is gastrointestinal bleeding. This can be ameliorated in high-risk patients by using a proton pump inhibitor. Major bleeding on aspirin is generally managed with drug withdrawal, tranexamic acid and, rarely, platelet transfusions.

P2Y12 receptor antagonists: Clopidogrel, prasugrel, ticagrelor and cangrelor

The purinergic receptors P2Y1 and P2Y12 are receptors for extracellular ATP and ADP. These G-protein-coupled receptors

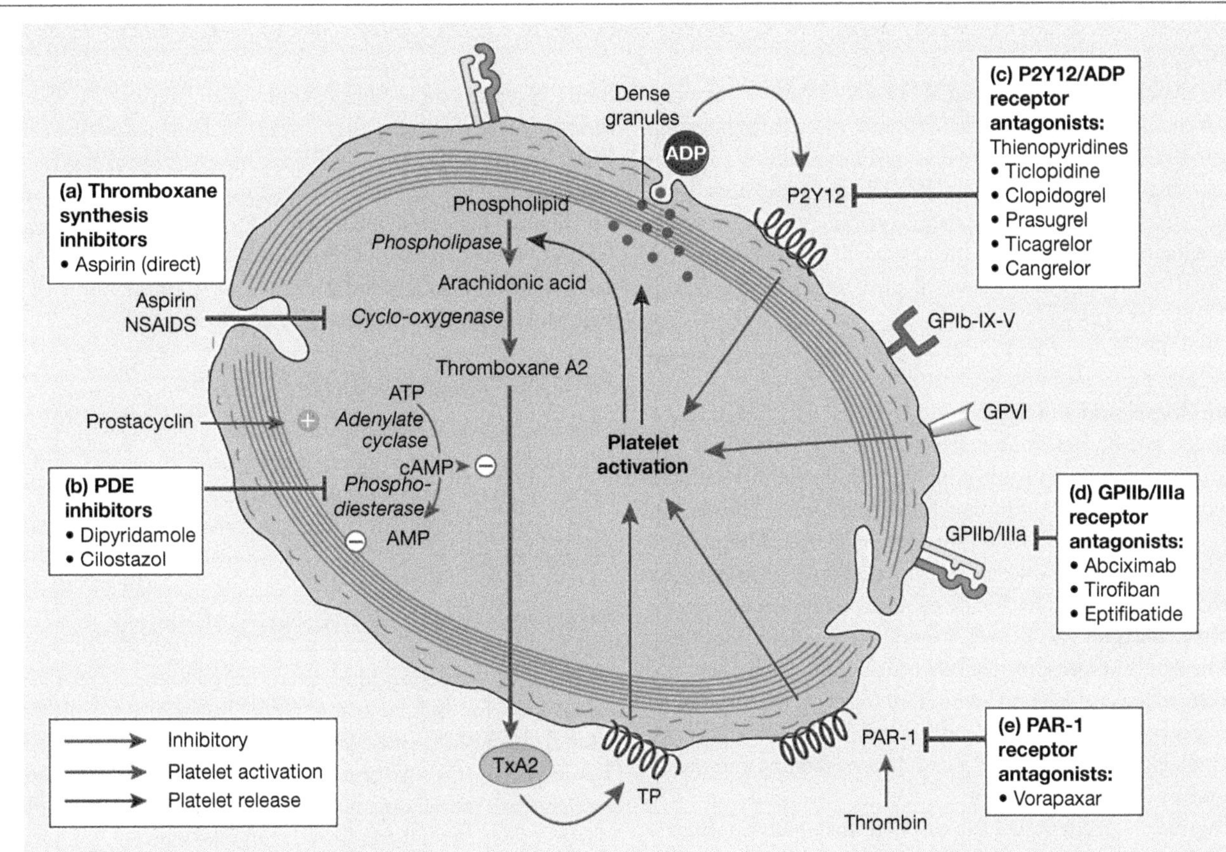

Figure 31.5 Sites of action of antiplatelet drugs. **(a)** Aspirin acetylates the enzyme cyclo-oxygenase irreversibly. **(b)** Phosphodiesterase (PDE) inhibitors inhibit phosphodiesterase, increase cyclic adenosine monophosphate (cAMP) levels and inhibit aggregation. **(c)** Clopidogrel and other P2Y12 inhibitors prevent signalling through the platelet ADP receptor, preventing direct activation of the platelet. **(d)** Glycoprotein (GP) IIb/IIIa receptor inhibitors prevent platelet aggregation. **(e)** PAR-1 inhibitors inhibit activation by thrombin. Others (not shown) include prostacyclin (epoprostenol), which stimulates adenylate cyclase and dextrans, which coat the surface, interfering with adhesion and aggregation. ADP, adenosine diphosphate; AMP, adenosine monophosphate; cAMP, cyclic adenosine monophosphate; NSAIDs, non-steroidal anti-inflammatory drugs; $P2Y_{12}$, purinergic receptor P2Y12; PAR1, protease-activated receptor 1; TXA2, thromboxane A2; TP, G-protein-coupled receptor which binds TXA2.

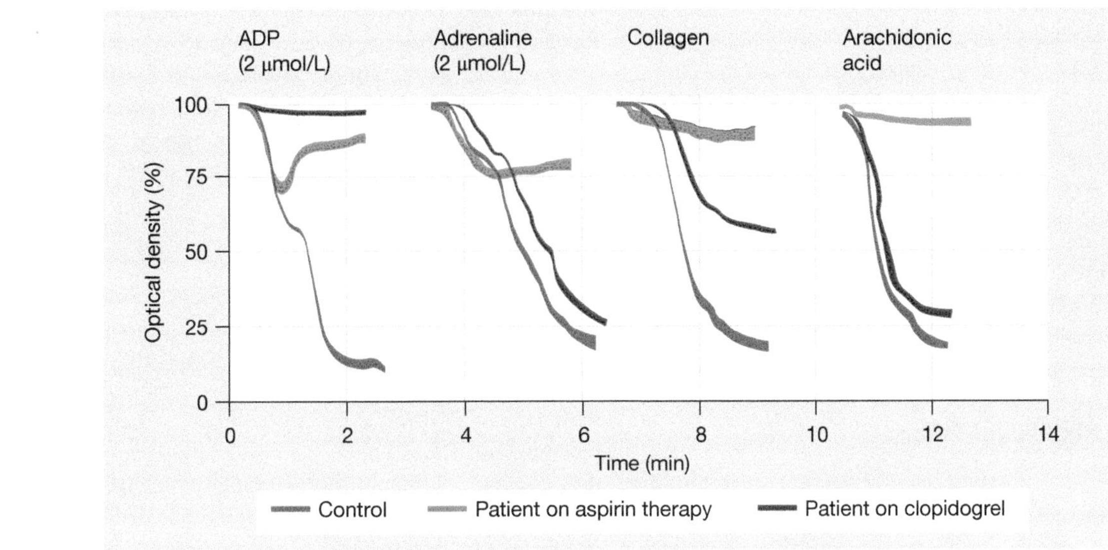

Figure 31.6 Defective platelet aggregation in patients on aspirin or clopidogrel therapy. With aspirin, there is no secondary phase of platelet aggregation with adenosine diphosphate (ADP) and reduced responses to arachidonic acid, adrenaline and collagen. With clopidogrel, the defect is mainly in ADP-induced aggregation.

on the platelet surface are essential for autocrine and paracrine activation. P2Y1 initiates ADP-induced platelet aggregation via stimulation of phospholipase C and mobilization of intracellular calcium that is reversible. P2Y12 mediates platelet activation by inhibiting adenylate cyclase and decreasing intracellular cAMP levels. This results in the activation of GPIIb/IIIa receptors and increased production of TXA2 and stable platelet aggregation.

Oral inhibitors of P2Y12 include thienopyridines (ticlopidine, clopidogrel and prasugrel) and ticagrelor.

Clopidogrel and prasugrel are pro-drugs, generating short-lived active metabolites that irreversibly inactivate the P2Y12 receptor, thus blocking ADP-induced platelet activation. Platelets are inhibited for their lifespan. The generation of active metabolites is related to the cytochrome P450 enzyme system and levels for prasugrel are 10-fold higher than clopidogrel. Specific cytochrome variants result in the slow metabolism of clopidogrel with poor response. Prasugrel is more effective but associated with an increased risk of major bleeding than clopidogrel. The clopidogrel effect lasts 3–10 days; prasugrel lasts 7–10 days.Clopidogrel is stopped a minimum of 5 days before surgery, and prasugrel a minimum of 7 days.

Ticagrelor is an adenosine triphosphate analogue that directly and reversibly binds the P2Y12 receptor, preventing ADP-induced P2Y12 activation. The inhibition lasts 3–5 days, and the drug is usually discontinued three days before non-acute surgery.

Cangrelor is a direct reversible inhibitor of the P2Y12 receptor, with a short half-life of 3–6 minutes and given as an intravenous infusion. It is used as a bridge around primary coronary intervention or in-stent thrombosis in patients not receiving a P2Y12 inhibitor. Its effect on platelet function disappears within 60 minutes of discontinuation.

Significant bleeding or emergency surgery in patients on P2Y12 antagonists can be remedied by tranexamic acid and platelet transfusions, although platelet transfusions have not demonstrated improvement in clinical outcomes.

Protease-activated receptor 1 inhibitor: vorapaxar

Thrombin-mediated platelet activation occurs via protease-activated receptors (PARs). PAR-1 activation results in TXA2 generation, dense granule release, platelet activation and platelet procoagulant response. Vorapaxar is a selective, competitive, potent and reversible PAR-1 antagonist. Vorapaxar disrupts intraplatelet signalling following activation by thrombin.

Glycoprotein IIb/IIIa inhibitors

Intravenous GPIIb/IIIa inhibitors prevent fibrinogen binding to activated GPIIb/IIIa receptors and inhibit platelet aggregation. Three GPIIb/IIIa inhibitors are available: abciximab, eptifibatide and tirofiban. Abciximab is a chimeric monoclonal antibody fragment with a plasma half-life of 10–30 minutes. It binds receptors non-competitively and irreversibly. Platelet function only recovers after 24 to 48 hours. Eptifibatide, a cyclic heptapeptide, and tirofiban, a non-peptide mimetic molecule, inhibit fibrinogen binding competitively and reversibly. Eptifibatide has a short plasma half-life of 2.5 hours, and platelets recover within 4 hours. Similarly, tirofiban has a half-life of 2 hours, and platelets recover between 4 and 8 hours. They require loading bolus followed by continuous infusion.

Phosphodiesterase (PDE) inhibitors

Dipyridamole and cilostazol are (PDE) inhibitors with vasodilator and antiplatelet effects. They increase intraplatelet cAMP and cGMP levels and reduce cellular adenosine uptake into red blood cells, platelets and endothelial cells. They are rarely used as single agents.

Thrombolytic (fibrinolytic) therapy

Blood flow reduction due to obstruction by thrombus is responsible for ischemia and tissue necrosis, particularly in arterial occlusion and less so with venous thrombosis. Thrombolytic therapy aims to rapidly restore blood flow by accelerating the endogenous proteolysis of the thrombus, which, under normal conditions, can take days.

Thrombolytic drugs

Several fibrinolytic drugs are available; some appear restricted to specific geographical locations. The commonly used fibrinolytic drugs include non-fibrin specific streptokinase and urokinase and the fibrin-specific recombinant tissue plasminogen activators (tPAs), e.g. alteplase and tenecteplase.

First-generation thrombolytics

The first generation of thrombolytics includes streptokinase and urokinase. They do not require the presence of cross-linked fibrin for plasminogen activation, and are non-fibrin-specific. Streptokinase was the most extensively used agent before the advent of recombinant tPA. It is not an enzyme; the 1:1 stoichiometric binding converts plasminogen to plasmin, with depletion of circulating fibrinogen, plasminogen and factors V and VIII. Urokinase is a naturally occurring plasminogen activator with slightly better efficacy than streptokinase.

Second-generation thrombolytics

Tissue plasminogen activator (tPA) is a serine protease that activates plasminogen on the surface of cross-linked fibrin, with which it forms a ternary complex (Chapter 26). The recombinant tPA, alteplase, has a circulating plasma half-life of 4–6 minutes. Although fibrin-specific, in therapeutic doses, it can cause activation of circulating plasminogen with a reduction of plasma fibrinogen. The reduction is related to the dose and duration of therapy. It is the most often used fibrinolytic agent. Systemic thrombolysis involves the administration of a loading intravenous bolus followed by an infusion over 60–90 minutes.

Modified versions of streptokinase (anisoylated plasminogen streptokinase activator complex, APSAC) and urokinase (single-chain urokinase plasminogen activator, SCU-PA) are also in clinical use.

Third-generation thrombolytics

Third-generation agents include modified tPA to improve the half-life and increase fibrin specificity. Increased resistance to plasminogen activator inhibitor 1 (PAI-1) inhibition is also seen with some molecules, which improves the half-life and allows bolus administration. Reteplase resembles human wild tPA, with a few missing domains. The most widely used third-generation agent is tenecteplase. It is derived from tPA but contains a three amino acid substitutions conferring an increase in fibrinolytic potency, higher resistance to PAI-1 and enhanced relative fibrin specificity. Tenecteplase has a longer half-life (20 minutes), enabling a bolus infusion.

Indications for thrombolytic therapy

Thrombolysis can be administered systemically or may be catheter-directed. A significant complication of thrombolytic therapy is bleeding, which can be fatal. This is related to the systemic activation of plasminogen and reductions in fibrinogen and alpha-2 antiplasmin. Excess plasmin generation can also affect platelets, FV and FVIII. Intracranial bleeding was seen in just under 1% of patients when thrombolysis was used to manage myocardial infarction, with a higher risk when used in ischemic stroke of approximately 5%. Patient selection for fibrinolytic therapy thus requires a careful risk-benefit analysis. The tolerance for bleeding complications is related to the indication; notably in arterial thrombosis when treatment is life-saving or limits disability.

In contrast, the benefits are less clear in venous thrombosis, and the risk-benefit analysis is against systemic therapy. Catheter-directed use of thrombolytics for PE and proximal DVT can be considered in selected situations. These bear less risk of systemic side effects due to localized use and lower systemic exposure from leakage.

1. Acute myocardial infarction (AMI) within 12 hours of onset
2. Acute ischemic stroke within 4.5 hours of symptom onset
3. Pulmonary embolism, massive or submassive, with hemodynamic compromise
4. Iliofemoral deep vein thrombosis – catheter-directed thrombolysis
5. Acute peripheral arterial occlusion – not amenable to surgery
6. Occlusion of indwelling catheters
7. Splanchnic vein thrombosis – systemically before insertion of a transjugular intrahepatic portosystemic shunt (TIPS)
8. Neonatal – for recanalization of large vessel thrombosis

Contraindications for thrombolytic therapy

The contraindications for thrombolytic therapy look at the potential for fatal bleeding. Further, over the years, some absolute contraindications have become relative. In addition to the general contraindications, there are also contraindications by indication.

Arterial thrombosis

The management of arterial thrombosis is designed to restore blood flow rapidly to alleviate ischemia-related damage. Treatment should also prevent reocclusion and promote healing. Further, rapidity of reperfusion is as important as achieving patency of the infarct-related artery to minimize tissue damage. Thus, the overall approach includes thrombolytic therapy, anticoagulants, antiplatelet agents and mechanical approaches (such as mechanical thrombectomy in stroke).

The pathophysiology of arterial thrombosis and risk factors have been discussed in Chapter 30. The scope of the specific management of acute coronary syndrome, acute stroke and acute lower limb ischemia is beyond the scope of this book, and an overview has been provided.

Acute arterial thrombotic occlusion requires emergency treatment, especially for small-calibre arteries. Systemic anticoagulation with a parenteral anticoagulant, e.g., heparin, or a direct thrombin inhibitor, e.g., bivalirudin, is given for coronary artery occlusion. Percutaneous interventions with thrombectomy and the placement of stents to maintain vessel patency in the setting of atherosclerotic plaque and thrombosis are also used to prevent or limit myocardial ischemia and infarction. For central nervous system thromboembolic stroke, systemic thrombolysis is used unless there are contraindications (Table 31.11), followed by a period of parenteral anticoagulation. Following acute management, patients are discharged on antiplatelet agents, often aspirin plus a platelet ADP receptor inhibitor such as clopidogrel if coronary artery stents are placed. Aspirin alone is given if the patient has a simple ischemic stroke.

Other individual arterial thrombosis syndromes can be managed with endovascular interventions (thrombectomy/clot retrieval, stenting), antiplatelet agents and/or anticoagulants. For arterial thrombosis in larger vessels, such as in a lower extremity, acute interventional thrombectomy is often performed to prevent limb ischemia, followed by systemic anticoagulation. The combination of aspirin and low-dose rivaroxaban has significant benefits for patients with peripheral arterial disease. There is an added benefit of reduction in other cardiovascular complications such as stroke and MI.

Atherosclerotic arterial events also require aggressive management of underlying risk factors such as smoking, diabetes, dyslipidaemia and hypertension. Statins are commonly used universally. Patients with embolic arterial thrombi due to atrial fibrillation are treated with systemic anticoagulation.

Table 31.11 General contraindications for thrombolytic therapy.

Absolute contraindications	Relative contraindications
Significant head trauma or prior stroke in the previous three months	Traumatic cardiopulmonary resuscitation
Active internal bleeding	Arterial puncture at a noncompressible site in previous 7 days
Elevated blood pressure (systolic > 185 mmHg or diastolic > 110 mmHg) that cannot be lowered safely	Untreated intracranial arteriovenous malformation
Aortic arch dissection	Untreated giant intracranial aneurysm
Intracerebral neoplasm	Recent major surgery or serious trauma (within the previous 14 days)
Symptoms suggestive of subarachnoid haemorrhage	Recent gastrointestinal or urinary tract haemorrhage (within the previous 21 days)
Intracranial/spinal surgery in the previous 3 months	Ischemic stroke within the previous 3 months
Previous intracranial haemorrhage	Pregnancy
Bleeding diathesis	Recent acute myocardial infarction (within the previous three months)
Proliferative diabetic retinopathy	

SUMMARY

- Antithrombotics are used for the prevention and treatment of thrombosis. Anticoagulants and antiplatelets prevent the formation of a thrombus or impair the growth of newly formed clots. Fibrinolytics and interventional techniques such as angioplasty and stenting ensure rapid recanalization.
- Anticoagulant drugs are used to prevent or treat venous or arterial thrombosis. They include parenteral and oral agents.
- Heparin is a naturally occurring polysaccharide belonging to the family of glycosaminoglycans. Unfractionated heparin is the least processed glycosaminoglycan usually obtained from porcine intestinal mucosa and has a short half-life.
- Low-molecular-weight heparins inhibit FXa more than thrombin. They have more predictable pharmacokinetics and are given subcutaneously. They are now first line for the prophylaxis of hospital-acquired VTE.
- Direct-acting oral anticoagulants (DOACs) include the FXa inhibitors rivaroxaban, apixaban and edoxaban and the FIIa (thrombin) inhibitor dabigatran. They have the advantage of fixed dosage, monitoring is not usually needed, and compared with warfarin, there are fewer drug and food interactions.
- DOACs are considered first-line treatment for patients with VTE and prevention of systemic embolism and stroke in patients with non-valvular atrial fibrillation.
- LMWH is the initial treatment for DVT or PE in pregnancy or if warfarin or some of the DOACs are to be used subsequently.
- Warfarin is mainly used for high-risk patients, e.g. with mechanical heart valves or antiphospholipid syndrome.
- The warfarin dose is usually aimed to raise the international normalized ratio (INR) to between 2.0 and 3.0. There are frequent drug and food interactions that affect the dose.
- Antiplatelet drugs, aspirin, clopidogrel, prasugrel, ticagrelor, cangrelor and dipyridamole are used to prevent and manage arterial thrombosis secondary to atherosclerosis.
- Thrombi, if acute, may be lysed by fibrinolytic agents, e.g. streptokinase or recombinant tissue plasminogen activator.

Now visit **www.wiley.com/go/haematology9e** to test yourself on this chapter.

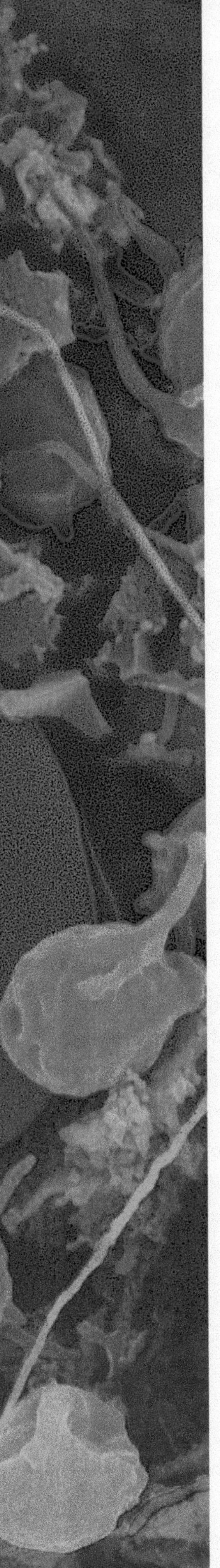

CHAPTER 32

Haematological changes in systemic diseases

Key topics

Hoffbrand's Essential Haematology, Ninth Edition. A. Victor Hoffbrand, Pratima Chowdary, Graham P. Collins, and Justin Loke.

© 2024 John Wiley & Sons Ltd. Published 2024 by John Wiley & Sons Ltd.

Companion website: www.wiley.com/go/haematology9e

Anaemia of chronic disease (inflammation)

Many of the anaemias seen in clinical practice occur in patients with systemic disorders and are the result of a number of contributing factors. The anaemia of chronic disease (ACD; also discussed on p. xx) can occur in patients with a variety of chronic inflammatory and malignant diseases (Table 32.1). Usually, both the erythrocyte sedimentation rate (ESR) and C-reactive protein (CRP) are raised, since inflammation contributes to suppression of erythropoiesis. ACD may be complicated by additional haematological changes due to the disease. The serum iron and total iron binding capacity (transferrin) are typically both low, while serum ferritin is normal or raised. The characteristic features and pathogenesis are described in Chapter 3.

ACD is corrected by the successful treatment of the underlying disease. It does not respond to iron therapy despite the low serum iron, since iron is typically present in the body in normal or elevated levels, but due to inflammation the developing erythroid cells cannot access it. Responses to recombinant erythropoietin therapy may be obtained, but ACD alone is not an approved indication. In many conditions ACD is complicated by concomitant anaemia from other causes, e.g. iron or folate deficiency, renal failure with decreased erythropoietin secretion, bone marrow infiltration by neoplastic cells or hypersplenism.

Haematological problems in the elderly

Anaemia

The World Health Organization defines anaemia as a haemoglobin less than 130 g/L in adult men and less than 120 g/L in non-pregnant women. Using these criteria, the incidence of anaemia is substantial in the elderly, e.g. more than 25% in men and more than 20% in women over 85 years old. The incidence is higher in people of sub-Saharan African ancestry, increases with age and predicts for shorter survival. In the United States about 10% of subjects over 65 years old are anaemic, and this is associated with increased hospitalization, disability and mortality.

Table 32.1 Causes of anaemia of chronic disease (ACD).

Chronic inflammatory diseases
Infectious, e.g. pulmonary abscess, tuberculosis, osteomyelitis, pneumonia, bacterial endocarditis
Non-infectious, e.g. rheumatoid arthritis, systemic lupus erythematosus and other connective tissue diseases, sarcoid, Crohn disease or ulcerative colitis
Malignant disease
e.g. carcinoma, lymphoma, sarcoma

The three main causes of anaemia in the elderly are ACD, iron or vitamin B_{12} deficiency and renal disease, but about a third of cases are unexplained after initial evaluation. Possibly some of the patients with unexplained anaemia have myelodysplasia. Clones with molecular mutations characteristic of myeloid neoplasms are increasingly present with advancing age in the bone marrow, without morphological changes, and their contribution to anaemia is often unclear (Chapter 16). The elderly also have reduced marrow reserve and develop more severe and prolonged anaemia, neutropenia and thrombocytopenia after chemotherapy than younger subjects.

Thrombosis

There is a greater incidence of arterial and venous thrombosis with advancing age (Chapter 30). This is partly due to increase in plasma levels of some of the clotting factors as well as reduced fibrinolysis. Relative immobility due to degenerative arthritis and frailty may also contribute. For arterial thrombosis, atheromatous plaques are a major contributor. Elderly subjects tend to be more sensitive than younger patients to anticoagulants and need careful monitoring to avoid haemorrhage.

Malignant disease (other than primary bone marrow disease)

Anaemia

Contributing factors to anaemia in cancer include ACD, blood loss and iron deficiency (especially in uterine, gastric or colorectal tumours), marrow infiltration (Fig. 32.1), haemolysis and marrow suppression from radiotherapy or chemotherapy (Table 32.2). Marrow infiltration may be associated with a leuco-erythroblastic blood film (p. 108).

Microangiopathic haemolytic anaemia (Chapter 6) occurs with mucin-secreting adenocarcinoma (Fig. 32.2), particularly of the stomach, lung and breast. Less common forms of anaemia with malignant disease include autoimmune haemolytic anaemia with malignant lymphoma and rarely with other tumours; pure red cell aplasia with thymoma or lymphomas; and myelodysplasia secondary to chemotherapy. There is also an association of pernicious anaemia with carcinoma of the stomach.

The anaemia of malignant disease may respond partly to erythropoiesis-stimulating agents, but care must be taken not to accelerate tumour growth (Chapter 2). Folic acid should only be given if there is definite megaloblastic anaemia caused by folate deficiency.

Polycythaemia

Secondary polycythaemia is occasionally associated with renal, hepatic, cerebellar and uterine tumours, which can secrete erythropoietin (Chapter 15).

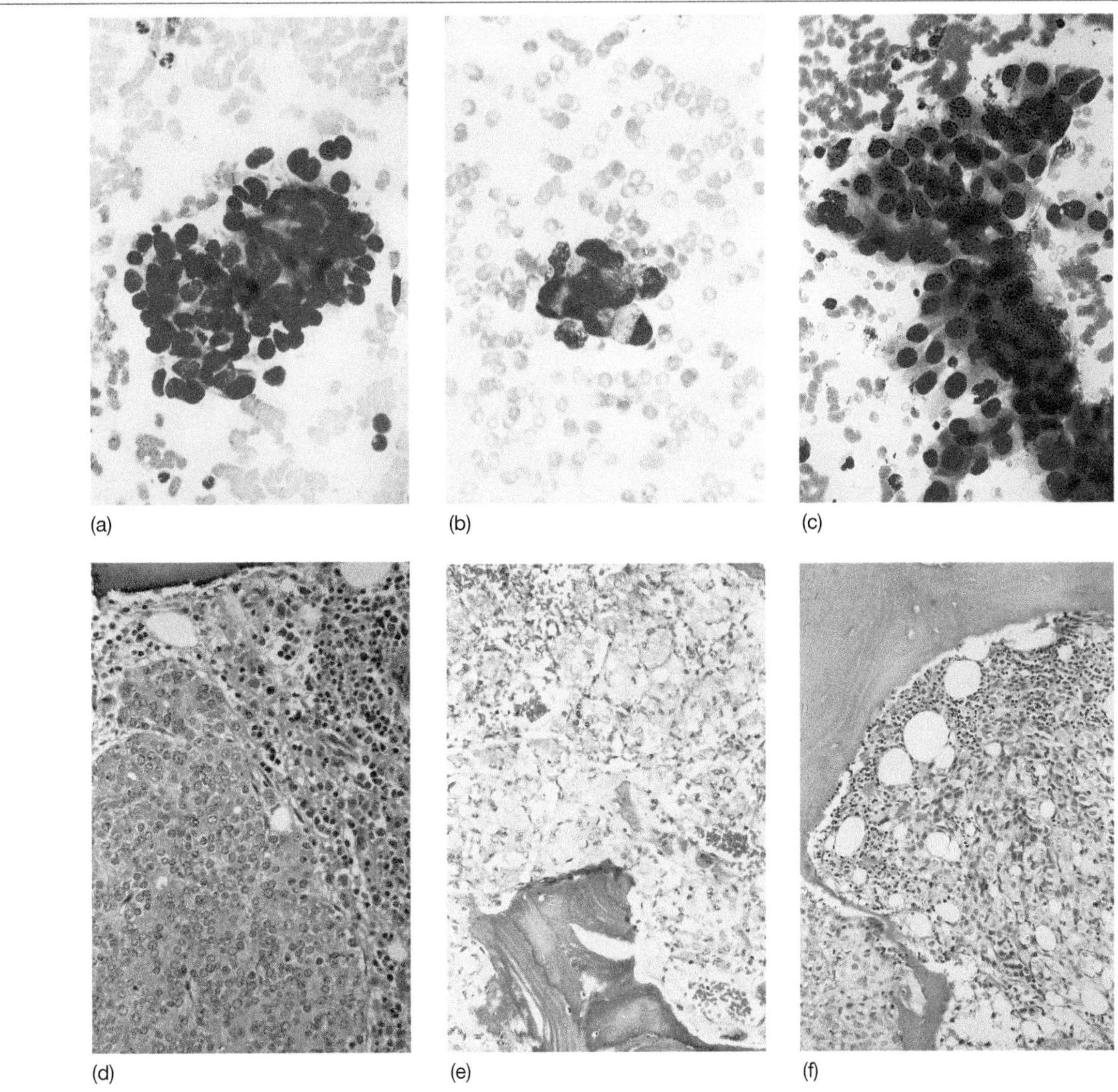

Figure 32.1 Metastatic carcinoma in bone marrow aspirates: **(a)** breast; **(b)** stomach; **(c)** colon; bone marrow trephine biopsies: **(d)** prostate; **(e)** stomach; **(f)** kidney.

White cell changes

Leukaemoid reactions (p. xxx) may occur, with tumours showing widespread necrosis and inflammation. Use of granulocyte colony-stimulating factor (G-CSF) to prevent chemotherapy-induced neutropenia can also cause a leukaemoid reaction. Hodgkin lymphoma is associated with a variety of secondary white cell abnormalities, including eosinophilia, monocytosis and leucopenia. In non-Hodgkin lymphoma, malignant cells may circulate in the blood (p. xxx).

Platelet and blood coagulation abnormalities

Patients with malignant disease may show either thrombocytosis or thrombocytopenia. Disseminated tumours, particularly mucin-secreting adenocarcinomas, are associated with disseminated intravascular coagulation (DIC; p. xxx) and generalized haemostatic failure due to thrombocytopenia and consumption of coagulation factors. Activation of fibrinolysis occurs in some patients with carcinoma of the prostate or urinary bladder. Occasional patients with malignant disease have spontaneous bruising or bleeding caused by an acquired inhibitor of one or other coagulation factor, most frequently factor VIII.

Cancer patients have a high incidence (estimated at 15%) of venous thromboembolism. This risk is increased by surgery and by some drugs, e.g. thalidomide. Thrombosis is most common in ovarian, brain, pancreatic and colon cancers. Thrombosis may be difficult to manage with vitamin K antagonists because of bleeding, interruptions with chemotherapy and

Table 32.2 Haematological abnormalities in malignant disease.

Haematological abnormality	Tumour or treatment associated
Pancytopenia	
Marrow hypoplasia	Chemotherapy, radiotherapy
Myelodysplasia	Chemotherapy, radiotherapy
Leuco-erythroblastic	Metastases in marrow
Megaloblastic	Folate deficiency
	B_{12} deficiency (carcinoma of stomach)
Red cells	
Anaemia of chronic disorders	Most forms
Iron deficiency anaemia	Especially gastrointestinal, uterine
Pure red cell aplasia	Thymoma
Immune haemolytic anaemia	Lymphoma, ovary, other tumours
Microangiopathic haemolytic anaemia	Mucin-secreting carcinoma
Polycythaemia	Kidney, liver, cerebellum, uterus
White cells	
Neutrophil leucocytosis	Most forms
Leukaemoid reaction	Disseminated tumours (with necrosis)
Eosinophilia	Hodgkin lymphoma, others
Monocytosis	Various tumours
Platelets and coagulation	
Thrombocytosis	Gastrointestinal tumours with bleeding,
Thrombocytopenia	Multiple causes
Disseminated intravascular coagulation	Mucin-secreting carcinoma
Activation of fibrinolysis	Prostate
Acquired inhibitors of coagulation	Most forms
Tumour cell procoagulants – tissue factor and other cancer procoagulants	Especially ovarian, pancreas, brain, colon

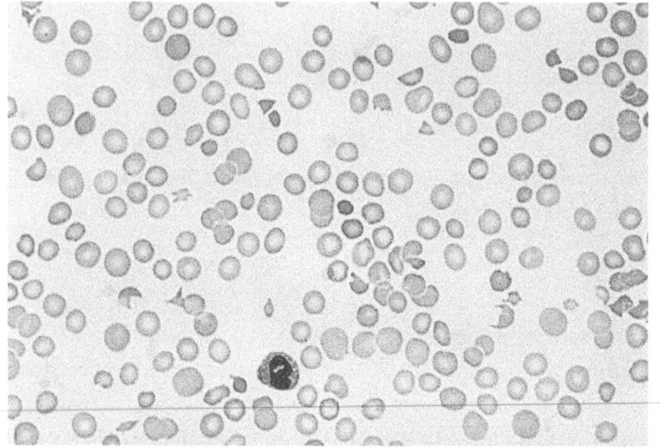

Figure 32.2 Peripheral blood film in metastatic mucin-secreting adenocarcinoma of the stomach showing red cell polychromasia and fragmentation and thrombocytopenia. The patient had disseminated intravascular coagulation.

thrombocytopenia, anorexia or vomiting (Chapter 30). Liver disease and drug interactions can cause further complications, so daily low-molecular-weight heparin injections are preferable and increasingly direct-acting oral anticoagulants are used.

Rheumatoid arthritis (and other connective tissue disorders)

In patients with rheumatoid arthritis, ACD is proportional to the activity and severity of the disease. Connective tissue disorders are complicated in some patients by iron deficiency caused by gastrointestinal bleeding related to therapy with salicylates, non-steroidal anti-inflammatory agents or corticosteroids. Bleeding into inflamed joints may rarely contribute to anaemia. Marrow hypoplasia may follow therapy with gold salts.

In **Felty syndrome**, splenomegaly is associated with neutropenia and increased large granular lymphocyte numbers (Fig. 32.3). Anaemia and thrombocytopenia may also be present.

In systemic lupus erythematosus (SLE), 50% of patients are leucopenic with reduced neutrophil and lymphocyte counts, often associated with circulating immune complexes. Renal impairment and drug-induced gastrointestinal blood loss also contribute to the ACD. Autoimmune haemolytic anaemia – typically with immunoglobulin (Ig) G and complement (C3d) on the surface of the red cells – occurs in 5% of patients and may be the presenting feature of the syndrome. There also may be autoimmune thrombocytopenia.

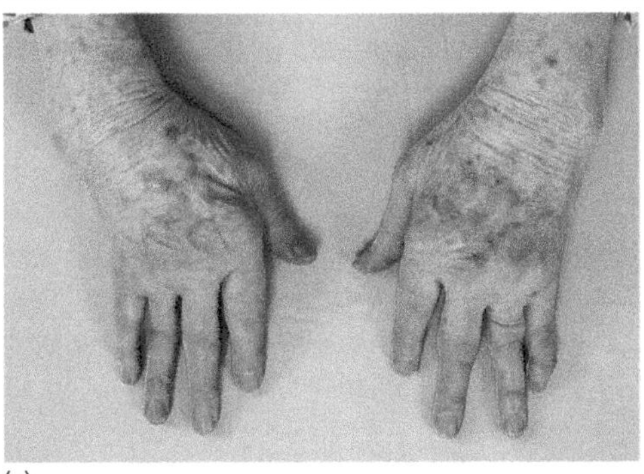

(a)

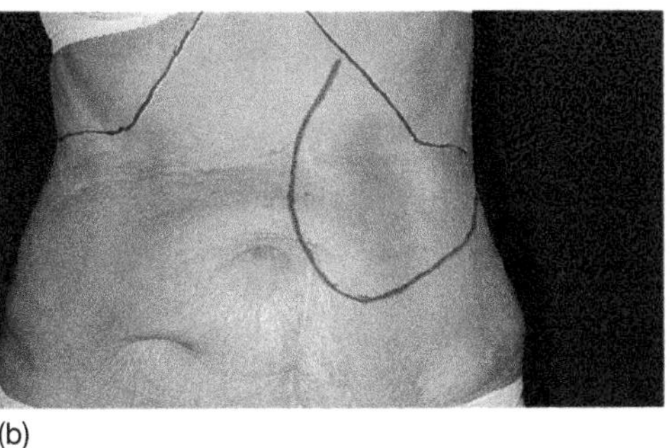

(b)

Figure 32.3 Felty syndrome: **(a)** the typical deformities of rheumatoid arthritis of the hands and **(b)** splenomegaly.

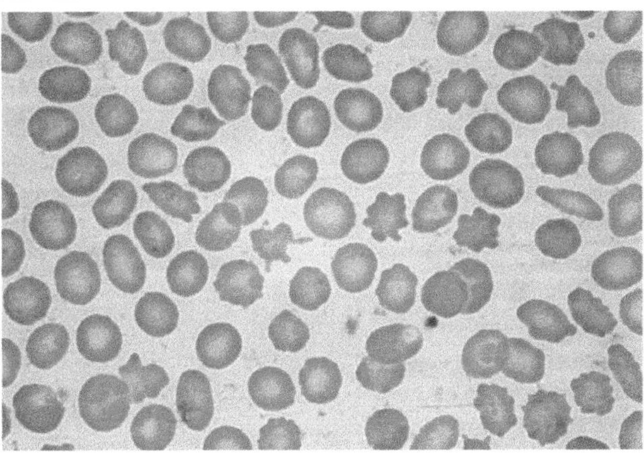

Figure 32.4 Peripheral blood film in chronic renal failure showing numerous 'burr' cells (echinocytes). With haemodialysis these typically are reduced in number, indicating their cause by a toxin normally cleared by the kidneys.

The lupus anticoagulant is described on page xxx. This circulating anti-cardiolipin interferes with blood coagulation by altering the binding of coagulation factors to platelet phospholipid and predisposes to both arterial and venous thrombosis and recurrent abortions. Tests for antinuclear antibodies (ANA) and anti-DNA antibodies are usually positive in SLE.

Patients with temporal arteritis and polymyalgia rheumatica have a markedly elevated ESR, pronounced red cell rouleaux in the blood film and a polyclonal immunoglobulin response. These and other vasculitides can also be associated with ACD.

Renal failure

Anaemia

A normochromic anaemia is present in most patients with chronic renal failure. Generally, there is a 20 g/L fall in haemoglobin level for every 10 mmol/L rise in blood urea, though there is wide variation. The dominant pathological mechanism is impaired red cell production as a result of defective erythropoietin secretion (Fig. 2.6). Variable shortening of red cell lifespan also occurs and, in severe uraemia, the red cells show abnormalities including 'burr' cells (Fig. 32.4). Increased red cell 2,3-diphosphoglycerate (DPG) levels in response to the anaemia and hyperphosphataemia result in decreased oxygen affinity and a shift of the haemoglobin–oxygen dissociation curve to the right (p. xx), which is augmented by uraemic acidosis. The patient's symptoms are therefore relatively mild for the degree of anaemia.

Other factors may complicate the anaemia of chronic renal failure (Table 32.3): ACD, iron deficiency from blood loss during dialysis or caused by bleeding because of defective platelet function, and folate deficiency in some chronic dialysis patients. Folic acid is usually given prophylactically.

Patients with polycystic kidneys usually have relatively retained erythropoietin production and have less severe anaemia for the degree of renal failure.

Table 32.3 Haematological abnormalities in renal failure.
Anaemia
Reduced erythropoietin production
Anaemia of chronic disorders
Iron deficiency
Blood loss, e.g. dialysis, venesection, defective platelet function
Folate deficiency
Chronic haemodialysis without replacement therapy
Microangiopathic haemolytic anaemia
Abnormal platelet function
Thrombocytopenia: immune complex-mediated, e.g. systemic lupus erythematosus, polyarteritis nodosa, acute nephritis, following allograft, haemolytic uraemic syndrome, thrombotic thrombocytopenic purpura
Thrombosis
Nephrotic syndrome
Polycythaemia
In renal allograft recipients
Rarely in renal cell carcinoma, cysts, arterial disease

Treatment

Recombinant erythropoietin corrects the anaemia in patients on dialysis or in chronic renal failure, providing that iron and folate deficiency have been corrected. The dosage of epoetin usually required is 50–150 units/kg three times a week, with a target haemoglobin of 120 g/L. Longer-acting preparations such as darbepoetin are increasingly used. Complications of therapy have included initial transient flu-like symptoms, hypertension and clotting of the dialysis lines.

A poor response to recombinant erythropoietin suggests iron or folate deficiency, infection or hyperparathyroidism. A regimen of intravenous iron sucrose 400 mg given prophylactically every month provided the serum ferritin is <700 μg/L and transferrin <40% has been found to reduce the need for erythropoietin compared with giving intravenous iron to correct iron deficiency, shown by low-serum ferritin and percentage saturation of total iron-binding capacity (TIBC), and increased percentage of hypochromic red cells in the blood. Trials are in progress of the prolyl hydroxylate inhibitors daprodustat, molidustat and vadadustat (Chapter 2) for treatment of the anaemia of patients with chronic renal failure including those receiving dialysis. In the short term, these drugs seem non-inferior to erythropoietin but longer term studies are needed.

Platelet and coagulation abnormalities

A bleeding tendency with purpura, gastrointestinal or uterine bleeding occurs in 30–50% of patients with chronic renal failure and is marked in patients with acute renal failure. The bleeding may be out of proportion to the degree of thrombocytopenia and has been associated with abnormal platelet or vascular function, which can be reversed by dialysis. Correction of the anaemia with recombinant erythropoietin also improves the bleeding tendency.

Immune complex-mediated thrombocytopenia occurs in some patients with acute nephritis, SLE and polyarteritis nodosa and also following renal allografts. Renal allografts may also lead to polycythaemia in 10–15% of patients.

The haemolytic uraemic syndrome and thrombotic thrombocytopenic purpura are discussed on page xxx. Patients with the nephrotic syndrome have an increased risk of venous thrombosis due to loss of anticoagulant proteins in the urine.

Congestive heart failure

Anaemia is present in 30–50% of patients with congestive heart failure due to chronic kidney disease, haemodilution and release of cytokines increasing hepcidin synthesis (reducing iron absorption and recycling of iron from macrophages) and reducing erythropoietin secretion. Iron deficiency may be caused by gastrointestinal or genitourinary bleeding related to anti-platelet or anticoagulation therapy, poor nutrition, impaired iron absorption (due to the raised hepcidin and congestion). Treatment with oral or better tolerated intravenous iron in those with a serum ferritin <100 μg/L or transferrin saturation <20% may improve left ventricular ejection fraction, lower CRP and brain natriuretic peptide (BNP) levels, reduce fatigue and increase exercise capacity and quality of life.

Liver disease

The haematological abnormalities in liver disease are listed in Table 32.4. Chronic liver disease can be associated with anaemia that is mildly macrocytic and often accompanied by target cells, mainly as a result of increased cholesterol in the membrane (Fig. 32.5a). Contributing factors to the anaemia may include blood loss, e.g. bleeding varices with iron deficiency, dietary folate deficiency and direct suppression of haemopoiesis by alcohol.

Haemolytic anaemia may occur in patients with alcohol intoxication (Zieve syndrome; Fig. 32.5b) and in Wilson disease (caused by copper oxidation of red cell membranes). Autoimmune haemolytic anaemia is found in some patients with chronic immune hepatitis. Haemolysis may also occur in end-stage liver disease because of abnormal red cell membranes resulting from lipid changes; 'spur' cells (acanthocytes) are common in advanced cirrhosis and are associated with a poor prognosis. Viral hepatitis may be associated with aplastic anaemia (Chapter 24).

The acquired coagulation abnormalities associated with liver disease are described on page xxx. There are deficiencies of vitamin K-dependent factors (II, VII, IX and X) and, in severe disease, of factor V and fibrinogen. Thrombocytopenia may

Table 32.4 Haematological abnormalities in liver disease.

Liver failure ± obstructive jaundice ± portal hypertension
Refractory anaemia – usually mildly macrocytic, often with target cells; may be associated with: Blood loss and iron deficiency Alcohol (± ring sideroblastic change) Folate deficiency Haemolysis, e.g. Zieve syndrome, Wilson disease, immune, hypersplenism from portal hypertension
Bleeding tendency Deficiency of vitamin K-dependent factors; also of factor V and fibrinogen Thrombocytopenia, immune platelet function defects Functional abnormalities of fibrinogen Increased fibrinolysis Portal hypertension – haemorrhage from varices
Viral hepatitis Aplastic anaemia
Hepatic tumours Polycythaemia due to erythropoietin secretion by the cancer cells Neutrophil leucocytosis and leukaemoid reactions

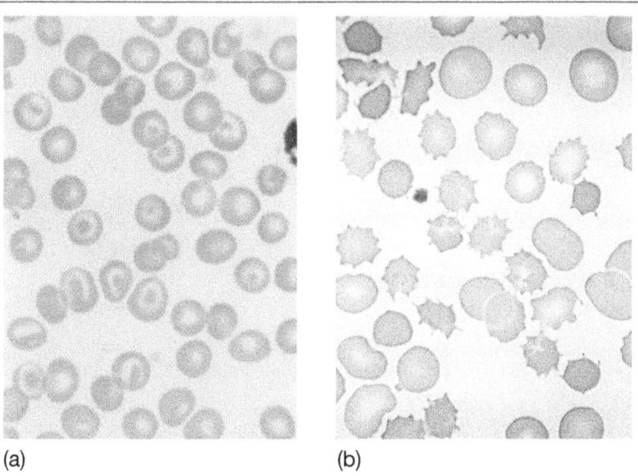

Figure 32.5 Liver disease: peripheral blood film showing: **(a)** macrocytosis and target cells; and **(b)** marked acanthocytosis and echinocytosis in Zieve syndrome. There may also be blue-green crystals of precipitated proteins in the neutrophils in severe liver disease.

occur from hypersplenism resulting from portal hypertension, or from immune complex-mediated platelet destruction. Abnormalities of platelet function may also be present. Dysfibrinogenaemia with abnormal fibrin polymerization may occur as a result of excess sialic acid in the fibrinogen molecules. A consumptive coagulopathy may be superimposed. These haemostatic defects may contribute to major blood loss from bleeding varices caused by portal hypertension.

Hypothyroidism

In mild hypothyroidism, there are typically no haematological changes. In more severe hypothyroidism, a moderate anaemia is common, as triodothyronine (T3) and thyroxine (T4) potentiate the action of erythropoietin. There is also a reduced oxygen need from the hypometabolic state and thus reduced erythropoietin secretion. The anaemia is often macrocytic and the mean corpuscular volume (MCV) falls with thyroxine replacement therapy.

Autoimmune thyroid disease, especially Hashimoto disease, is associated with pernicious anaemia. Iron deficiency may also be present, particularly in women with menorrhagia.

Infections

Haematological abnormalities are usually present in patients with infections of all types (Table 32.5). The effect of inflammation as a prothrombotic stimulus is also discussed on page xxx.

Bacterial infections

Acute bacterial infections are the most common cause of neutrophil leucocytosis. Toxic granulation, Döhle bodies and metamyelocytes may be present in the blood (Chapter 8). Leukaemoid reactions with a white cell count above 50×10^9/L and early granulocyte precursors in the blood may occur in severe infections, particularly in infants and young children. Mild anaemia is common if the infection is prolonged, such as in untreated tuberculosis. Severe haemolytic anaemia occurs in bacterial septicaemias, particularly those caused by Gram-negative organisms, where there is usually associated DIC (p. xx).

DIC dominates the clinical picture in certain infections, e.g. bacterial meningitis. The acute phase response to infections is accompanied by a rise in coagulation factors and a fall in natural anticoagulants.

Clostridium perfringens organisms produce an α toxin, a lecithinase acting directly on the circulating red cells (Fig. 32.6). Haemolysis in bartonellosis (Oroya fever) is caused by direct red cell infection. *Mycoplasma pneumoniae* infections are associated with autoimmune haemolytic anaemia of the 'cold' type (Chapter 6). With severe acute bacterial infections there may be thrombocytopenia. Chronic bacterial infections are associated with the ACD.

In tuberculosis, additional factors in the pathogenesis of anaemia include marrow replacement and fibrosis associated with miliary disease and reactions to anti-tuberculous therapy (e.g. isoniazid is a pyridoxine antagonist and may cause sideroblastic anaemia). Disseminated tuberculosis is associated with leukaemoid reactions and patients with involvement of bone marrow may show leuco-erythroblastic changes in the peripheral blood film.

Viral infections

Acute viral diseases are often associated with a mild anaemia. An immune haemolytic anaemia with an anti-i autoantibody is associated with infectious mononucleosis (Chapter 24). Viral infections, as well as syphilis, have been associated with paroxysmal cold haemoglobinuria (p. xx). Viruses have also been linked to the pathogenesis of the haemolytic uraemic syndrome, thrombotic thrombocytopenic purpura (Chapter 29) and the haemophagocytic syndrome (Chapter 8). Aplastic anaemia may occur with viral A hepatitis or more usually non-A, non-B, non-C hepatitis, due to an unknown virus. Transient red cell aplasia is associated with human parvovirus infection, and this may result in severe anaemia in subjects with a haemolytic anaemia (Chapter 24).

Acute thrombocytopenia is frequent in rubella and varicella infections, and in dengue fever. Rubella, cytomegalovirus (CMV) and other viral infections may cause a reactive lymphocytosis similar to that found in infectious mononucleosis. CMV infections in infants are associated with massive hepatosplenomegaly. In haemopoietic stem cell transplant recipients or other immunosuppressed patients, CMV infections may cause pancytopenia as well as other severe disorders (Chapter 25).

Table 32.5 Blood abnormalities associated with infections.

Haematological abnormality	Infection associated
Anaemia	
ACD	Chronic infections, especially tuberculosis
Aplastic anaemia	Viral hepatitis
Transient red cell aplasia	Human parvovirus
Marrow fibrosis	Tuberculosis
Immune haemolytic anaemia	Infectious mononucleosis, *Mycoplasma pneumoniae*
Direct red cell damage or microangiopathic haemolytic anaemia	Bacterial septicaemia (associated DIC), *Clostridium perfringens*, malaria, bartonellosis Viruses *Escherichia coli* and *Streptococcus pneumoniae* – haemolytic uraemic syndrome and TTP
Hypersplenism	Chronic malaria, tropical splenomegaly syndrome, leishmaniasis, schistosomiasis
White cell changes	
Neutrophil leucocytosis	Acute bacterial infections
Leukaemoid reactions	Severe bacterial infections particularly in infants
Monocytosis	Tuberculosis, listerosis
Eosinophilia	Parasitic diseases, e.g. hookworm, filariasis, strongyloidiasis, schistosomiasis, trichinosis
Lymphocytosis	Acute viral infections, e.g. HIV, influenza, infectious mononucleosis, cytomegalovirus, rubella, viral hepatitis Bacterial infections, e.g. pertussis, tuberculosis, rickettsia, brucellosis Toxoplasmosis
Neutropenia	Salmonella, rickettsia, brucellosis, overwhelming septicaemia
Lymphopenia	TB, acute bacterial infections, brucellosis, acute viral infections including SARS-CoV-2,chronic HIV
Thrombocytopenia	*Legionella pneumonophilia, rickettsia*
Megakaryocytic depression, immune complex mediated and direct interaction with platelets	Acute viral infections particularly in children, e.g. measles, varicella, rubella, malaria, severe bacterial infection, SARS-Cov-2 especially with DIC, HIV
Prothrombotic state	All with prolonged inflammation

ACD, anaemia of chronic disorders; DIC, disseminated intravascular coagulation; HIV, human immunodeficiency virus; TTP, thrombotic thrombocytopenic purpura.

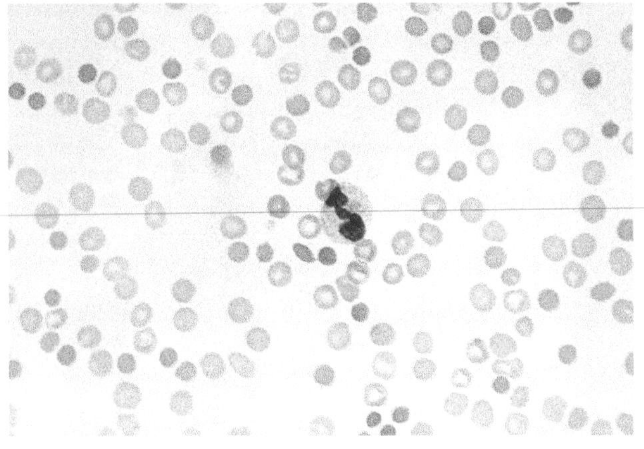

Figure 32.6 Peripheral blood film in a patient with haemolytic anaemia in clostridial septicaemia showing red cell contraction and spherocytosis.

Severe acute respiratory syndrome)-CoV (coronavirus)-2 infection

SARS -CoV -2 infection causes a wide variety, severity and chronicity of pathology in humans. The infection may be symptomless in some, but rapidly fatal in others. Recovery may be complete within a few days or weeks; in about one third of patients, symptoms persist beyond 90 days-the post-COVID19 syndrome. The infection most frequently causes chest problems with cough, breathing difficulties and hypoxia related to pneumonitis with pulmonary endothelialitis, microthrombi, pulmonary thrombosis or venous thromboembolism (Chapter 29). Arterial thrombosis with myocardial infarction or limb ischemia is less frequent. Fatigue and muscle or body aches are frequent. Features of gastro-intestinal or renal damage may be dominant.

Haematological complications

Anaemia is common. There may be haemolysis with or without a positive IgG direct antiglobulin test. Anaemia may also be due to renal dysfunction and the anaemia of chronic inflammation. The CRP, ferritin and LDH are all raised related to the severity. **There is a fall in lymphocytes also related to the severity of the disease; a progressive decline predicts the need for intensive care and for death.** Large lymphocytes with increased pale cytoplasm are always present, and large granular lymphocytes and lymphoplasmacytoid cells are often present (Fig. 32.7). The neutrophils may be raised with a left shift. Morphological abnormalities include dark, clumped nuclear chromatin with absent or hypolobation and hyper- or hypo-granulation of the cytoplasm with basophilic inclusions (Fig. 32.7). Large vacuolated monocytes with irregular nuclear outline are also frequent.

The platelet count is reduced, related to the severity of the disease. It is due to multiple causes. Hypergranular and giant, vacuolated platelets are described (Fig. 32.7). Clinical and laboratory features of DIC, the haemophagocytic lymphohistiocytosis (HLH) or the macrophage activation syndrome (Chapter 8) are often present. Factor VIII and plasminogen-activator inhibitor type 1 levels are raised predisposing to thrombosis. Increasing PT, APTT and D-dimer levels are additional markers of disease severity (Chapter 29).

Vaccine-induced immune thrombotic thrombocytopenia (VITT) may occur very rarely in individuals following vaccination with adenovirus vector-based vaccines. This is discussed in Chapter 29.

Human immunodeficiency virus (HIV) infection

HIV is associated with a wide range of haematological changes, which tend to be worse in more advanced disease. These are caused by marrow defects including dysplasia (Fig. 32.8) and immune cytopenias directly resulting from HIV infection, the effects of opportunistic infections or lymphoma, and the side effects of drugs used to treat HIV itself or drugs for the complicating infection or lymphoma.

Anaemia is common and more severe as the disease progresses. It is usually multifactorial in origin. The virus can

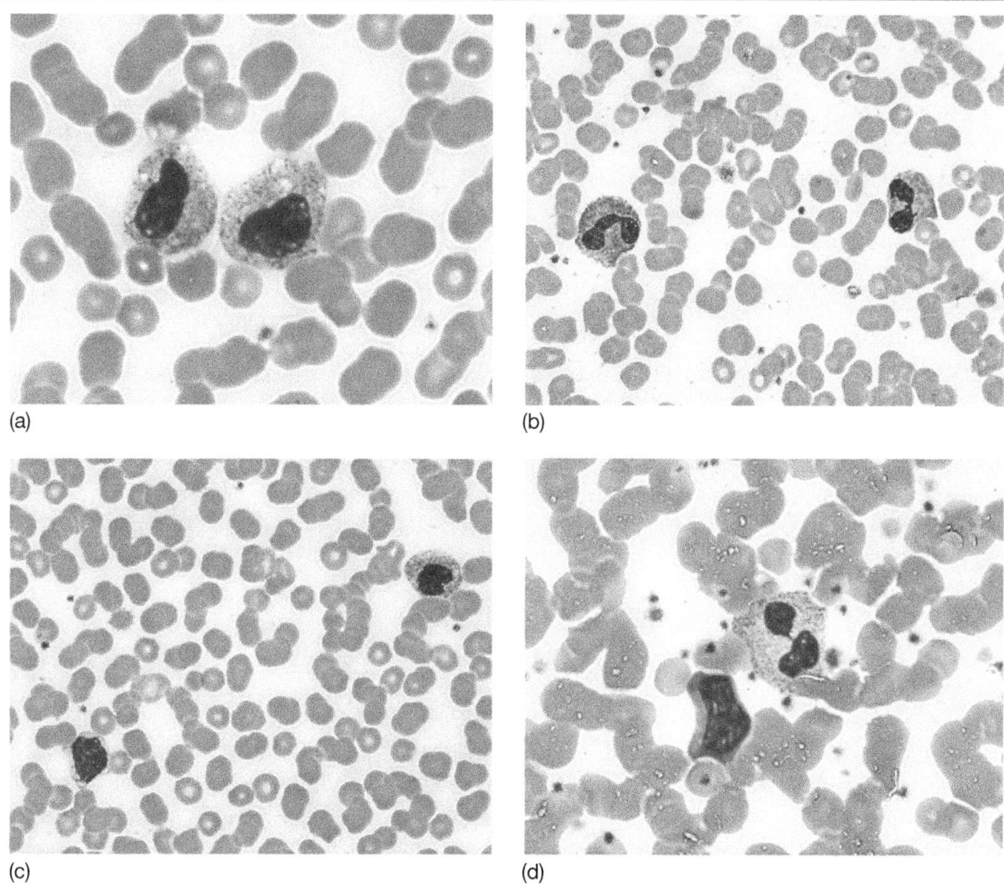

Figure 32.7 SARS-CoV-2 infection. Peripheral blood films from severe cases showing: **(a)** two neutrophils with clumped chromatin, toxic granulation, cytoplasmic vacuolation **(b)** two neutrophils with pseudo-Pelger-Huët appearances and toxic granulation; a large vacuolated platelet is also present **(c)** neutrophil with condensed nuclear chromatin, irregular areas of cytoplasmic basophilia (Döhle bodies), vacuolation and toxic granulation; and a large granular lymphocyte (**d**) an activated (pleomorphic) lymphocyte and a bi-lobed neutrophil with toxic granulation. Source: **(a–d)** Courtesy of Professor Gina Zini.

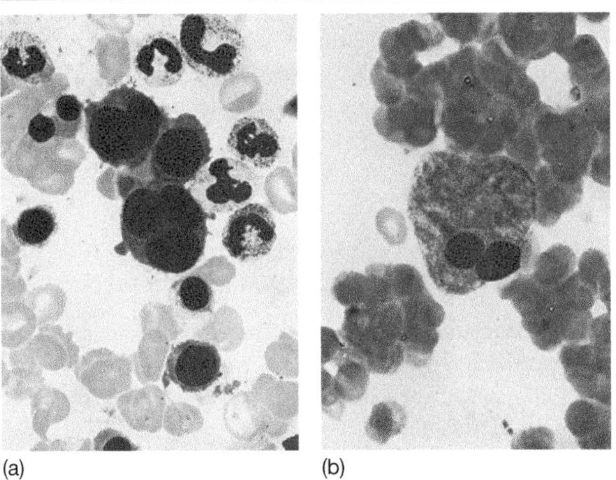

Figure 32.8 **(a)** HIV infection: bone marrow showing dyserythropoiesis. **(b)** HIV infection: bone marrow showing a dysplastic megakaryocyte. Source: A.V. Hoffbrand *et al.* (2019) *Color Atlas of Clinical Hematology,* 5th edn. Reproduced with permission of John Wiley & Sons.

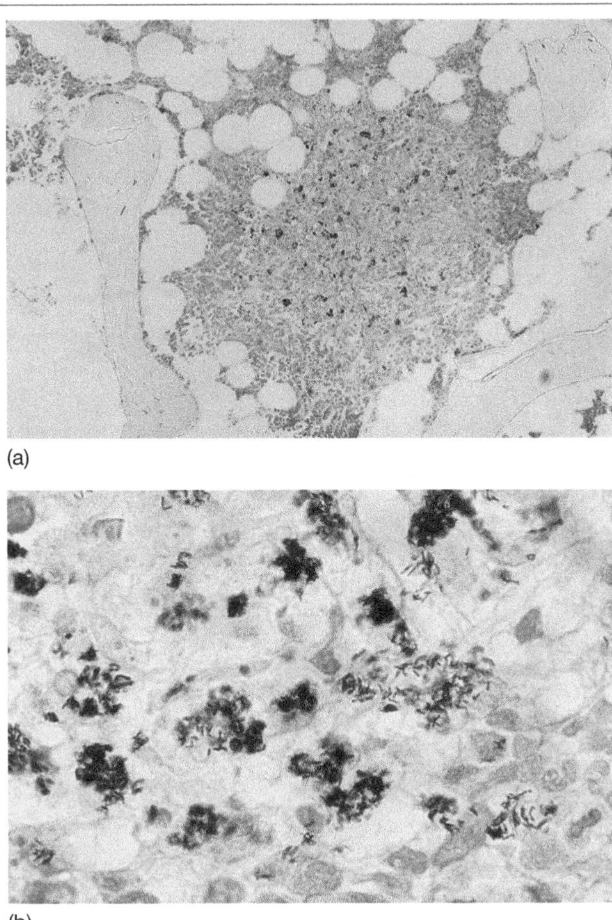

Figure 32.9 Human immunodeficiency virus (HIV) infection: bone marrow trephine biopsy. **(a)** Granuloma showing positivity with Ziehl-Nielsen stain. **(b)** Higher power shows large numbers of acid-fast bacilli.

directly suppress haemopoiesis. ACD, marrow dysplasia (Fig. 32.8), secondary infections, autoimmune haemolysis and drug therapy are other causes of anaemia. Serum vitamin B_{12} is often low, most likely because of intestinal malabsorption, but the anaemia does not respond to vitamin B_{12} therapy. Blood transfusions or recombinant erythropoietin injections are needed.

Thrombocytopenia and neutropenia may be immune or secondary to marrow dysfunction (Fig. 32.8). The marrow may be hypercellular with prominent plasma cells and lymphocytes, normocellular, hypocellular or fibrotic. Dysplastic features are common, with ineffective thrombopoiesis or granulocyte formation accounting at least in part for the cytopenia. The dysplastic marrow cells do not show the chromosome abnormalities found in myelodysplasia, however, and are not pre-leukaemic. Thrombocytopenia is treated if necessary by corticosteroids, high-dose gammaglobulin infusions or by other therapies for immune thrombocytopenia (Chapter 27), or by anti-retroviral therapy.

Increased plasma cells in the marrow and polyclonal increase in immunoglobulins are frequent. A paraprotein is present in 5–10% of cases, but appears benign and usually resolves with highly active anti-retroviral therapy.

Non-Hodgkin lymphoma, in over 90% high grade, both systemically and in the central nervous system, occurs in HIV-infected individuals with over 100 times the frequency expected in the general population. Diffuse large B-cell lymphoma is the most common, with 20% confined to the central nervous system. A substantial minority are Burkitt lymphoma, and HIV should always be sought in new cases of Burkitt and Burkitt-like lymphoma. Hodgkin lymphoma, usually of poor prognosis type, is also increased in frequency. EBV infection appears to underlie this as well as Burkitt lymphoma and multicentric Castleman disease with HHV8 infection (p. 285).

Treatment of lymphomas in the setting of HIV is with combination chemotherapy and immunotherapy, e.g. rituximab. Continuation of the necessary anti-retroviral therapy exaggerates the tendency to cytopenia induced by chemotherapy, so prophylaxis against opportunistic infections is important. The bone marrow may indeed reveal the presence of opportunistic infection (Fig. 32.9).

Other infections

Malaria

Some degree of haemolysis is seen in all types of malarial infection (Chapter 6). The most severe abnormalities are found in *Plasmodium falciparum* infections (Fig. 32.10). In the most severe cases, DIC occurs and intravascular haemolysis is

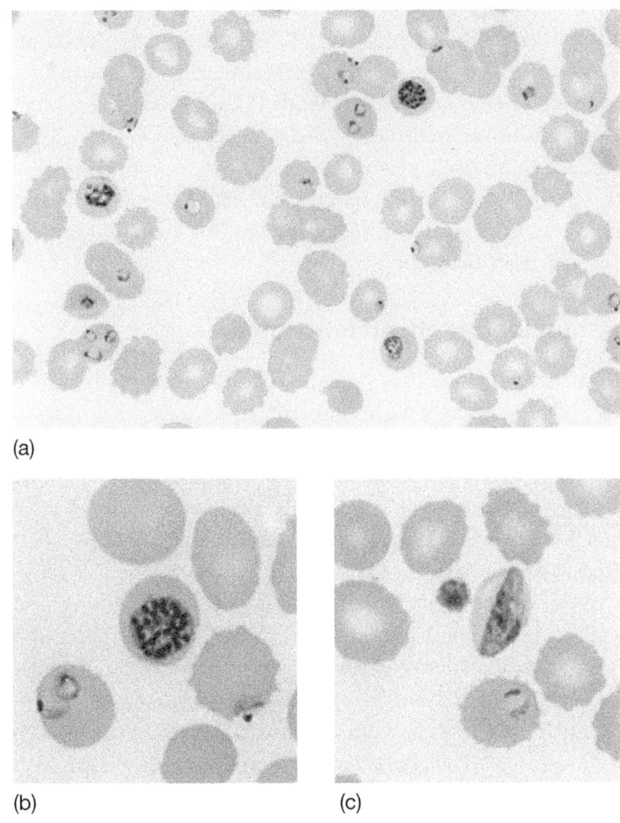

Figure 32.10 Malaria: peripheral blood in severe *Plasmodium falciparum* infection showing **(a)** many ring forms and a merozoite; and at higher magnification: **(b)** a merozoite; and **(c)** a gametocyte.

marked with haemoglobinuria. This may be associated with quinine therapy ('blackwater fever'). Thrombocytopenia is commonly found in acute malaria. Patients with chronic malaria have an anaemia of chronic disorders; hypersplenism may contribute to the anaemia and result in moderate thrombocytopenia and neutropenia. Tropical splenomegaly is probably a chronic immune reaction to malaria (Chapter 10). Dyserythropoiesis in the marrow, folate deficiency and protein-calorie malnutrition may contribute to anaemia.

Toxoplasmosis

Toxoplasmosis in children and adults is associated with lymphadenopathy and large numbers of atypical lymphocytes in the blood. Congenital disease may cause a syndrome resembling hydrops fetalis with severe anaemia, a hydropic infant with gross hepatosplenomegaly and thrombocytopenia.

Kala-azar (visceral leishmaniasis)

The visceral form of leishmaniasis is associated with pancytopenia, hepatosplenomegaly and lymphadenopathy. Bone marrow or splenic aspirates may show large numbers of parasitized macrophages (Fig. 32.11).

Other parasitic diseases

Chronic schistosomiasis (bilharzia) affects over 200 million people worldwide. It is one of the most frequent causes of iron deficiency due to bleeding from the bowel or bladder. Hypersplenism follows splenic enlargement associated with portal hypertension due to liver infestation. In the acute phase of both African and South American trypanosomiasis,

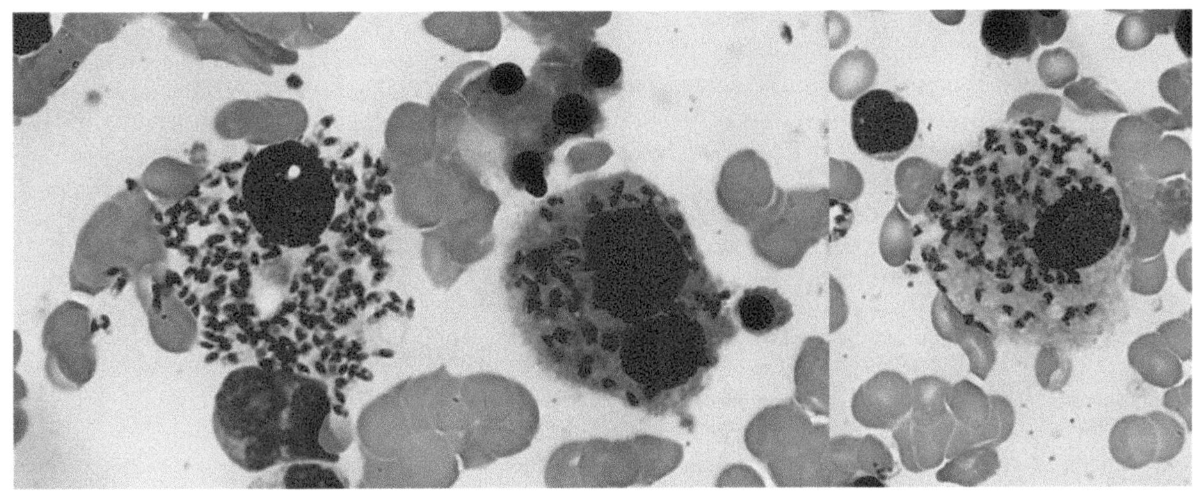

Figure 32.11 Kala-azar: bone marrow aspirates showing macrophages containing Leishman–Donovan bodies.

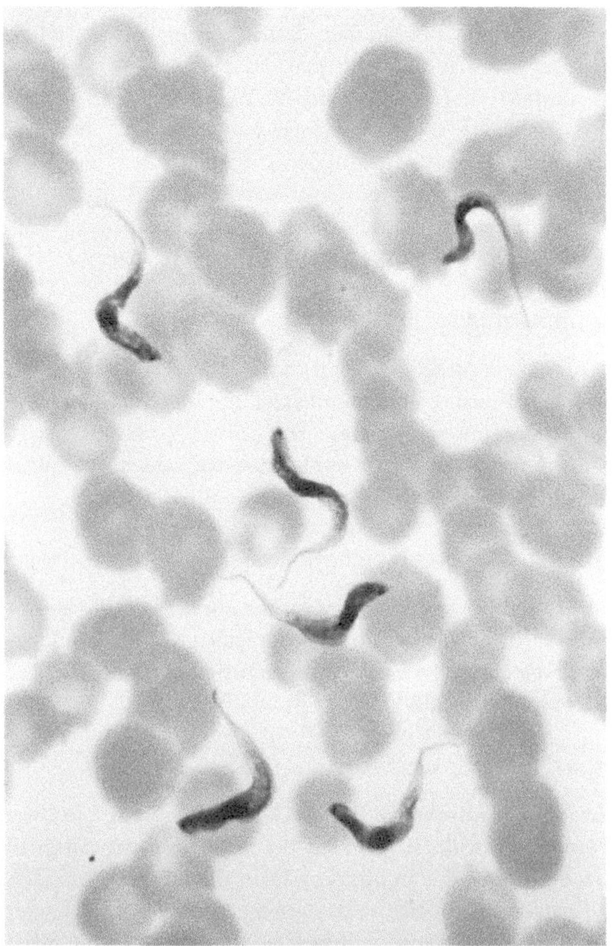

Figure 32.12 African trypanosomiasis: blood film showing *Trypanosoma brucei*.

organisms are found in the peripheral blood (Fig. 32.12). Microfilariae of bancroftian filariasis and loiasis are also detected during blood film examination (Fig. 32.13). In many parasitic diseases, there is eosinophilia.

Non-specific monitoring of systemic disease

The inflammatory response to tissue injury includes changes in plasma concentrations of proteins known as acute phase proteins. These include fibrinogen, other clotting factors, complement components, CRP (see below), haptoglobin, serum amyloid A (SAA) protein, ferritin and others. The rise in these liver derived proteins is part of a wider response, which includes fever, leucocytosis and increased immune reactivity. The acute phase response is mediated by cytokines, e.g. IL-1and TNF released from macrophages and other cells (Fig. 8.4). Quantitative measurements of acute phase proteins are valuable indicators of the presence and extent of inflammation and of its response to treatment. **When short-term (less than 24 hours) changes in the inflammatory response are expected, CRP is the test of choice (Table 32.6). Long-term changes in the acute phase proteins are monitored by either the ESR or plasma viscosity**. These tests are influenced by plasma proteins, which are either slowly responding acute-phase reactants, e.g. fibrinogen, or are not acute-phase proteins, e.g. immunoglobulins.

Erythrocyte sedimentation rate

This commonly used but non-specific test measures the speed of sedimentation of red cells in plasma over a period of 1 hour. The speed is mainly dependent on the plasma concentration of large proteins, e.g. fibrinogen and immunoglobulins. The normal range in men is 1–5 mm/hour and in women 5–15 mm/hour, but there is a progressive increase with age. The ESR is raised in a wide variety of systemic inflammatory and neoplastic diseases and in pregnancy. It is useful for diagnosing and monitoring temporal arteritis and polymyalgia rheumatica and for monitoring patients with Hodgkin lymphoma. High values (>100 mm/hour) have a 90% predictive value for serious disease, including infections, collagen vascular disease or malignancy, particularly myeloma. A raised ESR is associated with marked rouleaux formation of red cells in the peripheral blood film (Fig. 22.7). Changes in the ESR can be used to monitor the response to therapy.

Lower than expected ESR readings occur in polycythaemia vera because of the high red cell concentration. Higher than expected values may occur in severe anaemia because of the low red cell concentration.

Plasma viscosity

Plasma viscosity is affected by the concentration of plasma proteins of large molecular size, especially those with pronounced axial asymmetry: fibrinogen and some immunoglobulins. Normal values at room temperature are usually in the range of 1.50–1.70 mPa/s. Lower levels are found in neonates because of lower levels of proteins, particularly fibrinogen. Viscosity increases only slightly in the elderly as fibrinogen increases. There is no difference in values between men and women. Other advantages over the ESR test include independence from the effects of anaemia and results that are available within 15 minutes.

C-reactive protein (CRP)

Phylogenetically CRP is a crude 'early' immunoglobulin which initiates the inflammatory reaction. CRP–antigen complexes can substitute for antibody in the fixation of Clq and trigger the complement cascade, initiating the inflammatory response to antigens or tissue damage. Subsequent binding of C3b on the surface of microorganisms opsonizes them for phagocytosis.

(a)

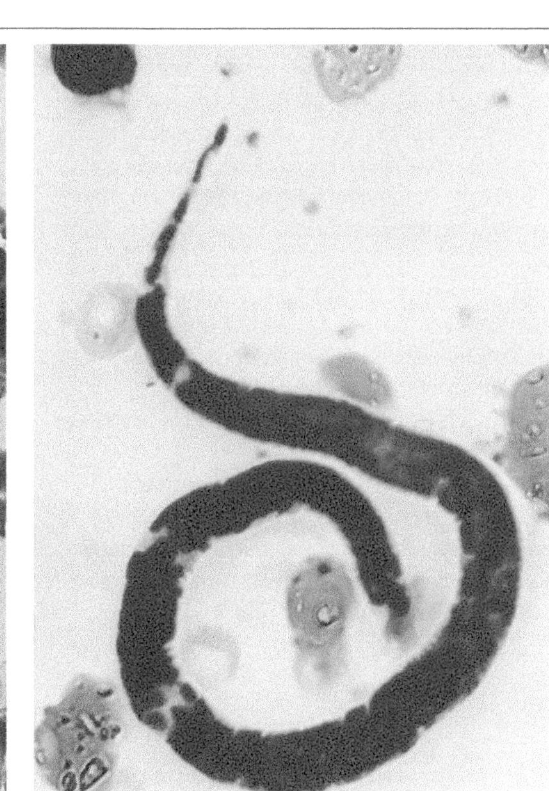

(b)

Figure 32.13 Peripheral blood films showing microfilariae of **(a)** *Wuchereria bancrofti*; and **(b)** *Loa loa*.

Table 32.6 Advantages and disadvantages of the tests used to monitor the acute phase response.

Advantages	**Disadvantages**
*CRP**	CRP is sensitive to interleukin-6 but less to other proinflammatory molecules
Specific test of acute phase protein	Costly when assayed in small numbers
Fast response (6 hours) to change in disease activity	Sophisticated equipment and antisera required
High sensitivity – owing to large incremental change	
Can be measured on stored serum	
Small sample volumes	
Automated analysis	
ESR and plasma viscosity	Not sensitive to acute changes (<24 hours)
Useful in chronic disease	Not specific for acute phase response
ESR inexpensive, easy, no electrical power required	Slow to change with alteration in disease activity and insensitive to small changes in activity
Plasma viscosity—result obtained quickly (15 minutes)	Fresh samples (<2 hours) required for ESR
Plasma viscosity not affected by anaemia	

* C-reactive protein (CRP) is normally present in plasma at low concentrations (<5 mg/L). Levels are not influenced by anaemia, pregnancy or heart failure. During severe acute infection the plasma concentration may rise 100-fold. ESR, erythrocyte sedimentation rate.

After tissue injury, an increase in CRP, serum amyloid A (SAA) protein and other acute phase reactants, synthesized in the liver, may be detected within 6–10 hours. Immunoassays of CRP are widely used for early detection of acute inflammation or tissue injury and for the monitoring of remission, e.g. response of infection to an antibiotic.

Table 32.6 lists the advantages and disadvantages of some of the tests used to assess the acute phase response.

SUMMARY

- Chronic inflammation or malignant disorders cause anaemia with low serum iron and iron-binding capacity, normal or raised serum ferritin, an inadequate response to erythropoietin and reduced red cell life span. The degree of anaemia relates to the severity of the underlying disease. It does not respond to iron therapy.
- This anaemia may be complicated in systemic diseases by other causes of anaemia, e.g. iron or folate deficiencies, renal failure, bone marrow infiltration, haemolysis, hypersplenism.
- Polycythaemia is a much less frequent complication of systemic diseases, e.g. renal.
- White cell changes are also frequent in systemic diseases. These include neutrophil leucocytosis, especially in bacterial infections, leuco-erythroblastic or leukaemoid reactions, and, in viral and connective tissue diseases, neutropenia.
- Eosinophilia occurs with certain infections, particularly parasitic and allergic disease.
- Monocytosis is associated with chronic bacterial infections, e.g. tuberculosis, brucellosis.
- Lymphocytosis is a feature of viral infections and some bacterial infections, e.g. *Bordetella pertussis*. SARS-CoV-2 infection causes anaemia, lymphopenia and thrombocytopenia as well as, in severe cases, DIC with thrombosis especially in the pulmonary vasculature.
- Platelets may be increased or low in malignant, infectious and other systemic diseases. DIC is a major cause of thrombocytopenia and a fall in coagulation factors in systemic diseases.
- C-reactive protein can be used for non-specific monitoring of systemic disease in the short term (hours or days) and erythrocyte sedimentation rate (or plasma viscosity) over weeks or months.

Now visit **www.wiley.com/go/haematology9e** to test yourself on this chapter.

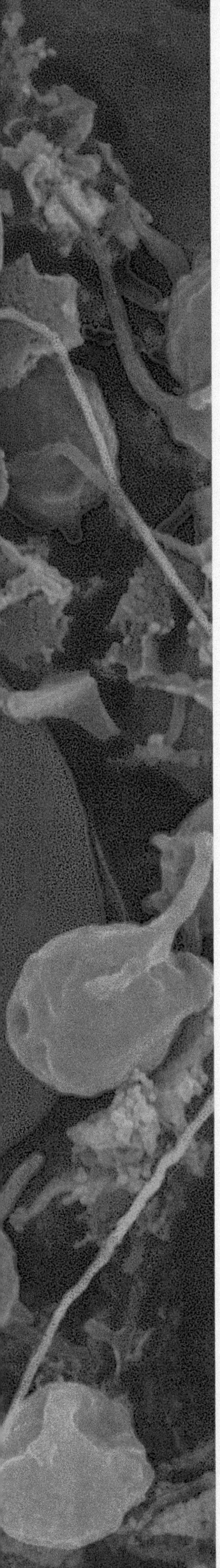

CHAPTER 33

Blood transfusion

Key topics

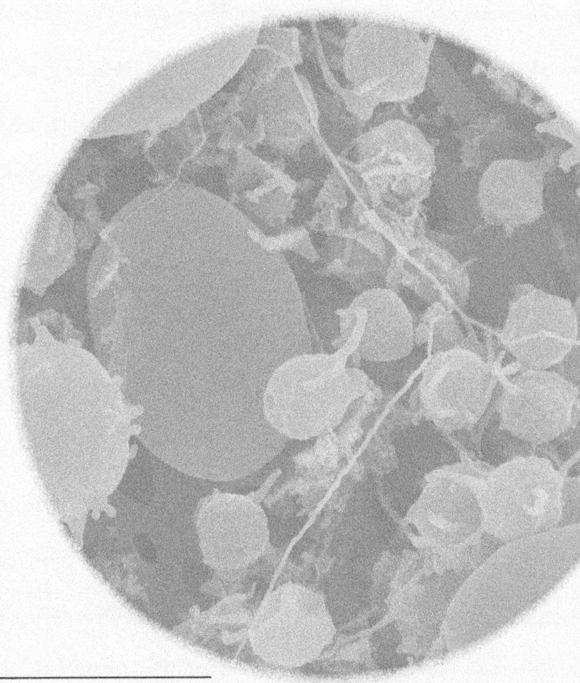

Hoffbrand's Essential Haematology, Ninth Edition. A. Victor Hoffbrand, Pratima Chowdary, Graham P. Collins, and Justin Loke.

© 2024 John Wiley & Sons Ltd. Published 2024 by John Wiley & Sons Ltd.

Companion website: www.wiley.com/go/haematology9e

Blood transfusion consists of the 'safe' transfer of blood components (Fig. 33.1) from a donor to a recipient. Blood product collection, processing and transfusion are tightly regulated. The World Health Organization and the Council of Europe have defined a code of ethical principles. In the United States blood banks are under the jurisdiction of the Food and Drug Administration (FDA), whereas in the United Kingdom, of the Medicines and Healthcare Regulatory Agency (MHRA).The FDA and the MHRA inspect all blood facilities at least once every two years (more frequently if problems are detected) and quality standards are similar to those imposed on pharmaceutical manufacturers. All adverse events involving UK blood products must be reported to the online Serious Adverse Blood Reactions and Events (SABRE) scheme, and similar reporting mechanisms exist in other countries.

In the United States, more than 5 million individual patients receive blood products annually, with at least 15 million blood products dispensed. In England and North Wales, more than 500 000 patients receive a cumulative ~2 million blood products annually. Blood transfusion is dominantly based in hospitals but blood transfusion at home for anaemic patients with other illnesses if essential can been safely practised.

Blood donor selection

In most countries blood donors contribute on a voluntary basis and this is generally preferable in terms of product safety. The measures to protect donors and for donor selection are listed in Table 33.1. Prospective blood donors are asked a series of specific, direct questions about risk factors for infection with blood-transmissible diseases, and this screening is estimated to eliminate more than 90% of unsuitable donors. The donor's haemoglobin is checked by a gravimetric method with a drop of blood in a copper sulphate solution or more accurately by a haemoglobinometer.

Red cell antigens and blood group antibodies

The clinical significance of blood groups in blood transfusion is that individuals who lack a particular blood group antigen may have preformed antibodies or may produce antibodies reacting with that antigen, which may lead to a transfusion reaction. Approximately 400 red blood cell group antigens have been described. The different blood group antigens vary greatly in their clinical significance, with the ABO and Rh groups being the most important. Some other systems are listed in Table 33.2.

Blood group antibodies

The ABO blood group antigens are unusual in that naturally occurring antibodies – usually immunoglobulin M (IgM) and rarely IgG – occur in the plasma of subjects who lack the corresponding antigen, even if they have not been

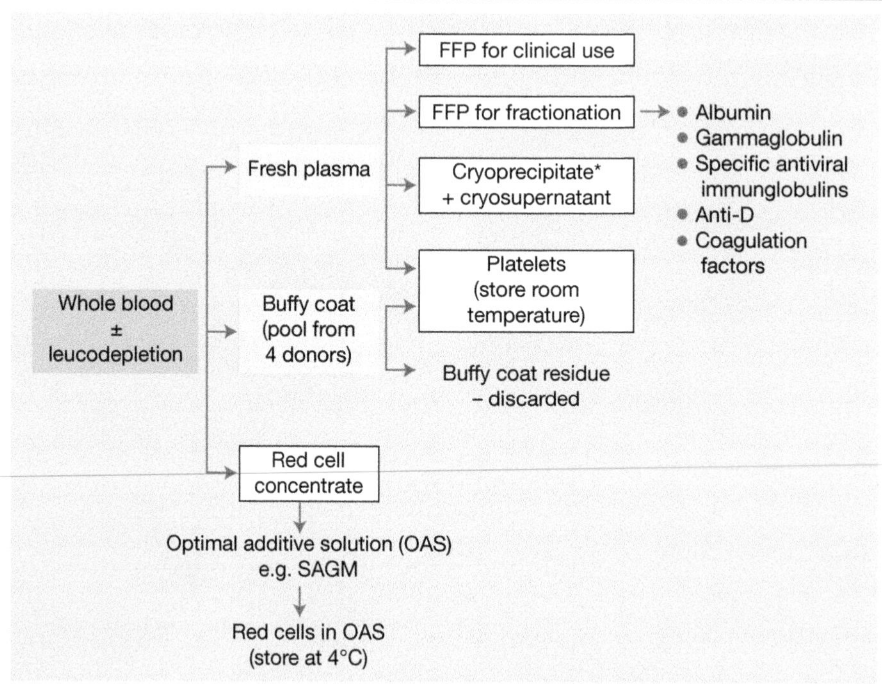

Figure 33.1 The preparation of blood components from whole blood. FFP, fresh frozen plasma; SAGM, saline-adenine-glucose-mannitol. *Cryoprecipitate is mainly a source of fibrinogen. Cryosupernatant is used for plasma exchange in thrombotic thrombocytopenic purpura. Leucodepletion – see text.

Table 33.1 Measures used to protect the donor and for donor selection.

Donor selection
Age 17–70 years (maximum 65 at first donation)
Weight above 50 kg
Haemoglobin >135 g/L for men, >125 g/L for women
Minimum donation interval of 12 weeks for males, 16 weeks for females
Apheresis for platelets or plasma up to 24 times in 12 months
Pregnant and lactating women excluded because of high iron requirements; donation deferred for 9 months post pregnancy
Exclusion of those with: Known cardiovascular disease, including hypertension Significant respiratory disorders Epilepsy and other CNS disorders Inflammatory bowel disease Insulin-dependent diabetes Chronic renal disease Cancer Ongoing medical investigation or clinical trials
Exclusion of any donor returning within a short period to occupations such as driving a bus, plane or train, heavy machine or crane operator, mining, scaffolding etc. because delayed faint would be dangerous
Defer for 12 months after body piercing or tattoo, paid sex, after acupuncture, 3 months after homosexual sex with the same partner and no others
Defer for 2 months after live vaccinations such as measles, mumps
Defer if travel history suggests risk of infection

NB. Individuals with genetic haemochromatosis (Chapter 4) accepted provided they meet the other donor selection criteria.
There is no evidence that SARS-CoV-2 can be transmitted by transfusion.

Table 33.2 Donor testing in England and Wales.

1. Blood group, Rh status (D, C, E, c, e), K
2. Screen for red cell alloantibodies
3. *Microbiological tests* Human immunodeficiency virus (HIV) 1 and 2; antibody and RNA Hepatitis B virus (HBV) – antibody and RNA Hepatitis C virus (HCV) – antibody and RNA Hepatitis E virus (HEV) – RNA Human T-cell lymphotropic viruses (HTLV-1 and -2) – antibody (on pools of samples) Cytomegalovirus (CMV) – antibody, for immunosuppressed recipients Malaria – antibody screening of potentially exposed donors Chagas' disease – antibody screening of potentially exposed donors Bacteria – all donations tested for antibody to syphilis (*Treponema pallidum*);platelets by culture methods

At the current time there is no reliable test for detecting prions in blood products. In the United States, blood products are tested for eight microbial pathogen types: bacterial contamination (blood culture), hepatitis B (core antibody and surface antigen), hepatitis C (antibody and nucleic acid amplification testing), HIV-1 and HIV-2 (antibody testing for both, and nucleic acid testing for HIV-1), HTLV-I and HTLV-2 (antibody testing for both), *Treponema pallidum* (anti-treponemal antibody testing) and West Nile Virus (nucleic acid testing). In 2018, universal testing for Zika virus (a nucleic acid test) was added. Although prions are not tested for, anyone who lived in the United Kingdom for at least 3 months between 1980 and 1996, or in Europe or Saudi Arabia for 5 years after 1980, is permanently barred from blood donation in the United States, because of a perceived risk of variant Creutzfeldt–Jacob disease.

transfused or been pregnant (Tables 33.3 and 33.4). The origin of these antibodies is thought to be immunological recognition of bacterial cell wall glycoproteins in the gut that are similar to AB antigens. Consistent with this hypothesis, antibodies typically arise in the first few months of life as the bowel is colonized by normal bacterial flora. The most important of these natural antibodies are anti-A and anti-B. They are usually IgM and react optimally at cold temperatures (4°C) so, although reactive at 37°C, they are called cold antibodies.

Immune antibodies against non-ABO system antigens, in contrast, develop in response to the introduction – by transfusion or by transplacental passage during pregnancy – of red cells possessing antigens that the subject lacks. These antibodies are commonly IgG, although some IgM antibodies may also develop, usually in the early phase of an immune response. Immune antibodies react optimally at 37°C (warm antibodies). Only IgG antibodies are capable of transplacental passage from mother to foetus and the most important immune antibody is the Rh antibody, anti-D.

ABO system

The protein that defines the ABO antigens is a glycosyltransferase that is encoded from a single gene for which there are three major alleles, A, B and O. The A and B alleles catalyse the addition of different carbohydrate residues (*N*-acetyl galactosamine for group A and galactose for group B) to a basic antigenic glycoprotein or glycolipid with a terminal sugar L-fucose on the red cell, known as the H substance (Fig. 33.2). The O allele is non-functional and so does not modify the H substance. Although there are six common genotypes, the absence of a specific anti-H prevents the serological recognition of more than four phenotypes (Table 33.4). The A allele actually itself has two variants, A1 and A2, but these are of minor clinical significance. A2 cells react more weakly than A1 cells with anti-A, and patients who are A2B can be wrongly grouped as B.

The A, B and H antigens are present on most body cells, including white cells and platelets. In the 80% of the population

Table 33.3 Clinically important blood group systems.

Systems	Frequency of antibodies	Cause of haemolytic transfusion reaction	Cause of haemolytic disease of newborn
ABO	Almost universal	Yes (common)	Yes (usually mild)
Rh	Common	Yes (common)	Yes
Kell	Occasional	Yes (occasional)	Anaemia not haemolysis
Duffy	Occasional	Yes (occasional)	Yes (occasional)
Kidd	Occasional	Yes (occasional)	Yes (occasional)
Lutheran	Rare	Yes (rare)	No
Lewis	Occasional	Yes (rare)	No
P	Occasional	Yes (rare)	Yes (rare)
MNS	Rare	Yes (rare)	Yes (rare)
Li	Rare	Unlikely	No

Table 33.4 The ABO blood group system.

Phenotype	Genotype	Antigens	Naturally occurring antibodies	Frequency (UK, %)
O	OO	O	Anti-A, anti-B	46
A	AA or AO	A	Anti-B	42
B	BB or BO	B	Anti-A	9
AB	AB	AB	None	3

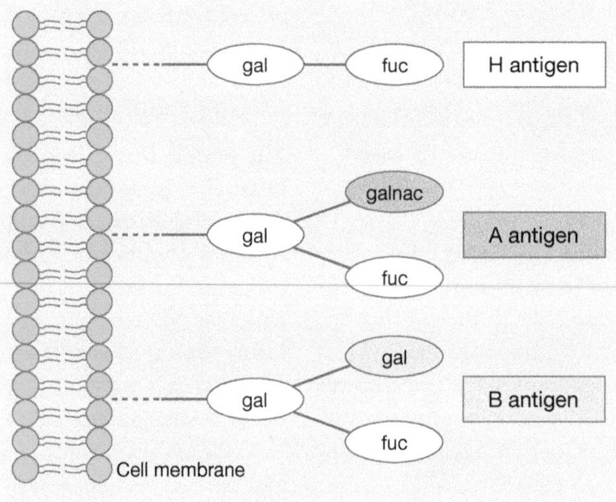

Figure 33.2 Structure of ABO blood group antigens. Each consists of a chain of sugars attached to lipids or proteins which are an integral part of the cell membrane. The H antigen of the O blood group has a terminal fucose (fuc). The A antigen has an additional *N*-acetyl galactosamine (galnac), and the B antigen has an additional galactose (gal). glu, glucose.

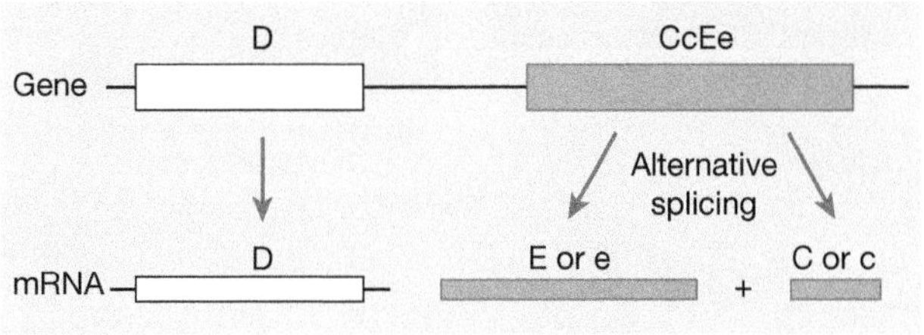

Figure 33.3 Molecular genetics of the Rh blood group. The locus consists of two closely linked genes, *RhD* and *RhCcEe*. The *RhD* gene codes for a single protein which contains the RhD antigen, whereas *RhCcEe* mRNA undergoes alternative splicing to three transcripts. One of these encodes the E or e antigen, whereas the other two (only one is shown) contain the C or c epitope. A polymorphism at position 226 of the *RhCcEe* gene determines the Ee antigen status, whereas the C or c antigens are determined by a four amino acid allelic difference. Some individuals do not have an *RhD* gene and are therefore RhD–.

who possess **secretor genes**, these antigens are also found in soluble form in secretions and body fluids, e.g. plasma, saliva, semen and sweat.

Rh system

The Rh blood group locus is composed of two related structural genes, *RhD* and *RhCE*, which encode the membrane proteins that carry the D and the Cc and Ee antigens. The *RhD* gene may be either present or absent, giving the Rh D+ or Rh D– phenotype, respectively. Alternative RNA splicing from the *RhCE* gene generates two proteins, which encode the C or c and the E or e antigens (Fig. 33.3). A shortened nomenclature for the Rh phenotype is commonly used (Table 33.5).

Rh antibodies rarely occur naturally and are therefore immune antibodies that result from previous transfusion or pregnancy. Anti-D is responsible for most of the clinical problems associated with the system and a simple subdivision of subjects into Rh D+ and Rh D– using anti-D antibody is sufficient for routine clinical purposes. About 85% of the European population is Rh D+; some ethnic groups such as Basques have a lower proportion of Rh D+ persons. Anti-C, anti-c, anti-E and anti-e are occasionally seen and may cause both transfusion reactions and haemolytic disease of the newborn. Anti-d does not exist. Rh haemolytic disease of the newborn is described in Chapter 34.

Other blood group systems

Other blood group systems are less frequently of clinical importance. Although naturally occurring antibodies of the P, Lewis and MNS systems are not uncommon, they usually only react at low temperatures and hence are of no clinical consequence. Immune antibodies against antigens of these systems are detected infrequently. Many of the antigens are of low antigenicity and others, e.g. Kell (K), although comparatively immunogenic, are of relatively low frequency and therefore provide few opportunities for isoimmunization, except in multiply transfused patients.

Hazards of allogeneic blood transfusion

A large number of measures are taken to protect the recipient (Table 33.6).

Transfusion-transmitted infection

Donor selection and testing of all donations are designed to prevent transmission of diseases (Tables 33.1 and 33.2). The main

Table 33.5 The most common Rh genotypes in the UK population.

CDE nomenclature	Short symbol	Frequency in white people (%) Rh	Rh D status
cde/cde	Rr	15	Negative
CDe/cde	R^1r	31	Positive
CDe/CDe	R^1R^1	16	Positive
cDE/cde	R^2r	13	Positive
CDe/cDE	R^1R^2	13	Positive
cDE/cDE	R^2R^2	3	Positive
Other genotypes		9	Positive (almost all)

Table 33.6 Measures to protect recipient

Measures to protect recipient
Donor selection (see Table 33.1)
Donor deferral/exclusion (see Table 33.1)
Stringent arm cleaning
Microbiological testing of donations (Table 33.2)
Immunohaematological testing of donations
Discarding the first 20–30 mL of blood collected from the donor in case of contamination by skin bacteria
Leucodepletion of cellular products (filtration at collection of whole blood or of components individually)
Post-collection viral inactivation of FFP
Monitoring and testing for bacterial contamination
Pathogen inactivation of cellular components
Safest possible sources of donor for plasma products

FFP, fresh frozen plasma.

Table 33.7 Infectious agents reported to have been transmitted by blood transfusion.

Viruses	
Hepatitis viruses	Hepatitis A virus (HAV) **Hepatitis B virus (HBV)** **Hepatitis C virus (HCV)** Hepatitis D virus (HDV) (requires co-infection with HBV) Hepatitis E virus (HEV)
Retroviruses	**Human immunodeficiency virus (HIV) 1 + 2** **Human T-cell lymphotropic virus (HTLV) I + 2**
Herpes viruses	**Cytomegalovirus (CMV)** Epstein–Barr virus (EBV)
Other viruses	Parvovirus B19 West Nile virus Dengue Zika
Bacteria	
Endogenous	***Treponema pallidum* (syphilis)** *Yersinia enterocolitica*/*Salmonella* spp.
Exogenous	Environmental species – staphylococcal spp./*Pseudomonas*/*Serratia* spp.
Protozoa	
	***Plasmodium* spp. (malaria)** ***Trypanosoma cruzi* (Chagas' disease)**
Prions	
	New variant Creuzfeldt–Jacob disease (nvCJD)

risk is from viruses that have long incubation periods, especially where these are asymptomatic. Recent viral infections can be transmitted in the pre-symptomatic viraemic phase, if blood has been collected during that short period (Table 33.7).

Hepatitis

Donors with a history of hepatitis are deferred for 12 months. If there is a history of jaundice, they can be accepted if markers for HBV and HCV are negative and liver tests have normalized. Hepatitis B is the most important transfusion-transmitted virus because it is readily transmitted by transfusions or body fluids and because there is a window period after infection in which tests for the antigen and antibody are negative. Hepatitis E can cause serious clinical disease so a screening approach testing pools of 24 donations for HEV RNA has been introduced in the United Kingdom.

Human immunodeficiency virus (HIV)

This can be transmitted by cells or plasma. Men who have sex with men, intravenous drug users and sex workers are currently excluded from donation, as are their sexual partners and partners of haemophiliacs. Inhabitants of large areas of sub-Saharan Africa and South-East Asia where HIV infection is particularly common are also excluded in the United Kingdom, but not from donating in their home countries. Very rarely transmission may occur when the donor is incubating the infection but is not yet positive for the antigen–antibody test used ('window period transmission'), but this is extremely rare now that all blood is screened with nucleic acid testing for HIV-1.

Human T-cell lymphotropic viruses

Human T-cell lymphotropic virus type 1 (HTLV-1) is associated with adult T-cell leukaemia/lymphoma or tropical spastic paraparesis. Human T-cell lymphotropic virus type 2 (HLTV 2) has no known association with any clinical condition. Screening for both is mandatory in the United Kingdom and United States, despite the low prevalence of approximately 1 in 50 000 untested donors.

Cytomegalovirus

Post-infusion cytomegalovirus (CMV) infection is usually subclinical, but may cause an infectious mononucleosis syndrome. Immunosuppressed individuals are at risk of pneumonitis and a potentially fatal disease. These are premature babies (less than 1500 g), stem cell and other organ transplant recipients, patients who have received alemtuzumab (anti-CD52) and pregnant women (where the foetus is at risk). For such recipients, CMV-negative blood or blood components must be given, if they are CMV negative.

West Nile virus

This is an arthropod-borne infection of birds with humans and horses as incidental hosts. Transmission by transfusion especially in United States and Canada has led to serious illness and deaths in the elderly and immunosuppressed.

Other infections

Syphilis and other bacterial infections are more likely to be transmitted by platelets (stored at room temperature) than blood (stored at 4°C). However, all donations are tested. Malarial parasites are viable in blood stored at 4°C, so in endemic areas all recipients are given antimalarial drugs. In non-endemic areas, donors are carefully vetted for travel to tropical areas and in some centres tests for malarial antibodies are performed. Chagas' disease is a significant problem with blood transfusion in Latin America. Bacterial infections resulting from skin commensals are most frequently transmitted by platelets stored for more than 3 days. In the United States, all blood is now screened for Zika virus.

Prions

The risk of new variant Creuzfeldt–Jacob disease (nvCJD) is considered a threat to blood safety in the United Kingdom. There are four reports of possible transmission by blood transfusion in the United Kingdom all before 2007. Recipients of blood or blood components or tissue or organ transplants since 1980 are now excluded as blood donors in the United Kingdom. Also those who have received human pituitary-derived hormones or grafts of human dura or ocular tissue. Universal leucocyte depletion of all blood donations reduces the risk. No screening tests for prions are available.

Techniques in blood group serology

The most important technique is based on the agglutination of red blood cells. Saline agglutination is important in detecting IgM antibodies, usually at room temperature or at 4°C, e.g. anti-A, anti-B (Fig. 33.4). Addition of colloid to the incubation or proteolytic enzyme treatment of red cells increases the sensitivity of the indirect antiglobulin test (see below), as does low ionic strength saline (LISS). These latter methods can detect a range of IgG antibodies.

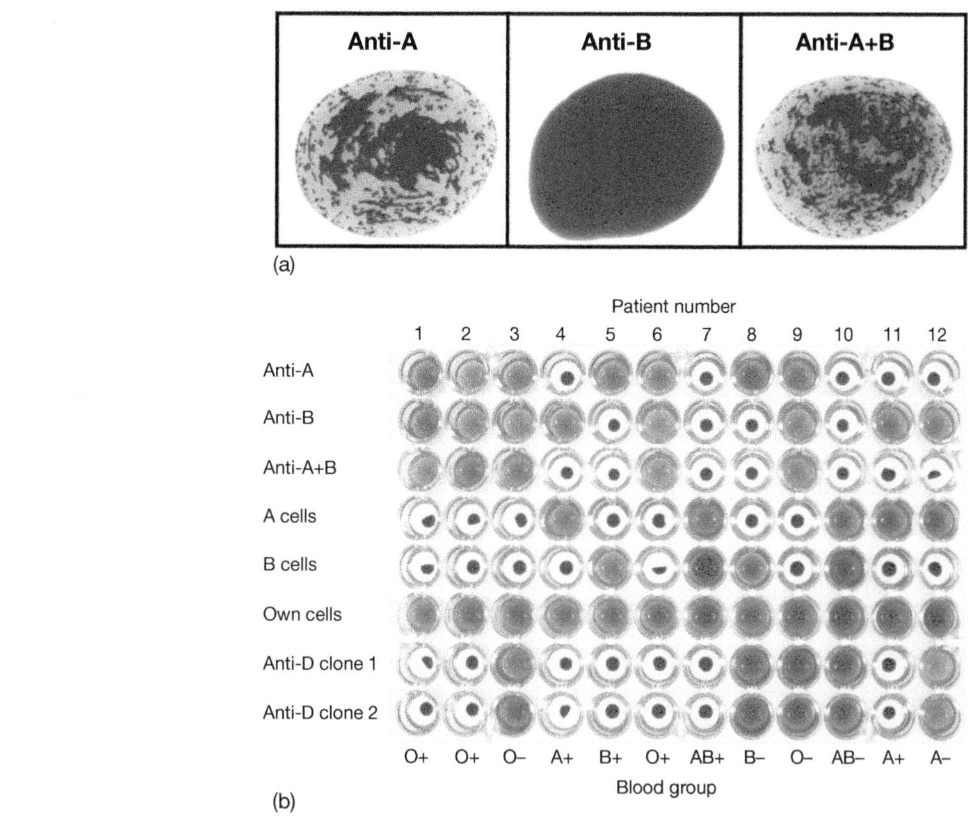

Figure 33.4 **(a)** The ABO grouping in a group A patient. The red cells suspended in saline agglutinate in the presence of anti-A or anti-A + B (serum from a group O patient). **(b)** Routine grouping in a 96-well microplate. Positive reactions show as sharp agglutinates; in negative reactions the cells are dispersed. Rows 1–3, patient cells against antisera; rows 4–6, patient sera against known cells; rows 7–8, anti-D against patient cells.

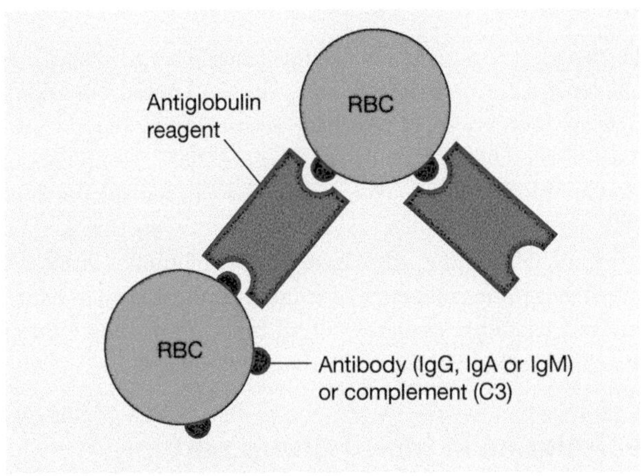

Figure 33.5 The antiglobulin test for antibody or complement on the surface of red blood cells (RBC). The antihuman globulin (Coombs') reagent may be broad spectrum or specific for immunoglobulin G (IgG), IgM, IgA or complement (C3).

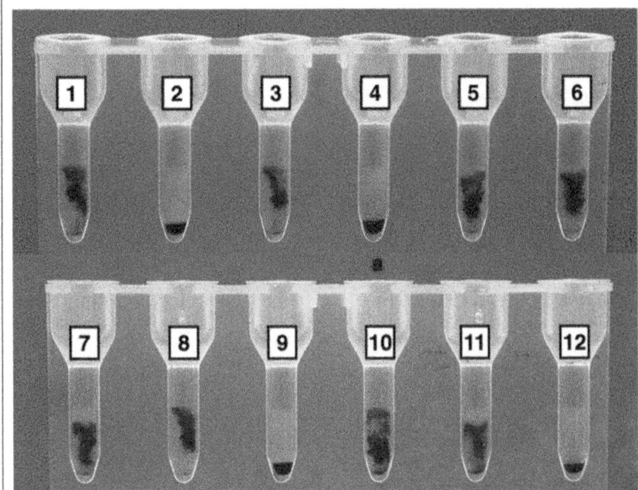

Figure 33.6 Patient antibody screening using the microcolumn (gel) system: 10 tests with two controls (tube 11 is the positive control and tube 12 the negative control) are shown. The patient's serum is tested against screening cells with known red cell phenotype. Tubes 1, 3, 5–8 and 10 show positive results. The patient's serum contained anti-Fya. Source: Courtesy of Mr G. Hazlehurst.

The antiglobulin (Coombs') test is a fundamental and widely used test in both blood group serology and general immunology. Antihuman globulin (AHG) is produced in animals following the injection of human globulin, purified complement or specific immunoglobulin, e.g. IgG, IgA or IgM. Monoclonal preparations are also now available. **When AHG is added to human red cells coated with immunoglobulin or complement components, agglutination of the red cells indicates a positive test (Fig. 33.5).**

The antiglobulin test may be either direct or indirect. The direct antiglobulin test (DAT) is used for detecting antibody or complement already on the red cell surface where sensitization has occurred *in vivo*. The AHG reagent is added to washed red cells and agglutination indicates a positive test. A positive test occurs in haemolytic disease of the newborn, autoimmune or drug-induced immune haemolytic anaemia and haemolytic transfusion reactions.

The indirect antiglobulin test (IAT) is used to detect antibodies that have coated the red cells *in vitro*. It is a two-stage procedure: the first step involves the incubation of test red cells with serum; in the second step, the red cells are washed and the AHG reagent is added. Agglutination implies that the original serum contained antibody which has coated the red cells *in vitro*. This test is used as part of the routine antibody screening of the recipient's serum prior to transfusion and for detecting blood group antibodies in a pregnant woman.

Most of the above methods were originally developed for tube techniques. These were replaced by 96-well microplates, but most laboratories now use gel-based technology (Fig. 33.6).

Typing of ABO, RhD and other Rh antigens (C, E, c and e) and for K is performed on all donations. Phenotyping for other red cell antigens such as Duffy, Kidd, MNSs is performed on some units to provide suitable blood for alloimmunized patients and those likely to make antibodies, e.g. sickle cell patients. In the United Kingdom, K negative blood is given to women of child-bearing age to minimize the formation of anti-K.

Cross-matching and pre-transfusion tests

A number of steps are taken to ensure that patients receive compatible blood at the time of transfusion. Although group O blood could be given to group A, B or AB recipients since the recipients will not haemolyse the donor red cells, this choice of donor blood should usually be avoided because of the danger of haemolysis of recipient red cells by A and B antibodies in the donor's plasma. The problems in transfusing red cells in the early weeks and months after allogeneic stem cell transplantation when the patient's blood group will be changing to that of the stem cell donor are discussed in Chapter 12.

From the patient

1 The ABO and Rh blood group is determined.
2 Serum is screened for important antibodies by an indirect antiglobulin test on a large panel of antigenically-typed group O red cells.

If a red cell alloantibody is discovered in the recipient, donor blood is selected lacking the relative antigen. The most common antibodies are against Rh D, C, c, E, e and K.

From the donor

An appropriate ABO and Rh unit is selected.

Table 33.8 Techniques used in compatibility testing. Donor cells tested against recipient serum and agglutination detected visually or microscopically after mixing and incubation at the appropriate temperature.

For detecting clinically significant IgM antibodies
Saline 37°C
For detecting immune antibodies (mainly IgG)
Indirect antiglobulin test at 37°C Low ionic strength saline at 37°C Enzyme-treated red cells at 37°C

Ig, immunoglobulin.

The cross-match

The techniques that may be used are described in Table 33.8.

Electronic issue

In this, a patient has group and antibody screens performed on two separate occasions. If both antibody screens are negative and no blood has been transfused between the test, ABO and Rh compatible blood is issued directly, without further laboratory testing.

Antibody screening of patients' sera need only consist of a well-controlled sensitive IAT, using a low ionic strength solution (LISS), commonly with microcolumns. If the antibody screening is positive, antibody identification against a panel of 8–12 fully phenotyped red cells should be performed. For identification, in addition to the IAT, a second sensitive technique, e.g. using enzyme-treated cells, polyethylene glycol or manual polybrene test, is recommended. Saline tests are not essential for antibody screening or identification and all tests should be performed at 37°C, as antibodies reacting at lower temperatures only are generally of no clinical importance.

Molecular techniques for blood grouping

Most blood group polymorphisms are due to single nucleotide polymorphisms in the respective genes. Molecular techniques, ranging from low to high-throughput microarray technology and DNA sequencing, have been used blood group testing and extended red cell genotyping. Molecular typing is usually performed when a blood group phenotype is required but a suitable red cell sample is not available.

1 The most important indication is the antenatal determination of foetal blood groups, especially RhD when there is a risk of haemolytic disease of the newborn because the mother has a blood group antibody with this potential. Cell-free foetal DNA in the maternal plasma is the usual source of foetal DNA.
2 Molecular methods are also useful in transfusion-dependent patients where serological methods are not possible because of the presence of transfused red cells in the patient's blood. The molecular tests are carried out on DNA isolated from whole blood of the transfused patient.
3 Alloimmunization is a frequent complication of chronic transfusion in especially those with sickle cell anaemia and thalassaemia major. Extended blood grouping before the first unit is transfused is recommended for these patients. Genotyping improves accuracy. Subsequent transfusions can then be matched for an extended list of antigens. Molecular testing of large numbers of blood donors for multiple blood groups is being introduced to establish a database of donors typed for all clinically significant groups. This will be useful especially for transfusion-dependent patients.
4 Another group of patients who can benefit from blood group genotyping are those with autoimmune haemolytic anaemia, whose red cells are coated with immunoglobulin, or have received monoclonal antibody therapy, e.g. daratumumab making serological typing difficult.

Complications of blood transfusion

Haemolytic transfusion reactions

Haemolytic transfusion reactions may be immediate or delayed (Table 33.9). Immediate life-threatening reactions associated with massive intravascular haemolysis are the result of complement-activating antibodies in the recipient plasma of IgM or IgG classes, almost always of ABO specificity. Delayed reactions associated with extravascular haemolysis, e.g. immune antibodies of the Rh system, which are unable to activate complement are generally less severe, but may still be life-threatening. The cells become coated with IgG and are removed in the reticuloendothelial system (Fig. 33.7). In mild cases, the only signs of a transfusion reaction may be a progressive unexplained anaemia with or without jaundice. In some cases where the pre-transfusion level of an antibody was too low to be detected in a cross-match, a patient may be reimmunized by transfusion of incompatible red cells, and this will lead to a delayed transfusion reaction with accelerated clearance of the red cells. There may be rapid appearance of anaemia with mild jaundice.

Clinical features of a major haemolytic transfusion reaction

Haemolytic shock phase This may occur after only a few millilitres of blood have been transfused or up to 1–2 hours after the end of the transfusion. Clinical features include urticaria, pain in the lumbar region, flushing, headache, precordial pain, shortness of breath, vomiting, rigors, pyrexia and a fall in blood pressure. If the patient is anaesthetized, this shock phase is masked. There is increasing evidence of red cell destruction, and haemoglobinuria, jaundice and disseminated intravascular coagulation (DIC) may all become apparent. Moderate leucocytosis, e.g. $15–20 \times 10^9$/L, is usual.

Table 33.9 Complications of blood transfusion.

Early (hours)	Late (days or years) delayed transfusion reaction
Acute intravascular IgM haemolytic reaction	Delayed haemolysis due to red cell alloantibodies Post-transfusion purpura
Reactions caused by infected blood	Immune sensitization, e.g. to red cells, platelets or Rh D antigen
Allergic reactions to white cells, platelets or proteins	Transfusion-associated graft-versus-host disease
Pyrogenic reactions (to plasma proteins or caused by HLA antibodies)	Transfusional iron overload (Chapter 4)
Circulatory overload	
Hypothermia	
Bacterial contamination (acute sepsis, endotoxin shock)	
Air embolism	
Thrombophlebitis	
Citrate toxicity	
Hyperkalaemia	
Hypocalcaemia (infants, massive transfusion)	
Clotting abnormalities (after massive transfusion)	
Transfusion-related acute lung injury (TRALI)	
Anaphylaxis (in IgA-deficient subjects)	

CMV, cytomegalovirus; HIV, human immunodeficiency virus; HLA, human leucocyte antigen; Ig, immunoglobulin.

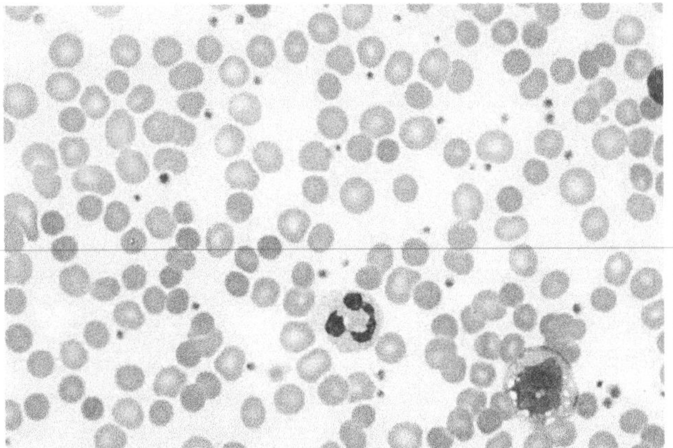

Figure 33.7 Blood transfusion: delayed transfusion reaction. Peripheral blood film showing microspherocytes and polychromasia. Source: A.V. Hoffbrand *et al.* (2019) *Color Atlas of Clinical Hematology*, 5th edn. Reproduced with permission of John Wiley & Sons. Courtesy of Dr W. Erber.

The oliguric phase In some patients with a haemolytic reaction, there is renal tubular necrosis with acute renal failure.

Diuretic phase Fluid and electrolyte imbalance may occur during the recovery from acute renal failure.

Investigation of an immediate transfusion reaction

If a patient develops features suggesting a severe transfusion reaction, the transfusion should be stopped and investigations for blood group incompatibility and bacterial contamination of the blood must be initiated.

1 **Most severe reactions occur because of clerical errors in the handling of donor or recipient blood specimens.** Therefore it must be established that the identity of the recipient (from the patient's wristband) is the same as that on the compatibility label and that this corresponds with the actual unit being transfused.
2 The unit of donor blood and post-transfusion samples of the patient's blood should be sent to the laboratory who will:
   (a) repeat the group on pre- and post-transfusion samples and on the donor blood, and repeat the cross-match;
   (b) perform a direct antiglobulin test on the post-transfusion sample;
   (c) check the plasma for haemoglobinaemia;
   (d) perform tests for DIC; and
   (e) examine the donor sample directly for evidence of gross bacterial contamination and set up blood cultures from it at 20°C and 37°C. If the clinical picture is suggestive of bacterial infection, blood cultures must be taken from the patient and broad-spectrum intravenous antibodies started.
3 A post-transfusion sample of urine must be examined for haemoglobinuria.
4 Further samples of blood are taken 6 hours and/or 24 hours after transfusion for a blood count and bilirubin, free haemoglobin and methaemalbumin (p.xx) estimations.
5 In the absence of positive findings, the patient's serum is examined 5–10 days later for red cell or white cell antibodies.

Management of patients with major haemolysis

The principal object of initial therapy is to maintain the blood pressure and renal perfusion. Intravenous dextran, plasma or saline and furosemide are sometimes needed. Hydrocortisone 100 mg intravenously and an antihistamine may help to alleviate shock. In the event of severe shock, support with intravenous adrenaline 1: 10 000 in small incremental doses may be required. Further compatible transfusions may be required in severely affected patients. If acute renal failure occurs this is managed in the usual way, if necessary with dialysis until recovery occurs.

Other transfusion reactions

Hyperhaemolysis syndromes Some patients, particularly with sickle cell anaemia, haemolyse donor blood even though no alloantibodies to red cells can be detected. The haemolysis appears to be due to overactivity of the recipient's macrophages. It is treated by infusions of gammaglobulin, corticosteroid therapy and eculizumab (anti-complement C5, see p. xxx).

Febrile reactions because of white cell antibodies Human leucocyte antigen (HLA) antibodies (see below and Chapter 25) are usually the result of sensitization by pregnancy or a previous transfusion. They produce rigors, pyrexia and, in severe cases, pulmonary infiltrates. They are minimized by giving leucocyte depleted (filtered) packed cells (see below).

Febrile or non-febrile non-haemolytic allergic reactions. These are usually caused by hypersensitivity to donor plasma proteins and, if severe, can result in anaphylactic shock. The clinical features are urticaria, pyrexia and, in severe cases, dyspnoea, facial oedema and rigors. Immediate treatment is with antihistamines and hydrocortisone. Adrenaline is also useful. Washed red cells or frozen red cells may be needed for further transfusions if the majority of plasma-removed blood, e.g. saline, adenine, glucose, mannitol (SAGM) blood, causes reactions.

Post-transfusion acute circulatory overload (TACO) The management is that of cardiac failure. These reactions are prevented by a slow transfusion of packed red cells or of the blood component required, accompanied by diuretic therapy.

Transfusion of bacterially contaminated blood This is very rare, but may be serious. It can present with circulatory collapse. It is a particular problem with platelet packs that are stored at 20–24°C.

Graft-versus-host disease (GVHD) This potentially fatal complication may occur when live lymphocytes are transfused to an immunocompromised patient. It is prevented by irradiation of the blood products for susceptible recipients (Table 33.10). Irradiation does increase plasma potassium and shorten red cell but not platelet shelf life. The increased use of immunological therapies has complicated the issue of exactly when irradiation of blood components is needed. In an emergency, if irradiation is not possible, transfusion of leucocyte depleted red cells >14 days old is recommended.

Transfusion related acute lung injury (TRALI) This presents within 6 hours of an infusion with cough, breathlessness, fever and rigors, depending on severity. Pulmonary infiltrates are seen on chest X-ray (Fig. 33.8). Management is in a high-dependency/intensive care unit with ventilator support if needed. It is caused by transfer of leucoagglutins HLA antibodies in donor plasma or platelets, which cause endothelial and epithelial injury. Most of the donors are multiparous women, so in the United Kingdom and United States FFP and plasma to support platelet pools (see below) are now from male donors.

Severe anaphylactic reactions This life-threatening reaction in an IgA-deficient subject may result from transfusion of any blood product, most frequently fresh frozen plasma. It is characterized by shock, bronchospasm, laryngeal oedema and widespread skin and mucous membrane angioedema. Intramuscular epinephrine is recommended immediately, followed by parenteral steroids.

Table 33.10 Indications for irradiated blood products.
Recipients of allogeneic stem cell transplantation
Recipients of autologous stem cell transplantation
Bone marrow or stem cell allogeneic or autologous donors: for 7 days prior to harvest and during harvest
Recipients of solid organ transplants when receiving immune suppressive therapy
Patients with Hodgkin lymphoma
Patients with acute leukaemia
Patients treated with fludarabine, bendamustine, cladribine, pentostatin, other purine antagonists
Patients with haematological (but not those with other diseases or after solid organ transplants) treated with anti-CD52 or anti-thymocyte globulin (ATG)
Patients for 7 days before and for 3 months or more after CAR-T cell therapy (Chapter 9)
Inherited immunodeficiency
Intrauterine and neonatal exchange blood transfusions

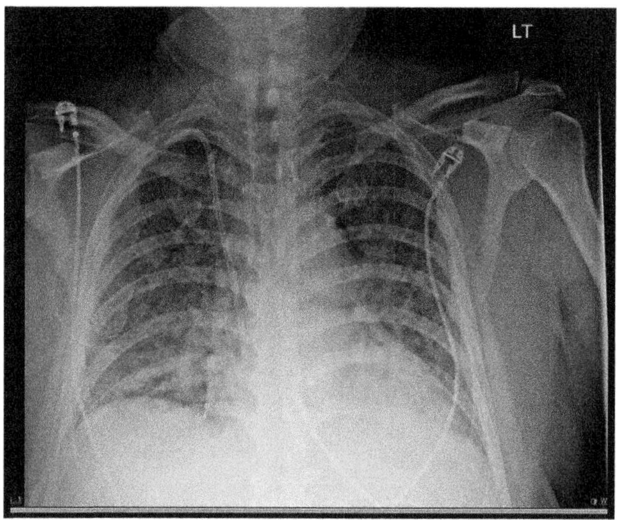

Figure 33.8 Chest X-ray of a 57-year-old man who developed dyspnoea and hypoxia several hours after transfusion of 2 units of red blood cells. Diffuse bilateral airspace infiltrates consistent with transfusion related acute lung injury (TRALI) are present. One of the blood donors was a multiparous woman. Infection and circulatory overload were excluded.

Post-transfusion purpura This is a rare problem of severe thrombocytopenia 7–10 days after transfusion of a platelet-containing product, usually red cells. It is caused by an antibody in the recipient (resulting from previous transfusion or pregnancy) which is usually directed against a platelet specific antigen HPA-Ia (PIAI). Both the transfused and recipient platelets are destroyed by the immune complexes. It is usually self-limiting, but immunoglobulin or plasma exchange may be needed.

Viral transmission Post-transfusion hepatitis may be caused by one of the hepatitis viruses, although CMV and Epstein–Barr virus (EBV) have also been implicated. Post-transfusion viral hepatitis, HTLV or HIV infection is very rarely seen because of routine screening of all blood donations.

Other infections Toxoplasmosis, malaria and syphilis may be transmitted by blood transfusion. Transfusion-transmitted nvCJD has probably occurred in three cases in the United Kingdom.

Post-transfusional iron overload Repeated red cell transfusions over many years, in the absence of blood loss, cause deposition of iron initially in reticuloendothelial macrophages at the rate of 200–250 mg/unit of red cells. After 30–50 units in adults, and lesser amounts in children, the liver, myocardium and endocrine glands are damaged, with clinical consequences. This becomes a major problem in thalassaemia major and other severe chronic refractory anaemias (Chapter 4).

Reduction of blood product use

In the light of transfusion risks and limited resources, appropriate use of blood components is of ever-increasing importance.

Preoperative correction of anaemia (particularly iron deficiency) and cessation of anti-platelet therapies, e.g. aspirin, where possible, together with lower trigger levels for red cell transfusions (haemoglobin 70–80 g/L in most surgical and critical care unit patients), can all help to reduce blood use.

In surgery, the use of alternative fluid replacement, intra-operative or post-operative cell salvage and biological alternatives e.g. erythropoietin, recombinant clotting factors, recombinant activated clotting factor VII (VIIa) or fibrin glue all may help. After major non-cardiac surgery tranexamic acid reduces the transfusion need by about 25%.

Blood components and storage

A blood donation is taken by an aseptic technique into plastic bags containing an appropriate amount of anticoagulant sodium citrate, citric acid and dextrose. Some also contain phosphate (CPD) into which most whole blood is collected and adenine. Optimal additive solutions aimed at prolonging red cell life are discussed below. The citrate anticoagulates the blood by combining with blood calcium. Three components are made by initial centrifugation of whole blood: red cells, buffy coat and plasma (Fig. 30.1). Platelets and plasma may also be collected by apheresis and centrifuging. Donors of platelets may undergo apharesis up to 24 times a year.

Leucodepletion

In many countries, including the United Kingdom and United States, blood products are now routinely filtered to remove the majority of white cells, a process known as leucodepletion. This is usually performed soon after collection and prior to processing and is more effective than filtration of blood at the bedside (Table 33.1). A blood component is defined as leucocyte-depleted if there are less than 5×10^6/L white cells present.

Leucodepletion reduces the incidence of febrile transfusion reactions and HLA alloimmunization. It is effective at preventing transmission of CMV infection and in addition should reduce the theoretical possibility of transmission of nvCJD in countries where this has been reported.

Red cells

Red cells are stored at 4–6°C for up to 35 days, depending on the preservative. After the first 48 hours there is a slow progressive potassium (K+) loss from the red cells into the plasma. In cases where infusion of K+ could be dangerous, fresh blood should be used, e.g. for exchange transfusion in haemolytic disease of the newborn. During red cell storage there is a fall in 2,3-diphosphoglycerate (2,3-DPG), but after transfusion 2,3-DPG levels return to normal within 24 hours. Optimum additive solutions (OASs) have been developed to increase the shelf life of plasma-depleted red cells by maintaining both adenosine triphosphate (ATP) and 2,3-DPG levels. SAG-M the usual OAS contains saline, adenine, glucose and mannitol.

Packed (plasma depleted) red cells are the treatment of choice for most transfusions (Fig. 33.9a). In older subjects, a diuretic is often given simultaneously and the infusion should be sufficiently slow to avoid circulatory overload. Washed red cells for which plasma has been exchanged for a SAG-M solution may be needed to reduce allergic reactions, especially in those with IgA deficiency. Freezing red cells (in glycerol) is used for prolonged storage of red cells of rare phenotypes, e.g. Bombay blood.

Recombinant erythropoietin is widely used to reduce transfusion requirements, e.g. in patients with renal failure on dialysis, cancer patients and in myelodysplastic neoplasias.

Intraoperative cell salvage is also used to reduce donor blood consumption.

Red cell substitutes are under development, but have not yet proven clinically valuable. These synthetic oxygen-carrying substitutes are often fluorinated hydrocarbons and stromal-free pyridoxylated and polymerized haemoglobin solutions.

Patients with religious objections to red blood cell transfusion such as Jehovah's Witnesses vary in their willingness to receive recombinant erythropoietin and non-red-cell blood products such as plasma and platelets.

Granulocyte concentrates

These are prepared as buffy coats or on blood cell separators from normal healthy donors or from patients with chronic myeloid leukaemia. They have been used in patients with

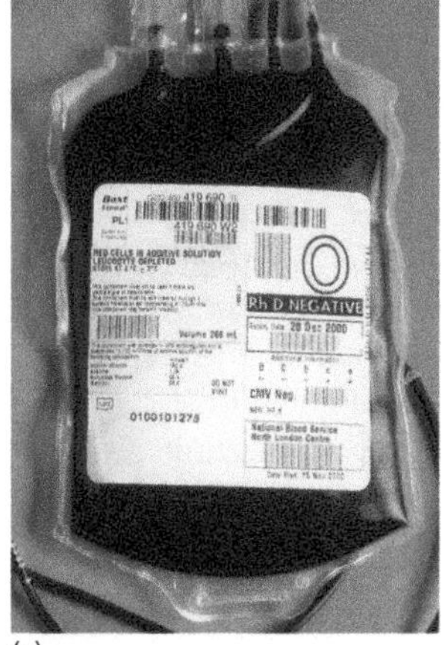

(a)

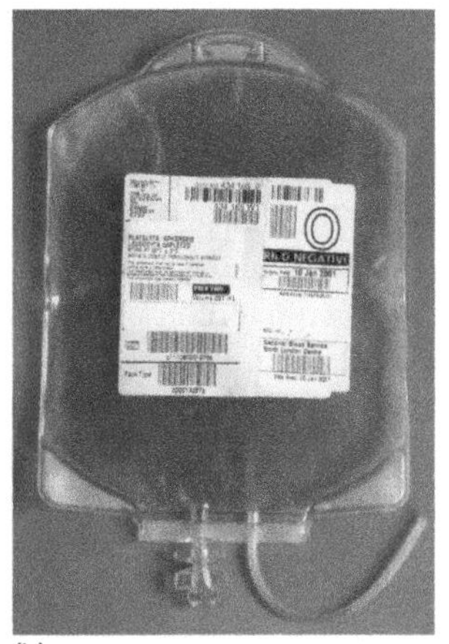

(b)

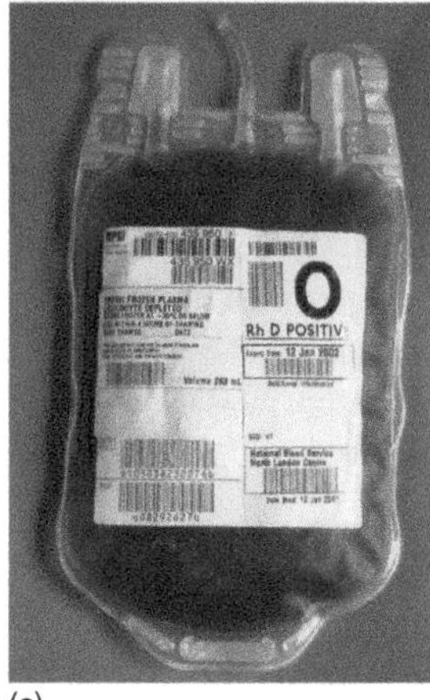

(c)

Figure 33.9 Blood components: **(a)** plasma-depleted red cells; **(b)** platelets; and **(c)** fresh frozen plasma.

severe neutropenia (<0.5×10^9/L) and life-threatening infection, e.g. bacterial sepsis or angioinvasive fungu) who are not responding to antibiotic therapy and are expected to eventually recover blood counts. It is not usually possible to give sufficient granulocytes quickly enough to alter the course of the infection. Granulocytes may transmit CMV infection and must be irradiated to eliminate the risk of causing GVHD. Administration of G-CSF or steroids increases the yield of granulocytes by apharesis but is not permitted for routine donors in the United Kingdom.

Platelet concentrates

These are harvested by apharesis or from individual donor units of blood (Fig. 33.9b). Four buffy coats with platelet additive solution and plasma from one of the donors (preferably male) are processed to make a pool of approximately 3×10^{11} platelets. They are stored at room temperature with a shelf life of 5–7 days. Donors are allowed to undergo apharesis up to 24 times a year. Apharesis of one donor produces 2–3 adult doses of platelets. Platelet transfusion is used in patients who are thrombocytopenic, or have disordered platelet function and who are actively bleeding (therapeutic use) or are at serious risk of bleeding (prophylactic use).

For prophylaxis the platelet count should be kept above 10×10^9/L unless there are additional risk factors such as sepsis, drug use or coagulation disorders for which the threshold should be above 20×10^9/L. For insertion of a venous catheter the platelet count should be > 20×10^9/L, for lumbar puncture > 40×10^9/L. For invasive procedures e.g. liver biopsy, major surgical procedures > 50×10^9/L, for insertion or removal of epidural catheters > 80×10^9/L. For brain or eye surgery other than cataract removal, the count should be > 100×10^9/L.

Therapeutic use is indicated in bleeding associated with platelet disorders. In massive haemorrhage the count should be kept above 50×10^9/L (Chapter 29).

Platelet transfusions should be avoided in autoimmune thrombocytopenic purpura unless there is serious haemorrhage. They are contraindicated in heparin-induced thrombocytopenia, thrombotic thrombocytopenic purpura and haemolytic uraemic syndrome (Chapter 29).

Refractoriness to platelet transfusions is defined by a poor platelet increment post transfusion (less than 7.5×10^9/L per platelet unit transfused at 1 hour or less than 4.5×10^9/L at 24 hours). The causes are either immunological (mostly HLA alloimmunization) or non-immunological (sepsis, hypersplenism, DIC, drugs). Platelets express HLA class I but not class II antigens. HLA-matched or cross-match-compatible platelets are needed for patients with HLA antibodies.

The need for platelet transfusions has been reduced with the introduction of direct stimulators of platelet production such as romiplostim or eltrombopag.

Preparations from human plasma

Fresh frozen plasma (FFP)

Rapidly frozen plasma separated from fresh blood or obtained by apharesis is stored at less than –30°C (Fig. 33.9c). Frozen plasma is usually prepared from single donor units, although pooled products are also available. Male donors are preferred to reduce the risk of passive transfer of donor white cell antibodies that can cause TRALI (see above). Its main use is for the replacement of coagulation factors, e.g. when specific concentrates are unavailable or after massive transfusions, in liver disease and DIC, after cardiopulmonary bypass surgery, to reverse a warfarin effect, and in thrombotic thrombocytopenic purpura (see Chapter 29). Virally inactivated forms of FFP are now available.

Human albumin solution (4.5%)

This is a useful plasma volume expander when a sustained osmotic effect is required prior to the administration of blood, but it should not be given in excess. It is also used for fluid replacement in patients undergoing plasmapheresis and sometimes for fluid replacement in selected patients with hypoalbuminaemia. For routine volume repletion, there is no benefit from colloidal solutions such as human albumin compared with crystalloid solutions such as normal saline or Lactated Ringer's fluid.

Human albumin solution (20%) (salt-poor albumin)

This may be used in severe hypoalbuminaemia when it is necessary to use a product with minimal electrolyte content. Principal indications for its use are patients with nephrotic syndrome or liver failure.

Cryoprecipitate

This is obtained by thawing FFP at 4°C and contains concentrated factor VIII and fibrinogen and factor XIII. It is stored at less than –30°C or, if lyophilized, at 4–6°C, and was used widely as replacement therapy in haemophilia A and von Willebrand disease before more purified preparations of factor VIII became available. Its main use is in fibrinogen replacement in DIC or massive transfusion or hepatic failure.

Fibrinogen

Concentrates are available for patients with congenital or acquired hypofibrinogenaemia who are bleeding.

Freeze-dried factor VIII concentrates

These are also used for treating haemophilia A or von Willebrand disease. The small volume makes them ideal for children, surgical cases, patients at risk from circulatory overload and for those on home treatment. Their use is declining as recombinant forms of factor VIII become widely available.

Freeze-dried factor IX–prothrombin complex concentrates

A number of preparations are available that contain variable amounts of factors II, VII, IX and X. They are mainly used for treating factor IX deficiency (haemophilia B), but are also used in patients with liver disease or in haemorrhage following overdose with oral anticoagulants or in patients with factor VIII inhibitors. There is a risk of thrombosis.

Immunoglobulin

Pooled immunoglobulin is a valuable source of antibodies against common viruses. It is used in hypogammaglobulinaemia for passive protection against viral and bacterial disease. Repeated doses are needed, for example in the winter months at 3–4-week intervals. It may also be used in immune thrombocytopenia and other acquired immune disorders, e.g. post-transfusion purpura or alloimmune neonatal thrombocytopenia.

Specific immunoglobulin

This may be obtained from donors with high titres of antibody, e.g. anti-RhD, anti-hepatitis B, anti-herpes zoster or anti-rubella.

Acute blood loss and massive haemorrhage

After a single episode of blood loss, there is initial vasoconstriction with a reduction in total blood volume. The plasma volume rapidly expands and the haemoglobin and packed cell volume fall, and there is a rise in neutrophils and platelets. The reticulocyte response begins on the second or third day and lasts 8–10 days. The haemoglobin begins to rise by about the seventh day but, if iron stores have become depleted, the haemoglobin may not subsequently rise to normal. Clinical assessment is needed to gauge whether blood transfusion is needed. This is usually unnecessary in adults at losses less than 500 mL unless haemorrhage is continuing. **The management of massive blood loss when there is loss of 30-40% of blood volume, e.g. after major trauma, with red cell, clotting factor and platelet support, is described on p xxx.**

SUMMARY

- Blood transfusion involves the safe transfer of blood components from a donor to a recipient. Most commonly this is red cells and the red cells must be matched between recipient and donor.
- Careful donor selection and microbiological testing help to protect both donor and recipient.
- Red cells contain over 400 antigens. The ABO and Rh systems are most important in transfusion. Subjects lacking an antigen, e.g. group A or B may develop a naturally occurring antibody to it, usually IgM. These antibodies in a recipient may haemolyse or opsonize donor red cells if these contain the antigen.
- Antibodies may also develop from exposure to the antigen by a transfusion or pregnancy. Cross-matching of donor red cells with recipient plasma is therefore carried out to ensure they are compatible.
- Complications of blood transfusion may be acute (within hours) or late (after days or years). They include haemolytic reactions, febrile reactions to white cells or proteins, circulatory overload, shock due to bacterial contamination or anaphylactic reaction, lung injury, transmission of infections, especially viral, transfusion-associated graft-versus-host disease and, in the longer term, iron overload.
- Blood components other than red cells can also be transfused. These include platelets and protein products including fresh frozen plasma, albumin solutions, coagulation factor concentrates and immunoglobulin.

Now visit **www.wiley.com/go/haematology9e** to test yourself on this chapter.

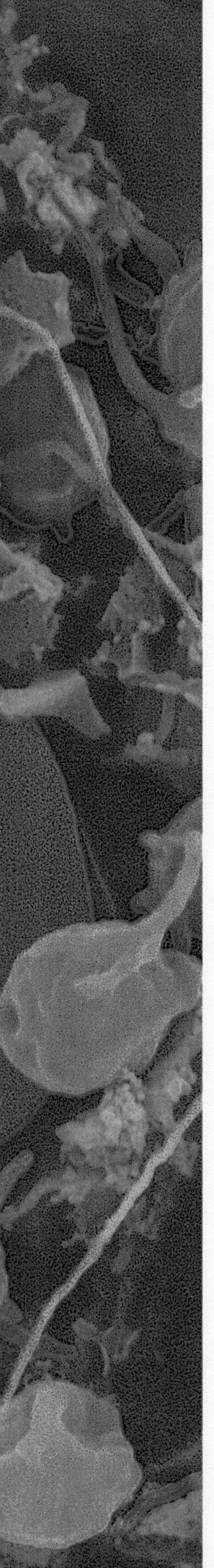

CHAPTER 34

Pregnancy and neonatal haematology

(Written with Professor Irene Roberts)

Key topics

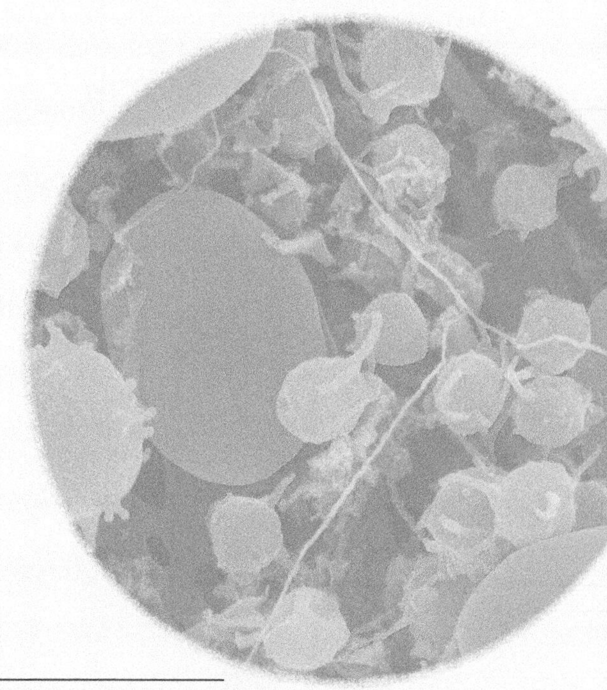

Hoffbrand's Essential Haematology, Ninth Edition. A. Victor Hoffbrand, Pratima Chowdary, Graham P. Collins, and Justin Loke.

© 2024 John Wiley & Sons Ltd. Published 2024 by John Wiley & Sons Ltd.

Companion website: www.wiley.com/go/haematology9e

Haematology of pregnancy

Pregnancy places extreme stresses on the haematological system and an understanding of the physiological changes that result is obligatory in order to interpret any need for therapeutic intervention.

Definition of anaemia in pregnancy

Physiological anaemia is a term sometimes used to describe the fall in haemoglobin (Hb) concentration that occurs during normal pregnancy (Fig. 34.1), but it is not a true anaemia. Blood plasma volume increases by approximately 1250 mL, or 45%, above normal by the end of gestation and although the red cell mass itself increases by some 25%, this difference still leads to a fall in Hb concentration.

The World Health Organization (WHO) classifies pregnant women with haemoglobin levels of 110 g/L or more as normal. The US Centers for Disease Control (CDC) consider pregnant women with haemoglobin levels of at least 110 g/L in the first and third trimesters and at least 105 g/L in the second trimester as normal. In the UK Guidelines anaemia is defined as below 110 g/L in the first trimester, below 105 g/L in the second and third trimesters and below 100 g/L post-partum are considered to show anaemia and to require investigation.

Iron deficiency anaemia

Up to 600 mg iron is required for the mother's increase in red cell mass and a further 300 mg for the foetus and placenta. In addition, a median of 250 mg of iron is lost due to bleeding during delivery. Despite a physiological increase in iron absorption, few women avoid depletion of iron reserves by the end of pregnancy

In uncomplicated pregnancy, the mean corpuscular volume (MCV) typically rises by approximately 4 fL. A fall in red cell MCV is the earliest sign of iron deficiency. Later, the mean corpuscular haemoglobin (MCH) falls and finally anaemia results. The prevalence of maternal anaemia in low- and middle-income countries is nearly 50% due to combinations of iron and folate deficiency, infectious disease and a haemoglobin disorder either thalassaemia or a haemoglobin variant. The anaemia, if severe, is associated with an increased risk of perinatal and neonatal mortality. The prevalence in the United Kingdom of iron deficiency anaemia in pregnancy has been estimated at 30% and in the puerperium 20%. Women from ethnic minorities were more likely to be anaemic.

Early iron deficiency is likely if the serum ferritin is below 30 μg/L but higher levels do not exclude iron deficiency. The deficiency should be treated with oral iron supplements. Routine iron supplementation in pregnancy is not carried out in the United Kingdom, but is recommended for women with a previous history of anaemia in pregnancy, those with multiparity of 3 or more, those with twin or higher order multiple pregnancy, inter-pregnancy <1 year, and those with poor, vegetarian or vegan diets. The CDC in the United States and the WHO recommend iron for all pregnant women.

Ferrous iron salts are used to give 40–80 mg iron each morning on an empty stomach with water alone or with vitamin C. Pregnant patients prescribed oral iron are prone to discontinue treatment due to gastrointestinal adverse effects, as they have decreased bowel motility caused by elevated progesterone, and also have compression of the rectum by the enlarged uterus. Alternate day therapy or lower doses may be needed. The haemoglobin should be measured 2–3 weeks after starting iron to check compliance. Intravenous iron infusion is effective (p. xxx) and is considered in the second or third trimesters for women

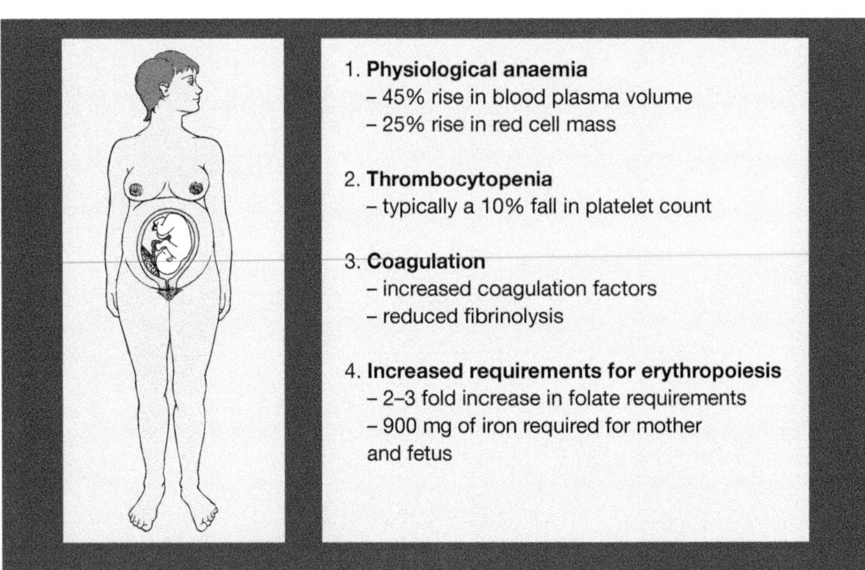

Figure 34.1 Haematological changes during pregnancy.

with confirmed iron deficiency who are intolerant of oral iron or do not respond to it. It is avoided in the first trimester.

Women with blood loss >500 mL, with uncorrected antenatal anaemia or with suggestive symptoms, should have their FBC checked and if the haemoglobin level is <100 g/L should take iron 40–80 mg daily for 3 months or be considered for intravenous iron. Red cell transfusion also needs careful consideration and informed consent.

Folate and vitamin B_{12} deficiency

Folate requirements are increased approximately two-fold in pregnancy and serum folate levels fall to approximately half the normal range, with a less dramatic fall in red cell folate. In some parts of the world, megaloblastic anaemia during pregnancy is common because of a combination of poor diet and exaggerated folate requirements. **Given the protective effect of folate against neural tube defects (NTDs), folic acid should be taken periconceptually and throughout pregnancy (Chapter** 5). Food fortification with folic acid is now being practised in over 80 countries and has been associated with a fall in incidence of NTDs. Vitamin B_{12} deficiency has historically been considered rare during pregnancy, but the incidence is increasing in some countries due to the frequency of bariatric surgery. Serum vitamin B_{12} levels fall to below normal in 20–30% of pregnancies and may cause diagnostic confusion. They recover to normal after the pregnancy.

Thrombocytopenia

The platelet count falls by an average of 10% in an uncomplicated pregnancy. The specific cause of this drop is unclear, but there is evidence for both reduced production and increased platelet destruction. In approximately 7% of women this fall is more severe and can result in thrombocytopenia (platelet count less than 140×10^9/L).

In over 75% of cases this is mild and of unknown cause, referred to as incidental or gestational thrombocytopenia of pregnancy. Approximately 21% of cases are secondary to a hypertensive disorder and 4% are associated with immune thrombocytopenic purpura (ITP; Fig. 34.2).

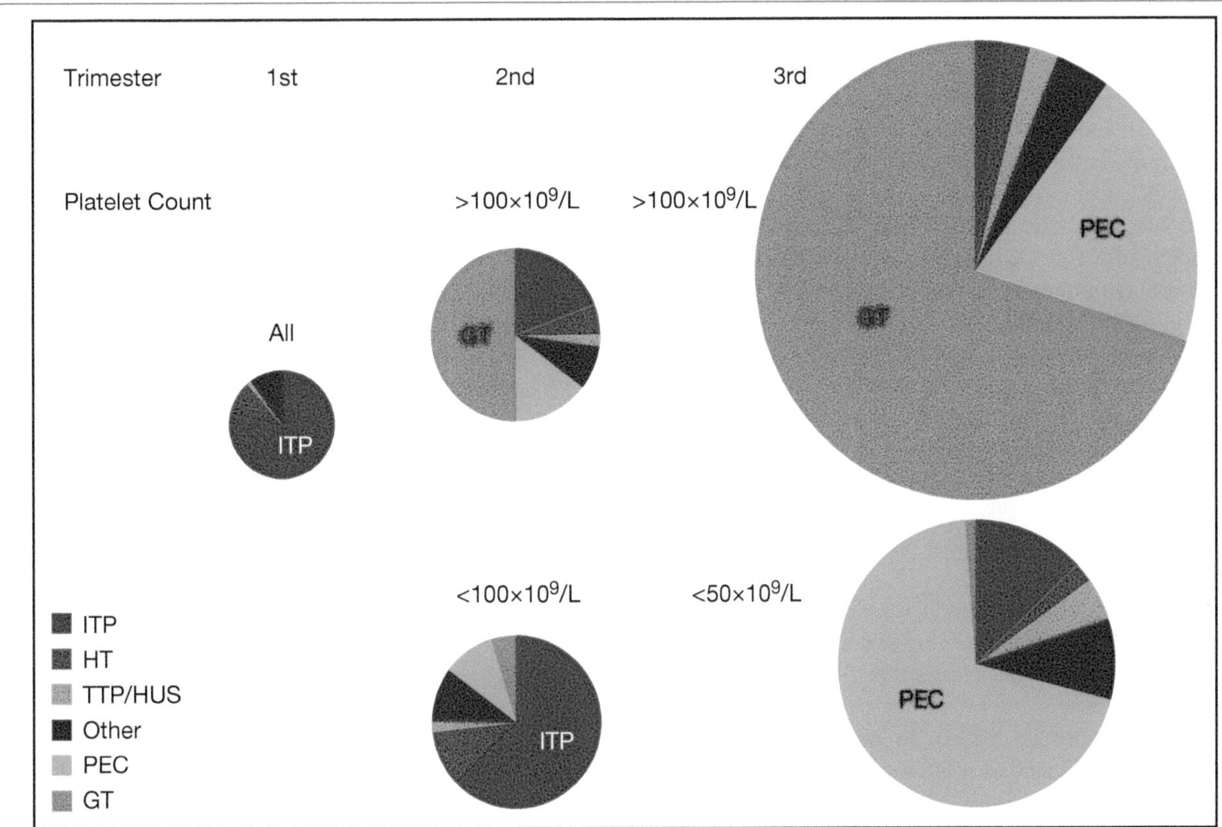

Figure 34.2 Relative prevalence of causes of thrombocytopenia in pregnancy based on trimester of presentation. 'Other' indicates miscellaneous disorders, including infection, disseminated intravascular coagulation (DIC), type IIB von Willebrand disease, immune and non-immune drug-induced thrombocytopenia, paroxysmal nocturnal haemoglobinuria, bone marrow failure syndromes (aplastic anaemia, myelodysplasia, myeloproliferative disorders, leukaemia/lymphoma and marrow infiltrative disorders), among others. GT, gestational thrombocytopenia; HT, hypertension HUS, haemolytic-uraemic syndrome; ITP, immune thrombocytopenia; PEC, pre-eclampsia/HELLP (haemolysis, elevated liver enzymes and low platelets); TTP, thrombotic thrombocytopenic purpura. Source: Based on D.B. Cines *et al.* (2017) *Blood* 130: 144–51.

Incidental (gestational) thrombocytopenia of pregnancy

This is a diagnosis of exclusion, usually detected at the time of delivery. If the platelet count falls to the range 100–140 × 10^9/L, it can confidently be attributed to gestational. It recovers within 6 weeks of delivery. No treatment is needed and the infant is not affected.

Thrombocytopenia of hypertensive disorders

This is variable in severity, with the platelet count usually <100 × 10^9/L. The platelet count rarely falls to below 40 × 10^9/L except in the setting of severe microangiopathy. It is more severe when associated with pre-eclampsia; the primary treatment is as rapid a delivery as possible. The HELLP syndrome (haemolysis, elevated liver enzymes and low platelets) falls into this category. It is associated with prolongation of prothrombin time (PT) and activated partial thromboplastin time (APTT).

Immune thrombocytopenic purpura

In pregnancy, ITP (p. xxx) represents a particular problem, both to the mother and to the foetus, as the antibody crosses the placenta and the foetus may become severely thrombocytopenic. Like other adults, pregnant women with ITP and platelet counts higher than 50 × 10^9/L do not usually need treatment. Treatment is required for women with platelet counts below 10 × 10^9/L and for those with platelet counts of 10–30 × 10^9/L who are in their second or third trimester or who are bleeding. Treatment is with steroids, intravenous immunoglobulin (Ig) G, rituximab or rarely splenectomy as appropriate. Thrombopoietin receptor antagonists are avoided because of potential teratogenetic side effects.

At delivery, umbilical vein blood sampling or foetal scalp vein sampling to measure the foetal platelet count may be offered, although their exact role is unclear. In general, caesarean section is not indicated when the maternal platelet count is above 50 × 10^9/L, unless the foetal platelet count is known to be less than 20 × 10^9/L. Platelet transfusion may be given to mothers in labour with very low platelet counts or who are actively bleeding.

Newborns of mothers with ITP should have a blood count measured for the first 5 days of life, as the platelet count may progressively drop. A count greater than 50 × 10^9/L is reassuring. Cerebral ultrasonography may be performed to look for intracranial haemorrhage (ICH). In newborns without evidence of ICH, treatment with intravenous IgG is appropriate if the infant's platelet count is less than 20 × 10^9/L. Neonates with thrombocytopenia and ICH should be treated with steroids and intravenous IgG therapy.

Haemostasis and thrombosis

Pregnancy leads to a hypercoagulable state with consequent increased risks of thromboembolism and disseminated intravascular coagulation (DIC; p.xxx). There is an increase in plasma factors VII, VIII, X and fibrinogen, with shortening of PT and APTT; fibrinolysis is suppressed. These changes last for up to 2 months into the puerperal period and the incidence of thrombosis during this period is increased. There is an association between thrombophilic conditions in the mother and recurrent foetal loss (p. xxx). This is presumed to result from placental thrombosis and infarction. In women with recurrent foetal loss and inherited thrombophilia, however, giving LMW heparin does not increase live births.

Treatment of thrombosis

Warfarin has no role in management. It crosses the placenta and in addition is associated with embryopathy, especially between 6 and 12 weeks' gestation. **Low-molecular-weight heparin is now the treatment of choice**, because it can be given once daily and is less likely than unfractionated heparin to cause osteoporosis. Fixed low-dose LMWH is the standard prophylaxis regimen for pregnant women with prior VTE.

Neonatal haematology

Neonatal is defined as within 28 days of birth, infants 28 days to <1 year.

Haemoglobin and MCV are higher at birth than in adults (Table 34.1). The cord blood Hb varies between approximately 165 and 170 g/L and is influenced by the timing of cord clamping. At birth the haemoglobin ranges from 149 to 23.7 g/L (Table 34.1). The reticulocyte count is initially high (2–6%), but falls to below 0.5% at 1 week as erythropoiesis is suppressed in response to the marked increase in the oxygenation of tissues after birth (Fig. 34.3). This is associated with a progressive fall in Hb to a range of 94–130 g/L at 2 months, from which point it recovers to a mean of 125 g/L at around 6 months. **The lower limit of normal during childhood is 110 g/L.** Preterm infants have a more dramatic fall in Hb to 70–90 g/L at 8 weeks and are more prone to iron and folate deficiency in the first few months of life. Switching of globin types is discussed in Chapter 7.

In the blood film, nucleated red cells will be seen for the first 4 days and for up to 1 week in preterm infants. Numbers are increased in cases of hypoxia, haemorrhage or haemolytic disease of the newborn (HDN).

MCV averages 119 fL at birth (range 100–125 fL) and is even higher in preterm newborns, but falls to normal adult values by 2 months (Table 31.1). By 1 year, the MCV has fallen to around 70 fL and rises throughout childhood again to reach adult levels at puberty.

Anaemia in the neonate

This should be considered for Hb below 140 g/L at birth. The clinical significance of anaemia is compounded by the high (70–80%) levels of HbF at birth, as this is less effective

Table 34.1 Impact of gestational age at birth on the principal blood count parameters in healthy neonates.

Gestation at birth	Term (≥37 weeks)	30–36 weeks	26–29 weeks	<26 weeks
Erythropoiesis				
Hb (g/L)	140–215	130–215	115–200	115–185
Hct (L/L)	0.43–0.65	0.40–0.42	0.30–0.58	0.30–0.57
MCV (fL)	98–115	100–117	103–130	104–133
MCH (pg)	32.5–39	33.5–40.5	33.5–43	34.5–44.5
NRBC				
/100 WBC	≤5	≤25	≤25	≤25
× 10^9/L	<1.0	1.0–2.0	2.0–3.0	2.0–3.0
Leucocytes (× 10^9/L)				
Neutrophils				
0–72 hours	3.0–28.0	1.0–25.0	1.0–25.0	1.0–25.0
72–240 hours	2.7–13.0	1.0–12.5	1.3–15.3	1.3–15.3
Monocytes	0.45–3.3	0.20–2.50	0.2–2.20	0.2–2.50
Eosinophils	0.12–1.20	0.06–1.10	0.03–0.90	0.01–0.80
Lymphocytes	3.0–11.0	3.0–11.0	2.5–11.0	3.0–12.0
Blast cells (%)	<5	<8	<8	<8
Platelet count (× 10^9/L)	140–450	140–450	140–450	140–450

Hb, haemoglobin concentration; Hct, haematocrit; MCH, mean cell haemoglobin; MCV, mean cell volume; NRBC, nucleated red blood cell.
Source: I. Roberts, B.J. Bain (2022) *Neonatology Haematology – A Practical Guide*, 1st edn. Hoboken, NJ: Wiley-Blackwell, p. 12. Reproduced with permission of John Wiley & Sons.

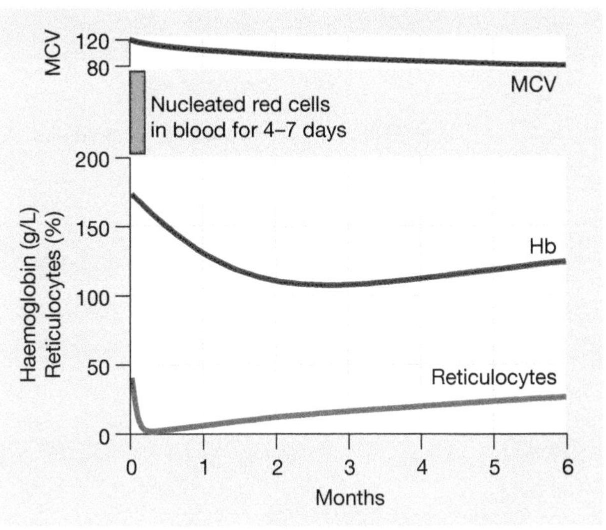

Figure 34.3 Typical profile of the blood count in the neonatal period.

than HbA at releasing oxygen to the tissues (p. xx). Causes include the following (Fig. 34.4):

1 ***Haemorrhage*** Foetomaternal, twin–twin, cord, internal, placenta.
2 ***Increased destruction*** Haemolysis (immune or nonimmune) or infection.
3 ***Decreased production*** Congenital red cell aplasia, infection e.g. parvovirus. Anti-K causes alloimmune anaemia of the foetus and newborn with decreased erythropoiesis.

Generally, anaemia at birth is usually secondary to immune haemolysis or haemorrhage; non-immune causes of haemolysis may present later. Impaired red cell production is often not apparent for at least 3 weeks. Haemolysis is often associated with severe jaundice and the main causes include HDN and congenital disorders of the red cell membrane or red cell enzymes.

Red cell transfusion may be needed for symptomatic anaemia with Hb less than 10–12 g/L if oxygen-dependent, or a lower threshold if oxygen-independent and/or age > 15 days (H.V. New *et al.* (2016) Guidelines on transfusion for fetuses, neonates and older children. *Br. J. Haematol.* 175: 784–828).

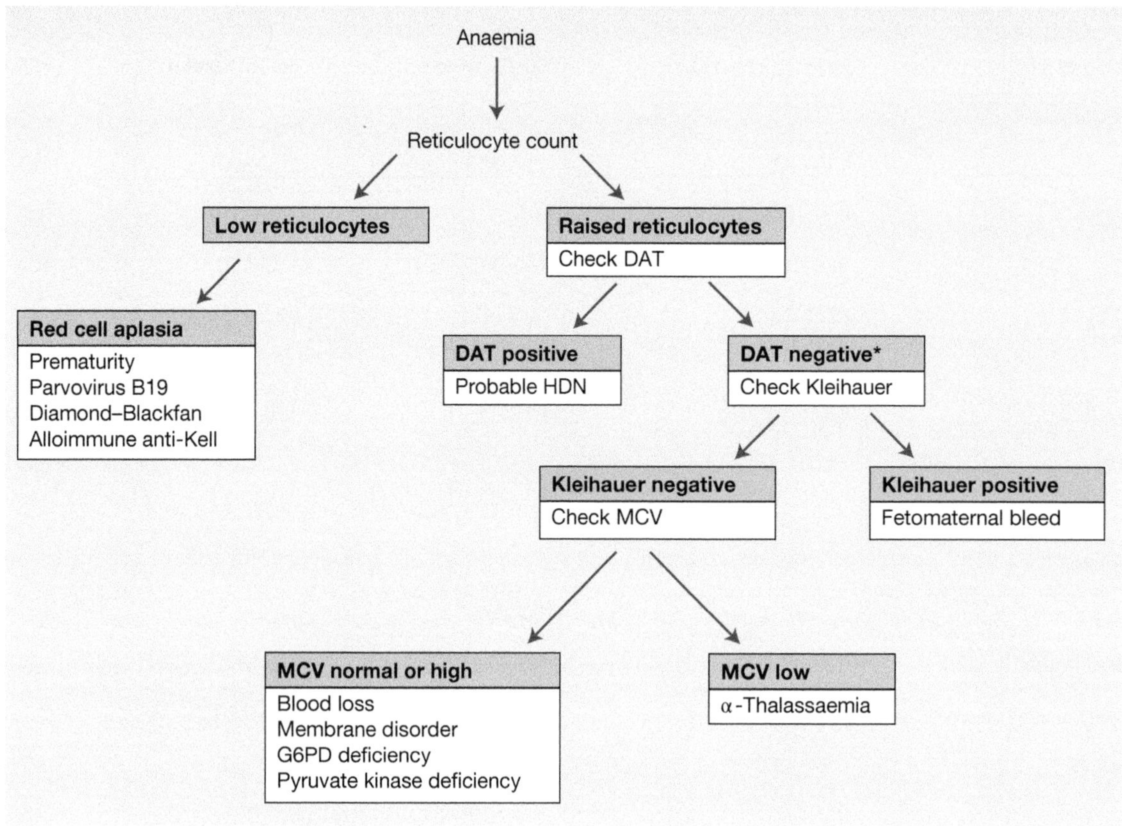

Figure 34.4 The investigation of neonatal anaemia. *The DAT test may be negative in HDN due to ABO incompatibility. DAT, direct antiglobulin test; HDN, haemolytic disease of the newborn; MCV, mean corpuscular volume.

Anaemia of prematurity

Premature infants are among the most widely transfused patients. The ABO blood groups and the corresponding antibodies may be poorly expressed in the first 4 months of life and transfer of maternal antibodies may also complicate blood grouping the infant. **Premature infants have a more marked fall in Hb after birth and this is termed physiological anaemia of prematurity (Table 34.2).** Features include a slowly falling Hb, normal blood film and reticulocytopenia. It can be minimized by late (after 1 minute) clamping of the cord and by ensuring adequate iron and folate replacement and limiting phlebotomy. Erythropoiesis-stimulating agents are used in some centres. A single unit of donor blood can be aliquoted into six or eight 'paedi' packs for repeated transfusions.

Table 34.2 Impact of postnatal age on Hb and Hct values in healthy term and preterm neonates.

	Postnatal age		
	Birth	2 weeks	4 weeks
Gestation at birth 35–42 weeks			
Hb (g/L)	140–215	110–180	100–170
Hct (L/L)	0.43–0.65	0.32–0.55	0.27–0.48
Gestation at birth 29–34 weeks			
Hb (g/L)	130–215 g/L	100–170	80–135
Hct (L/L)	0.40–0.42	0.30–0.48	0.24–0.42

Hb, haemoglobin concentration; Hct, haematocrit.
Source: I. Roberts, B.J. Bain (2022) L/L, litre cells/litre blood. *Neonatology Haematology – A Practical Guide*, 1st edn. Hoboken, NJ: Wiley-Blackwell, p. 13. Reproduced with permission of John Wiley & Sons.

Neonatal polycythaemia

This is defined as a venous haematocrit over 0.65 and can occur with twin–twin transfusion, intrauterine growth restriction and maternal hypertension or diabetes. If symptoms are present, it should be treated with partial exchange transfusion using a crystalloid solution.

Neonatal neutropenia

The neutrophil count falls in the first few weeks of life and then rises slowly to adult values by one year. Neutrophil function is also impaired in the first weeks, increasing the risk of infection. From the age of a few weeks, the lymphocyte count is higher than neutrophils throughout childhood.

Foetal-neonatal alloimmune thrombocytopenia

Foetal-neonatal alloimmune thrombocytopenia (FNAIT) results from a process similar to that of HDN. Foetal platelets that possess a paternally inherited antigen (HPA-1a in 80%) that is not present on maternal platelets can sensitize the mother to make antibodies which cross the placenta, coat the platelets, which are then destroyed by the reticuloendothelial system and lead to serious bleeding, including intracranial haemorrhage. Alloimmune thrombocytopenia differs from HDN in that 50% of cases occur in the first pregnancy. Its incidence is approximately 1 in 1000–5000 births.

Thrombocytopenia can lead to serious, sometimes fatal, bleeding *in utero* or after birth. Most experts recommend that all cases of suspected FNAIT should undergo cranial ultrasound scanning to exclude intracranial haemorrhage. Severe neonatal thrombocytopenia (platelet count $<30 \times 10^9/l$) should be treated with transfusion of HPA-compatible platelets. Weekly maternal administration of IVIg is the most appropriate first-line antenatal treatment of FNAIT; foetal platelet transfusion is rarely performed.

Other causes of neonatal thrombocytopenia include perinatal infection, placental insufficiency and congenital genetic causes.

Coagulation

Standard tests need to be interpreted with caution in the neonate. The APTT and PT are prolonged because of reduced levels of the vitamin K-dependent factors II, VII, IX and X, which become normal at around 6 months. Neonates have an increased risk of thrombosis. This is a result of physiologically low levels of inhibitors of coagulation and the use of indwelling vascular catheters. Antithrombin (AT) and protein C levels are approximately 60% of normal for the first 3 months. Homozygous protein C deficiency is associated with fulminant purpura fulminans in early life. Therapeutic protein C concentrates are now available. Homozygous AT deficiency usually presents later in childhood, but arterial and venous thrombosis may also occur in the neonate.

Fresh frozen plasma may be of benefit in neonates with clinically significant bleeding or prior to invasive procedures with a risk of bleeding, if there is an abnormal coagulation profile. Haemorrhagic disease of the newborn is discussed in Chapter 29.

Haemolytic disease of the newborn

HDN is the result of red cell alloimmunization, in which IgG antibodies passage from the maternal circulation across the placenta into the circulation of the foetus, where they react with foetal red cells and lead to their destruction. Anti-D antibody is responsible for most cases of severe HDN, although anti-c, anti-E, anti-K and a wide range of other antibodies are found in occasional cases (see Table 30.3). Intrauterine transfusion if needed for HDN, parvovirus or other causes of foetal anaemia should only be undertaken at a specialized centre. Irradiated fresh blood of extended matching genotype is needed. Although antibodies against the ABO blood group system are the most frequent cause of HDN, this is usually mild.

Rh haemolytic disease of the newborn

When an Rh D-negative (p. 376) woman has a pregnancy with an Rh D-positive foetus, Rh D-positive foetal red cells cross into the maternal circulation (especially at parturition and during the third trimester) and sensitize the mother to form anti-D. The mother could also be sensitized by a previous miscarriage, amniocentesis or other trauma to the placenta or by blood transfusion. Anti-D crosses the placenta to the foetus during the next pregnancy, coats Rh D-positive foetal red cells and results in reticuloendothelial destruction of these cells, causing anaemia and jaundice. If the father is heterozygous for D antigen, and mother Rh D negative, there is a 50% probability that the foetus will be D-positive. The foetal Rh D genotype can be established by polymerase chain reaction (PCR) analysis for the presence of Rh D in a maternal blood sample.

The main aim of management is to prevent anti-D antibody formation in Rh D-negative mothers. This can be achieved by the administration of small amounts of anti-D antibody, which 'mop up' and destroy Rh D-positive foetal red cells before they can sensitize the immune system of the mother to produce anti-D.

Prevention of Rh immunization

At the time of booking, all pregnant women should have their ABO and Rh group determined and serum screened for antibodies at least twice during the pregnancy. **All non-sensitized Rh D-negative women should be given at least 500 units (100 μg) of anti-D at 28 and 34 weeks' gestation** to reduce the risk of sensitization from foeto-maternal haemorrhage. Foetal Rh D molecular typing from DNA in maternal blood can be used before 28 weeks. If the foetus is Rh D-negative, no further anti-D prophylaxis is needed. In addition, at birth the babies of Rh D-negative women who do not have antibodies must have their cord blood grouped for ABO and Rh. If the baby's blood is Rh D-negative, the mother will require no further treatment. If the baby is Rh D-positive, prophylactic anti-D should be administered to the mother at a minimum dose of 500 units intramuscularly within 72 hours of delivery.

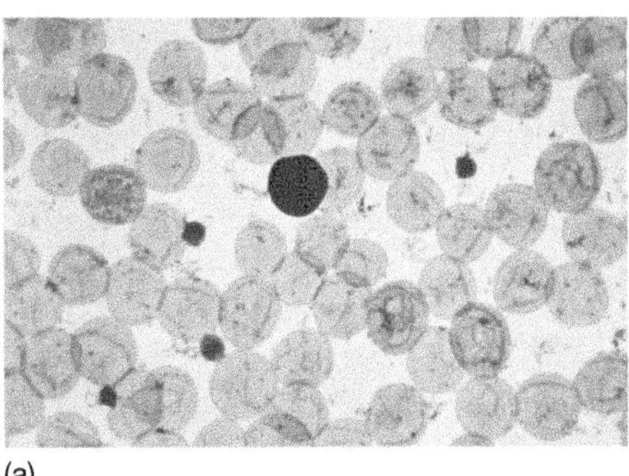

(a)

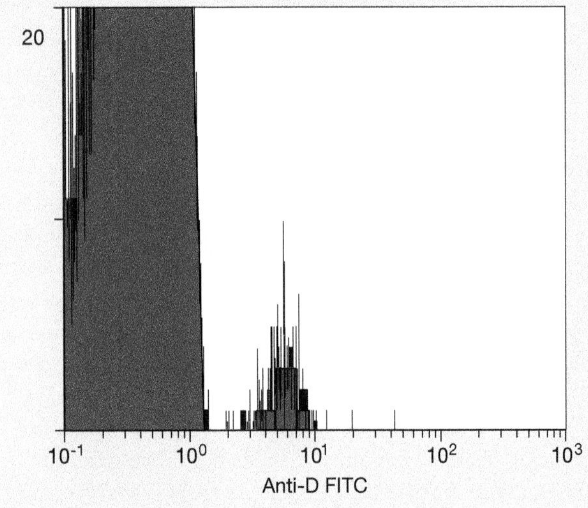

(b)

Figure 34.5 **(a)** Kleihauer test for foetal red cells; a deeply eosin-staining cell containing foetal haemoglobin is seen at the centre. Haemoglobin has been eluted from the other red cells by an incubation at acid pH and these appear as colourless ghosts. **(b)** Determination by flow cytometry of the number of RhD foetal cells in maternal blood using fluorescent-labelling of antibody to RhD, the mother being RhDd. Source: Courtesy of Dr W. Erber.

A **Kleihauer test** is performed. This uses differential staining to estimate the number of foetal cells in the maternal circulation (Fig. 34.5a). If the Kleihauer is positive, many centres will perform flow cytometry for a more accurate estimate of the volume of foeto-maternal haemorrhage (FMH; Fig. 34.5b). The chance of developing antibodies is related to the number of foetal cells found. The dose of anti-D is increased if there is greater than 4 mL transplacental haemorrhage. Anti-D IgG (125 units) is given for each 1 mL of FMH greater than 4 mL.

Sensitizing episodes during pregnancy

Anti-D IgG should be given to Rh D-negative women who have potentially sensitizing episodes during pregnancy: 250 units is given if the event occurs up to week 20 of gestation and 500 units thereafter, followed by a Kleihauer test. Potentially sensitizing events as well as delivery are listed in Table 34.3.

Table 34.3 Potentially sensitizing events in pregnancy (from British Committee for Standards in Haematology (BCSH) Guidelines 2014: https://b-s-h.org.uk/guidelines).
Amniocentesis, chorionic villus biopsy and cordocentesis
Antepartum haemorrhage/per vaginal bleeding in pregnancy
External cephalic version
Fall or abdominal trauma (sharp/blunt, open/closed)
Ectopic pregnancy
Evacuation of molar pregnancy
Intrauterine death and stillbirth
In utero therapeutic interventions (transfusion, surgery, insertion of shunts, laser)
Miscarriage, threatened miscarriage
Therapeutic termination of pregnancy
Delivery – normal, instrumental or caesarean section
Intraoperative cell salvage

Source: S. Allard, M. Contreras. In A.V. Hoffbrand *et al.* (eds) (2016) *Postgraduate Haematology*, 7th edn. Reproduced with permission of John Wiley & Sons.

Treatment of established anti-D sensitization

If anti-D antibodies are detected during pregnancy, they should be quantified at regular intervals. The clinical severity is related to the strength of anti-D present in maternal serum, but is also affected by such factors as the IgG subclass, rate of rise of antibody and past history. The development of haemolytic disease in the foetus can be assessed by velocimetry of the foetal middle cerebral artery by Doppler ultrasonography, as increased velocities correlate with foetal anaemia (Fig. 34.6). If anaemia is detected, foetal blood sampling and intrauterine transfusion of irradiated Rh D-negative packed red cells may be indicated.

Clinical features of HDN

1. ***Severe disease*** **Intrauterine death from hydrops fetalis (Fig. 34.7a).**
2. ***Moderate disease*** **The baby is born with anaemia and jaundice and may show pallor, tachycardia, oedema and hepatosplenomegaly.** If the unconjugated bilirubin is not controlled and reaches levels exceeding 250 µmol/L, bile pigment deposition in the basal ganglia may lead to **kernicterus** – central nervous system damage with generalized spasticity and possible subsequent mental deficiency, deafness and epilepsy. This problem becomes acute after birth as maternal clearance of foetal bilirubin ceases and conjugation of bilirubin by the neonatal liver has not yet reached full activity.
3. ***Mild disease*** **Mild anaemia with or without jaundice.**

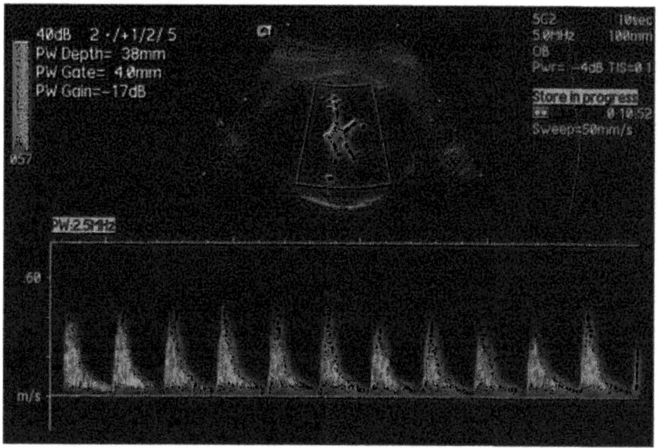

Figure 34.6 Doppler ultrasonography of the circle of Willis in a foetus. The cursor is placed over the middle cerebral artery and an increased blood velocity correlates with anaemia. Source: S. Kumar, F. Regan (2005) Management of pregnancies with RhD alloimmunisation. *BMJ* 330: 1255. Reproduced with permission of BMJ Publishing Group Ltd.

Investigations will reveal variable anaemia with a high reticulocyte count; the baby is Rh D-positive, the direct antiglobulin test is positive and the serum bilirubin raised. In moderate and severe cases, many erythroblasts are seen in the blood film (Fig. 34.7b).

Treatment

Exchange transfusion may be necessary; the indications for this include severe anaemia (Hb <100 g/L at birth) and severe or rapidly rising hyperbilirubinaemia. More than one exchange transfusion may be required and 500 mL is usually sufficient for each exchange. The donor blood should be less than 5 days old, CMV negative, irradiated, Rh D-negative and ABO compatible with the baby's and mother's serum. Phototherapy (exposure of the infant to bright light of appropriate wavelength) degrades bilirubin and reduces the likelihood of kernicterus.

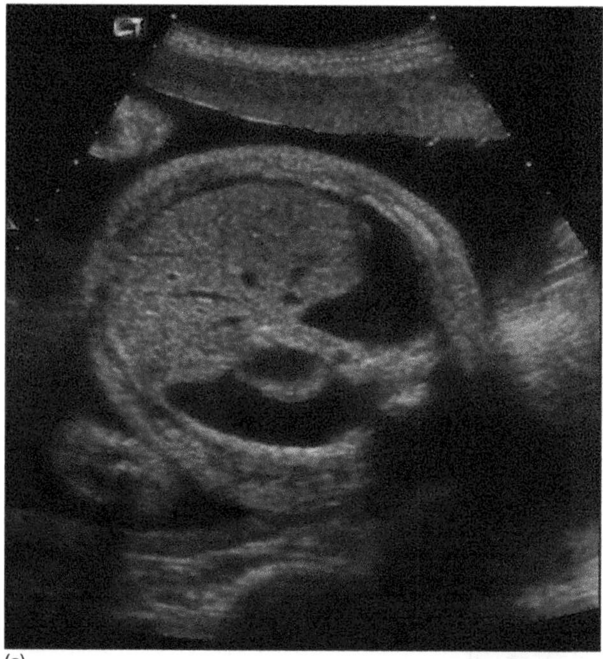

(a)

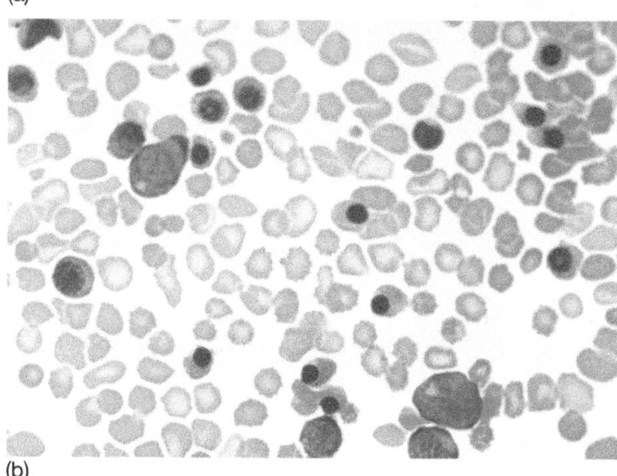

(b)

Figure 34.7 (a) Ultrasound features of hydrops fetalis showing skin oedema, hepatomegaly and ascites. Source: S. Kumar, F. Regan (2005) Management of pregnancies with RhD alloimmunisation. *BMJ* 330: 1255. Reproduced with permission of BMJ Publishing Group Ltd. **(b)** Rh haemolytic disease of the newborn (erythroblastosis fetalis): peripheral blood film showing large numbers of erythroblasts, polychromasia and crenated cells.

ABO haemolytic disease of the newborn

In 20% of births, a mother is ABO incompatible with the foetus. Group A and group B mothers usually have only IgM ABO antibodies (p. xxx). **The majority of cases of ABO HDN are caused by 'immune' IgG antibodies in group O mothers.** Although 15% of pregnancies in white people involve a group O mother with a group A or group B foetus, most mothers do not produce IgG anti-A or anti-B and most affected babies have only mild-moderate jaundice which may require phototherapy. Exchange transfusions are needed in only 1 in 3000 infants. The mild course of ABO HDN is partly explained by the A and B antigens not being fully developed at birth and by partial neutralization of maternal IgG antibodies by A and B antigens on other cells, in the plasma and tissue fluids.

In contrast to Rh HDN, ABO disease may be found in the first pregnancy and may or may not affect subsequent pregnancies. The direct antiglobulin test on the infant's cells is occasionally negative or only weakly positive. Examination of the blood film shows autoagglutination spherocytosis, polychromasia and erythroblastosis.

SUMMARY

- Pregnancy results in multiple changes in the haematological systems.
- There is a fall in haemoglobin because of an increased plasma volume that is proportionally greater than a 25% increase in red cell mass.
- Iron deficiency is frequent; folate deficiency is associated with maternal anaemia and also with neural tube defects (NTDs) in the foetus.
- Serum vitamin B_{12} levels fall in pregnancy, but recover post-partum.
- Platelets counts fall on average by 10%. If the count falls below 100 × 109/L other causes than gestational thrombocytopenia are sought, e.g. immune thrombocytopenia, hypertensive disorders.
- Pregnancy is a hypercoagulable state with increased levels of coagulation factors and risk of thrombosis or disseminated intravascular coagulation.
- Neonates have higher haemoglobin levels than adults. Anaemia at birth is usually caused by haemorrhage or immune haemolysis.
- Haemolytic disease of the newborn is brought about by Rh D IgG antibodies, made by a Rh D-negative mother, crossing the placenta. It may cause death of the foetus (hydrops fetalis) or haemolytic anaemia. It is now rare because of administration of Rh anti-D to Rh D-negative mothers at the time of exposure to Rh D-positive foetal cells or blood products.
- ABO haemolytic disease of the newborn is more frequent. It is usually mild and may occur in the first pregnancy. It is most frequently caused by group O mothers making immune IgG antibodies (which cross the placenta) against a group A or B foetus.

Now visit **www.wiley.com/go/haematology9e** to test yourself on this chapter.

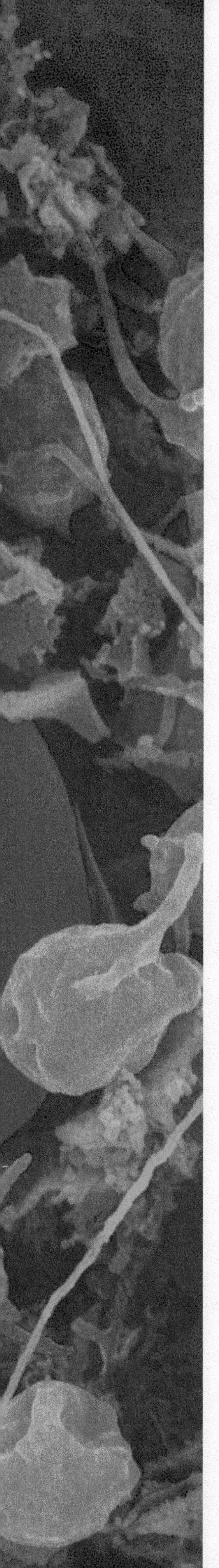

APPENDIX

5th edition (2022) of the World Health Organization Classification of Haematolymphoid Tumours

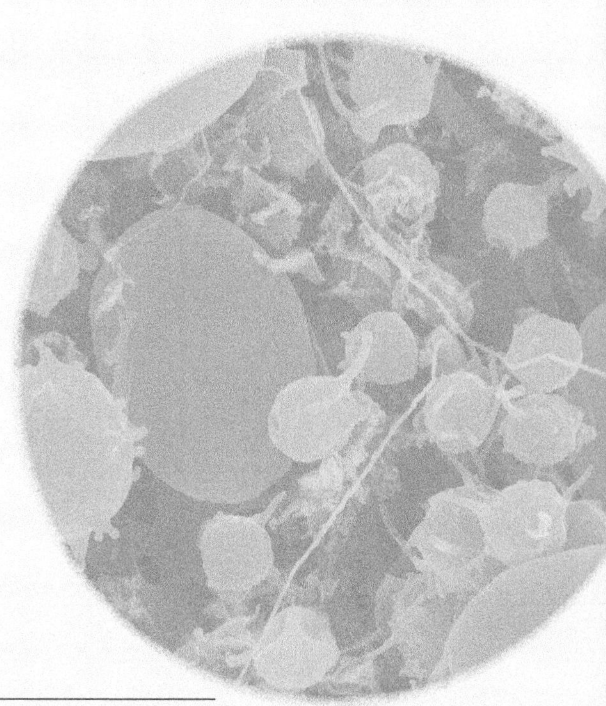

Hoffbrand's Essential Haematology, Ninth Edition. A. Victor Hoffbrand, Pratima Chowdary, Graham P. Collins, and Justin Loke.
© 2024 John Wiley & Sons Ltd. Published 2024 by John Wiley & Sons Ltd.
Companion website: www.wiley.com/go/haematology9e

A. Myeloid and Histiocytic/Dendritic Neoplasms

J.D. Khoury et al. (2022) Leukemia 36: 1703–19

Table A.1 Subtypes of myeloid neoplasms associated with germline predisposition.

Myeloid neoplasms with germline predisposition without a pre-existing platelet disorder or organ dysfunction
■ Germline *CEBPA* P/LP variant (CEBPA-associated familial AML)
■ Germline *DDX41* P/LP variant[a]
■ Germline *TP53* P/LP variant[a] (Li-Fraumeni syndrome)
Myeloid neoplasms with germline predisposition and pre-existing platelet disorder
■ Germline *RUNX1* P/LP variant[a] (familial platelet disorder with associated myeloid malignancy, FPD-MM)
■ Germline *ANKRD26* P/LP variant[a] (Thrombocytopenia 2)
■ Germline *ETV6* P/LP variant[a] (Thrombocytopenia 5)
Myeloid neoplasms with germline predisposition and potential organ dysfunction
■ Germline *GATA2* P/LP variant (GATA2-deficiency)
■ Bone marrow failure syndromes
■ Severe congenital neutropenia (SCN)
■ Shwachman–Diamond syndrome (SDS)
■ Fanconi anaemia (FA)
■ Telomere biology disorders
■ RASopathies (Neurofibromatosis type 1, CBL syndrome, Noonan syndrome or Noonan syndrome-like disorders[a])
■ Down syndrome[a]
■ Germline *SAMD9* P/LP variant (MIRAGE Syndrome)
■ Germline *SAMD9L* P/LP variant (SAMD9L-related Ataxia Pancytopenia Syndrome)[b]
■ Biallelic germline *BLM* P/LP variant (Bloom syndrome)

[a]Lymphoid neoplasms can also occur.
[b]Ataxia is not always present.
LP, likely pathogenic; P, pathogenic.

Table A.2 Acute leukaemias of ambiguous lineage.

Acute leukaemia of ambiguous lineage with defining genetic abnormalities
Mixed-phenotype acute leukaemia with *BCR::ABL1* fusion
Mixed-phenotype acute leukaemia with *KMT2A* rearrangement
Acute leukaemia of ambiguous lineage with other defined genetic alterations
Mixed-phenotype acute leukaemia with ZNF384 rearrangement
Acute leukaemia of ambiguous lineage with BCL11B rearrangement
Acute leukaemia of ambiguous lineage, immunophenotypically defined
Mixed-phenotype acute leukaemia, B/myeloid
Mixed-phenotype acute leukaemia, T/myeloid
Mixed-phenotype acute leukaemia, rare types
Acute leukaemia of ambiguous lineage, not otherwise specified
Acute undifferentiated leukaemia

Table A.3 Lineage assignment criteria for mixed-phenotype acute leukaemia.

	Criterion
B lineage	
CD19 strong[a]	1 or more also strongly expressed: CD10, CD22, or CD79a[c]
or,	
CD19 weak[b]	2 or more also strongly expressed: CD10, CD22, or CD79a[c]
T lineage	
CD3 (cytoplasmic or surface)[d]	Intensity in part exceeds 50% of mature T-cell levels by flow cytometry or, immunocytochemistry positive with non-zeta chain reagent
Myeloid lineage	
Myeloperoxidase	Intensity in part exceeds 50% of mature neutrophil level
or,	
Monocytic differentiation	2 or more expressed: Non-specific esterase, CD11c, CD14, CD64 or lysozyme

[a] CD19 intensity in part exceeds 50% of normal B-cell progenitor by flow cytometry.
[b] CD19 intensity does not exceed 50% of normal B-cell progenitor by flow cytometry.
[c] Provided T lineage not under consideration, otherwise cannot use CD79a.
[d] Using anti-CD3 epsilon chain antibody.

B. Lymphoid Neoplasms

R. Alaggio et al. (2022) Leukemia 36: 1720–48

B.1. The International Consensus Classification (ICC)

This classification from the US Society of Hematopathology, the European Association of Hematopathology and several Clinical Advisory Committees composed of geneticists and oncologists also appeared in 2022. It is generally identical to the WHO 5 classification but differs mainly for some of the more unusual diseases and sub-types. For example, the diseases prolymphocytic leukaemia and hairy cell leukaemia variant are deleted in WHO 5 but retained from WHO 4 by The ICC.

The WHO 5 classification has been used throughout this edition. The reader can find the ICC classification in the following references.

D.A. Arber *et al.* (2022) The international consensus classification of myeloid neoplasms and acute leukemias: integrating morphological, clinical and genomic data. *Blood* 140: 1200–28.

E. Campo *et al.* (2022) The international consensus classification of mature lymphoid neoplasms: a report from the clinical advisory committee. *Blood* 140: 1229–53.

B.2. European Leukemia Network (ELN)

A third international classification of the myeloid neoplasms was also published in 2022.This includes the classification and management of the myeloid leukaemias.

H. Döhner *et al.* (2022) Diagnosis and management of AML in adults: 2022 recommendations from an international expert panel on behalf of ELN. *Blood* 140: 1345–77.

Index

Hoffbrand's Essential Haematology 9E, 2024

Note: Page locators in **bold** indicate tables. Page locators in *italics* indicate figures. This index uses letter-by-letter alphabetization.

Hoffbrand's Essential Haematology, Ninth Edition. A. Victor Hoffbrand, Pratima Chowdary, Graham P. Collins, and Justin Loke.
© 2024 John Wiley & Sons Ltd. Published 2024 by John Wiley & Sons Ltd.
Companion website: www.wiley.com/go/haematology9e